Oxford Textbook of

Cognitive Neurology and Dementia

Oxford Textbooks in Clinical Neurology

Oxford Textbook of
Cognitive Neurology and Dementia

Edited by

Masud Husain

Professor of Neurology & Cognitive Neuroscience, Nuffield Department of
Clinical Neurosciences, University of Oxford,
John Radcliffe Hospital, UK

Jonathan M. Schott

Professor of Neurology, Dementia Research Centre, Department of
Neurodegenerative Diseases, UCL Institute of Neurology, UK

Series Editor

Christopher Kennard

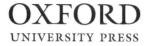

OXFORD
UNIVERSITY PRESS

Great Clarendon Street, Oxford, OX2 6DP,
United Kingdom

Oxford University Press is a department of the University of Oxford.
It furthers the University's objective of excellence in research, scholarship,
and education by publishing worldwide. Oxford is a registered trade mark of
Oxford University Press in the UK and in certain other countries

Published in the United States of America by Oxford University Press
198 Madison Avenue, New York, NY 10016, United States of America

British Library Cataloguing in Publication Data

Data available

Library of Congress Cataloging in Publication Data

Data available

ISBN 978-0-19-965594-6 (Hbk.)
ISBN 978-0-19-883108-2 (Pbk.)

Printed in Great Britain by
Ashford Colour Press Ltd, Gosport, Hampshire

Preface

Cognitive neurology, or behavioural neurology as it is known in the United States, has a reputation of being a complex subspecialty. To the outsider it presents a formidable challenge, seemingly requiring knowledge of several different areas of expertise ranging from basic aspects of neuroscience—molecular, cognitive, and neuroimaging—through to neuropsychology, neuropsychiatry, and bedside neurological assessment. Even for experts, the dramatic growth of basic neuroscience research in these areas has meant that it can be extremely difficult to keep up with new developments or key conceptual advances. Perhaps more challenging still is to know how such advances can best be applied in practice when confronted with a patient with a cognitive complaint.

Our aim in producing this textbook is to bring some order to the apparent chaos for both the novice and those established in the field. While there are several excellent texts that selectively cover either dementia or the neuroscience underlying cognitive disorders, we wanted to produce a modern, pragmatic resource that covers both these areas in an accessible manner for clinicians. Our second objective was to produce a textbook that spans diverse areas of expertise in an *integrated* fashion. Wherever possible, therefore, we have tried to link information in chapters on basic sciences to those on clinical syndromes.

The text is firmly based on the clinical approach to the patient with cognitive impairment and dementia, but it also provides essential background knowledge that is fundamental to clinical practice. It is written for those who want to learn more about cognition and dementia, including neurologists, geriatricians, and psychiatrists who are involved in assessing and treating such patients, but also for others curious to find out about cognitive disorders and their underlying neurobiology. We hope that, whatever your background, you will find this the one essential textbook that you want to revisit.

Bringing together such a diverse range of information has been a challenge for us. We are extremely grateful to our contributors for being so considerate in taking up our suggestions for changes to their manuscripts and for their patience. Finally, we acknowledge with thanks the forbearance of our families who observed our involvement in this project with much more than tolerance and grace.

Masud Husain
Jonathan M. Schott

Contents

SECTION 3
Cognitive impairment and dementia

Abbreviations

3C	Three-City Study	ATP	Adenosine 5'-triphosphate
5-CSRTT	5-choice serial reaction time task	ATXN	Ataxin
5-HIAA	5-hydroxyindoleacetic acid	AWD	Alcohol-withdrawal delirium
5-HT	Serotonin	BACE	Beta secretase
Aβ	amyloid β	BIBD	Basophilic inclusion body disease
ABCA	ATP-binding cassette	BIC	Binding of item and context
ACA	Anterior cerebral artery	BIN	Bridging integrator
ACC	Anterior cingulate circuit	BIRT	Brain Injury Rehabilitation Trust
ACE–R	Addenbrooke's Cognitive Examination Revised	BMIPB	BIRT Memory and Information Processing Battery
Ach	Acetylcholine	BOLD	Blood oxygenation level dependent
AChE	Acetylcholinesterase inhibitors	BORB	Birmingham Object Recognition Battery
AD	Alzheimer's disease	BPSD	Behavioural and psychological symptoms of dementia
ADC	Apparent diffusion coefficient		
ADEAR	Alzheimer's Disease Education & Referral Center	BSE	Bovine spongiform encephalopathy
		bvFTD	Behavioural variant frontotemporal dementia
ADHD	Attention deficit/hyperactivity disorder		
ADL	Activities of daily living	CAA	Cerebral amyloid angiopathy
AE	Autoimmune encephalitis	CAA-RI	CAA-related inflammation
AEDs	Antiepileptic drugs	CADASIL	Cerebral autosomal dominant arteriopathy with subcortical infarcts and leukoencephalopathy
AF	Arcuate fasciculus		
AG	Argyrophilic grains		
AGD	Argyrophilic grain disease	CAG	Cytosine–adenine–guanine
AI	Anterior insula	CAM	Confusion Assessment Method
AIP	Anterior intraparietal sulcus	CAMCOG–R	Cambridge Cognition–Revised
ALS	amyotrophic lateral sclerosis	CAMDEX	Cambridge mental disorders of the older population examination
AMACR	α-Methylacyl-CoA		
aMCI	amnesic mild cognitive impairment	CANTAB	Cambridge Automatic Neuropsychological Test Battery
AMPA	α-amino-3-hydroxy-5-methyl-4-isoxazolepropionic acid		
		CARASIL	Cerebral autosomal recessive arterioapthy with subcortical infarcts and leukoencephalopathy
AMTS	Abbreviated Mental Test Score		
Ang	Angular gyrus		
ANI	Asymptomatic neurocognitive impairment	CASPR2	Contactin-associated protein 2
AOS	Apraxia of speech	CASS	Cas scaffolding
APA	American Psychiatric Association	CAT	Computed axial tomography
APGBD	Adult polyglucosan body disease	CBD	Corticobasal degeneration
APO	Apolipoprotein	cblC	Cobalamin C disease
APP	Amyloid precursor protein	CBS	Corticobasal syndrome
ARSACS	Autosomal recessive spastic ataxia of Charlevoix–Saguenay	CBT	Cognitive behaviour therapy
		CC75C	Cambridge City over-75s Cohort Study
ART	Antiretroviral therapy		
ASYMAD	Asymptomatic AD	CCAS	Cerebellar cognitive affective syndrome

CERAD	Consortium to Establish a Registry of Alzheimer's Disease
CFS–NMT	Cramp-fasciculation syndrome–neuromyotonia
ChE-Is	Cholinesterase inhibitors
CI	Confidence interval
CIS	Clinically isolated syndrome
CJD	Creutzfeld–Jakob disease
CLS	Complementary learning system
CLU	Clusterin
CMB	Cerebral microbleed
CNS	Central nervous system
CoA	Coenzyme A
CPAP	Continuous positive airway pressure
CPE	CNS penetration effectiveness
CR	Complement component receptor
CRAFT	Convergence, Recollection, and Familiarity Theory
CRF	Corticotrophic releasing factor
CRT	Cognitive remediation therapy
CS	Contention scheduler
CS	Contrast sensitivity
cSAH	Subarachnoid blood in the convexity
CSHA	Canadian Study of Health and Aging
CSF	Cerebrospinal fluid
CT	Computed tomography
CTE	Chronic traumatic encephalopathy
CTSD	Cathepsin D
CVLT	California verbal learning test
DA	Dopamine
DAI	Diffuse axonal injury
DALY	Disability-adjusted life years
DAN	Dorsal attentional network
DAT	Dopamine transporter
DDA	Direct detection assay
DHA	Docosahexanoic acid
DIAN	Dominantly Inherited Alzheimer Network
DIR	Double inversion recovery
DIs	Dystrophic neurites
DLB	Dementia with Lewy bodies
DL-PFC	Dorsolateral prefrontal circuit
DM	Decision making
DMN	Default mode network
DMTs	Disease modifying therapies
DMTS	Delayed-matching-to-sample
DPVS	Dilated perivascular spaces
DRPLA	Dentatorubral-pallidoluysian atrophy
DRS	Dementia rating scale
DSM	Diagnostic and Statistic Manual
DTI	Diffusion tensor imaging
DTX	Dendrotoxin
DWI	Diffusion-weighted imaging
EC	Entorhinal cortex
ECF	Extracytoplasmic function
EClipSE	Epidemiological Clinicopathological Studies in Europe
ECT	Electroconvulsive therapy
EDS	Excessive daytime sleepiness
EEG	Electro-encephalography
EF	Executive functions
EL	Encephalitis lethargica
ELSA	English Longitudinal Study of Ageing
EMEA	European Medicines Agency
EMG	Electromyogram
EPESE	Established Populations for Epidemiologic Studies of the Elderly
EMP	Epilepsy, progressive myoclonus
ESCRT	Endosomal-sorting complex required for transport
ETV	Endoscopic third ventriculostomy
EWS	Ewing's sarcoma protein
FA	Fractional anisotropy
FAB	Frontal assessment battery
FAD	Flavin adenine dinucleotide
FBD	Familial British dementia
FBDS	Faciobrachial dystonic seizures
FCSRT	Free and Cued Selective Reminding Test
FDA	Food and Drug Administration
FDD	Familial Danish dementia
FDG	Fluorodeoxyglucose
FDOPA	18F-fluorodopa
FEF	Frontal eye fields
FEP	First episode psychosis
FERM	Fermitin
FFA	Fusiform face area
FFI	Fatal familial insomnia
FIQ	Full-scale IQ
FLAIR	Fluid-attenuated inversion recovery
fMRI	Functional magnetic resonance imaging
FMRIB	Functional MRI of the Brain
FRDA	Friedreich's ataxia
FSL	FMRIB Software Library
FTA-Abs	Fluorescent treponemal antibody-absorption
FTD	Frontotemporal dementia
FTLD	Frontotemporal lobar degeneration
FTLD-t	Frontotemporal degeneration-tau
FTLD-u	Frontotemporal degeneration-ubiquitin
FUS	Fused-in-sarcoma
GABA	Gamma aminobutyric acid
GAD	Glutamic acid decarboxylase
GBA	Glucoserebrosidase
GBD	Global Burden of Disease
GBE	Glycogen brancher enzyme
GCIs	Glial cytoplasmic inclusions
GCL	Granule cell layer
GCS	Glasgow Coma Scale
GDNF	Glial-derived neurotrophic factor
GFAP	Glial fibrillary acidic protein
GHD	Growth hormone deficiency
GLM	General linear model
Gpe	Global pallidus external
Gpi	Globus pallidus internal
GMS/AGECAT	Geriatric Mental State Examination/Automated Geriatric Examination Computer Assisted Taxonomy
GRE	Gradient-recalled echo
GSS	Gerstmann–Sträussler syndrome
GWAS	Genome-wide association studies

^{1}H-MRS	Proton magnetic resonance spectroscopy	MCI	Mild cognitive impairment
HAD	HIV-associated dementia	MCS	Minimially conscious state
HADS	Hospital Anxiety and Depression Scale	MD	Multiple demand
HANDs	HIV-associated neurocognitive disorders	MEF	Myocyte enhancer factor
HCV	Hepatitis C virus	MEG	Magnetoencephalography
HD	Huntington's disease	MELAS	Mitochondrial encephalopathy lactic acidosis and stroke-like episodes
HDL	Huntington's disease-like syndrome		
HIC	High-income countries	MERRF	Myoclonic epilepsy with ragged red fibres
HIV	Human immunodeficiency virus	MIBG	Metaiodobenzylguanidine
HIVE	HIV encephalopathy	MID	Multi-infarct dementia
HMG-CoA	Hydroxy-3-methylglutaryl-coenzyme A	mIPS	Medial intraparietal sulcus
HR	Hazard ration	MMA	Methylmalonic acid
HRT	Hormone replacement therapy	MMSE	Mini-Mental State Examination
HSV	Herpes simplex virus	MND	Mild neurocognitive impairment
HTLV	Human T-lymphotropic virus	Mnd	Motor neurone disease
IBMPFD	Inclusion body myopathy with Paget disease of the bone and frontotemporal dementia	MNI	Montreal Neurological Institute
		MoCA	Montreal Cognitive Assessment
IBVM	^{123}I-iodobenzovesamicol	mOPJ	Medial occipitoparietal junction
ICA	Independent component analysis	MoS	Morvan's syndrome
ICD	International Classification of Diseases	MP	Methylphenidate
ICDs	Impulse control disorders	MRC	Medical Research Council
ICH	Intracerebral haemorrhages	MRC CFAS	Medical Research Council's cognitive function and ageing study
iCJD	Iatrogenic CJD		
ICN	Intrinsic connectivity networks	MRI	Magnetic resonance imaging
ICU	Intensive care unit	MRS	Magnetic resonance spectroscopy
IDED	Intra- and extra-dimensional	MS	Multiple sclerosis
IFOF	Inferior fronto-occipital fasciculus	MSA	Multiple system atrophy
IGF-II	Insulin-like growth factor II	MSE	Mental state examination
Ig	Immunoglobulin	MSUD	Maple-syrup urine disease
IGT	Iowa Gambling Task	MTG	Middle temporal gyrus
ILF	Inferior longitudinal fasciculus	MTHFR	Methylenetetrahydrofolate reductase
ILSA	Italian Longitudinal Study of Ageing	MTL	Medial temporal lobes
IPD	Inherited prion disease	NAA/Cr	N-acetyl aspartate/Creatinine
IPL	Inferior parietal lobule	NA	Noradrenaline
IPS	Intraparietal sulcus	NART	National Adult Reading Test
IRIS	Immune reconstitution inflammatory syndrome	NAWM	Normal-appearing white matter
		NBIA	Neurodegeneration with brain iron accumulation
IT	Inferotemporal		
IWG	International Working Group	nbM	Nucleus basalis of Meynert
JC	John Cunningham	NCIs	Neuronal cytoplasmic inclusions
LAMIC	Low and medium-income countries	NE	Norepinephrine
LDX	Lisdexanphetamine dimesylate	nfvPPA	Non-fluent variant primary progressive aphasia
LE	Limbic encephalopathy		
LGI1	leucine-rich glioma inactivated 1	NGF	Nerve growth factor
LOC	Lateral occipital cortex	NICE	National Institute for Health and Care Excellence
LP	Lumbar puncture		
LPA	Logopenic progressive aphasia	NIFID	Neuronal intermediate filament inclusion disease
LTD	Long-term depression		
LTM	Long-term memory	NIIs	Neuronal intranuclear inclusions
LTOCs	long-term observational controlled studies	NINCDS–ADRDA	National Institute of Neurological and Communicative Disorders and Stroke and the Alzheimer's Disease and Related Disorders Association
LTP	Long-term potentiation		
M4PA	Methyl-4-piperidyl acetate		
MAPT	Microtubule-associated tau		
MATRICS	Measurement and Treatment Research for Improving cognition in schizophrenia	NINDS	National Institute of Neurologic Disease and Stroke
MB	Microbleeds	NMDA	N-methyl-D-asparate
MBD	Marchiafava–Bignami disease	NMDAR	NMDA receptor
MCA	Middle cerebral artery	NMT	Neuromyotonia
MCCB	MATRICS consensus cognitive battery	NPI	Neuropsychiatric Inventory

NPH	Normal pressure hydrocephalus	PVS	Persistent vegetative state
NSAbs	Neuronal surface-directed antibody	PVS	Prominent perivascular spaces
OFC	Orbitofrontal circuit	RA	Retrograde amnesia
OMPFC	Orbitomedial prefrontal cortex	RAVLT	Rey auditory verbal learning test
OMS	Opsoclonus-myoclonus syndrome	RBD	REM sleep behaviour disorder
OPRI	Octapeptide repeat insertion mutation	rCBF	Regional cerebral blood flow
OR	Odds ration	RCT	Randomized controlled trial
OTC	Ornithine transcarbamylase	REM	Rapid eye movement
PACS	Primary angiitis of the central nervous system	RMT	Recognition memory test
		ROI	Regions of interest
PANDA	Parkinson neuropsychometric dementia assessment	ROS	Reactive oxygen species
		RPD	Rapidly progressive dementia
Paquid	Personnes âgées QUID	RPR	Rapid plasma reagin
PAS	Periodic acid–Schiff	RRMS	Relapsing and remitting MS
PASAT	Paced auditory serial addition test	RSN	Resting state network
PCA	Posterior cerebral artery	rtQUIC	Real-time Quaking-Induced Conversion Assay
PCA	Posterior cortical atrophy		
PCA	Principal component analysis	SAG	Supervisory attentional gateway
PCR	Polymerase chain reaction	SAS	Supervisory attentional system
PD-CRS	PD Cognitive Rating Scale	SCA	Spinocerebellar ataxia
PDD	Parkinson's disease with dementia	sCJD	sporadic CJD
PEF	Parietal eye fields	SCLC	Small cell lung cancer
PERM	Progressive encephalomyelitis with rigidity and myoclonus	SCOPA-Cog	SCales for Outcomes of PArkinson's disease-cognition
PET	Positron emission tomography	SD	Semantic dementia
PFC	Prefrontal cortex	SDAT	Senile dementia of Alzheimer type
PFNA	Progressive nonfluent aphasia	SE	status epilepticus
PiB	Pittsburgh Compound-B	SEC	Structured event complex
PICALM	Phosphatidylinositol binding clathrin assembly protein	SI	Stimulus-independent
		SLC	Solute carrier
PiD	Pick's disease	SLF	Superior longitudinal fasciculus
PIGD	Postural-instability gait difficulty	SMA	Supplementary motor area
PIQ	Performance IQ	Smg	Supramarignal gyrus
PLEDS	Periodic lateralizing epileptiform discharges	SN	Salience network
PML	Progressive multifocal leukoencephalopathy	SNP	Single nucleotide polymorphism
PNFA	Progressive non-fluent aphasia	SNpc	Substantia nigra pars compacta
PNS	Peripheral nerve hyperexcitability	SNpr	Substantia nigra pars reticulata
PPA	Parahippocampal place area	SNr	Substantia nigra
PPA	Primary progressive aphasia	SNRIs	Serotonin-norepinephrine reuptake inhibitors
PPC	Posterior parietal cortex		
PPMS	Primary progressive MS	SO	Stimulus-oriented
PPN	Pedunculopontine nucleus	SOL	Space-occupying lesion
PPT-1	Palmitoyl-protein thioesterase 1	SORL	Sortilin-related receptor
PPVT	Peabody picture vocabulary test	SPECT	Single photon emission computed tomography
PrP	Prion protein		
PSA	Potential support ratio	SPL	Superior parietal lobule
PSEN	Presenilin	SPM	Statistical parametric mapping
PSIR	Phase-sensitive inversion recovery	SPMS	Secondary progressive MS
PSP	Progressive supranuclear palsy	SPS	Stiff-person syndrome
PSP–CBS	PSP–corticobasal syndrome	SPSMQ	Short portable mental status questionnaire
PSP–CSTD	PSP–corticospinal tract dysfunction	Spt	Sylvian parietotemporal
PSP–P	PSP–parkinsonism	SS	Superficial siderosis
PSP–PAGF	PSP–pure akinaesia with gait freezing	SSI	Small subcortical infarct
PSP–PPAOS	PSP–primary progressive apraxia of speech	SSPE	Subacute sclerosing panencephalitis
PSP–RS	PSP–Richardson's syndrome	SSRI	Selective serotonin reuptake inhibitors
PSTI	Pancreatic secretory trypsin inhibitor	SSRT	Stop-signal reaction time
PTA	Post-traumatic amnesia	STG	Superior temporal gyrus
PTK	Protein tyrosine kinase	STM	Short-term memory
PTSD	Post-traumatic stress disorder	STN	Subthalmic nucleus

STRIVE	STandards for ReportIng Vascular changes on nEuroimaging	VaMCI	MCI of vascular origin
STS	Superior temporal sulcus	VAN	Ventral attentional network
SVD	Small vessel disease	VBM	Voxel-based morphometry
svPPA	Semantic variant primary progressive aphasia	VCD	Vascular cognitive disorder
		VCI	Vascular cognitive impairment
SWI	Susceptibility-weighted images	vCJD	variant CJD
tACS	Transcranial alternating current stimulation	VDRL	Venereal disease research laboratory
TAF	TATA-binding protein-associated factor	VENs	Von Economo neurons
TCA	Tricarboxylic acid	VFD	Visual field disorders
TCMA	Transcortical motor aphasia	VGKC	Voltage-gated potassium channel
tDCS	Transcranial direct current stimulation	VIP	Vasoactive intestinal polypeptide
TDP	TAR DNA-binding protein	vIPS	Ventral intraparietal sulcus
TFND	Transient focal neurological deficits	VIQ	Verbal IQ
TMS	Transcranial magnetic stimulation	VL	Ventrolateral
ToM	Theory of Mind	VLSM	Voxel-based lesion symptom mapping
TPHA	treponema pallidum haemaglutination assay	VOSP	Visual object and space perception
TPPA	treponema pallidum particle agglutination	VTA	Ventral tegmental area
TPI	treponema pallidum immobilization	VVS	Ventral visual stream
TPJ	Temporoparietal junction	VWFA	Visual word form area
TRD	Treatement-resistant depression	WAIS	Wechsler Adult Intelligence Scale
TREM	Triggering receptor expressed on myeloid cells	WCST	Wisconsin Card Sorting Test
		WHO	World Health Organization
Uf	Uncinate fasciculus	WHOSIS	WHO Statistical Information Systems
UHDRS	Unified Huntington's Disease Rating Scale	WMH	White matter MRI hyperintensities
V1	Primary visual cortex	WRAT	Wide Range Achievement Test
VA	Ventral anterior	YLD	Years lost due to disability
VaD	Vascular dementia	YLL	Years of healthy life lost

Contributors

Dalia Abou Zeki, Johns Hopkins University School of Medicine, Baltimore, USA

Morgan D. Barense, University of Toronto, Canada; Rotman Research Institute, Baycrest Hospital, Toronto, Canada

Paolo Bartolomeo, INSERM U 1127, CNRS UMR 7225, Sorbonne Universités, and Université Pierre et Marie Curie-Paris 6, UMR S 1127, Institut du Cerveau et de la Moelle épinière (ICM), Pitié-Salpêtrière Hospital, Paris, France

Geert Jan Biessels, Department of Neurology, Brain Centre Rudolf Magnus, University Medical Centre, Utrecht, The Netherlands

Başar Bilgiç, Associate Professor of Neurology, Istanbul University, Istanbul Faculty of Medicine, Department of Neurology, Behavioral Neurology and Movement Disorders Unit, Istanbul, Turkey

Christopher R. Bowie, Departments of Psychology and Psychiatry, Queens University Kingston, Ontario, Canada

Jose Bras, Dementia Research Institute, University College London, UK

Carol Brayne, Department of Public Health & Primary Care, University of Cambridge, UK

Timothy J. Bussey, Department of Psychology, University of Cambridge, UK; MRC and Wellcome Trust Behavioural and Clinical Neuroscience Institute, University of Cambridge, UK

Diana Caine, Department of Neuropsychology, National Hospital for Neurology and Neurosurgery, London, UK

Marinella Cappelletti, Department of Psychology, Goldsmiths College, University of London, UK; UCL Institute of Cognitive Neuroscience, UK

Marco Catani, NatBrainLab, Institute of Psychiatry, Psychology and Neuroscience, King's College London, UK

John Collinge, MRC Prion Unit, Department of Neurodegenerative Disease, University College London (UCL) Institute of Neurology and NHS National Prion Clinic, National Hospital for

Neurology and Neurosurgery, UCL Hospitals NHS Foundation Trust, UK

Elizabeth A. Coon, Assistant Professor and Consultant of Neurology, Division of Autonomic Neurology, Mayo Clinic, Rochester, USA

Timothy M. Cox, Department of Medicine, University of Cambridge, UK

Sebastian J. Crutch, Dementia Research Centre, UCL Institute of Neurology, UK

Jeffrey L. Cummings, Cleveland Clinic Lou Ruvo Center for Brain Health, Las Vegas, USA

Rachelle S. Doody, Professor, Baylor College of Medicine, Department of Neurology, Houston, USA

Bruno Dubois, Dementia Research Center (IM2A) and Behavioral Unit, Salpêtrière University Hospital, Université Pierre et Marie Curie, Paris, France

Murat Emre, Professor of Neurology, Istanbul University, Istanbul Faculty of Medicine, Department of Neurology, Behavioral Neurology and Movement Disorders Unit, Istanbul, Turkey

Simon Fleminger, Department of Neuropsychiatry, Institute of Psychiatry, King's College London, UK

Tom Foltynie, Senior Lecturer & Honorary Consultant Neurologist, Sobell Department of Motor Neuroscience, UCL Institute of Neurology, UK

Nick C. Fox, Dementia Research Centre, Department of Neurodegenerative Diseases, UCL Institute of Neurology, UK

Ezequiel Gleichgerrcht, Department of Neurology and Neurosurgery, Medical University of South Carolina, USA

Georg Goldenberg, Department of Neurology, Technical University Munich, Germany

Steven M. Greenberg, Hemorrhagic Stroke Research Program, Massachusetts General Hospital, USA

Charles Gross, Department of Psychology and Princeton Neuroscience Institute, Princeton University, USA

Rita Guerreiro, Dementia Research Institute, University College London, UK

Haşmet A. Hanağası, Professor of Neurology, Istanbul University, Istanbul Faculty of Medicine, Department of Neurology, Behavioral Neurology and Movement Disorders Unit, Istanbul, Turkey

Lara Harris, King's College London, Institute of Psychiatry, Psychology and Neuroscience, UK

Philip D. Harvey, Leonard M. Miller Professor of Psychiatry and Behavioral Sciences, University of Miami Miller School of Medicine, USA

Davina J. Hensman Moss, Clinical Fellow, Department of Neurodegenerative Disease, UCL Institute of Neurology and National Hospital for Neurology and Neurosurgery, UK

Argye E. Hillis, Professor of Neurology, Executive Vice Chair, Dept. of Neurology, Director, Cerebrovascular Division, Johns Hopkins University School of Medicine, Baltimore, USA

Janice L. Holton, Queen Square Brain Bank for Neurological Disorders, UCL Institute of Neurology, UK

Kate Humphreys, South London and Maudsley NHS Foundation Trust, UK

Masud Husain, Professor of Neurology & Cognitive Neuroscience, Nuffield Department of Clinical Neurosciences, University of Oxford, John Radcliffe Hospital, UK

Agustin Ibañez, Institute of Translational and Cognitive Neuroscience (ITCN), Ineco Foundation, Favaloro University, Buenos Aires, Argentina; University Adolfo ibañez, Chile; Centre of Excellence in Cognition and its Disorders, Australian Research Council (ACR), Sydney, Australia

Sharon K. Inouye, Aging Brain Center, Institute for Aging Research, Hebrew SeniorLife, Boston, USA; Department of Medicine, Beth Israel Deaconess Medical Center, Harvard Medical School, Boston, USA

Sarosh R. Irani, Honorary Consultant Neurologist and Senior Clinical Fellow, Nuffield Department of Clinical Neurosciences, University of Oxford, UK

Keith A. Josephs, Professor and Consultant of Neurology, Divisions of Behavioural Neurology & Movement Disorders, Mayo Clinic, Rochester, USA

Georg Kerkhoff, Saarland University Department of Psychology, Clinical Neuropsychology Unit and Neuropsychological Outpatient Service, Campus Saarbrücken, Germany

Michael D. Kopelman, King's College London, Institute of Psychiatry, Psychology and Neuroscience, UK

Tammaryn Lashley, Queen Square Brain Bank for Neurological Disorders, UCL Institute of Neurology, UK

Alexander P. Leff, Professor of Cognitive Neurology and Honorary Consultant Neurologist, Institute of Neurology & National Hospital for Neurology and Neurosurgery, University College London, UK

Facundo Manes, Institute of Translational and Cognitive Neuroscience (ITCN), Ineco Foundation, Favaloro University, Buenos Aires, Argentina; UDP-INECO Foundation Core on Neuroscience (UIFCoN), Diego Portales University, Santiago, Chile; Australian Research Council (ACR) Centre of Excellence in Cognition and its Disorders, Sydney, Australia, National Scientific and Technical Research Council (CONICET), Buenos Aires, Argentina

Sergi Martinez-Ramirez, Hemorrhagic Stroke Research Program, Massachusetts General Hospital, USA

Simon Mead, MRC Prion Unit, Department of Neurodegenerative Disease, University College London (UCL) Institute of Neurology and NHS National Prion Clinic, National Hospital For Neurology and Neurosurgery, UCL Hospitals NHS Foundation Trust, UK

Benedict Daniel Michael, Post-Doctoral Research Fellow, Massachusetts General Hospital, Harvard Medical School; Institute of Infection and Global Health, University of Liverpool, UK; Walton Centre for Neurology and Neurosurgery, Liverpool, UK

Raffaella Migliaccio, INSERM U 1127, CNRS UMR 7225, Sorbonne Universités, and Université Pierre et Marie Curie-Paris 6, UMR S 1127, Institut du Cerveau et de la Moelle épinière (ICM), and Department of Neurology, Institute of memory and Alzheimer's disease, Pitié-Salpêtrière Hospital, Paris, France

Ellen M. Migo, King's College London, Institute of Psychiatry, Psychology and Neuroscience, UK

Bruce Miller, Department of Neurology, UCSF School of Medicine, San Francisco, USA

Thomas D. Miller, Patrick Berthoud/Encephalitis Society Clinical Research Fellow, Nuffield Department of Clinical Neurosciences, University of Oxford, UK; Specialist Registrar in Neurology, National Hospital For Neurology and Neurosurgery, University College London, London, UK

Thais Minett, Specialty Registrar in Radiology, Academic Clinical Fellow, Department of Radiology, University of Cambridge, UK

Barbara C. van Munster, Department of Internal Medicine, Academic Medical Centre, Amsterdam, The Netherlands; Department of Geriatrics, Gelre Hospitals, Apeldoorn, The Netherlands

Peter J. Nestor, German Centre for Neurodegenerative Diseases (DZNE), Magdeburg, Germany

Sam Nightingale, Institute of Infection and Global Health, University of Liverpool, UK

Jane Powell, Goldsmiths, University of London, UK

Geraint Rees, UCL Institute of Cognitive Neuroscience, UK

Tamas Revesz, Queen Square Brain Bank for Neurological Disorders, UCL Institute of Neurology, UK

Timothy Rittman, Clinical Research Fellow, University of Cambridge, UK

Trevor W. Robbins, Professor of Cognitive Neuroscience and Experimental Psychology Director, Behavioural and Clinical Neuroscience Institute Head of Dept. Psychology, University of Cambridge, UK

Jonathan D. Rohrer, Dementia Research Centre, UCL Institute of Neurology, UK

Maria A. Ron, Emeritus Professor of Neuropsychiatry, UCL Institute of Neurology, UK

Sophia E. de Rooij, Department of Internal Medicine, Academic Medical Centre, Amsterdam, The Netherlands; Department of Internal Medicine, University Medical Centre Groningen, The Netherlands

Martin N. Rossor, Dementia Research Centre, Department of Neurodegenerative Diseases, UCL Institute of Neurology, UK

Susan Rountree, Associate Professor, Baylor College of Medicine, Department of Neurology, Houston, USA

James Rowe, Professor of Cognitive Neurology, University of Cambridge, UK

Peter Rudge, MRC Prion Unit, Department of Neurodegenerative Disease, University College London (UCL) Institute of Neurology and NHS National Prion Clinic, National Hospital For Neurology and Neurosurgery, UCL Hospitals NHS Foundation Trust, UK

Lisa M. Saksida, Department of Psychology, University of Cambridge, UK; MRC and Wellcome Trust Behavioural and Clinical Neuroscience Institute, University of Cambridge, UK

Seyed Ahmad Sajjadi, Neurology Department, Addenbrooke's Hospital, Cambridge, UK

Anna Katharina Schaadt, Saarland University Department of Psychology, Clinical Neuropsychology Unit and Neuropsychological Outpatient Service, Campus Saarbrücken, Germany

Philip Scheltens, Alzheimer Centre and Department of Neurology, VU University Medical Centre, Neuroscience Campus Amsterdam, the Netherlands

Jonathan M. Schott, Professor of Neurology, Dementia Research Centre, Department of Neurodegenerative Diseases, UCL Institute of Neurology, UK

David J. Sharp, National Institute of Health (NIHR) Professor and Consultant Neurologist, The Computational, Cognitive and Clinical Neuroimaging Laboratory, Division of Brain Sciences, Imperial College London, UK

Tom Solomon, Institute of Infection and Global Health, University of Liverpool, UK; Walton Centre for Neurology and Neurosurgery, Liverpool, UK

Nicholas J.C. Smith, Department of Neurology, Women's and Children's Health Network and Discipline of Paediatrics, School of Medicine, University of Adelaide, Australia

Sarah J. Tabrizi, Professor of Clinical Neurology, Honorary Consultant Neurologist, Department of Neurodegenerative Disease, UCL Institute of Neurology and National Hospital for Neurology and Neurosurgery, UK

Teresa Torralva, Institute of Translational and Cognitive Neuroscience (ITCN), Ineco Foundation, Favaloro University, Buenos Aires, Argentina; UDP-INECO Foundation Core on Neuroscience (UIFCoN), Diego Portales University, Santiago, Chile; Australian Research Council (ACR) Centre of Excellence in Cognition and its Disorders, Sydney, Australia

Olga Uspenskaya-Cadoz, Quintiles; CNS Medical Strategy and Science; Levallois-Perret, France

Angela Vincent, Professor of Neuroimmunology and Honorary Clinical Immunologist, Nuffield Department of Clinical Neurosciences, University of Oxford, UK

Anand Viswanathan, Hemorrhagic Stroke Research Program, Massachusetts General Hospital, USA

Jason D. Warren, Dementia Research Centre, UCL Institute of Neurology, UK

Dylan Wint, Cleveland Clinic Lou Ruvo Center for Brain Health, Las Vegas, USA

Nicholas W. Wood, Galton Chair of Genetics, Vice Dean Research Faculty of Brain Sciences, NIHR UCLH BRC Neuroscience Programme Director, UCL Institute of Neurology, UK

Soo Jin Yoon, Associate Professor, Department of Neurology, Eulji University Hospital, Eulji University School of Medicine, Daejeon, Korea

Giovanna Zamboni, Nuffield Department of Clinical Neurosciences (NDCN), University of Oxford, UK

Ludvic Zrinzo, Professor of Neurosurgery, Sobell Department of Motor Neuroscience, UCL Institute of Neurology, UK

SECTION 1

Normal cognitive function

CHAPTER 1

Historical aspects of neurology

Charles Gross

Before science

The oldest known neurological procedure is trepanning or trephining, the removal of a piece of bone from the skull. It was practised from the late Palaeolithic period onwards and throughout the world. The motivation for trephining in non-literate cultures is obscure but may have been related to the treatment of epilepsy or headaches caused by skull injury, or relief of symptoms thought to have been caused by demonic forces. From classical Greece to the Renaissance, trephining was used to treat such maladies as head injury, epilepsy, and mental disease.[1,2]

The first written reference to the brain is in the *Edwin Smith Surgical Papyrus* written in about 1700 BCE but a copy of an older treatise dated to about 3000 BCE. It appears to be a handbook for a battlefield surgeon and consists of a coolly empirical description of 48 cases from the head down to the shoulders, when the text breaks off. For each case the author describes the examination, diagnosis, and feasibility of treatment.[3,4] The *Smith* papyrus stands out as a rock of empiricism in the ocean of magic and superstition in which Egyptian medical writings swim for about the next twenty-four centuries. It reflects craft and some empirical knowledge but it is not what we today call medical science.

Classical neuroscience

The Presocratics and the beginning of science

What we mean by 'science' today is the contribution of the Presocratic philosophers. They were responsible for the idea that the physical and biological universe is governed by consistent and universal laws that are amenable to understanding by human reason. This was a revolutionary change from the previous prevailing view of the universe as a plaything of gods and ghosts who acted in an arbitrary and capricious fashion. The Presocratics lived from the sixth to the fourth centuries BCE in various Greek city-states. They conceived their inquiries on the universe as demanding rational criticism and public debate and involving observation and measurement. (Systematic experimentation, especially in biology, was almost unknown for several centuries).[5-11]

Among the major Presocratics were Thales, Anaximander, Anaximenes, Heraclitus, Pythagoras, Empedocles, Zeno, and Democritus. Many of them were interested in sensory processes as sources of knowledge and several were physicians. One such physician was Alcmaeon (~570–500 BCE), head of a medical school in southern Italy. He was the first writer to advocate the brain as the site of sensation and cognition. He is said to have written:

> The seat of sensations is in the brain. This contains the governing faculty. All the senses are connected in some way with the brain;

consequently they are incapable of action if the brain is disturbed or shifts its position, for this stops up the passages through which senses act. This power of the brain to synthesize sensations makes it also the seat of thought: the storing up of perceptions gives memory and belief, and when these are stabilized you get knowledge.[12]

Alcmaeon is reported to have been the first to use dissection as a tool for intellectual inquiry. He dissected the eye and described the optic nerves and chiasm and suggested they brought light to the brain.[7-12]

The Hippocratic school

The other centre of Greek medicine was the island of Cos in the Aegean Sea and its most famous inhabitant Hippocrates (~425 BCE). The Hippocratic corpus of writing is the first large body of Western scientific writings that has survived. It consists of over 60 treatises of unknown authorship and date, perhaps a remnant of the library which once existed on Cos.[8]

The Hippocratic treatise of greatest relevance to neurology is the famed essay 'On the Sacred Disease' (i.e. epilepsy). The author of this treatise has no doubt that the brain is the seat of epilepsy; on the general functions of the brain he is equally clear:

> It ought to be generally known that the source of our pleasure, merriment, laughter and amusement, as of our grief, pain, anxiety and tears is none other than the brain. It is specially the organ which enables us to think, see, and hear and to distinguish the ugly and the beautiful, the bad and the good, pleasant and unpleasant . . . it is the brain too which is the seat of madness and delirium.[13]

Neurological and other disorders were explained and treated in terms of the theory of the four humours: phlegm (from the brain), blood (from the heart), yellow bile (from the liver), and black bile (from the spleen). These ideas, as elaborated later by Galen (129–210), pervaded medicine and were central to medical education well into the nineteenth century.[7-10,13,14]

Curiously, Aristotle (384–322 BCE) argued against the brain and in favour of the heart as the dominant organ for sensation, cognition, and movement. He systematically attacked the encephalocentric views of Alcmaeon and the Hippocratic doctors on a number of anatomical and embryological grounds, but the critical evidence available at this time was from the clinic, the study of brain-injured humans, and clinical medicine held no interest for Aristotle.[15]

Galen

Galen of Pergamon (129–213) was by far the most important physician, anatomist, and physiologist in classical antiquity.[14] Furthermore, he was the first to carry out systematic experiments on the nervous system, thereby initiating experimental neurology.[16] Galen's descriptions of the gross anatomy of the brain were

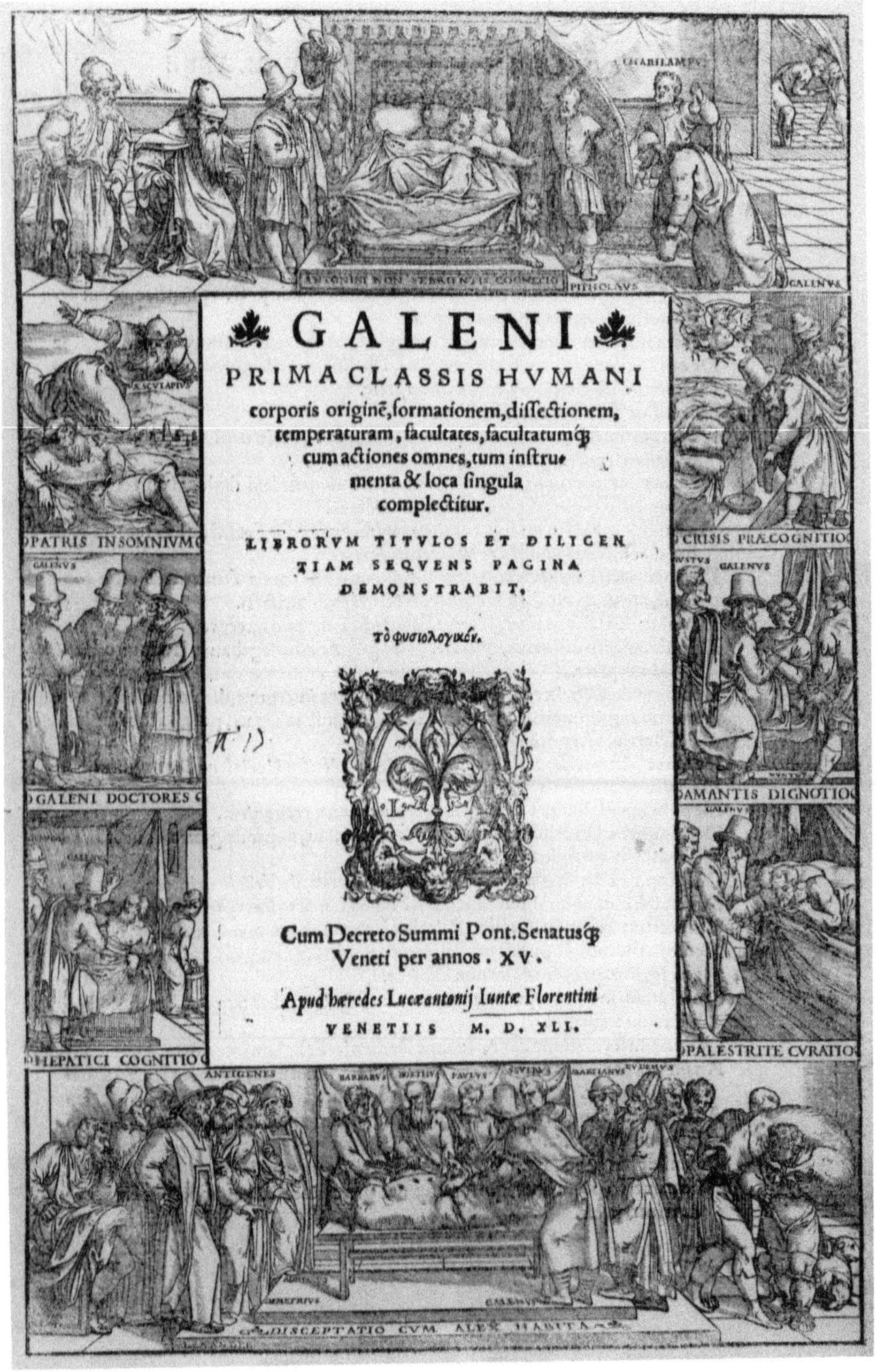

Fig. 1.1 Title page of Galen's *Omnia Opera* published in 1541 in Venice by Junta. The eight scenes, clockwise from the top, are: Galen bowing to a wealthy patient; Galen predicting the crisis in a patient's sickness; Galen diagnosing lovesickness; Galen bleeding a patient; Galen demonstrating the effect of cutting the recurrent laryngeal nerve in a pig; Galen palpating the liver; Galen and his teachers; Aesculpaius in a dream urging Galen's father to send him to medical school.
Reproduced from Gross CG, *Brain, Vision, Memory: Tales in the History of Neuroscience,* Copyright (1999), with permission from MIT Press.

very accurate, particularly with respect to the ventricles and cerebral circulation, both important in his physiological system. He usually presented his dissections as if they were of the human, but in fact, because of the taboo on dissecting the human body, they were invariably of animals, usually the ox in the case of brain anatomy.[17]

Galen's truly revolutionary work was to carry out the first systematic experiments on the functions of the nervous system. He used piglets in his experiments on brain lesions. He found that anterior brain damage had less deleterious effects than posterior. He viewed sensation as a central process since he knew from his clinical observations and animal experiments that sensation could be impaired by brain injury even when the sense organs were intact. Since animals could survive lesions that penetrated to the ventricles, Galen thought the soul was not located there but rather in the cerebral substance. He taught that all mental diseases were brain diseases.[16,18,19]

Galen's most famous experiment was the public demonstration of the effects of cutting the recurrent laryngeal nerve on squealing in a pig. Although the encephalocentric view that the brain controlled sensation, movement, and cognition remained strong in the Greco–Roman medical community, the opposing cardiocentric view, that the heart was the centre of sensation and cognition, was also active in Rome at this time, being advocated by the Stoic school and its leader Chrysippus (280–207 BCE). In order to refute the Stoics' view that the heart and not the brain controlled cognition, Galen arranged this public demonstration.[16,19]

He showed that cutting the recurrent laryngeal nerve would eliminate vocalization. Since vocalization was seen as reflecting the cognitive activity language, Galen's demonstration that cutting a nerve originating in the brain would eliminate squealing in a pig was the first, and most famous, demonstration that the brain controls cognition. The Renaissance edition of Galen's works included an engraving of him carrying out the experiment on a huge pig in front of a very distinguished audience (Fig. 1.1).

Medieval and Renaissance neuroscience

The medieval doctrine of brain function

At about the time of Galen's death, classical science and medicine seem to disappear. People prefer to believe rather than to discuss, critical faculty gives way to dogma, interest in this world declines in favour of the world to come, and worldly remedies are replaced by prayer and exorcism. The world view of medieval Christendom found Galen's teleology congenial to its own and by a smothering of critical facility froze Galen's research and all biology into a sterile system for over 1500 years. Galen was not to blame. Rather than develop his discoveries and methods, the European medieval world chose to accept his views as fixed and unchangeable facts in every branch of medicine.

The central feature of the medieval view of brain function was the localization of the mental faculties in the ventricles (Fig. 1.2). The faculties of the mind (derived from Aristotle) were distributed among the spaces within the brain (derived from the ventricles described by Galen). The anterior ventricle received input from the sense organs and was the site of the *common sense*, which integrated across modalities. The sensations yielded images and thus fantasy and imagination were also located in the anterior ventricle. The middle ventricle was the site of cognition: reasoning, judgement, and thought. The posterior ventricle was the site of memory. These specific localizations seem to have come from the fourth-century Byzantine physician Poseidon on the basis of his observations of human brain injury.[20,21]

The Islamic transmission

Greek medical learning was largely preserved in Islamic centres in the early Middle Ages. Hippocratic, Galenic, and other medical writings were largely lost to Europe both because of lack of familiarity with Greek and loss of the manuscripts themselves. This began to change in the tenth and eleventh centuries when translations from the Greek medical works into Syriac, Arabic, and Hebrew, and then into Latin finally reached Europe.[21] With the birth of universities, first in Bologna, anatomical dissections began, initially for forensic

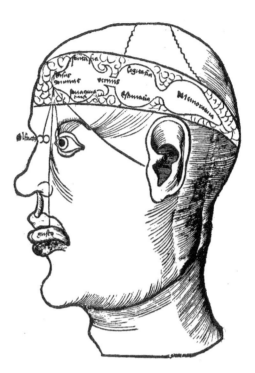

Fig. 1.2 Ventricular doctrine. Messages from the nose, tongue, eye, and ear go to the first ventricle in which common sense, fantasy, and imagination are found. The second ventricle contains thought and judgment; memory is in the third ventricle. Reproduced from Reish G, *Margarita Philosophica (Pearls of Philosophy)*, Copyright (1503), Johannes Schott.

purposes and following translations of Galen. However, it was not until Vesalius (1514–1564) that anatomy became largely free from the dominance of Galen. His *On the Fabric of the Human Body* (Fig. 1.3) along with Copernicus's (1473–1543) *On the Revolutions of the Celestial Spheres* mark the beginning of the scientific revolution, the revival in Europe of science.

Thomas Willis and 'neurology'

Thomas Willis (1621–74) wrote the first comprehensive text on the brain, *Cerebri Anatomie*, which dealt not only with brain anatomy but also with neurophysiology, neurochemistry, and clinical neurology, and introduced, in its English translation, the term 'neurology'.[22] *Cerebri Anatomie* actually involved the collaboration of a group of savants known as the Virtuosi, such as Robert Boyle and Christopher Wren, who later became founding members of the new Royal Society (see Fig. 1.4).

Willis rejected the still pervasive belief in the ventricles as the seats of higher psychological functions and instead implicated 'the critical and grey part of the cerebrum' in memory and will. Sensory signals came along sensory pathways into the corpus striatum where common sense was located. They were then elaborated into perception and imagination in the overlying white matter (then called the corpus callosum), and finally passed onto the cortex where they were stored as memories. Willis ascribed voluntary movements to the cortex but involuntary ones to the cerebellum. His ideas on brain function came from his own experiments on brain lesions in animals, from the correlation of the effects of human brain damage with post-mortem pathology, and from the comparison of the brains of various animals with those of humans.[22–24]

Although Willis was a major figure in his time, his ideas on the cerebral cortex soon fell out of favour and theories of the cortex

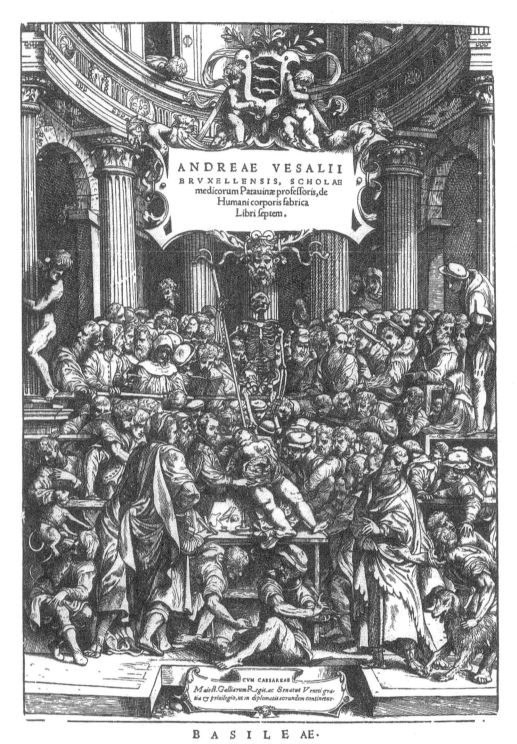

ANDREAE VESALII
BRVXELLENSIS, SCHOLAE
medicorum Patauinæ professoris, de
Humani corporis fabrica
Libri septem.

CVM CAESAREAE
Maiest. Galliarum Regis, ac Senatus Veneti gra-
tia & priuilegio, ut in diplomatis eorundem continetur.

B A S I L E AE·

Fig. 1.3 Title page of Andreas Vesalius's *De Humani Corpori Fabrica* (*On the Structure of the Human Body*), 2nd edn.1543 Basel: Oporinus. It shows a public dissection by Vesalius (centre). His assistant is relegated to sharpening knives (front). The bodies were from executions and usually males, unlike here. The dissection is being held outdoors with a wooden structure for spectators. For further details of the symbols and details in this famous woodcut from Titian's workshop, see CG Gross, *Brain, Vision, Memory: Tales in the History of Neuroscience* 1998. Cambridge, MA: MIT Press.

as glandular or vascular became dominant. Marcello Malpighi (1628–94), the discoverer of capillaries, was the first to examine the cortex under the microscope.[24–25] He saw it as made up of little glands or 'globules', and Antoni van Leewenhoek (1632–1723) and others followed suit. This was a common view in the seventeenth and eighteenth centuries, perhaps because it fit with the much earlier view of Aristotle that the brain was a cooling organ and the Hippocratic theory that it was the source of phlegm.[5,15] The other common view was that the cortex was largely made up of blood vessels; as Frederik Rusch (1628–1731) put it: '[t]he cortical

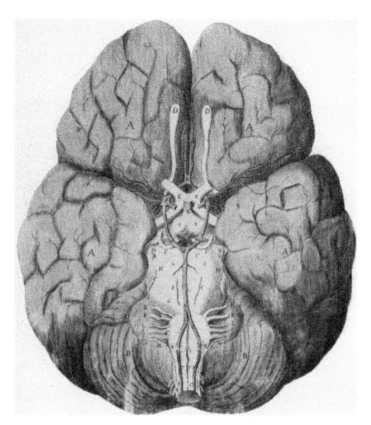

Fig. 1.4 Ventral view of the brain.
Reproduced from Willis T, *Cerebri Anatomie*, Copyright (1664), Martyn and Allestry, drawn by Christopher Wren.

substance of the cerebrum is not glandular, as many anatomists have described it ... but highly vascular'.[26] Albrecht von Haller (1708–77), who dominated physiology in the eighteenth century, also held a vascular view of the cortex. He found mechanical and chemical stimulation to be without effect throughout the cortex and declared it completely insensitive.[27]

The beginning of modern neuroscience

Gall and phrenology: Localization of function in the cortex

The revolutionary idea that different regions of the cerebral cortex have different function began with Franz Joseph Gall (1748–1828) and his collaborator, JC Spurzheim (1776–1832) and their system of phrenology.[28–30]

The central aim of phrenology was to correlate brain structure and function. Phrenology had five basic assumptions:

1. The brain is an elaborately wired machine for producing behaviour, thought, and emotions

2. The cerebral cortex is a set of organs each corresponding to an affective or intellectual function

3. Differences in traits among people and within individuals depend on differential development of different cortical areas

4. Development of a cortical area is reflected in its size

5. Size of a cortical area is correlated with the overlying skull ('bumps')

These otherwise reasonable hypotheses had one fatal flaw: the nature of the evidence. Gall and Spurzheim relied almost entirely on obtaining supportive or confirmatory evidence. They collected large numbers of skulls of people whose traits and abilities were known, examined the heads of distinguished savants and inhabitants of mental hospitals and prisons, and studied portraits of the high and low born on various intellectual and affective dimensions (Fig. 1.5). Throughout, they were seeking confirmation of their initial hypothesis usually deriving from a few cases. For example, the idea for a language organ in the frontal lobes comes from Gall's experience of a classmate who had a prodigious verbal memory and protruding eyes (being pushed out by a well-developed frontal lobe, Gall thought). The idea for an organ of destructiveness came from the skulls of a parricide and of a murderer, from noticing its prominence in a fellow student 'who was so fond of torturing animals that he became a surgeon', and from examining the head of a meat-loving dog he owned.[28]

They sought confirmations; contradictions were dismissed. Gall and Spurzheim's cortical localizations were of 'higher' intellectual and personality traits. They accepted the prevailing view that the highest sensory functions were in the thalamus and the highest motor functions in the corpus striatum.[29,30]

Phrenology met with considerable opposition from political and religious authorities, particularly on the Continent, largely because it was viewed as implying materialism and determinism and denied the unity of the mind (and soul) and the existence of free will. On the other hand, phrenology spread widely particularly in the United States and Great Britain both as a medical doctrine and as a form of

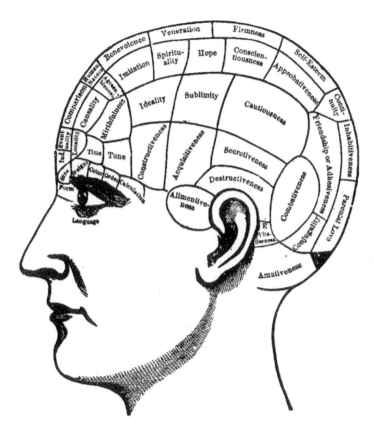

Fig. 1.5 The phrenological organs.
Reproduced from Human Nature Library, New York, Copyright (1887).

'pop' psychology. It generated widespread interest both among the general populace and among such writers and savants as Honore de Balzac, Charles Baudelaire, George Eliot, August Comte, Horace Mann, Alfred Russell Wallace, and George Henry Lewis. It rapidly became a fad and drawing-room amusement, particularly in Great Britain and the US. Phrenological societies and journals continued to flourish in both countries well into the twentieth century.[31]

Gall's mistaken assumption of a correlation between the skull and brain morphology was soon recognized, at least in the scientific community. In spite of its absurdities and excesses, phrenology became a major spur for the development of modern neuroscience in a variety of ways. It generated an interest in the brain and behaviour. It directed attention to the cerebral cortex. It stimulated study of both human brain damage and of experimental lesions in animals. It inspired tracing pathways from sense organs and to the muscles in order to identify 'organs' of the cerebral cortex. It spurred the anatomical subdivision of the cerebral cortex (cytoarchitectonics, myeloarchitectonics) to find organs of the brain.[29,30]

The cytoarchitectonic, positron emission tomography (PET), functional magnetic resonance imaging (fMRI), and other maps of the cerebral cortex that are now ubiquitous in neuroanatomy, neurophysiology, and neuropsychology textbooks bear more than a coincidental resemblance to phrenological charts. They are the direct descendants of the iconoclastic, ambitious, and heavily flawed programme of phrenology seeking to relate brain structure and behaviour.

Language and the brain

In the middle of the nineteenth century, Gall's theory of punctate localization of function in the cerebral cortex continued to be debated. Reports of correlations between the site of brain injury and specific psychological deficits in patients as well as experimental animals were published and actively discussed in both phrenological and mainstream medical publications.

The debate about localization reached a climax at a series of meetings of the Paris *Societé d'Anthropologie* in 1861. At the April meeting, Paul Broca (1824–80), professor at the Sorbonne and founder of the society, announced that he had a critical case on this issue. A patient with long-standing language difficulties—nicknamed 'Tam', because that was all he could say—had just died. The next day, Broca displayed Tam's brain at the meeting and it had widespread damage in the left frontal lobe. Over the next few months Broca presented several similar cases of difficulty in speaking, all with left frontal lesions. This discovery was the first clear evidence for a specific psychological defect after a specific brain lesion. Not only did these cases finally establish the principle of discrete localization of function in the cortex, but in addition, the discovery was hailed as a vindication of Gall: both of his idea of punctate localization and his localization of language in the frontal lobes.[29,30,32]

By 1865, Broca had accumulated enough cases to notice that all his brains from aphasic patients had their frontal damage on the left side and he described the left hemisphere as *dominant* for language.[32,34] (An obscure country doctor, Max Dax, apparently made the same observations in 1836, and his son Gustave Dax fought Broca over the priority for this claim.)[33]

In 1874, Carl Wernicke reported another type of language disturbance after left hemisphere lesions in which speech is fluent but nonsensical, often known as sensory or Wernicke's aphasia, as opposed to motor or Broca's aphasia. Whereas Broca's aphasia usually followed lesions of the third frontal convolution or Broca's area, Wernicke's aphasia usually followed damage to the posterior temporal lobe. Today a variety of aphasias have been described with more sophisticated descriptive analysis than 'motor' versus 'sensory'.[34]

It was generally assumed that language localization in left-handed individuals was the opposite of that in right-handers; that is, that language was in the right hemisphere in left-handed individuals. However, as pointed out by Alexander Luria on the basis of his large sample of head injuries in the Second World War, language is primarily in the right hemisphere in roughly half of all left-handers. This was confirmed by the Wada test (unilateral hemispheric anaesthesia), and fMRI and PET brain imaging. Today we know that language localization in left-handers is some kind of complex function of genetics and prenatal trauma, and that bilateral representation of language is much more common in left-handers (and females). Furthermore, even in right-handers, a variety of language functions exist in the right hemisphere. Finally, left hemisphere damage before puberty can be compensated by right hemisphere function.[35-37]

The discovery of motor cortex

Modern neurophysiology began with Gustav Fritsch (1838–1927) and Edmund Hitzig's (1838–1907) discovery in 1870 that stimulation of the motor cortex produces movement. Their discovery was the first experimental evidence that the cortex was involved in movement, the first demonstration that the cortex was electrically excitable, the first strong experimental evidence for functional localization in the cortex, and the first experimental evidence for somatotopic representation in the brain.

In their now classic experiment, Fritsch and Hitzig strapped their dogs down on Frau Hitzig's dressing table. They stimulated the cortex with 'galvanic stimulation': brief pulses of monophasic direct current from a battery. The usual response to this stimulation was a muscle twitch or spasm. Their central findings were that: a) the stimulation evoked contralateral movements, b) only stimulation of the anterior cortex elicited movements, c) stimulation of specific parts of the cortex consistently produced the activation of specific muscles, and d) the excitable sites formed a repeatable, if rather sparse, map of movements of the body laid out on the cortical surface (Fig. 1.6). They went on to show that lesion of a particular site impaired the movements produced by stimulation of that site. The loss of function was not complete, suggesting to them that there were other motor centres that had not been impaired by the lesion.[39]

Fritsch and Hitzig had no hesitation in announcing the general significance of their discovery:

> By the results of our own investigations, the premises for many conclusions about the basic properties of the brain are changed not a little . . . some psychological functions, and perhaps all of them . . . need circumscribed centers of the cerebral cortex.[39]

Soon after their paper appeared, the young Scottish physician David Ferrier set out to follow up their work.[40] Ferrier had been heavily influenced by John Hughlings Jackson, and he realized that Fritsch and Hitzig had confirmed Jackson's ideas. In a variety of species, including macaques, Ferrier replicated their basic findings that stimulation of the cortex can produce specific movements and that there is a topographic 'motor map' in the cerebral cortex.[41-44]

Both Fritsch and Hitzig's and Ferrier's papers on the motor cortex were initially greeted with considerable and equal scepticism. Their results went against the generally accepted views that the striatum was the highest motor centre and that the cortex was inexcitable. The critics usually interpreted the results of Fritsch and Hitzig and of Ferrier as artefactual due to 'spread of current' to the striatum, then considered the highest motor centre. To overcome these criticisms,

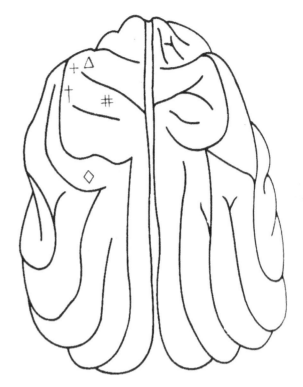

Fig. 1.6 Movements produced by electrical stimulation of the cerebral cortex of the dog.
Notes: Δ, twitching of neck muscles; +, abduction of foreleg; †, flexion of foreleg; #, movement of foreleg; ☐, facial twitching.
Reproduced from Fritsch GT, and Hitzig E, On the electrical excitability of the cerebrum [1870]. In: von Bonin G, trans., *Some Papers on the Cerebral Cortex*, Copyright (1960), with permission from Charles C Thomas.

Victor Horsley, Charles S Sherrington, and others began meticulous 'punctate' mapping of the cortex using the minimum current to elicit the smallest discernable movement.[e.g. 45-47] Sherrington's map of the motor cortex in the chimpanzee, followed by Wilbur Penfield's human motor homunculus and Clinton Woolsey's maps of monkeys and other animals, became the standard picture of the motor cortex.[48-50] Ferrier's maps of the motor cortex in the macaque were applied surprisingly quickly to human brain surgery. Starting in 1876, the Scottish surgeon William McEwen and the London surgeon RJ Godlee used Ferrier's maps to successfully locate and remove tumours.[51]

Recently, Michael Graziano has revisited Ferrier's idea that the motor cortex may control complex, highly integrated behaviour.[52]

The neuron doctrine

The neuron doctrine—the idea that the nervous system is made up of discrete nerve cells that are the anatomical, physiological, genetic, and metabolic bases of its functions—may be viewed as the single-most important development in the entire history of neuroscience. The work of two men was crucial to the final acceptance of the doctrine: Camillo Golgi (1843–1926) and Santiago Ramón y Cajal (1852–1934).[53]

Although Theodor Schwann suggested, in 1838, that all animal tissues are made up of cells, the nervous system resisted interpretation in terms of cell theory for about another 50 years. This was because with the stains and microscopes available, the nervous system often looked like an anastomosing network or 'reticulum'. The resolution of this enigma came, eventually, from the discovery by

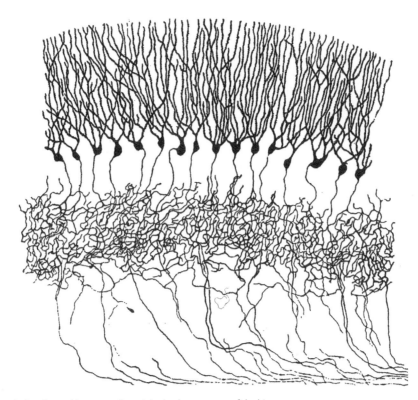

Fig. 1.7 Golgi's drawing of the reticulum formed by axon collaterals in the dentate gyrus of the hippocampus.
Reproduced from Golgi C, The neuron doctrine–theory and facts. Nobel Lecture, 11 December 1906. In: *Nobel Lectures Physiology or Medicine 1901–1921*. Copyright (1999), with permission from the Nobel Foundation.

Golgi in 1873 of a new silver stain that stained only a small proportion of cells but did so in their entirety.[53]

Using this stain, Golgi a) confirmed Otto Deiters's earlier observation of a single axon ('axis cylinder') coming from each nerve cell, b) found that dendrites ('protoplasmic prolongations') ended freely, c) discovered axon collaterals and thought they merged with the axon collaterals of other nerve cells to form a diffuse reticulum, and d) classified nerve cells by their processes. Golgi believed that the function of dendrites was nutritive and not the conducting of messages. He had a holistic view of brain function and thought that the reticulum, made up of anastomosing axon collaterals, was the basic mechanism of brain function (Fig. 1.7). This, he thought, accounted for such phenomena as recovery from brain damage. His holism led him to disbelieve the localization results of Fritsch and Hitzig and of Ferrier.[53]

Fourteen years later, Ramón y Cajal came across the Golgi silver stain and immediately began making the often-capricious Golgi method more reliable, particularly by working with younger animals who have less myelin, since myelin is resistant to silver staining. Unlike Golgi, Cajal concluded that axon collaterals did not anastomose but ended freely: neurons were separate independent units. Although microscopes were not able to visualize the gap between neurons, Cajal inferred (intuited might be a better term) its existence on several grounds. One was by using immature or even foetal animals where he observed axons growing out of cell bodies before approaching other neurons or muscles. Another was that when cutting a nerve fibre it would degenerate, but only up to the border with the next cell.[53] (See Fig. 1.8).

Beyond confirming the idea of the neuron as an independent unit, Cajal developed the 'Law of Dynamic Polarization', the idea that information transmission was from the dendrites to the cell body and out along the axon. He then used this 'law' to work out several neural circuits that began with sensory receptors in the retina or in the olfactory bulb.[53]

In 1906, Golgi and Cajal shared the Nobel Prize. Golgi's Nobel address was a vigorous defense of the reticular theory with the claim that the neuron theory 'is generally recognized as going out of favor'.[53,54] Over 100 years later, the neuron doctrine still stands as the bedrock of neuroscience. Its fundamental tenet of the discontinuity between neurons was finally confirmed by the electron microscope in the 1950s only to be soon modulated by the discovery of a very small number of gap junctions in which the cell membranes of adjacent neurons are immediately opposed and synaptic transmission is electrical.[55,56] The Law of Dynamic Polarization is still considered to be a fundamental property of neural circuits, although the existence of axon-less neurons, dendro-dendritic and axon–axonal synapses has complicated the picture.[53]

Twentieth-century neuroscience

Prefrontal cortex

The association of the prefrontal cortex with the higher intellectual faculties has a long history. Classical busts of gods, heroes, and famous writers and artists usually show a high forehead in contrast to both lower-class individuals and women, both of whom were usually depicted to have retreating foreheads.[57] The eighteenth-century Swedish theoretical neuroscientist and philosopher, Emanuel Swedenborg, attributed imagination, memory, thought, and will to the anterior regions of the brain.[58] Gall and Spurzheim placed the 'intellectual' faculties in the most anterior brain regions. When the

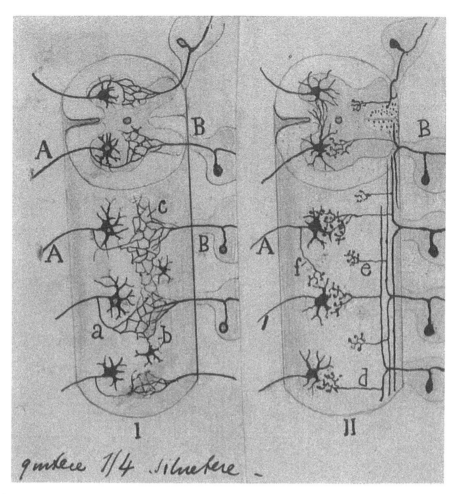

Fig. 1.8 Cajal's drawing of the sensory-motor connections of the spinal cord according to his neuron theory (right) and to Golgi's reticular theory (left). A: anterior roots; B; posterior roots. According to Golgi, collaterals of the motor axon (a) anastomose forming part of a diffuse interstitial network (c). According to Cajal, the axon collaterals (f) do not.

Reproduced from Cajal S Ramon y. *Recollections of My Life*, Trans. EH Craigie, Copyright (1937), American Philosophical Society.

systematic study of human brain injury and of experimental lesions in monkeys began in the nineteenth century, intellectual function was usually located in the prefrontal cortex. For example, from their observations of frontal lobe damage, the frontal lobes were thought by Hitzig to contain the highest intellectual centre, by Ferrier to be the centre of attention and therefore of ideation and perception, by Paul Flechsig to be the area for volition and the higher levels of personality, by Giovanni Bianchi to be the centre of centres, and by Wilhelm Wundt to be an 'apperception' centre.[59]

In 1848, one of the most notable cases of prefrontal injury occurred in a man working with explosives on the railroad, whose skull was accidentally pierced by an iron bar pierce. Remarkably, Phineas Gage survived the accident but his personality and behaviour changed irrevocably. From being a considerate, responsible foreman, he became 'fitful, indulging at times in the grossest profanities … manifesting but little deference for his fellows, impatient of restraint or advice when it conflicts with his desires, at times pertinaciously obstinate, yet capricious and vacillating, devising many plans of future operation, which are no sooner arranged that they are abandoned'.[60] Gage's case was not widely reported and its true importance was not fully appreciated until much later, but it stands as a landmark case in the history of observations of human prefrontal function.[61]

In the first objective tests of prefrontal function in animals, after prefrontal lesions, monkeys and chimpanzees were found to be severely and permanently impaired on performance of the 'delayed response test' in which the animal is required to remember, after a brief delay, at which of two sites a bait is hidden.[62] This was considered to be a test of 'recent memory'[62] and later one of 'working memory'.[63] The dorsolateral prefrontal cortex was subsequently shown to be crucial for performance of this task.[59,64]

An incidental observation on a single chimpanzee's behaviour during this task led directly to the widespread clinical use of frontal lobe surgery to treat a variety of psychiatric disorders. Prior to lesion of its frontal lobe, this animal would have temper-tantrums whenever she made an error on the delayed response test. She no longer did so following the operation.[62] When the Portuguese neurologist Egas Moniz heard of this observation at the International Congress of Neurology in London in 1935, he was inspired to initiate a series of frontal 'leucotomies' (cutting the white matter under the frontal cortex) to treat mental illness, and versions of the procedure technique were rapidly adopted elsewhere. In 1949, Moniz received the Nobel Prize for the introduction of frontal leucotomy. This and other psychosurgical procedures on the frontal lobe were carried out on an estimated 60 000 people in the US alone (Fig. 1.9). The practice radically declined in the 1980s largely

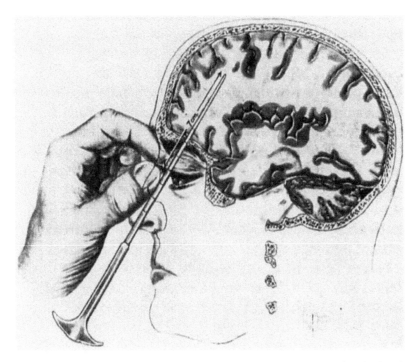

Fig. 1.9 W. Transorbital lobotomy used extensively by Walter Freeman: 'A transorbital leucotome is inserted through the orbital roof into the brain and the handle is swung medially and laterally to sever fibers at the base of the frontal lobe.'
Reproduced from *Proc. R. Soc. Med.* (Suppl.). 42, Freeman W, Transorbital leucotomy: the deep frontal cut. pp. 8–12, Copyright (1949), with permission from SAGE Publications.

because of the introduction of chlorpromazine and other psychoactive drugs.[65–67]

Assessment of the effects of frontal lobotomies is difficult because very few patients were studied objectively before and after surgery by independent investigators. Elliot Valenstein, who investigated the efficacy of the older lobotomies, summarized the situation as follows:

> In general, there seems to be strong suggestive evidence (if not absolutely convincing) that some patients may have been significantly helped by psychosurgery. There is certainly no grounds for either the position that all psychosurgery necessarily reduces people to a 'vegetable status' or that is has a high probability of producing marvelous cures ...There is little doubt, however, that many abuses existed. Quite apart from the effectiveness of the surgery there were always some risks. Patients did occasionally die from the operation, epilepsy was not an uncommon aftermath and various symptoms from infections and neurological damage could be attributed directly to the surgery.[68]

A small number of limited psychosurgical procedures are still carried out on the frontal lobe but they appear to be much more efficacious than the older procedures.[65]

Today, the prefrontal cortex is often divided into several systems with different functions and damage to each system tending to produce a different set of symptoms. To summarize (and simplify) one parcellation, damage to the dorsolateral system produces executive dysfunction, to the orbitofrontal system, disinhibition, and to the medial frontal system, apathetic motivation.[66] Another, more integrative theory has been offered by Earl Miller and Jonathan Cohen[69] (see also chapter 3).

Visual cortex

Bartolemo Panizza (1785–1867) was the first individual to produce detailed experimental and clinicopathological evidence for a visual area in posterior cerebral cortex. He carried out anatomical and lesion experiments on a variety of species as well as observations on brain-injured humans. His work was largely ignored, perhaps because it was published in Italian in a local journal, and because, following both Gall and Pierre Flourons, visual functions were considered subcortical, the cortex being reserved for 'higher psychic' functions.[70]

Soon after Fritsch and Hitzig's publication on the motor cortex, David Ferrier confirmed their results (see section on discovery of motor cortex above). Ferrier then applied their electrical stimulation methods to search for sensory cortices in monkeys. He found that stimulation of the angular gyrus produced eye movements and inferred that this area was the seat of visual perception. He supported this by showing that bilateral lesions of this area produced blindness (for the few post-operative days that the infected animals lived). Apparently confirming this view, he found that large occipital lesions had no visual effects unless they encroached on the angular gyrus.[71]

By contrast, soon after, Hermann Munk found that large occipital lesions produced blindness in both dogs and monkeys. Sanger Brown and Edward Schafer then confirmed Munk's report of total blindness after total occipital lesions in monkeys.[72] (We now know that Ferrier's failure to produce blindness after occipital lesions was because his lesions spared the representation of the fovea, whereas those of Munk and Brown and Schaeffer did not.)

By the turn of the century, anatomical, clinico-pathological, and experimental data were converging on the identity of a visual area in the posterior cerebral cortex corresponding to the region of the stripe of Gennari, described by Francisco Gennari in 1782 and named by G Elliot Smith as *area striata*.[72]

In 1941, SA Talbot and Wade Marshall, using visually evoked responses, mapped the visual topography of striate cortex in cats and monkeys (i.e. the projection or 'map' of the retina onto cortex). David Hubel and Torsten Wiesel, recording from single neurons, subsequently confirmed this retinotopic organization. Through the brilliant use of single neuron physiology, they revealed the functional architecture of striate cortex. They showed that single striate cells integrated binocular input and were sensitive to oriented lines and edges. Their research promised the possibility of understanding perception in terms of neurons and became the model for subsequent explorations of the visual cortex and for all of contemporary neurophysiology. They shared the Nobel Prize with Roger Sperry in 1961. Hubel and Wiesel then showed a second and third retinotopic area (V2 and V3) adjacent to striate cortex (V1) in the regions previously called para- and prestriate cortex.[73]

A new phase of cortical visual physiology began in the 1970s when John Allman and Jon Kass described a multiplicity of extra-striate visual areas in the squirrel monkey.[74] Even more visual areas were subsequently discovered in the macaque and human by Semir Zeki, Van Essen, and Charles Gross and their colleagues, a total of over 30 having been found to date.[75] Leslie Ungerleider and Mortimer Mishkin showed that these areas were organized into two main processing streams: a dorsal stream extended into posterior parietal cortex and was specialized for the analysis of space and movement, and a ventral stream extended into the temporal lobe and was specialized for pattern recognition, that is, for form and colour.[76] Proceeding down each stream, the successive visual areas tend to have larger receptive fields, less topographic organization, and neurons with more specialized properties.[77–79]

The inferior temporal cortex lies at the terminus of the ventral stream. Its neurons are no longer retinotopically organized and they respond selectively to complex shapes. In both monkeys and humans, the inferior temporal cortex contains several areas that selectively respond to images of faces.[76,77] There are also areas that specialize in representing locations and body parts. In both macaques and humans, these specialized areas were delineated with imaging methods.[78] The later stages in both the dorsal and ventral hierarchy of visual areas send projections to the hippocampus by way of perirhinal and parahippocampal cortex.[77,79]

Brain laterality

Broca and Wernicke's discoveries that left-hemisphere damage, at least in right-handers, resulted in deficits in producing and understanding language respectively, led to the idea that the left hemisphere was the *dominant* hemisphere and the right hemisphere was the non-dominant or *minor* hemisphere. At first, the dominant hemisphere was thought to be the most important hemisphere not only for language but also for other cognitive functions. For example, Hugo Liepmann (1863–1925) attributed 'purposeful' movements to the dominant hemisphere,[57] and his classification of limb apraxia remains highly influential to this day.

As early as 1865, John Hughlings Jackson, the 'father' of English neurology suggested that the so-called minor hemisphere might be more important than the major hemisphere for perceptual functions. However, it was not until the 1930s that evidence from the study of human patients showed that a variety of disorders in non-language functions were more common or more severe after right- than after left-hemisphere damage.[79,80] These sequelae of

right-hemisphere lesions included perceptual deficits (such as in object and face recognition and in visuo-constructive tasks), attentional deficits, and emotional disorders. Thus it became clear that the left hemisphere was the major one for language and related functions, whereas the right hemisphere was dominant for a variety of perpetual, attentional, and emotional functions. This lateralization of cognitive functions could also be shown in intact subjects by the unilateral anaesthetization of one hemisphere, a procedure know as the 'Wada' test, developed by the neurologist JA Wada in 1949.[80]

A new and powerful method of comparing the functions of the two hemispheres was developed by Roger Sperry and his colleagues in the 1950s. The clinical literature on patients with damage or agenesis of the corpus callosum had been contradictory, with many studies reporting no effect of a damaged or absent callosum. For example, Andrew Akelatis had sectioned the corpus callosum for treatment of epilepsy in a number of patients and reported a total absence of any cognitive effects of this surgery.[57]

By contrast, Sperry and his students showed, first in cats and monkeys and then in human patients, that section of the corpus callosum resulted in each hemisphere having 'its own mental sphere— that is, its own independent perceptual, learning, memory and other mental processes'.[81] Suddenly, it became possible to compare the functions of the two hemispheres directly. The key to Sperry's discovery was, in subjects with the corpus callosum sectioned, to direct sensory input into each hemisphere independently. For example, in the visual modality, he sectioned the optic chiasm sagitally so that information from the left eye went only to the left hemisphere and information from the right eye only to the right hemisphere. In humans, he achieved the same result by having the subject with sectioned corpus callosum fixate so that information presented to each visual half-field went to the contralateral hemisphere.[82] Sperry received the Nobel Prize in Medicine/Physiology for this work in 1981.

It should be mentioned that this important work became rather distorted in the popular literature by its neglecting the fact that although the hemispheres have specialized functions, in fact they work together in the intact individual.

Functions of the hippocampus in memory

A major advance in the neurology of memory came from the study of Patient HM who received bilateral lesions of the hippocampus and adjacent tissues to alleviate epileptic seizures in frankly experimental surgery by William Scoville in 1953. After the surgery, as studied primarily by Brenda Milner and later her student Suzanne Corkin, HM had very severe anterograde amnesia: he appeared to be unable to store any new information for more than a few minutes, and his short-term memory never became long term.[83]

Subsequent research indicated that only his 'declarative' memory (memory for facts and events) was impaired, whereas his 'procedural' memory (such as memory for motor and perceptual skills, and classical conditioning) was intact.[84,85] Similar dissociations between the two types of memory have been found in other patients after hippocampal damage (but see also chapter 13). The hippocampus is necessary for the formation of long-term declarative memories, which appear to be stored in portions of the cerebral cortex.[85]

Imaging

The most important advance in neurology in the last half-century has been the development of brain imaging, both structural (anatomical) and functional.

Structural imaging

CAT scanning (computed axial tomography), introduced in 1971, involves first X-raying the brain (or other body part) at different angles from which is produced a three-dimensional image reconstructed by computer. This was a remarkable advance in neurology replacing inferior techniques for estimating brain lesions or tumours such as pneumoencephalography, cerebral angiography, and clinical examination. MRI (magnetic resonance imaging) of the brain was developed at about the same time as CAT scanning but has much higher resolution. It derives from a technique developed in chemistry in the 1970s, 'nuclear magnetic resonance', involving the properties of hydrogen atoms in a magnetic field. MR techniques also permit visualization of white-matter connections in the brain using diffusion-weighted imaging and tractography (see chapter 8).

Functional imaging

Functional imaging of the brain measures changes in local activity in different brain structures as functions of cognitive activity. The first to do this was Angelo Mosso in 1881. He observed brain pulsations through skull openings in human patients, noted that they increase locally during cognitive tasks, and inferred increased blood flow with increased brain function.[86] A few years later, Charles C Roy and Sherrington, from their animal experiments, suggested 'automatic mechanisms' that regulated blood flow depending on variations in neural activity. In the 1920s, John Fulton studied a relationship of increased blood flow with the act of reading in a human patient.[86]

After the Second World War, several techniques were developed that enabled blood flow to be locally measured as a function of brain activity. In PET, a radioactive isotope such as ^{15}O is introduced into the bloodstream and its emitted gamma rays can be detected by the PET scanner. A reconstructed image will then show the distribution of blood flow and, presumably, regional difference in brain activity.[87]

fMRI is also a method of measuring local blood flow in the brain. It is based on the same technique as MRI except that the imaging is focused on measuring the ratio of oxygenated to deoxygenated haemoglobin known as the 'blood oxygenation level dependent' or BOLD effect. The BOLD response is a slightly delayed index of local brain activity. fMRI is today largely replacing PET for studies of brain activation because it is has much better spatial and temporal resolution, individuals can be safely studied repeatedly, activity on single trials can be measured, and it does not require a large medical centre for its use.[87]

fMRI studies have provided numerous new insights into cognitive neuroscience and promise many more in the future.

References

1. Gross CG. A hole in the head: a history of trepanation. In: CG Gross, *A Hole in the Head: More Tales in the History of Neuroscience*. Cambridge, MA: MIT Press, 2009, pp. 1–23.
2. Arnott R, Finger S, and Smith CUM. *Trepanation: Discovery, History, Theory*. Lisse: Swets & Zeitlinger, 2003.
3. Gross CG. Ancient Egyptian surgery and medicine. In: CG Gross *Brain, Vision Memory: Tales in the History of Neuroscience*. Cambridge, MA: MIT Press, 1998, pp. 1–7.
4. Breasted JH. *The Edwin Smith Surgical Papyrus*. Chicago, IL: The University of Chicago Press, 1930.
5. Gross CG. Greek Philosopher–Scientists and the Beginning of Brain Science. In: CG Gross, *Brain, Vision, Memory: Tales in the History of Neuroscience*. Cambridge, MA: MIT Press, 1998, pp. 8–29.
6. Freeman K. *The Pre-Socratic Philosophers*. Oxford: Blackwell, 1954.
7. Longrigg J. *Greek Rational Medicine: Philosophy and Medicine from Alcmaeon to the Alexandrians*. New York, NY: Routledge, 1993.
8. Lloyd GER. *Early Greek Science: Thales to Aristotle*. London: Chatto & Windus, 1970.
9. Sigerist H. *A History of Medicine, Vol. II: Early Greek, Hindu and Persian Medicine*. New York, NY: Oxford University Press, 1961.
10. Farrington B. *Greek Science, Its Meaning for Us*. New York, NY: Penguin Books, 1994.
11. Schrödinger E. *Nature and the Greeks*. Cambridge: Cambridge University Press, 1954.
12. Theophrastus [4th century BCE]. On the Senses. In: Stratton GM (trans.), *Theophrastus and the Greek Physiological Psychology Before Aristotle*. London: Allen & Unwin, 1917.
13. Hippocrates [4th century BCE]). *The Medical Works of Hippocrates*. Chadwick J (trans.), Springfield, IL: Charles C. Thomas, 1950.
14. Temkin O. *Galenism: Rise and Decline of a Medical Philosophy*. Ithaca, NY: Cornell University Press, 1973.
15. Gross CG. Aristotle on the Brain. *Neuroscientist*, 1:245–50, 1995.
16. Gross CG. Galen and the Squealing Pig. *Neuroscientist*.4:216–21, 1998.
17. Rocca J. *Galen on the Brain: Anatomical Knowledge and Physiological Speculation in the Second Century ad*. Leiden: Brill, 2003.
18. Galen[2nd century]. *On Anatomical Procedures:The Later Books*. Duckworth WLH, Towers B (trans.), Cambridge: Cambridge University Press, 1962.
19. Galen [2nd century]. *Galen On the Usefulness of the Parts of the Body*. May M.T. (trans.), Ithaca, NY: Cornell University Press, 1968.
20. Gross CG. The medieval cell doctrine of brain function. In: CG Gross, *Brain, Vision, Memory: Tales in the History of Neuroscience*. Cambridge, MA: MIT Press, 1998, pp. 30–5.
21. Russell GA. After Galen: late antiquity and the islamic world. In: S Finger, F Boller, and KL Tyler (eds).*History of Neurology*. New York, NY: Elsevier, 2010, pp. 61–78.
22. Willis T. *Cerebri anatomie*. London: Dring, 1664.
23. Isler H. The development of neurology and the neurological sciences in the 17th century. In: S Finger, F Boller, and KL Tyler (eds). *History of Neurology*. New York, NY: Elsevier, 2009, pp. 91–106.
24. Gross CG. The rebirth of brain science. In: CG Gross, *Brain, Vision, Memory: Tales in the History of Neuroscience*. Cambridge, MA: MIT Press, 1998, pp. 36–51.
25. Malpighi M (quotation). In: E Clarke and CD O'Malley (eds). *The Human Brain and Spinal Cord: A Historical Study Illustrated by Writings from Antiquity to the Twentieth Century*. San Francisco, CA: Norman, 1996, pp. 417.
26. Rusch F (quotation). In: E Clarke and CD O'Malley (eds). *The Human Brain and Spinal Cord: A Historical Study Illustrated by Writings from Antiquity to the Twentieth Century*. San Francisco, CA: Norman, 1996, p. 420.
27. Neuberger M. *The Historical Development of Experimental Brain and Spinal Cord Physiology Before Flourens*. Baltimore, MD: Johns Hopkins University Press, 1981.
28. Gall FJ and Spurzheim JC. *On the Function of the Brain and Each of Its Parts: With Observations on the Possibility of Determining the Instincts, Propensities and Talents, or the Moral and Intellectual Disposition of Men and Animals, by the Configuration of the Brain and Head*. Boston, MA: Marsh, Capen and Lyon, 1835.
29. Young RM. *Mind, Brain and Adaptation in the Nineteenth Century, Cerebral Localization and Its Biological Context from Gall to Ferrier*. Oxford: Clarendon Press, 1970.

30. Gross CG. The beginning of the modern era of cortical localization. In: CG Gross, *Brain, Vision, Memory: More Tales in the History of Neuroscience*. Cambridge, MA: MIT Press, 1998, pp. 52–64.

31. Cooter RS. *The Cultural Meaning of Popular Science: Phrenology and the Organization of Consent in Nineteenth-Century Britain*. Cambridge: Cambridge University Press, 1985.

32. Broca P [1861]. Remarks on the seat of the faculty of articulate language, followed by an observation of aphemia. In: G Von Bonin (ed.). *Some Papers on the Cerebral Cortex*. Springfield, IL: Charles C Thomas, 1960, pp. 49–72.

33. Finger S and Roe D. Does Gustave Dax deserve to be forgotten? The temporal lobe theory and other contributions of an overlooked figure in the history of language and cerebral dominance. *Brain Lang*. 1999;69:16–30.

34. Eling P and Whitaker H. History of aphasia: from brain to language. In: S Finger, F Boller, and KL Tyler (eds). *History of Neurology*. New York, NY: Elsevier, 2010, pp. 571–82.

35. Luria AR. *Basic Problems in Neurolinguistics*. The Hague: Mouton, 1976.

36. Knecht S, Drager B, Deppe M, *et al*. Handedness and hemispheric language dominance in healthy humans. *Brain*. 2000;123:2512–18.

37. Springer SP and Deutsch G. *Left Brain, Right Brain: Perspectives from Cognitive Neuroscience*. New York, NY: Freeman, 1997.

38. Magner LN. *A History of Medicine*. New York, NY: Dekker, 1992.

39. Fritsch GT and Hitzig E [1870]. On the electrical excitability of the cerberum. In: G Von Bonin (ed.). *Some Papers on the Cerebral Cortex*. Springfield, IL: Charles C Thomas, 1960, pp. 73–96.

40. Viets HR. West Riding, 1871–1876. *Bull. Hist. Med*. 1938;6:477–87.

41. Ferrier D. Experimental Researches in Cerebral Physiology and Pathology. *West Riding Lunatic Asylum Medical Reports*. 1873;3:30–96.

42. Ferrier D. Experiments on the brain of monkeys: No. 1. *Phil Trans R Soc Lond*. 1874–75;23:409–30.

43. Ferrier D. The Croonian lecture: experiments on the brain of monkeys (Second Series). *Phil Trans R Soc Lond*. 1875;165:433–88.

44. Taylor CS and Gross CG. Twitches versus movements: a story of motor cortex. *Neuroscientist*. 2003;9:332–42.

45. Horsley V and Schäfer EA. A record of experiments upon the functions of the cerebral cortex. *Phil Trans R Soc Lond B*. 1888;179:1–45.

46. Beevor CE and Horsley V. A minute analysis (experimental) of the various movements produced by stimulating in the monkey different regions of the cortical centre for the upper limb, as defined by Professor Ferrier. *Phil Trans R Soc Lond B*. 1887;178:153–67.

47. Brown TG and Sherrington CS. Studies in the physiology of the nervous System. XXII. On the phenomenon of facilitation. 1. its occurrence in reactions induced by stimulation of the 'motor' cortex of the cerebrum in monkeys. *Quart J Exp Physiol*. 1915;9:81–100.

48. Leyton ASF and Sherrington CS. Observations on the excitable cortex of the chimpanzee, orang-utan, and gorilla. *Q J Exp Physiol*. 1916;11:135–222.

49. Penfield W and Rasmussen T. *The Cerebral Cortex of Man: A Clinical Study of Localization of Function*. New York, NY: MacMillan, 1950.

50. Woolsey CN, Settlage PH, Meyer DR, *et al*. Pattern of localization in precentral and 'supplementary' motor cortex and their relation to the concept of a premotor area. In: *Association for Research in Nervous and Mental Disease*, Vol 30. New York, NY: Raven Press, 1952, pp. 238–64.

51. Finger S. *Minds Behind the Brain: The Pioneers and Their Discoveries*. New York, NY: Oxford University Press, 2000.

52. Graziano MSA. The organization of behavioral repertoire in motor cortex. *Ann Rev Neurosci*. 2006;29:105–34.

53. Shepherd GM. *Foundations of the Neuron Doctrine*, 1991. New York, NY: Oxford University Press, 1991.

54. Golgi C. The neuron doctrine—theory and facts. Nobel Lecture, 11 December 1906. In: *Nobel Lectures Physiology or Medicine 1901–1921*, 1967. New York, NY: Elsevier, 1906, pp. 189–217.

55. Robertson JD. Recent electron microscope observations on the ultrastructure of the crayfish median-to-motor giant Synapse. *Exp Cell Res*. 1955;8:226–29.

56. Furshpan EJ and Potter DD. Transmission at the giant motor synapses of the crayfish. *J Physiol*. 1959;145:289–325.

57. Finger S. *Origins of Neuroscience: A History of Explorations Into Brain Function*. New York, NY: Oxford University Press, 1994.

58. Gross CG. Emanuel Swedenborg: a neuroscientist before his time. *Neuroscientist*. 1997;3:142–47.

59. Gross CG and Weiskrantz L. Some changes in behavior produced by lateral frontal lesions in the macaque. In: JM Warren and K. Akert (eds). *The Frontal Granular Cortex and Behavior*. New York, NY: McGraw-Hill, 1964, pp. 74–98.

60. Harlow JM. Recovery from the passage of an iron bar through the head. *Publications of the Massachusetts Medical Society*. 1868;2:327–47.

61. Damasio A. *Descarte's Error*. London: Vintage Books, 2006.

62. Jacobsen CF, Wolfe JB, and Jackson TA. An experimental analysis of the functions of the frontal association areas in primates. *J Nerv Mental Dis*. 1935;82:1–14.

63. Pribram KH, Ahumada A, Hartog J, *et al*. A progress report on the neurological processes disturbed by frontal lesions in primates. In: EE Walker and K Akert (eds). *The Frontal Granular Cortex and Behavior*. New York, NY: McGraw-Hill, 1964, pp. 28–55.

64. Mishkin M. Effects of small frontal lesions on delayed alternation in monkeys. *J. Neurophysiol*. 1957;20:615–22.

65. Anderson CA and Arciniegas DB. Neurosurgical interventions for neuropsychiatric syndromes. *Curr Psychiat Rep*. 2004;6:355–63.

66. Filley CM. The frontal lobes. In: S Finger, F Boller, and KL Tyler (eds). *History of Neurology*. New York, NY: Elsevier, 2010, pp. 557–70.

67. Valenstein ES. *Great and Desperate Cures: The Rise and Decline of Psychosurgery and Other Radical Treatments for Mental Illness*. New York, NY: Basic Books, 1986.

68. Valenstein ES. *Brain Control*. New York, NY: John Wiley & Sons, 1973.

69. Miller EK and Cohen JD. An integrative theory of prefrontal cortex function. *Ann Rev Neurosci*. 2001;24:167–202.

70. Colombo M, Colombo A, and Gross CG. Bartolomeo Panizza's *Observations on the Optic Nerve (1855)*. *Beh Brain Res Bull*. 2002;58:529–39.

71. Ferrier D. *Functions of the Brain*, 2nd edn, London: Smith and Elder, 1886.

72. Gross CG. Beyond striate cortex: how large portions of the temporal and parietal cortex became visual areas. In: CG Gross. *Brain, Vision, Memory: Tales in the History of Neuroscience*. Cambridge, MA: MIT Press, 1998, pp. 180–210.

73. Hubel DH.*Eye, Brain and Vision*. New York, NY: Freeman, 1988.

74. Kaas JH. Theories of extrastriate cortex. In: JH Kaas, K Rockland, and A Peters (eds).*Cerebral Cortex, Vol. 12, Extrastriate Cortex in Primates*. New York, NY: Plenum Press, 1997, pp. 91–125.

75. Van Essen D. Organization of visual areas in macaque and human cerebral cortex. In: LM Chalupa and JS Werner (eds). *The Visual Neurosciences*, Vol. 1. Cambridge, MA: MIT Press, 2003, pp. 507–21.

76. Ungerleider LG and Mishkin M. Two cortical visual systems. In: D Ingle, M Goodale, and R Mansfield (eds). *Analysis of Visual Behavior*. Cambridge, MA: MIT Press, 1982, pp. 549–86.

77. Gross CG, Rodman HR, Gochin PM, *et al*. Inferior temporal cortex as a pattern recognition device. In: *Computational Learning and Cognition: Proceedings of the Third NEC Research Symposium*. EB Baum (ed.). Philadelphia, PA: SIAM, 1993, pp. 44–73.

78. Gross CG (2007). Single Neuron Studies of Inferior Temporal Cortex. *Neuropsychologia*. 2007;45:841–52.

79. Kravitz DJ, Saleem KS, Baker CI, *et al*. The ventral visual pathway: an expanded neural framework for the processing of object quality. *Trends Cogn Sci*. 2013;17:26–49.

80. Hecaen H and Albert ML. *Human Neuropsychology*. New York, NY: Wiley, 1978.

81. Sperry RW. Cerebral organization and behavior. *Science*. 1961;133: 1749–57.

82. Sperry RW. Hemisphere deconnection and unity in conscious awareness. *Am Psychol*. 1968;23:723–33.

83. Corkin S. *Permanent Present Tense: The Unforgettable Life of the Amnesic Patient, H.M.* New York, NY: Basic Books, 2013.

84. Corkin S. What's new with the amnesic patient H.M.? *Nat Rev Neurosci.* 2002;3:153–60.

85. Squire LR. Memory and the hippocampus: a synthesis from findings with rats, monkeys, and humans. *Psychol Rev.* 1992;99:195–231.

86. Posner MI and Raichle ME. *Images of Mind.* New York, NY: Scientific American Library, 1994.

87. Raichle ME. The Origins of Functional Brain Imaging in Humans. In: S Finger, F Boller, and KL Tyler (eds). *History of Neurology.* New York, NY: Elsevier, 2010, pp. 257–70.

CHAPTER 2

Functional specialization and network connectivity in brain function

Giovanna Zamboni

Do mental processes depend from 'localized' brain regions or are they 'global' resulting from the integrated functioning of the brain as a whole? Brain lesion studies and neuroimaging methods have given evidence of both interpretations, allowing contemporary neuroscience to reach the conclusion that localized regions of the brain do carry out specific cognitive functions but they do so through multiple and complex interactions with many other brain regions forming large-scale networks.

Focal nature of cognitive functions

Evidence for functional specialization from lesion cases

Historically, the notion that different cognitive abilities are related to the function of specific brain regions took a relatively long time to become widely accepted by the scientific community (see chapter 1). Such a concept was long resisted by 'holistic' perspectives of the brain which viewed each part as contributing to all functions. It was only with the anatomo-clinical works of Broca and Wernicke on language disorders in the 1860s and 1870s that that the concept of functional specialization was put on a sure footing.[1] Prior to this, the first intuition that mental functions were based in the brain had been advanced by Franz Joseph Gall in his controversial doctrine of phrenology.[2]

In 1861, Broca described a patient who lost the ability to speak following a stroke. Although able to understand language and repeat single words, and free of significant limb weakness, this individual could not articulate sentences or express himself in writing. Post-mortem examination revealed a lesion in the left posterior lateral region of the frontal lobe, subsequently termed Broca's area.[3] Broca described other similar cases, and by inferring the correlation between post-mortem anatomical lesions and language disorders (anatomo-clinical correlation method), he concluded that language is localized in the left hemisphere.

About a decade later, Carl Wernicke described another case of language disturbances following a stroke. This patient could speak fluently but in a meaningless way and could not understand spoken or written language. After his death, the damaged area was found to be in the posterior left temporal lobe at the junction with the parietal lobe, subsequently termed Wernicke's area. On the basis of his and Broca's findings, Wernicke proposed a model of language as a multi-component process, in which each component would have a specific, distinct anatomical localization.[4] He distinguished a centre for motor–verbal functions, localized in the left frontal regions, responsible for language articulation and production, from a centre for auditory–verbal functions, localized in the left temporal region, responsible for language perception. Lesions to the former would cause a non-fluent aphasia with intact comprehension (Broca's aphasia), while lesions to the latter would cause a fluent aphasia with impaired comprehension (Wernicke's aphasia).

In the same decades, studies by Fritsch and Hitzig in dogs further reinforced the notion that different functions are localized in different cortical regions by demonstrating that the stimulation of anterior regions of the cerebral cortex causes contralateral movements, and that their disruption causes contralateral paralysis.[5] Functional specialization was further supported by animal studies identifying oculor-motor centres in the frontal lobes,[6] auditory centres in the temporal lobes,[7] and visual centres in the occipital lobes (see also chapter 1).[8]

Many other cognitive functions were localized by investigating patients who had suffered from focal brain lesions. One of the most famous cases was reported by Harlow in 1848 who described Phineas Gage who, after having sustained a frontal lobe injury, presented profoundly altered social and interpersonal skills, to the point that people who knew him beforehand described him as 'no longer being Gage'. This first suggested that frontal brain regions are involved in social behaviour.[9]

Another landmark case was described by Scoville and Milner in 1957. Following bilateral temporal lobe resection in the attempt to treat his epilepsy, a patient named Henry Molaison (famously known as HM) became severely amnesic. He had permanently lost the ability to acquire new information (anterograde amnesia) and recall memories of the years immediately prior to surgery (retrograde amnesia), despite having normal reasoning skills, language, and short-term/working memory.[10] HM provided the first evidence that the hippocampus and surrounding medial temporal structures are essential for the consolidation of information in long-term memory.[11]

Following these single case studies, the study of lesions in humans evolved and expanded. Large groups of patients were assessed to establish correspondences between the brain and symptoms in a more quantitative, robust way, permitting statistical inference at the level of population.[12,13] Standardized scales to measure cognitive abilities were developed and used to compare patients' performance to healthy controls.[14]

The lesion method is based on the assumption that if a certain brain region is necessary for a certain function, then a lesion to that area should lead to a deficit in that function, whereas this should not occur when the brain region is undamaged (simple dissociation). Further expansion of the lesion method came with the concept of *double dissociation*, considered to be the strongest evidence for functional specialization and segregation. It requires the comparison between two patients (or groups of patients) different in terms of lesion localization: if one patient is significantly more impaired in function A, while the other is significantly more impaired in function B, then it is concluded that the two functions are independently associated with the two damaged areas.

Using the double dissociation technique, several investigators including Ennio De Renzi in stroke-lesioned patients,[14,15] Freda Newcombe in soldiers who had sustained focal and stable brain wounds during the Second World War,[16] Brenda Milner in surgical patients who had had lobectomies,[17] Gazzaniga in patients who had undergone callosotomy,[18] all demonstrated differential deficits following left and right hemisphere lesions and specialization of the right hemisphere for visual–perceptual and spatial tasks and left hemisphere for speech and skilled movements. Newcombe, for example, provided the first evidence of dissociated visual–perceptual and spatial deficits following, respectively, temporal-posterior lesions and dorsal-parietal lesions of the right hemisphere,[19] supporting the concept of a dorsal and ventral visual stream.

Through the study of lesion cases, the concept of functional specialization became a dominant theme in neuroscience. It is mainly thanks to this approach that today we are able to localize deficits such as aphasia, unilateral neglect, and impaired executive function at the bedside.

Evidence for functional specialization from structural imaging

The need to study large groups of patients together with the advent of computer tomography (CT) and magnetic resonance imaging (MRI) encouraged development of methods that allow comparison of lesions across different patients,[20] including transposition of brains into common, stereotactic spaces.[21] One common method consisted of identifying regions of lesion overlap. The extent and location of damage in a group of patients could be visualized in a colour-coded 'lesion density map', in which the region damaged in the highest number of patients would be surrounded by regions damaged by a progressively decreasing numbers of patients.[22,23]

Two approaches have been used to relate symptoms to lesions. One groups patients by location of their brain lesions and then examines differences in symptoms. For example, a study by Grafman and colleagues on veterans who suffered penetrating head injuries in Vietnam showed that soldiers with lesions in the ventromedial regions of the frontal lobes were more aggressive and violent than those with lesions in other brain areas.[24] The second approach groups patients by symptoms and then examines lesion location. For example, Damasio and colleagues classified patients with focal brain lesions according to whether they had selective deficits in naming famous persons, animals, or tools. By using lesion density maps, they showed that each of these category-specific deficits was associated with overlapping of lesions in different temporal lobe regions, arguing for a role of higher-order association areas outside of classic language areas in word retrieval.[25]

MRI offers a higher spatial resolution than CT and allows for more comprehensive characterization of lesions by 'dividing' the brain into three-dimensional units of volume (voxels). In one of the first studies that used a *voxel-based* approach, Adolphs and colleagues demonstrated involvement of somatosensory cortices as well as the amygdala in emotion recognition, by comparing the voxel-based lesion density map of patients with impaired emotion recognition with that of unimpaired cases. The resulting *difference map* revealed that voxels within the somatosensory cortex were significantly associated with impairment.[26]

Building on statistical approaches used in functional imaging (see next section), recently developed techniques such as *voxel-based lesion symptom mapping* (VLSM)[27,28] allow for improved symptom mapping by computing statistical tests iteratively for each and every voxel. The technique relies on comparison of continuous or discrete behavioural variables on patients grouped according to whether they have damage in that given voxel and then correcting for multiple comparisons. This is an example of a 'mass-univariate' approach because each voxel is assumed to be independent of another. Importantly, VLSM does not require patients to be grouped a priori according to lesion location or performance cut-offs, but produces statistical values for each given voxel indicating whether damage to that voxel has a significant effect on the cognitive variable of interest.[29–33]

Although fundamental to study symptom–lesion associations, voxel-based symptoms mapping methods are limited by their assumption that each voxel can be damaged independently of other voxels. It has been recently argued that this assumption is not biologically valid, as lesions in the human brain tend to follow patterns depending, for example, on vascular supply in the case of stroke. It is possible that 'collaterally damaged' voxels may be always associated with voxels that are instead critical for a certain deficit and therefore may systematically confound lesion–symptom associations, suggesting that multivariate rather than mass-univariate approaches may be better suited to identify true anatomical correlates of deficits/symptoms.[34]

Structural MRI data can also be analysed with procedures that provide subject-specific estimated maps of grey matter volume or thickness,[35–38] which are more suitable for studying subtle structural changes and, differently from VLMS, do not rely on 'radiologically visible' and discrete lesions. Among them, *voxel-based morphometry* (VBM) involves segmentation of the grey matter, spatial transposition of all the subjects' images to the same stereotactic space, and 'modulation' to obtain voxel-specific values of grey matter density (or volume). These values can then be used in regression analyses to compare groups of individuals or perform correlations with continuous variables of behavioural/cognitive performance. This is achieved with voxel-based statistical analysis aimed at identifying, for example, distribution of voxels of significant volumetric differences between two groups, or voxels whose grey matter density significantly correlates with performance.

VBM has been particularly useful in identifying brain–symptom associations in neurodegenerative diseases, in which pathological processes causing grey matter loss or atrophy are widespread and involve different brain regions to a variable degree. They are therefore are better represented by continuous variables rather than binary measurements, which are more suited to define discrete lesions. In patients with dementia or other neurodegenerative diseases, VBM has been reliably used to identify patterns of grey matter atrophy. For example, several VBM studies[39–41] have found that patients with Alzheimer's disease (AD) have focal atrophy in the medial temporal lobes, posterior cingulate/precuneus, and other association areas in a pattern that mirrors the spread of neurofibrillary tangles,[42] while the behavioural variant of frontotemporal dementia (FTD) is associated with atrophy in the frontal lobes.[43,44] Semantic dementia is associated with asymmetrical anterior temporal lobe atrophy. By contrast, progressive nonfluent aphasia is associated with left perisylvian atrophy.[45] In addition, VBM has also been extensively used to make inferences on the association of focal atrophy with specific cognitive deficits.[46-49] As an example, a VBM correlational analysis in patients with frontotemporal dementia reported that severity of apathy correlated with atrophy in the right dorsolateral prefrontal cortex, whereas severity of disinhibition correlated with atrophy in mesolimbic structures.[50]

Several other MRI-based tools have been used to study volumes of a priori defined regions of interest (ROIs) or rates of atrophy over time in neurodegenerative diseases. In AD, ROI-based measures of hippocampal volumes are significantly reduced compared to age-matched controls,[51-54] and the rate of change measured from serial MRIs obtained six months or one year apart significantly increased.[55-58]

By the use of correlational analyses, VBM and ROI-based methods allow for indirect inferences about the localization of specific symptoms in patients with dementia. However, differently from lesion–symptom mapping techniques, they do not prove the *necessity* of a brain region for a specific cognitive function.

Evidence for functional specialization from functional imaging in healthy subjects

Functional imaging has revolutionized the field of brain function mapping over the last 20 years. Activation-based positron emission tomography (PET) and task-based functional MRI (task fMRI) detect changes in metabolism or blood flow while subjects are engaged in sensorimotor or cognitive tasks and can be used to produce activation maps revealing which parts of the brain are engaged. These functional techniques have allowed extension of the concept of functional localization from the study of brain-injured patients to the study of healthy people.

PET activation studies measure focal variations in cerebral blood flow. A radiotracer is injected in the bloodstream while the subject is engaged in different tasks (usually an experimental condition and a control condition), with the assumption that blood flow will increase in brain regions where there is increased neural activity.[59] Task-based fMRI relies on the Blood Oxygen Level Dependent (BOLD) contrast, which is dependent on local changes in cerebral blood flow, cerebral blood volume, deoxyhaemoglobin concentration, local haematocrit, and changes in oxygen consumption. When a brain area is more active, it consumes more oxygen, causing an increase of blood flow and a change in the BOLD signal.[60,61] PET activation studies and task-based fMRI do not directly measure neural activity, but instead measure changes in parameters (metabolism and BOLD) correlated with neural activity that occur with a delay, limiting the temporal resolution of these techniques.

PET activation studies and task-based fMRI studies do not provide absolute measurements of physiological parameters but measure changes that occur in response to a task relative to another task, used as a control condition. By subtracting signal changes occurring during the control task from those occurring during the experimental task, it is possible to identify areas of increased activation associated with the task of interest, assuming that areas active in both control and experimental conditions have been cancelled out. To establish localization and strength of the association between the experimental condition and the measured brain changes, the functional images that have been acquired over time during different conditions and across different subjects need to be realigned and mapped into standard stereotactic, voxel-based spaces. Then, methods allowing statistical inference need to be used.

The most commonly used method to identify functionally specialized brain responses is statistical parametric mapping (SPM), which allows use of standard statistical tests on each voxel and assembles the resulting statistical parameters into images.[62] These are then used to compare different conditions and to identify regionally specific changes of signal attributable to the experimental task (Fig. 2.1).[63] Importantly, if a significant associations is found, this does not mean that the identified area is *necessary* for the specific function or cognitive process, nor that it is *specific* for it, because it may also be involved in other functions or tasks.

Since the advent of functional imaging techniques in the late 1980s and early 1990s, a huge number of studies have reported focal activations in response to specific tasks across a range of cognitive domains,[64] providing striking evidence for the concept of functional specialization. A review of these studies is outside the focus of the present chapter but a few early studies are worth considering as examples.

In a PET activation experiment, Zeki and colleagues showed that occipital area V4 is specific for colour vision, by comparing activations obtained during presentation of multicolour abstract images with those obtained during presentation of the same images in black and white, and that V5 or area MT is specific for motion perception, by comparing activations obtained during presentation of moving relative to stationary black and white patterns (see also chapter 6 for further examples).[65]

One important limitation of the subtraction method used in the early functional activation studies is that it depends on the assumption of 'pure insertion', that is, that a component process can be added into a task without affecting other processes. To modulate possible interactions between different cognitive components in neuroimaging experiments and disentangle the effect that one component has on the other, more sophisticated experimental techniques such as *factorial design* were implemented.[66] For language, a factorial design was used, as an example, to compare object naming with colour naming. It allowed identification of modality-independent naming areas in prefrontal and posterior temporal regions, and areas involved in object recognition in bilateral anterior temporal regions.[67]

The results of several functional imaging studies have challenged the traditional view of a one-to-one correspondence between brain regions and cognitive processes. On the one hand, single cognitive processes frequently elicit activation of several brain regions or distributed patterns of activations.[64,68] On the other hand, activations of single brain regions are frequently elicited by a wide range of cognitive tasks, even when these have been carefully modulated with factorial experimental designs.[68,69] Thus, although extensively supported by lesion cases and functional imaging studies, the concept of functional specialization alone may not be sufficient to explain brain functioning and organization in human.

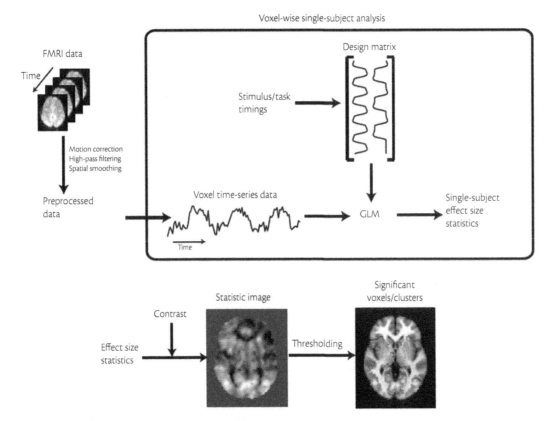

Fig. 2.1 Schematic representation of single-session analysis of fMRI data. fMRI data are acquired while stimuli are presented to the subject, who performs a task in the scanner. Data are then pre-processed (including motion correction, temporal filtering, and spatial smoothing) and entered into a regression model (general linear model, GLM) that expresses the observed BOLD response in terms of a linear combination of explanatory variables (in the design matrix) derived from stimulus/task timings and the haemodynamic response function (HRF), together with an error term. Voxel-specific effect-size statistics describe how well the modelled responses to the stimulus/task (explanatory variables) explain the continuous data. Thresholding is performed in a way that accounts for multiple comparison correction.
Courtesy of the Analysis Group of the Centre for Functional MRI of the Brain (FMRIB) from the FSL (FMRIB Software Library) course.

Network organization of cognitive functions

Towards the concept of distributed functional networks

Wernicke had first suggested that complex cognitive functions such as language result from distributed systems of linked focal brain regions. He proposed a model of language as a multi-component process, in which each component has a specific anatomical localization but is connected to the other components, reconciling evidence for functional specialization that he and others had provided with the notion that cognitive functions depend on integrated functioning across brain regions.[4] He even hypothesized the existence of a *conduction aphasia* that would be associated with a lesion of the pathways connecting the left hemisphere frontal and temporal lobe centres, characterized by preserved fluency and comprehension but impaired repetition and paraphasic speech (the use of incorrect words or phonemes while speaking).

In addition to conduction aphasia, other 'disconnection syndromes' resulting from damage of white matter tracts between cortical areas were described. As an example, alexia without agraphia, in which patients are able to write and speak but cannot read, was first described by Dejerine 1891 and associated with lesions to the white matter in proximity of the angular gyrus that interrupt the connections between the visual cortex and language areas. In 1965, the anatomical bases of disconnection syndromes were reviewed by Geschwind[70,71] who provided a theoretical framework that paved the road for modern concepts of distributed brain networks.[72] Around the same time, Alexander Luria, one of the founders of neuropsychology, proposed a model of human mental processes based on complex functional systems or 'functional units' that involved groups of brain areas working in a coordinated, hierarchical, and organized way.[73]

Related to this ideas is the notion that a lesion can cause functional damage 'remote' from the anatomical site of the lesion. This concept was extensively studied by Monakow who coined the term *diaschisis*—loss of function due to transient, indirect damage to remote parts of the brain not anatomically close to the site of the primary injury but functionally connected to it.[74] His work fostered the view of the brain as a complex, dynamic system in which function could be lost transiently. Evidence for diaschisis comes from functional imaging studies that show hypometabolism in regions remote from the cortical lesion,[75] demonstrating directly the existence of remote functional effects.[76]

These ideas led to the refutation of functional localization as the sole and sufficient explanation of brain function. Brain–symptom correlations started to be searched not only in specific, single brain regions but also in larger-scale networks connecting different regions across the brain. With the additional benefit of knowledge about anatomical structural connections from tracing methods in the autopsied brain, Mesulam proposed a model of brain function based on distinct, multifocal large-scale functional systems.[77] In his scheme, there is a spatial attention network anchored in the posterior parietal and dorsolateral frontal regions, a language network involving Wernicke's and Broca's areas, a memory network linking the hippocampus and inferior parietal cortex, a face/object recognition network anchored in temporal cortices, and a working-memory/executive-function network connecting prefrontal and inferior parietal cortices.[78]

Subsequently, McIntosh demonstrated the existence of networks by measuring the covariance of activity between regions in PET activation studies, thus identifying patterns of co-variation or *functional connectivity*.[79] For example, he studied people who had learned that an auditory stimulus signalled a visual event and found activation in left occipital visual areas when auditory stimuli were presented alone. He then showed that this occipital activation correlated with activation in the prefrontal cortex and that it accounted for most of the change in occipital activity.[80]

It is now widely accepted that the brain functions through large-scale networks including multiple specialized cortical areas reciprocally connected with parallel, bidirectional, and multisynaptic pathways. Thus deficits can be caused either by damage to specialized cortical areas, by damage to their connecting pathways, or both.[72,81,82]

Neuroimaging methods to study brain connectivity

Several methodological advances have allowed study of brain connectivity and large-scale brain networks from different perspectives. *Functional connectivity* refers to the functional relationship between brain regions inferred by searching for correlations in the fMRI signal between two or more brain regions (functional covariance). The structural bases of this relationship are ultimately assumed to exist through mono- or multisynaptic pathways.[83,84]

Correlations in the fMRI signal (BOLD signal) can be studied among regional changes occurring in response to cognitive tasks but also among regional changes that occur in the absence of tasks,

while participants are simply at rest (resting fMRI). In fact, it has been shown that the BOLD signal not only changes as a consequence of cognitive or 'task-related' demand, but also shows low frequency spontaneous fluctuations (0.01–0.1 Hz) that are temporally correlated and organized within specific spatial patterns in the brain.[85,86] The networks of brain regions whose spontaneous activity rises and falls coherently have been termed *resting state networks*.

To study functional correlation, a 'seed' voxel or anatomical ROI is 'seeded' to generate a correlation map showing all other regions in which signal changes significantly correlate with those within the seed region (seed-based correlation analysis). This approach is *hypothesis-driven* and requires a priori selection of the ROI or 'seed'. Alternatively, a more exploratory, *data-driven* approach can be used to create a matrix of correlations across each voxel/region with all other voxels/regions in the brain. Correlation matrices can be decomposed into spatial modes using, for instance, principal component analysis (PCA) or independent component analysis (ICA) to identify large-scale networks or maps of spatially independent and temporally correlated functional signals.[87–89]

Among the several resting state networks identified with ICA-based approaches, the *default mode network* (DMN, Fig. 2.2A)—which includes posterior cingulate cortex and precuneus, the medial prefrontal cortex, and lateral parietal regions—is considered to be specifically engaged during task-independent introspection or self-referential thought. The DMN was fist identified in task-related fMRI by studying task-induced *deactivations* (i.e. decreases in BOLD signal during experimental conditions compared to baseline or resting conditions).[90] It can also be identified with 'seed-based' methods examining correlations from regions such as the posterior cingulate.[91,92]

In addition to the DMN, other commonly identified networks are the 'executive control' networks linking dorsofrontal and parietal regions, the 'salience' network linking anterior cingulate to insular and limbic regions, and networks related to primary visual, auditory, and sensorimotor regions (Fig. 2.2).[86,88,89,93,94] Resting state networks (RSN) have been shown to be consistent across subjects[95] and to match activations found in task-based fMRI

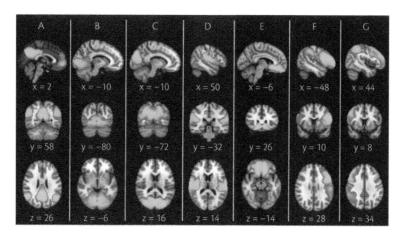

Fig. 2.2 Resting state networks (RSNs). Spatial maps of resting state networks (RSNs) obtained using independent component analysis (ICA). The three most informative orthogonal slices for each RSN are shown. A) DMN; B) ventromedial visual RSN; C) dorsolateral visual RSN; D) auditory RSN; E) orbitofrontal RSN; F) left frontoparietal RSN; G) right frontoparietal RSN. Coordinates are in MNI.

studies, suggesting that they reflect functionally significant brain networks.[96–98]

Effective connectivity represents another way to study functional correlations and network function. Different from functional connectivity, this method incorporates additional information such as anatomical constraints and considers interactions of several brain regions simultaneously. It is aimed at explicitly quantifying the influence that one region has on another and establish whether their connections are causal and have a specific directionality (from region A to area B rather than B to A).[100] Effective connectivity approaches include *dynamic causal modelling* (DCM) that allows testing of specific models of how different parts of a functional network are dynamically linked and coupled. DCM is less 'model-free' and more hypothesis-driven (and more computationally sophisticated) than functional connectivity. It tests dynamic interactions and is therefore task-dependent and condition-specific, and has been mainly applied to task-based fMRI studies, although it has been recently extended to modelling of resting-state data and comparing multiple different models.[101,102]

The principles used to investigate functional and effective connectivity from fMRI data can also be applied to data obtained with neurophysiological techniques such as electro-encephalography (EEG) and magnetoencephalography (MEG), allowing mapping of networks at high temporal resolution as well as studying frequency band-specific interactions.[103,104]

Structural connectivity refers to the white matter connections between brain regions. These can be visualized with tracing methods in animals or *ex vivo* methods in autopsied human brains, or inferred *in vivo* with structural imaging techniques such as diffusion tensor imaging (DTI). DTI can be used to estimate the structural integrity of brain connections (i.e. axons and fibre tracts) by measuring diffusion of water molecules through tissues.[105] It provides measures of fractional anisotropy (FA), a particularly sensitive index of microstructural integrity of cerebral white matter, and of radial and axial diffusivity, which give indications of axonal damage and demyelination, respectively. Common methods to assess structural disruption are voxel-wise[106] or diffusion tensor imaging tractography (see chapter 8).[107] Structural connectivity can also be estimated by studying the correlation among regional structural measures such as local cortical thickness and volume across subjects (anatomical covariance), in a way similar to functional connectivity.[108,109] Structural covariance does not demand existence of a direct anatomical connection between the regions whose structural measures are correlated. As with functional covariance, the identified connections might not reflect axonal pathways and caution is required in interpreting the results. Nevertheless, networks identified using this approach have been found to reflect genetic influences as well as experience-related plasticity reliably.[110]

Brain networks derived from all the methods described above can be examined using *graph theory* in which connectivity elements (single brain regions or maps of resting state networks) are defined as *network nodes* and their mutual relationships as *network edges*. In this way, brain networks can be mathematically described as graphs which, in their simplest form, correspond to correlations matrices representing the strength of edges between pairs of nodes. At the highest level of abstraction, even the whole brain can be defined as a network and its properties described in terms of number of edges per node, resistance to damage, efficiency, hierarchy, and sub-networks, among other graph theory measures.[111,112]

Although graph-theoretical approaches have several limitations, including the high dependence on how nodes are initially defined (with structural atlas-based or functional parcellations) and their high degree of abstraction, they have the potential of becoming more meaningful and interpretable in the near future.[113]

Large-networks abnormalities in neurodegenerative diseases

Connectivity methods have now been applied to neurological diseases. This has been particularly promising in the context of neurodegenerative diseases, which are associated with gradual and specific patterns of progression of pathology across the brain. Indeed, it has been increasingly suggested that different pathologies target specific large-scale networks.[114,115]

Since its identification, the DMN has been shown to be particularly relevant for AD, since it includes regions know to be vulnerable to atrophy, amyloid deposition, and reduced metabolism in patients with AD.[116] DMN functional connectivity is reduced in patients with AD compared to healthy controls.[117] Similarly, ROI-based studies using the hippocampus or the posterior cingulate as 'seeds' show decreased functional connectivity with regions of the DMN such as the medial prefrontal cortex, but increased functional connectivity with frontal and frontoparietal regions.[118–121]

More recent studies that used ICA-based methods confirm that patients with AD have significant decreased functional integrity and connectivity in regions of the DMN.[122–125] Among them, the few studies that also explored other resting state networks[99] found that that functional connectivity within frontal and frontoparietal networks is increased in patients with AD relative to controls, thus having the opposite connectivity effect than the DMN.[99,123,124,126] Importantly, these most recent studies examined changes in functional connectivity occurring over and above the structural changes that occur in neurodegenerative diseases by including VBM measures of atrophy as a covariate of no interest.

A number of resting-state fMRI studies have explored functional connectivity in other neurodegenerative diseases. For example, in patients with behavioural variant of frontotemporal dementia, functional connectivity was decreased in the salience network and increased in the DMN, a pattern opposite to the one found in patients with AD.[127] In patients with Parkinson's disease, functional connectivity is reduced in a network involving basal ganglia, and normalizes upon administration of dopaminergic medication.[128]

Do resting state networks identified with resting fMRI relate to actual brain functioning in response to cognitive demand? In healthy people, it has been increasingly shown that functional networks at rest reflect those utilized 'actively' during execution of tasks.[96–98] A recent study which combined resting and task-based fMRI also showed that this is true in patients, suggesting changes in functional connectivity secondary to neurodegenerative disease might directly reflect residual cognitive functioning in patients.[99] Effective connectivity has also been used in neurodegenerative diseases.[129]

In a seminal study combining anatomical covariance and functional connectivity,[130] Seeley and colleagues investigated patterns of atrophy of five different neurodegenerative syndromes (Alzheimer's disease, corticobasal degeneration, and the three variants of frontotemporal dementia) shown in blue in Figure 2.3). Using the identified regions of greater atrophy in each disease as a 'seed', they then showed that in healthy people, seed-based

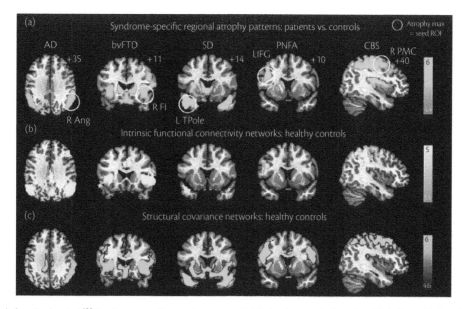

Fig. 2.3 Results of the study from Seeley, *et al.*[130] Syndrome-specific atrophy patterns (in blue), whose cortical maxima (circled) provided seed ROIs for functional (in yellow) and structural (in green) covariance analyses in a group of healthy controls.

Reproduced from *Neuron*, 62(1), Seeley WW, Crawford RK, Zhou J, Miller BL, Greicius MD, Neurodegenerative diseases target large-scale human brain networks, pp. 42–52, Copyright (2009), with permission from Elsevier.

covariance patterns of structural (Fig. 2.3, green) and functional (Fig. 2.3, yellow) measures mirrored syndrome-specific patterns of atrophy. This suggested that networks of functional and structural connectivity in the healthy brain are differentially vulnerable to specific neurodegenerative disease. More precisely, AD affects the DMN, the behavioural variant of frontotemporal dementia affects the salience network, semantic dementia targets the left temporal polar network, progressive non-fluent aphasia the left frontoparietal network, and corticobasal degeneration the sensory-motor network.

In a subsequent study, the same authors further explored network properties of each region found to be atrophic in the five neurodegenerative diseases to identify regions whose normal functional connectivity profile best overlapped with disease-specific patterns of atrophy (which they termed 'epicentres'). They then used graph-theoretical methods to explore possible models of disease spread and reported evidence for a model of trans-neuronal spread from highly vulnerable disease epicentres that, in healthy people, represent highly connected nodes or network hubs.[131]

Graph theory principles have also been applied to measures of cortical thickness covariance to explore network properties in patients with AD. Patients with AD have increased local connectivity of nodes (increased clustering) but decreased global efficiency (increased edges length between connected nodes), suggesting that AD is characterized by a deficit in long-range connectivity and associated with a reversion to less optimal connectivity and more localized connections.[132] AD patients also showed changes in the efficiency of specific nodes, with significant decreased efficiency in heteromodal temporal and parietal regions, and increased efficiency in frontal and occipital regions, in line with findings from functional connectivity.

One recent study specifically tested if network hubs, identified using DTI, in the normal brain are indeed vulnerable to specific brain disorders.[133] Analysis of data from published MRI studies

suggests these hubs are atrophic across twenty-six different neurological and psychiatric conditions. More precisely, nine diseases including AD and schizophrenia have atrophy located in specific highly connected regions; that is, temporal lobe hubs were specifically associated with AD, whereas frontal and temporal cortical hubs were associated with schizophrenia. Similar results were obtained when highly connected hubs were derived from functional connectivity calculated from a meta-analysis of task-related functional imaging studies, rather than from DTI. The authors concluded that highly connected regions within networks identified with different connectivity modalities are more likely to be anatomically affected by brain disorders.

Future directions

The contraposition between the concepts of functional specialization and connectivity has been a major theme in the history of neuroscience. While evidence discussed in the first part of this chapter demonstrates the existence of functionally specialized areas, a growing body of knowledge discussed in the second part shows the importance of connections for brain functioning. Network approaches account for connectivity and nodal or regional specialization, offering the promise to reconcile these seemingly opposing perspectives.[134] Several worldwide initiatives have been recently set up with the aim of describing comprehensively all macroscopic functional and structural connections of the healthy brain, by mapping what has been termed 'human connectomes'[135] (for a complete list of current research projects into macroscale connectomics, see reference 136). Some argue that this will help to attain a fundamental understanding of brain architecture and its relation with cognition and behaviour. Ultimately, it is hoped that it will be clinically useful to obtain individual-relevant reliable indices that can be used for identification of people at risk of specific diseases, prognostication, and measurement of treatment response.

References

1. Broca P. Localisations des fonctions cérébrales. Siège de la faculté du langage articulé. *Bulletin de la Société d'Anthropologie.* 1863; tome IV:200–08.

2. Gall FJ and Spurzheim G. *Anatomie et Physiologie du Système nerveux en général et du cerveau en particulier avec des observations sur la possibilité de reconnaître plusieurs dispositions intellectuelles et morales de l'homme et des animaux par la configuration de leur têtes.* Paris: Schoell, 1810.

3. Broca P. Perte de la parole, ramollissement chronique et destruction partielle du lobe antérieur gauche [Sur le siège de la faculté du langage.] *Bulletin de la Société d'Anthropologie.* 1861;tome II:235–8.

4. Wernicke C. *Der aphasische Symptomencomplex: Eine psychologische Studie auf anatomischer Basis.* Breslau: Cohn und Weigert, 1874.

5. Fritsch G and Hitzig E. Über die elektrische Erregbarkeit des Grosshirn. *Archive für Anatomie, Physiologie und wissenschaftliche Medicin.* 1870:300–32.

6. Ferrier D. Experimental researches in cerebral physiology and pathology. *West Riding Lunatic Asylum Med Rep.* 1973:30–96.

7. Luciani L. On the sensorial localization in the cortex cerebri. *Brain.* 1884;26:145–61.

8. Munk H. Weitere Mittheilungen zur Physiologie der Grosshirnrinde. *Verhandlungen der Physiologischen Gesellschaft zu Berlin.* 1878.

9. Damasio H, Grabowski T, Frank R, *et al.* The return of Phineas Gage: Clues about the brain from the skull of a famous patient. *Science.* 1994;264:1102–05.

10. Scoville WB and Milner B. Loss of recent memory after bilateral hippocampal lesions. *J Neurol Neurosur Ps.* 1957;20:11–21.

11. Squire LR and Zola-Morgan S. The medial temporal lobe memory system. *Science.* 1991;253:1380–6.

12. De Renzi E. Caratteristiche e problemi della neuropsicologia. *Archivio di psicologia, neurologia e psichiatria.* 1967;28:422–40.

13. Benton AL. The Fiction of the 'Gerstmann Syndrome'. *J Neurol Neurosur Ps.* 1961;24:176–81.

14. De Renzi E and Nichelli P. Verbal and non-verbal short-term memory impairment following hemispheric damage. *Cortex.* 1975;11:341–54.

15. De Renzi E. Asimmetrie emisferiche nella rappresentazione non verbali. Atti del XVI Congresso Nazionale di Neurologi. Rome 1967.

16. Newcombe F. *Missile Wounds of the Brain: A Study of Psychological Deficits.* London: Oxford University Press, 1969.

17. Milner B. Interhemispheric differences in the localization of psychological processes in man. *Brit Med Bull.* 1971;27:272–7.

18. Gazzaniga MS and Sperry RW. Language after section of the cerebral commissures. *Brain.* 1967;90:131–48.

19. Newcombe F. Dissociated visual perceptual and spatial deficits in focal lesions of the right hemisphere. *J Neurol Neurosur Ps.* 1969;32:73–81.

20. Damasio H and Damasio AR. *Lesion Analysis in Neuropsychology.* Oxford: Oxford University Press, 1989.

21. Talairach J and Tournoux P. *Co-planar stereotaxic atlas of the human brain: 3-dimensional proportional system: An approach to medical cerebral imaging.* Stuttgart: Thieme Medical, 1988.

22. Frank RJ, Damasio H, and Grabowski TJ. Brainvox: An interactive, multimodal visualization and analysis system for neuroanatomical imaging. *Neuroimage.* 1997;5:13–30.

23. Damasio H and Frank R. Three-dimensional in vivo mapping of brain lesions in humans. *Arch Neurol–Chicago.* 1992;49:137–43.

24. Grafman J, Schwab K, Warden D, *et al.* Frontal lobe injuries, violence, and aggression: a report of the Vietnam Head Injury Study. *Neurology.* 1996;46:1231–8.

25. Damasio H, Grabowski TJ, Tranel D, *et al.* A neural basis for lexical retrieval. *Nature.* 1996;380:499–505.

26. Adolphs R, Damasio H, Tranel D, *et al.* A role for somatosensory cortices in the visual recognition of emotion as revealed by three-dimensional lesion mapping. *J Neurosci.* 2000;20:2683–90.

27. Bates E, Wilson SM, and Saygin AP, *et al.* Voxel-based lesion-symptom mapping. *Nature Neurosci.* 2003;6:448–50.

28. Karnath HO, Fruhmann Berger M, Kuker W, *et al.* The anatomy of spatial neglect based on voxelwise statistical analysis: A study of 140 patients. *Cereb Cortex.* 2004;14:1164–72.

29. Walker GM, Schwartz MF, Kimberg DY, *et al.* Support for anterior temporal involvement in semantic error production in aphasia: New evidence from VLSM. *Brain and Lang.* 2011;117:110–22.

30. Baldo JV, Katseff S, and Dronkers NF. Brain Regions Underlying Repetition and Auditory-Verbal Short-term Memory Deficits in Aphasia: evidence from Voxel-based Lesion Symptom Mapping. *Aphasiology.* 2012;26:338–54.

31. van Asselen M, Kessels RP, Frijns CJ, *et al.* Object-location memory: A lesion-behavior mapping study in stroke patients. *Brain Cognition.* 2009;71:287–94.

32. Barbey AK, Colom R, Solomon J, *et al.* An integrative architecture for general intelligence and executive function revealed by lesion mapping. *Brain.* 2012;135:1154–64.

33. Knutson KM, Rakowsky ST, Solomon J, *et al.* Injured brain regions associated with anxiety in Vietnam veterans. *Neuropsychologia.* 2013;51:686–94.

34. Mah YH, Husain M, Rees G, *et al.* Human brain lesion-deficit inference remapped. *Brain.* 2014;137:2522–31.

35. Thompson PM, Mega MS, Woods RP, *et al.* Cortical change in Alzheimer's disease detected with a disease-specific population-based brain atlas. *Cereb Cortex.* 2001;11:1–16.

36. Ashburner J and Friston KJ. Voxel-based morphometry—the methods. *Neuroimage.* 2000;11:805–21.

37. Ashburner J and Friston KJ. Why voxel-based morphometry should be used. *Neuroimage.* 2001;14:1238–43.

38. MacDonald D, Kabani N, Avis D, *et al.* Automated 3-D extraction of inner and outer surfaces of cerebral cortex from MRI. *Neuroimage.* 2000;12:340–56.

39. Scahill RI, Schott JM, Stevens JM, *et al.* Mapping the evolution of regional atrophy in Alzheimer's disease: Unbiased analysis of fluid-registered serial MRI. *Proc Natl Acad Sci USA.* 2002;99:4703–07.

40. Busatto GF, Diniz BS, and Zanetti MV. Voxel-based morphometry in Alzheimer's disease. *Expert Rev Neurother.* 2008;8:1691–702.

41. Fennema-Notestine C, Hagler DJ, Jr, *et al.* Structural MRI biomarkers for preclinical and mild Alzheimer's disease. *Hum Brain Mapp.* 2009;30:3238–53.

42. Braak H and Braak E. Neuropathological staging of Alzheimer-related changes. *Acta Neuropathol.* 1991;82:239–59.

43. Rosen HJ, Gorno-Tempini ML, Goldman WP, *et al.* Patterns of brain atrophy in frontotemporal dementia and semantic dementia. *Neurology.* 2002;58:198–208.

44. Rosen HJ, Kramer JH, Gorno-Tempini ML, *et al.* Patterns of cerebral atrophy in primary progressive aphasia. *Am J Geriatr Psychiat.* 2002;10:89–97.

45. Gorno-Tempini ML, Dronkers NF, Rankin KP, *et al.* Cognition and anatomy in three variants of primary progressive aphasia. *Ann Neurol.* 2004;55:335–46.

46. Rosen HJ, Allison SC, Schauer GF, *et al.* Neuroanatomical correlates of behavioural disorders in dementia. *Brain.* 2005;128:2612–25.

47. Whitwell JL, Sampson EL, Loy CT, *et al.* VBM signatures of abnormal eating behaviours in frontotemporal lobar degeneration. *Neuroimage.* 2007;35:207–13.

48. Sarazin M, Chauvire V, Gerardin E, *et al.* The amnestic syndrome of hippocampal type in Alzheimer's disease: an MRI study. *J Alzheimers Dis.* 2010;22:285–94.

49. Boddaert N, Chabane N, Gervais H, *et al.* Superior temporal sulcus anatomical abnormalities in childhood autism: a voxel-based morphometry MRI study. *Neuroimage.* 2004;23:364–9.

50. Zamboni G, Huey ED, Krueger F, *et al.* Apathy and disinhibition in frontotemporal dementia: Insights into their neural correlates. *Neurology.* 2008;71:736–42.

51. Kesslak JP, Nalcioglu O, and Cotman CW. Quantification of magnetic resonance scans for hippocampal and parahippocampal atrophy in Alzheimer's disease. *Neurology.* 1991;41:51–4.

52. Jack CR, Jr., Petersen RC, O'Brien PC, *et al.* MR-based hippocampal volumetry in the diagnosis of Alzheimer's disease. *Neurology.* 1992;42:183–8.

53. Jack CR, Jr, Petersen RC, Xu YC, *et al.* Medial temporal atrophy on MRI in normal aging and very mild Alzheimer's disease. *Neurology.* 1997;49:786–94.

54. Chan D, Fox NC, Scahill RI, *et al.* Patterns of temporal lobe atrophy in semantic dementia and Alzheimer's disease. *Ann Neurol.* 2001;49:433–42.

55. Fox NC, Freeborough PA, and Rossor MN. Visualisation and quantification of rates of atrophy in Alzheimer's disease. *Lancet.* 1996;348:94–7.

56. Jack CR, Jr., Petersen RC, Xu Y, *et al.* Rates of hippocampal atrophy correlate with change in clinical status in aging and AD. *Neurology.* 2000;55:484–9.

57. Barnes J, Boyes RG, Lewis EB, *et al.* Automatic calculation of hippocampal atrophy rates using a hippocampal template and the boundary shift integral. *Neurobiol Aging.* 2007;28:1657–63.

58. Barnes J, Foster J, Boyes RG, *et al.* A comparison of methods for the automated calculation of volumes and atrophy rates in the hippocampus. *Neuroimage.* 2008;40:1655–71.

59. Fox PT and Mintun MA. Noninvasive functional brain mapping by change-distribution analysis of averaged PET images of H215O tissue activity. *J Nucl Med.* 1989;30:141–9.

60. Ogawa S, Menon RS, Tank DW, *et al.* Functional brain mapping by blood oxygenation level-dependent contrast magnetic resonance imaging. A comparison of signal characteristics with a biophysical model. *Biophys J.* 1993;64:803–12.

61. Ogawa S, Tank DW, Menon R, *et al.* Intrinsic signal changes accompanying sensory stimulation: functional brain mapping with magnetic resonance imaging. *Proc Natl Acad Sci USA.* 1992;89:5951–5.

62. Friston KJ, Ashburner JT, Stefan JK, *et al. Statistical Parametric Mapping: The Analysis of Functional Brain Images,* 1st edn. London: Academic Press, 2007.

63. Friston KJ, Holmes A, Poline JB, *et al.* Detecting activations in PET and fMRI: levels of inference and power. *Neuroimage.* 1996;4:223–35.

64. Cabeza R and Nyberg L. Imaging cognition II: An empirical review of 275 PET and fMRI studies. *J Cognitive Neurosci.* 2000;12:1–47.

65. Zeki S, Watson JD, Lueck CJ, *et al.* A direct demonstration of functional specialization in human visual cortex. *J Neurosci.* 1991;11:641–9.

66. Friston KJ, Price CJ, Fletcher P, *et al.* The trouble with cognitive subtraction. *Neuroimage.* 1996;4:97–104.

67. Price CJ, Moore CJ, Humphreys GW, *et al.* The neural regions sustaining object recognition and naming. *Proc Roy Soc Lond (Biol).* 1996;263:1501–07.

68. Price CJ and Friston KJ. Functional ontologies for cognition: The systematic definition of structure and function. *Cognitive Neuropsych.* 2005;22:262–75.

69. Fedorenko E, Duncan J, and Kanwisher N. Broad domain generality in focal regions of frontal and parietal cortex. *Proc Natl Acad Sci USA.* 2013;110:16616–21.

70. Geschwind N. Disconnexion syndromes in animals and man. II. *Brain.* 1965;88:585–644.

71. Geschwind N. Disconnexion syndromes in animals and man. I. *Brain.* 1965;88:237–94.

72. Catani M and Ffytche DH. The rises and falls of disconnection syndromes. *Brain.* 2005;128:2224–39.

73. Luria AR and Haigh B. *The Working Brain: An Introduction to Neuropsychology.* New York: Basic Books, 1973.

74. Monakow CV. *Die Lokalisation im Grosshirn und der Abbau der Funktion durch kortikale Herde.* Wiesbaden: J.F. Bergmann, 1914.

75. Price CJ, Warburton EA, Moore CJ, *et al.* Dynamic diaschisis: anatomically remote and context-sensitive human brain lesions. *J Cognitive Neurosc.* 2001;13:419–29.

76. Carrera E and Tononi G. Diaschisis: past, present, future. *Brain.* 2014;137:2408–22.

77. Mesulam MM. Large-scale neurocognitive networks and distributed processing for attention, language, and memory. *Ann Neurol.* 1990;28:597–613.

78. Mesulam MM. From sensation to cognition. *Brain.* 1998;121 (Pt 6):1013–52.

79. McIntosh AR, Grady CL, Ungerleider LG, *et al.* Network analysis of cortical visual pathways mapped with PET. *J Neurosci.* 1994;14:655–66.

80. McIntosh AR, Cabeza RE, and Lobaugh NJ. Analysis of neural interactions explains the activation of occipital cortex by an auditory stimulus. *J Neurophysiol.* 1998;80:2790–6.

81. Sporns O, Chialvo DR, Kaiser M, *et al.* Organization, development and function of complex brain networks. *Trends Cogn Sci.* 2004;8:418–25.

82. Bressler SL and Menon V. Large-scale brain networks in cognition: Emerging methods and principles. *Trends Cogn Sci.* 2010;14:277–90.

83. Honey CJ, Sporns O, Cammoun L, *et al.* Predicting human resting-state functional connectivity from structural connectivity. *Proc Natl Acad Sci USA.* 2009;106:2035–40.

84. Greicius MD, Supekar K, Menon V, *et al.* Resting-state functional connectivity reflects structural connectivity in the default mode network. *Cereb Cortex.* 2009;19:72–8.

85. Gusnard DA and Raichle ME. Searching for a baseline: functional imaging and the resting human brain. *Nature Rev Neurosci.* 2001;2:685–94.

86. Fox MD and Raichle ME. Spontaneous fluctuations in brain activity observed with functional magnetic resonance imaging. *Nature Rev Neurosci.* 2007;8:700–11.

87. Beckmann CF and Smith SM. Probabilistic independent component analysis for functional magnetic resonance imaging. *IEEE T Med Imaging.* 2004;23:137–52.

88. Beckmann CF, DeLuca M, Devlin JT, *et al.* Investigations into resting-state connectivity using independent component analysis. *Philos Trans R Soc Lond B Biol Sci.* 2005;360:1001–13.

89. De Luca M, Beckmann CF, De Stefano N, *et al.* fMRI resting state networks define distinct modes of long-distance interactions in the human brain. *Neuroimage.* 2006;29:1359–67.

90. Raichle ME, MacLeod AM, Snyder AZ, *et al.* A default mode of brain function. *Proc Natl Acad Sci USA.* 2001;98:676–82.

91. Greicius MD, Krasnow B, Reiss AL, *et al.* Functional connectivity in the resting brain: a network analysis of the default mode hypothesis. *Proc Natl Acad Sci USA.* 2003;100:253–8.

92. Andrews-Hanna JR, Reidler JS, Sepulcre J, *et al.* Functional-anatomic fractionation of the brain's default network. *Neuron.* 65:550–62.

93. Seeley WW, Menon V, Schatzberg AF, *et al.* Dissociable intrinsic connectivity networks for salience processing and executive control. *J Neurosci.* 2007;27:2349–56.

94. Damoiseaux JS, Beckmann CF, Arigita EJ, *et al.* Reduced resting-state brain activity in the 'default network' in normal aging. *Cereb Cortex.* 2008;18:1856–64.

95. Yeo BT, Krienen FM, Sepulcre J, *et al.* The organization of the human cerebral cortex estimated by intrinsic functional connectivity. *J Neurophysiol.* 2011;106:1125–65.

96. Smith SM, Fox PT, Miller KL, *et al.* Correspondence of the brain's functional architecture during activation and rest. *Proc Natl Acad Sci USA.* 2009;106:13040–5.

97. Laird AR, Eickhoff SB, Rottschy C, *et al.* Networks of task co-activations. *Neuroimage.* 2013;80:505–14.

98. Laird AR, Fox PM, Eickhoff SB, *et al.* Behavioral interpretations of intrinsic connectivity networks. *J Cognitive Neurosci.* 2011;23:4022–37.

99. Zamboni G, Wilcock GK, Douaud G, *et al.* Resting functional connectivity reveals residual functional activity in Alzheimer's disease. *Biol Psychiat.* 2013;74:375–83.

100. Friston KJ. Functional and effective connectivity: a review. *Brain Connectivity.* 2011;1:13–36.

101. Friston KJ, Li B, Daunizeau J, *et al.* Network discovery with DCM. *Neuroimage.* 2011;56:1202–21.

102. Stephan KE, Weiskopf N, Drysdale PM, *et al.* Comparing hemodynamic models with DCM. *Neuroimage.* 2007;38:387–401.

103. Varela F, Lachaux JP, Rodriguez E, *et al.* The brainweb: phase synchronization and large-scale integration. *Nature Rev Neurosci.* 2001;2:229–39.

104. Stam CJ. Use of magnetoencephalography (MEG) to study functional brain networks in neurodegenerative disorders. *J Neuro Sci.* 2010;289:128–34.

105. Moseley ME, Cohen Y, Kucharczyk J, *et al.* Diffusion-weighted MR imaging of anisotropic water diffusion in cat central nervous system. *Radiology.* 1990;176:439–45.

106. Smith SM, Jenkinson M, Johansen-Berg H, *et al.* Tract-based spatial statistics: voxelwise analysis of multi-subject diffusion data. *Neuroimage.* 2006;31:1487–505.

107. Catani M and Thiebaut de Schotten M. A diffusion tensor imaging tractography atlas for virtual in vivo dissections. *Cortex.* 2008;44:1105–32.

108. He Y, Chen ZJ, and Evans AC. Small-world anatomical networks in the human brain revealed by cortical thickness from MRI. *Cereb Cortex.* 2007;17:2407–19.

109. Mechelli A, Friston KJ, Frackowiak RS, *et al.* Structural covariance in the human cortex. *J Neurosci.* 2005;25:8303–10.

110. Evans AC. Networks of anatomical covariance. *Neuroimage.* 2013;80:489–504.

111. Bullmore E and Sporns O. Complex brain networks: Graph theoretical analysis of structural and functional systems. *Nature Rev Neurosci.* 2009;10:186–98.

112. Rubinov M and Sporns O. Complex network measures of brain connectivity: Uses and interpretations. *Neuroimage.* 2010;52:1059–69.

113. Smith SM, Vidaurre D, Beckmann CF, *et al.* Functional connectomics from resting-state fMRI. *Trends Cogn Sci.* 2013;17:666–82.

114. Pievani M, de Haan W, Wu T, *et al.* Functional network disruption in the degenerative dementias. *Lancet Neurol.* 2011;10:829–43.

115. Rowe JB. Connectivity Analysis is Essential to Understand Neurological Disorders. *Frontiers in Systems Neuroscience.* 2010;4.

116. Buckner RL, Snyder AZ, Shannon BJ, *et al.* Molecular, structural, and functional characterization of Alzheimer's disease: Evidence for a relationship between default activity, amyloid, and memory. *J Neurosci.* 2005;25:7709–17.

117. Greicius MD, Srivastava G, Reiss AL, *et al.* Default-mode network activity distinguishes Alzheimer's disease from healthy aging: Evidence from functional MRI. *Proc Natl Acad Sci USA.* 2004;101:4637–42.

118. Wang L, Zang Y, He Y, *et al.* Changes in hippocampal connectivity in the early stages of Alzheimer's disease: evidence from resting state fMRI. *Neuroimage.* 2006;31:496–504.

119. Allen G, Barnard H, McColl R, *et al.* Reduced hippocampal functional connectivity in Alzheimer disease. *Arch Neurol–Chicago.* 2007;64:1482–7.

120. Zhang HY, Wang SJ, Xing J, *et al.* Detection of PCC functional connectivity characteristics in resting-state fMRI in mild Alzheimer's disease. *Behav Brain Res.* 2009;197:103–8.

121. Zhang HY, Wang SJ, Liu B, *et al.* Resting brain connectivity: changes during the progress of Alzheimer disease. *Radiology.* 2010;256:598–606.

122. Gili T, Cercignani M, Serra L, *et al.* Regional brain atrophy and functional disconnection across Alzheimer's disease evolution. *J Neurol Neurosur Ps.* 2011;82:58–66.

123. Agosta F, Pievani M, Geroldi C, *et al.* Resting state fMRI in Alzheimer's disease: Beyond the default mode network. *Neurobiol Aging.* 2012; Aug;33(8):1564–78.

124. Damoiseaux JS, Prater KE, Miller BL, *et al.* Functional connectivity tracks clinical deterioration in Alzheimer's disease. *Neurobiol Aging.* 2012 Apr;33(4):828.e19–30.

125. Binnewijzend MA, Schoonheim MM, Sanz-Arigita E, *et al.* Resting-state fMRI changes in Alzheimer's disease and mild cognitive impairment. *Neurobiol Aging.* 2011;33:2018–28.

126. Jones DT, Machulda MM, Vemuri P, *et al.* Age-related changes in the default mode network are more advanced in Alzheimer disease. *Neurology.* 2011;77:1524–31.

127. Zhou J, Greicius MD, Gennatas ED, *et al.* Divergent network connectivity changes in behavioural variant frontotemporal dementia and Alzheimer's disease. *Brain.* 2010;133:1352–67.

128. Szewczyk-Krolikowski K, Menke RA, Rolinski M, *et al.* Functional connectivity in the basal ganglia network differentiates PD patients from controls. Neurology. 2014 Jul 15;83(3):208–14.

129. Rowe JB, Hughes LE, Barker RA, *et al.* Dynamic causal modelling of effective connectivity from fMRI: Are results reproducible and sensitive to Parkinson's disease and its treatment? *Neuroimage.* 2010;52:1015–26.

130. Seeley WW, Crawford RK, Zhou J, *et al.* Neurodegenerative diseases target large-scale human brain networks. *Neuron.* 2009;62:42–52.

131. Zhou J, Gennatas ED, Kramer JH, *et al.* Predicting regional neurodegeneration from the healthy brain functional connectome. *Neuron.* 2012;73:1216–27.

132. He Y, Chen Z, and Evans A. Structural insights into aberrant topological patterns of large-scale cortical networks in Alzheimer's disease. *J Neurosci.* 2008;28:4756–66.

133. Crossley NA, Mechelli A, Scott J, *et al.* The hubs of the human connectome are generally implicated in the anatomy of brain disorders. *Brain.* 2014;137:2382–95.

134. Sporns O. Structure and function of complex brain networks. *Dialogues in Clinical Neuroscience.* 2013;15:247–62.

135. Sporns O, Tononi G, and Kotter R. The human connectome: A structural description of the human brain. *PLoS Computational Biology.* 2005;1:e42.

136. Craddock RC, Jbabdi S, Yan CG, *et al.* Imaging human connectomes at the macroscale. *Nature Methods.* 2013;10:524–39.

CHAPTER 3

The frontal lobes

Teresa Torralva, Ezequiel Gleichgerrcht, Agustin Ibañez, and Facundo Manes

The frontal lobes are pivotal in the management of higher-level behavioural functions, such as the planning and execution of intentional motor behaviour including but not limited to limb and eye movements and speech articulation. They are also responsible for major information-processing operations, such as mnemonic functions. Among these are the short term, on-line maintenance and manipulation of information in working memory, which allows for an idea to be weighed up against alternatives,[1] the organization of information for encoding and retrieval within long-term memory,[2] and the establishment of abstract relationships and mental flexibility.[3] Furthermore, the frontal lobes have a role in various components of attention,[4] the processing of emotions,[5] social cognition,[6] and future-oriented thought.[7]

In light of the plethora of important functions mediated by the frontal lobes, impairment of frontal functions can be found, although in varying degrees, in many neurological and psychiatric disorders, predominantly in traumatic brain injury,[8] fronto-temporal dementia,[9,10] bipolar disorder,[11,12] schizophrenia,[13] and depression.[14]

An exceptionally large area of the brain, the frontal lobes account for approximately one-third of the human cerebral cortex. While it has been classically accepted that this area is larger in humans than in non-human primates, more recent studies suggest the frontal lobes are of comparable size throughout the primate lineage.[15] Instead, it is proposed that the human neural architecture is more sophisticated or perhaps organized differently than among non-human primates, thus allowing for a similarly sized cerebral cortex to accommodate the more advanced cognitive processes that characterize human but not other primates.[16] In particular, Semendeferi and colleagues supported this assumption by suggesting higher-level cognition in humans may be attributed to differences in individual cortical areas and a richer interconnectivity rather than a greater overall size (Fig. 3.1a and b).[17]

Besides sharing cerebral cortices that may be proportionally similar in size, humans and monkeys have distinct architectonic regions within their prefrontal cortex. Experimental and anatomical studies in monkeys have identified that each region is distinct in its connections with cortical and subcortical structures.[18] Connections are classified as either afferent or efferent and are mediated via specific fibre pathways. Critical information about perceptual and mnemonic processes occurring in posterior association cortical areas and subcortical structures is passed to particular prefrontal regions by means of afferent connections. Efferent connections deliver information from the prefrontal cortical areas to post-Rolandic cortical association areas and subcortical structures, thus enabling selective information processing.[19]

Each frontal lobe takes the form of a pyramid, with the frontal pole, central sulcus, and lateral, medial, and orbital walls contributing to its shape. All functional types of cortex are represented within the frontal lobes. The limbic cortex is represented in the form of an inconspicuous sliver of pyriform cortex at the most caudal end of the orbital surface, primary motor and motor association areas are located on the lateral and dorsomedial surfaces, the heteromodal cortex covers most of the lateral surfaces, and the paralimbic cortex is located on the caudal regions of the medial and orbital surfaces. The paralimbic component of the frontal lobe is continuous with the cingulate gyrus on the medial surface and with the insula and temporal pole on the orbital surface.[20]

The prefrontal cortex (PFC) occupying the rostral pole of the brain was once described as the area responsible for intelligence; however, damage to this part of the cortex does not result in intellectual deficits but, rather, PFC lesions have detrimental effects on executive and social functioning. The prefrontal cortex has been identified as an action-orientated region which plays an important role in the decision to carry out an action, the type of action to be carried out, and appropriate timing for such action.[21]

Frontal lobe functions can be grouped into five cortical-subcortical circuits, based on their function and anatomical makeup (Fig. 3.2). Each circuit is made up of equal component structures, including the cerebral cortex, a portion of the striatum, a station in the globus pallidus or substantia nigra, and, finally, the thalamus. These circuits project from and to the frontal lobes.[22] Each circuit contains a direct and indirect pathway that includes the subthalamic nucleus. This chapter will focus on three of these circuits, those principally related to non-motor cognition and behaviour.

The dorsolateral prefrontal circuit (DL-PFC)

This circuit originates in Brodmann's areas 9 and 46 on the dorsolateral surface of the anterior frontal lobe. The *mid-dorsolateral* prefrontal region is considered to be critical for the monitoring of information in working memory, which is necessary for high level planning and manipulation of information. This function may be exercised via the dorsal limbic pathways that link this region to the PFC with the hippocampal system via the posterior cingulate rostrosplenial region. The *posterior* dorsolateral frontal cortex appears to underlie what are sometimes referred to as attentional processes. These areas receive input from medial and lateral parieto-occipital

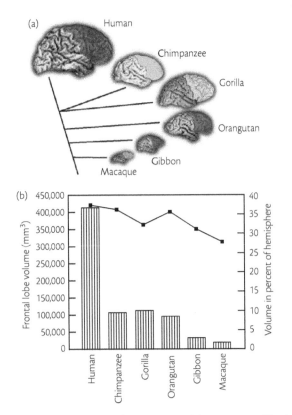

Fig. 3.1 (a) Relative size of the prefrontal cortex in different primates. (b) Volume of the frontal lobe across species. Values include both hemispheres.

(a) Adapted from *Journal of Human Evolution*, 32(4), Semendeferi K, Damasio H, Frank R, and Van Hoesen GW, The evolution of the frontal lobes: a volumetric analysis based on three-dimensional reconstructions of magnetic resonance scans of human and ape brains, pp. 375–88, Copyright (1997), with permission from Elsevier. (b) Adapted from *Nat Neurosci*, 5(3), Semendeferi K, Lu A, Schenker N, and Damasio H, Humans and great apes share a large frontal cortex, pp. 272–6, Copyright (2002), with permission from Nature Publishing Group.

cortical regions, as well as from the adjacent caudal superior temporal gyrus via the superior longitudinal, the occipito-frontal. and the arcuate fasciculi.[23]

Sequential connections are to the striosomes of the dorsolateral head of the caudate nucleus,[24] lateral aspect of the dorsomedial globus pallidus interna (Gpi), and rostrolateral sustancia nigra (SNr) via the direct pathway. The indirect pathway through the dorsal

globus palllidus externa (GPe) and the ventromedial subthalmic nucleus (STN) preserves some anatomical segregation from the motor and limbic circuits. The mediodorsal thalamus closes this loop by connecting back to areas 9 and 46 of the dorsolateral frontal lobe. Projections from the ventralis anterior nucleus also terminate in the inferotemporal cortex.[25]

The dorsolateral circuit is principally considered to subserve executive functions (EF), which include the mental capacities necessary for goal formulation, as well as the planning and achievement of these goals.[26] This circuit also plays a part in guiding behaviour, set-shifting, motor planning, strategy generation, and activation of remote memories.[27]

Lesions to the aforementioned frontal lobe circuit often result in a recognizable and distinct frontal lobe syndrome: the dorsolateral frontal syndrome (executive dysfunction syndrome). This syndrome specifically results in the impairment of executive functions with patients presenting with poor organizational strategies (e.g. Tower tests), reduced inhibition (e.g. Hayling test), lack of planning and motor programming deficits (e.g. frontal assessment battery or INECO frontal screening). Furthermore, damage to this area can result in difficulties generating hypotheses and impaired flexibly for maintaining or shifting sets, among others.[28]

The orbitofrontal circuit (OFC)

Originating in Brodmann's areas 10 and 11, the *orbitofrontal* circuit consists of medial and lateral sub-circuits. The medial orbitofrontal circuit sends fibres to the ventral striatum and to the dorsal part of the nucleus accumbens.[29] The lateral orbitofrontal circuit sends projections to the ventromedial caudate. These sub-circuits continue to the most medial portion of the caudomedial GPi and to the rostromedial SNr. Axons are sent from the GPi/SNr to the medial area of the magnocellular parts of the ventralis anterior thalamic nucleus. The circuit closes with projections back to the medial or lateral orbitofrontal cortex.[30] The orbitofrontal cortex has extensive connections with other cortical areas, especially in the inferior temporal and insular cortices, with the amygdala and hippocampus. It also receives auditory information from the secondary and tertiary auditory areas, somatosensory information from the secondary somatosensory and parietal cortex, and heteromodal inputs from the superior temporal cortex.[31]

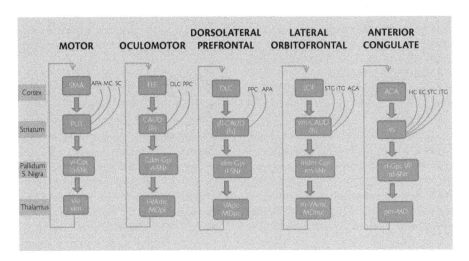

Fig. 3.2 Cortical-subcortical circuits of the frontal lobes.

Lesions to this circuit often result in the typically called orbito-frontal syndrome which is linked to personality changes, including emotional lability, irritability, outspokenness, reduced concerns or worries, and, at times, presenting with imitation and utilization behaviours (the act of grasping objects that are within reach or in the field of vision in a context that is inappropriate),[32] Eslinger and Damasio[5] used the term 'acquired sociopathy' when describing patients with previously normal personalities who, following damage to the ventromedial frontal cortex, developed decision-making and planning difficulties, which presented in the form of challenging, inappropriate, or maladaptive social behaviours. This was also observed in the famous case of the young man called Phineas Gage (Fig. 3.3).

This is one of the most famous cases in behavioural neurology, neuropsychiatry, and neuropsychology. It was pivotal in identifying a link between brain damage and behavioural deficits. Gage sustained a frontal lobe injury in a railroad construction accident while he was using explosives to excavate rocks. After an unplanned explosion, a large tamping iron used to pack sand over the explosive charge entered through the left side of his skull. This injury surprisingly did not cause immediate death and Gage survived, but sustained profound behavioural changes: a man previously described as proper, well organized, responsible, and serious now exhibited poor judgment, difficulties with decision-making, planning, and organizational skills, inappropriate emotional outbursts, and lack of inhibitory control.

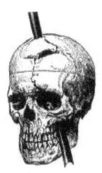

Fig. 3.3 Passage of the bar through the skull of Phineas Gage, as reconstructed by Harlow in 1868.
Reproduced from Publication of the Massachusetts Medical Society, 2, Harlow JM, Recovery after severe injury to the head, pp. 327–46, Copyright (1868), Massachusetts Medical Society.

The anterior cingulate circuit (ACC)

Neurons in the *anterior cingulate cortex* (Brodmann's area 24) serve as the origin of the anterior cingulate-subcortical circuit. Efferent projections include those to the ventral striatum, involving the ventromedial caudate, ventral putamen, nucleus accumbens, and olfactory tubercle, usually named *limbic striatum*. Fibres from the ventral striatum project to the rostromedial GPi, rostrodorsal SNr, and ventral pallidus inferior to the anterior commisure. The GPe connects to the medial STN, which returns to the ventral pallidum, which connects to the magnocellular mediodorsal thalamus. The circuit closes with projections to the anterior cingulate. This circuit is considered to mediate motivated behaviour, reversal learning,[34] reward processes and evaluation,[35] and it also functions, in part, to signal the occurrence of conflicts in information processing, thereby triggering compensatory adjustments in cognitive control.[36]

Lesions to this circuit often result in a syndrome, the anterior cingulate syndrome, characterized by reduced spontaneous activity, evident in disorders such as akinetic mutism and transient abulic hypokinesia or abulia.[37] A typical presentation of this syndrome is that of an apathetic individual with reduced emotional responses. The patient may require prompting to initiate verbal communication and, when verbal responses are elicited, they are likely to be monosyllabic in form. Assistance with feeding is often required due to lack of spontaneous movement, which may also lead to incontinence and other problems typically caused by lesions to areas outside the PFC.

Neurotransmitter circuits

Neurotransmitters modulate the signaling in neural networks and affects cognition and behaviour (see also chapter 9). Different neurotransmitter circuits are involved in the frontal lobes, given their dense interconnectivity with the rest of the brain. In particular, the PFC projections to subcortical arousal systems modulate monoamine and cholinergic inputs to other regions as well as onto itself.[38] Glutamatergic excitatory circuits project from frontal cortex to specific regions of the striatum. GABAergic inhibitory fibres project to the globus pallidus/substantia nigra, then to thalamus, and finally from the thalamus back to the prefrontal cortex. As such, the fast-acting transmitters of the frontal-subcortical circuits, namely GABA and glutamate, affects frontostriatal connections.

In addition to these projections, executive functions are affected by major ascending monoamines (dopamine, norepinephrine, serotonin, histamine, orexin, as well as acetylcholine), spread out to several forebrain regions (hippocampus, striatum, amygdala, and thalamus), as well as to the neocortex.[39] For instance, it comes as no surprise that several neuropsychiatric conditions associated with abnormal catecholaminergic (dopamine, serotonin, and noradrenalin) and cholinergic modulation[40] present with widespread frontal deficits. Monoamine modulators have strong influences on prefrontal cognitive functioning (Fig. 3.4). Several of these influences seem to affect cognitive functioning and self-control in healthy normal individuals, and more evidently so in neuropsychiatric conditions.

Asymmetries of the frontal lobes

In this section, we will briefly revise the few findings that have been reported in the literature about structural and functional

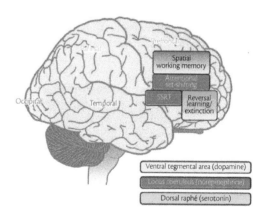

Fig. 3.4 Schematic summary of the differential impact of ascending monoamine systems on different tasks mediated by different sectors of the PFC. SSRT: stop-signal reaction time task.
Source data from *Annu Rev Neurosci*, 32, Robbins TW, Arnsten AF, The neuropsychopharmacology of fronto-executive function: monoaminergic modulation, pp. 267–87, Copyright (2009), Annual Reviews.

asymmetries of the frontal lobes. It is often assumed that anatomical asymmetries invariably reflect functional asymmetries, but this may not always be the case. Language functions have been the most widely studied asymmetries of the frontal lobes, with a left-hemisphere superiority and proficiency for the majority of vocal, motor, and language production functions.[41] Nevertheless, some language capacities exist in most right hemispheres[42] such as prosody, as well as the expression of the emotional content of language. In patients with brain injury, left frontal lobe damage also typically leads to more profound verbal fluency and working memory deficits than right-sided damage whereas right frontal damage causes deficits primarily in the use and representation of visuospatial data in a variety of tasks.

It has been also reported that the right prefrontal cortex has a predominant role in attentional mechanisms,[43] with studies showing a striking increase in blood flow and metabolic activity in the right prefrontal cortex including Brodman areas 8, 9, 44, and 46 during selective attention tasks in different sensory modalities (e.g. see reference 44). In relation to memory, Tulving and his colleagues proposed that the left and right frontal lobes may play different roles in memory processing: encoding information into memory seems to be 'the' role of the left prefrontal cortex whereas retrieval is related to the right prefrontal cortex.[45] One of the most remarkable asymmetries in the anterior cingulate is at the morphological level: there are two cerebral sulci in the left hemisphere and sometimes only one in the right hemisphere. This has been related to certain aspects of effortful versus automatic vocalization.[46] In spite of the large numbers of frontal functions that appear to be lateralized, the only functional asymmetry related strongly to an *anatomical* asymmetry is that of language and Broca's area in particular.

Frontal lobe functions

Executive functions (EF)

EF refers to a complex set of processes consisting of various higher-level cognitive functions. There is a general consensus regarding the type of functions that are grouped under this term. Welsh and Pennington[47] define EF as 'the ability to maintain an appropriate problem solving set for attainment of a future goal', comprising the capacity to inhibit a response, to plan future actions strategically, and to maintain a mental representation of the desired goal stated and the information presented. Furthermore, the EF has also been implicated in emotional and behavioural processes.[48] Zelazo, Qu, and Muller[49] have conceptualized the involvement of the EF in either 'cool', purely cognitive executive processes, or 'hot' executive processes, which involve affect and motivation. Mitchell and Phillips[50] suggest that not only does the PFC have a role in cognition and emotion, but that it is also responsible for coordinating the two processes. Laboratory-based executive functions tests have been criticized as lacking in ecological validity since the coordination between the two processes is poorly measured in any currently available test.

Executive dysfunction or impaired EF may involve cognitive deficits such as an inability to focus or maintain attention, impulsivity, disinhibition, reduced working memory, difficulties regulating performance, difficulties with advanced planning, poor reasoning ability, difficulties generating or implementing strategies, perseverative behaviour, inflexibility, and failure to learn from mistakes. Furthermore, in regards to behaviour, maladaptive affect, poor decision-making, and social behavioural problems have also been identified.[51]

Working memory

This process is essential for effective executive functioning and engagement in everyday activity.[52] Within Baddeley's model of working memory, working memory is defined as a limited capacity system that allows the temporary storage and manipulation of information necessary for such complex tasks as comprehension, learning, and reasoning. An integrated neural network consisting of the dorsolateral prefrontal cortex, anterior cingulate, parietal and temporal cortices, hippocampus, and basal ganglia all have a role in working memory.[53] Patients with working memory deficits can have difficulties in remembering information presented only a few minutes earlier and tend to lose track of what they are doing. They can miss important information during a conversation and can feel overwhelmed and frustrated. The most widely used tests to evaluate this function are the reverse digits span test and the 'letters and numbers' subtest of the Wechsler Adult Intelligence Scale (WAIS),[54] among others (for more information, see chapter 11).

Selective and sustained attention

Selective attention is the ability to attend solely to one type of stimuli while ignoring competing, non-essential stimuli. Sustained attention or vigilance refers to the ability to maintain concentration on a task. The frontal lobes in collaboration with the posterior parietal system and the anterior cingulate gyrus play a role in both types of attention.[55] Many researchers use simple tests that measure performance over time to detect sustained attention deficits.

Inhibitory control

This term refers to the ability to suppress or interrupt a previously activated response and resist distraction from external stimuli,[56] therefore patients with poor inhibitory control can be impulsive, careless, and intrusive. A network, which includes the lateral PFC, anterior cingulate, and basal ganglia, are responsible for this function.[57] Go–no go tests and the Hayling test[58] are the most widely used measures for detecting deficits in the inhibitory control domain. The Stroop test[59] is also used for measuring this capacity.

Mental flexibility

This refers to the ability to respond to differential environmental demands and to implement different problem-solving strategies by switching between thoughts and actions.[60] The lateral PFC, the orbitofrontal and parietal cortices, basal ganglia, and cerebellum are areas associated with this function.[61] Patients with problems in this domain may appear inflexible and rigid, with difficulties changing between activities and adapting to new situations. The well-known WCST (Wisconsin Card Sorting Test)[62] is *the* test for measuring mental flexibility.

Planning abilities

Planning is the ability to set future goals, to plan, problem solve, and organize time and resources in order to achieve a task.[60] The dorsolateral PFC, anterior cingulate, and caudate nucleus all have a role in planning.[63] Frontal lobe lesions can result in planning deficits, difficulties initiating activity, and difficulty coping with complex situations. The most frequently used tests for detecting planning abilities are the tower tests[64] and more ecological valid tests such as the hotel task.[65]

Multitasking

The term 'multitasking' refers to an individual's ability to simultaneously perform tasks in order to achieve goals and sub goals. The anterior PFC, specifically Brodmann's area 10, is associated with the abilities necessary for affective multitasking. Damage to the frontopolar cortex has been linked to severe disruption of multitasking ability and this disruption is exacerbated by a greater degree of damage.[66] Several studies have also demonstrated the presence of anterior frontal activity during multitasking[67,68] and when switching between different cognitive contexts.[69] A recent study supports the idea of the potential pivotal role of BA10 in higher order cognitive functions.[68]

Metacognition

This is another important frontal lobe function and refers to the ability to think about one's own mental processes and state of knowledge. Patients with frontal lobe lesions can demonstrate metacognitive deficits, such as overestimating their performance and capacity to learn.[70]

Memory systems

Memory refers to the acquisition, storage, retention, and retrieval of information. Within memory, there are three major processes: encoding, storage, and retrieval. Memory is fundamental for learning as it allows an individual to retain knowledge in order to form associations between behaviour and outcome. Although it has generally been associated with the temporal lobes and specifically the hippocampus, later research studies focused on the involvement of the PFC in memory. Wheeler and colleagues[71] performed a meta-analysis of existing memory studies concerned with recall, cued recall, and recognition. This research indicated that frontal lobe damage disrupted performance in all three areas of memory, with the greatest impairment found in free recall, followed by cued recall and then recognition. Furthermore, investigators found that frontal lobe patients have difficulties encoding semantic information,[72] determining the temporal order of remembered events,[73] and identifying the source of the encoded information.[74]

It is generally agreed that the frontal lobes do not play a substantial role in the consolidation, storage, and retention of new information,[75,76] however they are considered important in the organizational and strategic aspects of episodic memory, essential in encoding, retrieval, and verification of memory output.[76] Typically, frontal lobe patients have trouble utilizing encoding strategies, which results in a weaker memory trace and subsequent retrieval deficits.

Time travel or chronestaesia

The ability to link the past and the future is known as time travel,[77] or chronestaesia.[78] It is an important frontal lobe function, essential for autobiographical and prospective memory, and planning. Autobiographical memory is an awareness of the self, held as continuous over time, with an awareness of the past and future. It is mediated by a neural system that includes the anteromedial PFC, which integrates sensory and specific information.[79] Prospective memory is the recall of the intention to act at a certain time or in a certain situation. Planning requires a consideration of present and future actions in order to achieve a goal. Planning activates PFC areas 9, 46, and 10.[80] From visual perception to social cognition, the frontal regions of the brain make predictions about incoming actions based on contextual information available and on previous experiences.[81,82] Frontal regions provide early feed forward-feedback integration with temporal and visual areas.[83] Thus, the frontal lobes integrate experiences and memory stored in temporal regions in order to make predictions. For instance, the frontal prediction of actions and thoughts can become memories for the future.[84]

Language

In 1861, Paul Broca performed a post-mortem examination on a patient who had suffered severe speech/language problems for many years, with speech output limited to the word 'tan'. At post-mortem, a lesion centred in the left posterior-inferior frontal cortex was detected.[85] This case led to an acceptance of the correlation between inferior lateral frontal lobe damage and language disorder. Certain connections are considered to play a specific role in language, particularly Brodmann areas 6 and 4 are responsible for motor output and areas 44, 46, and 6, and their subcortical connections integrate motor output. It has been proposed that the dorsal lateral frontal and sensory association interconnections are involved in controlling cognition, and the prefrontal and medial frontal connections to the limbic system are involved in response to internal drives.[86]

Alexander[87] suggested that different types of language disorders could emerge from frontal lobe lesions:

1. With medial frontal lobe lesions but predominantly to the left lobe, reduction in speech activation or reduced overall ability to utilize speech can be observed. The severity can range from mutism, or delayed verbal initiations, to brief, unsustain responses.

2. Following left frontal injury specifically in the dorsolateral area, disorders such as transcortical motor aphasia (TCMA) can result. This type of lesion leads to imprecise, unconstrained language with limited, repetitive word use.

3. Lesions to the anterior left frontal lobes can result in more simplistic verbal abilities.

4. Finally, with right lateral and anterior frontal lesions, deficits can include poor organization of language, with socially inappropriate confabulations.

Although abnormal verbal output can result from lesions in either the right or left frontal lobes, the type of deficits reported differ widely. Damage to the right hemisphere does not cause aphasia, word finding, or grammatical deficits. Lexical, syntactic comprehension, and articulation are intact. Impairment, instead, is related to prosody, such as in the intonations used when asking a question, or making a statement.[88]

In addition to the role in cognitive processes, the frontal lobes play a critical role in mediating social behaviour. Some of the following abilities are central to developing and maintaining interpersonal relationships and have been strongly associated with the PFC.

Decision-making (DM)

DM involves weighing up possible positive and negative outcomes associated with a specific choice of action. A specific option can then be selected dependent on what the individual considers most beneficial. The Iowa Gambling Task (IGT) was developed to assess how individuals make decisions when faced with real-life situations[89] and to detect orbitofrontal cortex dysfunction. However, recent research[90,91,92] has further associated performance of this task with other regions, including the dorsolateral prefrontal cortex, the amygdala, the basal ganglia, and the anterior cingulate cortex, among others. Classical frontal lobe patients favour decisions related to high immediate rewards with longer-term punishments.[89]

The performance of frontal lobe patients on this assessment has been linked to an impairment of somatic markers, which results in an 'insensitivity to future rewards' and therefore instant gratification is preferred even when paired with longer-term negative consequences.[93] Torralva and colleagues[94] demonstrated that a group of early behavioural-variant frontotemporal dementia patients presented with abnormal decision-making as measured specifically by the IGT, despite a normal performance on standard cognitive tasks. Consistently, patients with behavioural variant FTD (bvFTD) as well as other diseases including Alzheimer's, primary progressive aphasia, Parkinson's, and Huntington's disease patients can exhibit disadvantageous DM due to involvement of different portions of the complex circuitry feeding DM.[95–97]

Theory of mind (ToM)

Theory of mind refers to the ability to account for the thoughts, beliefs, intentions, and desires of others while understanding that they may differ from our own. This information is used to form judgments about the likely behaviour and response of another person.[98] It has been suggested, although not without controversy,[99] that ToM is a cognitive module in its own, with an innate neural basis,[100] which may in fact be dissociated from other higher functions of the PFC such as decision-making.[10,94] Studies indicate that patients with orbitofrontal lesions perform worse than those with dorsolateral prefrontal lesions when attempting to identify deception, cheating, faux pas, and empathy.[101–103]

Moral behaviour

This refers to the ideals of human behaviour based on shared societal values, incorporating concepts of deed and duty, fairness, and self-control.[104] Previous studies[105] have suggested that the orbital and medial regions of the PFC are responsible for moral judgment. Furthermore, a 'morality network' consisting of the right ventromedial PFC, orbitofrontal cortex, and amygdala has been suggested (for a review see reference 106). The right ventromedial PFC was included in this morality network for its role in linking external stimuli with socio-emotional value, which in turn could affect moral judgment. The orbitofrontal cortex appears to inhibit immediate/automatic responses and enables consideration of social prompts, and the amygdala is involved in moral learning and threat response (for review see reference 106). Moll, de Oliveira-Souza, and Eslinger[107] expanded on these structures and proposed a brain–behaviour relationships model focused on the interactions between emotional, behavioural, and cognitive components. Accordingly, the authors suggested, amongst other structures, the importance of the anterior cingulate cortex, the superior temporal sulcus, the insula, the precuneus, the thalamus, and the basal forebrain. Consistently, studies both in neurodegenerative (e.g. reference 95) and neuropsychiatric populations (e.g. reference 97) affecting OFC functions, namely empathy/ToM, show patterns of moral judgment that deviate from the norm.

Empathy

Empathy is a means of demonstrating appropriate social behaviours and responses in complex or difficult situations. There are dozens of definitions of empathy. Baron-Cohen[108] defined empathy as 'our ability to identify what someone else is thinking or feeling, and to respond to their thoughts and feelings with an appropriate behaviour'. This definition suggests two stages in the empathy process: recognition phase and the response action. Empathy therefore requires not only identifying another person's feeling or thoughts (which overlaps for many authors with the concept of ToM), but providing an emotional response to it. One of the most important regions involved in the empathy circuit is the medial prefrontal cortex, which appears to play an important role for social information processing and for comparing our own perspective to that of others. Damage to this area, as well as other regions involved in this circuit, such as the inferior frontal gyrus, the frontal operculum, the anterior cingulated, the anterior insula, and the temporo-parietal junction, amongst others, can cause a lower degree of empathy.[108]

Personality changes

Changes in personality and psychosocial function following prefrontal lesions have been reported from Gage (see Fig. 3.3) to the present. Damage to the orbital and medial PFC leads to emotional lability as well as to deficits in social and emotional functioning.[109]

Theories of frontal lobe function

Many theories about the functioning of the frontal lobes have been developed with the intention of gaining a better understanding of this complex region. There is no consensus on which of these theories best captures frontal function. Indeed, many of them are not mutually incompatible. Some of the main PFC models are briefly addressed in this chapter in an attempt to introduce some of the most prominent contemporary models and frameworks to understand frontal lobe functions.

Multiple demand system and adaptative coding model

Based on functional neuroimaging (fMRI) and lesion studies that have shown that large parts of the frontal lobe are involved in very diverse cognitive task, some authors have proposed the existence of a multiple-demand (MD) system,[110] which comprises circumscribed regions of lateral and dorsomedial frontal cortex, anterior insula, and the intraparietal sulcus. Following results from single-cell electrophysiology studies in the behaving monkey, this model proposes that neurons of the MD system have the ability to adapt to the current task in order to code the specific information required for that task.[111] Also, recent evidence coming from human neuroimaging studies have supported this view, demonstrating an adaptive change in the patterns of activation coding task-relevant stimulus distinctions in the frontoparietal. These and other results have led some authors to suggest that the main function of the MD system is to construct the mental control programmes of organized behaviour.[110]

Attentional control model

This model[112] proposes the existence of two major mechanisms involved in behavioural regulation: the contention scheduler (CS) and the supervisory attentional system (SAS). The CS is concerned with automatic or well-learnt/well-established responses. This process schedules action while also inhibiting conflicting schemata, which structure and organize routine tasks. However, with novel or complex tasks, schemata are unlikely to have developed and, therefore, additional attentional control is required, hence initiating the SAS. The SAS sets priority for actions and brings conscious awareness and reflection to the forefront, rather than solely relying on simple automatic responses originated in the CS. In a three-step process, a strategy is generated: first, it incorporates a temporary schema for this complex or novel task; second, the schema is implemented and monitored; and finally, the schema is either rejected or modified. The SAS is proposed to be located in the PFC and the CS has been linked to the basal ganglia.

Somatic marker hypothesis

Although not without controversy, this model specifically focuses on the role of emotion in decision-making.[113] It proposes that when a difficult situation is encountered, in order to make a choice or decision, somatic markers stored as memories of past specific behavioural experiences and outcomes are activated. This system can be in effect even without the conscious awareness of the past event. Somatic markers are proposed to be stored in the ventromedial PFC and the model surmises that damage to this area can result in an inability to access somatic markers, which thus results in decision-making skill deficits.[114]

Temporal organization model

This model proposes that the PFC temporally organizes behaviour with that process constrained by short-term memory, motor attention, and the inhibition control of interference.[115] The framework describes mechanisms for monitoring and memory and attentional selection that prioritize goals and ensure that behavioural sequences are performed in the correct order. Temporal integration is mediated by the activity of PFC neurons and also by interactions between the PFC and posterior cortex—the specific posterior cortical areas that are involved in these interactions are determined by the modalities of the sensory and motor information. This model emphasizes processes of attention, short-term memory, and inhibitory control, however, the author also describes PFC function in terms of 'motor memory' (schemata), with a hierarchy of motor representations within the PFC. Attention and working memory are properties of the representations (neural networks), rather than explicit 'processes' in terms of computational procedures. Fuster's model is a hybrid of the representational and processing approaches and is consistent with the evolution and neurophysiology of the PFC. Motor memories that are stored in the PFC become more complex or abstract in anterior frontal regions. Fuster proposes that the functions of the ventromedial PFC parallel those of the dorsolateral PFC, but with the addition of emotional information, given the connectivity between ventromedial PFC and limbic regions (such as the amygdala). He supports the idea that automatic actions are stored in the basal ganglia and the premotor cortex, with PFC representation reserved for actions or behaviours that are not habitual or well learned. Consistent with this viewpoint, the premotor cortex and basal ganglia are known to be important in movement preparation; however, the PFC has been implicated in both novel and well-learned tasks.

Anterior attentional functions

Stuss[4] further developed Fuster's[115] model regarding the association between the frontal lobe and basic schemas, by incorporating a theory of the executive system. According to Stuss, a schema is a network of multiple, connected neurons that can be activated by sensory input, by other schemata, or by the executive control system (Fig. 3.5). Also, it has been suggested that schemata provide feedback to the executive system and compete to control of thought and behaviour. This process is governed by the contention scheduling process described in Norman and Shallice's attentional control model. Once activated, schemas can remain active for varying periods of time depending on the goal and whether further input is received from the executive control system. This

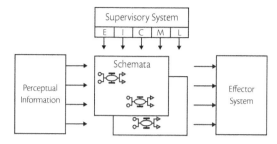

Fig. 3.5 Supervisory systems in human attention.
Adapted from *Annals of the New York Academy of Science*, 769, Stuss DT, Shallice T, Alexander M, and Picton T, A multidisciplinary approach to anterior attentional functions, pp. 191–211, Copyright (1995), with permission from John Wiley and Sons.

might be seconds sometimes or for longer periods, and activation has to be maintained by repeated input from the executive control system. Attention is the main focus in Stuss's theory. This theory proposed seven types of attentional functions, each of which has its neural correlates: sustaining (right frontal), concentrating (cingulate), sharing (cingulate plus orbitofrontal), suppressing (DL-PFC), switching (DL-PFC plus medial frontal), preparing (DL-PFC), and setting (left DL-PFC).

Working memory model

When an individual engages in complex cognitive tasks such as language comprehension, learning, and reasoning, the information is simultaneously and temporarily stored and manipulated within the brain in a system that has been termed working memory. Originally, according to the model advanced by Baddeley and Hitch,[116] there were three components to working memory, the most important of which was the central executive, accompanied by the visuospatial sketchpad and the phonological loop as 'slave' subsystems. Recently, in response to criticisms of the model, a fourth system named the episodic buffer was incorporated.[52] The central executive is capable of controlling the attention afforded to two or more activities occurring simultaneously, whilst also controlling the access to information in long-term memory store. The visuospatial sketchpad holds visual images whilst the phonological loop contains information about speech-based information (Fig. 3.6).

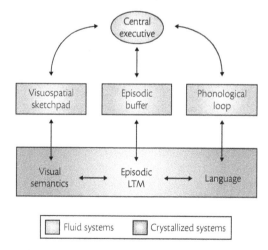

Fig. 3.6 Working memory model.
Reproduced from *Trends Cogn Sci.*, 4(11), Baddeley A, The episodic buffer: a new component of working memory? pp. 417–23, Copyright (2000), with permission from Elsevier.

Structured event complex (SEC) framework

The SEC is considered a sequential set of events that are goal orientated and represent the performance of a functional activity.[117] The SEC contains a set of linked memories that represent thematic knowledge, morals, abstractions, concepts, and social rules, among others. The SEC has been described as a 'memory engine'. Although the different components within a SEC are stored in different parts of the PFC and are represented uniquely, they are encoded and retrieved in unison. Anatomically, SEC components have connections to the posterior (temporal-parietal) or subcortical regions (basal ganglia, hippocampus, amygdala). The model proposes that damage to the SEC results in behavioural problems, as the individual has difficulty processing behavioural and social information, and thus in anticipating future episodes. Damage to specific areas of the PFC would result in specific difficulties. For example, with ventromedial PFC damage, social behavioural problems can arise,[118] whereas with dorsolateral PFC damage, impairment of reflective and mechanistic behaviour has been reported.[119]

Hierarchical organization of the prefrontal cortex

The PFC enables us to select specific actions or thoughts in relation to internal goals, which is the underlying core process behind executive control. For this reason, PFC functions are usually understood from the point of view of phenomenological events, including concepts such as goals, tasks, or intentions. Based on neuroimaging data, however, Koechlin and Summerfield[120] propose a quantitative model in which action selection is guided by hierarchically ordered control signals and processed in a network of brain regions organized along the anterior–posterior axis of the lateral prefrontal cortex. The theory clarifies how executive control can operate as a unitary function, despite the requirement that information be integrated across multiple distinct, functionally specialized prefrontal regions.

The 'gateway' hypothesis

The 'gateway' hypothesis[121] of rostral PFC developed by Burgess and collaborators proposes that lateral and medial regions of rostral PFC are differentially sensitive to changes in demands for stimulus-oriented (SO) or stimulus-independent (SI) attending. According to this model, four interlinked propositions support its central idea: first, some forms of cognition are triggered by perceptual experience (i.e. input through basic sensory systems), whereas other forms of cognition occur in the absence of sensory input; second, some central representations are activated both when a person witnesses an external stimulus and when they merely imagine it; third, if the first and second are true, then it is plausible that there is some brain system that can determine, when required, the source of activation of the central representations, which they refer to as the 'supervisory attentional gateway' (SAG). Proposition four is that rostral PFC plays a part in this mechanism.

This hypothesis assumes that there is, normally, continuous competition for activation of central representations between (i) input from sensory systems, (ii) reciprocal or associative activation from within the system, and (iii) 'top-down' influence from other supervisory systems. Thus many well-specified and/or familiar situations will require minimal operation of the SAG system. The proposal suggests that the SAG system affects the coordination of SI and SO cognition, specifically in situations where selection by this competition fails or is producing maladaptive behaviour and operates as a 'gateway' between the *internal* mental life that occurs independently of environmental stimuli and the mental life that is associated with interaction with *the external* world.

Conclusions

Given the complexity of the human frontal lobes and their intricate, expansive neural connections, a complete appreciation of the wide range of functions associated with these areas is fundamental in order to understand human cognition fully in both health and disease conditions.

New approaches have been developed from disciplines such as social cognition and studies of decision-making, theory of mind, empathy and moral behaviour providing a broader and ecologically valid approach to the understanding of the frontal lobe functions.

Our identity as autonomous human beings, our drives, ambitions, and essence are greatly dependent on our frontal lobes and further research is required to deepen our understanding of such complex cerebral region. With this in mind, the near future is likely to be an exciting time for the field of cognitive and social neurosciences, as our knowledge continues to develop in regards to perhaps the most uniquely human of all brain structures, our frontal lobes.

Acknowledgements

We appreciate the assistance of Clara Pinasco in formatting and referencing the manuscript.

This research was partially supported by grants CONICYT/ FONDECYT Regular (1130920 and 1140114), Foncyt-PICT 2012-0412, Foncyt-PICT 2012-1309, CONICET, and INECO Foundation.

References

1. Mesulam M. The human frontal lobes: Transcending the default mode through contingent encoding. In: D Stuss and R Knight (eds). *Principles of Frontal Lobe Function*. New York, NY: Oxford University Press, 2002, pp. 8–30.

2. Fletcher PC and Henson RN. Frontal lobes and human memory: insights from functional neuroimaging. *Brain*. 2001;124:849–81.

3. Dias R, Robbins TW, and Roberts AC. Dissociation in prefrontal cortex of affective and attentional shifts. *Nature*. 1996;380:69–72.

4. Stuss DT, Shallice T, Alexander M, *et al*. A multidisciplinary approach to anterior attentional functions. *Ann NY Acad Sci*. 1995;769:191–211.

5. Eslinger PJ and Damasio AR. Severe disturbance of higher cognition after bilateral frontal lobe ablation: patient EVR. *Neurology*. 1985;35:1731–41.

6. Iacoboni M and Dapretto M. The mirror neuron system and the consequences of its dysfunction. *Nature Neurosci*. 2006;7(12):942–51.

7. Schacter DL, Addis DR, and Buckner RL. Remembering the past to imagine the future. *Nature Neurosci*. 2007;8(9):657–61.

8. Stuss DT and Gow CA. 'Frontal dysfunction' after traumatic brain injury. *Neuropsy, Neuropsy Be*. 1992;5(4):272–82.

9. Neary D, Snowden JS, Gustafson L, *et al*. Frontotemporal lobar degeneration: a consensus on clinical diagnostic criteria. *Neurology*. 1998;51(6):1546–54.

10. Torralva T, Roca M, Gleichgerrcht E, *et al*. A neuropsychological battery to detect specific executive and social cognitive impairments in early frontotemporal dementia. *Brain*. 2009;132:1299–309.

11. Townsend JD, Sugar CA, Walshaw PD, *et al*. Frontostriatal neuroimaging findings differ in patients with bipolar disorder who have or do not have ADHD comorbidity. *J Affect Disord*. 2013;147:389–96.

12. Torralva T, Strejilevich S, Gleichgerrcht E, *et al.* Deficits in tasks of executive functioning that mimic real-life scenarios in bipolar disorder. *Bipolar Disord.* 2012;14(1):118–25.

13. Cohen JD and Servan-Schreiber D. A theory of dopamine function and its role in cognitive deficits in schizophrenia. *Schizophrenia Bulletin.* 1993;19(1):85–104.

14. Mayberg HS, Liotti M, Brannan SK, *et al.* Reciprocal limbic-cortical function and negative mood: Converging PET findings in depression and normal sadness. *Am J Psychiatry.* 1999;156(5):675–82.

15. Semendeferi K, Lu A, Schenker N, *et al.* Humans and great apes share a large frontal cortex. *Nature Neurosci.* 2002;5:272–6.

16. Rilling JK and Insel TR. The primate neocortex in comparative perspective using magnetic resonance imaging. *J Hum Evol.* 1999;37(2):191–223.

17. Semendeferi K, Damasio H, Frank R, *et al.* The evolution of the frontal lobes: a volumetric analysis based on three-dimensional reconstructions of magnetic resonance scans of human and ape brains. *J Hum Evol.* 1997;32:375–88

18. Jones EG. *The Thalamus.* New York: Plenum Press, 1985.

19. Yeterian EH, Pandya DN, Tomaiuolo F, *et al.* The cortical connectivity of the prefrontal cortex in the monkey brain. *Cortex.* 2012; 48(1):58–81.

20. Petrides M and Pandya DN. Comparative architectonic analysis of the human and macaque frontal cortex. In: F Boller and J Grafman (eds). *Handbook of Neuropsychology*, Vol 8. Amsterdam: Elsevier, 1994, pp. 17–57.

21. Barbas H. Organization of the principal pathways of prefrontal lateral, medial, and orbitofrontal cortices in primates and implications for the collaborative interaction in executive functions. In: J Risberg and J Grafman (eds). *The Frontal Lobes. Development, Function and Pathology.* New York, NY: Cambridge University Press; 2006, pp. 21–68.

22. Cummings JL. Anatomic and behavioral aspects of frontal-subcortical circuits. In: J. Grafman, KJ Holyoak, and F Boller (eds). *Structure and Functions of the Human Prefrontal Cortex*, Vol 769. New York, NY: New York Academy of Sciences, 1995, pp. 1–13.

23. Petrides M and Pandya D. Association Pathways of the Prefrontal Cortex and Functional Observations. In: D Stuss and R Knight (ed.). *Principles of Frontal Lobe Functions.* Oxford: Oxford University Press, 2002, pp. 31–50.

24. Selemon LD, Rajkowska G, and Goldman-Rakic PS. Abnormally high neuronal density in the schizophrenic cortex: A morphometric analysis of prefrontal area 9 and occipital area 17. *Archiv Gen Psychiat.* 1995; 52:805–18.

25. Middleton FA and Strick PL. Basal ganglia and cerebellar loops: Motor and cognitive circuits. *Brain Res.* 2000;31(2–3):236–50.

26. Lezak MD. The problem of assessing executive functions. *Int J Psychol.* 1982; 17(2–3): 281–97.

27. Stuss DT and Alexander MP. Executive functions and the frontal lobes: a conceptual view. *Psychol Res.* 2000;63(3–4):289–98. Review.

28. Saint-Cyr JA, Bronstein YL, and Cummings J. Neurobehavioral Consequences of Neurosurgical Treatments and Focal Lesions of Frontal-Subcortical Circuits. In: D Stuss and R Knight (eds). *Principles of Frontal Lobe Functions.* Oxford: Oxford University Press, 2002, pp. 408–27.

29. Haber SN, Kunishio K, Mizobuchi M, *et al.* The orbital and medial prefrontal circuit through the primate basal ganglia. *J Neurosci.* 1995;15(7 Pt 1):4851–67.

30. Ilinsky LA, Jouandet ML, and Goldman-Rakic PS. Organization of the nigrothalamocortical system in the rhesus monkey. *Journ Comp Neurol.* 1985;236:315–30.

31. Price JL. Architectonic structure of the orbital and medial prefrontal cortex. In: DH Zald and SL Rauch (eds). *The Orbitofrontal Cortex.* New York, NY: Oxford University Press, 2006, pp. 3–17.

32. Cummings JL. Frontal-subcortical circuits and human behaviour. *Archiv Neurol.* 1993;50:873–80.

33. Harlow JM. Recovery after severe injury to the head. *Publication of the Massachussetts Medical Society.* 1868;2:327–46.

34. Hampshire A, Chaudhry AM, Owen AM, *et al.* Dissociable roles for lateral orbitofrontal cortex and lateral prefrontal cortex during preference driven reversal learning. *Neuroimage.* 2012;59(4):4102–12.

35. Baker TE and Holroyd CB. Dissociated roles of the anterior cingulate cortex in reward and conflict processing as revealed by the feedback error-related negativity and N200. *Biol Psychol.* 2011;87(1):25–34.

36. Botvinick M, Cohen JD, and Carter CS. Conflict monitoring and anterior cingulate cortex: an update. *Trends Cogn Sci.* 2004;8(12):539–46.

37. Holroyd CB and Yeung N. Motivation of extended behaviors by anterior cingulate cortex. *Trends Cogn Sci.* 2012 Feb;16(2):122–8.

38. Gamo NJ and Arnsten AF. Molecular modulation of prefrontal cortex: rational development of treatments for psychiatric disorders. *Behav Neurosci.* 2011;125(3):282–96.

39. Robbins TW and Arnsten AF. The neuropsychopharmacology of fronto-executive function: monoaminergic modulation. *Annu Rev Neurosci.* 2009;32:267–87.

40. Chudasama Y and Robbins TW. Functions of frontostriatal systems incognition: comparative neuropsychopharmacological studies in rats, monkeys and humans. *Biol Psychol.* 2006;73(1):19–38.

41. Geschwind N. The organization of language and the brain. *Science.* 1970 Nov 27;170(3961):940–4.

42. Iacoboni M and Zaidel E. Hemispheric independence in word recognition: evidence from unilateral and bilateral presentations. *Brain Lang.* 1996 Apr;53(1):121–40.

43. Heilman KM, Bowers D, Valenstein E, *et al.* Disorders of visual attention. *Baillieres Clin Neurol.* 1993 Aug;2(2):389–413.

44. Lewin JS, Friedman L, Wu D, *et al.* Cortical localization of human sustained attention: detection with functional MR using a visual vigilance paradigm. *J Comput Assist Tomogr.* 1996 Sep–Oct;20(5):695–701.

45. Tulving E. Episodic memory: from mind to brain. *Annu Rev Psychol.* 2002;53:1–25.

46. Paus T, Koski L, Caramanos Z, *et al.* Regional differences in the effects of task difficulty and motor output on blood flow response in the human anterior cingulate cortex: a review of 107 PET activation studies. *Neuroreport.* 1998 Jun 22;9(9):R37–47. Review.

47. Welsh MC and Pennington BF. Assessing frontal lobe functioning in children: views from developmental psychology. *Dev Psychol.* 1988;4(3):199–230.

48. Gioia GA, Isquith PK, and Guy SC. Assessment of executive functions in children with neurological impairment. In: RJ Simeonsson and L Rosenthal (eds). *Children with Disabilities and Chronic Conditions.* New York, NY: Guilford Press, 2001, pp. 317–56.

49. Zelazo PD, Qu L, and Muller U. Hot and cool aspects of executive function: Relations in early development. In: W Shneider, R Schumann-Hengsteler, and B Sodian (eds). *Young Children's Cognitive Development: Interrelationships among Executive Functioning, Working Memory, Verbal Ability, and Theory of the Mind.* Mahwah, NJ: Lawrence Erlbaum Associates Publishers, 2004, pp. 71–93.

50. Mitchell RL, and Phillips LH. The psychological, neurochemical and functional neuroanatomical mediators of the effects of positive and negative mood on executive functions. *Neuropsychologia.* 2007;45(4):617–29. Review.

51. Muscara F, Catroppa C, and Anderson V. The impact of injury severity on executive function 7–10 years following pediatric traumatic brain injury. *Dev Neuropsychol.* 2008;33(5):623–36.

52. Baddley A. Fractioning the central executive. In: D Stuss and R Knight, (eds). *Principles of the Frontal Lobe Function.* New York, NY: Oxford University Press, 2002, pp. 246–60.

53. Curtis CE, Zald DH, and Pardo JV. Organization of working memory within the human prefrontal cortex: a PET study of self-ordered object morking memory. *Neuropsychologia.* 2000;38(11):1503–10.

54. Wechsler D. *Wechsler Intelligence Scales for Children*, 3rd edn. San Antonio, TX: The Psychological Corporation, 1991.

55. Fan J, McCandliss BD, Fossella J, *et al.* The activation of attentional networks. *Neuroimage.* 2005;26(2):471–9.

56. Barkley RA. Behavioral inhibition, sustained attention, and executive functions: Constructing a unifying theory of ADHD. *Psychological Bulletin.* 1997;121(1):65–94.

57. Tamm L, Menon V, and Reiss AL. Maturation of brain function associated with response inhibition. *J Am Acad Child Psy.* 2002;41(10):1231–8.

58. Burgess PW and Shallice T. The Hayling Test and Brixton Tests. Thurston, Suffolk: Thames Valley Test Company, 1997.

59. Golden CJ. *Stroop Color and Word Test. A Manual for Clinical and Experiemental Uses.* Wood Dale, IL: Stoelting Co, 1978.

60. Lezak M. *Neuropsychological Assesment.* New York, NY: Oxford University Press, 1993.

61. Buchsbaum BR, Creer S, Wei-Li C, et al. Meta-analisys of neuroimaging studies of the Wisconsin Card-Sorting Task and component processes. *Hum Brain Mapp.* 2005;25:35–45.

62. Nelson H. A modified card sorting response sensitive to frontal lobe defects. *Cortex.* 1976;12:313–24.

63. Dagher A, Owen AM, Boecker H, et al. Mapping the network for planning: A correlational PET activation study with the Tower of London task. *Brain.* 1999;122:1973–87.

64. Shallice T. Specific impairments of planning. *Philos Trans R Soc Lond B Biol Sci.* 1982;298(1989):199–209.

65. Manly T, Hawkins K, Evans J, et al. Rehabilitation of executive function: A facilitation of effective goal management on complex tasks using periodic auditory alerts. *Neuropsychologia.* 2002;40:2671–81.

66. Dreher JC, Koechlin E, Tierney M, et al. Damage of the frontal-polar cortex is associated with impaired multitasking. *PLoS One.* 2008;3(9):e3227.

67. Burgess PW, Quayle A, and Frith CD. Brain regions involved in prospective memory as determined by positron emission tomography. *Neuropsychologia.* 2001;39:545–55.

68. Badre D and D'Esposito M. Functional magnetic resonance imaging evidence for a hierarchical organization of the prefrontal cortex. *J Cognitive Neurosci.* 2007;19:2082–99.

69. Roca M, Torralva T, Gleichgerrcht E, et al. The role of Area 10 (BA10) in human multitasking and in social cognition: a lesion study. *Neuropsychologia.* 2011;49 (13):3525–31

70. Shimamura AP and Squire LR. Memory and metamemory: a study of the feeling-of-knowing phenomenon in amnesic patients. *J Exp Psychol Learn Mem Cogn.* 1986;12(3):452–60.

71. Wheeler MA, Stuss DT, and Tulving E. Frontal lobe damage produces episodic memory impairment. *J Int Neuropsychol Soc.* 1995;1(6):525–36.

72. Moscovitch M. Multiple dissociations of function in amnesia. In: L Cermak (ed.). *Human Memory and Amnesia.* Hillsdale, NJ: Erlbaum, 1982, pp. 337–70.

73. Shimamura AP. Memory and amnesia. *West J Med.* 1990;152(2):177–8.

74. Janowsky JS, Shimamura AP, and Squire LR. Source memory impairment in patients with frontal lobe lesions. *Neuropsychologia.* 1989;27:1043–56.

75. Petrides M. Dissociable roles of mid-dorsolateral prefrontal and anterior inferotemporal cortex in visual working memory. *J Neurosci.* 2000;20:7496–503.

76. Wincour G, McDonald RM, and Moscovitch M. Anterograde and retrograde amnesia in rats with large hippocampal lesions. *Hippocampus.* 2001;11:18–26.

77. Fuster JM. Executive frontal functions. *Exp Brain Res.* 2000;133(1):66–70. Review.

78. Tulving E. Chronestesia: Conscious awareness of subjective time. In: D Stuss and R Knight (eds). *Principles of Frontal Lobe Function.* New York, NY: Oxford University Press, 2002, pp. 311–25

79. Levine B. Autobiographical memory and the self in time: brain lesion effects, functional neuroanatomy, and lifespan development. *Brain Cognition.* 2004;55:54–68.

80. Cabeza R and Nyberg L. Imaging cognition II: an empirical review of 275 PET and fMRI studies. *J Cognitive Neurosci.* 2000;12:1–47.

81. Bar M. The proactive brain: memory for predictions. *Philos Trans R SocLond B Biol Sci.* 2009;364(1521):1235–43.

82. Ibañez A and Manes F. Contextual social cognition and the behavioral variant of frontotemporal dementia. *Neurology.* 2012;78(17):1354–62.

83. Kveraga K, Ghuman AS, Kassam KS, et al. Early onset of neural synchronization in the contextual associations network. *Proc Natl Acad Sci USA.* 2011;108(8):3389–94.

84. Fuster JM. The prefrontal cortex—an update: time is of the essence. *Neuron.* 2001;30(2):319–33.

85. Signoret JL, Castaigne P, Lhermitte F, et al. Rediscovery of Leborgne's brain: anatomical description with CT scan. *Brain Lang.* 1984;22(2):303–19.

86. Alexander MP, Benson DF, and Stuss DT. Frontal lobes and language. *Brain Lang.* 1989;37(4):656–91.

87. Alexander MP. Disorders of language after frontal lobe injury: Evidence of the neural mechanisms of assembling language. In: D Stuss and R Knight (eds). *Principles of Frontal Lobe Function.* New York, NY: Oxford University Press, 2002, pp. 159–67.

88. Weintraub S, Mesulam MM, and Kramer L. Disturbances in prosody. A right-hemisphere contribution to language. *Arch Neurol.* 1981;38(12):742–44.

89. Bechara A, Damasio AR, Damasio H, et al. Insensitivity to future consequences following damage to human prefrontal cortex. *Cognition.* 1994;50:7–15.

90. Clark L, Manes F, Antoun N, et al. The contributions of lesion laterality and lesion volume to decision-making impairment following frontal lobe damage. *Neuropsychologia.* 2003;41(11):1474–83.

91. Seymour B and Dolan R. Emotion, decision making, and the amygdala. *Neuron.* 2008;58(5):662–71.

92. Kable JW and Glimcher PW. The neurobiology of decision: consensus and controversy. *Neuron.* 2009;63(6):733–45.

93. Bechara A, Damasio H, and Damasio AR. Emotion, decision making and the orbitofrontal cortex. *Cereb Cortex.* 2000;10(3):295–307. Review.

94. Torralva T, Kipps CM, Hodges JR, et al. The relationship between affective decision-making and theory of mind in the frontal variant of fronto-temporal dementia. *Neuropsychologia.* 2007;45:342–9.

95. Gleichgerrcht E, Ibáñez A, Roca M, et al. Decision-making cognition in neurodegenerative diseases. *Nat Rev Neurol.* 2010;6(11):611–23. Epub 2010 Oct 12. Review.

96. Manes F, Torralva T, Ibáñez A, et al. Decision-making in frontotemporal dementia: clinical, theoretical and legal implications. *Dement Geriatr Cogn.* 2011;32(1):11–17.

97. Gleichgerrcht E, Torralva T, Roca M, et al. Decision making cognition in primary progressive aphasia. *Behav Neurol.* 2012; 25(1):45–52.

98. Bibby H and McDonald S. Theory of mind after traumatic brain injury, *Neuropsychologia.* 2005;43:99–114.

99. Mar RA. The neural bases of social cognition and story comprehension. *Annu Rev Psychol.* 2011;62:103–34.

100. Happe F, Brownell H, and Winner E. Acquired 'theory of mind' impairments following stroke. *Cognition.* 1999;70(3):211–40.

101. Stuss DT, Gallup GG, and Alexander MP. The frontal lobes are necessary for 'theory of mind'. *Brain.* 2001;124:279–86.

102. Shamay-Tsoory SG, Tomer R, Berger BD, et al. Characterization of empathy deficits following prefrontal brian damage: the role of the right ventromedial prefrontal cortex. *J Cogn Sci.* 2003;15:324–37.

103. Stone V, Baron-Cohen S, Calder A, et al. Acquired theory of mind impairments in individuals with bilateral amygdala lesions. *Neuropsychologia.* 2003;41(2):209–20.

104. Wilson MS. Social dominance and ethical ideology: the end justifies the means? *J Soc Psychol.* 2003;143(5):549–58.

105. Moll J, de Oliveira-Souza, R, Eslinger PJ, et al. The neural correlates of moral sensivity: a functional magnetic resonance imaging investigation of basic and moral emotions. *J Neurosci.* 2002; 22:2730–6.

106. Mendez MF. What frontotemporal dementia reveals about the neurobiological basis of morality. *Med Hypotheses.* 2006;67(2):411–8.

107. Moll J, de Oliveira-Souza R, and Eslinger PJ. Morals and the human brain: a working model. *NeuroReport.* 2003;14:299–305.

108. Baron-Cohen, S. *Zero Degrees of Empathy: A New Theory of Human Cruelty.* London: Clays Ltd., 2011.

109. Eslinger PJ, Flaherty-Craig CV, and Benton AL. Developmental outcomes after prefrontal cortex damage. *Brain Cognition*. 2004; 22:84–103.

110. Duncan J. The multiple-demand (MD) system of the primate brain: mental programs for intelligent behaviour. *Trends Cogn Sci*. 2010 Apr;14(4):172–9.

111. Freedman DJ, Riesenhuber M, Poggio T, *et al*. Categorical representation of visual stimuli in the primate prefrontal cortex. *Science*. 2001 Jan 12;291(5502):312–6.

112. Norman DA and Shallice T. Attention to action: Willed and automatic control of behaviour. In: RJ Davidson, GE Schwartz, and DE Shapiro (eds). *Conciousness and Self-Regulation*, Vol 4. New York, NY: Plenum Press, 1986, pp. 1–14.

113. Damasio AR. The somatic marker hypothesis and the possible functions of the prefrontal cortex. *Philos Trans R Soc Lond B Biol Sci*. 1996;351(1346):1413–20. Review.

114. Bechara A, Damasio H, and Damasio AR. The somatic marker hypothesis and Decision Making. In: F Boller, J Grafman (eds). *Handbook of Neuropsychology: Frontal Lobes*, 2nd edn. Amsterdam: Elsevier, 2002, pp. 117–43.

115. Fuster JM. Network Memory. *Trends Neurosci*. 1997;20(10):451–9. Review.

116. Baddeley A. The episodic buffer: a new component of working memory? *Trends Cogn Sci*. 2000;4(11):417–23.

117. Grafman J. The human prefronal cortex has evolved to represent components of structured event complexes. In: J Grafman (ed.). *Handbook of Neuropsychology*. Amsterdam: Elsevier, 2002, pp. 157–74.

118. Grafman J, Schwab K, Warden D, *et al*. Frontal lobe injuries, violence and agression: A report of the Vietnam head injury study. *Neurology*. 1996;46:1231–8.

119. Burgess PW, Veitch E, De Lacy Costello A, *et al*. The cognitive and neuroanatomical correlates of multitasking. *Neuropsychologia*. 2000;38:848–63.

120. Koechlin E and Summerfield C. An information theoretical approach to prefrontal executive function. *Trends Cogn Sci*. 2007 Jun;11(6):229–35.

121. Burgess PW, Dumontheil I, and Gilbert SJ. The gateway hypothesis of rostral prefrontal cortex (area 10) function. *Trends Cogn Sci*. 2007 Jul;11(7):290–8.

CHAPTER 4

The temporal lobes

Morgan D. Barense, Jason D. Warren,
Timothy J. Bussey, and Lisa M. Saksida

Introduction to the temporal lobes

The temporal lobes are essential for our memory and understanding of the world, including our knowledge about our very selves, and our ability to communicate effectively with other human beings. As a result, the consequences of damage to the temporal lobes—as can occur following insults including surgery, stroke, viral infection, or Alzheimer's disease—can be devastating (see Boxes 4.1 and 4.2 for some key historical examples). As we will see, however, the temporal lobe is not a unitary structure with a single function. How therefore can we understand how these different functions are organized within the temporal lobes? We start by considering the anatomy.

Temporal lobe circuitry

The temporal lobe is the region of cerebral cortex that lies inferior to the Sylvian (lateral) fissure (Fig. 4.2a). Posteriorly, the temporal lobe is bounded by the ventral edge of the parietal lobe and the anterior edge of the occipital lobe. The temporal lobes comprise approximately 20 per cent[5,6] of total cerebral cortex volume in humans. Regions on the lateral surface can be divided into those that represent auditory information (Brodmann areas 41, 42, 22) and those that represent visual information (Brodmann areas 20, 21, 37, 38) (Fig. 4.2b and c).

The first sulcus inferior to the Sylvian fissure is the superior temporal sulcus (STS), which contains multimodal cortex receiving inputs from visual, auditory, and somatic regions in addition

---

Box 4.1 Case study 1: Dense global amnesia

In 1953, a 27-year-old man, known to researchers by the initials HM, underwent experimental brain surgery—bilateral removal of his medial temporal lobes (MTL) (Fig. 4.1)—to treat his severe epilepsy. HM emerged from the surgery profoundly, and irrevocably, amnesic. Until his death in 2008, each new experience he had and each new person he met was destined to be forgotten, leaving his existence in an eternal present. In the words of HM himself, 'Every day is alone in itself, whatever enjoyment I've had and whatever sorrow I've had.'[1]

During neuropsychological examination he would look up between tests and anxiously say, 'Right now, I'm wondering. Have I done or said anything amiss? You see, at this moment everything looks clear to me, but what happened just before? That's what worries me. It's like waking from a dream; I just don't remember.'[2]

HM did not know that decades had elapsed since his surgery, he did not know his age, or whether he had grey hair.[3] He knew about the Second World War and the crash of the stock market in 1929, but he could not remember the scientists that worked with him continuously until his death. Mercifully, his personality and intellect were unchanged, and he was a gracious and patient man who generously devoted himself to a life as an object of intensive scientific study, making him likely the most important single case study in the history of brain science.

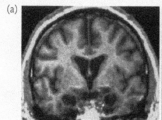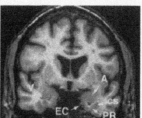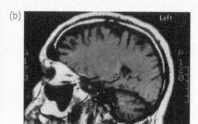

Fig. 4.1 HM's medial temporal lobe lesion. (a) Coronal image depicting the temporal lobe of HM (shown on left) and an age-matched control (shown on right). A = amygdala; H = hippocampus; cs = collateral sulcus; PR = perirhinal cortex; EC = entorhinal cortex. (b) Sagital section from the left side of HM's brain. The asterisk depicts the resected portion of the anterior temporal lobes. The arrow depicts the remaining intraventricular portion of the hippocampus.

Box 4.2 Case study 2: Wernicke's aphasia

In 1874, a young psychiatrist, Carl Wernicke, working in Breslau, recorded the clinical details of his patient, SA, a 59-year-old woman who had suddenly lost all ability to understand speech.[4] She gave 'completely absurd' answers to questions, and her conversation (though grammatical) was frequently garbled and marred by neologisms. She had difficulty naming familiar items, even though she remained able to use them competently.

After a more detailed assessment, Wernicke found that she had no other evidence of 'profound mental deterioration': he concluded instead that she had a selective impairment in comprehending speech signals, a 'sensory aphasia'. SA's language disturbance resolved steadily over the next few months, but her case prompted Wernicke to review the clinical records of his previous patients. These included one patient with a similar language syndrome who had come to post-mortem showing focal infarction of the first and second temporal convolutions within the left cerebral hemisphere.

Wernicke proposed that the culprit lesion in such cases, involving temporal lobe areas in proximity to auditory cortex, produces a fundamental defect of the 'sound images' for words. This insight led him to develop the first coherent model of a distributed, dominant hemisphere language circuit, linking speech perception ultimately with speech output. Wernicke's model provided a framework for understanding various selective disorders of language due to acute brain lesions or focal cerebral degenerations. Though first clearly described over a century ago, these disorders continue to inspire debate today.

to polymodal input from frontal and parietal regions. The middle and inferior temporal gyri (corresponding to Brodmann areas 20 and 21; also called area TE) comprise inferotemporal (IT) cortex, a region critical for visual object recognition. The medial temporal lobes (MTL) are a collection of heavily interconnected structures, which include allocortical structures such as the hippocampus and adjacent entorhinal, perirhinal, and parahippocampal cortex (Fig. 4.2d), and are traditionally believed to form a system devoted to long-term memory. At the tip of the temporal lobe is the temporal pole, a region critical for conceptual knowledge and social conceptual information processing.

However, brain regions do not operate in isolation but are interconnected in functional circuits comprising a number of cortical and allocortical regions. Of course, the connectivity between brain regions is rich and complex, and the temporal lobes are no exception in this regard. Nevertheless, when considering function it is useful to think in terms of three major pathways associated with this region (Fig. 4.3).

1. Cortical *modality-specific* sensory streams (devoted to only one sensory modality). Although the temporal lobes receive inputs from all modalities, for the present purposes we will focus on the visual and auditory pathways (Fig. 4.3a).

2. The continuation of these streams into cortical regions of the superior temporal sulcus (STS) and middle temporal gyrus (MTG) (Fig. 4.3b).

3. The continuation of these streams into the structures within the medial portion of the temporal lobes (MTL) (Fig. 4.3c).

Functions of the temporal lobes

Circuit 1. Cortical *modality-specific* sensory streams for vision and audition

The ventral visual stream (VVS)

As visual information leaves the striate cortex in the occipital lobes, it is organized into two functionally specialized hierarchical processing pathways. The 'dorsal stream' courses dorsally towards parietal regions and is crucial for processing the spatial locations of objects, as well for visually guiding actions towards objects in space.[7] The 'ventral visual stream' (VVS) extends ventrally through IT cortex towards anterior temporal regions and is crucial for the visual identification of objects (8) (Fig. 4.4a). These pathways have been dubbed the 'where/how' (dorsal) and 'what' (ventral) pathways. This section will focus on the ventral stream, the dorsal stream is discussed further in chapter 5.

The organization of the ventral stream is hierarchical, such that low-level inputs are transformed into more complex representations through successive stages of processing. As information progresses through the stream, receptive field size and neuronal response latencies increase, and the neurons increase the complexity of their tuning, with neurons in posterior regions of the stream firing in response to relatively simple stimuli and anterior regions of the stream firing to more complex and specific stimuli. For example, whereas neurons in V1 and V2 fire in response to simpler stimulus properties such as colour, orientation, and spatial frequency (Fig. 4.4b), cells in IT cortex respond to much more complex stimuli.[9] Indeed, cells in IT cortex are usually selective for a very specific stimulus, such as a hand (Fig. 4.4c).[10,11] Moreover, this selectivity is usually invariant over changes in stimulus size, orientation, contrast, and colour, that is, neural responses are not altered by changes in these parameters. Not surprisingly, lesions to this area of the brain lead to severe deficits in identifying and naming different categories of objects, a condition known as visual agnosia.

Evidence from neuroimaging indicates that distinct areas within the ventral temporal cortex may be specialized for specific categories of stimuli. The fusiform face area (FFA) responds more strongly to faces than to other non-face objects,[12] whereas the parahippocampal place area (PPA) responds more to images of buildings and scenes than to faces and other objects.[13] Other category-specific regions have been identified for inanimate objects, body parts, and letter strings,[14–16] There is currently a debate regarding whether these regions should be treated as modules for the representation of specific categories[17] or whether they should be considered as parts of a more general object-recognition system critical for recognizing fine-grained distinctions among well-known objects.[18,19]

In the context of memory systems, the structures of the VVS have been considered to comprise a 'perceptual representation system' which mediates perceptual priming, discrimination, and categorization of stimuli.[20] This so-called *non-declarative memory* system is contrasted with a declarative memory system for facts and events, thought to reside in the temporal lobe proper. These putative memory systems will be discussed in more detail below.

The cortical auditory stream

The organization of the human cortical auditory system is less well understood than the cortical visual system and much information has been obtained from animal models, in particular the macaque

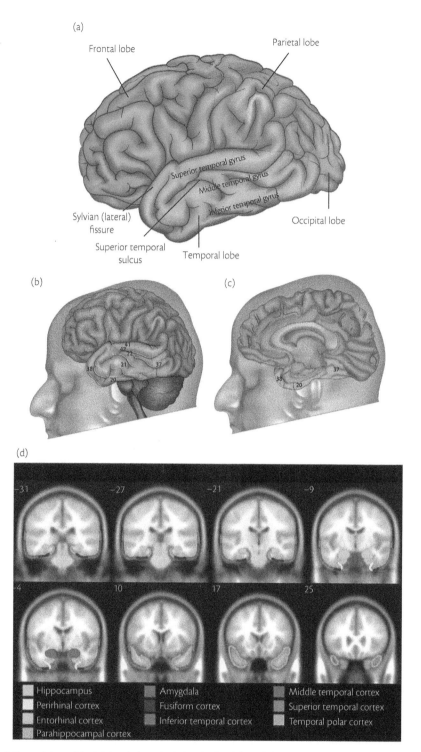

Fig. 4.2 Temporal lobe anatomy. (a) Lateral view of the left hemisphere depicting the four lobes of the cerebral cortex and major gyri and sulci. (b) Lateral view of the left hemisphere showing Brodmann's areas in the temporal lobes. (c) Medial view of the right hemisphere showing Brodmann's areas in the temporal lobes. (d) Coronal sections depicting different temporal lobe regions, superimposed on a Montreal Neurological Institute average brain template.

monkey.[21] However, certain basic principles of auditory cortical anatomical and functional organization have been identified. As is the case for visual information, cortical analysis of auditory information is distributed among multiple cortical areas, hierarchically organized into overlapping but separable processing streams (Fig. 4.5).

Primary auditory cortex is located in the medial portion of each Heschl's gyrus and can be identified from histoanatomical features and to some extent by functional properties such as tonotopic coding of pitch information. Higher-order areas relatively specialized for auditory processing are located in the surrounding superior

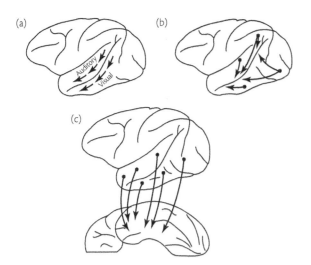

Fig. 4.3 Major functional circuits in the temporal lobes of the rhesus monkey. (a) Modality-specific streams devoted to either audition or vision progress from primary sensory regions towards the temporal pole. (b) Modality-specific auditory, visual, and somatic information inputs to multimodal regions of the superior temporal sulcus. (c) Auditory and visual information inputs to the medial temporal lobe.

Reproduced from Kolb B and Whishaw IQ, *Fundamentals of Human Neuropsychology*, 7th edn, Copyright (2015), with permission from Macmillan Higher Education.

temporal gyrus (STG), extending anteriorly to the temporal pole and posteriorly into planum temporale, posterior STG, and the temporoparietal junction (TPJ). Candidate homologues of these areas in the macaque and other species can be differentiated on anatomical and electrophysiological grounds; however, information about human auditory cortical subregions remains limited.

Analogous with the 'what/where' cortical processing streams in the visual system, auditory cortical organization appears to be broadly dichotomous, comprising a ventral stream directed along anterior STG, and a dorsal stream directed into the TPJ and projecting to parietal and frontal cortical areas. The ventral stream is concerned chiefly with representing information about auditory object identity whereas the dorsal stream is concerned with representing sound location and movement.[21,22]

Successive stages within these processing hierarchies are associated with increasing integration and abstraction of auditory information and the streams communicate widely with higher-order multimodal cortical areas in STS, MTG, and parietal lobe. Again analogous with the visual cortical system, fundamental tasks of cortical auditory processing include the representation of invariant object features and the association of these representations with meaning based on prior experience of the sensory world.

In the case of the most widely studied auditory signal, speech, it has been shown that acoustic properties of speech sounds as discrete auditory objects are encoded in more posterior areas in posterior and mid STG, whereas speech intelligibility—the meaning associated with the sounds—is extracted in more anterior areas in STG in the dominant cerebral hemisphere,[21] ultimately linking spoken language with other modalities of semantic knowledge. Similar organizational principles are likely to govern the processing of non-verbal environmental sounds.

In contrast, preparation to produce speech and other vocal sounds via the dorsal auditory pathway is initiated by mechanisms in the vicinity of planum temporale and posterior STG: a putative 'sensori-motor

interface' that lies within the compass of 'Wernicke's area' in classical aphasiology.[21,22] Specific agnosias for pre- or non-linguistic auditory phenomena are uncommon but well-documented: examples include so-called pure word deafness and agnosias for different aspects of music. Specific syndromes of this kind suggest underlying neural mechanisms that are functionally dissociable.[23]

Analogies between the visual and auditory cortical systems should not be overemphasized. The visual and auditory modalities present the brain with specific computational problems (in the auditory modality, for example, the problem of resolving multiple 'transparent' sound sources overlaid in the auditory environment and the requirement to integrate information dynamically over time); these problems are likely to be solved by modality-specific neural mechanisms. The peripheral visual and auditory processing pathways are organized along different lines: processing of information over subcortical relays is more extensive for auditory than for visual stimuli, and in addition, whereas visual information is relayed to the contralateral cerebral hemisphere, auditory information is distributed to both hemispheres.

The status of auditory spatial processing in the dorsal processing stream is less straightforward than the status of visuospatial processing in the dorsal visual stream:[21,22] there is extensive interaction between the dorsal and ventral auditory streams when processing sound identity and location, and it has been suggested that the dorsal auditory stream is not primarily a 'where' pathway but, rather, a 'how' pathway (processing dynamic changes in the auditory environment) or a 'do' pathway (programming motor responses based on relevant sound information).

Furthermore, the human cortical auditory system shows a unique specialization in the processing of speech sounds, and this may be partly based on distinctive neural mechanisms that are differentiated between the cerebral hemispheres. In particular, it has been suggested that the left hemisphere may preferentially process auditory signals that (like speech) contain frequent, rapid spectro-temporal transitions whereas the right hemisphere may preferentially process slower spectro-temporal variations or information unfolding over longer timescales (e.g. in musical melodies). However, any such dichotomy is likely to be an oversimplification.[24]

Circuit 2. Superior temporal sulcus, middle temporal gyrus, and afferent connections

A key principle of temporal lobe function is the *integration* of information from different sensory modalities and across processing stages to create unified representations of the world. Cortical areas in STS and MTG have extensive reciprocal anatomical communications with *modality-specific* (e.g. purely visual or purely auditory) superior, inferior, and posterior temporal cortices. Functionally, these regions have been implicated in the processing of visual, auditory, and somatic information and in the *cross-modal integration* of sensory information when resolving inter-modal incongruities or building coherent multimodal perceptual and semantic representations.[25–27]

Cognitive processing stages such as 'perceptual' and 'semantic' have been distinguished neuroanatomically as well as neuropsychologically.[27] However, the anatomical organization of temporal lobe circuitry suggests that modality-specific and multimodal cortical areas cooperate with mutual information exchange during the perceptual and semantic analysis of sensory objects. The existence of such cooperation has been supported by functional imaging

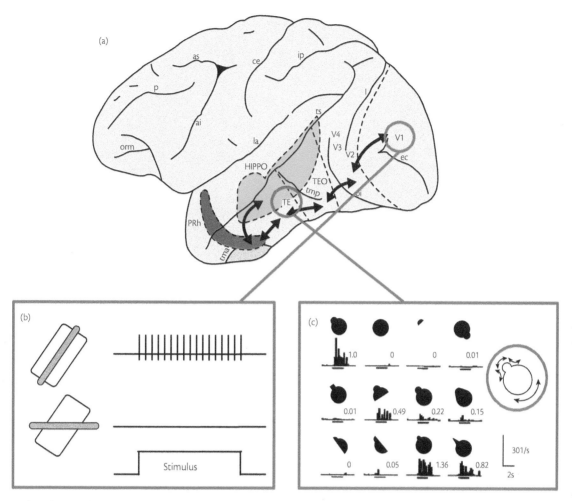

Fig. 4.4 The ventral visual stream. (a) The ventral visual stream is a processing pathway critical for the perceptual analysis of objects. It originates in primary visual cortex (V1) and progresses along the ventral surface of the temporal lobe towards anterior temporal regions. Information processing in this stream is organized hierarchically, such that early regions process version simple information and more anterior regions process more complex information. (b) For example, here we illustrate a V1 neuron that is tuned to a bar of light oriented in a particular direction and fires maximally (vertical lines correspond to action potentials) when a bar of light in its preferred orientation hits the cell's receptive field but not at all when the bar is dissimilar to its preferred orientation. (c) By contrast, anterior VVS regions are tuned to more complex features. Here we demonstrated a TE neuron that fires maximally (firing rates illustrated on the bar graph) to the shape circled in red. The preferences of these cells are remarkably selective and show weaker response rates as the image deviates from the preferred shape. Cells in TE are thought to respond to 'moderately complex' features.

(a) Adapted from *Philos Trans R Soc Lond B Biol Sci.*, 298(1089), Mishkin M, A Memory System in the Monkey, pp. 83–95, Copyright (1982), with permission from The Royal Society, Figure courtesy of Mort Mishkin. (b) Reproduced from Dowling, John E, *Neurons and Networks. An Introduction to Neuroscience*, Copyright (1992), with permission from Harvard University Press. (c) Reproduced from *Annu Rev Neurosci.*, 19, Tanaka K., Inferotemporal Cortex and Object Vision, pp. 109–39, Copyright (1996), with permission from Annual Reviews.

evidence in both healthy subjects and in defined clinical populations such as patients with semantic dementia.[28,29]

Indeed, one view is that the temporal poles—structures heavily damaged in semantic dementia—comprise an amodal semantic 'hub' that mediates communication across various sensory, motor, linguistic, and affective domains.[30] Damage to this temporal pole hub results in a dissolution of semantic knowledge across all conceptual domains and all modalities of testing.[31] This hub is thought to become especially critical when the semantic system must extract conceptual similarity structure that is not directly reflected in any single modality (e.g. sensory, motor, linguistic, affective).

For example, items that are very similar in kind may vary enormously in terms of their surface details: a penguin and a hummingbird are very different in terms of how they look and how they move, but they are classed as similar kinds of things.[32] In contrast,

light bulbs and pears share many surface similarities but are classed as very different kinds of objects. Thus, critical to any semantic system is the capacity to represent conceptual similarity structure that is not reflected in any single surface modality (e.g. shape or movement), and this cross-modal associative conceptual knowledge may be subserved by the temporal pole.

There are many instances where integration of cross-modal information is required to make sense of the environment. One key example is the representation of attributes of particular people, which generally entails conjoint processing of face and voice identity.[33] Functional imaging studies have shown that such processing engages multimodal cortical areas in STS and MTG as well as modality-specific visual and auditory areas. In addition to involvement of higher-order multimodal areas, there are likely to be direct connections between modality-specific auditory and visual areas,[34] underlining the potential for cross-modal interactions at multiple

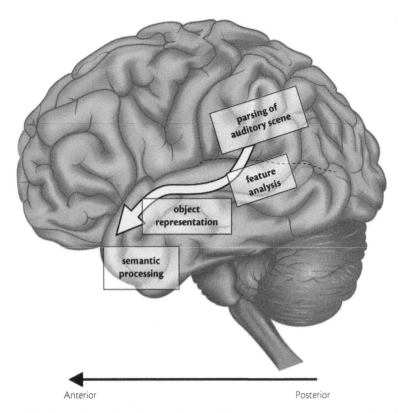

Anterior

Posterior

Fig. 4.5 Cortical auditory stream. A simplified schematic showing key processing stages in the putative ventral cortical stream for auditory object processing in the human brain. The auditory scene is initially parsed into constituent sound sources by non-primary cortex in the planum temporale and posterior superior temporal lobe, and adjacent cortical areas in and surrounding the superior temporal sulcus analyse the features of these sources and build auditory object representations. These auditory object representations become associated with meaning as a result of higher order semantic processing in the anterior temporal lobe and beyond.

levels of the processing hierarchy. Such interactions might be particularly relevant for resolving identity under ambiguous listening or viewing conditions. Analogous cross-modal interactions are likely to facilitate speech recognition from observation of lip movements and other non-auditory cues.[35]

Circuit 3. The medial temporal lobe and its afferent connections

Case study 1 (Box 4.1) introduces the famous patient, HM, who suffered profound amnesia following damage to the temporal lobes. One of the most remarkable features of HM's disorder (and that of other cases like him) was its seeming selectivity to the learning of new facts and events.[36] Patients with MTL resections showed severe anterograde amnesia, together with some retrograde amnesia for at least the immediate pre-operative period, but they manifested no other obvious changes in perceptual abilities, intellect, or personality.

Furthermore, all patients were able to remember relatively small amounts of information perfectly for seconds or minutes, so long as they were not interrupted. The instant their attention was diverted to a new topic, however, the material was lost. For example, one report[37] describes an occasion on which HM was asked to remember the number '584' and was then allowed to sit quietly with no interruption for several minutes. At the end of this interval he was able to recall the number correctly without any hesitation, stating, 'It's easy. You just remember 8. You see, 5, 8, 4, add to 17. You remember 8; subtract it from 17 and it leaves 9. Divide 9 in half and you get 5 and 4, and there you are: 584. Easy.'

Despite this elaborate mnemonic device, as soon as HM's attention was diverted to another topic, he was unable to remember, approximately one minute later, either the number '584' or the fact that he had been given a number to remember in the first place. This suggested that the structures in the MTL were critical to consolidate new long-term memories, but were not important for the rehearsal and maintenance of information over short time periods (a cognitive ability termed working memory).

Working memory was not the only form of memory that appeared to be spared in amnesic subjects. Numerous studies demonstrated that amnesia spared knowledge that was based on rules or procedures, but dramatically affected declarative memory—knowledge that was available as conscious recollections about facts (semantic memory) and events (episodic memory) (see, for example, references 3 and 38). For example, MTL amnesics could acquire selected motor skills (e.g. mirror drawing) over a period of days, despite having no recollection of having carried out the task. Subsequent studies expanded the collection of preserved abilities in amnesia to include memory for skills and habits, simple forms of conditioning, which eventually fell under the umbrella term of non-declarative memory and refer to a collection of abilities that are unconscious and expressed through performance rather than conscious recollection.

These findings led to the idea of an MTL declarative memory system containing several anatomically distinct structures, namely those damaged in HM: the hippocampus, together with the adjacent, anatomically related entorhinal, perirhinal, and parahippocampal cortices (see references 36 and 39). According to this

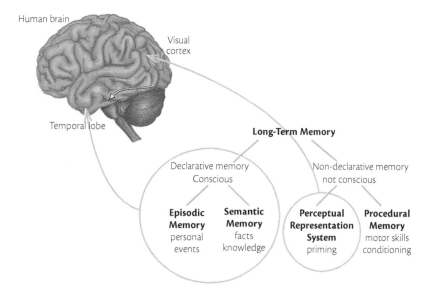

Fig. 4.6 Traditional taxonomy of memory systems. Declarative (implicit) memory refers to conscious memory for facts (semantic memory) and events (episodic memory), whereas non-declarative (implicit) memory refers to a collection of abilities that operate outside of conscious awareness.[39] The prevailing view in cognitive neuroscience is that the brain can be best understood as consisting of modules specialized for distinct cognitive functions. In this example, two different expression of long-term memory—conscious declarative memory and unconscious non-declarative memory—are presumed to have different neuroanatomical loci. Declarative memory is traditionally believed to be dependent on the medial temporal lobes, whereas priming (a form of non-declarative memory) is thought to be dependent on a perceptual representation system in more posterior neocortex.

view, the regions in the MTL work in concert, as a highly integrated system, to *bind* together the distributed elements of memory that are processed and represented by distinct cortical sites. This system is proposed to work in the service of declarative memory only, with no role in other cognitive functions, such as perception or working memory (Fig. 4.6). According to this account, injury to any component of the MTL memory system will result in a deficit on any type of declarative memory, and only declarative memory. According to this view, the process of consolidating the distributed elements of memory into a coherent and stable ensemble can take years, but eventually, memories are thought to become independent of the MTL memory system (reference 40, although see too reference 41).

Thus with respect to the pathway currently under discussion—the MTL and its afferents—the view had emerged of a *discontinuous* pathway containing two qualitatively different 'modules': the declarative memory system in the MTL, and the perceptual representation system in the VVS, which mediates the putatively non-declarative functions of visual priming, categorization, and perceptual discrimination. This modular view has recently come into question, as will be discussed below.

More recent ideas regarding the functional organization of the VVS–MTL stream

Despite the popularity of the putative MTL memory system, there were several findings that contradicted this view. These findings support two different but related ideas:

1. The heterogeneity of function within the putative MTL system, and
2. The VVS–MTL pathway as a continuous, rather than discontinuous, system.

Functional heterogeneity within the MTL

Beginning in the 1960s, researchers sought to understand the functions of the separate structures *within* the MTL. Many of these studies focused on *recognition memory*, indicated by the ability to judge whether an item has been seen previously. Despite the fact that recognition memory is considered a canonical example of declarative memory, damage to the hippocampus appears to be neither necessary nor sufficient to produce recognition memory deficits.[42–44] However, lesions that damaged one MTL cortical structure, the perirhinal cortex, consistently impaired recognition memory.[45–49] In addition, with the advent of more detailed anatomical techniques, investigations into the mnemonic contribution of the hippocampus alone—unconfounded by concomitant perirhinal damage—became possible. Using a precise excitotoxic lesion technique, it was shown that lesions to the hippocampus (without damage to underlying cortical regions) produced no recognition memory impairment.[50]

A subsequent meta-analysis of three studies in monkeys with hippocampal lesions demonstrated that whereas greater rhinal cortex damage was associated with worse performance on a recognition memory task, greater hippocampal damage was associated with *better* performance on the same task.[51] Further work indicated that the hippocampus and perirhinal cortex could be doubly dissociated.[52] These different structures, therefore, must contribute to memory in very different ways. Some of the most prominent ideas regarding division of labour between the hippocampus and other MTL structures are discussed below.

In a seminal review, Aggleton and Brown[53] addressed the neural substrates of two distinct memory processes, *recollection* (the 'remembering' of an event, associated with the retrieval of contextual details) and *familiarity* (the feeling of 'knowing' that an item has been experienced, in the absence of other associated details).[54,55] They proposed that the hippocampus, together with the fornix, mamillary bodies, and anterior thalamic nuclei, form a system that supports recollection, whereas familiarity reflects an independent process that depends on a distinct system involving the perirhinal cortex and the medial dorsal nucleus of the thalamus.

A closely related model, the Convergence, Recollection, and Familiarity Theory (CRAFT),[56] also contrasts hippocampal and cortical function. Under this view, recollection is thought to be supported by the hippocampus through *pattern separation*, a mechanism by which similar memories are differentiated into distinct, non-overlapping representations,[57] This computation is considered to be qualitatively different from the object/item familiarity and contextual familiarity computations supported by cortical MTL structures such as the perirhinal and parahippocampal cortices.

In a similar vein, the complementary learning system (CLS) is a network model that also makes important distinctions between hippocampal and MTL cortical contributions to memory.[58] Under this framework, the MTL neocortex has a slow learning rate and uses overlapping distributed representations to extract the shared structure of events (e.g. generalities based on accumulated experience, such as the best strategy for parking a car). Thus, because it does not sufficiently differentiate the representations of different information, this cortex is unable to support recall of information that has only been encountered on one or two occasions. In contrast, the hippocampus learns rapidly, using pattern separated representations to encode the details of specific events while minimising interference (e.g. the memory for where the car is parked today is kept separate from the representation of where the car was parked yesterday).

Other prominent views of MTL function argue that the engagement of different MTL structures is best characterized by the *type* of information being processed (e.g. items, contexts, or the associations between items and their contexts), rather than the processes themselves. One theory posits that the hippocampus has a critical role in *binding* together arbitrarily-related associations (termed *relational memory*), whereas MTL cortical structures maintain representations for individual items.[59,60]

This theory has subsequently been developed into a three-component model, termed the 'binding of item and context' (BIC) model.[61,62] Rather than proposing a simple mapping between different MTL structures and familiarity and recollection, this view posits that MTL subregions differ in terms of the information they process and represent. More specifically, the perirhinal cortex is thought to represent information about specific items (e.g. who and what), the parahippocampal cortex is thought to represent information about the context of these items (e.g. where and when), and the hippocampus represents the *associations* between these items and contexts. Thus, each region has a functionally distinct role, but collectively, MTL regions support memory by binding item and context information.

In summary, the wealth of recent evidence suggests that, in contrast to the idea of a unitary memory system, different MTL structures make functionally dissociable contributions to memory and as such, differing patterns of MTL damage will lead to distinct profiles of memory impairment.

The VVS–MTL pathway as a continuous, rather than discontinuous, system

A second assumption of the historical view of the VVS–MTL pathway has also recently been questioned, namely the assumption that this system is best thought of as discontinuous, containing two qualitatively different modules, the MTL memory system and the VVS perceptual representation system. However, beginning in the mid-1990s, experimental data began to suggest that structures within the MTL contribute not just to declarative memory but are also important for perceptual and other functions such as perceptual discrimination (e.g. being able to identify whether there are differences between visually similar objects).[48,63]

To account for these data, it was proposed that structures within the MTL such as perirhinal cortex may be best understood as an extension of the representational hierarchy within the VVS (Fig. 4.7).[64,65] In other words, rather than characterizing the function of MTL structures in terms of psychological labels like 'memory' and 'perception', it may be better to consider them in terms of the representations that they contain and the computations that they perform.[66] Under this view, MTL structures are thought to contain the rich neural representations of objects and scenes that are necessary for *both* memory and perception. Thus, damage to these representations causes deficits on both mnemonic and perceptual tasks.

This notion was encapsulated in a computational/theoretical framework[64,67] referred to as the 'representational-hierarchical' view.[68] In accord with the prevailing view in the VVS literature,[9,69] posterior regions in the VVS are assumed to represent simple features, whereas more anterior regions in the VVS and MTL are

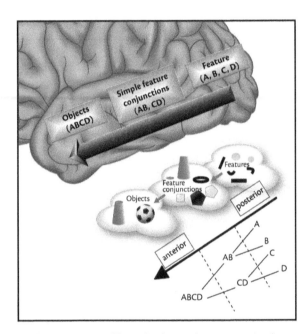

Fig. 4.7 The representational-hierarchical view. The representational-hierarchical view suggests that a given brain region could be useful for multiple cognitive functions, rather than being specialized exclusively for functions such as memory or perception.[64,65,84] Representations of visual stimulus features are organized hierarchically throughout the ventral visual stream, such that simple features are represented in more posterior regions and conjunctions of these features are represented in more anterior regions.[9,69] The representational-hierarchical view proposes that highly complex conjunctions of these features— at approximately the level of an everyday object—are represented in the perirhinal cortex. These object-level representations are important for both memory and perception, and thus, damage to the perirhinal cortex will impair both these cognitive functions.

assumed to represent more complex conjunctions of these features. According to the representational-hierarchical view (Fig. 4.7), because damage to the perirhinal cortex destroys or compromises highly complex visual representations, one must rely on the representations of simple features housed in more posterior regions of VVS to solve cognitive tasks. Thus, impairments in perception (as well as memory) are caused by perirhinal cortex damage because such damage leads to impoverished representations of complex stimuli, and the remaining representations of simple features are inadequate for making certain types of discrimination between visual objects.

To test the model, a 'lesion' was made by removing the layer of the computational network corresponding to perirhinal cortex, and the effects of this lesion were compared with previously reported effects of lesions in perirhinal cortex in monkeys.[64] The model was able to simulate the effects of lesions of perirhinal cortex on visual discrimination behaviour in a range of different experimental contexts (see, for example, references 70 and 71). Central to the model is the notion of 'feature ambiguity'. An ambiguous feature—for example, one that is rewarded as part of one stimulus but not as part of another stimulus—will not contribute towards the solution of a task such as a visual discrimination. In order to solve a problem that contains ambiguous features, more complex conjunctions of features (such as those represented in perirhinal cortex), which are much less likely to be ambiguous, are required.

Subsequent work therefore manipulated feature ambiguity explicitly to test this prediction of the model. A number of studies provided support for the prediction that perirhinal cortex is required for any visual discrimination task that necessitates resolution of feature ambiguity at the object level in monkeys[63,70–72] and humans,[73–78] although there have been some conflicting reports.[79–82] More recently, this work has been extended to show that impoverished visual representations following MTL damage cause deficits not only in complex discrimination tasks. For example, McTighe and colleagues[83] showed that the classical deficit in object recognition memory seen in animals with perirhinal cortex damage may be accounted for by *interference* due to feature ambiguity, and removing such interference can completely rescue memory. Similar findings have recently been reported in humans: individuals with memory disorders (from either focal damage to the MTL that included perirhinal cortex, and individuals with mild cognitive impairment) were also vulnerable to object-based interference, and when this interference was controlled, their performance was recovered to normal levels.[84-86]

A similar argument would apply to other regions in the MTL such as the hippocampus, albeit in the context of more complex stimulus representations such as spatial scenes.[66,68,87] Initial evidence supports this view: individuals with hippocampal damage were impaired on tasks requiring the rich representation of information, irrespective of timescales. For example, hippocampal amnesics were impaired on working memory tasks requiring maintenance of scenes,[88,89] topographical maps,[90] and objects in spatial arrays.[91,92] Even more strikingly, damage to the hippocampus also impaired performance on tasks that simultaneously presented all information necessary to make a correct response.[75,76,93,94]

What all these tasks had in common was the requirement to form a representation of the relationships between complex stimuli—either in terms of comparisons across complex objects,[93,94] or in terms of the relationships of the objects that comprise a scene.[75,76] These findings challenge the longstanding assumption that the hippocampus is uniquely involved in long-term memory, and suggest instead that this structure—along with the rest of the MTL—should best be understood in terms of the information it represents, rather than in terms of cognitive modules or circumscribed processes.

References

1. Milner B, Corkin S, and Teuber HL. Further analysis of the hippocampal amnesic syndrome: 14-year follow-up of HM. *Neuropsychologia.* 1968;6:215–34.

2. Milner B. Amnesia following operation on the temporal lobes. In: CWM Whitty and OL Zangwill (eds). *Amnesia.* London: Butterworths, 1966, pp. 109–33.

3. Corkin S. What's new with the amnesic patient H.M.? *Nat Rev Neurosci.* 2002 Feb;3(2):153–60.

4. Wernicke C. Der aphasische Symptomenkomplex: Eine psychologische Studie auf anatomischer Basis. In: Breslau, Cohn, Weigert (eds). *Wernicke's Works on Aphasia: A Sourcebook and Review.* The Hague: Mouton, 1874.

5. Kiernan JA. Anatomy of the temporal lobe. *Epilepsy Res Treat.* 2012. <http://dx.doi.org/10.1155/2012/176157>.

6. Kennedy DN, Lange N, Makris N, *et al.* Gyri of the human neocortex: An MRI-based analysis of volume and variance. *Cereb Cortex.* 1998 Jun;8(4):372–84.

7. Goodale MA. Transforming vision into action. *Vision Res.* 2011 Jul 1;51(13):1567–87.

8. Ungerleider L and Mishkin M. Two cortical visual streams. In: D Ingle, M Goodale, and R Mansfield (eds). *Analysis of Behavior.* Cambridge, MA: MIT Press, 1983, pp. 549–86.

9. Desimone R and Ungerleider LG. Neural mechanisms of visual processing in monkeys. In: F Boller and J Grafman (eds). *Handbook of Neuropsychology.* New York, NY: Elsevier Science, 1989, pp. 267–99.

10. Gross CG. Single neuron studies of inferior temporal cortex. *Neuropsychologia.* 2008 Feb 12;46(3):841–52.

11. Tanaka K. Inferotemporal cortex and object vision. *Annu Rev Neurosci.* 1996;19:109–39.

12. Kanwisher N, McDermott J, and Chun MM. The fusiform face area: A module in human extrastriate cortex specialized for face perception. *J Neurosci.* 1997 Jun 1;17(11):4302–11.

13. Epstein R and Kanwisher N. A cortical representation of the local visual environment. *Nature.* 1998 Apr 9;392(6676):598–601.

14. Kourtzi Z and Kanwisher N. Cortical regions involved in perceiving object shape. *J Neurosci.* 2000 May 1;20(9):3310–18.

15. Downing PE, Jiang Y, Shuman M, *et al.* A cortical area selective for visual processing of the human body. *Science.* 2001 Sep 28;293(5539):2470–3.

16. McCandliss BD, Cohen L, and Dehaene S. The visual word form area: expertise for reading in the fusiform gyrus. *Trends Cogn Sci.* 2003 Jul;7(7):293–9.

17. Kanwisher N. Functional specificity in the human brain: a window into the functional architecture of the mind. *Proc Natl Acad Sci USA.* 2010 Jun 22;107(25):11163–70.

18. McGugin RW, Gatenby JC, Gore JC, *et al.* High-resolution imaging of expertise reveals reliable object selectivity in the fusiform face area related to perceptual performance. *Proc Natl Acad Sci USA.* 2012 Oct 16;109(42):17063–8.

19. Gauthier I, Tarr M, and Bub D (eds). *Perceptual Expertise: Bridging Brain and Behavior.* Oxford: Oxford University Press, 1990.

20. Tulving E and Schacter DL. Priming and human memory systems. *Science.* 1990 Jan 19;247(4940):301–6.

21. Rauschecker JP and Scott SK. Maps and streams in the auditory cortex: nonhuman primates illuminate human speech processing. *Nat Neurosci.* 2009 Jun;12(6):718–24.

22. Warren JE, Wise RJ, and Warren JD. Sounds do-able: auditory-motor transformations and the posterior temporal plane. *Trends Neurosci.* 2005 Dec;28(12):636–43.

23. Goll JC, Crutch SJ, and Warren JD. Central auditory disorders: toward a neuropsychology of auditory objects. *Curr Opin Neurol.* 2010 Dec;23(6):617–27.

24. McGettigan C and Scott SK. Cortical asymmetries in speech perception: what's wrong, what's right and what's left? *Trends Cogn Sci.* 2012 May;16(5):269–76.

25. Noppeney U, Josephs O, Hocking J, *et al.* The effect of prior visual information on recognition of speech and sounds. *Cereb Cortex.* 2008 Mar;18(3):598–609.

26. Naumer MJ, Doehrmann O, Muller NG, *et al.* Cortical plasticity of audio-visual object representations. *Cereb Cortex.* 2009 Jul;19(7):1641–53.

27. Binder JR, Desai RH, Graves WW, *et al.* Where is the semantic system? A critical review and meta-analysis of 120 functional neuroimaging studies. *Cereb Cortex.* 2009 Dec;19(12):2767–96.

28. Martin A and Chao LL. Semantic memory and the brain: Structure and processes. *Curr Opin Neurobiol.* 2001 Apr;11(2):194–201.

29. Goll JC, Ridgway GR, Crutch SJ, *et al.* Nonverbal sound processing in semantic dementia: a functional MRI study. *Neuroimage.* 2012 May 15;61(1):170–80.

30. Patterson K, Nestor PJ, and Rogers TT. Where do you know what you know? The representation of semantic knowledge in the human brain. *Nat Rev Neurosci.* 2007 Dec;8(12):976–87.

31. Hodges JR, Patterson K, Ward R, *et al.* The differentiation of semantic dementia and frontal lobe dementia (temporal and frontal variants of frontotemporal dementia) from early Alzheimer's disease: a comparative neuropsychological study. *Neuropsychology.* 1999 Jan;13(1):31–40.

32. Rogers TT and Cox CR. The neural bases of conceptual knowledge: Revisiting a Golden Age hypothesis in the era of cognitive neuroscience. In: A Duarte, MD Barense, and DR Addis (eds). *The Cognitive Neuroscience of Memory.* Oxford: Wiley, 2015.

33. Campanella S and Belin P. Integrating face and voice in person perception. *Trends Cogn Sci.* 2007 Dec;11(12):535–43.

34. Blank H, Anwander A, and von Kriegstein K. Direct structural connections between voice- and face-recognition areas. *J Neurosci.* 2011 Sep 7;31(36):12906–15.

35. McGettigan C, Faulkner A, Altarelli I, *et al.* Speech comprehension aided by multiple modalities: Behavioural and neural interactions. *Neuropsychologia.* 2012 Apr;50(5):762–76.

36. Squire LR and Wixted JT. The cognitive neuroscience of human memory since H.M. *Annu Rev Neurosci.* 2011 Jul 21;34:259–88.

37. Milner B. The memory defect in bilateral hippocampal lesions. *Psychiatr Res Rep Am Psychiatr Assoc.* 1959 Dec;11:43–58.

38. Cohen NJ and Squire LR. Preserved learning and retention of pattern-analyzing skill in amnesia: dissociation of knowing how and knowing that. *Science.* 1980 Oct 10;210(4466):207–10.

39. Squire LR and Zola-Morgan S. The medial temporal lobe memory system. *Science.* 1991 Sep 20;253(5026):1380–6.

40. Squire LR and Bayley PJ. The neuroscience of remote memory. *Curr Opin Neurobiol.* 2007 Apr;17(2):185–96.

41. Moscovitch M, Rosenbaum RS, Gilboa A, *et al.* Functional neuroanatomy of remote episodic, semantic and spatial memory: a unified account based on multiple trace theory. *J Anat.* 2005 Jul;207(1):35–66.

42. Mishkin M. Memory in monkeys severely impaired by combined but not by separate removal of amygdala and hippocampus. *Nature.* 1978;273(5660):297–8.

43. Murray EA and Mishkin M. Severe tactual as well as visual memory deficits follow combined removal of the amygdala and hippocampus in monkeys. *J Neurosci.* 1984 Oct;4(10):2565–80.

44. Mayes AR, Holdstock JS, Isaac CL, *et al.* Relative sparing of item recognition memory in a patient with adult-onset damage limited to the hippocampus. *Hippocampus.* 2002;12(3):325–40.

45. Meunier M, Bachevalier J, Mishkin M, *et al.* Effects on visual recognition of combined and separate ablations of the entorhinal and perirhinal cortex in rhesus monkeys. *J Neurosci.* 1993 December;13(12):5418–32.

46. Suzuki WA, Zola-Morgan S, Squire LR, *et al.* Lesions of the perirhinal and parahippocampal cortices in the monkey produce long-lasting memory impairment in the visual and tactual modalities. *J Neurosci.* 1993 June;13(6):2430–51.

47. Zola-Morgan S, Squire LR, Clower RP, *et al.* Damage to the perirhinal cortex exacerbates memory impairment following lesions to the hippocampal formation. *J Neurosci.* 1993 January;13(1):251–65.

48. Eacott MJ, Gaffan D, and Murray EA. Preserved recognition memory for small sets, and impaired stimulus identification for large sets, following rhinal cortex ablations in monkeys. *Eur J Neurosci.* 1994 Sep 1;6(9):1466–78.

49. Bowles B, Crupi C, Mirsattari SM, *et al.* Impaired familiarity with preserved recollection after anterior temporal-lobe resection that spares the hippocampus. *Proc Natl Acad Sci USA.* 2007 Oct 9;104(41):16382–7.

50. Murray EA and Mishkin M. Object recognition and location memory in monkeys with excitotoxic lesions of the amygdala and hippocampus. *J Neurosci.* 1998;18(16):6568–82.

51. Baxter MG and Murray EA. Opposite relationship of hippocampal and rhinal cortex damage to delayed nonmatching-to-sample deficits in monkeys. *Hippocampus.* 2001;11(1):61–71.

52. Winters BD, Forwood SE, Cowell RA, *et al.* Double dissociation between the effects of peri-postrhinal cortex and hippocampal lesions on tests of object recognition and spatial memory: heterogeneity of function within the temporal lobe. *J Neurosci.* 2004 Jun 30;24(26):5901–8.

53. Aggleton JP and Brown MW. Episodic memory, amnesia, and the hippocampal-anterior thalamic axis. *Behav Brain Sci.* 1999 Jun;22(3):425–44; discussion 44–89.

54. Mandler G. Recognizing: The judgement of previous occurrence. *Psychol Rev.* 1980;87:252–71.

55. Jacoby LL. A process dissociation framework: separating automatic from intentional uses of memory. *J Memory Lang.* 1991;30:513–41.

56. Montaldi D and Mayes AR. The role of recollection and familiarity in the functional differentiation of the medial temporal lobes. *Hippocampus.* 2010 Nov;20(11):1291–314.

57. Norman KA and O'Reilly RC. Modeling hippocampal and neocortical contributions to recognition memory: A complementary-learning-systems approach. *Psychol Rev.* 2003 Oct;110(4):611–46.

58. Norman KA. How hippocampus and cortex contribute to recognition memory: Revisiting the complementary learning systems model. *Hippocampus.* 2010 Nov;20(11):1217–27.

59. Eichenbaum H and Cohen NJ. *From Conditioning to Conscious Recollection: Memory Systems of the Brain.* New York, NY: Oxford University Press, 2001.

60. Eichenbaum H, Otto T, and Cohen NJ. Two functional components of the hippocampal memory system. *Behav Brain Sci.* 1994;17:449–518.

61. Diana RA, Yonelinas AP, and Ranganath C. Imaging recollection and familiarity in the medial temporal lobe: a three-component model. *Trends Cogn Sci.* 2007 Sep;11(9):379–86.

62. Eichenbaum H, Yonelinas AP, and Ranganath C. The medial temporal lobe and recognition memory. *Annu Rev Neurosci.* 2007;30:123–52.

63. Buckley MJ and Gaffan D. Perirhinal cortex ablation impairs visual object identification. *J Neurosci.* 1998 Mar 15;18(6):2268–75.

64. Bussey TJ and Saksida LM. The organization of visual object representations: A connectionist model of effects of lesions in perirhinal cortex. *Eur J Neurosci.* 2002 Jan;15(2):355–64.

65. Murray EA and Bussey TJ. Perceptual-mnemonic functions of the perirhinal cortex. *Trends Cogn Sci.* 1999 April;3(4):142–51.

66. Bussey TJ and Saksida LM. Object memory and perception in the medial temporal lobe: an alternative approach. *Curr Opin Neurobiol.* 2005 Dec;15(6):730–7. Review.

67. Cowell RA, Bussey TJ, and Saksida LM. Why does brain damage impair memory? A connectionist model of object recognition memory in perirhinal cortex. *J Neurosci*. 2006 Nov 22;26(47):12186–97.

68. Saksida LM and Bussey TJ. The representational-hierarchical view of amnesia: Translation from animal to human. *Neuropsychologia*. 2010 Jul;48(8):2370–84.

69. Riesenhuber M and Poggio T. Hierarchical models of object recognition in cortex. *Nat Neurosci*. 1999 Nov;2(11):1019–25.

70. Bussey TJ, Saksida LM, and Murray EA. Perirhinal cortex resolves feature ambiguity in complex visual discriminations. *Eur J Neurosci*. 2002 Jan;15(2):365–74.

71. Bussey TJ, Saksida LM, and Murray EA. Impairments in visual discrimination after perirhinal cortex lesions: Testing 'declarative' vs. 'perceptual-mnemonic' views of perirhinal cortex function. *Eur J Neurosci*. 2003 Feb;17(3):649–60.

72. Buckley MJ, Booth MC, Rolls ET, *et al*. Selective perceptual impairments after perirhinal cortex ablation. *J Neurosci*. 2001 Dec 15;21(24):9824–36.

73. Barense MD, Bussey TJ, Lee AC, *et al*. Functional specialization in the human medial temporal lobe. *J Neurosci*. 2005 Nov 2;25(44):10239–46.

74. Barense MD, Gaffan D, and Graham KS. The human medial temporal lobe processes online representations of complex objects. *Neuropsychologia*. 2007 Jul 2;45(13):2963–74.

75. Lee AC, Buckley MJ, Pegman SJ, *et al*. Specialization in the medial temporal lobe for processing of objects and scenes. *Hippocampus*. 2005 July;15(6):782–97.

76. Lee AC, Bussey TJ, Murray EA, *et al*. Perceptual deficits in amnesia: challenging the medial temporal lobe 'mnemonic' view. *Neuropsychologia*. 2005;43(1):1–11.

77. Barense MD, Ngo JK, Hung LH, *et al*. Interactions of memory and perception in amnesia: the figure-ground perspective. *Cereb Cortex*. 2012 Nov;22(11):2680–91.

78. Barense MD, Rogers TT, Bussey TJ, Saksida LM, and Graham KS. Influence of conceptual knowledge on visual object discrimination: insights from semantic dementia and MTL amnesia. *Cereb Cortex*. 2010 Nov;20(11):2568–82.

79. Shrager Y, Gold JJ, Hopkins RO, *et al*. Intact visual perception in memory-impaired patients with medial temporal lobe lesions. *J Neurosci*. 2006 Feb 22;26(8):2235–40.

80. Kim S, Jeneson A, van der Horst AS, *et al*. Memory, visual discrimination performance, and the human hippocampus. *J Neurosci*. 2011 Feb 16;31(7):2624–9.

81. Knutson AR, Hopkins RO, and Squire LR. Visual discrimination performance, memory, and medial temporal lobe function. *Proc Natl Acad Sci USA*. 2012 Aug 7;109(32):13106–11.

82. Levy DA, Shrager Y, and Squire LR. Intact visual discrimination of complex and feature-ambiguous stimuli in the absence of perirhinal cortex. *Learn Mem*. 2005 Jan-Feb;12(1):61–6.

83. McTighe SM, Cowell RA, Winters BD, *et al*. Paradoxical false memory for objects after brain damage. *Science*. 2010 Dec 3;330(6009):1408–10.

84. Barense MD, Groen, II, Lee AC, *et al*. Intact memory for irrelevant information impairs perception in amnesia. *Neuron*. 2012 Jul 12;75(1):157–67.

85. Newsome RN, Duarte A, and Barense MD. Reducing perceptual interference improves visual discrimination in mild cognitive impairment: Implications for a model of perirhinal cortex function. *Hippocampus*. 2012 Oct;22(10):1990–9.

86. Yeung LK, Ryan JD, Cowell RA, and Barense MD. Recognition Memory Impairments Caused by False Recognition of Novel Objects. *J Exp Psychol Gen*. 2013 Nov;142(4):1384–97.

87. Lee AC, Yeung LK, and Barense MD. The hippocampus and visual perception. *Front Hum Neurosci*. 2012;6:91.

88. Ryan JD and Cohen NJ. The nature of change detection and online representations of scenes. *J Exp Psychol Hum Percept Perform*. 2004 Oct;30(5):988–1015.

89. Hannula DE, Tranel D, and Cohen NJ. The long and the short of it: Relational memory impairments in amnesia, even at short lags. *J Neurosci*. 2006 Aug 9;26(32):8352–9.

90. Hartley T, Bird CM, Chan D, *et al*. The hippocampus is required for short-term topographical memory in humans. *Hippocampus*. 2007;17(1):34–48.

91. Pertzov Y, Miller TD, Gorgoraptis N, *et al*. Binding deficits in memory following medial temporal lobe damage in patients with voltage-gated potassium channel complex antibody-associated limbic encephalitis. *Brain*. 2013 Aug;136(Pt 8):2474–85.

92. Olson IR, Page K, Moore KS, *et al*. Working memory for conjunctions relies on the medial temporal lobe. *J Neurosci*. 2006 Apr 26;26(17):4596–601.

93. Warren DE, Duff MC, Jensen U, *et al*. Hiding in plain view: lesions of the medial temporal lobe impair online representation. *Hippocampus*. 2012 Jul;22(7):1577–88.

94. Warren DE, Duff MC, Tranel D, *et al*. Observing degradation of visual representations over short intervals when medial temporal lobe is damaged. *J Cogn Neurosci*. 2011 Dec;23(12):3862–73.

CHAPTER 5

The parietal lobes

Masud Husain

Gross anatomy

On its lateral surface, the human parietal lobe consists of an anterior and a posterior portion. The anterior part, bounded by the central sulcus in front and postcentral sulcus behind, has largely been implicated in basic sensorimotor functions. The posterior parietal lobe, which lies between the postcentral sulcus and the occipital and temporal lobes, has a far greater role in cognitive function. It is divided by the intraparietal sulcus (IPS) into the superior parietal lobule (SPL) and the inferior parietal lobule (IPL) (Fig. 5.1).

The IPL consists of the angular and supramarginal gyrus (Brodmann's areas 39 and 40 respectively). The nearby border zone between the temporal and parietal lobes is referred to as the temporoparietal junction (TPJ). In humans, parts of the IPL and TPJ appear to have distinctly different functions in the left and right hemisphere, with limb apraxia, language, and number processing disorders more often associated with left-sided lesions and visuospatial, attentional, and social (e.g., theory of mind) deficits associated with right-sided ones.[1-6] The portion of the lateral parietal cortex that lies deep to the temporal lobe within the insula is referred to as the parietal operculum and posterior insula.

On its medial surface (Fig. 5.2) the parietal lobe consists of a large cortical area, the precuneus,[7] which lies adjacent to the posterior cingulate cortex[8] and retrosplenial cortex.[9] In recent years, these medial regions have become the focus of much interest in Alzheimer's disease. Indeed, several investigators have reported that atrophy and hypometabolism in these areas is closely associated with mild cognitive impairment and early Alzheimer's disease.[10-13]

Functional network connectivity

Although we have known about the connections of parietal cortex at a gross anatomical level for over a century, our understanding of its detailed connectivity has, until relatively recently, been based largely on studies in non-human primates.[14] However, there is considerable debate about whether the parietal lobes in human and monkey are homologous structures.[15,16] The IPL in humans is proportionately much larger, and it has been argued that it may have both a different structure and function to the IPL in monkey. Conversely, there is much evidence to suggest that there might be some homologous sub-regions across the two species (see references 5 and 16 for discussion).

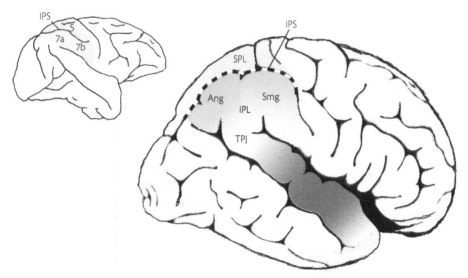

Fig. 5.1 Lateral view of parietal cortex of human and macaque monkey. The human parietal cortex consists of an anterior portion (uncoloured) situated in front of the postcentral sulcus, and a posterior portion behind this. The posterior parietal cortex is divided by the intraparietal sulcus (IPS) into two parts: the superior parietal lobule (SPL) and the inferior parietal lobule (IPL). The IPL consists of the angular gyrus (Ang) and supramarignal gyrus (Smg), and borders the superior temporal gyrus (purple) at a region that is often referred to as the temporo-parietal junction (TPJ). In macaque monkeys, the posterior parietal cortex consists of an SPL (Brodmann's area 5) and an IPL (Brodmann's areas 7a and 7b) but, according to Brodmann, the homologues of these macaque regions are all confined to the human SPL (shaded in yellow), so he considered that the IPL in humans consists of novel cortical areas. Subsequent anatomists disagreed with this scheme, considering the IPL to be similar across both species. It remains to be established whether there are new functional sub-regions within the human IPL.

Adapted from *Trends Cogn Sci.* 11(1), Husain M and Nachev P. Space and the parietal cortex, pp. 30–6, Copyright (2007), with permission from Elsevier,

Recent human neuroimaging studies which have examined structural and functional connectivity suggest that both these views might be correct: there appear to be novel regions within the human IPL as well as conserved ones that are homologous to those in the rhesus monkey.[17,18] In addition, as noted previously, there is abundant evidence to suggest that the IPL in humans is strongly lateralized between the hemispheres, while the case for such hemispheric specialization in monkeys is weak.

The main projections to parietal cortex in non-human primates come from areas involved in sensory processing (e.g. visual, somatosensory, and vestibular), while the major outputs are to premotor regions (frontal eye fields and superior colliculus, which control saccadic eye movements, and premotor cortex, which controls reaching and grasping). In turn, these premotor areas project back to parietal cortex, which also sends projections back to brain regions involved in sensory processing. Thus, the parietal cortex is an important location for the convergence of information from different sensory modalities, as well as for the association of sensory and motor signals.[19] These findings also appear to hold for human parietal regions.[20,21] The parietal cortex appears to be a major hub in cortical organization, operating on 'bottom-up' inputs from sensory regions as well as 'top-down' control signals from the frontal lobe.

In the monkey, the anterior parietal lobe is the site of primary somatosensory processing. This region projects heavily to the SPL, whereas visual signals project from occipital cortex predominantly to the IPL. The occipital visual projection to the IPL in the monkey is considered to be part of a 'dorsal visual stream' of pathways involved in spatial perception, or visual control of eye and limb movement,[22–24] The IPS appears to be an extremely important site for the convergence of information from the SPL and IPL, as well as from premotor centres. Regions within the IPS encode sensory, motor, attention and short-term memory information in both monkeys and humans.[20,21] The medial parietal cortex appears to receive both visual and somatosensory inputs and also has reciprocal connections to premotor cortex.

In humans, the dorsal visual stream emanating from occipital regions appears to project more heavily to the SPL, IPS, and precuneus rather than to the IPL.[5,25,26]. Parts of the more ventral parietal regions in humans—the IPL and TPJ—may instead have evolved to subserve higher cognitive functions, including language, number processing, and praxis in the left hemisphere, and spatial, attentional, and 'social' cognitive functions in the right hemisphere.[1–6] Human neuroimaging studies that have assessed resting state function connectivity and functional activation now implicate both IPL/TPJ and medial parietal regions as key network hubs—cortical areas where there is massive convergence of information from many different brain regions.[12,27,28]

Medial parietal areas and more posterior parts of the IPL have been implicated as part of the so-called default mode network. This set of brain regions is strongly *deactivated* during goal-directed tasks, but is active when an individual is at wakeful rest, thinking but not focusing on a problem in the outside world.[13] In contrast, more anterior parts of the IPL and adjacent TPJ in the right hemisphere have been identified as part of a ventral attention network[4,29] which is active during attentive states, while in the left hemisphere, homologues of these regions appear to form part of a language network (Fig. 5.3).[29] Both IPL and TPJ have high degrees of functional and structural connectivity with *ventrolateral* frontal regions, including Broca's area in the left hemisphere and its homologue in the right hemisphere (see also chapter 8).[29,30]

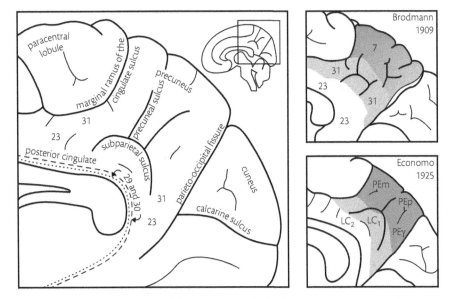

Fig. 5.2 Medial view of the parietal cortex of human. The human medial parietal cortex includes the precuneus, the posterior cingulate cortex (Brodmann's area 23), the retrosplenial cortex embedded in the posterior callosal sulcus (Brodmann's areas 29 and 30), and the transitional zone (area 31) which separates precuneus from cingulate cortex. The precuneus is located between the marginal ramus of the cingulate sulcus anteriorly and the parieto-occipital fissure posteriorly. The two insets on the right show two different parcellations of these regions according to Brodmann and von Economo subsequently.
Adapted from *Proc Natl Acad Sci USA*. 106(47), Margulies DS, Vincent JL, Kelly C, Lohmann G, Uddin LQ, Biswal BB, *et al*. Precuneus shares intrinsic functional architecture in humans and monkeys, pp. 20069–74, Copyright (2009), with permission from *Proc Natl Acad Sci USA*.

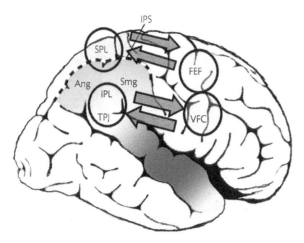

Fig. 5.3 Dorsal and ventral attention networks. The ventral frontoparietal attention network extends from the IPL (inferior parietal lobule) and TPJ (temporoparietal junction) to the VFC (ventral frontal cortex) and is considered to be lateralized to the right hemisphere. Homologous regions in the left hemisphere are considered to form part of a language network. The dorsal attention network, by contrast, is considered to be bilateral. It extends from the SPL (superior parietal lobe) and IPS (intraparietal sulcus) to the FEF (frontal eye fields).

Adapted from *Trends Cogn Sci.* 11(1), Husain M and Nachev P. Space and the parietal cortex, pp. 30–6, Copyright (2007), with permission from Elsevier, reproduced under the Creative Commons CC BY License.

By contrast, the SPL and IPS appear to be heavily connected to *dorsolateral* frontal regions. These parietal and frontal areas are considered to be part of a dorsal attention network which, unlike the ventral attention network, appears to be symmetric across both hemispheres (Fig. 5.3).[4] The dorsal frontoparietal attention network (not to be confused with the 'dorsal visual stream' which connects occipital regions to dorsal parietal areas—see chapter 6) may play a role in directing attention to locations or objects of interest in the environment.

The IPL and medial parietal regions, particularly posterior cingulate and retrosplenial cortex, also have strong connections to the medial temporal lobe (MTL),[24,25,31] accessing the hippocampus via the parahippocampal region.[32] The functional role of parieto-hippocampal interactions is yet to be established but these may play an important role in episodic memory. Intriguingly, atrophy and hypometabolism in medial parietal regions that connect to the MTL and are part of the default mode network is closely associated with mild cognitive impairment and early Alzheimer's disease.[10–13] Some have argued that it is the strong network connectivity of these parietal regions to MTL areas affected in Alzheimer's pathology that makes them particularly vulnerable relatively early in the course of the illness.[12]

Next, the functional anatomy of the parietal cortex in the context of disorders of perception, action, language, and number processing that follow damage to the human parietal lobe is considered. Where possible, the anatomy of lesion localization is related to the deficits observed.

Perception and attention

Parietal regions play a crucial role in perception, integrating information from different sensory modalities and directing attention, particularly for localizing or attending to objects at different spatial locations.[19,20,33,34,35–38] Some of the most prominent disorders that follow damage to the posterior parietal lobe are characterized by a spatial component,[39] although non-spatial functions also contribute.[40] At one end of the spectrum are sensory defects; for example, in the visual domain, inferior quadrantanopias which arise because of damage to part of the optic radiations as they pass through the parietal white matter from the lateral geniculate nucleus to the calcarine sulcus. At the other end of the spectrum are complex disorders of attention that can have devastating consequences for a patient, presenting an enormous challenge for rehabilitation.

It is important to appreciate that many perceptual disorders that follow parietal damage are difficult to explain simply in terms of deficits in sensory processes alone. Thus, for example, visual disorientation, mislocalization, and constructional apraxia (discussed below) have all been attributed to deficits of 'spatial remapping'.[41,42] This may be due to difficulties in updating representations that combine visual information and motor commands sent to the eye muscles to produce a dynamic, spatial 'map' of the body and the external world.[19,43] Not knowing which way the eyes were pointing in the orbit when the retinal 'snapshot' was taken can lead to poor integration of the relative locations of items around us, a factor that probably contributes to several parietal disorders of perception and attention.

It is also the case that many perceptual deficits (e.g. unilateral neglect syndrome) are not confined to one sensory modality but are multimodal, involving vision, audition, and touch. Indeed, some have considered the parietal lobe to be essential in forming a multimodal representation of the body schema,[44,45] consistent with the known convergence of different types of sensory input to parietal regions. Many of the studies that have been performed in patients, however, have focused on disturbances of vision and touch because these are often the most clinically conspicuous findings.

Visual disorientation and mislocalization

Holmes first described in detail a syndrome of '*visual disorientation*' in cases of bilateral posterior parietal damage following gunshot wounds.[46,47] Typically, when asked to touch an object in front of him, a patient would reach in the wrong direction and grope hopelessly until his hand came into contact with it, almost as if he was searching for a small object in the dark, and experience great difficulty in walking through a room without bumping into objects. Less dramatic impairments have been demonstrated in unilateral lesions. Patients with parietal lesions misreach when pointing to visual targets presented on a perimeter.[48] However, a potential confound is that parietal damage may lead to a disorder of visually guided reaching (see optic ataxia below) in addition to visual mislocalization.

To circumvent this issue, Warrington developed a perceptual test, first briefly presenting a dot and then a card on which appeared numbers at different locations. She asked patients to report the number which best approximated the dot's location.[49] *Visual mislocalization* on such tasks is more prominent following posterior lesions of the right hemisphere.[49,50] A version of this dot localization test, without brief visual presentation, continues to be used in neuropsychological batteries today (e.g. visual object and space perception or VOSP battery). Depth perception and judgment of line orientation may also be impaired after unilateral (right?) parietal lesions.[39]

Disorders of touch and proprioception

Classically, parietal lesions lead to 'discriminative' sensory loss.[44] Two-point discrimination, position sense, texture discrimination, stereognosis (ability to identify by touch objects placed in the hand), and graphesthaesia (recognition of numbers scratched on the hand) may all be impaired. Usually, this 'cortical sensory loss' is limited to one or two body parts, is more prominent in the arm than the leg, and follows damage to the contralateral anterior parietal lobe or its connections. However, there are also reports of *astereognosis* following damage to the SPL or IPL. One patient with a large SPL cyst complained that she kept 'losing' her arm if she did not look at it: she could not maintain a representation of the limb in the absence of vision.[51] In contrast to astereognosis, *tactile agnosia* refers to selective impairment of tactile object recognition in the absence of a clinically demonstrable basic sensory impairment. With their eyes closed, patients with tactile agnosia are unable to recognize familiar objects placed in the hand contralateral to the lesion which often involves the IPL and or posterior insula.[52]

Constructional apraxia

A common way to demonstrate visuospatial impairments following parietal damage is to ask patients to copy a drawing (e.g. a complex figure such as the Rey–Ostrrieth figure, or equivalent) or a three-dimensional block design. Typically, they encounter difficulty in understanding the spatial relationships of the drawing or block design and produce poor reproductions. Such an inability to use visual information to guide acts which require an understanding of the spatial relationship of objects is referred to as *constructional apraxia*, a syndrome most often associated with right IPL damage.[53,54] Paterson and Zangwill gave a particularly clear account of a young man with a focal lesion of the right IPL.[55] They observed that the patient drew complex objects or scenes detail by detail, and appeared to lack any real grasp of the object as a whole. They characterized this problem as a 'piecemeal approach'—a fragmentation of the visual contents with deficient synthesis.[55] It is as if snapshots of the visual scene fail to be integrated correctly, so the relative locations of different parts of the scene or an object are not correctly perceived.

Disorders of attention

Parietal regions appear to play a crucial role in deploying selective attention to spatial locations or objects as well as sustaining attention over time.[5,33,34,38] For example, neurons that are selective for a region of space increase their firing when monkeys attend more closely to that location.[33,38] Three disorders of attention follow damage to the posterior parietal lobes: *extinction, neglect*, and *simultagnosia*. The first two often occur after unilateral damage, whereas the last is less common and is observed in its full-blown form after bilateral parietal lesions or atrophy often as part of Bálint's syndrome.[56] None of them can be adequately explained as simple sensory impairments.

Extinction is the failure to report a contralesional stimulus (one presented to the side opposite the brain lesion) in the presence of a competing ipsilesional stimulus (on the same side of space as the brain lesion). It can occur in visual, tactile, or auditory domains. For example, patients acknowledge the presence of a single visual stimulus (e.g. the examiner's finger) when it is presented briefly in either left or right visual hemifields. However, when both stimuli are simultaneously presented transiently, one in each hemifield, they report seeing only the ipsilesional one. Extinction can occur with either left or right parietal lesions, and has been associated with damage to the IPS or TPJ,[21] but might also occur with lesions to other brain regions.

Neglect (also referred to as unilateral neglect or hemispatial neglect) is a failure to acknowledge a contralesional stimulus—regardless of the presence or absence of a competing stimulus in ipsilesional space—which cannot be explained simply by sensory loss or motor deficit.[4,57] It is often multimodal, involving visual, tactile, and auditory domains. If neglect is very dense it can be difficult to distinguish from sensory deficits, and some patients with large lesions suffer from both (e.g. a visual field deficit and neglect). However, the clinician is often alerted to the presence of neglect by the patient's persistent turning of eyes and head towards the ipsilesional side (without an associated gaze palsy), by finding that unawareness of contralesional stimuli can vary and is not absolute, by observing in the visual domain that the apparent field loss does not obey the vertical meridian (unlike homonymous hemianopia), and by the patient's failure to orient fully into contralesional space on simple pen-and-paper tasks such as line bisection and cancellation. Some patients also fail to draw the contralesional side of objects. A patient with hemianopia (without neglect) may be slow in performing these tasks but will usually explore contralesional space.

Finally, an important clinical clue comes from the patient's history. Most patients with neglect are not aware they have a problem (see anosognosia below), whereas those with a hemianopia (without neglect) complain bitterly that they have difficulty seeing on one side of space. Neglect is most severe and most long-lasting following right parietal/TPJ lesions, particularly stroke, although it can also occur after right inferior frontal, basal ganglia, and thalamic damage.

Simultagnosia (or simultanagnosia) refers to a disorder of vision in which individuals have difficulty apprehending the entire scene, in visualizing its separate elements simultaneously. Although they may describe some of the details meticulously, individuals with simultagnosia may still not appreciate what is happening overall in a picture (e.g. the Boston cookie theft scene). Their perception appears piecemeal, as if they have snapshots of different items in a scene but cannot integrate these into a coherent whole.[58] Simultagnosia is one component of Bálint's syndrome.[56] Previously, simultagnosia was most commonly associated with massive bilateral lesions of temporoparieto-occipital cortex (e.g. from watershed infarctions). Nowadays, it is most commonly observed as a feature of posterior cortical atrophy[59] (see chapter 15) which is usually a posterior variant of Alzheimer's disease.

Anosognosia

Unawareness of illness is referred to as anosognosia. Patients may steadfastly deny they have suffered a stroke or hemiparesis, even if the examiner demonstrates that one limb is weak. The condition is often, but not invariably, associated with unilateral neglect, with many such patients denying they have a visual disorder. Anosognosia appears most commonly after right-hemisphere lesions. Although it is traditionally associated with right IPL damage,[60] recent studies of anosognosia for hemiparesis suggest involvement of right posterior insula or premotor frontal regions.[61,62]

Visuomotor and motor control

Neurons in the parietal cortex integrate sensory information (e.g. location of a visual object) with motor commands (e.g. to the eyes or limbs) and, together with premotor regions in frontal cortex, appear to play a crucial role in directing gaze and the hand to objects—including tools—around us.[20,63,64] Imaging studies have identified several regions within dorsal and dorsomedial parietal cortex involved in directing the eyes and the hands to reach, as well as action observation (e.g. when people view others using tools) (Fig. 5.4). Some of the disorders that follow parietal damage reflect such functions.[16,65]

Optic ataxia

Bálint first used the term 'optic ataxia' to refer to an impairment of visually guided reaching that he observed following bilateral posterior cortical damage. Since then, many reports have followed of patients with unilateral or bilateral parietal lesions. The term Bálint's syndrome is used to refer to a combination of optic ataxia, simultagnosia, and ocular apraxia,[56] most commonly observed nowadays in cases of posterior cortical atrophy.[59] However, many patients have been reported with optic ataxia alone. The most commonly described defect appears to be a 'field effect': inaccurate reaching with either hand to visual targets located in the visual hemifield contralateral to the lesion. However, an 'arm effect' has also been reported: misreaching with the contralesional arm to targets in either visual field. This may also occur in combination with a 'field effect'.[66]

At the bedside, the disorder is best demonstrated by asking the patient to fixate centrally (e.g. on the examiner's nose) and point to a target presented peripherally (e.g. the examiner's finger). If the patient is allowed to move his eyes and look at the target, the disorder may not be evident. As well as misdirecting their reaches, optic ataxic patients may also encounter difficulty in planning the appropriate grasp required to pick up an object.[66] Lesions in either hemisphere appear to cause the syndrome, with the critical lesion site being the SPL and adjacent IPS, consistent with functional imaging studies in healthy people which demonstrate these regions play a crucial role in reaching and grasping (Fig. 5.4).[20,64]

Impairments of gaze control or ocular apraxia

In addition to simultagnosia and optic ataxia, patient's with Bálint's syndrome experience difficulty in shifting gaze to objects in peripheral vision.[56] They seem to lock their gaze on the item they are fixating and have difficulty initiating saccades to other objects—*ocular apraxia*. Holmes described a similar problem in his cases with visual disorientation, but in addition reported other disorders of oculomotor control.[46,47] Typically, when one of his patients was asked to look at something or was spoken to, he would stare in the wrong direction and then move his eyes awkwardly until he found, often as if by chance, the object he was looking for. Some of Holmes' cases also failed to accommodate and converge their eyes correctly, and smooth pursuit could also be impaired. Holmes considered these problems to be secondary to visual perceptual deficits. However, these disorders may be accounted for by loss of neurons associated with maintaining fixation, directing saccades, or pursuit eye movements, all of which have been demonstrated in monkey posterior parietal cortical neurons.[19] Functional imaging studies in humans suggest that there are several parietal eye fields located within the dorsal IPS (Fig. 5.4).[35,67]

Limb apraxia

Limb apraxia refers to an impairment in the ability to perform skilled movements which cannot be attributed to weakness,

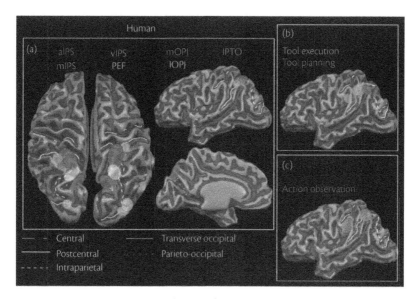

Fig. 5.4 Parietal regions activate in imaging studies of action control. (a) Schematic of parietal regions implicated in functional imaging studies of directing saccades, pointing or grasping. The parietal eye fields (PEF) are now known to consist of several different regions that are activated by eye movements. Area AIP (anterior intraparietal sulcus) has been considered to play a role in grasping while areas mIPS (medial intraparietal sulcus) and mOPJ (medial occipitoparietal junction) have been implicated in reaching. Area vIPS (ventral intraparietal sulcus) responds to multimodal moving stimuli. (b) Lateral inferior parietal regions in the left hemisphere active during tool use or thinking about tool use. (c) Left parietal regions active during action observation.
Adapted from *Curr Opin Neurobiol.* 16(2), Culham JC and Valyear KF. Human parietal cortex in action, pp. 205–12, Copyright (2006), with permission from Elsevier.

sensory disturbance, or involuntary movements such as tremor,[1] It may occur in up to 50 per cent of unselected patients with left-hemisphere damage, but frequently goes unrecognized either because patients may not be aware of a problem in daily life, or because praxis is commonly not tested, or because many left-hemisphere patients are dysphasic.

Liepmann, at the turn of the last century (see reference 68), originally proposed that there are three types of apraxia: ideational, ideomotor, and limb-kinetic (or melokinetic). He considered that inadequate formulation of a motor programme would result in *ideational apraxia*. Traditionally, this is considered to be best observed when a patient is asked to produce a *sequence of gestures* on command, rather than when the examiner performs a gesture for him to imitate. By contrast, in *ideomotor apraxia*, a patient may know what to do but cannot produce the correct actions either on verbal request or when asked to imitate gestures. He is aware of his poor performance and may try to correct it, so the problem is one of defective execution rather than ideation. This is the most common type of limb apraxia for which clinicians usually test. Finally, limb-kinetic apraxia consists of loss of control of fine finger movements and often follows damage to the corticospinal pathways, and will not be considered further in this discussion.

In *ideomotor apraxia*, the representation of the gesture to be performed is considered to be intact but its execution is defective. Traditionally, an important piece of evidence in favour of this distinction is the failure of patients to produce correct gestures even when asked to imitate the examiner's movements. Thus, these patients perform poorly regardless of whether they have to produce a gesture on verbal command (by recalling a movement representation) or imitate it. Typically, however, their performance is better when imitating movements or using objects than when they are asked to pantomime transitive acts (i.e. mime the use of a tool or instrument). Intransitive movements (communicative gestures such as waving goodbye) may be relatively well preserved. Thus, ideomotor apraxia appears to spare movements that are automatic or habitual such as waving, or repetitive as in finger-tapping.

Some patients with ideomotor apraxia may use a body part as a tool, such as using their fingers to act like scissor blades, when asked to pantomime using scissors. This type of error may have been overemphasized, since even neurologically normal individuals will sometimes do this. Other patients produce inappropriate movements about multiple joints. For example, when asked to pantomime the use of a screwdriver, they may rotate their arm at the shoulder rather than at the elbow.

The localization of apraxia appears in many ways to be the mirror image of the neglect syndrome, involving inferior parietal and frontal regions in the left hemisphere.[69] Liepmann considered ideomotor apraxia to be a disconnection syndrome, in which sensory visual and audioverbal representations (in the posterior left hemisphere) were disconnected from kinesthetic-motor 'engrams' (around the central sulcus). The critical anatomical site of the disconnection, he suggested, was the white matter underlying the left IPL. Liepmann was quite clear that his model did not envisage a centre for 'gesture control' within the IPL, but subsequent investigators have challenged this scheme, arguing that movement representations encoding the spatial and temporal patterns of skilled movements, are stored within the left IPL (see reference 68 and Fig. 5.4).

The use of the term *ideational apraxia* has been extremely confusing. It is often used to refer to an impairment in the ability to perform a series of motor acts. For example, when asked to make a cup of tea, a patient may perform each element of the sequence but in an incorrect order. However, De Renzi has argued that ideational apraxia refers to an inability to recall previously well-established actions, for example, object use, an 'amnesia of usage'.[70] There are certainly examples of patients who have difficulty using a single object without having to perform a sequence of acts using multiple objects. For example, Pick originally reported a case who used a razor as a comb! Some favour a different term—*conceptual apraxia*—to specify a defect in the knowledge required to select and use tools and objects.[71] This appears most frequently to follow lesions of the left posterior parietal lobe. Functional imaging studies in healthy people have delineated left parietal regions involved in tool use and observing the actions of others.[64]

Language and number processing

In functional imaging studies, part of the left IPL (angular gyrus) is activated by tasks that require semantic processing including comprehension during reading,[72] while a region around the left TPJ (known as area Spt: Sylvian parietotemporal, within the planum temporale) has been implicated in auditory sensorimotor processing and phonological short-term or working memory.[73] By contrast, neuroimaging has implicated the left IPS in number processing.[74]

Conduction aphasia

Lesions of the left parietal lobe have been associated with the syndrome of *conduction aphasia* which is characterized by fluent speech but with phonemic errors, intact comprehension but poor repetition. Classically this has been considered to be a 'disconnection syndrome' in which the arcuate fasciculus is affected, thereby disconnecting superior temporal lobe language zones from Broca's area. More recent lesion analysis suggests that damage to cortical area Spt might be sufficient without having to invoke white matter disconnection,[73] although this is contested.

Dyscalculia and Gerstmann's syndrome

There is now considerable evidence that lesions of the left parietal lobe can lead to deficits in number processing and *dyscalculia* (see chapter 17). The existence of Gerstmann's syndrome (dyscalculia, dysgraphia, finger agnosia, or the inability to distinguish between fingers and left-right disorientation) —has, however, been disputed. When reported, it has been associated with left parietal lesions near the TPJ.

Memory

It is generally agreed that the parietal lobes play a role in short-term or working memory. Imaging studies have repeatedly demonstrated this with verbal material more likely to activate left parietal regions more than right, and vice versa for spatial material. Most often the IPS has been implicated.[75] Lesion studies too have implicated posterior parietal areas in the left hemisphere in phonological working memory and right hemisphere regions in spatial working memory.[76,77] Some recent studies suggest that parietal areas, which project heavily to the medial temporal lobe, might also play a role in aspects of episodic memory largely on the basis of imaging data,[78] but this proposal remains controversial.

References

1. Goldenberg G. Apraxia and the parietal lobes. *Neuropsychologia*. 2009 May;47(6):1449–59.
2. Henseler I, Regenbrecht F, and Obrig H. Lesion correlates of patholinguistic profiles in chronic aphasia: comparisons of syndrome-, modality- and symptom-level assessment. *Brain*. 2014 Mar;137(Pt 3):918–30.
3. Grafman J, Passafiume D, Faglioni P, *et al.* Calculation disturbances in adults with focal hemispheric damage. *Cortex*. 1982 Apr;18(1):37–49.
4. Corbetta M and Shulman GL. Spatial neglect and attention networks. *Annu Rev Neurosci*. 2011;34:569–99.
5. Singh-Curry V and Husain M. The functional role of the inferior parietal lobe in the dorsal and ventral stream dichotomy. *Neuropsychologia*. 2009 May;47(6):1434–48.
6. Decety J and Lamm C. The role of the right temporoparietal junction in social interaction: how low-level computational processes contribute to meta-cognition. *Neuroscientist*. 2007 Dec;13(6):580–93.
7. Cavanna AE and Trimble MR. The precuneus: a review of its functional anatomy and behavioural correlates. *Brain*. 2006 Jan 3;129(3):564–83.
8. Leech R and Sharp DJ. The role of the posterior cingulate cortex in cognition and disease. *Brain*. 2014 Jan;137(Pt 1):12–32.
9. Vann SD, Aggleton JP, and Maguire EA. What does the retrosplenial cortex do? *Nat Rev Neurosci*. 2009 Nov;10(11):792–802.
10. Pengas G, Hodges JR, Watson P, *et al.* Focal posterior cingulate atrophy in incipient Alzheimer's disease. *Neurobiol Aging*. 2010 Jan;31(1):25–33.
11. Karas G, Scheltens P, Rombouts S, *et al.* Precuneus atrophy in early-onset Alzheimer's disease: a morphometric structural MRI study. *Neuroradiology*. 2007 Dec;49(12):967–76.
12. Buckner RL, Sepulcre J, Talukdar T, *et al.* Cortical hubs revealed by intrinsic functional connectivity: mapping, assessment of stability, and relation to Alzheimer's disease. *J Neurosci*. 2009 Feb 11;29(6):1860–73.
13. Buckner RL, Andrews-Hanna JR, and Schacter DL. The brain's default network: anatomy, function, and relevance to disease. *Ann NY Acad Sci*. 2008 Mar;1124:1–38.
14. Schmahmann JD and Pandya D. *Fiber Pathways of the Brain*. Oxford University Press, 2009.
15. Husain M and Nachev P. Space and the parietal cortex. *Trends Cogn Sci*. 2007;11:30–6.
16. Caminiti R, Chafee MV, Battaglia-Mayer A, *et al.* Understanding the parietal lobe syndrome from a neurophysiological and evolutionary perspective. *Eur J Neurosci*. 2010 Jun;31(12):2320–40.
17. Mars RB, Jbabdi S, Sallet J, *et al.* Diffusion-weighted imaging tractography-based parcellation of the human parietal cortex and comparison with human and macaque resting-state functional connectivity. *J Neurosci*. 2011 Mar 16;31(11):4087–100.
18. Mantini D, Corbetta M, Romani GL, *et al.* Evolutionarily novel functional networks in the human brain? *J Neurosci*. 2013 Feb 20;33(8):3259–75.
19. Andersen RA. Multimodal integration for the representation of space in the posterior parietal cortex. *Philos Trans R Soc Lond B*. 1997;1997(352):1421–8.
20. Culham JC and Valyear KF. Human parietal cortex in action. *Curr Opin Neurobiol*. 2006 Apr;16(2):205–12.
21. Vandenberghe R and Gillebert CR. Parcellation of parietal cortex: convergence between lesion-symptom mapping and mapping of the intact functioning brain. *Behav Brain Res*. 2009 May 16;199(2):171–82.
22. Ungerleider LG and Mishkin M. *Two Cortical Visual Systems. Analysis of Visual Behaviour*. Cambridge, MA: MIT Press, 1982.
23. Milner AD and Goodale MA. *The Visual Brain in Action*. Oxford: Oxford University Press, 1995.
24. Kravitz DJ, Saleem KS, Baker CI, *et al.* A new neural framework for visuospatial processing. *Nat Rev Neurosci*. 2011 Apr;12(4):217–30.
25. Margulies DS, Vincent JL, Kelly C, *et al.* Precuneus shares intrinsic functional architecture in humans and monkeys. *Proc Natl Acad Sci USA*. 2009 Nov 24;106(47):20069–74.
26. Katzner S and Weigelt S. Visual cortical networks: of mice and men. *Curr Opin Neurobiol*. 2013 Apr;23(2):202–6.
27. Cabeza R, Ciaramelli E, and Moscovitch M. Cognitive contributions of the ventral parietal cortex: an integrative theoretical account. *Trends Cogn Sci*. 2012 Jun;16(6):338–52.
28. Carter RM and Huettel SA. A nexus model of the temporal-parietal junction. *Trends Cogn Sci*. 2013 Jul;17(7):328–36.
29. Laird AR, Fox PM, Eickhoff SB, *et al.* Behavioral interpretations of intrinsic connectivity networks. *J Cogn Neurosci*. 2011 Dec;23(12):4022–37.
30. Thiebaut de Schotten M, Dell'Acqua F, *et al.* A lateralized brain network for visuospatial attention. *Nat Neurosci*. 2011 Oct;14(10):1245–6.
31. Kahn I, Andrews-Hanna JR, Vincent JL, *et al.* Distinct cortical anatomy linked to subregions of the medial temporal lobe revealed by intrinsic functional connectivity. *J Neurophysiol*. 2008 Jul;100(1):129–39.
32. Ranganath C and Ritchey M. Two cortical systems for memory-guided behaviour. *Nat Rev Neurosci*. 2012 Oct;13(10):713–26.
33. Colby C and Goldberg ME. Space and attention in parietal cortex. *Annu Rev Neurosci*. 1999;22:319–49.
34. Culham JC and Kanwisher N. Neuroimaging of cognitive functions in human parietal cortex. *Curr Opin Neurobiol*. 2001;11:157–63.
35. Sereno MI and Huang R-S. Multisensory maps in parietal cortex. *Curr Opin Neurobiol*. 2014 Feb;24(1):39–46.
36. Driver J and Spence C. Multisensory perception: beyond modularity and convergence. *Curr Biol*. 2000 Oct 19;10(20):R731–5.
37. Macaluso E. Orienting of spatial attention and the interplay between the senses. *Cortex*. 2010 Mar;46(3):282–97.
38. Bisley JW and Goldberg ME. Attention, intention, and priority in the parietal lobe. *Annu Rev Neurosci*. 2010;33:1–21.
39. De Renzi E. *Disorders of Space Exploration and Cognition*. New York, NY: Wiley, 1982.
40. Husain M and Rorden C. Non-spatially lateralized mechanisms in hemispatial neglect. *Nat Rev Neurosci*. 2003;4(1):26–36.
41. Pisella L, Alahyane N, Blangero A, *et al.* Right-hemispheric dominance for visual remapping in humans. *Philos Trans R Soc Lond B Biol Sci*. 2011 Feb 27;366(1564):572–85.
42. Russell C, Deidda C, Malhotra P, *et al.* A deficit of spatial remapping in constructional apraxia after right-hemisphere stroke. *Brain*. 2010 Apr;133(Pt 4):1239–51.
43. Duhamel JR, Colby C, and Goldberg ME. The updating of the representation of visual space in parietal cortex by intended eye movements. *Science*. 1992;1992:90–2.
44. Head H and Holmes G. Sensory Disturbances from Cerebral Lesions. *Brain*. 1911 Jan 11;34(2–3):102–254.
45. Haggard P and Wolpert DM. Disorders of Body Scheme. In: HJ Freund, M Jeannerod, M Hallett, and R Leiguarda (eds). *Higher-Order Motor Disorders*. Oxford University Press: Oxford, 2005.
46. Holmes G. Disturbances of visual orientation. *Br J Ophthalmol*. 1918 Sep;2(9):449–68.
47. Holmes G. Disturbances of visual orientation. *Br J Ophthalmol*. 1918 Oct;2(10):506–16.
48. Ratcliff G and Davies-Jones GA. Defective visual localization in focal brain wounds. *Brain*. 1972;95(1):49–60.
49. Warrington EK and Rabin P. Perceptual matching in patients with cerebral lesions. *Neuropsychologia*. 1970 Nov;8(4):475–87.
50. Hannay HJ, Varney NR, and Benton AL. Visual localization in patients with unilateral brain disease. *J Neurol Neurosur Ps*. 1976 Apr;39(4):307–13.
51. Wolpert DM, Goodbody SJ, and Husain M. Maintaining internal representations: the role of the human superior parietal lobe. *Nat Neurosci*. 1998 Oct;1(6):529–33.
52. Caselli RJ. Ventrolateral and dorsomedial somatosensory association cortex damage produces distinct somesthetic syndromes in humans. *Neurology*. 1993 Apr;43(4):762–71.
53. Hier DB, Mondlock J, and Caplan LR. Behavioral abnormalities after right hemisphere stroke. *Neurology*. 1983 Apr;33(3):337–44.

54. Ruessmann K, Sondag HD, and Beneicke U. On the cerebral localization of constructional apraxia. *Int J Neurosci*. 1988 Sep;42(1–2):59–62.

55. Patterson A and Zangwill OL. Disorders of visual space perception associated with lesions of the right cerebral hemisphere. *Brain*. 1944;67:331–58.

56. Rizzo M and Vecera SP. Psychoanatomical substrates of Bálint's syndrome. *J Neurol Neurosur Ps*. 2002 Feb;72(2):162–78.

57. Parton A, Malhotra P, and Husain M. Hemispatial neglect. *J Neurol Neurosur Ps*. 2004 Jan;75(1):13–21.

58. Dalrymple KA, Barton JJS, and Kingstone A. A world unglued: simultanagnosia as a spatial restriction of attention. *Front Hum Neurosci*. 2013;7:145.

59. Crutch SJ, Lehmann M, Schott JM, et al. Posterior cortical atrophy. *Lancet Neurol*. 2012 Feb;11(2):170–8.

60. Vossel S, Weiss PH, Eschenbeck P, et al. The neural basis of anosognosia for spatial neglect after stroke. *Stroke J Cereb Circ*. 2012 Jul;43(7):1954–6.

61. Karnath H-O, Baier B, and Nägele T. Awareness of the functioning of one's own limbs mediated by the insular cortex? *J Neurosci*. 2005 Aug 3;25(31):7134–8.

62. Berti A, Bottini G, Gandola M, et al. Shared cortical anatomy for motor awareness and motor control. *Science*. 2005 Jul 15;309(5733):488–91.

63. Andersen RA and Cui H. Intention, action planning, and decision making in parietal-frontal circuits. *Neuron*. 2009 Sep 10;63(5):568–83.

64. Vingerhoets G. Contribution of the posterior parietal cortex in reaching, grasping, and using objects and tools. *Front Psychol*. 2014;5:151.

65. Andersen RA, Andersen KN, Hwang EJ, et al. Optic ataxia: from Balint's syndrome to the parietal reach region. *Neuron*. 2014 Mar 5;81(5):967–83.

66. Perenin M-T and Vighetto A. Optic ataxia: a specific disruption in visuomotor mechanisms. I. Different aspects of the deficit in reaching for objects. *Brain*. 1988;111:643–74.

67. Konen CS and Kastner S. Representation of eye movements and stimulus motion in topographically organized areas of human posterior parietal cortex. *J Neurosci*. 2008 Aug 13;28(33):8361–75.

68. Goldenberg G. *Apraxia: The Cognitive Side of Motor Control*. Oxford: Oxford University Press, 2013.

69. Haaland KY, Harrington DL, and Knight RT. Neural representations of skilled movement. *Brain*. 2000 Nov;123 (Pt 11):2306–13.

70. De Renzi E and Lucchelli F. Ideational apraxia. *Brain*. 1988 Oct;111 (Pt 5):1173–85.

71. Heilman KM, Maher LM, Greenwald ML, et al. Conceptual apraxia from lateralized lesions. *Neurology*. 1997 Aug;49(2):457–64.

72. Binder JR, Desai RH, Graves WW, et al. Where is the semantic system? A critical review and meta-analysis of 120 functional neuroimaging studies. *Cereb Cortex*. 1991. 2009 Dec;19(12):2767–96.

73. Hickok G and Poeppel D. The cortical organization of speech processing. *Nat Rev Neurosci*. 2007 May;8(5):393–402.

74. Nieder A and Dehaene S. Representation of number in the brain. *Annu Rev Neurosci*. 2009;32:185–208.

75. Baddeley A. Working memory: looking back and looking forward. *Nat Rev Neurosci*. 2003 Oct;4(10):829–39.

76. Shallice T and Warrington EK. Independent functioning of verbal memory stores: a neuropsychological study. *Q J Exp Psychol*. 1970 May;22(2):261–73.

77. Hanley JR, Young AW, and Pearson NA. Impairment of the visuospatial sketch pad. *Q J Exp Psychol A*. 1991 Feb;43(1):101–25.

78. Cabeza R, Ciaramelli E, Olson IR, et al. The parietal cortex and episodic memory: an attentional account. *Nat Rev Neurosci*. 2008 Aug;9(8):613–25.

CHAPTER 6

The occipital lobes

Geraint Rees

Introduction

In the human brain, the occipital lobe is a pyramidal shaped structure located at the most posterior point of each cerebral hemisphere. Traditionally it is defined as extending from the occipital pole to the parieto-occipital fissure, and in primate brains it is a structure involved in processing visual information. The discovery and functional characterization of different visual areas of the occipital lobe is one of the major achievements of twentieth-century neurology and visual neuroscience and has helped clarify and understand the clinical presentation of many sensory disorders caused by occipital lobe damage or dysfunction.

At the end of the nineteenth century, it was noted that unilateral lesions of the striate cortex of the occipital lobe in monkeys lead to hemianopia.[1] This identification of the occipital lobe with visual function was extended to humans in clinical observations[2] that suggested that the calcarine sulcus, which extends anteriorly from the occipital pole on the medial aspect of the occipital lobe, was the crucial location which when damaged produced contralateral hemianopia. These clinical observations established that the occipital lobe received input from the contralateral hemiretina, but the precise correspondence between how the visual field was represented on the retina and how it was represented in the calcarine sulcus remained obscure because of the relatively large size of the lesions in the patients who were studied, which limited the ability to localize function.

The invention and subsequent utilization of the high-velocity rifle in the armed conflicts that swept the world at the beginning of the twentieth century produced new opportunities to discover the functional anatomy of visual cortex. In soldiers with head injuries that were associated with visual field defects, it proved possible to determine the intracerebral trajectory of the bullet that caused such a defect because its velocity meant that it took a straight course between entry and exit wounds. Inouye[3] studied such brain-injured patients from the Russo–Japanese war, and deduced that the visual fields were represented in striate cortex in the form of a map. Specifically, he proposed that the central visual field was represented more posteriorly in the contralateral occipital lobe. Moreover, he suggested from careful consideration of the different patients that the cortical maps were distorted, with the central visual field occupying a larger area of occipital cortex than the peripheral visual fields.

The British neurologist Gordon Holmes subsequently studied over 2000 brain-injured British soldiers in the First World War,[4] confirming and extending these observations to propose an antero-posterior organization with central vision located more posteriorly and peripheral vision more anteriorly in the calcarine sulcus.

Holmes also concluded that cortical lesions resulted in homonymous (congruous) defects and produced a more detailed description of the representation in the visual cortex of the horizontal and vertical axes of the retina.

These clinical observations thus firmly established the correspondence between the gross anatomy of the human occipital lobe and the deficits in vision that resulted from brain injury. In particular, they proposed a retinotopic organization of the visual cortex whereby there is a topographic correspondence between locations in the retina and corresponding locations in the early visual cortex that represent a particular part of the visual field. Specifically, nearby regions on the retina project to nearby cortical regions and in the cortex, neighbouring positions in the visual field are represented by groups of neurons that are adjacent in the grey matter. This primary visual cortex (subsequently known as V1) was located in the calcarine sulcus in the posterior occipital lobe.

Using non-invasive brain imaging to measure retinotopic maps

In the 1980s and early 1990s, investigators realized that the topographic organization of visual areas in humans that had been revealed almost a century earlier could now be studied using non-invasive methods. The use of positron emission tomography (PET) and then the advent of functional magnetic resonance imaging (MRI) allowed signals to be recorded from healthy volunteers that reflected local neuronal activity in the human brain. Some of the first studies to demonstrate this new technique employed activation of the occipital lobe in response to visual field stimulation with a flashing checkerboard.[5] By asking participants to fixate and presenting visual stimuli at particular locations rather than throughout the visual field, investigators devised efficient approaches that could map topographic cortical representations of the visual field in the occipital lobe.[6–8] This technique became known as retinotopic mapping and is now a standard procedure (Fig. 6.1).

These early studies showed, as suspected from earlier clinico-pathological investigation, that the mapping from the retina to the visual cortex was not only topographic but could be best described by a log-polar transformation. Such a transformation results in the standard x/y (Cartesian) axes in the retina being modified into a polar coordinate system in the cortex, where position on the retina (corresponding to position in the visual field) is represented on the cortical surface in terms of eccentricity (the difference from the centre of vision) and polar angle (relative to a horizontal or vertical axis). The logarithmic nature of the transformation is such that

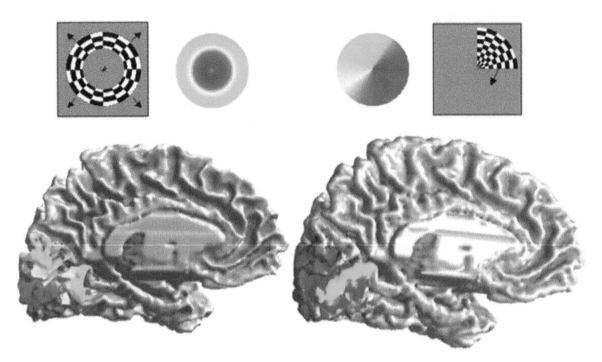

Fig. 6.1 Retinotopic maps in the early visual cortex. Two different stimuli used to delineate retinotopic maps in the human occipital lobe are expanding rings (left) and rotating wedges (right). Each stimulus traverses the visual field repeatedly while brain activity is measured using fMRI. Analysis allows each point on the cortical surface that responds to the visual stimuli to be labelled according to the location in the visual field that when stimulated produces the maximal activation. When the colour labels correspond to visual field eccentricity (left panels) or phase/angle (right panels), two different types of macroscopic organization are visible. On the left, regions responding to more central portions of the visual field are located more posteriorly; while on the right, a pattern of stripes orthogonal to the organization shown in the right panels illustrates a series of visual field representations that when analysed more closely correspond to the organization shown in Fig. 6.2.
Reproduced from *J Vis*. 3(10), Dougherty RF *et al*. Visual field representations and locations of visual areas V1/2/3 in human visual cortex, pp. 586–98, Copyright (2003), with permission from the Association for Research in Vision and Ophthalmology.

representations of the central retina (visual field) are expanded relative to those of the more peripheral retina (visual field).

The elegance of this log-polar transformation in accounting for the topographic cortical representations in human visual cortex is evident when inspecting such retinotopic maps (Fig. 6.1). A variety of visualization methods have been developed in the last 25 years that computationally separate the grey and white matter, and often make responses from sulcal regions visible by computationally 'inflating' or 'flattening' representations of the cortical surface (see Fig. 6.4). By examining the activations produced by retinotopic mapping using functional MRI on such surface representations, the topographic relationship between visual field stimulation and the locations that respond on the cortical surface becomes apparent. In particular, examining the angle (phase) component of retinotopic maps reveals a stripey pattern on the medial occipital cortex whereby representations of the horizontal and vertical meridians are arranged in parallel stripes on the cortical surface (Fig. 6.1 right-hand panel). These alternating bands correspond to the borders between what are now known to be multiple retinotopic maps whose representations lie alongside each other in the occipital lobe.

A complementary organizational principle is revealed when examining the eccentricity map, where stripes at right angles to the angle (phase) map show that there is a gradient of representations of eccentricity (Fig. 6.1 left-hand panel), with more central regions of the visual field being represented more posteriorly in the retinotopic map and more peripheral regions anteriorly.

Organization of retinotopic maps in human early visual cortex

This organization of the early visual cortex has now been repeatedly confirmed and is summarized in Fig. 6.2 (also see Fig. 6.6). A complete representation of the visual field is contained within the primary visual cortex or V1, which is consistently located in the depths of the calcarine sulcus extending superiorly and anteriorly onto the medial surface of the occipital lobe, and posteriorly to the occipital pole. Its boundaries superiorly and inferiorly are representations of the vertical meridian; the lower vertical meridian lies superiorly and represents the boundary between V1 and dorsal V2. Inferiorly the upper vertical meridian lies between V1 and ventral V2. V2 therefore contains a complete representation of the contralateral visual field, but split between an anatomically dorsal portion (representing the contralateral lower visual quadrant) and a ventral portion (representing the contralateral upper visual quadrant). Similarly V3 is also split into dorsal and ventral portions, so V1–V3 form a concentric arrangement in occipital cortex.

This organization elegantly complements and accounts for previous clinical observations and deductions of cortical anatomy from those observations. For example, the split representation of V2 and V3 can account for the clinical observation that homonymous quadrantic field defects arising from cortical lesions can have sharp horizontal edges. Although it was thought initially that such field defects might arise from lesions to primary visual cortex in the calcarine sulcus, this appeared inconsistent with the often irregular

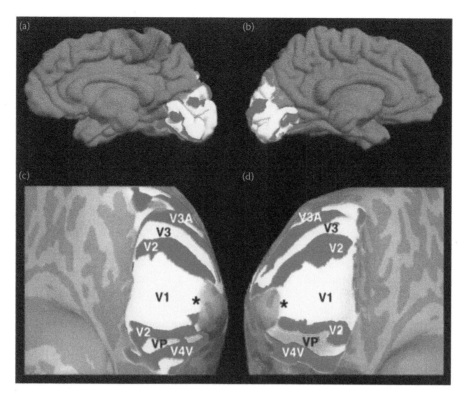

Fig. 6.2 Topography of human primary visual cortex and surrounding areas. The functional anatomy of early visual areas is overlaid on an anatomical MRI image from a single participant for right and left hemispheres respectively. Panels (a) and (b) show occipital cortex from right and left hemispheres; panels (c) and (d) present the same data in a cortically 'inflated' view and from a posterior vantage point. Human brain areas revealed by retinotopic mapping are displayed in false (blue/yellow) colour and labelled. A concentric arrangement of V1, V2, and V3 is apparent.

Reproduced from *Proc Natl Acad Sci USA*. 95(3), Tootell RBH, Hadjikhani NK, Vanduffell W, *et al*. Functional analysis of primary visual cortex (V1) in humans, pp. 811–17, Copyright (1998), with permission from PNAS.

borders of cortical lesions because the representation of the horizontal meridian runs along the depths of the calcarine sulcus, and in order to produce a sharp edge to the field defect the lesion would need to run exactly along such a boundary. But the split representation of V2/V3 provides an elegant answer to this conundrum, as proposed by Horton and Hoyt.[9] Specifically, even if a lesion has irregular boundaries, if it is located in V2/3 and crosses the boundary of the horizontal meridian between V3 and V2 or V2 and V1, then it will produce a quadrantic field defect because of the split representation of the upper and lower visual fields in V2 and V3. Thus the retinotopic organization of early human visual cortices has localizing power for clinical practice.

Damage to the early visual cortex generally results in a visual field defect. Profound bilateral cortical damage such as that caused by bilateral cerebral infarction in the territory of the posterior cerebral arteries can also cause Anton's syndrome, albeit rarely.[10] Patients with Anton's syndrome have no functional vision and sometimes cannot even distinguish light and dark; they have normal pupillary responses to light. However, despite being profoundly cortically blind, strikingly they deny having any visual difficulty. Anton's syndrome is therefore an anosognosia. A variety of explanations have been advanced but without a clear consensus on the underlying mechanisms.[11] Typically the cortical damage associated with Anton's syndrome involves early (retinotopic) visual cortices bilaterally. However, the syndrome has also been described following bilateral optic nerve damage and frontal contusions,[12] so can also be caused by peripheral lesions to the early visual system.

Retinotopic mapping has further revealed a multiplicity of visual maps in humans, extending throughout occipital cortex. In contrast to the V1—V3 retinotopic maps, the precise number, extent, and organization of such maps remains a topic of debate (see reference13 for a review). These may include areas known as hV4, VO-1, and VO-2 on the ventral occipital surface next to the ventral portion of V3; maps that have been labelled LO-1, LO-2, TO-1, and TO-2 on the lateral occipital surface that are coextensive with object-selective cortices discussed below; and V3A/V3B on the dorsal surface plus further maps running into parietal cortex (see reference 14 for a review).

Technically these maps are often much smaller and their responses harder to measure, so their precise functional properties and exact characterization remain often controversial. Nevertheless, the sheer multiplicity of maps in the human occipital lobe suggests that they must be important for visual processing, but a demonstration that such a topographic organization is critical for normal visual function remains elusive. Clinically, neurodevelopmental disorders that massively disrupt topographic visual field maps such as albinism[15] or failure of development of the optic chasm (see e.g. reference 16) have relatively little effect on spatial vision. Finally, position in the visual field is not the only feature that is mapped on the cortical surface. Consistent with observations in monkeys, it appears that ocular dominance and orientation[17] can be mapped on the occipital cortical surface though the spatial scale of such mapping is sufficiently fine that measurement with contemporary neuroimaging remains challenging.

Functional segregation in the human occipital lobe

Alongside the use of non-invasive brain imaging to delineate spatial maps in the occipital lobe has come parallel investigation of whether different areas of the occipital lobe respond differentially to the many features that make up a visual scene. Early clinical investigators such as Holmes' suggested that selective disturbances of motion perception could not be distinguished from more general disorders of the perception of objects and that purely cortical lesions did not cause loss of colour vision.[18] Subsequent clinical observations showed that selective disturbances of colour[19] and motion[20] could result from focal damage to the occipital lobe.

In humans, these observations following brain damage were complemented by pioneering work using positron emission tomography to visualize changes in blood flow associated with neural activity during perception of different visual features (Fig. 6.3). This demonstrated an area of extrastriate cortex on the lateral surface of the occipital lobe close to the boundary with the temporal lobe that responded more strongly to moving than stationary stimuli.[21] This area is now known as V5/MT, reflecting its apparent homology with similar motion-responsive regions in monkey. A second region on the ventral surface of the occipital lobe responded more to coloured patterns than to matched grayscale patterns, considered to be consistent with a colour-responsive region in monkey cortex known as area V4.[22]

These early observations demonstrated the principle of functional specialization in the extrastriate visual cortex; different cortical regions process different aspects of the visual scene. Such functionally specialized areas, when damaged, give rise to corresponding clinical deficits in, for example, colour or motion perception. Further investigation has revealed that some of these functionally specialized regions also contain spatial maps. For example, the colour-responsive region in the ventral visual cortex has retinotopic organization[23] although the precise nature of that organization has remained a topic of vigorous debate. Similarly the

motion-responsive region V5/MT, although smaller, also appears to contain visual field maps (e.g. see reference 24).

Functional specialization is not restricted to simple features of visual scenes such as colour and motion, and subsequent investigation has revealed specialization for the categories of visual objects (see reference 25 for a review and Fig. 6.4 for a summary). Anterior and lateral to early retinotopic cortices lie areas that respond more strongly when healthy humans view pictures of objects compared to scrambled objects or textures.[26] Such object-selective areas are particularly centred in lateral occipital cortex (LOC) where a large area demonstrates relatively non-specific responses to all types of objects. Damage focused on this region, such as that seen in patient DF,[27] can be associated with visual agnosia. Also, close to area V5/MT is a cortical region whose responses show selectivity for visually presented body parts.[28] This 'extrastriate body area' appears to play a causal role in perceiving people in real-world scenes, as transient inactivation of the area with transcranial magnetic stimulation causes impairments in tasks that require identification of people (compared to cars) in visually presented scenes.[29]

In contrast, more ventrally in occipital (and occipito-temporal) cortex lie regions that appear to be selective for particularly types of object such as faces[30] or houses and scenes of particular places. Similarly, damage to this region is associated with difficulties in discriminating the spatial configuration of different elements of a face,[32] as well as the association of prosopagnosia with more medial temporo-occipital lesions close to regions also showing face-selective responses. There are also more dorsal object-selective regions along the transverse occipital sulcus thought to be involved in the context of grasping and object manipulation whose functional role is less well understood (e.g. see reference 33). Selectivity of this kind for visual responses appears to be remarkably robust. Even following bilateral destruction of primary visual cortices (and accompanying cortical blindness), some measure of selective responses to faces and body parts remains in different cortical regions.[34] This indicates that the inputs from which such selectivity derive come not just from early retinotopic visual cortices but also from subcortical pathways.

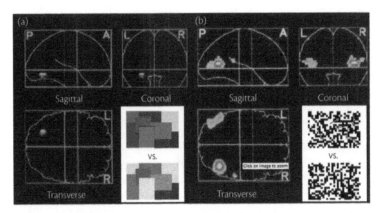

Fig. 6.3 Functional specialization. Responses to moving and coloured stimuli, relative to control stimuli that lack motion or colour, produce distinct spatial patterns of activation in occipital cortex. (a) Activity in the brain measured using PET when participants view a coloured Mondrian (inset) compared to a grey Mondrian is seen on the left ventral occipital surface. Activated regions are projected onto a 'glass brain' in sagittal, coronal, and tranverse sections. (b) Similar plotting conventions are used to display regions in lateral occipital cortex that respond more strongly when participants view moving random dots compared to static dots. Note that earlier visual cortical areas (see Fig. 6.2) are not activated in these comparisons because they respond roughly equally to both moving and static dots, thus indicating the selectivity of visual areas later in the anatomical hierarchy.

Adapted from *J Neurosci.* 11(3), Zeki S, Watson JD, Lueck CJ, *et al.* A direct demonstration of functional specialization in human visual cortex, pp. 641–9, Copyright (1991), with permission from the Society for Neuroscience.

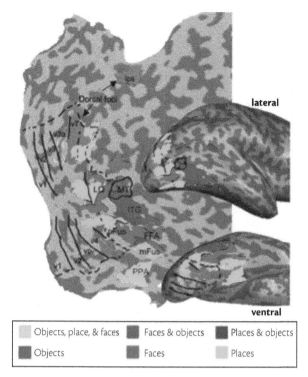

lateral

ventral

Objects, place, & faces	Faces & objects	Places & objects
Objects	Faces	Places

Fig. 6.4 Object-selective areas in the human occipital lobe. This figure summarizes a number of different studies that have used functional MRI to describe different areas in human occipital cortex and adjoining areas that respond selectively to different types of objects. The colour code indicates the type of object that an area responds to and the colours are overlaid on either computationally 'inflated' lateral or ventral views of the left hemisphere, or a left hemisphere that has been computationally 'cut' and 'flattened'. The early visual areas V1–V3 (see Fig. 6.2 and text) are not selective for particular objects or object classes, but the lateral occipital (LO) area is selective for objects, the fusiform face area (FFA) for faces, and the parahippocampal place area (PPA) for places.
Reproduced from *Annu Rev Neurosci*. 27, Grill-Spector K and Malach R, The human visual cortex, pp. 649–77, Copyright (2004), with permission from Annual Reviews.

Organizational principles of occipital cortex

We have already seen that there are two dominant features of the functional organization of the occipital cortex in humans that correspond to clinical observations following occipital damage. The first is functional specialization; different areas process different aspects of the visual scene, and so focal cortical damage can produce remarkably specific deficits in visual perception as well as more general disorders of object vision such as agnosia. The second is that most occipital regions contain a multiplicity of topographic maps of the visual field, and even functionally specialized regions are often also topographically mapped. Thus focal damage, particular to early cortical regions V1–V3, produces visual deficits that are mapped to the corresponding region of the visual field, but are there any more general organizing principles that govern the relationship between all these visual field maps and functionally specialized areas?

The patterns of anatomical connectivity between different regions have been proposed as one way to uncover organizational principles, in particular distinguishing between feed-forward and feed-back connections established through anatomical fibre tracing in monkeys. This suggested a hierarchical organization of visual cortex based on anatomy (see reference 35; Fig. 6.5). One

influential framework proposes that visual cortical areas within this anatomical hierarchy are segregated into *dorsal and ventral processing streams*.[36]

Ungerleider and Mishkin observed that lesions to inferotemporal cortex in monkey led to deficits in their ability to distinguish between different visual objects on the basis of their appearance, but did not affect their performance on a task that required knowledge only of the spatial locations of different objects. Conversely, posterior parietal cortex lesions produced deficits in tasks requiring knowledge of spatial relations but not on visual discrimination tasks. They thus proposed that the anatomical distinction between dorsal and ventral streams is mirrored in a simple distinction between spatial and object vision—'where' and 'what' respectively (Fig. 6.6).

The simple distinction that Ungerleider and Mishkin made between 'what' and 'where' has become progressively more complicated as clinical syndromes have been more fully considered. For example, damage to the human parietal cortex can lead to optic ataxia where patients have difficulty reaching and grasping objects placed in the contralateral visual field. However, such patients also have difficulties with aspects of vision less obviously spatial, such as the size and shape of objects they are able to grasp correctly.[37] This, and other observations, has led to proposals[38] that the functional distinction between dorsal and ventral streams may reflect a subtler distinction between a system that uses visual information for skilled action ('vision for action'—the dorsal stream) and 'vision-for-perception' (ventral stream). More broadly, it is recognized that even with such functional distinctions, coordinated and goal-directed action requires the integrated operation of both streams.

Such schemes have proven very useful heuristically in terms of understanding and integrating a large amount of neuroscientific data on the occipital lobe, but in isolation they cannot always tell the whole story. For example, while an anatomical hierarchy is apparent,[35] it is equally clear that signals from the retina reach different points in the anatomical hierarchy and at different times, which do not always correspond.[39] Thus some areas 'higher' in the proposed anatomical hierarchy might receive signals earlier than other areas apparently 'lower' in the hierarchy. In the context of a highly dynamic system where signals associated with visual perception pass backwards and forwards,[40] the idea of a simple linear progression of stages of the analysis of a visual scene is likely to be an oversimplification.

Comparisons between humans and other species

The existence of visually responsive areas in the occipital lobe of non-human primates has been known for over a century,[1] and pioneering work using single unit electrophysiology (see e.g. reference 41) delineated many of the principles of functional specialization at the level of single neurons that have subsequently been elaborated and elucidated using functional imaging techniques in humans. Combining electrophysiology with other tools including cytoarchitectural and anatomical connectivity analyses has led to the parcellation of extra striate cortex in non-human primate into a number of different visual areas. More recently it has been possible to use functional MRI (fMRI) methods in both humans and non-human primates to compare the organization of visual maps (see e.g. reference 42) and functionally specialized regions (e.g. reference 43).

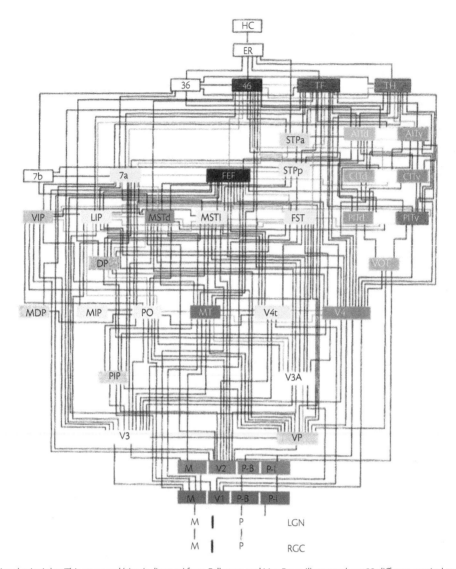

Fig. 6.5 Possible organizational principles. This proposed 'circuit diagram' from Felleman and Van Essen illustrates how 32 different cortical areas responding to visual stimulation in the macaque are connected anatomically, and sets out a proposed hierarchy of areas.

Reproduced from *Cereb Cortex.* 1(1), Felleman DJ and Van Essen DC, Distributed hierarchical processing in the primate cerebral cortex, pp. 1–47, Copyright (1991), with permission from Oxford University Press.

While there are strong similarities across species, it has also become increasingly apparent that there are important differences. For example, topographic maps in humans are substantially larger than in macaque; and homology of areas beyond V1–V3 and V5/MT is significantly more difficult to establish with clarity.

Cytoarchitecture of human occipital cortex

This chapter has focused on relatively macroscopic measurements of occipital lobe structure and function, and how they correspond to clinicopathological syndromes following brain damage. However, it has also been known for over a century that the detailed histological structure—the cytoarchitecture and myeloarchitecture—of the human brain differs across the cortical surface. This led to the publication of classic cytoarchitectonic maps of the human cerebral cortex (e.g. reference 44), and in particular the distinction between striate and extra striate cortex touched upon above. More recently there has been substantial progress in the computerized image

analysis of histological specimens and the introduction of markers that reflect different architectonic aspects of cortical organization (such as receptor autoradiography). Together with developments in image analysis techniques that allow for inter-subject variability in macroscopic anatomy, this has enabled new insights into the detailed structure of human visual cortex.[45] For example, probabilistic cytoarchitectonic maps are now available of occipital cortex.[46] Signals obtained from structural MRI sequences, including high-resolution MRI, reflect the myeloarchitecture and cytoarchitecture found in histological sections (e.g. reference 47) which has led to renewed interest in using structural MRI to identify specific regions of human visual cortex such as V5/MT (e.g. reference 48).

Individual variability in human occipital cortex anatomy

Most investigations of the occipital lobe focus on the commonalities in structure and function across individuals and how these

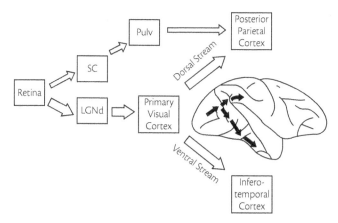

Fig. 6.6 Schematic illustration of how visual signals from the retina reach dorsal and ventral processing streams. The dorsal and ventral pathways are schematically illustrated on an outline of a macaque monkey brain, but the organizational principles are broadly consistent in humans. The broad functional distinction between dorsal and ventral streams may reflect the use of visual information for action (dorsal stream) or perception (ventral stream) but goal-directed action usually requires the coordinated action of both streams.
Reproduced from Goodale M and Milner D, *The Visual Brain in Action*, Copyright (1995), with permission from Oxford University Press.

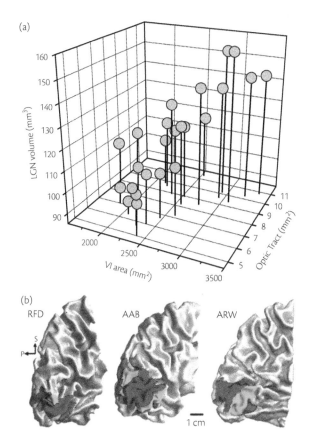

Fig. 6.7 Individual variability. (a) Each point represents data from a single post-mortem human. There is correlated variability in the surface area of the primary visual cortex (V1), the volume of the lateral geniculate nucleus and the surface area of the optic tract. Note the variation of almost twofold in the surface area of primary visual cortex across individuals. (b) Three example right hemispheres in which the central 2–12 degrees of the visual field representation in V1–V3 have been mapped. While in each individual the macroscopic concentric organization of V1–V3 demonstrated in Fig. 6.2 is apparent, there is also substantial individual variability in the surface area of V1 (magenta), V2 (cyan), and V3 (red).
(a) Reproduced from *J Neurosci*. 17(8), Andrews TJ *et al.* Correlated size variations in human visual cortex, lateral geniculate nucleus, and optic tract, pp. 2859–68, Copyright (1997), with permission from the Society for Neuroscience. (b) Reproduced from *J Vision*. 3(10), Dougherty *et al.* Visual field representations and locations of visual areas V1/2/3 in human visual cortex, pp. 586–98, Copyright (2003), with permission from the Association for Research in Vision and Ophthalmology.

differ following brain damage, but it has long been noted informally that the precise sulcal and gyral anatomy can vary somewhat across individuals [e.g. Fig. 6.7]. For example, while there are regularities, such as the position of the calcarine sulcus running anteriorly from the occipital pole, the precise direction and shape of the sulcus varies across individuals (e.g. reference 49). Similarly, at a histological level, the architectonic features that delineate striate (primary) visual cortex extend for a variable distance above and below the calcarine sulcus, presumably accounting for the variability that can be observed macroscopically in non-invasive estimates of the spatial extent of primary visual cortex [Fig. 6.7].

Indeed, in normal human subjects the range of interindividual variation in V1 area is approximately threefold.[50] Importantly, this variability in V1 area in humans is correlated with the cross-sectional area of the optic tract and the volumes of the magnocellular and parvocellular layers of the lateral geniculate nucleus (reference 51; Fig. 6.7). This coordinated variation indicates that development of the different parts of the human visual system are interdependent. Notably, the range of variability in the size of these visual system components is substantially greater than the variability of the overall size of the human brain, which is about 30 per cent.[52] It has been suggested that such coordinated variation in size might be associated with differences in visual ability across individuals, and this has recently become the focus of renewed investigation (see reference 53 for a review).

One recent investigation studied how variability in cortical magnification and overall size of V1 was related to fine visual acuity. Individuals with a larger overall cortical area in V1 had lower overall Vernier acuity thresholds; they were able to make finer perceptual judgements.[54] This relationship between objective measures of visual perception and individual differences in visual cortex size extends also to the subjective qualities of visual perception. Although it is difficult to compare the subjective visual experiences of different people directly, inter-individual differences in the perceived strength of a perceptual illusion—whereby physically

identical stimuli produce perceptually different appearances depending on their local context—can be quantitatively compared. In a study that compared individuals' susceptibility to geometrical visual illusions (the Ponzo and Ebbinghaus illusions), just such variability in illusion strength was found.[55] Moreover, the strength of the illusion correlated negatively with the size of early retinotopic visual area V1, but not visual area V2 and visual area V3.

Summary

The fundamental organization and the macroscopic anatomy that gives rise to clinicopathological correlations between brain damage and visual behaviour have been known in outline for over a century. However, recent advances in brain imaging technology and the ability to integrate information from many different sources has led to dramatic advances in our understanding of the relationship between structure and function in the human visual system. This in turn clarifies the anatomical basis for many clinical syndromes but also lays the foundation for a mechanistic understanding of the relationship between structure, function, and the effects of damage to the human visual system.

References

1. Munk H. *Über die Functionen der Grosshirnrinde.* Hirschwald, Berlin, 1881.
2. Henschen S. *Klinische und Anatomische Beiträge zur Pathologie des Gehirns* (Pt 1). Almquist & Wiksell, Upsala, 1890.
3. Inouye T. (1909) Die Sehstörungen bei Schssverletzungen der Kortikalen Sehsphäre nach Beobachtungen an Verwundeten der Letzten Japanischen Kriege, W. Engelmann (English trans.); visual disturbances following gunshot wounds of the cortical visual area. *Brain (Suppl).* 2000;123.
4. Holmes G and Lister WT (1916) Disturbances of vision from cerebral lesions, with special reference to the cortical representation of the macula. *Brain.* 1916;39:34–73.
5. Belliveau JW, Kennedy DN Jr, McKinstry RC, *et al.* Functional mapping of the human visual cortex by magnetic resonance imaging. *Science.* 1991;254(5032):716–9.
6. DeYoe EA, Carman GJ, Bandettini P, *et al.* Mapping striate and extrastriate visual areas in human cerebral cortex. *Proc Natl Acad Sci USA.* 1996;93:2382–6.
7. Engel SA, Rumelhart DE, Wandell BA, *et al.* fMRI of human visual cortex. *Nature.* 1994;369:525.
8. Sereno MI, Dale AM, Reppas JB, *et al.* Borders of multiple visual areas in humans revealed by functional magnetic resonance imaging. *Science.* 1995;268:889–93.
9. Horton JC and Hoyt WF. Quadrantic visual field defects. A hallmark of lesions in extrastriate (V2/V3) cortex. *Brain.* 1991;114 (Pt 4):1703–18.
10. Anton G. Herderkrankungen des Gehirnes, welche vom Patienten selbst nicht wahrgenommen werden. *Wiener klinische Wochenschrift.* 1898;11;227–9.
11. Prigatano G and Schacter DL (eds). *Awareness of Deficit after Brain Injury.* Oxford: Oxford University Press, 1991.
12. McDaniel KDK and McDaniel LD. Anton's Syndrome in a Patient With Posttraumatic Optic Neuropathy and Bifrontal Contusions *Arch Neurol.* 1991;48(1):101–05. doi:10.1001/archneur.1991.00530130113028.
13. Wandell BA and Winawer J. Imaging retinotopic maps in the human brain. *Vision Res.* 2011;51(7):718–37. doi:10.1016/j.visres.2010.08.004. Epub 6 August 2010.
14. Sereno MI and Huang RS. Multisensory maps in parietal cortex. *Curr Opin Neurobiol.* 2014;24(1):39–46. doi:10.1016/j.conb.2013.08.014.
15. Hoffmann MB, Tolhurst DJ, Moore AT, *et al.* Organization of the visual cortex in human albinism. *J Neurosci.* 2003;23(26):8921–30.
16. Victor JD, Apkarian P, Hirsch J, *et al.* Visual function and brain organization in non-decussating retinal-fugal fibre syndrome. *Cereb Cortex.* 2000;10(1):2–22.
17. Yacoub E, Harel N, and Ugurbil K. High-field fMRI unveils orientation columns in humans. *Proc Natl Acad Sci USA.* 2008;105(30):10607–12. doi:10.1073/pnas.0804110105. Epub 18 July 2008.
18. McDonald I. Gordon Holmes and the neurological heritage. *Brain.* 2006;130(1), 288–98.
19. Meadows JC. Disturbed perception of colours associated with localised cerebral lesions. *Brain.* 1974;97:615–32.
20. Zihl J, von Cramon D, and Mai N. Selective disturbance of movement vision after bilateral brain damage. *Brain.* 1983;106:313–40.
21. Lueck CJ, Zeki S, Friston KJ, *et al.* The colour centre in the cerebral cortex of man. *Nature.* 1989;340(6232):386:3863.
22. Zeki SM, Watson JD, Lueck CJ, *et al.* A direct demonstration of functional specialization in human visual cortex. *J Neurosci.* 1991;11(3):641–9.
23. McKeefry DJ and Zeki S. The position and topography of the human colour centre as revealed by functional magnetic resonance imaging. *Brain.* 1997;120(12): 2229–42.
24. Amano K, Wandell BA, and Dumoulin SO. Visual field maps, population receptive field sizes, and visual field coverage in the human MT+ complex. *J Neurophysiol.* 2009;102(5):2704–18.
25. Grill-Spector K and Malach R. The human visual cortex. *Annu Rev Neurosci.* 2004;27:649–77.
26. Malach R, Reppas JB, Benson RR, *et al.* Object-related activity revealed by functional magnetic resonance imaging in human occipital cortex. *Proc Natl Acad Sci USA.* 1995 Aug 29;92(18):8135–9.
27. Bridge H, Thomas OM, Minini L, *et al.* Structural and Functional Changes across the Visual Cortex of a Patient with Visual Form Agnosia. *J Neurosci.* 2013;33(31):12779–91.
28. Downing PE, Jiang Y, Shuman M, *et al.* A cortical area selective for visual processing of the human body. *Science* 2001;293:2470–3.
29. van Koningsbruggen MG, Peelen MV, and Downing PE. A causal role for the extrastriate body area in detecting people in real-world scenes. *J Neurosci.* 2013;17;33(16):7003–10.
30. Kanwisher N, McDermott J, and Chun MM. The fusiform face area: A module in human extrastriate cortex specialized for face perception. *J Neurosci.* 1997 Jun 1;17(11):4302–11.
31. Epstein R, Harris A, Stanley D, *et al.* The parahippocampal place area: Recognition, navigation, or encoding? *Neuron.* 1999 May;23(1):115–25.
32. Barton JJ, Press DZ, Keenan JP, *et al.* Lesions of the fusiform face area impair perception of facial configuration in prosopagnosia. *Neurology.* 2002 Jan 8;58(1):71–8.
33. Culham JC and Valyear KF. Human parietal cortex in action. *Curr Opin Neurobiol.* 2006 16(2):205–12.
34. Van den Stock J, Tamietto M, Zhan M, *et al.* Neural correlates of body and face perception following bilateral destruction of the primary visual cortices. *Front Behav Neurosci.* 2014 Feb 13;8:30. doi:10.3389/fnbeh.2014.00030. eCollection 2014.
35. Felleman DJ and Van Essen DC. Distributed hierarchical processing in the primate cerebral cortex. *Cereb Cortex.* 1991;1(1):1–47.
36. Ungerleider LG and Mishkin M. Two Cortical Visual Systems. In: MA Goodale and AD Milner (eds). *The Analysis of Visual Behavior.* Cambridge: Cambridge University Pess, 1982, pp. 549–86.
37. Perenin M -T and Vighetto A. Optic ataxia: A specific disruption in visuomotor mechanisms. 1. Different aspects of the deficit in reaching for objects. *Brain.* 1988;111:643–74.
38. Goodale MA and Milner AD. Separate visual pathways for perception and action. *Trends Neurosci.* 1992;15(1):20–5.
39. Schmolesky MT, Wang Y, Hanes DP, *et al.* Signal timing Across the Macaque Visual System. *J Neurophysiol.* 1988;79:3272–8.
40. Lamme VAF and Roelfsema PR. The distinct modes of vision offered by feed-forward and recurrent progressing. *Trends Neurosci.* 2000;23(11):571–9.
41. Hubel DH and Wiesel TN. Functional architecture of macaque visual cortex. *Proc. Roy Soc Ser B.* 1977;198:1–59.
42. Brewer AA, Press WA, Logothetis NK, *et al.* Visual areas in macaque cortex measured using functional magnetic resonance imaging. *J Neurosci.* 2002;22(23):10416–26.
43. Tsao DY, Freiwald WA, Tootell RB, *et al.* A cortical region consisting entirely of face-selective cells. *Science.* 2006;311(5761):670–4.
44. Brodmann K. Vegleichende Lokalisationslehre der Grosshirnde. Leipzig: Barth, 1909.
45. Amunts K, Schleicher A, and Zilles K. Cytoarchitecture of the cerebral cortex—More than localisation. *Neuroimage.* 2007;37:1061–5.
46. Amunts K, Malikovic A, Mohlberg H, *et al.* Brodmann's areas 17 and 18 brought into stereotaxic space Where and how variable? *Neuroimage.* 2000;11:66–84.
47. Eickhoff S, Walters NB, Schleicher A, *et al.* High-resolution MRI reflects myeloarchitecture and cytoarchitecture of human cerebral cortex. *Hum Brain Mapp.* 2005;24(3):206–15.

48. Walters NB, Egan GF, Kril JJ, *et al*. In vivo identification of human cortical areas using high-resolution MRI: an approach to cerebral structure-function correlation. *Proc Natl Acad Sci USA*. 2003;100(5):2981–6. Epub 24 February 2003.

49. Iaria G and Petrides M. Occipital sulci of the human brain: variability and probability maps. *Journ Comp Neurol*. 2007;501:243–59.

50. Stensaas SS, Eddington DK, and Dobelle WH. The topography and variability of the primary visual cortex in man. *J Neurosurg*. 1974;40:747–55.

51. Andrews TJ, Halpern SD, and Purves D. Correlated Size Variations in Human Visual Cortex, Lateral Geniculate Nucleus and Optic Tract. *J Neurosci*. 1997;17(8), 2859–68.

52. Boyd R. Tables of the weights of the human body and internal organs in the sane and insane of both sexes at various ages arranged from 2614 post-mortem examinations. *Philos Trans*. 1861;1:249–53.

53. Kanai R and Rees G. The structural basis of inter-individual differences in human behaviour and cognition. *Nature Neurosci*. 2011;12:231–42.

54. Duncan RO and Boynton GM. Cortical Magnification within Human Primary Visual Cortex Correlates with Acuity Thresholds. *Neuron*. 2003;38:659–71.

55. Schwarzkopf DS, Song C, and Rees G. The surface area of human V1 predicts the subjective experience of object size. *Nature Neurosci*. 2011;14:28–30.

CHAPTER 7

The basal ganglia in cognitive disorders

James Rowe and Timothy Rittman

Introduction

The basal ganglia are a vital set of forebrain nuclei, richly connected with the cortex, thalamus, and brainstem. As one of the oldest parts of the brain in evolutionary terms, it is not surprising that neurological disease affecting the basal ganglia has severe consequences for behaviour and cognition. In this chapter, we review the principles underlying the anatomy and connectivity of the basal ganglia because they illuminate the myriad clinical features of basal ganglia dysfunction across a broad range of disorders.

Thomas Willis is credited with the first description of the 'corpora striata' in 1664, correctly identifying their role in movement but also suggesting they receive sensory information. A century ago, Kinnier Wilson suggested that the basal ganglia were mainly concerned with inhibiting signals from the motor cortex.[1] Further work suggested the basal ganglia act as a 'funnel' for messages from motor association cortex, integrating information for delivery via the ventrolateral thalamus to motor cortex.[2] The idea that the basal ganglia were primarily concerned with motor function remained largely unchallenged until the 1980s. This motor chauvinism was reinforced by the false impression that significant cognitive impairment was uncommon in Parkinson's disease, whereas it is now recognized as a common and early feature of the disease.[3]

The basal ganglia are central to the understanding and treatment of many cognitive disorders, some of which are associated with movement disorders (e.g. akinetic rigidity, tremor, dystonia, and chorea). The separation of cognitive and movement disorders is artificial but still common in didactic teaching of neurology and neuroscience, contrary to the clinical evidence and functional anatomy of the basal ganglia. For example, dementias such as frontotemporal dementia (FTD) and dementia with Lewy bodies (DLB) are often associated with extrapyramidal motor dysfunction, and many diseases cause a syndrome in which cognitive and motor deficits have similar weighting, such as Huntington's disease (HD), progressive supranuclear palsy (PSP), corticobasal degeneration (CBD), neurodegeneration with brain iron accumulation, paediatric autoimmune neurological disorders associated with streptococci and encephalitis lethargica. Psychiatric disorders of addiction, obsessive–compulsive disorders and impulsivity are also associated with basal ganglia dysfunction and cognitive abnormalities, but lie outside the scope of this chapter.

The diversity of clinical disorders and cognitive functions associated with the basal ganglia reflects their unique functional anatomy and neurochemistry. We will first review the normal gross anatomy of the basal ganglia, and examine how this supports both *integration* and *segregation* of cognitive processes. We then consider the neurochemical organization and connectivity of the basal ganglia. Finally, we show how the basal ganglia contribute to cognitive disorders, revealed by neuropsychology, and structural and functional brain imaging.

Macroscopic anatomy

The macroscopic organization of the basal ganglia is intimately connected with that of the cortex and thalamus. The principal input nucleus is the striatum, comprising the caudate and putamen (see Fig. 7.1), but the subthalamic nucleus also receives direct cortical inputs. The striatum projects to the globus pallidus (also called the pallidum) which has two parts: internal and external. The substantia nigra and the subthalamic nuclei are smaller but critical nuclei in the basal ganglia complex. The inputs, connections, and outputs of these basal ganglia nuclei are arranged in a series of cortico-striato-thalamo-cortical loops, with gross structural homologies (Fig. 7.2). Studies injecting tracers, for example in premotor regions, first suggested a cognitive role for the basal ganglia by revealing connections from the pallidum via the thalamus to premotor cortex.[4,5] These connections were reciprocal, in a closed-loop system that could facilitate feedback from the basal ganglia to association cortex.[6] Further closed-loop systems were identified, suggestive of distinct motor, oculomotor, cognitive, and limbic functions.

At first glance, these loops suggest separate *parallel processing* of information by subdomains of the basal ganglia (Fig. 7.2). For example, the ventral striatum receives input from the orbital and medial prefrontal cortex and anterior cingulate. This loop is closely associated with reward, motivation, and reinforcement in a limbic system, with the clinical counterparts of apathy, learning deficits, addiction, and cognitive inflexibility. In contrast, the central regions of the striatum receive their main input from dorsolateral prefrontal cortex, forming a loop that has been linked to associative and executive functions underlying adaptive behaviours (e.g. planning, set-shifting, and working memory). Topographical mapping in the caudate preserves the differences between projections from, for example, dorsolateral cortical prefrontal areas 9, 46, and supplementary eye fields. The dorsal components form a further loop with inputs from premotor and motor cortex, and are most closely associated with motor control and action selection. The early dysexecutive syndrome in Parkinson's disease[3,7] is likely to reflect dysfunction of this associative (cognitive) loop.

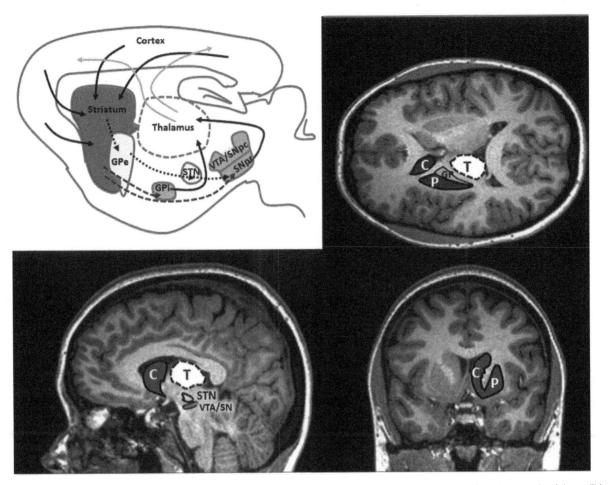

Fig. 7.1 The top left panel illustrates the relative size and position of the principal basal ganglia in the rat, connecting cortex via the striatum to the globus pallidus (with external part, Gpe, and internal part, GPi), subthalamic nucleus (STN), and substantia nigra pars reticulata (SNpr) and thalamus (T). Dopaminergic innervation of the striatum is from the ventral tegmental area (VTA) and substantia nigra pars compacta (SNpc). The other three panels illustrate the equivalent structures in an adult human brain on a structural magnetic resonance image in axial, saggital, and coronal sections and distinguishing the caudate (C) and putamen (P) that make up the striatum.

Human structural and functional neuroimaging confirms this functional anatomy. For example, diffusion-weighted magnetic resonance imaging (MRI) with tractography identifies the major corticostriatal pathways,[8] with limbic, associative, and motor pathways between cortex, striatum, and substantia nigra (and the adjacent ventral tegmental area of dopaminergic neurons). In addition, meta-analysis of PET imaging identifies analogous functional loops.[9] More recently, detailed analysis for the functional connectivity patterns of individual basal ganglia structures has been possible using seed-based connectivity in functional MRI scans.[10]

Despite the apparent parallel organization of these loops, they are not wholly segregated. Indeed, it is *a priori* necessary for limbic, associative, and motor systems to interact to enable goal-directed behaviours that develop or adapt appropriate responses, essential for tasks such as rule learning.

A revised model of basal ganglia function has been developed that proposes multiple mechanisms of *interaction* (Fig. 7.3). First, the axonal projections from cortex to the striatum can cross between limbic and associative areas, or between associative and motor areas, facilitating cross-talk between systems. Thus, the general topography outlined above has soft boundaries. In addition, adjacent cortical areas project on to smaller and partially overlapping basal ganglia regions so that there is approximately a ten-to-one reduction in the number of neurons receiving input in the basal ganglia. The onward projections back to the cortex terminate in wide terminal fields suggesting important processing and integration of information as it flows through the basal ganglia. Finally, the reciprocal connections between basal ganglia structures are not symmetric.[11] This asymmetry promotes a directional flow from limbic to associative to motor regions. Together, these mechanisms enable both segregation and integration of cognitive, motor, sensory, and affective information as it passes through the basal ganglia.

Connectivity within the basal ganglia: Direct and indirect pathways

Medium spiny neurons predominate in the striatum, making up 95 per cent of rat striatal neurons.[12] They receive the bulk of glutamatergic cortical inputs, and are the main striatal output cell, with GABAergic projections. Medium spiny neurons are densely dendritic, synapsing with other medium spiny neurons and interneurons within the striatum to create a complex internal structure. There is considerable plasticity within this densely connected network, arising from spike-timing-dependent processes that are dependent on glutamatergic NMDA receptors and the presence of dopamine receptor activation.[13]

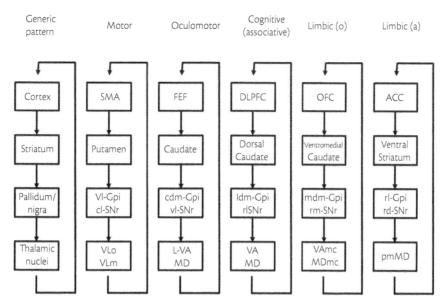

Fig. 7.2 The cortico-striato-thalamo-cortical loops follow a generic pattern (left), which is mirrored in parallel motor, oculomotor, cognitive, and limbic circuits.[4] Functional differences are related to the specific subregions of cortex, striatum, pallidum, nigra, and thalamus. Note that this model of basal ganglia connectivity emphasizes segregated information processing within each of the parallel loops. SMA, supplementary motor area; FEF, frontal eye fields; DLPFC, dorsolateral prefrontal cortex; OFC, orbitofrontal cortex; ACC, anterior cingulate cortex; Gpi, globus pallidus internal; SNr, substantia nigra pars reticulata; and thalamic nuclei including ventrolateral, VL, ventral anterior, VA, mediodorsal, MD.

Reproduced from *Prog Brain Res.*, 85, Alexander GE, Crutcher MD, DeLong MR, Basal ganglia-thalamocortical circuits: parallel substrates for motor, oculomotor, 'prefrontal' and 'limbic' functions, pp. 119–46, Copyright (1991), with permission from Elsevier.

The striatum is the main receiving centre of the basal ganglia, but it has complex projections to other parts of the basal ganglia, and on to thalamus and cortex. The 'dual circuit' model (also called the 'rate' model, or 'Albin DeLong' model: see Fig. 7.4) has been highly influential in clinical and pre-clinical analyses of basal ganglia function since the early 1990s. In this model, GABAergic outputs from the striatum form two main pathways which are associated with two types of dopaminergic neurones.

The *direct* pathway contains medium spiny neurons with predominant dopamine D1 receptors, which in response to glutamatergic cortical inputs and dopaminergic inputs from substantia nigra pars compacta (or ventral tegmental area, VTA) send inhibitory GABAergic projections directly to the globus pallidus interna and substantia nigra pars reticulata, which in turn send inhibitory connections to the thalamus.

The *indirect* pathway's medium spiny neurons have dopamine D2 receptors and send inhibitory projections to the globus pallidum externa, with onward inhibitory projections to the subthalamic nucleus. The subthalamic nucleus' projections to the globus pallidus interna and substantia nigra are excitatory. The result is antagonism between the direct and indirect pathways. In the motor loop, the direct pathway promotes movement and the indirect pathway inhibits movement, with analogous regulation of cognitive tasks in the cognitive (associative) loop and reward or punishment tasks in the limbic (affective) loop.

This dual-circuit model explains many experimental findings and clinical phenomena. For example, stimulation of D2 receptors preferentially expressed in the indirect pathway enhances activity in the external segment of the globus pallidus, inducing a net decrease in basal ganglia output. Conversely, loss of dopamine increases inhibitory output of the basal ganglia, and inhibition of thalamocortical activity. However, new anatomical, transgenic, and optogenetic investigations suggest a much more complex set of interactions within and even between the direct and indirect pathways (Fig. 7.4). It becomes once again much more difficult to predict the input–output function of the system. Moreover, recent evidence suggests coordination through transient co-activation of the direct and indirect pathways, rather than simple antagonism,[14] with heteromeric D1–D2 receptors and at best partial separation of D1 and D2 striatal projections to internal and external segments of the globus pallidus.[15] Nonetheless, the dual-circuit model remains a useful starting point for understanding the functional anatomy of the basal ganglia and the cognitive consequences of basal ganglia disorders.

Dopaminergic neurons of the substantia nigra and VTA project to the striatum and pallidum. The firing rate of these dopaminergic cells is not uniform: their background 'tonic' firing rate is supplemented by brief 'phasic' bursts of firing. The *phasic* dopaminergic signal is critical for cognitive function as it signals a prediction error in the brain. For example, animal studies show that an unexpected reward leads to phasic activity in dopaminergic projections to the striatum which gradually diminishes if the animal can learn to predict the reward.[16] Phasic reductions of firing can also occur if, for example, an expected reward is omitted or delayed. This dopaminergic signal is fundamental to learning, memory, the control of attention, and switching between behavioural strategies in response to environmental or internal feedback. *Tonic* firing rates affect the signal-to-noise for phasic firing: pharmacological enhancement of tonic dopaminergic firing might therefore paradoxically attenuate the behavioural benefits of dopamine dependent phasic rewards (reduced signal-to-noise) or phasic punishments.[17]

An interesting corollary of phasic dopaminergic responses is that they may contribute to the sense of agency (the sense that we control our own actions) which is affected by many neurological diseases.[18]

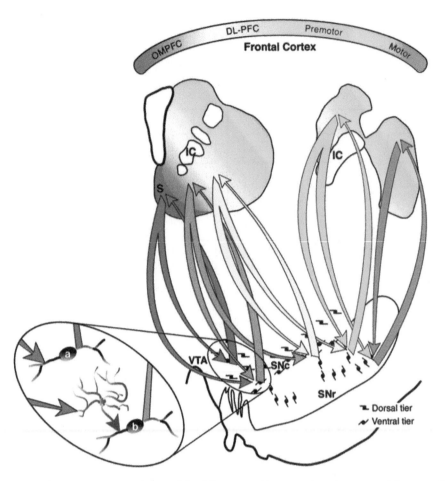

Fig. 7.3 Cortico-striatal and striato-nigral projections are not entirely parallel or fully segregated, but instead introduce cross-talk between affective, cognitive, and motor pathways. Striato-nigral projections illustrated here broadly follow a rostrocaudal gradient according to function (red = limbic, green = associative, blue = motor). As part of an affective loop, the accumbens shell (S) receives input from the amygdala, hippocampus, and orbitofrontal cortex; the accumbens core receives input from orbitomedial prefrontal cortex (OMPFC); as part of the cognitive loop, the dorsolateral prefrontal cortex (DLPFC) projects to the central striatum while as part of the motor loop premotor and motor cortex project to the dorsolateral striatum. Midbrain projections from the shell target both the ventral tegmental area (VTA) and ventromedial SNc (inset, red arrows). Midbrain projections from the VTA to the shell form a 'closed', loop (red arrow). Projections from the medial substantia nigra project to the core to form the first part of a spiral (orange arrow). The spiral of connectivity continues through the adjacent loops, illustrated by the yellow, green, and blue arrows. The magnified inset oval region shows the synaptic interactions in reciprocal loops: the reciprocal component terminates directly on a dopamine cell, resulting in inhibition, while the feedforward component terminates indirectly on a dopamine cell via a GABAergic interneuron (brown). This leads to disinhibition and facilitation of dopaminergic cell burst firing. IC, internal capsule; SNc, substantia nigra, pars compacta; SNr, substantia nigra, pars reticulata.

Reproduced from *J Neurosci.*, 20(6), Haber SN, Fudge JL, McFarland NR, Striatonigrostriatal pathways in primates form an ascending spiral from the shell to the dorsolateral striatum, pp. 2369–82, Copyright (2000), with permission from the Society for Neuroscience.

Whether a sensory event is perceived as being casued by one's own action as the 'agent' or perceived as externally caused depends on the harmony or discrepancy between sensory information and the sensory predictions made from precise internal models of the consequences of one's own actions.[19,20] Dopaminergic drugs and basal ganglia disorders such as Parkinson's disease and corticobasal degeneration affect the sense of agency, for example with alien limb phenomena.[21,22] Before reviewing the effects of such neurodegenerative disorders in detail, we turn next to the neuropsychological consequences of focal lesions to the basal ganglia.

Lesions of the basal ganglia

Ischaemic strokes, haemorrhage, tumours, and focal necrotic, metabolic, or immunological responses can lead to selective damage of basal ganglia nuclei, unilaterally or bilaterally. Motor syndromes have been widely described, such as hemiballismus after subthalamic nucleus stroke, and hemidystonia or hemi-parkinsonism after striatal lesions. However, cognitive syndromes and personality change are under-recognized in clinical practice. Many patients with basal ganglia lesions have significant and long-lasting cognitive change.[23]

The cognitive and behavioural effects of basal ganglia lesions should not be seen as mere disconnection of the cortical regions from which they receive afferents. Although there are often marked similarities between the effect of a cortical lesion and lesion of the part of the basal ganglia to which it projects, the basal ganglia are not passive conduits: the integration and compression of information through cortico-striato-thalamo-cortical loops, and the distinct pharmacology of the basal ganglia mean that basal ganglia lesions often have very widespread effects. Given the close proximity of functionally distinct circuits, and the heterogeneity of lesions,

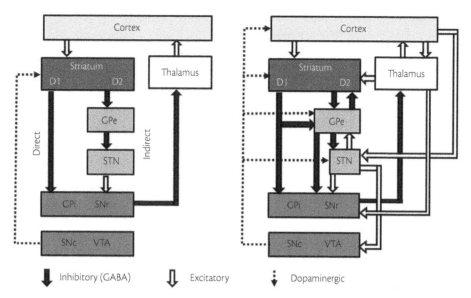

Inhibitory (GABA)   Excitatory   Dopaminergic

Fig. 7.4 The left panel illustrates the influential 'dual circuit model', in which the output of the basal ganglia is determined by the balance between the direct pathway, with striatonigral inhibitory connections that promote behaviour, and the indirect pathway, via the external globus pallidus (GPe) and subthalamic nucleus (STN), that suppress behaviour. The balance between these two pathways is modulated by dopaminergic inputs from the substantia nigra pars compacta (SNc) and the ventral tegmental area (VTA), which act on D1 and D2 dopamine receptors that are differentially expressed in the direct and indirect pathways. The right-hand panel brings together the evidence for a more complex connectivity, including dopaminergic modulation at multiple sites, and reciprocal connections among the globus pallidus pars externa, subthalamic nucleus, and globus pallidus pars interna (Gpi). SNr, substantia nigra pars reticulata.
Modified from *Nat Rev Neurosci.* 11(11), Redgrave P, Rodriguez M, Smith Y, Rodriguez-Oroz MC, Lehericy S, Bergman H, *et al.* Goal-directed and habitual control in the basal ganglia: implications for Parkinson's disease, pp. 760–72, Copyright (2010), with permission from Nature Publishing Group.

the neuropsychological approach to basal ganglia function has arguably not been as informative for functional mapping as it has been for cortical functions.

Bellebaum and colleagues studied the ability to learn new rules in ten patients with unilateral lesions, using probabilistic stimulus association task with differential rewards. Patients were able to learn the associations, but were impaired at learning the *reversal of associations*, especially with dorsal lesions, a deficit also observed in Parkinson's disease. Carry-over effects impaired learning of secondary tasks. Intriguingly, a patient with bilateral lesions showed superior performance compared to controls, due to an effective compensatory declarative memory strategy.[24]

The complex cognitive consequences of basal ganglia lesions are demonstrated in Benke and colleagues' description of two cases with haematomas affecting distinct regions of the left striatum and pallidum. Despite only having unilateral lesions, both patients were acutely abulic, with minimal spontaneous activity of speech, long response latencies, motivational deficits, and relative indifference to their illness.[25] A disabling lack of concern, motivation, and initiative persisted long term, without depression. On untimed tests, both patients had preserved arithmetic, reading, writing, naming, and comprehension but both manifested a dynamic aphasia with sparse delayed and reduced verbal output and reduced fluency. Cognitive flexibility, set-shifting, design fluency, and attention were severely affected, with difficulty initiating responses and responding to error feedback. These features overlap with the dysexecutive syndrome of frontal cortical lesions, as well as Huntington's and Parkinson's disease.

The syndrome manifested by these two patients did not, however, correspond to the separate predictions of affective, associative and motor functions in segregated parallel loops via ventral and dorsal striatum. This may be because the lesions were larger than were

seen by non-invasive brain imaging: more extensive overlapping changes in white matter connections might have been revealed by techniques such as diffusion-weighted imaging. However, there was a surprising similarity between the two patients' neuropsychological deficits, despite their lesions being in quite different places. This suggests extensive cross-talk between the basal ganglia circuits for affective, associative, and motor functions, confirming the extent to which the basal ganglia create an integrated system for complex goal-directed behaviours.[26]

Lesions to the ventral striatum and caudate nucleus may also affect social and emotional cognition,[27,28] while pallidal lesions may also lead to profound apathy.[29] This reflects the rich interconnections of this basal ganglia region with the orbitofrontal cortex and ventromedial prefrontal cortex, which are associated with social and emotional cognition in health,[30] and social cognitive impairments in degenerative neurological disease.[31] For example, Kemp and colleagues reported the effects of a haemorrhagic arteriovenous malformation in the left caudate nucleus of a 44-year-old man.[32] He gradually lost empathy and changed character, becoming 'mean', 'selfish', and paranoid. His abstract reasoning remained excellent, together with language, memory, visual attention, and most executive functions (except for some slowing). He could recognize basic emotions (e.g. anger, sadness) and accurately answer questions about scenarios pertaining to other people's knowledge or beliefs. However, he was greatly impaired in recognizing other people's complex mental states (e.g. desire) and could not understand the occurrence of social *faux pas*.[33] Although the only lesion was in the caudate nucleus, brain perfusion imaging suggested hypometabolism in the upstream and downstream connections of the caudate, specifically in the left thalamus, prefrontal and orbitofrontal cortex, highlighting the need to recognize cortico-striato-thalamo-cortical loops as a coherent system.

Some authors present Parkinson's disease as a model of basal ganglia dysfunction but this approach can be misleading. Parkinson's disease is associated with widespread pathology, in basal ganglia, brainstem nuclei, and cortex, and affects multiple neurotransmitter systems. Few studies have directly compared Parkinson's disease with focal basal ganglia lesions.[34] Both impair rule-based categorization tasks, but focal lesions selectively impair the learning of a complex discrimination task based on a conjunction of stimuli, not a simple categorization task. In contrast, Parkinson's disease affects the sustained performance of a simple one-dimensional task as well as causing suboptimal strategies on the more complex conjunction task.

In summary, even unilateral lesions of the basal ganglia can cause long-lasting and severe cognitive deficits, affecting executive functions, learning, and social cognition. However, human lesion data currently lack the anatomical specificity for precise functional mapping of the basal ganglia.

Neurodegenerative disorders of the basal ganglia

Much of the information available about the role of basal ganglia in cognition has come from the study of neurodegenerative disorders, especially Parkinson's disease and Huntington's disease, but also progressive supranuclear palsy and frontotemporal dementia. One must bear in mind that these disorders are not neuropathologically restricted to the basal ganglia, or to a single neurotransmitter such as dopamine. For example, serotonergic,[35] noradrenergic,[36] and extrastriatal dopamine[37] systems all contribute to cognitive deficits in Parkinson's disease. Nonetheless, striatal dysfunction is a major contributor the neuropsychological profile of these neurodegenerative disorders (see Fig. 7.5). Whilst the cognitive manifestations of these disorders are discussed in more detail in Section 3, a brief overview of each with particular focus on the basal ganglia, is provided below.

Parkinson's disease

Half of all people with Parkinson's disease have mild cognitive impairment soon after diagnosis,[3] and cognitive deficits may be present before diagnosis or the onset of motor symptoms. However, the cognitive impact of Parkinson's disease is multifaceted. The dual syndrome hypothesis[38,39] sets out the distinction between common early frontostriatal deficits and a later dementia. Early frontostriatal deficits are associated with loss of striatal dopamine (and loss of serotonin and noradrenaline) and are seen in about a third of patients at presentation, doubling after four years.[7,40] They are characterized by impairments in executive functions: cognitive flexibility including reversal learning, response inhibition, planning, attentional set-shifting, action selection, and decision-making according to risk or reward. Indeed, the impact of early Parkinson's disease on learning and memory is in part due to these executive function deficits.[41]

The dementia associated with Parkinson's disease is not merely a worsening of these frontostriatal deficits but rather a set of temporoparietal cortical deficits, most associated with cholinergic loss. These encompass poor episodic memory, visuospatial deficits, poor fluency, and risk of hallucination. Approximately one in ten people with Parkinson's disease develops dementia by three years and half by ten years.[97]

The ability to adapt behaviour to a novel or changing environment is central to the concept of executive functions. This has been widely studied in the context of visual discrimination learning, from the Wisconsin Card Sort Test and Montreal Card Sort Test through to translational models such as the Cambridge Automatic Neuropsychological Test Battery's (CANTAB) intra- and extra-dimensional shift task (IDED). During the IDED task, participants learn a series of visual discriminations based on compound stimuli. When a given discrimination is learned to criterion, the rules change and, in response to feedback, subjects must change their cognitive strategy and learn a new discrimination. Mild to

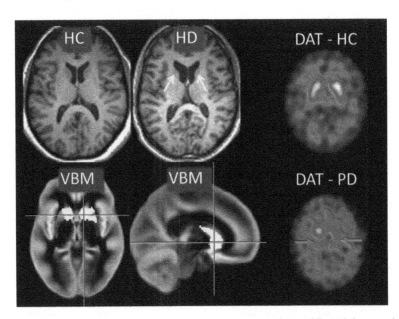

Fig. 7.5 In contrast to healthy adults (top left, HC), a carrier of CAG expansions in the Huntingtin gene (top middle, HD) shows marked atrophy of the caudate nucleus (yellow arrows) while still asymptomatic several years before Huntington's disease onset. Below, a voxel-based morphometry (VBM) analysis of 21 presymptomatic carriers confirms the significant degree of caudate atrophy (yellow cluster) in the absence of significant cortical atrophy. In contrast, the caudate is grossly preserved in early Parkinson's disease but dopamine transporter (DAT) imaging shows significant dopaminergic denervation of the striatum, especially the putamen (DAT-PD, red arrows), in contrast to a healthy adult (DAT-HC).
Courtesy of Prof. Roger Barker.

moderate Parkinson's disease does not affect the acquisition of simple discrimination, but it severely impairs the ability to make an attentional shift between two alternate perceptual dimensions in the stimuli, such as 'colour' and 'shape' (the 'extra-dimensional shift').[42–44]

This deficit in Parkinson's disease is ambiguous: it could be due to perseveration (the inability to disengage attention from a previously relevant dimension) or to learned irrelevance (the inability to attend and learn about information which has previously been shown to be irrelevant). People with Parkinson's disease are especially impaired when an extra-dimensional shift is accompanied by learned irrelevance.[45] However, the deficit in Parkinson's disease does not in itself indicate that it is due to striatal dopaminergic abnormalities. Indeed, dopaminergic medication makes little difference to extra-dimensional shift impairments.[46] In addition, severe dopamine depletion from the caudate in marmosets does not impair discrimination learning or extradimensional shifts. However, caudate dopamine depletion does impair shifting back to a previously reinforced dimension, suggesting that it is learned irrelevance which is affected by striatal dopamine depletion in Parkinson's disease.[47,48]

Parkinson's disease impairs *reversal learning*, in which reward contingencies are reversed across a set of stimuli. The striatum is implicated in reversal learning, from animal models and human neuroimaging.[49] People with Parkinson's disease are impaired on reversal learning, but dopaminergic medication may actually worsen this impairment. This paradoxical effect may result from the precision of normal dopaminergic firing, with phasic bursts against background tonic activity, such that dopaminergic medication reduces signal-to-noise of the ventral striatal phasic dopamine release that signals reversal.[17] Interestingly, the adverse effect of dopamine treatment is restricted to conditions in which the reversal is signalled by unexpected punishment, not reward.[50] The presence of cognitive impairment, including reversal learning deficits, depends on the stage of disease and the type of stimulus used, with a difference in the importance of cortex versus striatum according the use of abstract versus concrete rules.[50,51] The shift and reversal tasks described above relied on trial and error learning, according to feedback. However, Parkinson's disease also impairs cognitive flexibility when the required task shift is explicitly cued[52] or implied by a sequence of stimuli.[53,54]

To optimize behaviour, it is often necessary to weight different cognitive strategies according to recent experience and anticipated events, rather than make 'black and white switches' between cognitive strategies as in the IDED task and reversal paradigms. Rowe and colleagues studied such weighting between cognitive strategies, using a continuous performance task with two concurrent stimulus dimensions and a partial reward schedule.[55] People with Parkinson's disease were able to modulate the balance between alternate cognitive sets, according to the reward relevance of anticipated stimuli. However, the associated activations of the caudate nucleus and the ventrolateral prefrontal cortex were dependent on the severity of disease and dopaminergic treatment: there was a non-linear (inverted U-shaped) relationship between the activation and the disease severity. The deviation from normality of this inverted U-shape curve increased progressively across the cortex (from motor to premotor to dorsal then ventral prefrontal cortex) and striatum (from caudal putamen to ventral striatum). A similar U-shape function in caudate and ventral prefrontal cortical

activations in Parkinson's disease was observed for cognitive decisions regarding alternate manual responses,[56] and represents a generalized non-linear function of dopamine in human cognition.[55]

The non-linear U-shaped relationship between performance (or activation) and disease severity, or between performance (or activation) and dopaminergic drug dose, has major implications for treating cognitive function in Parkinson's disease. First, clinical decisions for dose escalation are typically made according to motor features (e.g. tremor, rigidity) and the levodopa dose is rarely chosen so as to optimize cognitive function even though cognitive impairments are a major determinant of patient and carer quality of life. Second, it may not be possible to optimize both cognitive and motor functions with a given dose using systemic medication. Instead, a combined approach with local basal ganglia therapies (such as deep brain stimulation or gene therapy) and systemic drugs may be required to approximate optimal treatment in different basal ganglia circuits for affective, cognitive, and motor functions. Third, since dopaminergic dysfunction in early Parkinson's disease mainly affects the dorsal striatum disease,[57] dopaminergic medication may effectively 'overdose' the ventral striatum and prefrontal cortex. Indeed, compensatory changes in the substantia nigra and VTA may lead to mild hyperdopaminergic states in the ventral striatum and mesocortex in early Parkinson's[58] in addition to pharmacotherapeutic overdose of the ventral striatum.

A striking consequence of ventral striatal dopamine 'overdose' is the induction of *impulse control disorders* (ICDs) in about one in seven patients on dopamine agonists. These include hypersexuality, paraphilias, pathological gambling, binge eating, and impulsive shopping which can be devastating in their long-term consequences even after medication is reduced and the behaviour abated. As explained above, dopaminergic neurons projecting from the ventral tegmental area signal unexpected rewards, or cues that have been associated with reward.[59] This dopamine reward signal in the striatum is exaggerated in relatively impulsive normal adults[60] and appears to be magnified in Parkinson's disease. For example, positron emission tomography (PET) studies reveal abnormally enhanced dopamine release in the ventral striatum of patients with pathological gambling.[61] However, extrastriatal dopamine may also contribute to the pathogenesis of ICDs in Parkinson's disease[62] including the cingulate and medial prefrontal cortical mechanisms by which actions are associated with reward. Functional MRI (fMRI) studies suggest that Parkinson's disease (even without ICDs) reduces the cingulate cortical response to reward anticipation, but increases the regional response to actual reward.[54]

This devaluation of anticipated future rewards in Parkinson's disease contributes to the preference for smaller immediate rewards over larger delayed rewards,[63] especially in those patients with ICDs and those taking dopamine agonists. For reversal learning, there is again a differential effect of Parkinson's disease on positive (rewarding) versus negative (punishment) feedback: patients at risk of ICDs become less responsive to negative feedback,[64] as well as more responsive to rewards. This distortion of the evaluation of outcomes, worsened by dopamine agonists, increases risk taking despite lower ventral striatal, orbitofrontal, and anterior cingulate activity.[65,66]

Huntington's disease

Huntington's disease (HD) is a complex, multifocal neurological disorder, caused by an inherited expansion of a trinucleatide cytosine–adenine–guanine (CAG) repeat in the Huntingtin gene. The disease causes progressive motor dysfunction, cognitive decline, and psychiatric disturbances starting usually between 30 and 50 years old. Cognitive symptoms or signs often develop prior to motor signs. Although the normal functions of this gene are not fully elucidated, striatal involvement is characteristic,[67] with severe loss of the caudate nuclei as one of the hallmarks of the disease (Fig. 7.5).

Huntington's disease impairs executive functions, emotion and social cognition, and memory. The autosomal dominant genetic aetiology of Huntington's disease allows one to study presymptomatic stages of disease, in the absence of medication or gross performance deficits. In addition, there are correlations between caudate volume and cognitive function and functional brain imaging by fMRI, pointing to the relevance of the striatum to cognitive function and cognitive decline in Huntington's disease.[68–70]

Caudate loss is evident in presymptomatic carriers (Fig. 7.5),[71,72] which progresses in severity and spatial extent during the symptomatic phase from the dorsal head of caudate to ventral striatum and putamen.[72–75] In contrast, cortical atrophy is more commonly associated with later stages of disease.[74] Within the body and head of the caudate, medium spiny neurons of the indirect pathway are especially affected. In keeping with the dual pathway model, this leads to disinhibition of the external globus pallidus, and downstream disinhibition of the thalamus. The direct pathway becomes overactive, exaggerating the thalamic disinhibition.

The imbalance between direct and indirect pathways can affect associative, affective, and motor loops through the basal ganglia. However, because of the topographical organization of neuropathology, there are trends towards differential times of onset of cognitive and behavioural impairments according to the functional anatomy of the cortico-striato-thalamo-cortical loops. For example, Holl and colleagues reported deficits in verbal fluency and Stroop interference,[76] but in contrast to Parkinson's disease, patients with Huntington's disease were unimpaired on a gambling task that required risk decision-making. The dissociation is likely because of the differential distribution of pathology across the ventromedial versus dorsolateral caudate nucleus and the respective connections of these regions. However, these clinicopathological correlations are only partial. Among patients ten or more years before estimated disease onset, there is evidence of caudate volume reduction in the absence of cognitive decline.[77–79] This suggests early compensation for the striatal changes, either within the striatum or the regions with which it is interconnected.

Cognitive changes in such presymptomatic cases or early stage disease are likely to be due to striatal involvement, and Huntington's disease has often been used as a model to study the role of the striatum in cognition, especially when supported by specific structure–function correlations. For example, early 'striatal'-stage disease impairs rule based language learning, in contrast to later cortical stages which affect other forms of learning.[80] Importantly, learning capacity correlates with the severity of caudate atrophy. Other early deficits include executive functions such as fluency, interference control, and Trail Making Test B,[78,81,82] emotion recognition,[83,84] and visuomotor integration.[85]

In symptomatic disease, the severity and range of cognitive deficits broadens, due to emerging cortical as well as extended striatal involvement. Planning, attention, and rule learning, psychomotor speed, episodic memory, and emotional or social cognition

progressively decline. However, some major cognitive domains remain relatively unaffected until late stages of disease, including semantic memory, language (not including fluency), visuospatial functions, and orientation.[82]

Further evidence for the striatal contribution to cognitive change comes from functional brain imaging with fMRI. For example, ventral striatal activity related to anticipated reward is blunted in gene carriers approaching disease onset.[86] However, changes in activation are not necessarily localized to the striatum, even in early disease. For example, the executive function of set-shifting activates extensive prefrontal, parietal and cingulate cortex, and basal ganglia in healthy adults. The putamenal and pallidal activations were *increased* in patients even in premanifest cases, but there were also extensive increases in cortical activations.[87]

Similarly, during working memory performance the activation differences observed in manifest and presymptomatic carriers include, but are not confined to, the caudate and putamen.[88] This should not be surprising, in view of the connectivity through cortico-striato-thalamo-cortical loops, as the effects of a lesion or perturbation in one node of the circuit are propagated throughout the circuit, including recurrent connections to the cortical regions that project to the striatum. The importance of this circuit-based understanding of cognitive dysfunction is underscored by the correlations between cognitive decline and (i) atrophy of cortex;[89] (ii) atrophy of caudate;[90] (iii) changes in the white matter structural connections between frontal cortex and the striatum;[91,92] and (iv) changes in frontostriatal functional connectivity.[70,86]

Progressive supranuclear palsy

Progressive supranuclear palsy (PSP) is sometimes still described as a 'Parkinson's plus' syndrome and movement disorder. However, this overlooks the marked clinical and pathological distinctions from Parkinson's disease,[93] and the extensive cognitive problems which are a major determinant of patient and carer quality of life.[94] 'Mental features' were noted in the original description 50 years ago,[95] and cognitive change remains part of the supportive diagnostic criteria. Indeed, one in ten patients present with cognitive symptoms,[96] and two-thirds will develop a dementia.[97,98]

PSP is caused by hyperphosphorylation and aggregation of the microtubule-associated protein tau, leading to cell dysfunction and death. It affects many parts of the basal ganglia, including the striatum, pallidum, substantia nigra, subthalamic nucleus (other affected regions include the red nucleus, pontine tegmentum, oculomotor nuclei, medulla, dentate nucleus and cortex[99]). Atrophy of the dorsal midbrain is severe with marked reductions in dopaminergic innervation of striatum and cortex. Caudate atrophy is evident on MRI,[100] together with severe striatal hypometabolism from FDG-PET[101] and abnormal striato-frontal connections.[102,103]

The cognitive effects of PSP include behavioural change (apathy, irritability, childishness, impulsivity), executive dysfunction, memory, visuospatial, language and social cognitive deficits. Cognitive slowing typically develops early in the disease. Executive deficits occur in about three quarters of patients. For example, Robbins and colleagues[105] identified deficits in short-term memory and spatial working memory with poor memory strategies, but also poor planning on the Tower of London task, and severe deficits in attentional set-shifting. However, simple rule acquisition remains relatively intact.[104,105] Others have reported deficits in tests of frontal lobe function such as the Trail Making B task[106] and a range of executive and non-verbal reasoning tasks.[98,107,108] Even verbal fluency, which requires executive as well as lexical functions, is profoundly impaired in PSP.[97] Recent work has also shown that emotional and social cognitive systems are abnormal in PSP.[31,109] Both emotion recognition and higher-order social inferences (known as Theory of Mind) are affected across visual and auditory domains. One-third of patients manifest poor episodic memory and poor visuospatial functions.[110–112] However, such deficits may be in part related to executive impairments, affecting retrieval or task strategies.

Despite the wide-ranging cognitive deficits in PSP and the severity of pathology in the basal ganglia, it is less clear to what extent the basal ganglia changes are the cause of the cognitive decline. Albert and colleagues used PSP to illustrate the concept of 'subcortical dementia', attributing the majority of cognitive change to subcortical pathology. This was distinguished from 'cortical dementias' such as Alzheimer's disease with amnesia, aphasia, apraxia, and agnosia. However, the extent of cortical pathology and of cortical neurotransmitter loss has become more widely recognized, and functional cognitive impairments shown to correlate with cortical atrophy[100,113] or cortical hypopmetabolism,[114] including global cognitive function and social cognitive deficits.[31] Nonetheless, dorsal striatal atrophy occurs in PSP,[113,115] and caudate atrophy can be severe, correlating with global cognitive decline in PSP,[104] hypometabolism,[101] and the presence of neuropathology in the majority of cases.[116] Further, albeit indirect, evidence comes from the observation that greater pathology in the caudate and substantia nigra is associated with a classical phenotype (also called PSP–Richardson's syndrome) with prominent cognitive and behavioural changes, as opposed to a syndrome more closely resembling Parkinson's disease.[117]

Frontotemporal dementia

Frontotemporal dementia (FTD) has long been associated with severe atrophy of the frontal, temporal, and insula cortex. However, the basal ganglia are also affected, especially in the behavioural variant of frontotemporal dementia, with hypometabolism and atrophy.[118,119] The non-fluent variant of primary progressive aphasia (progressive non-fluent aphasia) is also associated with atrophy in caudate, nucleus accumbens, and, to a lesser extent, the putamen. In the semantic variance of primary progressive aphasia (semantic dementia) the caudate is grossly preserved. In addition to atrophy, functional connectivity of the striatum is abnormal in FTD.[120] It has been suggested that cognitive deficits related to striatal dysfunction in FTD are lateralized, with right-sided changes associated with behavioural change, apathy, empathy, and stereotypies, whereas left-sided changes are associated with executive, language, and psychomotor features.[121]

However, the contribution of the striatal atrophy to cognitive impairment in FTD is not fully characterized. It may be that some of the observations reflect changes that are secondary to atrophy of the cortical areas with which striatal regions interconnect. It is necessary to try to uncouple the cortical from striatal contributions to cognitive impairment, for example by closer analysis of individual differences or longitudinal designs. For example, Dalton and colleagues used voxel-based morphometry to study the anatomical basis of the impairment of probabilities-associative learning in FTD. Performance variability within the patient group correlated with grey matter volume in the striatum, including ventral striatum, head of caudate, and rostral putamen.[122]

Conclusion

The basal ganglia are affected by diverse neurological disorders, with common cognitive and behavioural consequences including the impairment of executive functions (e.g. attentional shifts, reversal), apathy and impulse control disorders, disrupted learning, social and emotional cognition. The cognitive deficits are similar to the effects of lesions of the frontal cortical regions with which the striatum is densely connected. A set of 'frontostriatal' circuits has been proposed, in which the functional consequences of disease reflect the anatomy, pharmacology, and connectivity of the normal basal ganglia. These circuits are organized by two broad principles that facilitate integration and segregation of information processing: first, that there is homology between cortico-striato-thalamo-cortical loops for motor, cognitive, and limbic functions; second, that there is an anatomical and pharmacological distinction between direct and indirect pathways connecting the striatum, pallidum, subthalamic nucleus, and substantia nigra. Neurodegenerative disorders show partial selectivity within these networks, by region and by pharmacologically defined neuronal subtypes, leading to characteristic neuropsychological profiles in premanifest, early, and late stages of disease.

Acknowledgements

James Rowe is supported by the Wellcome Trust (103838) and Timothy Rittman is supported by the Medical Research Council.

References

1. Wilson S. An experimental research into the anatomy and physiology of the corpus striatum. *Brain*. 1914;36:427–92.
2. Heimer L, Switzer R, and Hoesen G. Ventral striatal and ventral pallidum: Additional copmonents of the motor system? *Trends Neurosci.* 1982;5:83–7.
3. Yarnall AJ, Breen DP, Duncan GW, *et al.* Characterizing mild cognitive impairment in incident Parkinson disease: The ICICLE–PD Study. *Neurology.* 2014;82(4):308–16. Epub 2013/12/24.
4. Alexander GE, Crutcher MD, and DeLong MR. Basal ganglia-thalamocortical circuits: Parallel substrates for motor, oculomotor, 'prefrontal' and 'limbic' functions. *Prog Brain Res.* 1990;85:119–46.
5. Alexander GE, DeLong MR, and Strick PL. Parallel organization of functionally segregated circuits linking basal ganglia and cortex. *Annu Rev Neurosci.* 1986;9(1–2):357–81.
6. Middleton FA and Strick PL. Basal ganglia and cerebellar loops: Motor and cognitive circuits. *Brain Res Rev.* 2000;31(2–3):236–50.
7. Williams-Gray CH, Foltynie T, Brayne CE, *et al.* Evolution of cognitive dysfunction in an incident Parkinson's disease cohort. *Brain.* 2007;130(Pt 7):1787–98.
8. Draganski B, Kherif F, Kloppel S, *et al.* Evidence for segregated and integrative connectivity patterns inthe human basal ganglia. *J Neurosci.* 2008;28:7143–52.
9. Postuma RB and Dagher A. Basal ganglia functional connectivity based on a metanalysis of 126 positron emission tomography and functional magnetic resonance imaging publications. *Cereb Cortex.* 2006;10:1508–21.
10. Choi EY, Yeo BTT, and Buckner RL. The organization of the human striatum estimated by intrinsic functional connectivity. *J Neurophysiol.* 2012;108(8):2242–63.
11. Haber SN, Fudge JL, and McFarland NR. Striatonigrostriatal pathways in primates form an ascending spiral from the shell to the dorsolateral striatum. *J Neurosci.* 2000;20(6):2369–82. Epub 2000/03/08.
12. Oorschot DE. Total number of neurons in the neostriatal, pallidal, subthalamic, and substantia nigral nuclei of the rat basal

ganglia: A stereological study using the cavalieri and optical disector methods. *Journ Comp Neurol*. 1996;366(4):580–99.

13. Pawlak V and Kerr JND. Dopamine receptor activation is required for corticostriatal spike-timing-dependent plasticity. *Journal of Neurosci*. 2008;28(10):2435–46.

14. Cui G, Jun S, Jin X, Pham M, *et al*. Concurrent activation of striatal direct and indirect pathways during action initiation. *Nature*. 2013;494(7436):238–42.

15. Calabrese P, Picconni B, Tozzi A, *et al*. Direct and Indirect pathways of basal ganglia: A critical reappraisal. *Nat Neurosci*. 2014;17(8):1022–30.

16. Schultz W and Dickinson A. Neuronal coding of prediction errors. *Annu Rev Neurosci*. 2000;23:473–500.

17. Cools R, Lewis SJ, Clark L, *et al*. L-DOPA disrupts activity in the nucleus accumbens during reversal learning in Parkinson's disease. *Neuropsychopharmacol*. 2007;32(1):180–9.

18. Wolpe N and Rowe J. Disorders of Volition from Neurological Disease. In: P Haggard (ed.). *Agency: Functions and Mechanisms*. Oxford: Oxford University Press, 2014, pp. 389–414.

19. Redgrave P, Vautrelle N, and Reynolds JNJ. Functional properties of the basal ganglia's re-entrant loop architecture: Selection and reinforcement. *Neuroscience*. 2011;198:138–51.

20. Redgrave P and Gurney K. The short-latency dopamine signal: a role in discovering novel actions? *Nature Rev Neuro*. 2006;7(12):967–75.

21. Wolpe N, Moore JW, Rae CL, Rittman T, Altena E, Haggard P, *et al*. The medial frontal-prefrontal network for altered awareness and control of action in corticobasal syndrome. *Brain*. 2013;137(1):208–20. Epub 2013/12/03.

22. Moore J, Schneider S, Schwingenshuhc P, Morettoa G, Bhatia KP, and Haggard P. Dopaminergic medication boosts action–effect binding in Parkinson's disease. *Neuropsychologia*. 2010;48:1125–32.

23. Bhatia K and Marsden C. The behavioural and motor consequences of focal lesions of the basal ganglia in man. *Brain*. 1994;117(4):859–76.

24. Bellebaum C, Koch B, Schwarz M, and Daum I. Focal Basal Ganglia lesions are associated with impairments in reward-based reversal learning. *Brain*. 2008;131(3):829–41.

25. Benke T, Delazer M, Bartha L, and Auer A. Basal Ganglia Lesions and the Theory of Fronto-Subcortical Loops: Neuropsychological Findings in Two Patients with Left Caudate Lesions. *Neurocase*. 2003;9(1):70–85.

26. Haber SN. The primate basal ganglia: parallel and integrative networks. *J Chem Neuroanat*. 2003;26(4):317–30.

27. Calder A, Keane J, Lawrence A, and Manes F. Impaired recognition of anger following damage to the ventral striatum. *Brain* 2004;127:1958–69.

28. Paulman S, Pell M, and Kotz S. Functional contributions of the basal ganglia to emotional prosody: Evidence from ERPs. *Brain Res*. 2008;1217:171–8.

29. Adam R, Leff A, Sinha N, Turner C, *et al*. Dopamine reverses reward insensitivity in apathy following globus pallidus lesions. *Cortex*. 2013 May;49(5):1292–303.

30. Amodio D and Frith C. Meeting of minds: The medial frontal cortex and social cognition. *Nat Rev Neurosci*. 2006;7(4):268–77.

31. Ghosh BC, Calder AJ, Peers PV, Law *et al*. Social cognitive deficits and their neural correlates in progressive supranuclear palsy. *Brain*. 2012;135(Pt 7):2089–102.

32. Kemp J, Berthel MC, Dufour A, *et al*. Caudate nucleus and social cognition: Neuropsychological and SPECT evidence from a patient with focal caudate lesion. *Cortex*. 2013;49(2):559–71. Epub 2012/02/14.

33. Baron-Cohen S, O'Riordan M, Stone V,. Recognition of faux pas by normally developing children and children with Asperger syndrome or high-functioning autism. *J AutismDev Disord*. 1999;29(5):407–18.

34. Ell S, Weinstein A, and Ivry R. Rule-Based Categorization Deficits in Focal Basal Ganglia Lesion and Parkinson's Disease Patients. *Neuropsychologia*. 2010;48(10):2974–86.

35. Ye Z, Altena E, Nombela C, *et al*. Selective serotonin reuptake inhibition modulates response inhibition in Parkinson's disease. *Brain*. 2014 Apr;137(Pt 4):1145–55.

36. Ye z, Altena E, Nombela C, Houseden C, *et al*. Improving impulsivity in Parkinson's disease with atomoxetine. *Biol Psychiat*. 2014. doi:10.1016/j.biopsych.2014.01.024.

37. Christopher L, Marras C, Duff-Canning S, , *et al*. Combined insular and striatal dopamine dysfunction are associated with executive deficits in Parkinson's disease with mild cognitive impairment. *Brain*. 2014;137:565–75.

38. Kehagia A, Barker R, and Robbins T. Neuropsychological and clinical heterogeneity of cognitive impairment and dementia in patients with Parkinson's disease. *Lancet Neurol*. 2010;9:1200–13.

39. Kehagia A, Barker R, and Robbins T. Cognitive impairment in Parkinson's disease: The dual syndrome hypothesis. *Neurodegener Dis*. 2013;11:79–92.

40. Foltynie T, Brayne CE, Robbins TW, *et al*. The cognitive ability of an incident cohort of Parkinson's patients in the UK. The CamPaIGN study. *Brain*. 2004;127(Pt 3):550–60.

41. Grahn JA, Parkinson JA, and Owen AM. The role of the basal ganglia in learning and memory: Neuropsychological studies. *Behav Brain Res*. 2009;199:53–60.

42. Owen AM, James M, Leigh PN, *et al*. Fronto-striatal cognitive deficits at different stages of Parkinson's disease. *Brain*. 1992;115(Pt 6):1727–51.

43. Owen AM, Roberts AC, Hodges JR, *et al*. Contrasting mechanisms of impaired attentional set-shifting in patients with frontal lobe damage or Parkinson's disease. *Brain*. 1993;116(Pt 5):1159–75.

44. Downes JJ, Roberts AC, Sahakian BJ, *et al*. Impaired extra-dimensional shift performance in medicated and unmedicated Parkinson's disease: Evidence for a specific attentional dysfunction. *Neuropsychologia*. 1989;27(11–12):1329–43.

45. Slabosz A, Lewis SJ, Smigasiewicz K, *et al*. The role of learned irrelevance in attentional set-shifting impairments in Parkinson's disease. *Neuropsychol*. 2006;20(5):578–88.

46. Cools R, Barker RA, Sahakian BJ, *et al*. Enhanced or impaired cognitive function in Parkinson's disease as a function of dopaminergic medication and task demands. *Cereb Cortex*. 2001;11(12):1136–43.

47. Crofts HS, Dalley JW, Collins P, *et al*. Differential effects of 6-OHDA lesions of the frontal cortex and caudate nucleus on the ability to acquire an attentional set. *Cereb Cortex*. 2001;11(11):1015–26.

48. Collins P, Roberts AC, Dias R, *et al*. Perseveration and strategy in a novel spatial self-ordered sequencing task for nonhuman primates. Effects Of excitotoxic lesions and dopamine depletions of the prefrontal cortex. *J Cogn Neurosci*. 1998;10(4):332–54.

49. Cools R, Clark L, Owen AM, *et al*. Defining the neural mechanisms of probabilistic reversal learning using event-related functional magnetic resonance imaging. *J Neurosci*. 2002;22(11):4563–7.

50. Cools R, Altamirano L, and D'Esposito M. Reversal learning in Parkinson's disease depends on medication status and outcome valence. *Neuropsychologia*. 2006;44(10):1663–73.

51. Cools R, Clark L, and Robbins TW. Differential responses in human striatum and prefrontal cortex to changes in object and rule relevance. *J Neurosci*. 2004;24(5):1129–35.

52. Cools R, Barker RA, Sahakian BJ, *et al*. L-Dopa medication remediates cognitive inflexibility, but increases impulsivity in patients with Parkinson's disease. *Neuropsychologia*. 2003;41(11):1431–41.

53. Rowe JB, Eckstein D, Braver T, *et al*. How does reward expectation influence cognition in the human brain? *J Cogn Neurosci*. 2008;20(11):1980–92.

54. Rowe JB, Hughes L, Ghosh BC, *et al*. Parkinson's disease and dopaminergic therapy—differential effects on movement, reward and cognition. *Brain*. 2008;131:2094–105.

55. Cools R and D'Esposito M. Inverted U-shaped dopamine aactions on human working memory and cognitive control. *Biol Psychiatry*. 2011;69(2):113–25.

56. Hughes LE, Altena E, Barker RA, *et al*. Perseveration and choice in parkinson's disease: The impact of progressive frontostriatal dysfunction on action decisions. *Cerebral Cortex*. 2013;23(7):1572–81.

57. Kish S, Shannak K, and Hornykiewicz O. Uneven pattern of dopamine loss in the striatum of patients with idiopathic Parkinson's

diease. Pathologic and clinical implications. *New Engl J Med.* 1988;318(14):876–80.

58. Rakshi JS, Uema T, Ito K, *et al.* Frontal, midbrain and striatal dopaminergic function in early and advanced Parkinson's disease A 3D [(18)F] dopa-PET study. *Brain.* 1999;122(Pt 9):1637–50.

59. Schultz W. Behavioral theories and the neurophysiology of reward. *Annu Rev Psychol.* 2006;57:87–115.

60. Buckholtz J, Treadway M, Cowan R, *et al.* Dopaminergic netwrok differences in human impulsivity. *Science.* 2010;329(5991):532.

61. Steeves T, Miyasaki J, Zurowski M, *et al.* Increased striatal dopaminergic release in Parkinson's patients with pathological gambling: A [11C] raclopride PET study. *Brain.* 2009;132(5):1376–85.

62. Ray N, Miyasaki J, Zurowski M, *et al.* Extrastriatal dopaminergic abnormalities of DA homeostasis in Parkinson's patients with medication-induced pathological gambling: A [11C] FLB-457 and PET study. *Neurobiol Dis.* 2012;48:519–28.

63. Housden C, O'Sullivan S, Joyce E, *et al.* Intact reward learning but elevated delay discounting in Parkinson's disease patients with impulsive-compulsive spectrum behaviors. *Neuropsychopharmacol.* 2010;35:2155–64.

64. van Eimeren T, Ballanger B, Pellecchia G, *et al.* Dopamine agonists diminish value sensitivity of the orbitofrontal cortex: A trigger for pathological gambling in Parkinson's disease? *Neuropsychopharmacolo.* 2009;34(13):2758–66.

65. Voon V, Gao J, Brezing C, *et al* H. Dopamine agonists and risk: Impulse control disorders in Parkinson's disease. *Brain.* 2011;134:1438–46.

66. Djamshidian A, O'Sullivan S, Wittmann B, *et al.* Novelty seeking behaviour in Parkinson's disease. *Neuropsychologia.* 2011;49:2483–8.

67. Vonsattel J. Huntington disease models and human neuropathology: Similarities and differences. *Acta Neuropathol.* 2008;115:55–69.

68. Georgiou-Karistianis N, Poudel G, Dominguez R, *et al.* Functional andconnectivity changes during working memory inHuntington's disease: 18-month longitudinal data from the IMAGE–HD study. *Brain Cognition.* 2013;83:80–91.

69. Zimbleman J, Paulsen J, Mikos A, *et al.* fMRI detection of early neural dysfunction in preclinical Huntington's disease. *J Int Neuropsychol Soc.* 2007;13(5):758–69.

70. Wolf R, Sambataro F, Vasic N, *et al.* Altered frontostriatal coupling in premanifest Huntington's disease: Effects of increasing cognitive load. *Eur J Neurol.* 2008;15(11):1180–90.

71. Majid DS, Stoffers D, Sheldon S, *et al.* Automated structural imaging analysis detects premanifest Huntington's disease neurodegeneration within one year. *Mov Disord.* 2011; 26(8):1481–8.

72. Aylward E, Codori A, Rosenblatt A, *et al.* Rate of caudate atrophy in presymptomatic and symptomatic stages of Huntington's disease. *Mov Disord.* 2000;15(3):552–60.

73. Aylward E, Li Q, Stine O, *et al.* Longitudinal change in basal ganglia volume in patients with Huntington's disease. *Neurology.* 1997;48:394–9.

74. Douaud G, Gaura V, Ribeiro M, *et al.* Distribution of grey matter atrophy in Huntington? s disease patients: A combined ROI-based and voxel-based morphometric study. *Neuroimage.* 2006;32:1562–75.

75. Tabrizi S, Reilmann R, and Roos R. Potential endpoints for clinical trials in premanifest and early Huntington's disease in the TRACK–HD study: Analysis of 24 month observational data. *Lancet Neurol.* 2012;11:42–53.

76. Holl A, Wilkinson L, Tabrizi S, *et al.* Selective executive dysfunction but intact risky decision-making in early Huntington's disease. *Mov Disord.* 2013;28(8):1104–9.

77. Tabrizi SJ, Scahill R, Durr A, *et al.* Biological and clinical changes in premanifest and early stage Huntington's disease in the TRACK–HD study: The 12-month longitudinal analysis. *Lancet Neurol.* 2011;10(1):31–42.

78. Stout J, Paulsen J, Queller S, *et al.* Neurocognitive signs in prodromal Huntington's diease. *Neuropsychol.* 2011;1(25):1–14.

79. Dominguez D, Egan G, Gray M, *et al.* Multimodal neuroimaging in premanifest and early Huntington's diease. 18 month longitudinal data from the IMAGE-HD study. *PLoS One.* 2013;8(9):e74131.

80. De Diego-Balaguer R, Couette M, Dolbeau G, *et al.* Striatal degeneration impairs language learning: Evidence from Huntington's disease. *Brain.* 2008;131:2870–81.

81. Holl A, Wilkinson L, Tabrizi SJ, *et al.* Selective Executive Dysfunction but Intact Risky Decision-Making in Early Huntington's Disease. *Mov Disord.* 2013;28:1104–9.

82. Dumas E, Van den Bogaard S, Middelkoop H, *et al.* A review of cognition in Huntington's disease. *Front Biosci (Schol Ed).* 2013;5:1–18.

83. Snowden J, Austin N, Sembi S, *et al.* Emotion recognition in Huntington's disease and frontotemporal dementia *Neuropsychologia.* 2008;46:2638–49.

84. Henley S, Novak M, Frost C, King J, Tabrizi S, and Warren J. Emotion recognition in Huntington's diease: A systematic review. *Neurosci Biobehav R.* 2012; 36:237–53.

85. Say M, Jones R, Scahill R, *et al.* Visuomotor Integration deficits precede clinical onset in Huntington's disease. *Neuropscyhologia.* 2011 49:264–70.

86. Enzi B, Edel M-A, Lissek S, *et al.* Altered ventral striatal activation during reward and punishment processing in premanifest Huntington's disease: A functional magnetic resonance study. *Exp Neurol.* 2012;235:256–64.

87. Gray M, Egan G, Ando A, *et al.* Prefrontal activity in Huntiongton's dieae reflects cognitive and neuropsychiatric disturbances: The IMAGE–HD study. *Exp Neurol.* 2013; 239:218–28.

88. Georgiou-Karistianis N, Stout JC, Dominguez D, *et al.* Functional magnetic resonance imaging of working memory in Huntington's disease: Cross-sectional data from the IMAGE–HD study. *Hum Brain Mapp.* 2013;35:1847–64.

89. Rosas H, Salat D, Lee S, *et al.* Cerebral cortex and the clinical expression of Huntington's disease: Complexity and heterogeneity. *Brain.* 2008;131:1057–68.

90. Peinemann A, Schuller S, Pohl C, *et al.* Executive dysfunction in early stages of Huntington's disease is associated with striatal and insular atrophy: A neuropsychological and voxel-based morphometric study. *J Neurol Sci.* 2005;239:11–9.

91. Rosas H, Tuch D, Hevelone ND, *et al.* Diffusion tensor imaging in presymptomatic and early Huntington's disease: Selective white matter pathology and its relationship to clinical measures. *Mov Disord.* 2006;21:1317–25.

92. Bohanna I, Georgiou-Karistianis N, Sritharan A, *et al.* Diffusion Tensor Imaging in Huntington's disease reveals distinct patterns of white matter degeneration associated with motor and cognitive deficits. *Brain Imaging and Behavior.* 2011;5:171–80.

93. Burrell J, Hodges J, and Rowe J. Cognition in corticobasal syndrome and progressive supranuclear palsy. *Mov Disord.* 2014;29(5):684–93.

94. Schrag A, Selai C, Davis J, *et al.* Health-related quality of life in patients with progressive supranuclear palsy. *Mov Disord.* 2003;18(12):1464–9.

95. Steele J, Richardson J, and Olszewski J. Progressive supranuclear palsy: A heterogeneous degeneration involving the brain stem, basal ganglia and cerebellum, with vertical gaze and pseudobulbar palsy, nuchal dystonia and dementia. *Arch Neurol.* 1964;10:333–59.

96. Bensimon G, Ludolph A, Agid Y, *et al.* Riluzole treatment, survival and diagnostic criteria in Parkinson plus disorders: The NNIPPS study. *Brain.* 2009;132(Pt 1):156–71. Epub 2008/11/26.

97. Rittman T, Ghosh BC, McColgan P, *et al.* The Addenbrooke's Cognitive Examination for the differential diagnosis and longitudinal assessment of patients with parkinsonian disorders. *J Neurol Neurosur Ps.* 2013;84(5):544–51.

98. Pillon B, Dubois B, and Agid Y. Severity and specificity of cognitive impairment in Alzheimer's, Huntington's, and Parkinson's diseases and progressive supranuclear palsy. *Ann NY Acad Sci.* 1991;640:224–7. Epub 1991/01/01.

99. Litvan I, Hauw JJ, Bartko JJ, *et al.* Validity and reliability of the preliminary NINDS neuropathologic criteria for progressive supranuclear palsy and related disorders. *J Neuropathol Exp Neurol.* 1996;55(1):97–105. Epub 1996/01/01.

100. Cordato NJ, Duggins AJ, Halliday GM, *et al.* Clinical deficits correlate with regional cerebral atrophy in progressive supranuclear palsy. *Brain.* 2005;128(Pt 6):1259–66.

101. Karbe H, Grond M, Huber M, *et al.* Subcortical damage and cortical dysfunction in progressive supranuclear palsy demonstrated by positron emission tomography. *J Neurol.* 1992;239(2):98–102. Epub 1992/02/01.

102. Whitwell JL, Avula R, Master A, *et al.* Disrupted thalamocortical connectivity in PSP: A resting-state fMRI, DTI, and VBM study. *Parkinsonism Relat Disord.* 2011;17(8):599–605. Epub 2011/06/15.

103. Gardner RC, Boxer AL, Trujillo A, *et al.* Intrinsic connectivity network disruption in progressive supranuclear palsy. *Ann Neurol.* 2013;73(5):603–16. Epub 2013/03/29.

104. Ghosh BC, Carpenter RH, and Rowe JB. A longitudinal study of motor, oculomotor and cognitive function in progressive supranuclear palsy. *PLoS One.* 2013;8(9):e74486. Epub 2013/09/24.

105. Robbins TW, James M, Owen AM, *et al.* Cognitive deficits in progressive supranuclear palsy, Parkinson's disease, and multiple system atrophy in tests sensitive to frontal lobe dysfunction. *J Neurol Neurosur Ps.* 1994;57(1):79–88.

106. Grafman J, Litvan I, Gomez C, *et al.* Frontal lobe function in progressive supranuclear palsy. *Arch Neurol.* 1990;47(5):553–8. Epub 1990/05/01.

107. Dubois B, Pillon B, Legault F, *et al.* Slowing of cognitive processing in progressive supranuclear palsy. A comparison with Parkinson's disease. *Arch Neurol.* 1988;45(11):1194–9. Epub 1988/11/01.

108. Lagarde J, Valabregue R, Corvol JC, *et al.* Are Frontal Cognitive and Atrophy Patterns Different in PSP and bvFTD? A Comparative Neuropsychological and VBM Study. *PLoS One.* 2013;8(11):e80353. Epub 2013/11/28.

109. O'Keeffe FM, Murray B, Coen RF, *et al.* Loss of insight in frontotemporal dementia, corticobasal degeneration and progressive supranuclear palsy. *Brain.* 2007;130(Pt 3):753–64. Epub 2007/03/10.

110. Brown RG, Lacomblez L, Landwehrmeyer BG, *et al.* Cognitive impairment in patients with multiple system atrophy and progressive supranuclear palsy. *Brain.* 2010;133(Pt 8):2382–93.

111. Pillon B, Blin J, Vidailhet M, *et al.* The neuropsychological pattern of corticobasal degeneration: Comparison with progressive supranuclear palsy and Alzheimer's disease. *Neurology.* 1995;45(8):1477–83. Epub 1995/08/01.

112. Bak TH, Crawford LM, Hearn VC, *et al.* Subcortical dementia revisited: Similarities and differences in cognitive function between progressive supranuclear palsy (PSP), corticobasal degeneration (CBD) and multiple system atrophy (MSA). *Neurocase.* 2005;11(4):268–73.

113. Cordato NJ, Pantelis C, Halliday GM, *et al.* Frontal atrophy correlates with behavioural changes in progressive supranuclear palsy. *Brain.* 2002;125(Pt 4):789–800.

114. Blin J, Baron JC, Dubois B, *et al.* Positron emission tomography study in progressive supranuclear palsy. Brain hypometabolic pattern and clinicometabolic correlations. *Arch Neurol.* 1990;47(7):747–52. Epub 1990/07/01.

115. Looi J, Macfarlane M, Walterfang M, *et al.* Morphometric analysis of subcortical structures in progressive supranuclear palsy: in vivo evidence of neostriatal and mesencephalic atrophy. *Psychiatry Res Neuroimaging.* 2011;194:163–75.

116. Verny M, Duyckaerts C, Agid Y, *et al.* The significance of cortical pathology in progressive supranuclear palsy. Clinico-pathological data in 10 cases. *Brain.* 1996;119 (Pt 4):1123–36. Epub 1996/08/01.

117. Williams DR, Holton JL, Strand C, *et al.* Pathological tau burden and distribution distinguishes progressive supranuclear palsy-parkinsonism from Richardson's syndrome. *Brain.* 2007;130:1566–76.

118. Halabi C, Halabi A, Dean DL, *et al.* Patterns of striatal degeneration in frontotemporal dementia. *Alzheimer Dis Assoc Disord.* 2013;27(1):74–83. Epub 2012/03/01.

119. Garibotto V, Borroni B, Agosti C, *et al.* Subcortical and deep cortical atrophy in frontotemporal lobar degeneration. *Neurobiol Aging.* 2011;32:875–84.

120. Seeley WW, Crawford RK, Zhou J, *et al.* Neurodegenerative diseases target large-scale human brain networks. *Neuron.* 2009;62(1):42–52.

121. O'Callaghan C, Bertoux M, and Hornberger M. Beyond and below the cortex: The contribution of striatal dysfunction to cognition and behaviour in neurodegeneration. *J Neurol Neurosur Ps.* 2014;85(4):371–8.

122. Dalton M, Weikert T, Hodge JR, *et al.* Impaired acquisition rates of probabilistic associative learning in frontotemporal dementia is associated with fronto-striatal atrophy. *NeuroImage: Clinical.* 2013;2:56–62.

CHAPTER 8

Principles of white matter organization

Marco Catani

Introduction

Connectional neuroanatomy delineates the origin, course, and termination of white matter pathways in the central nervous system. In clinical practice, understanding white matter anatomy can help to improve early diagnosis, optimize treatment strategies, and predict outcomes. In this chapter, the reader will be introduced to methods for studying white matter anatomy, a modern classification of the major brain pathways underlying cognition and behaviour, and principles of white matter organization and function. A particular emphasis is given to more recent tractography approaches and their application to the *in vivo* study of white matter anatomy in the healthy and pathological brain.

The study of white matter anatomy

The term *white matter* applies to the substance of the brain that contains axonal fibres connecting neurons located in the *grey matter*. In fresh tissue, white and grey matter appear different in colour due to the presence of a whitish myelin sheath around the axonal fibres. Myelinated axons tend to group together into small bundles and several bundles gather into larger tracts called *fasciculi*.

Several methods have been applied to the study of white matter connections in the animal and human brain (Table 8.1).[1-4] The techniques developed by early neuroanatomists for gross blunt dissections of white matter tracts led to important anatomical insights, including the identification of most of the white matter tracts contributing to higher cognitive functions.[5-7] Blunt dissections are performed on postmortem brains using specimens preserved in alcohol[5,6] or frozen for several days.[8,9] These procedures harden the white matter and permit manual separation of different tracts with the blunt back of a knife or a spatula. One of the limitations of these methods is the proneness to artefacts (i.e. often separation does not occur along natural cleavages) and the difficulty to obtain quantitative measurements. Also, blunt dissections require neuroanatomical knowledge, experience, and patience to achieve reliable results.

The study of white matter made a significant leap forward with the introduction of myelin staining methods for degenerating fibres (e.g. Weigert–Pal or Marchi staining).[10] The observation of serial sections of stained specimens permitted visualization of tracts in the brains of patients with cortico-subcortical lesions (mainly vascular) or in experimentally lesioned animal brains. Compared to blunt dissections, the histological methods are able to show the anatomy of fibres and their terminations in more detail. However, most of these methods have the same limitations as blunt dissections and the reconstruction of specific tracts in the human brain is highly dependent on the availability of pathological specimens with precisely localized lesions.

In the 1960s, a significant increase in knowledge about connectivity arose from the use of cellular transport mechanisms to detect connections between nerve cells.[11] Once injected, the tracers enter the neuron and are transported from the body of the neuron to its terminations (i.e. anterograde direction), or in the opposite direction (i.e. retrograde direction).[3] These methods show the anatomy of connections at the level of the single axons and remain the gold standard to understand connectivity of the animal brain. The possibility of combining multiple tracers offers also a unique advantage for depicting multiple pathways at the same time (e.g. feed-forward and feedback connections from and to a specific area).

In the 1990s, viruses were adopted as transneuronal tracers[12] with the possibility of visualizing different axonal pathways composing an entire functional system (e.g. first, second, and third order neurons). Unfortunately, these methods are invasive and cannot be applied to the human brain. Also, correlative analysis between anatomical features of individual connections and behavioural performances are difficult to perform.

In the last 15 years tractography based on diffusion magnetic resonance imaging has been developed for the *in vivo* quantification of certain microstructural characteristics of a tissue[13] and the virtual reconstruction of white matter trajectories.[14-17] Tractography studies are based on the measurement of water diffusion, typically within a cubic voxel in which the microstructural organization of the cerebral tissue hinders the free movement of water. In voxel-containing parallel axons, water diffusion is higher in the direction parallel to the fibres and restricted in the perpendicular direction. The diffusion tensor is a useful way to describe the three-dimensional displacement of water molecules and obtain an estimate of the microstructural organization of the fibres.[18]

Tractography is based on algorithms that link together the principal tensor orientation of adjacent voxels in a continuous trajectory. One advantage of this method is the possibility of quantifying diffusion properties of white matter in the living human brain that relate to underlying biological features (e.g. tract volume, myelination. etc.)[13] and correlate them with behavioural performances.[19-22] Like other methods, tractography suffers some limitations, including artefactual reconstructions and the difficulty of interpreting current diffusivity indices in relation to pathological changes.[4]

Table 8.1 Methods for studying brain connections

Method	Advantages	Limitations
Blunt dissections	◆ Applicable also to human brains ◆ Direct anatomical method ◆ Identify large tracts	◆ Only for postmortem tissue ◆ Operator-dependent ◆ Variable quality of the prepared sample ◆ Destructive ◆ Qualitative analysis only ◆ Limited ability to visualize crossing bundles and cortical projections (false negatives) ◆ Produce artefactual trajectories (false positives) ◆ Time consuming
Staining degenerating myelin (e.g. Marchi's method)	◆ Direct anatomical method ◆ Identify large and small tracts ◆ Operator-independent	◆ Only for postmortem tissue ◆ Fibre delineation limited to the lesion site and extension ◆ Variable quality of the prepared sample ◆ Destructive ◆ Qualitative analysis only ◆ Time consuming ◆ 3D reconstruction limited
Neurohistology	◆ Direct anatomical method ◆ Used to identify details of local networks ◆ Allows to distinguish the fibres' neurochemical properties (e.g. cholinergic vs dopaminergic)	◆ Only for postmortem tissue ◆ Small field of view ◆ 3D reconstruction limited ◆ Time consuming ◆ Destructive
Axonal tracing	◆ Direct anatomical method ◆ Identify large and small tracts ◆ Allow direct testing of specific hypotheses (e.g. connectivity of individual cortical regions) ◆ Can reveal fibre directionality ◆ Possibility to combine multiple tracers	◆ Not suitable for humans ◆ Fibre delineation depends on the injection site ◆ Variable quality of results depending on the tracer used ◆ Qualitative analysis is difficult ◆ Limited number of tracts per sample ◆ Destructive ◆ Time consuming ◆ 3D reconstruction limited
Viral tracers	◆ Visualization of multisynaptic pathways ◆ Can reveal fibre directionality	◆ Spurious labelling of neurons due to cell lysis (false positives) ◆ Weak labelling due to low viral concentration (false negatives) ◆ Tropism of viruses varies according to animal species ◆ Quantitative analysis is difficult
Tractography	◆ *In vivo* ◆ Applicable to human and animal brains ◆ Noninvasive ◆ Time efficient ◆ Allows the study of large populations ◆ Correlation with behavioural and other functional measures ◆ Quantitative ◆ Multiple hypothesis testing ◆ Not destructive	◆ Indirect anatomical method ◆ Low spatial resolution ◆ Presence of artefacts ◆ Operator-dependent ◆ Limited visualization of bending, merging, and crossing fibres ◆ Indirect quantitative indices of fibre volume and integrity

Classification of white matter pathways

White matter connections can be classified into three major groups: *association*, *commissural*, and *projection* pathways.[23] These three groups are composed of long-range connections mediating connectivity between distant regions. A fourth group of connections, the *U-shaped fibres*, is responsible for the local connectivity between neighbouring gyri, usually within the same lobe (intralobar) or between lobes (interlobar).[24] Additional tracts that do not fit into the classical nomenclature have been described.[24–27] These tracts are intermediate between long association pathways and short U-shaped fibres as they connect distant regions but within the same lobe (i.e. the vertical occipital tract of Wernicke or the frontal aslant tract in the frontal lobe).[24,25,28–30]

Association pathways

Association pathways connect cortical regions within the same hemisphere and their fibres have either a posterior–anterior or an anterior–posterior direction.[17] The terminology used to indicate the association tracts often refers to their shape (e.g. the uncinate from the Latin *uncinatus* meaning 'hook-like'), their origin and termination (e.g. inferior fronto-occipital fasciculus), or their course and location (e.g. inferior longitudinal fasciculus). Most of the long association tracts are composed of short and long fibres. The short fibres run more superficially, closer to the cortex, and connect neighbouring regions. These short fibres can also be classified separately as individual U-shaped tracts.[24,27] The long fibres run just underneath the U-shaped fibres and the depth of their course varies according to the distance they travel (the deepest fibres travel furthest distance).

The association tracts are involved in higher cognitive functions, such as language, praxis, visuospatial processing, memory, and emotion.[31] The major association tracts of the human brain are the arcuate fasciculus, the superior longitudinal fasciculus, the cingulum, the uncinate fasciculus, the inferior longitudinal fasciculus, and the inferior fronto-occipital fasciculus (Fig. 8.1).

The *arcuate fasciculus* (AF) is a dorsal association tract connecting perisylvian regions of the frontal, parietal, and temporal lobe. In humans two parallel pathways have been distinguished within the arcuate fasciculus. The medial direct pathway (i.e. the arcuate fasciculus *sensu strictu* or direct long segment) connects Wernicke's region in the

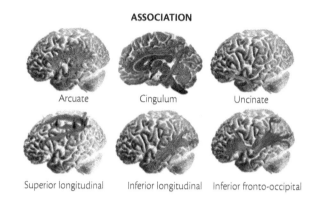

ASSOCIATION

Fig. 8.1 Tractography reconstruction of the major association pathways of the human brain.
Adapted from Catani, Marco, Thiebaut de Schotten, Michel, Atlas of Human Brain Connections, Copyright (2012), with permission from Oxford University Press..

temporal lobe (BA 41, 42, 22, 37) with Broca's region in the frontal lobe (BA 6, 44, 45). The indirect pathway consists of an anterior segment linking Broca's to Geschwind's region in the inferior parietal lobule (BA 39, 40) and a posterior segment linking Geschwind's to Wernicke's region.[32] The direct long segment of the arcuate fasciculus is larger on the left hemisphere compared to the right in about 80 per cent of the population. The remaining 20 per cent shows a bilateral distribution.[19]

Among the left lateralized people the degree of asymmetry is quite heterogeneous with 60 per cent of them showing an extreme degree of left lateralization and the remaining 20 per cent a moderate left asymmetry (Fig. 8.2). In general, those who have a more bilateral

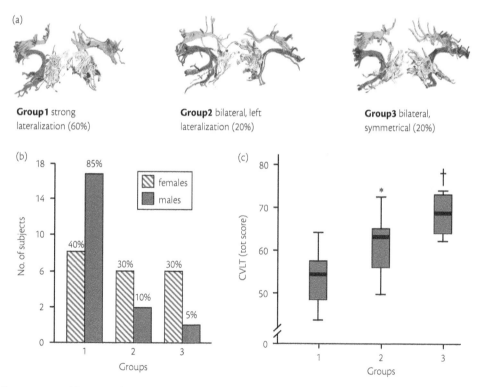

Fig. 8.2 Lateralization of long segment of the arcuate fasciculus and behavioral correlates. (a) Distribution of the lateralization pattern of the direct long segment (red). (b) Distribution of the lateralization groups between genders. (c) Performances in the CVLT according to the three lateralization groups (*, P = 0.01 versus Group 1; †, P = 0.001 versus Group 1).
Adapted from *Proc Natl Acad Sci USA*. 104(43), Catani M, Allin MP, *et al*. Symmetries in human brain language pathways correlate with verbal recall, pp. 17163–8, Copyright (2007), with permission from PNAS.

distribution of the long segment connections perform better on a verbal memory task that relies on semantic clustering for retrieval (i.e. California verbal learning test, CVLT).[19] Furthermore, the direct long segment in the left hemisphere mediates auditory-motor integration, which is crucial during early stages of language acquisition and word learning.[22] The role of the indirect pathway could be more complex and related to linking semantics and phonology,[33] processing syntactically complex sentences,[34,35] and various aspects of verbal working memory.[36] The role of the direct and indirect pathways in word repetition remains to be clarified.[37,38]

The *superior longitudinal fasciculus* (SLF) has three distinct branches as originally described in the monkey brain using axonal tracing methods.[39] In humans, the first branch of the superior longitudinal fasciculus (SLF I) connects the superior parietal lobule and precuneus (BA 5 and 7) to the superior frontal (BA 8, 9, 32) and perhaps to some anterior cingulate areas (BA 24). The SLF I processes the spatial coordinates of trunk and inferior limbs and contributes to the preparatory stages of movement planning (e.g. anticipation),[40] oculomotor coordination,[41] visual reaching,[42] and voluntary orientation of attention.[43]

The second branch (SLF II) originates in the anterior intraparietal sulcus and the angular gyrus (BA 39) and terminates in the posterior regions of the superior and middle frontal gyrus (BA 6, 8, 9). In the left hemisphere, the SLF II is involved in processing the spatial coordinates of the upper limbs, and in other functions similar to the SLF I.[40,44] In the right hemisphere the SLF II participates in attention,[45,46] visuospatial processing,[47] and spatial working memory.[48]

The third branch (SLF III) connects the intraparietal sulcus and inferior parietal lobule to the inferior frontal gyrus (BA 44, 45, 47). The SLF III corresponds to the anterior segment of the arcuate fasciculus and the two terms are currently used interchangeably.[24] Future studies will be necessary to establish whether, according to its functional role, the SLF III/anterior segment should be considered as part of the sensory-motor SLF system or the arcuate language network.

In the human brain the three branches have a different pattern of lateralization (Fig. 8.3).[21] In right-handed subjects the SLF I is symmetrically distributed between left and right hemispheres; the SLF II shows a trend of right lateralization and the SLF III is significantly right lateralized. Most importantly, the lateralization of the SLF II correlates with asymmetry in behavioural performances for visuospatial tasks (Figs 8.3c and d). In particular, the majority of the people have a larger SLF II volumes on the right hemisphere and show a greater deviation to the left (i.e. pseudo-neglect effect) in the line bisection, whereas those subjects deviating to the right show an opposite pattern of lateralization (i.e. larger volume of the left SLF II). Moreover, the same the correlation was found between the lateralization of SLF II volumes and the performances on a modified Posner paradigm, a task that measures spatial orienting of attention. Again, larger SLF II volumes in the right hemisphere corresponded to faster detection times of stimuli flashed in the left hemifield.

It is unknown how differences between the two hemispheres in SLF II volume can lead to asymmetrical processing of visual scenes. A larger tract in the right hemisphere could depend on several

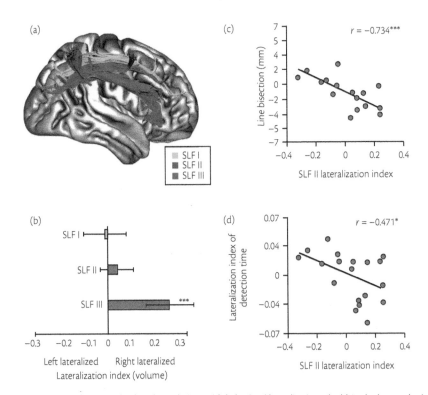

Fig. 8.3 Asymmetry of the superior longitudinal fasciculus (SLF) and correlations with behavioral lateralizations. (a–b) In the human brain the three SLF branches show varying degrees of asymmetry (95% confidence intervals). (c–d) The asymmetry of the SLF II correlates with the deviation on the line bisection task (c), and the lateralization of the detection time (d). *P < 0.05 and ***P < 0.001.

factors, including greater fibre myelination, more axons, and larger axonal diameter which are correlated with conduction speed or greater recruitment of cortical areas.[49,50] Similar results have been found with other visuospatial attentional tests.[104] Overall these findings suggest that right hemispheric specialization for spatial attention might, in part, be explained by an unbalanced speed of visuospatial processing along the SLF II.

The *cingulum* is a sickle-shaped tract composed of fibres of different length. The longest fibres run from the amygdala, uncus (BA35), and parahippocampal gyrus (BA36 and 30) to subgenual areas of the orbitofrontal lobe (BA 25 and 11).[51–53] Shorter fibres, that join and leave the cingulum along its length, connect to adjacent areas of the cingulate cortex (BA 23 and 24), superior medial frontal gyrus (BA 32, 6, 8, and 9), paracentral lobule (BA4), precuneus (BA 7), cuneus (BA 19), lingual (BA 18 and 19), and fusiform gyri (BA 19 and 37).

The cingulum can be divided into a dorsal and a ventral component.[54,55] The dorsal component connects areas of the dorsomedial default-mode network.[56,57] This consists of a group of medial regions whose activity decreases in the transition between a 'resting state' and the execution of goal directed tasks, irrespective of the nature of the task. The default-mode network has been linked to a number of functions including working memory, focusing attention to sensory-driven activities, understanding other people's intention (mentalising or theory of mind), prospective thinking (envisioning the future), and memory for personal events (autobiographic memory).[57–59] The ventral cingulum connects amygdala and parahippocampal cortex to retrosplenial regions and forms a network dedicated to spatial orientation.[60,61]

The *uncinate fasciculus* (UF) is a hook-shaped tract that connects the anterior part of the temporal lobe (BA 38) with the orbital (BA 11 and 47) and polar (BA 10) frontal cortex.[17] The fibres of the uncinate originate from the temporal pole (BA 38), uncus (BA 35), parahippocampal gyrus (BA 36 and 30), and amygdala. After a U-turn, the fibres of the uncinate enter the anterior floor of the external/extreme capsule between the insula and the putamen. Here, the uncinate runs inferiorly to the fronto-occipital fasciculus before entering the orbital region of the frontal lobe, where it splits into a ventro-lateral branch, which terminates in the lateral orbitofrontal cortex (BA 11 and 47), and an antero-medial branch that continues towards the cingulate gyrus (BA 32) and the frontal pole (BA 10).[51]

Whether the uncinate fasciculus is a lateralized bundle is still debated. An asymmetry of the volume and density of fibres of this fasciculus has been reported in a human postmortem neurohistological study in which the uncinate fasciculus was found to be asymmetric in 80 per cent of subjects, containing on average 30 per cent more fibres in the right hemisphere compared to the left.[62] However, diffusion measurements have shown higher fractional anisotropy in the left uncinate compared to the right in children and adolescents,[63] but not in adults.[21] The uncinate fasciculus connects the anterior temporal lobe to the orbitofrontal region and part of the inferior frontal gyrus and may play an important role in lexical retrieval, semantic association, naming, and social cognition.[35,65–67]

The *inferior longitudinal fasciculus* (ILF) does not constitute a single pathway, but contains fibres of different length. The occipital branches of the inferior longitudinal fasciculus connect with a number of regions dedicated to vision, including the extrastriate areas on the dorso-lateral occipital cortex (e.g. descending occipital gyrus), the ventral surface of the posterior lingual and fusiform gyri, and the medial regions of the cuneus.[64] These branches run

anteriorly parallel and lateral to the fibres of the splenium and optic radiation and, at the level of the posterior horn of the lateral ventricle, gather into a single bundle. In the temporal lobe, the inferior longitudinal fasciculus continues anteriorly and projects to the middle and inferior temporal gyri, temporal pole, parahippocampal gyrus, hippocampus, and amygdala.

An observation originally emphasized by Campbell,[68] and consistent with axonal tracing[2] and tractography findings, is that long associative fibres, such as those of the inferior longitudinal fasciculus, arise from the extrastriate cortex but not the calcarine striate cortex. The inferior longitudinal fasciculus carries visual information from occipital areas to the temporal lobe and plays an important role in visual object and face recognition, reading, and in linking object representations to their lexical labels.[69–71]

In humans, the *inferior fronto-occipital fasciculus* (IFOF) is a long-ranged bow-tie-shaped tract that originates from the inferior and medial surface of the occipital lobe (BA 19 and 18), with a minor contribution probably from the medial parietal lobe.[9,17,74] As it leaves the occipital lobe and enters the temporal stem, the inferior fronto-occipital fasciculus narrows in section and its fibres gather at the level of the external/extreme capsule just above the uncinate fasciculus. As it enters the frontal lobe, its fibres spread to form a thin sheet, curving dorsolaterally, that terminates mainly in the ventrolateral frontal cortex (BA 11) and frontal pole (BA 10).[17] Smaller bundles terminate in the rostral portion of the superior frontal gyrus (rostral portion of BA 9).[2,39]

There are significant simian–human differences in the anatomy of the inferior fronto-occipital fasciculus.[75,76] Axonal tracing studies in monkey suggest that frontal fibres running through the extreme capsule do not reach the occipital lobe. For this reason, the term extreme capsule tract is a preferred name for the monkey brain.[2] The inferior fronto-occipital fasciculus may have a role in reading, writing, and other semantic and syntactic aspects of language.[28,72–74]

Commissural Pathways

Commissural pathways are composed of fibres connecting the two halves of the brain. The major telencephalic commissures of the human brain include the corpus callosum, the anterior commissure, and the hippocampal commissure (Fig. 8.4). A general assumption underlying the concept of commissural connections is that the information is transferred between homologous cortical or subcortical regions. There are, however, a significant number of heterotopic commissural fibres connecting non-homologous regions, at least in the corpus callosum.[77]

The corpus callosum is the largest commissural tract in the human brain, consisting of 200–300 million axons of varying size and degrees of myelination.[78,79] The corpus callosum forms the roof of the lateral ventricles and its fibres are conventionally divided into an anterior forceps (or forceps minor) in the frontal lobe, a middle portion (body) in the frontoparietal region, and a posterior forceps (or forceps major) in the occipital lobe; on either side of the brain the tapetum stretches out into the temporal lobes. Other criteria have been adopted to subdivide the corpus callosum.

The most common methods segment the corpus callosum as seen in mid-sagittal section. Classical anatomical subdivisions of the corpus callosum include (from anterior to posterior) the rostrum (orbitofrontal cortex), genu (prefrontal cortex), body (motor and premotor cortex), isthmus (temporal cortex), and splenium

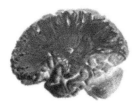
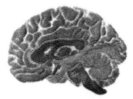

Corpus callosum   Anterior commissure

Fig. 8.4 Tractography reconstruction of the major commissural pathways of the human brain.
Adapted from Catani, Marco, Thiebaut de Schotten, Michel, Atlas of Human Brain Connections, Copyright (2012), with permission from Oxford University Press.

(occipital and temporal cortex). More recently, diffusion tensor imaging has been used to divide the corpus callosum into different subregions according to the pattern of its cortical projections.[80–84]

The anterior commissure is a small bundle of fibres shaped like the handlebars of an old bicycle straddling the midline. It is a familiar landmark in neuroradiology (e.g. distances in Talairach coordinates are measured from the anterior commissure as origin).[85] It crosses the midline as a compact cylindrical bundle between anterior and posterior columns of the fornix and runs laterally, at first through the anterior perforated substance, and then between the globus pallidus and putamen before dividing into an anterior and posterior branch. The more anterior fibres connect the amygdalae,[86] hippocampal gyri, and temporal poles,[87] while more posterior fibres connect the ventral temporal and occipital regions.

The commissural pathways allow the transfer of inputs between the two halves of the brain and play a significant role in the functional integration of motor, perceptual, and cognitive functions between the two hemispheres.[88,89] Several callosal disconnection syndromes have been described in neurology, from anarchic hand syndrome to alien hand syndrome.[54]

Projection pathways

Projection pathways connect the cortex to subcortical neurons and are usually divided into ascending and descending fibres (Fig. 8.5). The largest projection tracts of the cerebral hemispheres are the corona radiata and the fornix.

Within the hemispheres sensory information travels through a complex system of ascending thalamic projections. After a short course within the internal capsule, the thalamic radiations enter the corona radiata and terminate in the cortex of the ipsilateral hemisphere. The efferent thalamic projections to the cerebral cortex radiate anteriorly to the frontal cortex (anterior thalamic peduncle), superiorly to the precentral frontal regions and parietal cortex (superior thalamic peduncle), posteriorly to the occipito-temporal cortex (posterior thalamic peduncle), and infero-anteriorly to the temporal cortex and amygdala (inferior thalamic peduncle).

The three major descending cortico-subcortical projection systems of the corona radiata are the corticospinal and corticobulbar tracts, the cortical efferents to the basal ganglia and the cortical efferents, via the pons, to the cerebellum.[90,91] The projections to the basal ganglia and cerebellum are indirectly reciprocal, so that the cortex also receives projections from these centres via the thalamus, to create complex cortico-basal ganglion and cortico-cerebellar circuits. These projection systems are only partially segregated anatomically as they share several subcortical relay stations (e.g. the thalamus).[92]

The fornix is also considered as a projection tract for its projections to the hippocampus, mammillary bodies, and hypothalamic nuclei. The fornix is part of the limbic system dedicated to memory and its fibres connect the hippocampus with the mammillary body, the anterior thalamic nuclei, and the hypothalamus; it also has a small commissural component known as the hippocampal commissure.[17,51,60] Fibres arise from the hippocampus (subiculum and entorhinal cortex) of each side, run through the fimbria, and join beneath the splenium of the corpus callosum to form the body of the fornix. Other fimbrial fibres continue medially, cross the midline, and project to the contralateral hippocampus (hippocampal commissure). Most of the fibres within the body of the fornix run anteriorly beneath the body of the corpus callosum towards the anterior commissure.

Above the interventricular foramen, the anterior body of the fornix divides into right and left columns. As each column approaches the anterior commissure it diverges again into two components. One of these, the posterior columns of the fornix, curves ventrally in front of the interventricular foramen of Monroe and posterior to the anterior commissure to enter the mammillary body (postcommissural fornix), adjacent areas of the hypothalamus, and anterior thalamic nucleus. The second component, the anterior columns of the fornix, enters the hypothalamus and projects to the septal region and nucleus accumbens.[60] The fornix also contains some afferent fibres to the hippocampus from septal and hypothalamic nuclei.[52]

Short association pathways

A number of short U-shaped fibres and intralobar association tracts have been described in the human brain using postmortem dissections and, more recently, tractography.[107] The role of these tracts is largely unknown. Among the short intralobar association tracts connections, the frontal aslant tract, the frontal orbito-polar tract, and the vertical occipital bundle of Wernicke have been well characterized using tractography (Fig. 8.6).

The frontal aslant tract connects the most posterior part of Broca's territory (i.e. precentral cortex, BA 6, pars opercularis, BA 44) in the inferior frontal gyrus with the pre-supplementary motor area (SMA) in the superior frontal gyrus (BA 8 and 6), the medial prefrontal cortex, and the anterior cingulate cortex.[26,29,30] This tract is left lateralized in most right-handed subjects, suggesting a role in language. Medial regions of the frontal lobe facilitate speech initiation through direct connections to the pars opercularis and triangularis of the inferior frontal gyrus. Patients with lesions to these areas present with various degrees of speech impairment from a total inability to initiate

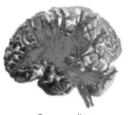
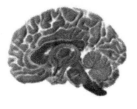

Corona radiata   Fornix

Fig. 8.5 Tractography reconstruction of the major projection pathways of the human brain.
Adapted from Catani, Marco, Thiebaut de Schotten, Michel, Atlas of Human Brain Connections, Copyright (2012), with permission from Oxford University Press.

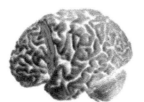 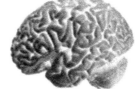 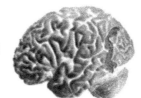

Frontal aslant tract   Fronto-orbitopolar tract   Vertical occipital tract

Fig. 8.6 Tractography reconstruction of three short intralobar fibres of the frontal and occipital lobe.

speech (i.e. mutism) to mild altered fluency.[93,94] The frontal aslant tract is damaged in patients with a non-fluent/agrammatic variant of primary progressive aphasia, PNFA,[67] and in traumatic brain injury patients with difficulties in response inhibition control.[105]

The frontal orbito-polar bundle is a ventral tract connecting posterior (BA 25 and 11) and anterior orbitofrontal gyri (BA 11) and the frontal pole (BA 10). The posterior orbital gyrus receives inputs from the limbic regions (i.e. amygdala, hippocampus, nucleus basalis of Meynert, olfactory cortex, and insula) and plays an important role in processing olfactory and gustatory inputs and integration of emotions and memories associated with sensory experiences.[95]

The anterior orbitofrontal cortex receives direct auditory and visual inputs from posterior occipital and temporal cortex through the inferior fronto-occipital and uncinate fasciculus.[74,96] The frontal orbito-polar tract represents a transmodal network for binding memories and emotions with olfactory, taste, visual, and auditory inputs. This multisensory association and limbic integration could guide more complex cognitive and behavioural functions, such as reward behaviour associated with sensory and abstract reinforcers (e.g. monetary gain and loss)[97] or response inhibition (e.g. go/no-go tasks).[98]

The vertical occipital bundle of Wernicke was originally described by Sachs in 1892 as an intralobar group of fibres connecting the inferior occipital gyrus (BA 19, 37) with dorsolateral occipital cortex (BA 19) and perhaps posterior parietal cortex (BA 39).[25] This tract links dorsal and ventral visual streams and is likely to be involved in reading.[27,28]

Contribution of white matter to cognition and behaviour

Optimal cognitive processes rely on an efficient propagation of the action potential along the axons.[99] Higher speed of conduction is important, for example, to guarantee a quick response to external stimuli or to propagate signal to distant regions without delay. The function of white matter tracts is not limited to information transmission but also includes aspects that impact on information processing. Collateral axons, for example, branch off the main axon and generally feed back onto their own neuronal bodies or cortical inhibitory neurons. Through these collateral axons, neurons mediate self-modulation of their own firing. Collateral axons and branching are also important to filter, amplify, and distribute signal to multiple cortical and subcortical targets.[100] Hence, in a modern view of white matter networks, axonal fibres constitute not only conducting devices but also nexuses of convergence and divergence, feedback loops, feed-forward connections, and transition points from serial to parallel processing.[101]

Historically, the study of white matter function has been hindered by the lack of methods for *in vivo* quantitative measurements of fibre anatomy in the central nervous system. Most of the properties of fibres have been derived from studies of peripheral nerves, but this may not apply directly to fibres of the central nervous system.[50] Tractography can indirectly measure properties of white matter bundles that influence the speed of signal propagation. Indeed, preliminary evidence of a direct correlation between diffusion-derived anatomical features of individual tracts and behavioural performances are forthcoming. The two most important biological axonal features affecting the speed of conduction of the nervous signal are the axonal diameter and its myelination. In general, axons with larger diameter offer a weaker resistance along the longitudinal axis and therefore facilitate faster conduction along a direction longitudinal to the main axis. Similarly, heavily myelinated axons increase the resistance across the membrane and expedite faster longitudinal conduction.[49,50]

While the axonal diameter of fibres is generally determined by maturational processes that occur during early brain development and plateau in adolescence, the degree of myelin produced by oligodendrocytes changes quite rapidly in relation, for example, to the frequency of firing of specific groups of fibres engaged in certain cognitive processes. This explains, for example, why changes in myelin can occur after intense training.[102]

Tractography can help advancing our understanding of cognitive disorders. In older age, white matter changes occur in relation to reduced number of myelinated fibres, gliosis, and ischaemic damage. Depending on the location, white matter changes have a significant impact on cognition.[103] The study of white matter connections with tractography is becoming an important tool for quantifying tissue damage, perhaps in regions where white matter changes are not visibile on conventional MRI. Furthermore, the use of tractography or tractography-derived atlases could improve localization of white matter damage along critical pathways. Finally, individual differences in tract anatomy (e.g. lateralization) could have important implications for understanding variability in cognitive and behavioural performances. It may also help to identify patterns of vulnerability and resilience to brain disorders.[106]

References

1. Vercelli A, Repici M, Garbossa D, *et al*. Recent techniques for tracing pathways in the central nervous system of developing and adult mammals. *Brain Res Bull*. 2000;51(1):11–28.
2. Schmahmann JD and Pandya DN. *Fiber Pathways of the Brain*. Oxford: Oxford University Press, 2006.
3. Morecraft RJ, Ugolini G, Lanciego JL, *et al*. Classic and Contemporary Neural Tract Tracing Techniques. In: H Johansen-Berg and

TE Behrens. *Diffusion MRI: From Quantitative Measurement to In Vivo Neuroanatomy.* London: Elsevier, 2009, pp. 273–308.

4. Dell'Acqua F and Catani M. Structural human brain networks: hot topics in diffusion tractography. *Curr Opin Neurol.* 2012;25(4):375–83.

5. Catani M and ffytche DH. The rises and falls of disconnection syndromes. *Brain.* 2005;128(10):2224–39.

6. Reil JC. Die vördere Commissur im großen Gehirn. *Archiv für die Physiologie.* 1812;11:89–100.

7. Burdach K. *Vom Baue und Leben des Gehirns und Rückenmarks.* Leipzig: Dyk, 1819–26.

8. Ludwig E and Klingler J. *Atlas Cerebri Humani. The Inner Structure of the Brain Demonstrated on the Basis of Macroscopical Preparations.* Boston, MA: Little Brown, 1956.

9. Martino J, Brogna C, Robles SG, *et al.* (2010). Anatomic dissection of the inferior fronto-occipital fasciculus revisited in the lights of brain stimulation data. *Cortex.* 2010;46(5):691–9.

10. Marchi V and Algeri EG. Sulle degenerazioni discendenti consecutive a lesioni in diverse zone della corteccia cerebrale. *Riv Sper Freniatr Med Leg Alien Ment.* 1886;141–59.

11. Lanciego JL and Wouterlood FG. Neuroanatomical tract-tracing methods beyond 2000: what's now and next. *J Neurosci Methods.* 2000;103(1):1–2.

12. Kuypers HG and Ugolini G. Viruses as transneuronal tracers. *Trends Neurosci.* 1990;13(2):71–5.

13. Beaulieu C. The Biological Basis of Diffusion Anisotropy. In: H Johansen-Berg and TE Behrens. *Diffusion MRI: From Quantitative Measurement to In Vivo Neuroanatomy.* London: Elsevier, 2009, pp. 105–26.

14. Conturo TE, Lori NF, Cull TS, *et al.* Tracking neuronal fiber pathways in the living human brain. *Proc Natl Acad Sci USA.* 96(18):10422–7.

15. Mori S, Crain BJ, Chacko VP, *et al.* Three-dimensional tracking of axonal projections in the brain by magnetic resonance imaging. *Ann Neurol.* 1999;45(2):265–9.

16. Basser PJ, Pajevic S, Pierpaoli C, *et al.* In vivo fiber tractography using DT-MRI data. *Magnet Resonance Med.* 2000;44(4):625–32.

17. Catani M, Howard RJ, *et al.* Virtual in vivo interactive dissection of white matter fasciculi in the human brain. *Neuroimage.* 2002;17(1):77–94.

18. Basser PJ, Mattiello J, and LeBihan D. MR diffusion tensor spectroscopy and imaging. *Biophysical Journal.* 1994;66(1):259–67.

19. Catani M, Allin MP, Husain M, *et al.* Symmetries in human brain language pathways correlate with verbal recall. *Proc Natl Acad Sci USA.* 2007;104(43):17163–8.

20. Kontis D, Catani M, Cuddy M, *et al.* Diffusion tensor MRI of the corpus callosum and cognitive function in adults born preterm. *Neuroreport.* 2009; 20(4):424–8.

21. Thiebaut de Schotten M, Dell'Acqua F, Forkel SJ, *et al.* A lateralized brain network for visuospatial attention. *Nat Neurosci.* 2011;14(10):1245–6.

22. Lopez-Barroso D, Catani M, Ripollés P, *et al.* Word learning is mediated by the left arcuate fasciculus. *Proc Natl Acad Sci USA.* 2013;110(32):13168–73.

23. Meynert T. *A Clinical Treatise on Diseases of the Fore-brain based upon a Study of its Structure, Functions, and Nutrition* (trans Bernard Sachs). New York, NY: GP Putnam's Sons, 1885.

24. Catani MF, Dell'acqua F, Bizzi A, *et al.* Beyond cortical localization in clinico-anatomical correlation. *Cortex.* 2012;48(10):1262–87.

25. Sachs H. *Das Hemisphärenmark des menschlichen grosshirns.* Leipzig: Verlag Von Georg Thieme, 1892.

26. Oishi K, Zilles Z, Amunts K, *et al.* Human brain white matter atlas: identification and assignment of common anatomical structures in superficial white matter. *NeuroImage.* 2008;43(3):447–57.

27. Guevara P, Poupon C, Rivière D, *et al.* Robust clustering of massive tractography datasets. *Neuroimage.* 2011;54(3):1975–93.

28. Yeatman JD, Rauschecker AM, Wandell BA, *et al.* (2013). Anatomy of the visual word form area: adjacent cortical circuits and long-range white matter connections. *Brain Lang.* 2013;125(2):146–55.

29. Lawes INC, Barrick TR, Murugam V, *et al.* Atlas-based segmentation of white matter tracts of the human brain using diffusion tensor tractography and comparison with classical dissection. *Neuroimage.* 2008;39(1):62–79.

30. Ford A, McGregor KM, Case K, *et al.* Structural connectivity of Broca's area and medial frontal cortex. *Neuroimage.* 2010;52(4):1230–7.

31. Catani M. Diffusion tensor magnetic resonance imaging tractography in cognitive disorders. *Curr Opin Neurol.* 2006;19(6):599–606.

32. Catani M, Jones DK, and ffytche DH. Perisylvian language networks of the human brain. *Ann Neurol.* 2005;57(1):8–16.

33. Newhart M, Trupe LA, Gomez Y, *et al.* Asyntactic comprehension, working memory, and acute ischemia in Broca's area versus angular gyrus. *Cortex.* 2012;48(10):1288–97.

34. Perani D, Saccuman MC, Scifo P, *et al.* Neural language networks at birth. *Proc Natl Acad Sci USA.* 2011;108(38):16056–61.

35. Wilson SM, Galantucci S, Tartaglia MC, *et al.* (2011). Syntactic processing depends on dorsal language tracts. *Neuron.* 72(2):397–403.

36. Jacquemot and Scott

37. Breier JI, Hasan K, Zhang W, *et al.* Language dysfunction after stroke and damage to white matter tracts evaluated using diffusion tensor imaging. *Am J Neuroradiol.* 2008;29(3):483–7.

38. Fridriksson J, Kjartansson O, Morgan PS, *et al.* Impaired speech repetition and left parietal lobe damage. *J Neurosci.* 2010;30(33):11057–61.

39. Petrides M and Pandya DN. Projections to the frontal cortex from the posterior parietal region in the rhesus monkey. *J Comp Neurol.* 1984;228(1):105–16.

40. Leiguarda RC and Marsden CD. Limb apraxias: Higher-order disorders of sensorimotor integration. *Brain.* 2000;123(Pt 5):860–79.

41. Anderson EJ, Jones DK, O'Gorman RL, *et al.* Cortical network for gaze control in humans revealed using multimodal MRI. *Cereb Cortex.* 2011.

42. Johnson PB, Ferraina S, Bianchi L, *et al.* Cortical networks for visual reaching: physiological and anatomical organization of frontal and parietal lobe arm regions. *Cereb Cortex.* 1996;6(2):102–19.

43. Corbetta M and Shulman GL. Control of goal-directed and stimulus-driven attention in the brain. *Nature Rev Neurosci.* 2002;3(3):201–15.

44. Goldenberg G and Karnath HO. The neural basis of imitation is body part specific. *J Neurosci.* 2006;26(23):6282–7.

45. Lynch JC and Mountcastle VB, Talbot WH, *et al.* Parietal lobe mechanisms for directed visual attention. *J Neurophysiol.* 1977;40(2):362–89.

46. Corbetta MF, Miezin FM, Gordon L, *et al.* A PET study of visuospatial attention. *J Neurosci.* 1993;13(3):1202–26.

47. Thiebaut de Schotten M, Urbanski M, Duffau H, *et al.* Direct evidence for a parietal-frontal pathway subserving spatial awareness in humans. *Science.* 2005;309(5744):2226–8.

48. Levy R and Goldman-Rakic PS. Segregation of working memory functions within the dorsolateral prefrontal cortex. *Exp Brain Res.* 2000;133(1):23–32.

49. Hursh JB. Conduction Velocity and diameter of nerve fibers. *Am J Physiol.* 1939;127:131–39.

50. Waxman SG and Bennett M. Relative conduction velocities of small myelinated and non-myelinated fibres in the central nervous system. *Nat New Biol.* 1972;238(85):217–9.

51. Crosby EC, Humphrey T, and Lauer EW. *Correlative Anatomy of the Nervous System.* New York, NY: Macmillian Co, 1962.

52. Nieuwenhuys R, Voogd J, Huijzen C van. *The Human Central Nervous System.* Berlin: Springer, 2008.

53. Catani MF, Dell'acqua F, and Thiebaut de Schotten. A revised limbic system model for memory, emotion and behaviour. *Neurosci Biobehav Rev.* 2013;37(8):1724–37.

54. Catani M and Thiebaut de Schotten M. *Atlas of Human Brain Connections.* Oxford: Oxford University Press, 2012.

55. Jones DK, Christiansen KF, Chapman RJ, *et al.* Distinct subdivisions of the cingulum bundle revealed by diffusion MRI fibre tracking: implications for neuropsychological investigations. *Neuropsychologia.* 2013;51(1):67–78.

56. Raichle ME, MacLeod AM, Snyder AZ, *et al.* A default mode of brain function. *Proc Natl Acad Sci USA.* 2001;98(2):676–82.

57. Raichle ME and Snyder AZ. A default mode of brain function: a brief history of an evolving idea. *Neuroimage*. 2007;37(4):1083–90; discussion 1097–9.

58. Amodio DM and Frith CD. Meeting of minds: the medial frontal cortex and social cognition. *Nat Rev Neurosci*. 2006;7(4):268–77.

59. Broyd SJ, Demanuele C, Debener S, et al. Default-mode brain dysfunction in mental disorders: a systematic review. *Neurosci Biobehav Rev*. 2009;33(3):279–96.

60. Aggleton JP. EPS Mid-Career Award 2006. Understanding anterograde amnesia: disconnections and hidden lesions. *Q J Exp Psychol (Colchester)*. 2008;61(10):1441–71.

61. Vann SD, Aggleton JP, Maguire EA, et al. What does the retrosplenial cortex do? *Nat Rev Neurosci*. 2009;10(11):792–802.

62. Highley JR, Walker MA, Esiri MM, et al. Asymmetry of the uncinate fasciculus: a post-mortem study of normal subjects and patients with schizophrenia. *Cereb Cortex*. 2002;12(11):1218–24.

63. Eluvathingal TJ, Hasan KM, Kramer L, et al. Quantitative diffusion tensor tractography of association and projection fibers in normally developing children and adolescents. *Cereb Cortex*. 2007;17(12):2760–8.

64. Catani M, Jones DK, Donato R, et al. Occipito-temporal connections in the human brain. *Brain*. 2003;126(Pt 9):2093–107.

65. Craig MC, Catani M, Deeley Q, et al. Altered connections on the road to psychopathy. *Molecular Psychiatr*. 2009;14(10):946–53.

66. Papagno C, Miracapillo C, Casarotti A, et al. What is the role of the uncinate fasciculus? Surgical removal and proper name retrieval. *Brain*. 2011;134(Pt 2):405–14.

67. Catani M, Mesulam MM, Jakobsen E, et al. A novel frontal pathway underlies verbal fluency in primary progressive aphasia. *Brain*. 2013;136(Pt 8):2619–28.

68. Campbell AW. *Histological Studies on the Localisation of Cerebral Function*. Cambridge, Cambridge University Press, 1905.

69. Epelbaum S, Pinel P, Gaillard R, et al. Pure alexia as a disconnection syndrome: new diffusion imaging evidence for an old concept. *Cortex*. 2008;44(8):962–74.

70. Fox C, Iaria G, and Barton J. Disconnection in prosopagnosia and face processing. *Cortex*. 2008;44(8):996–1009.

71. ffytche DH, Blom JD, and Catani M. Disorders of visual perception. *Journal of neurol, Neurosur Psych*. 2010;81(11):1280–7.

72. Duffau H, Gatignol P, Mandonnet E, et al. New insights into the anatomo-functional connectivity of the semantic system: a study using cortico-subcortical electrostimulations. *Brain*. 2005;128(Pt 4):797–810.

73. Anwander A, Tittgemeyer, von Cramon DY, et al. Connectivity-based parcellation of Broca's area. *Cereb Cortex*. 2007;17(4):816–25.

74. Forkel SJ, Thiebaut de Schotten M, Kawadler JM, et al. The anatomy of fronto-occipital connections from early blunt dissections to contemporary tractography. *Cortex*. 2014;56:73–84.

75. Catani M. From hodology to function. *Brain*. 2007;130(Pt 3):602–5.

76. Schmahmann JD, Pandya DN, Wang R, et al. Association fibre pathways of the brain: parallel observations from diffusion spectrum imaging and autoradiography. *Brain*. 2007;130(Pt 3):630–53.

77. Clarke S. *The Role of Homotopic and Heterotopic Callosal Connections in Humans*. Cambridge, MA: MIT Press, 2003.

78. Tomasch J. Size, distribution, and number of fibres in the human corpus callosum. *Anat Rec*. 1954;119(1):119–35.

79. Aboitiz F, Scheibel AB, Fisher RS, et al. (1992). Fiber composition of the human corpus callosum. *Brain Res*. 1992;598(1–2):143–53.

80. Huang H, Zhang J, Jiang H, et al. DTI tractography based parcellation of white matter: application to the mid-sagittal morphology of corpus callosum. *Neuroimage*. 2005;26(1):195–205.

81. Hofer S and Frahm J. Topography of the human corpus callosum revisited—comprehensive fiber tractography using diffusion tensor magnetic resonance imaging. *Neuroimage*. 2006;32(3):989–94.

82. Zarei M, Johansen-Berg H, Smith S, et al. (2006). Functional anatomy of interhemispheric cortical connections in the human brain. *J Anat*. 1006;209(3):311–20.

83. Park HJ, Kim JJ, Lee SK, et al. Corpus callosal connection mapping using cortical gray matter parcellation and DT-MRI. *Hum Brain Mapp*. 2008;29(5):503–16.

84. Chao YP, Cho KH, Yeh CH, et al. Probabilistic topography of human corpus callosum using cytoarchitectural parcellation and high angular resolution diffusion imaging tractography. *Hum Brain Mapp*. 2009;30(10):3172–87.

85. Talairach J and Tournoux P. *Co-planar Stereotaxic Atlas of the Human Brain: 3-Dimensional Proportional System—An Approach to Cerebral Imaging*. New York, NY: Thieme Medical Publishers, 1988.

86. Turner BH, Mishkin M, Knapp ME, et al. Distribution of the anterior commissure to the amygdaloid complex in the monkey. *Brain Res*. 1979;162(2):331–7.

87. Demeter S, Rosene DL, Van Hoesen GW, et al. Fields of origin and pathways of the interhemispheric commissures in the temporal lobe of macaques. *J Comp Neurol*. 1990;302(1):29–53.

88. Gazzaniga MS. Cerebral specialization and interhemispheric communication: does the corpus callosum enable the human condition? *Brain*. 2000;123(Pt 7):1293–326.

89. Glickstein M and Berlucchi G. Classical disconnection studies of the corpus callosum. *Cortex*. 2008;44(8):914–27.

90. Dejerine J. *Anatomie des Centres Nerveux*. Paris: Rueff et Cie, 1901.

91. Newton JM, Ward NS, Parker GJ, et al. Non-invasive mapping of corticofugal fibres from multiple motor areas—relevance to stroke recovery. *Brain*. 2006;129(Pt 7):1844–58.

92. Schmahmann JD and Pandya DN. Disconnection syndromes of basal ganglia, thalamus, and cerebrocerebellar systems. *Cortex*. 2008;44(8):1037–66.

93. Penfield W and Rasmussen T. Vocalization and arrest of speech. *Arch Neurol Psychiatry*. 1949;61(1):21–7.

94. Bizzi A, Nava S, Ferrè F, et al. Aphasia induced by gliomas growing in the ventrolateral frontal region: assessment with diffusion MR tractography, functional MR imaging and neuropsychology. *Cortex*. 2012;48(2):255–72.

95. Rolls E. *The Functions of the Orbitofrontal Cortex*. Oxford: Oxford University Press, 2002.

96. Price JL. Definition of the orbital cortex in relation to specific connections with limbic and visceral structures and other cortical regions. *Ann NY Acad Sci*. 2007;1121:54–71.

97. Kringelbach ML. The human orbitofrontal cortex: linking reward to hedonic experience. *Nature Rev Neurosci*. 2005;6(9):691–702.

98. Iversen SD and Mishkin M. Perseverative interference in monkeys following selective lesions of the inferior prefrontal convexity. *Exp Brain Res*. 1970;11(4):376–86.

99. Filley CM. Neurobiology of hite matter disorders. In: DJ Jones (ed.). *Diffusion MRI*. New York, NY: Oxford University Press, 2011, pp. 19–30.

100. Waxman SG. Regional differentiation of the axon: a review with special reference to the concept of the multiplex neuron. *Brain Research*. 1972;47:269–88.

101. Catani M and MM Mesulam. What is a disconnection syndrome? *Cortex*. 2008;44(8):911–3.

102. Scholz J, Klein MC, Behrens TE, et al. Training induces changes in white-matter architecture. *Nat Neurosci*. 2009;12(11):1370–1.

103. Lamar M, Catani M, et al. (2008). The impact of region-specific leukoaraiosis on working memory deficits in dementia. *Neuropsychologia*. 2008;46(10):2597–601.

104. Chechlacz M, Gillebert CR, Vangkilde SA, et al. Structural variability within frontoparietal networks and individual differences in attentional functions: an approach using the theory of visual attention. *J Neurosci*. 2015;35(30):10647–58.

105. Bonnelle V, Ham TE, Leech R, et al. Salience network integrity predicts default mode network function after traumatic brain injury. *Proc Natl Acad Sci USA*. 2012;109(12):4690–5.

106. Forkel SJ, Thiebaut de Schotten M, Dell'Acqua F, et al. Anatomical predictors of aphasia recovery: a tractography study of bilateral perisylvian language networks. *Brain*. 2014;137(7):2027–39.

107. Catani MF, Dell'Acqua F, Vergani F, et al. Short frontal lobe connections of the human brain. *Cortex*. 2012;48(2):273–91.

CHAPTER 9

Neurochemistry of cognition

Trevor W. Robbins

Introduction

Cognition and behaviour are among the more obvious outputs of brain functioning and are inextricably linked, not only to themselves, but to neuronal networks that depend ultimately on chemical neurotransmission.[1] In fact, less than 70 years ago it was considered controversial to believe that the brain used chemical neurotransmitters at all. It was shortly agreed that only two such substances existed (with excitatory and inhibitory functions), and we have now come to realize that the brain employs probably over 50 such molecules, sometimes in the same neurons.[2] The 1960s saw enthusiasm for the 'chemical coding' of behaviour, doubtless stimulated by the discovery of the triplet genetic code. However, this is now considered to be a rather naïve viewpoint, given that neurotransmitters can be dispersed in many different neuroanatomical locations in distinct neuronal circuitries with obviously different functions, including, for example, the peripheral nervous system, and the now common observation that the same molecule can function as a blood-borne hormone as well as a specific neurotransmitter. Incidentally, this does of course imply that a drug specifically affecting a single neurotransmitter is bound to affect more than one function, producing obvious side-effects of medications.

There are now agreed criteria for classifying chemical neurotransmitters, depending on considerations such as whether they are synthesized in neurons, released following action potentials into the synapse, where they may bind to receptor proteins and are eventually metabolized or recycled for example by so-called reuptake systems utilizing transporter molecules.[2]

Today, most classifications of neurotransmitters agree that there are 'fast signalling' molecules, generally working directly on ion channel ('ionotropic') membrane receptors and responsible for the functioning of large-scale neural networks such as those in the cerebral cortex, hippocampus, striatum, and cerebellum.[2,3] Glutamate is the most prevalent excitatory amino acid neurotransmitter and gamma aminobutyric acid (GABA) the major inhibitory amino acid transmitter employed in such networks. They have major functions in the control of cortical neuronal activity, including oscillations at various frequencies, and are implicated in such diverse functions as learning and memory and speech on the one hand, and the control of epileptiform activity on the other.

Although it is quite common for computational modelling of neural networks to operate on the assumption that nodes of connections may be switched on or off, corresponding to the likely modes of action of glutamate and GABA respectively, it is evident that these and other neurotransmitter systems function in a far more sophisticated way, often at multiple receptors, both pre- and postsynaptic and involving biochemical effects on G-proteins essential to cell

function. They may alternatively change voltages in ion channels so as to alter the excitability of the cell. Additionally, the concentration of neurotransmitter in the synaptic cleft is regulated not only by catabolic enzymes, for example, monoamine oxidases in the case of the monoamines and acetylcholine esterase in the case of acetylcholine, but also pre-synaptic transporters that enable reuptake of the released neurotransmitter back into the pre-synaptic cell.

Many factors contribute to the 'fidelity' of the signalling impinging on the post-synaptic cells and involve, for example, neuromodulatory neurotransmitters that act conditionally on the cell, depending on its current state (see reference 3). These neuromodulators, which include the classical monoamines dopamine (DA), noradrenaline (NA), and serotonin (or 5-hydroxytryptamine, 5-HT), usually tend to have a spatially and temporally less precise mode of action than the amino acid 'fast signalling neurotransmitters', and may operate over a longer timescale than glutamate or GABA. They too may work via several receptors, there being over 15 serotonin receptors, for example.[2]

It is also now clear that more than one neurotransmitter may be released from a single neuron, in contradistinction to Henry Dale's original principle. This principle of co-transmission, which generally involves a neuropeptide as the co-transmitter, has been shown to hold, for example, for dopamine cells (where the neuropeptide is cholescystokinin), noradrenaline (neuropeptide Y), and acetylcholine (Ach), vasoactive intestinal polypeptide (VIP). As these neuropeptides may also play some role in the peripheral nervous system, this exemplifies the principle of central and peripheral signalling by the same molecule acting as a hormone as well as a neurotransmitter. For more detail on basic neurochemistry and neuropharmacology the reader is urged to consult Cooper, Bloom, and Roth.[2] The main neurotransmitters mentioned above are listed in Table 9.1.

Functions of neurotransmitter systems and pathways

Although neurotransmitters may participate in a range of functions, their distribution nevertheless is not all random in the brain and their anatomical pathways may be quite specific, often for evolutionary reasons that are not entirely clear (Fig. 9.1). For example, there are two distinct ascending noradrenergic pathways, only one of which richly innervates the neocortex and forebrain. However, there is very sparse innervation of the basal ganglia by noradrenaline, which by contrast receive rich dopaminergic and serotoninergic inputs. Indeed, the discoveries concerning innervation of the caudate-putamen by the dopaminergic pathways of the substantia nigra and the production of Parkinson's disease by degeneration of

Table 9.1 Major chemical neurotransmitters

Classical neurotransmitters	
'Fast signalling'	**Receptors**
Glutamate (excitatory) (GLU)	NMDA, AMPA, Kainate
Gamma-aminobutyric acid (inhibitory) (GABA)	GABA-a, GABA-b
'Slow modulatory'	
Acetylcholine (Ach)	Nicotinic, muscarinic
Dopamine (DA)	D1–D5
Noradrenaline (NA) (norepinephrine)	alpha1,2; beta 1,2
Serotonin (5-hydroxytryptamine, 5-HT)	At least 15, including 5-HT1a, 5-HT1b, 5HT2a, 5-HT2c, 5-HT3, 5-HT6 etc.
Neuropeptides	
Very slow modulators/co-transmitters	
Cholecystokinin (CCK)—co-transmitter for DA	CCK-A, CCK-B
Neuropeptide Y—co-transmitter for NA	NPY1R, NPY2R
Vasoactive intestinal polypeptide (VIP)—co-transmitter for Ach	VPAC1, VPAC2
Oxytocin, Vasopressin, etc	OXTR, V1–V3

Reproduced from Robbins TW, Cognitive psychopharmacology. In: K Ochsner and S Kosslyn (eds). *Handbook of Cognitive Neuroscience*, Copyright (2014), with permission from Oxford University Press.

that pathway have led to a considerable research focus on the role of dopamine in motor control.

In experimental terms, the functions of these systems can be studied by the use of specific ligands, receptor agonists, and antagonists, and by the use of selective neurotoxins such as 6-hydroxydopamine (for DA- and NA-containing cells), 5,7 dihydroxytryptamine, (5-HT cells), and 192-IgG-saporin, the immunotoxin (Ach cells). Additionally, neurotransmitter systems can be studied in combination with other techniques to achieve correlative analyses with behaviour, including positron emission tomography, electrophysiology, microiontophoresis, *in vivo* microdialysis, *in vivo* voltammetry, optogenetics, and transgenic mice with knock-out or knock-in of specific receptor proteins.[1,4]

Glutamate systems: The neurochemistry of cognition and learning

Hebb[5] was among the first to consider the network properties of the brain and how neuronal circuits might participate in perception and learning. A major insight concerned the possible *plasticity* inherent in such networks and its contribution to learning and memory. In particular, he predicted that the coordinated firing of two or more neurons might result in the storage of a memory trace via transient, reverberating neuronal activity that somehow was converted to a longer-term structural change in the nerve cells, biasing them to fire in future to similar inputs. Indirect evidence for this type of change was later provided by the discovery of *long-term*

potentiation (LTP), the incremental response shown by neurons consequent upon prior experience of high-frequency, tetanizing stimulation.[6] (A decremental response is termed complementarily, *long-term depression* (LTD).)

These phenomena were originally found in hippocampal circuitry (dentate gyrus and CA1-3) but have now been characterized in many regions, including the neocortex (including both visual cortex and prefrontal cortex), the amygdala, parts of the striatum, and cerebellum. These brain regions are of course implicated in diverse aspects of perception and memory as well as other components of cognition. However, the question is to what extent LTP/LTD processes actually reflect behavioural learning?

This question was addressed in an important study in which it was shown that D-2-amino-5-phosphonopentanoic acid (AP-5), a competitive antagonist at the glutamate N-methyl-D-asparate (NMDA) receptor subtype, significantly impaired learning in a spatial navigation escape task sensitive to hippocampal damage in the rat when infused into the ventricle at doses also blocking LTP measured *in vitro* in tissue slices.[7] Pre-trained, established performance was unaffected, indicating that the effects could not be attributed to ancillary processes such as motivation, perception, or motor function. Thus it was concluded that the NMDA receptor, probably acting as a 'coincidence detector', mediated plasticity or associative learning mechanisms.

These results have now been confirmed for a number of other learning paradigms, from aversive contextual Pavlovian conditioning,[8] fear-potentiated startle,[9] discriminated approach behaviour[10] including 'autoshaping',[11] and experience shaping the development of the visual cortex[12] to conditioned taste aversion, and the chick imprinting response.[13] These observations are all consistent with a role for glutamate receptors in many forms of learning and memory, dependent on several distinct brain regions.[14]

The relative contributions of LTP and LTD to learning in different systems remains an interesting question. On the one hand, it appears that quite common molecular mechanisms may be implicated in superficially different forms of learning and memory. One intriguing possible exception may be stimulus-response habit learning, which is generally associated with circuits including the dorsal striatum (specifically, the putamen). Lovinger[15] has described possibly distinct forms of LTP/LTD implicated in striatal mechanisms of goal-directed, as compared to stimulus-response habit, learning.

The 'post-trial' paradigm, where drugs are administered to disturb the *consolidation* of memory at some time following training or experience, can be used to dissect the components of underlying memory processes.[16] The effect of such drugs on memory can be measured in a subsequent *retention* or *retrieval* test performed some time after (usually one to three days) initial training (see Fig. 9.2a). If a drug produces deficits—or improvements—in later retention when administered soon after training but not at a later time-point, including at the time of retention testing itself, this is good evidence for a specific effect on memory consolidation. However, if a drug only affects retention, then it is likely that it is producing general performance effects, although possibly on memory retrieval processes. A great deal of evidence indicates that NMDA receptors are implicated in the initial encoding and consolidation of the memory trace, but not in its subsequent retrieval.[14]

NMDA receptors are implicated in consolidation and also in a related, hypothetical process of '*reconsolidation*' (Fig. 9.2b), rediscovered through work in experimental animals that may have

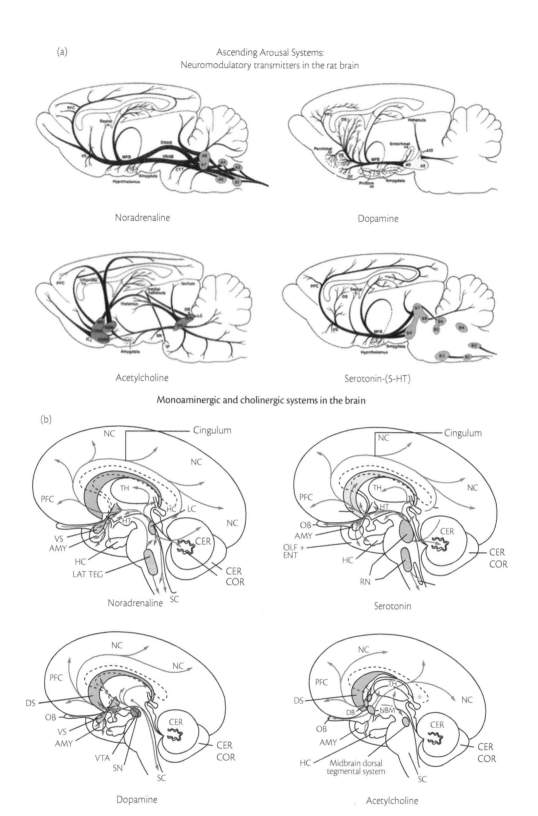

Fig. 9.1 Ascending monoaminergic and cholinergic arousal systems in the (a) rat and (b) human brain (sagittal section), based on histochemical and immunocytochemical analysis.[91,92] Similar systems are conserved in the primate, including human brain. Abbreviations: (a) PFC, prefrontal cortex; MFB, medial forebrain bundle; CTT, central tegmental tract; DNAB, dorsal noradrenergic ascending bundle; VNAB, ventral noradrenergic bundle. A1–A10, catecholamine cell groups. Cx, cortex. Ms, medial septum. VDAB, vertical limb of the diagonal band of Broca; HDAB, horizontal limb of the diagonal band of Broca. NBM, nucleus basalis magnocellularis (cell group Ch4); tpp, pedunculopontine tegmental nucleus (cell group Ch5); dltn, laterodorsal tegmental nucleus (cell group Ch6); ICj, islands of Calleja; SN, substantia nigra; IP, interpeduncular nucleus; DR, dorsal raphé nucleus. DS, dorsal striatum, VS, ventral striatum. B1–B9, indoleamine cell groups. (b) Monoaminergic and cholinergic systems in the human brain. Abbreviations: PFC, prefrontal cortex; NC, neocortex; OB, olfactory bulb; TH, thalamus; DS, dorsal striatum (caudate-putamen); VS, ventral striatum (nucleus accumbens); S, septum; DB, diagonal band of Broca; NBM, nucleus basalis of Meynert; AMY, amygdala; HC, hippocampus; HT, hypothalamus; SN, substantia nigra; VTA, ventral tegmental area; CER cerebellum (nuclei); CER COR, cerebellar cortex. OLF +ENT, olfactory and entorhinal cortex; LAT TEG, lateral tegmental nuclei; origin of the ventral noradrenergic bundle; LC, locus coeruleus; RN, raphé nuclei; SC, spinal cord.

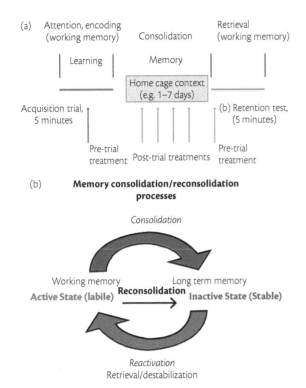

(a) Attention, encoding
(working memory)

Consolidation

Retrieval
(working memory)

Learning

Memory

Home cage context
(e.g. 1–7 days)

Acquisition trial,
5 minutes

(b) Retention test,
(5 minutes)

Pre-trial
treatment

Post-trial treatments

Pre-trial
treatment

(b)   **Memory consolidation/reconsolidation
processes**

Consolidation

Working memory
Active State (labile)   **Reconsolidation**   Long term memory
Inactive State (Stable)

Reactivation
Retrieval/destabilization

Fig. 9.2 (a) The one- trial learning, post-trial treatment memory design, in which manipulations are made post-trial to define time-limited memory consolidation processes, as measured during the memory retention test (see e.g. reference 16). (b) Symmetrical processes of memory consolidation and reconsolidation. Reactivating former consolidated memory traces (e.g. by reminder stimuli) can render their retrieval vulnerable to disruption, e.g. by NMDA receptor antagonists or protein synthesis inhibition, thus 'erasing' the memory trace (see also reference 17).

clinical implications in the treatment of neuropsychiatric disorders such as post-traumatic stress disorder and drug addiction. Reconsolidation is said to occur when a previously consolidated memory trace becomes 'active' upon a reminder cue. It is the process by which previously consolidated memories become *stabilized* at retrieval and then require '*restabilization*' to persist in the brain.[17]

In the destabilized state the memory trace is 'labile' and can be disrupted by treatment with protein synthesis inhibitors and other amnesic agents including NMDA receptor antagonists (infused into the amygdala), with the result that memory retention is impaired when tested a few days later. The implication is that when a memory trace becomes active, it undergoes updating and 'reconsolidation' or restabilization as an essentially new memory trace.

The reminder cue is necessarily presented in the absence of the event it signals, and so this is akin to one-trial '*extinction*', an active process by which an association is suppressed (often resulting in a reduction of behavioural output). Intriguingly, extinction is also NMDA-receptor-dependent. Thus NMDA antagonists are known to block the extinction of learned fear, again when infused into the amygdala.[18] In a complementary fashion, extinction is accelerated by a glutamate receptor agonist, D-cycloserine, a finding that has been used to enhance effects of behavioural therapy of patients with anxiety disorders.

Recent evidence suggests that both destabilization and restabilization implicate the NMDA receptor, but intriguingly these two processes can be dissociated pharmacologically by GluN2B and GluN2A receptor antagonists, respectively. Thus the former protects consolidated CS-fear memories from the effects of amnesic agents,[19,20] whereas it is the GluN2A receptor that is necessary for reconsolidation itself.[20]

Another important question is the role of other glutamate receptor subtypes. For example, the changes in neuronal plasticity effected by NMDA receptors are ultimately mediated by the fast depolarization of post-synaptic cells via the AMPA receptor subtype.[21] However, AMPA receptor antagonists generally cause more general impairments. Thus, for example, NMDA-receptor blockade within the hippocampus impaired encoding, but not retrieval of flavour-place associative learning in rats. Whereas AMPA receptor blockade using CNQX (6-cyano-7-nitroquinoline-2,3-dione) disrupted both encoding and retrieval.[22]

These differential effects of manipulating the NMDA and AMPA receptor have also been shown for potentially 'declarative' forms of memory such as recognition. Winters and Bussey[23] infused selective NMDA and AMPA receptor antagonists into the perirhinal cortex of rats at various stages of training and performance of an object recognition task. They found that the NMDA receptor antagonist did not impair initial encoding of the object but did impact on its consolidation into long-term memory. However, the same treatment had no effect when made just prior to the retention test, whereas the AMPA receptor antagonist (CNQX) disrupted retrieval, similar to the effects of these agents on associative memory in the hippocampus. Intriguingly, in the amygdala, AMPA receptor antagonism has been shown to have relatively little effect on memory destabilization or restabilization, despite also impairing retrieval of a CS-fear association.[20] Thus, the glutamate receptor subtypes have remarkably specific effects on different components of memory processes.

Studies with mice that lack the AMPA receptor subunit A have also been shown to have significant effects on spatial working memory tasks (though not in long-term spatial memory), adding to previous evidence of NMDA receptors in working memory functions.[24] This is of particular interest given that drugs such as the NMDA non-competitive antagonist (and dissociative anaesthetic) ketamine causes working memory deficits in humans.[24]

Roles in processes such as working memory for glutamate receptors raise the interesting issue of whether other cognitive functions, including so-called executive functions, are mediated by glutamate receptors. Thus, evidence in rats of apparent impairments in attentional set-shifting following acute or chronic treatment with NMDA receptor antagonists[26] may be related to similar difficulties with the Wisconsin Card Sorting test exhibited by patients with schizophrenia. It appears likely that most neocortical functions involving processing and plasticity are influenced by glutamatergic mechanisms; it is a challenging question whether this conclusion could lead to clinical application.

Potential cognitive enhancing effects of glutamate receptor agonists

Many important clinical disorders from epilepsy to schizophrenia and Alzheimer's disease involve disruptions of glutamatergic signalling and so it is logical to ask whether they could be remedied by drugs with appropriate glutamatergic mechanisms. Obvious and possibly insurmountable problems include the action of such drugs to produce epileptic seizures and neurodegeneration; however, there are some indications that such 'cognitive enhancing' effects might be feasible. Thus D-cycloserine, which acts at the strychnine-insensitive glycine recognition site of the NMDA receptor complex to boost NMDA signally, has been shown to improve learning and memory in several situations in rodents and primates. Small beneficial effects have also been reported in clinical studies of Alzheimer's disease and schizophrenia (see reference 14 for a review).

The discovery of another class of glutamate receptors, the metabotropic receptors, also offers some grounds for optimism in modulation of glutamate-mediated neurotransmission. For example, animal models of schizophrenia[27] and Rett's syndrome[28] have shown beneficial effects of both mGluR5 receptor potentiators (positive allosteric modulators) and mGluR receptor antagonists. An alternative approach depends on drugs causing positive allosteric modulations of the AMPA receptor, called 'AMPA-kines'. These agents have been tested in both human memory (verbal list learning), where a significant improvement was observed in elderly individuals with relatively low baseline levels of performance,[29] and also in studies of visual recognition memory in non-human primates. In the latter study, Porrino and colleagues[30] demonstrated impressive, dose- and delay-dependent improvements in recognition memory in rhesus monkeys (Fig. 9.3) that were accompanied by changes in cerebral blood flow in the temporal lobe and dorsolateral prefrontal cortex. However, to date, the use of AMPA-kines as cognitive enhancers has not been validated in a clinical trial.

GABA: Inhibitory neurotransmission and cognition

GABA is the key *inhibitory* neurotransmitter in the brain synthesised from glutamate by the enzyme glutamic acid decarboxylase (GAD). It is responsible for the efficient functioning of several types of inhibitory interneuron which prevent overactivity in many neural circuits, especially in the cerebral cortex, hippocampus, and striatum (for which GABA-containing medium spiny cells are the major outputs) (see reference 2). Although it is not logically necessary for neuronal inhibition to translate into behavioural inhibition, it is the case that drugs simulating effects of GABA-ergic agonists often have behavioural *disinhibitory* actions.

Benzodiazepine drugs such as chlordiazepoxide (Librium) and diazepam (Valium) are the best known anxiolytic agents, which also have sedative, amnesic, and anticonvulsant actions. These drugs act at those $GABA_A$ receptors with a particular constellation of GABA receptor subunits. Thus, they act as positive allosteric modulators and enhance phasic inhibition by improving the efficacy of GABA itself in opening inhibitory chloride channels. The sedative, anticonvulsant, anxiolytic, and amnesic effects of benzodiazepines appear to depend on different configurations of subunits at the benzodiazepine receptor which are prevalent in different brain regions.[31] For example, it is thought that the anxiolytic actions depend to a large extent on GABA receptors in the amygdala, which is classically associated with fear and anxiety.

By contrast, the amnesic actions appear to be linked to an alpha-5 subunit in GABA receptor subtypes mainly in the hippocampus. A drug acting specifically as an inverse agonist at this GABA receptor subtype has been shown to antagonize the amnesic effects of alcohol which partly depend on the activation of GABA receptors.[32]

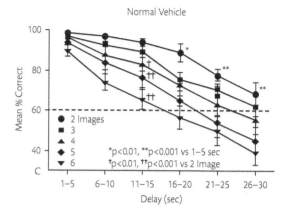

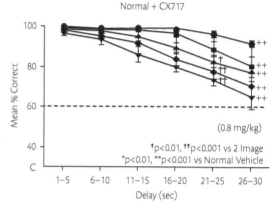

Fig. 9.3 Dose-dependent improvements in recognition memory in rhesus monkeys following treatment with an AMPA-kine (CX-717). Recognition memory was measured in a delayed non-matching to sample test that also varies memory load (the length of the list of visual objects that has to be remembered before retention testing). Monkeys were required to remember which of two visual discriminanda is more novel and choose it in a 2-choice test over a previously presented, and hence 'familiar' stimulus after various delays between presentation of the sample and the choice test.

Intriguingly, the amnesic effects of benzodiazepines do not appear to be secondary to the drugs' sedative actions as the sleep-inducing or hypnotic actions of certain benzodiazepines (such as triazolam or Halcion) are dependent on an independent GABA receptor subunit population in hind-brain sites distinct from the hippocampus.[31]

GABA in inhibitory neurons plays an important role in the generation of so-called *gamma oscillations* in the gamma rhythm components of the electro-encephalograph (EEG).[33] Gamma rhythms are observed in many brain regions during states of wakefulness and sleeping, yet their precise functions and mechanisms are still unknown. Gamma-band rhythms are produced by neuronal inhibition. Gamma oscillations are usually transient and are the product of a coordinated interaction of neuronal excitation and inhibition, detected as local field potentials. Gamma rhythm is generally correlated with the irregular firing of single neurons, and the network frequency of gamma oscillations varies extensively.

Gamma oscillations per se have to be distinguished from mere increases of gamma-band power and spiking activity, and their magnitude is modulated by slower rhythms which may serve to 'couple' activity in different cortical circuits. Gamma oscillations are thus thought to be important mechanisms for coordinating activity across widespread neural networks such as the hippocampus and prefrontal cortex in such behavioural processes as working memory.[34] Thus, cognitive deficits in disorders such as schizophrenia probably result from the disruption of neuronal population dynamics as a consequence of cortical pathology, including the loss of parvalbumin containing GABA-ergic cortical interneurons.[35]

Monoamines: Serotonin (5-hydroxytryptamine, 5-HT)

Serotonin is a ubiquitous and ancient neurotransmitter (even being present in invertebrates such as *Aplysia*) with over 15 distinct receptors. It ramifies extensively from cell bodies in the mid-brain dorsal and raphé nuclei to virtually all regions of the mammalian brain (see Fig. 9.1). It has been implicated as a neuromodulator in virtually all behavioural processes from sensory input to motor output, including motivation and cognition.[2]

Serotonin also plays a central role in mood and emotion, but it is part of major paradox in being sometimes associated with anxiety when up-regulated and depression when down-regulated, even though these two states overlap considerably.[36] Depression—and many anxiety disorders including panic—is often treated with selective serotonin reuptake inhibitors (such as fluoxetine or Prozac), their chronic effects being associated with up-regulation of serotoninergic function. By contrast, anxiety is sometimes treated with drugs that reduce serotonin release; for example, by acting as agonists at 5-HT autoreceptors (buspirone).

Classically, in animal studies serotonin has also been associated with enhancing the activity of a punishment system, as opposed to a hypothetical (dopamine-modulated) reward system, which mediates behavioural suppression or inhibition. This is also consistent with evidence that depletion of serotonin is also linked to behavioural disinhibition, in the form of both impulsive behaviour (i.e. premature or risky behaviour), and compulsive behaviour (in the form e.g. of obsessive–compulsive disorder (OCD); OCD is often treated with high doses of selective serotonin reuptake inhibitors (SSRIs)).[37]

These diverse effects of serotonin are generally considered to be explained by its modulation of distinct systems, perhaps via different receptors, but the evidence for this hypothesis is still quite fragmentary. The issue is complicated by the fact that serotonin is implicated in processes as diverse as sensory processing (modulated by 5-HT2A receptors, and sometimes hallucinogenic effects, via 5HT2A agonist drugs such as psilocybin and LSD),[38] and eating behaviour, probably mediated via 5-HT2C receptors in the hypothalamus.[39] These diverse and apparently non-specific effects may nevertheless result from rather specific modulatory roles of serotonin. For example, in explaining the sensory effects of serotonin modulation it is significant that the serotoninergic innervation of the neocortex is heavily biased towards layer 4, that is, the thalamic sensory input (contrasting, e.g. with that of noradrenaline which is mainly biased towards the deeper layers).[40]

Moreover, serotonin is especially implicated in functions of the ventral prefrontal cortex with its rich serotoninergic innervations. This perhaps explains the special role of serotonin in reversal learning which is especially linked to the orbitofrontal cortex (OFC) functioning. Thus, local depletion of serotonin in the OFC led to significant deficits in reversal learning in marmoset monkeys which had to learn to shift responding from one visual object to another (previously unrewarded) in order to gain reinforcement. This was accompanied by apparent perseverative behaviour and by a tendency to be biased in responding to particular cues.[41] Intriguingly, this 'stickiness' in behaviour did not extend to shifting attention between different visuoperceptual dimensions present in both stimuli.[42] It is possible that these deficits simulate some of the problems exhibited by patients with OCD.

Monoamines: Dopamine: Cognition and activation

Dopamine (DA) has striking links to behaviour, psychopathology, and neurological disease. The seminal mapping of the mesencephalic DA pathways into ramifying mesostriatal, mesolimbic, and mesocortical projections (see Fig. 9.1), as well as the identification of several DA receptors and their signalling pathways have raised important questions about the functions of this important neuromodulatory neurotransmitter.[43] The possibly misleading triadic division of these projections has suggested discrete and even parallel functions in movement (e.g. Parkinson's disease, dorsal striatum), reward (e.g. drugs of abuse, nucleus accumbens), and cognition (e.g. schizophrenia and attention deficit/hyperactivity disorder (ADHD), prefrontal cortex). However, although this tripartite parcellation is attractively parsimonious, there is considerable evidence for overlapping functions (e.g. of cognition in the caudate-putamen and reinforcement in OFC). Similarly, the mediation of reward by DA-dependent functions of the nucleus accumbens also entails an implication in learning and cognitive decision-making processes.

A key issue is under what states or conditions the central DA systems become active and how this activity affects cognition, behaviour, and movement. There are considerable neurochemical data indicating that central DA is affected by such factors as stress and arousal. A particularly useful principle, applied especially to the understanding of the relationship between DA activity and behavioural or cognitive output is the *Yerkes–Dodson Law*,[44] which generally takes the form of an inverted U-shaped function linking level of arousal (or 'stress') with behavioural performance (Fig. 9.4). Thus, whereas performance at low or high values of arousal is relatively poor, it is optimal at intermediate values.

When discussing the functions of the dopamine system, we have employed the term '*activation*' to describe a similar 'energetic' construct to that of arousal, which is however meant to capture how dopamine affects the rate and vigour of behavioural (and cognitive, e.g. thinking) output. Unlike 'arousal', activation does not connote a simple wakefulness construct associated with neocortical changes, for example in EEG (cf reference 45). As posited in Robbins and Everitt's review[45] of the considerable empirical data already then available, activation is induced by many related states or stimuli, including food deprivation, 'stress', psychomotor stimulant drugs, aversive stimuli such as tail-pinch and foot-shock, novelty and conditioned stimuli, including predictors of appetitive events such as food and also aversive events. The function of 'activation' is to enhance behaviour in preparation for the presentation of a goal or reinforcer (whether appetitive or aversive).

Activation affects processing in target structures innervated by the mesolimbic, mesocortical, and mesostriatal pathways,

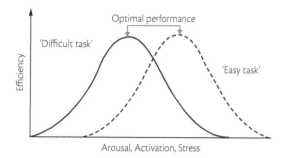

Fig. 9.4 The Yerkes–Dodson (1908) inverted U-shaped relationship between levels of arousal (or activation, or stress) and levels of performance on a variety of different tasks. Note that optimal performance is obtained at intermediate doses of the drug, Note also that optimal levels of arousal are higher for 'easy' than for 'more difficult' tasks.

Reproduced from Robbins TW, Cognitive psychopharmacology. In: K Ochsner and S Kosslyn (eds). *Handbook of Cognitive Neuroscience*. Copyright (2014), with permission from Oxford University Press.

essentially in 'gain-amplificatory' mode. In the mesolimbic projections, for example to the ventral striatum, including the nucleus accumbens, the role of enhanced DA activity is to increase responsiveness to cues paired with reinforcement and thus also to enhance appetitive *approach* to the goal. This is very similar to Berridge's concept of 'incentive salience'[46] and is related to other earlier writings on the role of DA in *motivation*.[47]

Another major empirical advance has been that the fast *phasic* firing of cells in the ventral tegmental area and substantia nigra appears to encode an error prediction signal.[48] Such a neural signal is highly relevant to some models (Pavlovian or temporal difference) about how we learn new information. Thus, with training, the phasic DA cell firing occurs in response to conditioned stimuli (e.g. visual flash) that are *predictive of reward* rather than to the reward itself (e.g. food). However, if the reward is omitted, there is a 'dip' in firing, as if the signal encodes an error in the prediction. This pattern of activity conforms to the changes in associative learning described by the Rescorla–Wagner rule.[48]

There is an evident need to understand the relative functional contribution of such *phasic* responses—implicated in plasticity and new, mainly appetitive learning of Pavlovian associations—with the *tonic* mode of action of the same DA systems assumed to underlie the activational (e.g. motivational) effects of DA.[49,50] It is also unclear at present precisely how DA contributes to *aversive* learning.

The Yerkes–Dodson principle has been often criticized in experimental psychology for its apparent capacity to account for diverse datasets rather too readily. However, it does conform to many dose-response relationships found for drug effects on behaviour, which often have characteristic inverted-U shape functions. The principle was applied initially to important data suggesting that the level of DA D1 receptor activity produced Yerkes–Dodson-like effects on working memory in both rats and monkeys.[51] A more recent manifestation of the principle was shown in work on the catechol-O-methyl transferase polymorphism which hypothetically modulates prefrontal DA function and produces a predictable pattern of effects on working memory performance.[52,53]

However, these data raise several important issues:

(i) Is the function relating DA to performance the same for all forms of behaviour? The finding of Yerkes and Dodson (1908) that easy tasks were optimally performed at higher levels of arousal than difficult tasks, suggests it might not be. Recent evidence from Parkinson's disease has shown that therapeutic doses of L-Dopa can improve some aspects of cognition, while impairing others, even in the same patient.[54]

(ii) Are there inverted-U shaped functions for the sub-cortical DA systems, as well as for prefrontal DA D1 receptors? Some recent evidence[55] suggests that this is the case.

(iii) And, relevant to other neuromodulators such as noradrenaline and acetylcholine to be reviewed below, are their actions on behaviour and cognition also to be described in terms of inverted-U-shaped functions, possibly in other brain regions than the prefrontal cortex or striatum?

Monoamines: Noradrenaline (NA): Cognition and arousal

The central noradrenergic (NA) systems arise from two major systems in the brain-stem, the dorsal and ventral noradrenergic ascending bundles (Fig. 9.1). The former, arising in the locus coeruleus, is more likely to be implicated in cognitive function, innervating as it does, among other structures, the cerebral cortex and hippocampus. This is of considerable clinical interest, given the implication of NA pathology in such varied disorders as Parkinson's and Alzheimer's diseases, Korsakoff's syndrome, post-traumatic stress disorder (PTSD), and attention deficit hyperactivity disorder (ADHD). The ventral noradrenergic bundle, by contrast, innervates the hypothalamus and portions of the limbic system and is implicated in vegetative functions. These systems, as for the other monoamines, are implicated in response to stress and arousal. The locus coeruleus itself plays an important role in sleep–waking and in the production of the EEG and the P300 cortical potential (see reference 56 for a recent review).

Electrophysiological investigations have shown that the locus coeruleus responds mainly to *salient* stimuli, regardless of their precise temporospatial characteristics. This salience is provided especially by the *novelty*, as well as the *intensity*, of stimuli from all of the sensory modalities, and also by conditioning. Thus, familiar stimuli, which lose salience by habituation, do not activate locus coeruleus NA cells. Overall, the coeruleo-cortical NA projections behave like a classical arousal system, being most active in waking, and least active during REM sleep.[57]

In view of its extensive forebrain projections, NA, like 5-HT, has been implicated in a variety of functions including arousal, stress responses, anxiety, executive control, and memory consolidation. An early theoretical proposal was that the the locus coeruleus functioned akin to the 'cognitive arm' of a central sympathetic ganglion.[58] The relationship between arousal (or the noradrenaline status) and cognition may also operate according to the inverted-U Yerkes–Dodson principle described above, as shown by Arnsten[59] in her studies of effects of adrenoceptor agents on working memory.

However, a notable hypothesis has been that the coeruleo-cortical NA system enhances selective attention by enhancing 'signal-to-noise' processing. Precisely how this is done is not absolutely clear, although many studies point to the general reduction in neuronal firing produced by microiontophoresis of NA onto cortical cells, which may have the effect of reducing 'noise'. Segal and Bloom[60] have shown that locus coeruleus stimulation can increase or decrease evoked cell firing within terminal regions of the dentate gyrus of the hippocampus, depending on the salience of the stimulus.

The evidence linking NA to attentional functions, including vigilance, has come from two main sources:

(i) Effects on attentional performance in a rodent test of sustained attention, the 5-choice serial reaction time task (5-CSRTT). Specifically, rats with profound forebrain NA deletion were impaired at detecting visual targets when these were temporally unpredictable or in the presence of distracting noise.[61]

(ii) Electrophysiological recording from locus coeruleus NA cells in monkeys during attentional performance. Here the finding was that optimal attentional performance occurred during tonic firing phases, whereas performance was suboptimal during heightened tonic firing.[62]

These effects on attention may underlie many of the other actions of central NA on functions such as learning, memory, and cognition. For example, considerable evidence links aversive memory consolidation to noradrenergic modulation of the amygdala;[16] moreover, memory reconsolidation in rats[63] and humans[64,65] is blocked by the beta adrenoceptor blocker propanolol.

Central NA also contributes importantly to performance by rats on an attentional set-shifting task where subjects are required to shift their attention from one aspect or dimension (such as its shape or colour) of a complex stimulus to another (a model of the human Wisconsin Card Sort Test of cognitive flexibility and prefrontal cortical functioning mentioned above).[66] Whether similar effects can be shown in humans will depend on whether drugs that selectively activate noradrenergic receptors can be employed. It is of interest that the psychomotor stimulant drug methylphenidate, used (as Ritalin) in the treatment of ADHD, acts not only to block the actions of the dopamine transporter but also the noradrenaline transporter, and so it is possible that both actions contribute to the effects of methylphenidate to improve attention and working memory, and also to enhance cognitive control or executive function (see review in reference 67).

Atomoxetine is a drug also used in the treatment of ADHD which has more selective actions in acting mainly to block the noradrenaline transporter, thus avoiding the up-regulation of striatal DA that potentially contributes to drug abuse following medication by methylphenidate. Atomoxetine has been shown to have notable actions in reducing impulsive behaviour, and thus enhancing cognitive control, in both rodents and humans.[68,69] Thus, even in healthy volunteers, atomoxetine speeded the stop-reaction time, a measure of the ability to cancel an already-initiated motor response. A similar action has been shown in ADHD.[70] Moreover, this apparent improvement in inhibitory control appears to depend on activation of the right inferior frontal gyrus, a cortical region previously implicated in cognitive control.[71] It is currently a matter of considerable research interest whether common effects on attention contribute to these effects on cognitive control, or whether both functions are independently modulated by central NA.

Acetylcholine (Ach): Roles in attention and cognition

Acetylcholine (Ach) has been considered as a neurotransmitter for almost a century. Subsequent research in both basic and human neuroscience has strongly implicated Ach in processes of attention and arousal, parallel to analogous roles for the catecholamines (dopamine and noradrenaline). There are three major cholinergic tracts, including the midbrain dorsal tegmental system with functions in the sleep–waking cycle, the basal forebrain (nucleus basalis) system, and the adjacent medial septo-hippocampal projections (Fig. 9.1). However, Ach also functions as a neurotransmitter in interneurons, for example, in the striatum.[2]

Early work showed beneficial effects of the anticholinesterase physostigmine on attention in rats as measured in a visual target detection procedure, whereas the antimuscarinic cholinergic receptor antagonist, scopolamine impaired it.[72,73] Nicotine was later shown to enhance performance in a sustained attention task in non-smoking humans that required detection of rapidly presented (100/min), specified sequences of digits at a single location.[74] Converging evidence in humans from studies of the effects of scopolamine on cognition also implicated possible effects of the drug on cholinergically mediated attentional processes.[75,76] Soon after these early behavioural demonstrations of Ach involvement in attention, electrophysiological studies of the V1 area of cat showed apparent effects of Ach to enhance signal processing in receptive fields of visual cortical neurons,[77] although some subsequent work[78] has failed to confirm this.

Damage to the nucleus basalis in rats using either excitotoxic or immunotoxic lesioning procedures, that typically produced substantial loss of cholinergic terminals in the frontal cortex, substantially disrupted 5-CSRTT performance by rats in terms of impaired detection of brief visual events presented randomly at one of five locations, deficits later shown to be especially evident at longer test sessions. Such impaired discrimination performance could be remedied by systemic administration of optimal doses of physostigmine or nicotine, as well as by cholinergically enriched neural transplants into the rodent cortex (see review by Everitt and Robbins, reference 79).

Further experiments using intracerebral monitoring of Ach with *in vivo* microdialysis showed the neurotransmitter to be released in the prefrontal cortex when attentional demands were increased.[80] Other experiments using different measures of attention in rats and mice have generally confirmed the importance of acetylcholine for attentional function. Sophisticated neurochemical studies involving the monitoring via *in vivo* voltammetry of choline release as a surrogate index of acetylcholine[81] have also been linked to target detection, and its improvement by alpha-4, beta-2 nicotinic agonists.[82] Indeed, the evidence implicating selective effects of Ach in attentional performance in rodents is perhaps more convincing than for any of the other major neurotransmitters.

Parallel evidence of cholinergic involvement in attention can be found from investigations of rhesus monkeys with lesions of the nucleus basalis that exhibit specific deficits in Posner's test of covert attentional orienting. This finding is consistent with evidence that nicotine enhances attentional orienting in both monkeys and humans, as well as from evidence of augmentation of responses of primary visual cortex neurons in their receptive fields to attended stimuli by iontophoretically applied Ach.[83]

The demonstration that the intellectual status of patients with Alzheimer's disease is related to cortical cholinergic loss.[84] has highlighted a possible role for cholinergic agents in its remediation. The possible relevance of the basic neuroscience findings on acetylcholine reviewed above was demonstrated by the improvements produced by the anticholinesterase drug tacrine on performance of patients with probable Alzheimer's disease on the same five-choice serial reaction time task as used in rodents, with concomitant improvements in clinical rating scales of attention 'alerting'.[85] Subsequent clinical experience has shown that such medications (e.g. rivastigmine) are also effective in the treatment of the fluctuating attentional capacities of patients with Lewy body dementia, who tend to have even more profound reductions of cholinergic function than do patients with Alzheimer's disease.[86]

Ach is also implicated in memory functions, including working memory, recognition memory, and semantic retrieval, but it remains to be resolved whether its effects on attention contribute to these actions, as seems plausible, for example, for memory encoding or resisting interference in working memory. There may be specific effects on memory-related processes, perhaps mediated by similar neuronal mechanisms to those of attention, but in brain regions more specialized for memory processing, such as the hippocampus.[87]

New vistas on novel neurotransmitters: Neuropeptides

This brief review has considered functions in cognition of the main 'fast signalling' (i.e. glutamate and GABA) and 'neuromodulatory' (i.e. the monoamines and acetylcholine) neurotransmitters. As mentioned in the introduction to this chapter, there are at least 50 substances that have neurotransmitter properties and more are being discovered by the year. The largest category that we have not considered in any detail are the neuropeptides, whose actions are generally slow but often specific and hormone-like.[2] Examples include the gut hormones cholescystokinin and vasoactive intestinal polypeptide, adrenaline, corticotrophic releasing factor (CRF), vasopressin, and the opioid peptides such as enkephalin and beta endorphin. Many of these substances have functions in aspects of memory, in conjunction, for example with NMDA receptors and central adrenoceptors. However, there is no very great evidence of major roles in cognitive functions per se, although possible roles, for example in stress, will have indirect actions on such cognitive functions as working memory via the Yerkes–Dodson like influence. Analogously, the discovery of orexin, a hypothalamic neuropeptide, has been shown to have functions in motivation and arousal that may similarly impinge indirectly on cognition.

Perhaps one of the most intriguing discoveries has been the possible role of oxytocin in social cognition. This peptide has been shown to improve social recognition memory not only in animals,[88] but also in human subjects, where there is evidence of selective improvement of memory for faces but not non-facial stimuli.[89] A classic study indicated that oxytocin administered to humans actually enhanced 'trust' in an economic game designed to measure this.[90] Such discoveries, with implications for the treatment of disorders such as autism and possibly even of some neurodegenerative conditions, indicate rich promise for the future study of the psychopharmacology of cognition, and its therapeutic application.

Further reading

Robbins TW. Cognitive psychopharmacology. In: K Ochsner and S Kosslyn (eds). *Handbook of Cognitive Neuroscience*. Oxford: Oxford University Press, 2013, pp 401–18.

Robbins TW. The neuropsychopharmacology of attention. In: K Nobre and S Kastner (eds). *Handbook of Attention*. Oxford: Oxford University Press, 2013, pp. 509–40.

References

1. Meyer J and Quenzer LF. *Psychopharmacology: Drugs, The Brain, and Behavior*. Sutherland, MA: Sinaeuer Associates, 2005.
2. Cooper JR, Bloom FE, and Roth RH. *Biochemical Basis of Neuropharmacology*, 8th edn. Oxford: Oxford University Press, 2003.
3. Iversen LL and Goodman EC (eds). *Fast and Slow Chemical Signalling in the Nervous System*. Oxford: Oxford University Press, 1986.
4. Squire, LR, Berg D, Bloom FE, *et al.* (eds). (2013) Section II. Cellular and Molecular Neuroscience in *Fundamental Neuroscience*, 4th edn. New York, NY: Elsevier, 2013.
5. Hebb DO. *The Organization of Behavior: A Neuropsychological Theory*. New York, NY: John Wiley and Sons, 1950.
6. Bliss TV and Collingridge GL. A synaptic model of memory: long-term potentiation in the hippocampus. *Nature*. 1993;361:31–3.
7. Morris RG. Selective impairment of learning and blockade of long-term potentiation by an N-methyl-D-aspartate receptor antagonist, AP5. *Nature*. 1986;319:774–6.
8. Young SL, Bohenek DL, Fanselow MS. NMDA processes mediate anterograde amnesia of contextual fear conditioning induced by hippocampal damage: Immunization against amnesia by context pre-exposure. *Behavioural Neuroscience*. 1994;108:19–29.
9. Miserendino MJD, Sananes CB, Melia KK, *et al.* Blocking of acquisition but not expression of conditioned fear-potentiated startle by NMDA antagonists in the amygdala. *Nature*. 1990;345:716–18.
10. Burns LH, Everitt BJ, Robbins TW. Intra-amygdala infusion of the N-methyl-Daspartate receptor antagonist AP5 impairs acquisition but not performance of discriminated approach to an appetitive CS. *Behavioural Neural Biology*. 1994;61:242–50.
11. Dalley JW, Lääne K, Theobald DEH, *et al.* Time-limited modulation of appetitive Pavlovian memory by D1 and NMDA receptors in the nucleus accumbens. *Proc Natl Acad Sci USA*. 2005;102:6189–94.
12. Carmignoto G and Vicini S. Activity-dependent decrease in NMDA receptor responses during development of the visual cortex. *Science*. 1992;258:1007–11.
13. McCabe BJ, Davey, JE, and Horn G. Impairment of learning by localized injection of an *N*-methyl-D-aspartate receptor antagonist into the hyperstriatum ventrale of the domestic chick. *Behav Neurosci*. 1992;106(6):947–53.
14. Robbins TW and Murphy ER. Behavioural pharmacology: +40 years of progress and a focus on glutamate receptors. *Trends Pharmacol Sci*. 2006;27:141–8.
15. Lovinger DM. Neurotransmitter roles in synaptic modulation, plasticity and learning in the dorsal striatum. *Neuropharmacol*. 2010;58:951–61.
16. McGaugh JL. Memory—a century of consolidation. *Science*. 2000;287:248–52.
17. Nader K. Memory traces unbound. *Trends Neurosci*. 2003;26(2):65–72.
18. Falls WA, Miserendino M, and Davis M. Extinction of fear-potentiated startle: Blockade by infusion of an NMDA antagonist into the amygdala. *J Neurosci*.1992;12:854–63.
19. Ben Mamou C, Gamache G, and Nader K. NMDA receptors are critical for unleashing consolidated auditory fear memories. *Nature Neurosci*. 2006;9:1237–9.
20. Milton AL, Merlo E, Ratano P, *et al.* Double dissociation of the requirement for GluN2B- and GluN2A-containing NMDA receptors in the destabilization and restabilization of a reconsolidating memory. *J Neurosci*.2013;16;33(3):1109–15.
21. Kew JN and Kemp, JA. Ionotropic and metabotropic glutamate receptor structure and pharmacology. *Psychopharmacol*. 2005;179:4–29.
22. Day M, Langston R, and Morris RGM. Glutamate-receptor-mediated encoding and retrieval of paired-associate learning. *Nature*. 2003;424:205–09.

23. Winters BD and Bussey TJ. Glutamate receptors in perirhinal cortex mediate encoding, retrieval, and consolidation of object recognition memory. *J Neurosci*. 2005;25:4243–51.

24. Schmitt WB, Deacon RM, Seeburg PH, *et al*. A within-subjects, within-task demonstration of intact spatial reference memory and impaired spatial working memory in glutamate receptor-A-deficient mice. *J. Neurosci*. 2003; 23: 3953–9.

25. Krystal JH, Karper LP, Selbyl JP, *et al*. Subanesthetic effects of the noncompetitive NMDA antagonist, ketamine, in humans. Psychotomimetic, perceptual, cognitive, and neuroendocrine responses. *Arch Gen Psychiatry*. 1994;51:199–214.

26. Stefani MR, Groth K, Moghaddam B. Glutamate receptors in the rat medial prefrontal cortex regulate set-shifting ability. *Behavioural Neuroscience*. 2003;117:728–37.

27. Gastambide F, Cotel MC, Gilmour G, *et al*. Remediation of reversal learning deficits in the neurodevelopmental MAM model of schizophrenia by a novel mGlu5 positive allosteric modulator. *Neuropsychopharmacol*. 2012;37:1057–66.

28. Zoghbi HY and Bear MF. Synaptic dysfunction in neurodevelopmental disorders associated with autism and intellectual disabilities. *Cold Spring Harbor Perspectives in Biology* 2012;4:a009886 1–22.

29. Lynch G. Memory enhancement: The search for mechanism-based drugs. *Nature Neurosci*. 2002;5(Suppl):1035 –8.

30. Porrino LJ, Daunais JB, Rogers GA, *et al*. Facilitation of task performance and removal of the eff ects of sleep deprivation by an ampakine (CX717) in nonhuman primates. *PLoS Biology*. 2005;3(9):e299.

31. Mohler H. (2007). Functional relevance of GABA-A receptor subtypes. In: S Enna and H Mohler (eds). *The Receptors: The GABA Receptors*, 3rd edn. Totowa, NJ: Humana Press, 2007, pp. 23–40.

32. Nutt DJ, Besson M, Wilson SJ, *et al*. Blockade of alcohol's amnestic activity in humans by an alpha5 subtype benzodiazepine receptor inverse agonist. *Neuropharmacol*. 2007;53(7):810–20.

33. Bartos M, Vida I, and Jonas P. Synaptic mechanisms of synchronized gamma oscillations in inhibitory interneuron networks. *Nature Rev Neurosci*. 2007;8:45–56.

34. Buczaki G. *Rhythms of the Brain*. New York, NY: Oxford University Press, 2006.

35. Lewis DA, Cho RY, Carter CS, *et al*. Sub-unit-selective modulation of GABA Type-A receptor neurotransmission in schizophrenia. *Am J Psychiat*. 2008;165:1585–93.

36. Cools R, Roberts AC, and Robbins TW. Serotoninergic regulation of emotional and behavioural control processes. *Trends Cogn Sci*. 2008;12:31–40.

37. Boureau YL and Dayan P. Opponency revisited: competition and co-operation between dopamine and serotonin. *Neuropsychopharmacol*. 2011;36:74–97.

38. Titler M, Lyon RA, and Glennon RA. Radioligand binding evidence implicates the brain 5HT2 receptor as a site of action for LSD and phenylisopylamine hallucinogens. *Psychopharmacol*. 1988;94:213–16.

39. Nonogaki K, Strack AM, Dallman MF, *et al*. Leptin-independent hyperphagia and type 2 diabetes in mice with a mutated serotonin 5-HT$_{2C}$ receptor gene. *Nature Med*. 1998;4:1152–6.

40. Morrison JH. , Foote SL, Molliver ME et al Noradrenergic and serotonergic fibers innervate complementary layers in monkey primary visual cortex: an immunohistochemical study Proc. Nat. Acad. Sci,1982: 79:2401–2405.

41. Clarke HF, Dalley JW, Crofts HS, *et al*. Cognitive inflexibility after prefrontal serotonin depletion. *Science*. 2004;304:878–80.

42. Clarke HF, Walker SC, Crofts HS, *et al*. Prefrontal serotonin depletion affects reversal learning but not attentional set shifting. *J Neurosci*. 2005;25:532–38.

43. Robbins TW. From behaviour to cognition: functions of mesostriatal, mesolimbic and mesocortical dopamine systems. In: LL Iversen, SD Iversen, SB Dunnett, *et al*. (eds). *Dopamine Handbook*. Oxford: Oxford University Press, 2010, pp. 203–14.

44. Yerkes RM and Dodson JD. The relation of strength of stimulus to rapidity of habit-formation. *Journal of Comparative Neurology and Psychology* 1908; 18: 459–82.

45. Robbins TW and Everitt BJ. Functions of dopamine in the dorsal and ventral striatum. In: TW Robbins (ed.). *Seminars in the Neurosciences*. London: Saunders, 1992, pp. 119–27.

46. Berridge KC. What is the role of dopamine in reward today? *Psychopharmacol*. 2006;191:391–432.

47. Crow TJ. Specific monoamine systems as reward pathways. In: A Wauquier and ET Rolls (eds). *Brain-Stimulation Reward*. Amsterdam: North-Holland, 1976, pp. 211–38.

48. Schultz W. Getting formal with dopamine and reward. *Neuron*. 2002;36:241–53.

49. Grace A. Phasic versus tonic dopamine release and the modulation of dopamine system responsivity: a hypothesis for the etiology of schizophrenia. *Neurosci*. 1991;41:1–24.

50. Niv Y, Daw ND, Joel D, *et al*. Tonic dopamine: Opportunity costs and the control of response vigor. *Psychopharmacol*. 2006;191:507–20.

51. Williams GV and Goldman-Rakic PS. Modulation of memory fields by DA D1 receptors in prefrontal cortex. *Nature*. 1995;376:572–5.

52. Egan MF, Goldberg TE, Kolachana BS, *et al*. Effect of COMT Val108/158 Met genotype on frontal lobe function and risk for schizophrenia. *Proc Natl Acad Sci USA*. 2001;98:6917–22.

53. Mattay VS, Callicott JH, Fera F, *et al*. Catechol-o-methyltransferase val (158)-met genotype and individual variation in the response to amphetamine. *Proc Natl Acad Sci USA*. 2003;100:6186–91.

54. Cools R, Barker R., Sahakian BJ, *et al*. Enhanced or impaired cognitive function in Parkinson's disease as a function of dopaminergic medication and task demands. *Cerebral Cortex*. 2001;11:1136–43.

55. Clatworthy PL, Lewis SJG, Brichard L, *et al*. Dopamine release in dissociable strital subregions predicts the different effects of oral methylphenidate on reversal learning and spatial working memory. *J Neurosci*. 2009;29:4690–6.

56. Chamberlain SR and Robbins TW. Noradrenergic modulation of cognition: Therapeutic considerations. *J Psychopharmacol*. 2013;27:694–718.

57. Aston-Jones G, Chiang G, and Alexinsky T. Discharge of norepinehrine locus coeruleus neurons in behaving rats and monkey suggest a role in vigilance. *Prog Brain Res*. 1991;8:501–20.

58. Amaral DG and Sinnamon HM. The locus coeruleus. Neurobiology of a central noradrenergic nucleus. *Prog Neurobiol*. 1977;9:147–96.

59. Arnsten AFT. Stress signalling pathways that impair prefrontal cortex structure and function. *Nature Neurosci*. 2009;10:410–22.

60. Segal M and Bloom FE. The actions of norepinephrine in the rat hippocampus. IV The effects of locus coeruleus stimulation on evoked hippocampal unit activity. *Brain Res*. 1976;107:513–25.

61. Carli M, Robbins TW, Evenden JL, *et al*. Effects of lesions to ascending noradrenergic neurones on performance of a 5-choice serial reaction task in rats; implications for theories of dorsal noradrenergic bundle function based on selective attention and arousal. *Behav Brain Res*. 1983;9:361–80.

62. Rajkowski J, Majczynski H, Clayton E, *et al*. Activation of Monkey locus coeruleus neurons varies with difficulty and performance in a target detection task. *J Neurophysiol*. 2004;92:361–71.

63. Debiec J and LeDoux JE. Disruption of consolidation but not consolidation of auditory fear conditioning by noradrenergic blockers in the amygdala. *Neurosci*. 2004;129:267–72.

64. Schwabe L, Nader K, Wolf OT, *et al*. Neural signature of reconsolidation impairments by propanolol in humans. *Biol Psychiat*. 2012;71:380–6.

65. Lonergan MH, Olivea-Figueroa LA, *et al*. Propanolol's effects on the consolidation and reconsolidation of long term emotional memory in healthy participants: a meta-analysis. *Journal of Psychiatry & Neuroscience* 2013;38:222–31.

66. Lapiz MD and Morilak DA. Noradrenergic modulation of cognitive function in rat medial prefrontal cortex as measured by attentional set shifting capability. *Neurosci*. 2006;137:1039–49.

67. Del Campo N, Chamberlain SR, Sahakian BJ, *et al*. The roles of dopamine and noradrenaline in the pathophysiology and treatment of attention-deficit hyperactivity disorder. *Biol Psychiat* 2011;69:145–57.

68. Robinson ESJ, Eagle DM, Mar AC, *et al*. Similar effects of the selective noradrenaline reuptake inhibitor atomoxetine on three distinct forms of impulsivity in the rat. *Neuropsychopharmacol*. 2008;33:1028–37.

69. Chamberlain SR, Müller U, Blackwell AD, *et al*. Neurochemical modulation of response inhibition and probabilistic learning in humans. *Science*. 2006;311:861–3.

70. Chamberlain SR, Del Campo N, Dowson J, *et al*. Atomoxetine improved response inhibition in adults with attention-deficit/hyperactivity disorder. *Biol Psychiat*. 2007;62:977–84.

71. Chamberlain SR, Hampshire A, Müller U, *et al*. Atomoxetine modulates right inferior frontal activation during inhibitory control: A pharmacological functional magnetic resonance imaging study. *Biol Psychiat*. 2009;65:550–55.

72. Warburton DM and Brown K. Attenuation of stimulus sensitivity induced by scopolamine. *Nature*. 1971;230:126–7.

73. Warburton DM and Brown K. Facilitation of discrimination performance by phsyostigmine sulphate. *Psychopharmacologia (Berl.)*. 1972;27:277–84.

74. Wesnes K and Warburton DM. Effects of scopolamine and nicotine on human rapid information processing performance. *Psychopharmacol*. 1984;82:147–50.

75. Broks P, Preston GC, Traub M, *et al*. Modelling dementia: effects of scopolamine on memory and attention. *Neuropsychologia*. 1988;26:685–700.

76. Sahakian BJ. Cholinomimetics and human cognitive performance. In: LL Iversen, SD Inversen, and SH Snyder (eds). *Handbook of Psychopharmacology*, Vol 20. New York, NY: Plenum, 1988, pp. 393–424.

77. Sillito AM and Kemp JA. Cholinergic modulation of the functional organization of the cat visual cortex. *Brain Res*. 1983;289:143–55.

78. Zinke W, Roberts MJ, Guo K, *et al*. Cholinergic modulation of response properties and orientation tuning of neurons in primary visual cortex of anaesthetized marmoset monkeys. *Eur J Neurosci*. 2006;24:314–28.

79. Everitt BJ and Robbins TW. Central cholinergic systems and cognition. *Annu Rev Psychol*. 1997;48:649–84.

80. Dalley JW, McGaughy J, O'Connell MT *et al*. Distinct changes in cortical acetylcholine and noradrenaline efflux during contingent and noncontinent performance of a visual attentional task. *J. Neurosci*. 2001;21:4908–14.

81. Parikh V, Kozak R, Martinez V, *et al*. Prefrontal acetylcholine release controls cue detection on multiple timescales. *Neuron*. 2007;56:141–54.

82. Hasselmo ME and Sarter M. Modes and models of forebrain cholinergic modulation of cognition. *Neuropsychopharmacol*. 2011;36:52–73.

83. Witte EA, Davidson MC, and Marrocco, RT. Effects of altering brain cholinergic activity on covert orienting of attention: comparison of monkey and human performance. *Psychopharmacol*. 1997;132:324–34.

84. Perry E, Walker M, Grace J, *et al*. Acetylcholine in mind: a neurotransmitter correlate of consciousness. *Trends in Neuroscience* 1999;22:273–80.

85. Sahakian BJ, Owen AM, Morant NJ, *et al*. Further analysis of the cognitive effects of tetrahydroaminoacridine (THA) in Alzheimer's disease: assessment of attentional and mnemonic function using CANTAB. *Psychopharmacol*. 1993;110:395–401.

86. Emre M, Aarsland D, Albanese A, *et al*. Rivastigmine for dementia associated with Parkinson's disease. *N Engl J Med*. 2004;351:2509–18.

87. Hasselmo ME. The role of acetylcholine in learning and memory. *Curr Opin Neurobiol*. 2006;16:710–15.

88. Bielsky IF and Young LJ. Oxytocin, vasopressin and social recognition in mammals. *Peptides* 2004;25(9):1565–74.

89. Rimmele U, Hediger K, Heinrichs M, *et al*. Oxytocin makes a face in memory familiar. *J Neurosci*. 2009;2(1):38–42.

90. Kosfeld M, Heinrichs M, Zak P, *et al*. Oxytocin increases trust in humans. *Nature*. 2005;435:673–6.

91. Dahlstrom A and Fuxe K Evidence for the existence of monoamine-containing neurons in the central nervous system. *Acta Physiol Scand* 1964;62:1–55.

92. Woolf NJ, Eckenstein F, and Butcher LL Cholinergic systems in the rat brain: I. projections to the limbic telencephalon. *Brain Res Bull*. 1984; 13:751–84.

SECTION 2

Cognitive dysfunction

CHAPTER 10

Bedside assessment of cognition

Seyed Ahmad Sajjadi and Peter J. Nestor

Introduction

As with any clinical problem, the history usually provides the most valuable information for assessing suspected cognitive disorders. The key difference with a history in suspected dementia, compared to other medical consultations, is that cognitive impairment can mean that history from the patient is incomplete or unreliable. For this reason, collateral history from an informant such as a spouse or other individual with close contact to the patient is essential. This is equally true for patients that fall into the 'worried well' category who, although cognitively intact and therefore able to tell their own story, may provide a distorted view of the severity of their symptoms. In such instances, an informant can help by providing independent observation of the patient's ability to manage in everyday life.

A bedside cognitive assessment complements the history and is used to test hypotheses emerging from the patient/informant interview regarding the suspected clinical syndrome. Bedside cognitive testing can be impossible to interpret if one does not have a clear understanding of how cognitive abilities in one domain can have knock-on effects to other domains. For instance, a test purporting to examine executive function may be impossible for an aphasic patient if the test depends on comprehension of instructions or detailed verbal responses. One must be aware, therefore, that a 'cognitive hierarchy' exists. In other words, relatively preserved function in particular cognitive domains can be a prerequisite for satisfactory performance of others.

The most striking example of this hierarchy is the necessity of adequate attention for the reliable assessment of all other cognitive domains. In the outpatient setting, it is seldom relevant to examine attention formally in order to decide if further testing can proceed because it is usually obvious from talking to the patient that a profound attention deficit is not present. It is also unlikely that, in the outpatient environment, a patient will attend who is suffering from a major delirium. Inpatient referrals for cognitive assessment, however, frequently have reduced arousal and attention deficits in the context of an acute confusional state (delirium) making further in-depth assessments futile. Severe aphasia should also be viewed as an exclusion to further testing in other domains that are language-dependent. Obviously, it is prudent to ensure satisfactory state of basic visual and auditory abilities prior to embarking upon assessments of those aspects of cognitive function that are reliant upon these sensory modalities.

Instruments for global assessment of cognition

Several cognitive assessment tools are available that provide a global score for cognition. Although more expansive batteries will provide more information, there will be a time penalty; the choice of which battery to use, therefore, mostly depends on local logistical factors—in other words how much time is available to administer a battery. Table 10.1 provides a summary of the briefer assessment tools that are possible to integrate into a standard consultation, and their main pros and cons.

Importantly, a bedside battery can provide invaluable information about the stage of illness. To this end, incorporating a global battery is particularly useful as it provides a numerical score that can be used to track change over time and provides a straightforward way of communicating severity to colleagues. The utility of these points cannot be overemphasized. Compiling a medical report in which cognitive assessment is communicated solely on the basis of what the patient could or could not do over a range of ad hoc bedside cognitive assessments can make it impossible for a third party to judge the severity of the impairment. It is important to stress, however, that the numerical summary scores derived from these batteries are not directly comparable across different dementia syndromes. For instance, a score of 25/30 on the Mini-Mental State Examination (MMSE)[1] in a typical presentation of Alzheimer's disease does not necessarily indicate the same level of impairment in everyday life as it would in a behavioural presentation of frontotemporal dementia. Using this example, a patient with Alzheimer's disease and an MMSE of 25/30 will typically have memory impairment but nonetheless, remains fairly independent, whereas a patient with behavioural variant frontotemporal dementia with this score, may require high levels of assistance. Within diagnostic categories, however, these scores can be very useful in forming a mental picture of where a patient stands in the course of the illness and, most helpfully, they can be repeated in individual patients to track change over time.

In many instances, a careful history and a global measure are all one needs to make a reasonably confident diagnosis. Moreover, in situations where the global measure is not adequate to reach a diagnosis, the *pattern* of the patient's performance provides a starting point to tailor cognitive tests of interest for the individual.

Problem oriented cognitive assessment

Attention and orientation

Preserved attention and orientation are prerequisites for normal cognitive function and impaired orientation is one of the hallmarks of delirium. Orientation is typically assessed by testing awareness of time and place (and person). Time orientation is specifically assessed by asking the date, time of day, day of the week, month, season, and year. Place orientation includes items such as town, state/county, name of the hospital, floor, ward, etc. Most of these questions are well covered by the global assessment instruments

Table 10.1 Popular global bedside cognitive assessment tools

Test	Description (cut-off point for dementia)	Advantage	Disadvantage
AMTS[1]	Brief 10-item assessment tool (6–8/10)	Short screening tool for identification of cognitive problems; easy to use on general medical wards and in primary care setting	Brevity means it can only be used for very crude staging
MMSE[2]	Scored out of 30, The most widely used cognitive assessment tool (24/30)	Widely recognized test; objective scoring criteria; very useful staging procedure; brief	Heavily biased to verbal domain; not suitable for differential diagnosis; not sensitive to very mild impairments
MoCA[3]	Scored out of 30, aimed at detection of early dementia (26/30)	Relatively comprehensive albeit brief assessment tool; not biased towards particular cognitive domain	Not suitable for patients at the more advanced stages of dementia
ACE[4]	Scored out of 100, ACE-III is the most recent version of the test (82–88/100)	Robust validation in various neurodegenerative conditions; appropriate for tracking change; sensitive to subtle cognitive impairment and differential diagnosis	Too long for some clinical environments

Source data from AMTS: Abbreviated Mental Test Score; MMSE: Mini-Mental State Examination; MoCA: the Montreal Cognitive Assessment; ACE-R: Addenbrooke's Cognitive Examination-revised.

discussed above. Typically, patients with early degenerative diseases are more impaired in time orientation than place, though the latter is also frequently impaired in more advanced stages especially if the assessment is being carried out far from their home (in which case, patients may often confuse the home town and local hospital with their present location).

One exception is the syndrome of semantic dementia in which one can occasionally encounter patients who are fully oriented in time, but, owing to the semantic deficit, cannot name town, state/county, name of hospital, etc. Person orientation (i.e. name) is seldom informative in the outpatient setting. When an individual cannot produce their own name in the context of an organic disorder, it typically indicates that they are so demented or delirious as to be unable to respond to any verbal instruction. Apparent ignorance of one's own name in someone who is otherwise capable of communicating typically indicates a psychogenic state.

Common bedside tests of attention include spelling a five-letter word, such as 'world', backwards (included in the MMSE), and serial 7s ('take 7 from 100 and keep going down by 7', included in both MMSE and MoCA). Forward and backward digit span and recitation of the months of the year or the days of the week in reverse order are further examples. The choice of the appropriate test is partly dictated by the presumed cognitive syndrome. For instance, in suspected dominant (left) hemisphere syndromes such as various types of aphasia one should opt for less language taxing tests such as digit span. Vigilance is another way of assessing attention and concentration. For instance, the examiner asks the patient to listen for a particular letter of the alphabet whilst they read out a list of random letters with the target letter appearing frequently but unpredictably in the list (included in the MoCA). The patient indicates the occurrence of the target letter by tapping each time the letter is read.

Attention testing is clinically useful to monitor change in patients with delirium, such as metabolic encephalopathies. For this purpose, digit span—which measures attention and working memory capacity—can be particularly helpful because it provides a quantifiable score. In testing digit span, individual numbers should be uttered separately in a monotonous way at a rate of one digit/second (in contrast to grouping numbers in clusters as one would in giving a telephone number). Normal digit span is at least six

forwards, with backward digit span being one or two digits less than the forward span.

Declarative memory

Episodic memory

Episodic memory refers to memory for specific events from one's past—such as what one did this morning, on one's last holiday, one's wedding day, and so on. Episodic memory impairment is a defining feature of early-stage typical Alzheimer's disease and is also frequently observed in non-Alzheimer dementias. It is the most common reported problem in a cognitive disorders clinic. It is, therefore, important to have a plan for how it should be examined.

Episodic memory can, in turn, be divided to *retrograde*, reflecting one's ability to remember events from before the onset of the memory-impairing disease, and *anterograde* meaning the ability to acquire new memories after disease onset. Except for rare examples of highly restricted mesial temporal lobe lesions causing relatively pure anterograde deficits, both anterograde and retrograde memory are affected simultaneously in most amnestic syndromes including Alzheimer's disease. This is an important and clinically useful point for assessing memory at the bedside. In clinic, one often hears statements from informants of the type 'it's his short-term memory, the long-term memory is perfect'. The first point to note is that this lay distinction between 'short-term' and 'long-term' is only a distinction between recent (e.g. recalling events from this morning) and remote (e.g. recalling events from school days) episodic memory. Furthermore, the lay usage should not be confused with the neuropsychological term 'short-term memory' which is often used as a synonym for working memory—the ability not only to hold information in mind but also to manipulate it. The key relevance of highlighting this point is that this frequently reported observation from informants is very often untrue—understanding the falsehood is particularly useful in bedside memory examination and, in turn, reaching an accurate diagnosis.

The reason that informants report a problem restricted to 'short-term memory' presumably relates to a couple of factors. First is that they were eye-witnesses to the events constituting the apparent 'short-term memory' deficit, so they have their own recollection to act as a control to the patient's forgetting. Second is that it is very easy to fool oneself and believe that remote episodic memory is intact based on the patient producing some generic or over-learned details. For example, a patient with a significant remote memory deficit, may have some frequently retold anecdotes from their past life that give the illusion of a good remote memory. Generic memories can also give this illusion; for instance, asking a patient what they did last Christmas can prompt responses about eating too much, seeing family, etc. In this example, the patient is not necessarily providing specific information about what they remember of the event; the information is generic as it could describe many Christmas days.

The relevance of this to episodic memory testing is that asking the patient for details of their past life can be very informative in detecting a deficit. The key is that the examiner sets the agenda rather than letting the patient discuss what *they* wish to recount. One should ask the patient for specific details from their past life such as name of their school, first and subsequent employment positions, where they were married, places they have lived, and so on. Although such examples are not true episodic memories (rather, they are personal semantic details), these simple questions will frequently expose memory gaps in even very early Alzheimer's disease and will often provoke a 'head-turning sign'; the patient turning repeatedly to their spouse hoping for assistance.

True episodic memories can be probed in a similar manner by asking for specific details of the events of their last holiday, last Christmas, last birthday, wedding day, birth of a child, etc. It takes little practice as an examiner to separate the generic information of a patient attempting to camouflage their deficit from true episodic memory impairment. For instance, using the last holiday example, imagine a patient who always spends their summer holiday at the same seaside resort. In this scenario, responding with generic information such as they went to the beach or ate at restaurants does not indicate true recollection. In contrast, true episodic recall involves recounting details specific to that trip, for example, 'one day it rained so we visited the art gallery, there was a photography exhibition', 'we took a boat trip to view a seal colony, the sea was rough and our friend became ill', etc. It is precisely this fine-grained, true episodic memory that people with early Alzheimer's disease struggle with, and, as such, the utility of including such questions in the examination routine cannot be overemphasized.

The other method of testing memory at the bedside is by giving the patient something to learn and then asking them to recall the information after a distraction period. Typical examples are word lists or a name/address, and examples exist as subtests in all of the bedside global assessment tools. There are a few points worth highlighting with this form of testing. First, the degree of difficulty in such tests is influenced by the amount one has to remember as well as the length of the distraction period. To this end, the memory component of the MMSE—three-word recall after a distraction period of only a few seconds (while one spells 'WORLD' backwards or does serial 7s)—is very easy for intelligent, mildly impaired patients. As such, a perfect score on this measure should not be interpreted as meaning there is no memory impairment.

Second, some of these tests include multiple encoding trials (i.e. repeat the information more than once to enhance learning) and recognition (i.e. after asking the patient to recall the information without cue—'free recall'—asking them to identify previously learned information that was not freely recalled, intermixed with foils that they did not learn earlier). The profile of deficits across these different components is sometimes helpful for differential diagnosis. For instance, in very mild Alzheimer's disease, the encoding trials can show no abnormality whereas delayed recall is typically very impaired. In contrast, in dementia with Lewy bodies, encoding is often impaired with patients unable to reach ceiling performance even after a third trial, yet they often show little, or no, decline from the third encoding trial to delayed recall (Fig. 10.1).

In general, bedside tests of learning and recall are quite sensitive surrogate markers for an episodic memory deficit, and this is even true for the three-word recall in the MMSE. Specificity, however, can be a problem as patients with non-degenerative causes of memory complaints, such as psychiatric disorders, also can score poorly on such measures. This is important because separating degenerative from non-degenerative causes is the commonest clinical problem encountered in a memory clinic. It is also one of the most difficult problems, particularly as a diagnosis of depression does not necessarily imply that depression is the primary cause of the symptoms; it is also a common co-morbidity in early dementia. It is important to stress that there is no foolproof examination technique to sort out this problem, and sometimes it is only with

		Trial 1	Trial 2	Trial 3	Delayed Recall
Normal	Joseph Barnes	✓✓	✓✓	✓✓	✓✓
	19 Woodland Close	✗✗✓	✓✓✓	✓✓✓	✗✓✓
	Browndale	✓	✓	✓	✓
	Yorkshire	✓	✓	✓	✓
Very early AD	Joseph Barnes	✓✓	✓✓	✓✓	✓✗
	19 Woodland Close	✗✗✓	✓✓✓	✓✓✓	✗✗✗
	Browndale	✓	✓	✓	✗
	Yorkshire	✓	✓	✓	✗
Mild DLB	Joseph Barnes	✓✓	✓✓	✓✓	✓✓
	19 Woodland Close	✗✗✗	✗✗✗	✗✗✗	✗✗✗
	Browndale	✗	✗	✓	✗
	Yorkshire	✓	✓	✓	✓

Fig. 10.1 Examples of performance seen in learning and recall of a name and address in very mild Alzheimer's disease (AD) and dementia with Lewy bodies (DLB).

follow-up that the diagnosis emerges. That said, the formal examination of personal milestones and episodes, as already described, can be particularly useful because patients suffering depression or anxiety are often better on these ecological measures.

These measures can also be very helpful where there is a suspicion that a patient's apparent poor performance on tests of learning and recall is an elaboration (due to a lack of effort). Such patients may return catastrophic performance when knowing their memory is being formally examined, but demonstrate good memory for real-life past events when questions are presented in what appears to be a general conversation. Another clue to look out for in such situations, is where the patient can go into incredibly fine-grained detail when recounting the circumstances (i.e. minute details of the events leading up to, and following on from, memory lapses), thereby demonstrating good episodic memory.

Semantic memory

Semantic memory refers to knowledge of facts, concepts, and objects. For instance, that Paris is the capital city of France, that an elephant is a large mammal with a trunk, that a 'hobby' is a pastime one indulges in for recreation, and so on. These examples demonstrate the distinction from episodic memory in that such examples are not recollected from a particular time and place. In other words, knowing that Paris is the capital of France is a fact that one encounters in various contexts; recalling the events of a specific trip that one made to Paris are episodic memories.

Semantic memory can be tested in many ways. Simply naming pictures or objects in the office is useful, but it is important to stress that while a semantic deficit will cause naming difficulty, a naming problem does not necessarily imply a semantic deficit. The latter can also result from a word-retrieval deficit. The examination can get at this by asking the patient questions about objects they cannot name. For instance, a patient with a word-retrieval deficit may not be able to name a 'stethoscope' yet can provide description: 'the thing the doctor uses to listen to your chest'. Patients with semantic deficit, as seen in the syndrome of semantic dementia (also known as semantic variant primary progressive aphasia), in contrast, will often respond that they have no idea when asked for a description. Another way to distinguish a semantic deficit from a word-retrieval problem is cueing. Performance of a patient with anomia due to a retrieval deficit will benefit from cueing ('it is a steth …?') whereas cueing typically is of less help to a patient with a semantic deficit.

Understanding how semantic knowledge deteriorates in neurodegenerative disease is crucial to understanding how to test it. Two, somewhat interrelated factors, namely, age of acquisition and word frequency, are important determinants of this process. The semantic material that is most robust is that acquired very early in life and that which occurs at the highest frequency in everyday life. Asking a patient to identify high-frequency items such as a pen or a dog can be done successfully in spite of a significant semantic decline. One must choose harder items, therefore, to expose the deficit. Even with no special equipment in a medical consultation, this can be achieved with objects such as the stethoscope, a stapler, a paperclip, etc.

Other examples of bedside semantic tests include naming to description (e.g. 'what do you call the Australian animal that hops and has a pouch?'). To take naming out of the equation, one can give semantically complex commands such as, 'point to an electronic communication device'. Note that traditional three-stage commands (e.g. 'take the paper in your left hand, fold it in half, and lay it on the table') are not good tests of semantic comprehension as they lack semantic complexity; these are typically taxing working memory by stringing together a sequence of commands but the semantic content ('paper', 'hand', 'table') is very simple.

Language

Naming and semantic knowledge are major components of language and were covered in the previous section. Other aspects that are useful to assess in reaching a clinical diagnosis include fluency and grammatical ability, repetition, and reading.

Speech fluency and grammar

Non-fluent aphasia is best identified by listening to the patient converse rather than by doing tests. When severe, the problem is obvious with severely laboured, slow speech. In the very earliest stages of a non-fluent aphasia, however, it can be difficult to pick up or can appear as though the patient is suffering from slight anxiety. In such circumstances, it is often the patient's own history—and not the informant's observations—that gives the clue in that they may complain of trouble forming sentences or mispronouncing words. Such complaints should be taken seriously even if they seem to be so subtle as to not be evident in the course of conversation; they are often the harbinger of a progressive non-fluent aphasia.

When non-fluent aphasia is evident, it manifests as slow, laboured utterances with reduced sentence length. Phonological and phonetic errors may be evident: the former being incorrect placement of real phonemes (caterpillar → capperpillar), the latter being sounds not corresponding to any normally articulated phonemes. The latter is a feature of so-called apraxia of speech.

Non-fluent aphasia in degenerative disease typically, does not give rise to the agrammatic 'telegraphic' speech described in stroke aphasia. Although grammar is impaired on formal tests, the manifestation in speech is typically to produce correct but very simplified grammar. The speech of Alzheimer-related progressive aphasia (logopenic aphasia) is usually fluent in grammatical terms but halting due to frequent word-finding pauses. In semantic dementia, speech is fluent and can sound remarkably normal. These patients often do not have word-finding difficulties apparent in conversation, presumably because word-finding difficulty implies that the individual knows the concept for which they are trying to retrieve the word; if the concept is lost, one does not search for it.

Bedside testing of grammar involves asking the patient grammatically complex, but semantically simple, questions such as reversible passive and centre-embedded sentences. Examples of the former include 'Jack was sacked by Jill; who was the boss?', 'John was hit by Sam; who got hurt?', and so on. Note here that the reversibility refers to the fact that the subject and object of the sentence give no clue as to the correct response, in contrast to a sentence such as 'the sheep was eaten by the wolf; who survived?' where, although passive, one could answer correctly simply by knowing that a sheep cannot eat a wolf. Also, note here that if one uses this testing approach, chance performance is 50 per cent, so one needs to present several examples to be sure of a problem. One could also look for a discrepancy between performance on passive constructions and easier active constructions ('Jill sacked Jack; who was the boss?'). Centre-embedded sentences mean embedding a clause between subject and simple predicate, for example 'the bowl the fish is in is red; what is red?'. The idea here is that the patient struggling with grammar might incorrectly answer 'the fish' because it occurs close to 'red' in the sentence.

Repetition

Impaired repetition can be either at the single-word level or a problem with sentence repetition. Impairment at the single-word level implies impairment also with sentences. Isolated sentence repetition can occur and implies problems with auditory–verbal working memory. This is thought to be the basis of sentence repetition deficits seen in association with Alzheimer pathology.

The repetition equivalent to testing semantics with lower-frequency items is to ask the patient to repeat long words—little can go wrong in repeating 'cat'! To create graded difficulty one can start with two syllable words 'gallop' and 'rapid' and proceed to complex multi-syllabic words such as 'perspiration' and 'literary'. Also, by combining repetition with definition, one has a quick screening test for both articulation and semantics; for example, ask the patient to repeat 'caterpillar' then ask for a definition of a caterpillar; other examples include 'rhinoceros', 'catastrophe', etc. Asking the patient to repeat one of the complex multisyllabic words such as 'catastrophe' a number of times over and looking specifically for inconsistent repetition mistakes from one trial to the next is considered a sign of apraxia of speech.

Reading

Reading orthographically regular and irregular words can also be very helpful and represents a simple bedside test to administer to expose semantic deficits through the phenomenon of 'surface dyslexia'. It is particularly useful in the English language, less so in languages with more transparent orthography to pronunciation rules. Irregular words refer to words that are not pronounced as they are written and in order to pronounce them correctly, one requires semantic knowledge. For instance, if knowledge of the word 'pint' is lost, it will be pronounced as it is written (to rhyme with 'hint'). In other words, it is read according to its 'surface structure' rather than its deeper meaning, hence, 'surface dyslexia'. Note that the rule about semantic dementia and high-frequency words applies here as well. One does not observe surface errors to ultra-high-frequency words such as 'was' even if it is not pronounced as written. One needs to test by having the patient read lower-frequency words of which, in English, at least, there are many: 'yacht', 'sew', etc.

Visual perception

Hemianopia and visual neglect are tested as part of the standard neurological examination. Deficits in higher-order visual processing, particularly spatial processing, are important to test for at the bedside in suspected posterior cortical atrophy. In fact, visuoperceptual testing in individuals suspected of having this syndrome is particularly useful because often patients and informants struggle to articulate the nature of the problem clearly. In contrast, the deficit can be quickly exposed with simple bedside tests. Visuoconstructive ability is a useful screening test (i.e. clock, wire-cube drawing, etc.). Deficits on such tasks are often referred to as constructional apraxia. Drawing such items also has a motor and planning component, so impairment does not necessarily imply a perceptual problem. The hallmark of posterior cortical atrophy is simultanagnosia and this is fairly easily demonstrated with simple bedside tests (Fig. 10.2).

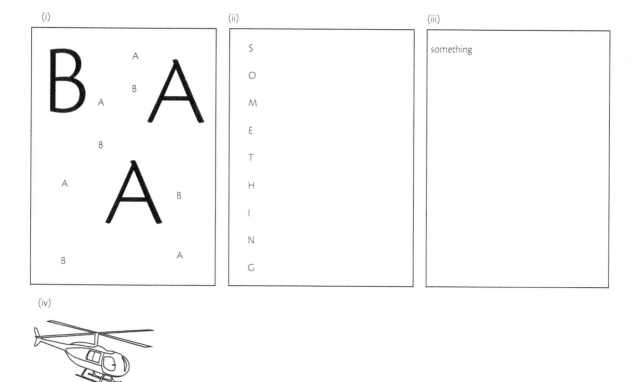

Fig. 10.2 Tests of simultanagnosia. Panels each represent an A4 sheet. (i) The patient is asked to point to the 'As' (then later 'Bs'). Typically they find the small letters, but miss the large ones. In (ii) the patient is asked to read the word. They typically struggle, having to read letter by letter down the page, or cannot manage it at all, whereas when the word is written normally (iii) it can be read. Note in both examples that the impairment cannot be attributed to a visual acuity problem as the patient fails to identify the larger items. (iv) simultanagnosia can mean that patients only pick details out of pictures when naming. In the example shown, a simultanagnosic patient (posterior cortical atrophy) named this item as 'chopsticks'. When asked to explain, it became evident that they were only noticing the rotor-blades of the helicopter. This is important to be aware of as apparently bizarre answers can lead to the incorrect belief that the patient is simulating their deficits.

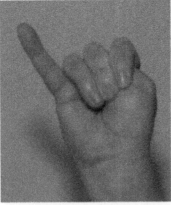

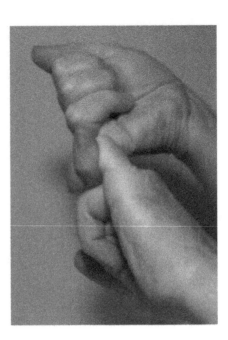

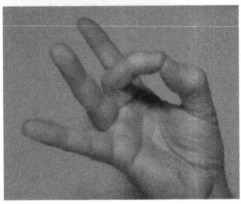

Fig. 10.3 Examples of meaningless gestures to test apraxia. Note that 'meaningless' is culture-specific, and items should be chosen to avoid offensive gestures in the target population!

Dressing apraxia is another useful bedside test that accompanies deficits in perception. It is easily assessed by asking the patient to put on a sweater or jacket that has had one of its sleeves turned inside out.

Limb apraxia

Limb apraxia is the inability to execute motor responses despite intact basic motor functions (see also chapter 6). It is therefore important to have first confirmed that basic motor (and sensory) functions are intact from the general neurological examination. Limb apraxia is a prominent feature of the corticobasal syndrome and can be examined by having the patient copy meaningless hand gestures (Fig. 10.3). Having the patient imitate meaningful actions (pretending to stir a cup of coffee or comb one's hair, etc.) can also be tested. This form of apraxia has a semantic and a motor component and, in the authors' experience, such testing does not add meaningfully to the assessment of apraxia.

Executive function and 'frontal' behaviour

Executive function covers problem solving, abstraction, multitasking, and so on. Impairments are often thought of as synonymous with frontal lobe dysfunction. While it is true that the frontal lobes are critical for these functions, these kinds of complex tasks really require the whole cognitive brain; they are the strongest example of needing all cognitive faculties working and this is seldom the case in degenerative disease.

There are a multitude of bedside tests purporting to test executive function. Popular examples include:

◆ Go–no go: 'When I tap the table once, you tap the table once; if I tap the twice, you do not tap', the idea being that the stimulus-bound patient cannot suppress the impulse to tap twice in the latter condition

◆ Proverb interpretation: the patient cannot abstract the proverbial message and provides a literal interpretation

◆ Cognitive estimates: asking questions in which one would not normally know the answer but could make a reasonable guess, e.g. 'How fast can a racehorse gallop?' or 'How far is London from Paris?', etc.

◆ Differences and similarities: 'In what way are a sculpture and a piece of music similar?' or 'What is the difference between a dwarf and a child'?

There are problems with all of these tests when used to aid diagnosis. Ideally, for example, they should be sensitive and specific to the behavioural form of frontotemporal dementia but they typically fail on both counts. One of the problems is the fact that tests such as proverbs, cognitive estimates, and differences/similarities tend to be influenced by premorbid intelligence. To this end, it is not uncommon to find members of the normal population who will explain the meaning of proverbs in a concrete manner or who may make grossly inaccurate cognitive estimates. There is also the consequential problem of deciding how figurative a response should be for it to be deemed non-literal. Perhaps the main problem is

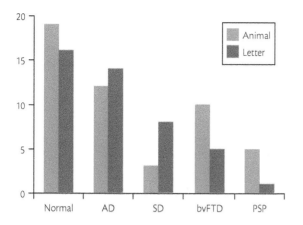

Fig. 10.4 Patterns of performance on letter fluency versus animal fluency (y-axis indicates words produces in one minute) in the *early* stages of the respective disorders: AD, Alzheimer's disease; SD, semantic dementia; bvFTD, behavioural variant frontotemporal dementia; PSP, progressive supranuclear palsy.

that the behavioural changes, associated most typically with frontal lobe degeneration, are extremely complex, and so, try as these tests might, they are just too simplified to capture this complexity.

A far more robust approach to identifying behavioural variant frontotemporal dementia and other frontal lobe conditions is to take note of the patient's actual behavior in the social setting of the consultation. Careful observation and recording of how the patient appears, interacts, and the content of their conversation are essential to reach an accurate diagnosis. In this regard, the examination is highly similar to the mental state examination (MSE) that forms a routine part of a psychiatric assessment. The reason this is important is because although the details of personality change will come from an informant—hence the informant's account is essential to identifying the characteristic changes of frontotemporal dementia—if one relies solely on the informant's account, there is a risk of making a false-positive diagnosis.

This risk is minimized by corroborating the informant's history with careful observation of the patient. The changes one might observe include restlessness, such as being unable to remain seated and preferring to get up and wander; impulsively wanting to terminate the consultation; not respecting personal space; being distracted by environmental stimuli such as going to the window to look at traffic or wanting to see what is on a computer monitor. At it most severe, utilization behaviour may be observed in which the patient will start using anything handed to them; giggling fatuously; repetitive use of a catchphrase or cliché in conversation; making disinhibited remarks about people in the clinic, and so on.

One final bedside test that has some utility in frontotemporal dementia and also for a range of other conditions is verbal fluency: asking the patient to produce as many different words as they can think of in one minute that begin with a certain letter and then

the same for a semantic category. For instance, words beginning with the letter 'P' and animals beginning with any letter. There is some variability in the number that healthy people can produce, but the pattern of the two tasks rather than the absolute score is often informative. Healthy people typically can produce at least 15 P-words and do slightly better than their letter fluency score in the animal fluency condition. In early Alzheimer's disease, one often sees a reversal of this pattern even if the absolute scores are not particularly low, perseverations are also common; in semantic dementia there is typically a profound reduction in animal word fluency; in behavioural variant frontotemporal dementia there is often a disproportionate reduction in letter fluency; in progressive supranuclear palsy this is usually extreme, often as few as only one P-word in one minute (Fig. 10.4).

Conclusion

In summary, much valuable diagnostic information can be gleaned from a thoughtful cognitive examination. If more detailed, quantitative information is needed across the cognitive domains, a formal neuropsychological evaluation is an appropriate next step. This is particularly true in clinically ambiguous situations, such as where deficits are so subtle as to be of uncertain significance. Neuropsychological scores in such instances can act as an invaluable baseline that can be repeated at a future time-point to assess change. Referral for neuropsychological assessment should not be used, however, as a substitute to a careful assessment. The best chance of making an accurate diagnosis lies in a careful history, and cognitive examination and this should be viewed as the foundation to inform interpretation for ancillary tests including neuropsychology, imaging, and laboratory investigations.

Further reading

Larner AJ (ed.). *Cognitive Screening Instruments: A Practical Approach*. London: Springer-Verlag, 2013.

Hodges JR. *Cognitive Assessment for Clinicians*, 2nd edn. Oxford: Oxford University Press, 2007.

References

1. Qureshi K and Hodkinson M. Evaluation of a 10 question mental test of the institutionalized elderly. *Age Ageing*. 1974;3:152–7.
2. Folstein M, Folstein S, and McHugh P. 'Mini-Mental State': A practical method for grading the cognitive state of patients for the clinician. *J Psychiatr Res*. 1975;12:189–98.
3. Nasreddine Z, Phillips N, Bédirian V, *et al*. The Montreal Cognitive Assessment (MoCA): A brief screening tool for mild cognitive impairment. *J Am Geriatr Soc*. 2005;53:695–9.
4. Mioshi E, Dawson K, Mitchell J, *et al*. The Addenbrooke's Cognitive Examination Revised (ACE-R): A brief cognitive test battery for dementia screening. *Int J Geriatr Psychiatry*. 2006;21:1078–85.

CHAPTER 11

Neuropsychological assessment

Diana Caine and Sebastian J. Crutch

Introduction

Neuropsychological assessment of patients presenting with cognitive disorders provides crucial information on which to base diagnosis as well as evaluate whether there have been changes in an individual's condition. For example, while 'dementia' is defined as a cognitive syndrome affecting memory, thinking, behaviour, and the ability to perform everyday activities, intensive neuropsychological research has resulted in the identification of differential and pathognomonic patterns of cognitive decline in different conditions.[1,2] Particularly in the early stages of disease, dementia syndromes with different underlying aetiologies often selectively affect specific functional systems, consistent with the characteristic sites and distribution patterns of the relevant pathology.[3] A number of dementia syndromes therefore have what might be regarded as a characteristic cognitive signature.

Neuropsychological assessment, especially in the earliest disease stages of disease, when a patient is first being investigated for cognitive failure in daily life, is directed towards (i) establishing whether or not the patient's complaints are more likely to be neurogenic than psychogenic; and (ii) characterizing a patient's cognitive status with a view to determining whether the cognitive profile is consistent with one or another of these cognitive signatures. This chapter will address how this assessment is done and will include some case studies. It also seeks to expand the 'psychological' in 'neuropsychological' to address, albeit briefly, the impact of those cognitive changes on the patients' sense of themselves and on their relations with others.

The aim of neuropsychological assessment is to demonstrate the presence or absence of cognitive decline on objective measures of cognitive function. In the context of dementia, notwithstanding advances in neuroimaging, the documentation of cognitive change on neuropsychological assessment not infrequently precedes positive findings on other investigative measures. The usefulness of neuropsychological testing for diagnosis rests on interpretation of the pattern of performance across tests of the different cognitive domains, rather than on the result of any particular test or any particular cognitive domain on its own. For that reason, neuropsychological assessment typically includes a range of measures including current general intellectual function as well as tests of performance in the major cognitive domains: memory, language comprehension and production, executive function, visuoperceptual and visuospatial function, attention, and processing speed. At the same time, while an assessment needs to be comprehensive it also needs to be efficient, in the interest of the patient's well-being and cooperation on the one hand, and practicality on the other.

Test selection, structure, and properties

The selection of neuropsychological tests for an assessment will depend on a variety of factors including the nature of the referral (e.g. evaluation for evidence of cognitive impairment, monitoring of disease progression), the patient's clinical status (e.g. under investigation, diagnosed, dementia type/syndrome, disease severity), the availability of information about their cognitive status (e.g. bedside cognitive screening, previous neuropsychological assessment), and the overall context of the assessment (e.g. clinical, research, clinical trial, medico-legal). Appropriate test selection is important in all contexts.

Within the standard clinical setting, there is freedom to choose tests but also pressure for the psychologist to work reactively, adapting the roster of assessments according to the patient's presentation and emerging cognitive pattern. Such responsive practice is essential to identify and verify apparent deficits and build up a meaningful profile of the individual within the time and other constraints of a given service. By contrast, group research studies and clinical trials usually involve the administration of a predetermined battery of tests. In this context, careful selection to ensure appropriateness of the tasks for the target population and the frequency they are administered is critical to ensure that patients are not repeatedly confronted with tasks which are too difficult and may cause frustration and distress, and to avoid practice effects (see section on practice effects).

Whilst test selection is often dictated by mundane factors such as test availability or local service traditions, familiarity with the structure and psychometric properties of different neuropsychological measures is critical in maximizing the validity and effectiveness of the assessment.

Task difficulty, and ceiling and floor effects

The difficulty of a particular task can determine its suitability for use in particular situations. For example, demanding uncued and cued recall tests of episodic memory may be required to discriminate between healthy individuals and those with pre-symptomatic Alzheimer's disease (AD) (e.g. free and cued selective reminding test (FCSRT)[4–5] (see also chapter 32). By contrast, evaluation or monitoring of memory impairment in mild to moderate AD patients may be more appropriately assessed using forced choice recognition procedures (e.g. recognition memory test).[6] Dedicated tools for the assessment of those with more severe cognitive impairment are also available (e.g. Severe Impairment Battery).[7] Some tasks offer alternate forms with different degrees of difficulty (e.g. long, short, and easy forms of the recognition memory test).

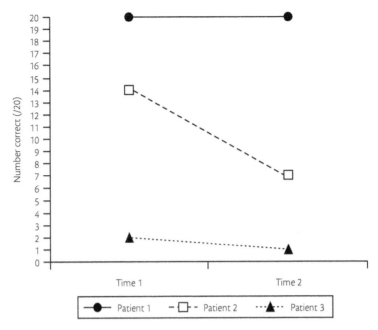

Fig. 11.1 Illustration of ceiling and floor effects and their impact on the interpretation of longitudinal assessment data. The figure describes the cases of three putative patients all administered an imagined test at two time-points. Patient 1 exhibits ceiling effects at both time 1 and time 2, making it impossible to assess from this data alone whether (a) there is any impairment in this function, (b) performance is worsening over time, or (c) the task is simply too easy to detect (a) and/or (b). Likewise, Patient 3's score at or near floor at both time-points, indicating a deficit but preventing any meaningful evaluation of further decline over time. Only the performance of Patient 2 is adequately captured within the difficulty level/dynamic range of this task.

Appropriate task difficulty (or use of tasks with a wide dynamic range or which are graded in difficulty; see section on dynamic range and graded difficulty test structure) limits the occurrence of ceiling effects (where maximal scores mask subtle deficits) and floor effects (where minimal scores mask residual abilities; see Fig. 11.1).

Dynamic range and graded difficulty test structure

Tasks with a wide dynamic range permit the evaluation of multiple levels of cognitive deficit through the use of continuous measures (e.g. response time) or through variability in the difficulty of discrete test items (see Fig. 11.2). As the term suggests, graded difficulty tasks order discrete items from easy to hard, so that discontinuation rules can be employed to prevent unnecessary administration of overly difficult items. Consequently, such tasks protect against ceiling and floor effects and are ideally suited to cognitive domains in which there is considerable inter-individual variability in the healthy population (e.g. vocabulary size, calculation skills), and where longitudinal evaluation of cognitive change over multiple time-points is required.

Confounding and collateral deficits

Few neuropsychological tests tap a single type of cognitive process; many tasks possess inherent sensory, linguistic, and attentional-executive demands such that poor performance may occur for a number of different reasons. Picture-naming tests are a simple example; nominally a measure of word-retrieval skills, the task also requires visuoperceptual, semantic, executive control, and articulatory skills. The impact of collateral cognitive deficits not only necessitates the interpretation of the target test in the context of the broader cognitive profile, but also motivates the test selection (e.g. evaluating word retrieval in posterior cortical atrophy by naming to verbal description rather than naming to visual confrontation).

Composite scores

Some neuropsychological assessment goals or research questions may be addressed best using composite scores rather than individual tests or between-test profiles. For example, the designers of outcome measures for some early-stage and preventative AD trials advocate use of composite measures (which may include a combination of tests such as the ADAS delayed word list recall,[8] logical memory delayed paragraph recall,[9] Wechsler Adult Intelligence Scale—Revised (WAIS–R) digit symbol substitution,[10] and mini-mental state examination[11]). Such composites require validation for use in phase 3 trials, but composites have a long pedigree in clinical neuropsychology (e.g. WAIS IQ scales are a composite of multiple subtests; see Fig. 11.2).

Practice effects

Many neuropsychological tasks are subject to practice effects when administered on more than one occasion. Whilst the magnitude of the effects has been evaluated for some tasks,[12] other tasks attempt to minimize practice effects by using parallel stimulus sets (e.g. Graded Difficulty Spelling Test).[13] In many longitudinal studies, disease effects are determined from the absence of practice effects rather than reductions in absolute tests scores (i.e. a divergence over time between patient and control groups). However, the interpretation of changes between initial and follow-up assessment performance in individual clinical patients (relative to a single set of cross-sectional normative data) is more problematic.

The strategy of neuropsychological assessment

Neuropsychological investigation begins with an evaluation of the patient's estimated optimal level of function prior to any recent

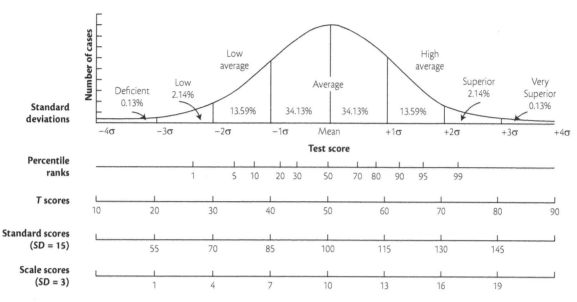

Fig. 11.2 Comparison of standardized scores [standard deviations (z scores), percentile ranks, T scores, standard scores (commonly termed 'IQ scores') and scale scores] across the normal distribution. Standardized scores provide a means for efficient comparison of performance levels across different tasks and domains. Note: not all neuropsychological tests yield normally distributed scores in healthy populations; the relative value or meaningfulness of standardized scores is reduced in tasks where the normative data are positively or negatively skewed.

change or decline. In addition to information elicited about the patient's education and employment history, which is very often a useful guide in this regard, an estimation of pre-morbid IQ is also based on performance on a reading test known to be highly correlated with IQ. The National Adult Reading Test (NART)[14] is such an instrument, comprising 50 words all of which have low sound–spelling correspondence. Performance on this test, in native English speakers—and in many, but not all, neurological conditions—is thought to be relatively robust to brain damage. The exception is any condition in which reading may itself be a prominent symptom; for instance, semantic dementia. The interpretation of test results depends crucially upon establishing whether the patient's performance is at variance with the level of performance expected based on this estimation of optimal functional level. Failure to do this risks underestimating decline in patients of better than average intellect or, conversely, overestimating deterioration in patients whose general intellectual function has always been lower than average.

Identification of cognitive deficits is accomplished in the first instance by comparing a patient's scores with those of age—and sometimes also education-matched—normative scores, taking into account the patient's premorbid IQ. In addition to the scores themselves, the qualitative features of a patient's performance and the nature of the errors can also be illuminating as to the nature of the deficit. Thus, for instance, errors on a test of object naming may arise from visuoperceptual problems (e.g. seeing a pair of handcuffs as 'spectacles' or 'a bicycle') or from semantic loss (e.g. calling a picture of an anteater 'a dog').

In describing our approach to neuropsychological assessment below mention is made of tests which represent just a small sample of the many tests currently available (for reference to specific tests see reference 15). A comprehensive neuropsychological assessment should include evaluation of the following:

General intellectual function

The neuropsychological assessment should evaluate the extent to which there may be a discrepancy between a patient's current level

of intellectual of function and the optimal pre-morbid level that has been estimated. The Wechsler Adult Intelligence Scale,[16] now in its fourth incarnation, has for decades been regarded as the gold standard for testing general intellectual function. The full battery of tests is very long but robust estimates of current IQ can be obtained from shortened versions, as recognized by the test-makers themselves in the form of the Wechsler Abbreviated Scale of Intelligence (WASI)[17] which comprises four subtests from which verbal, performance, and full-scale IQ (VIQ, PIQ, and FIQ) scores can all be generated. In addition to providing estimates of current global intellectual function, much useful information can be gathered from a patient's performance on individual subtests and/or discrepancies between scales or subtests. For example, individuals with semantic dementia typically exhibit significantly lower VIQ than PIQ (with especially weak performance on vocabulary and similarities; see case study 2 this chapter), whilst conversely individuals with posterior cortical atrophy typically struggle with the visual demands of many performance subtests (e.g. matrix reasoning, see case study 1 this chapter).

Memory

From a theoretical point of view, memory is a complex cognitive domain comprising a number of components including registration, encoding, retention, and retrieval. Memory complaints are by far the commonest reason for referral for neuropsychological assessment, although in the layperson's vocabulary 'memory' functions as a catch-all for almost any self-reported cognitive change. From the perspective of assessment, two aspects of memory are of particular importance: episodic memory, the encoding and recall of new information; and semantic memory, the knowledge of concepts, facts, and meanings, which is usually considered in the context of language rather than memory as such (see section on language). Episodic memory is typically assessed with tests of recognition (e.g. recognition memory test (RMT)[6] tests for words and faces, and recall of both verbal and visual information (e.g. BIRT Memory and Information Processing Battery BMIPB;[18] Doors and

People Test).[19] Impairment on tests of delayed recall is a particularly sensitive measure of memory decline and by far the most common presenting feature in typical AD.[20] Working memory can also be tested in both verbal and visuospatial domains using digit span or its analogue, spatial span (Wechsler Memory Scale–III).[21]

Language

In the context of dementia, language complaints are less common than concerns about memory but, as is very well documented, can be the symptom that heralds primary progressive aphasia.[22] Apart from attention to the patient's spontaneous speech for evidence of word-finding difficulty, paraphasic errors, or problems with articulation or speech production, screening for language deficits in the context of neuropsychological assessment of dementia usually relies on tests of naming and fluency in addition to verbal comprehension tasks within the general intellectual assessment (e.g. the vocabulary or similarities subtests of the WAIS).

The naming of line drawings of objects and animals (e.g. Graded Naming Test)[23] is a sensitive test of semantic knowledge[24] as well as being a test of lexical access.[25] Category fluency (commonly, the number of animal names a patient is able to produce in 60 seconds) is another easily administered task that has also been shown to be a robust measure of semantic memory.[26] Although not designed to do so, both are also liable to elicit phonological difficulties or problems with articulation or apraxia of speech, where they are present. Where deficits on these tests, in the context of relative preservation of performance on other tasks, suggest that language is a prominent early symptom of decline, other language tasks including tests of repetition, reading, spelling, and sentence comprehension are also administered. In the primary progressive aphasias a disturbance of one or another aspect of language is the most prominent feature early in the course of the disease, with the particular pattern of the disturbance indicating which progressive aphasic disorder is in question.

Visuospatial function

Deficits in visual processing can also sometimes be amongst the earliest presenting signs in a dementing process.[27-28] Elementary visuospatial function can be assessed using the 'visuospatial' components of the visual object and space perception (VOSP) battery:[29] position discrimination, dot counting, number location, or cube analysis. In addition, the copy condition of the BMIPB complex figure-recall task (or similar) also acts as a test of visuoconstructive task which might be a more sensitive measure of early visuospatial decline in some patients.

Visuoperceptual function

Inability correctly to name line drawings might arise from semantic memory loss—loss of knowledge of what a thing is—or from a failure of visual perception, sometimes a difficult distinction to make. A failure to perceive an object accurately may reflect loss of stored object-specific structural representations (e.g. inability to perceive common objects from unfamiliar angles) or because of more basic impairments of edge, form, and colour processing which deprive intact structural representations of the necessary input. The VOSP also comprises tests of visuoperceptual function (object decision, incomplete letters, silhouette naming) and of more basic visual processing (shape detection) which evaluate this domain. As suggested earlier, the nature of errors on other tasks with a perceptual component, such as object naming, represent further assessment of this function. Visual processing problems are characteristically the earliest signs of disease in posterior cortical atrophy, irrespective of the underlying pathogenesis.

Praxis

Apraxia refers to a loss of the ability to execute or carry out purposeful movements, whether meaningful or not, despite intact motor and sensory capacity. Although not usually part of routine neuropsychological assessment, it can constitute a significant component of a dementing syndrome (e.g. corticobasal degeneration, Creutzfeldt–Jakob disease), and where there are symptomatic complaints which suggest it may be present, it should be systematically evaluated (see, for example, reference 30 and chapter 16 for further details).

Frontal and executive function

The frontal lobes can be thought of as mediating two different aspects of behaviour: (i) the first is executive function, the ability to plan, organize, monitor, and voluntarily alter responses, in addition to abstract thinking, reasoning, and problem-solving; and (ii) social behaviour, the ability successfully to interact with others through empathy, understanding what others have in mind, conversational turn-taking, and so on. The first of these is assessed using tests which require cognitive flexibility (for example, Trail Making Test),[31] strategy formation (letter fluency); abstract concept formation (for example, modified card sorting test),[32] and the inhibition of prepotent responses in favour of alternative competing responses (for example, Stroop test,[33] Hayling sentence completion[34]). The latter is not so easily tested in a standard neuropsychological assessment but these are features that are readily elicited from the history or, indeed, from the patient's behaviour during testing. Tests of social cognition or theory of mind (e.g. The Awareness of Social Inference Test;[35] Reading the Mind in the Eyes[36]) can be useful where this is the most prominent feature of a presentation.

Information-processing speed

A reduction in the rate at which cognitive or psychomotor tasks are performed is a common feature of any kind of brain impairment, while psychomotor retardation is also a known feature of depression. Reduced information-processing speed may also be particularly prominent in individuals with pronounced subcortical damage (e.g. some forms of vascular dementia). While measures of speed are therefore not always helpful in differential diagnosis, they do help in understanding a patient's competencies and difficulties in daily life. There are numerous measures amongst the most common of which are timed-number or letter-cancellation tasks.

Mood

Mood, which can independently have an impact on the efficacy of cognition, can consequently also be a significant factor in the diagnostic process. In the first instance, differentiation of the impact of mood from possible organic causes of cognitive decline is frequently a crucial question in the early diagnostic work-up for dementia. Second, both anxiety in response to cognitive failure and depression in response to awareness of cognitive decline and its implications can exacerbate impaired performance. Thus, in addition to formal measures of cognition, the neuropsychological assessment should include evaluation, by both interview and questionnaire, of the patient's mood. Commonly used instruments include the Beck Depression Inventory,[37] Geriatric Depression Scale,[38] and the Cornell Scale for Depression in Dementia.[39] Here, the history of the symptomatology can be key in determining whether a mood disorder is the primary diagnosis or whether disturbed mood is a response to cognitive decline.

Interpretation of test results

In interpreting test results, both quantitative and qualitative features need to be considered. From the quantitative point of view, the pattern of results—the pattern of intact and impaired scores—across the whole range of tests administered is considered in addressing the question of whether the pattern obtained fits with one of the known dementia syndromes. Qualitatively, the patient's behaviour during testing (e.g. signs of impulsivity, restlessness, and agitation, level of insight and awareness, bewilderment, comprehension or recall of task instructions) as well as the nature of the errors made (e.g. evidence of semantic rather than visual errors on naming; phonological or semantic paraphasias; confabulation on memory tests) may contribute significantly to interpretation of test results.

A patient who presents with memory or other cognitive complaints of insidious onset often also presents with low mood. Here, again, the pattern of performance—for example, reduced scores on tests of attention, poor immediate recall without further loss over time—as well as the patient's behaviour during testing can both be helpful in discriminating between neurogenic and psychogenic disorders. Of course, these may not be mutually exclusive; frequently mood is low precisely because the person is aware that their cognition is failing.

Case studies

1. Case MC: Posterior cortical atrophy

MC was a 53-year-old, right-handed senior civil servant who presented with concerns about memory. She had a bachelor's degree in the humanities and the postgraduate certificate in education teaching qualification. She was able to give a clear and coherent account of her difficulties. There was no relevant past medical history and took no medication. About five years prior to presentation, she had gone through a very stressful period involving antisocial behaviour directed towards her home and family. She developed panic attacks and recalled an occasion when she was in a supermarket, feeling overwhelmed, nauseated, and disorganized. These symptoms recurred and progressed to the extent that over the six months prior to the initial neurology consultation she began to feel that she was not coping at work: she found her job—which she had been doing competently and comfortably to that point—stressful. She did not always get the gist of meetings. She had started trying to write things down but nonetheless felt she was always covering up for herself. She became concerned about her ability to multitask, or to understand e-mails. She missed a couple of appointments and was more reliant on her diary.

She was managing the housework without difficulties but reported that forgetfulness and losing things were an issue. Most notably, she found she became rather panicky whilst trying to follow routes, instructions, and maps. As well as difficulties with maps she had bumped the car on a few occasions and lost confidence somewhat whilst driving. She felt that her ability to do mental

arithmetic had perhaps declined. She reported no problems with speech, her sleep was normal, and she had no hallucinations. She did not smoke and drank alcohol occasionally. There was no family history of cognitive impairment. She described being stressed and feeling depressed particularly over the previous six months.

Her scores on neuropsychological assessment can be seen in Table 11.1 (see also Fig. 11.3). Estimated optimal level of premorbid function, based on education, employment history, and from her performance on the NART reading test was thought to be in the high-average range. From the scores in Table 11.1 it is clear that neither verbal (average) nor performance (impaired) IQ scores are at premorbid levels, but that the decrement is much more striking in the non-verbal domain, with scores poorer than expected on all three non-verbal tests administered. She scored in the impaired range on both recognition memory tests, confirming her subjective account of forgetfulness in daily life. Object naming, category fluency, and visuoperceptual function were all intact while visuospatial function

Table 11.1 Neuropsychology scores for patient MC

Test	Result
Estimated Premorbid Functioning	
NART FSIQ	115
Current Intellectual Functioning	
WAIS–III	
Verbal IQ	103
Vocabulary	Average
Similarities	High-average
Arithmetic	Average
Digit Span	Average
Performance IQ	67
Picture completion	Borderline
Block design	Impaired
Picture arrangement	Impaired
Memory	
WRMT—words	<5th %ile
WRMT—faces	<5th %ile
Language	
Graded naming test	50th %ile
Semantic fluency ('animals')	25–50th %ile
Visuoperceptual Skills	
VOSP inc. letters	>5th %ile cut-off
Visuospatial Skills	
VOSP position discrimin.	**<5% cut off**
AMIPB figure copy	**<10th %ile**
Executive Function	
Fluency—'S'	90th %ile
Stroop test	72nd %ile
Processing Speed	
Counting backwards	NAD

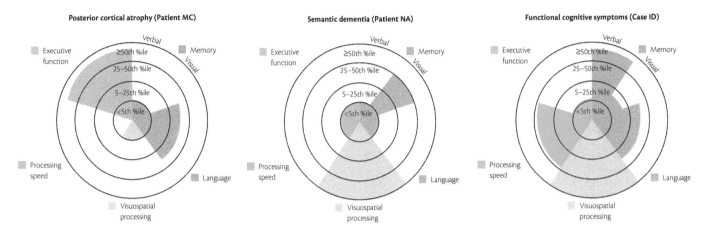

Fig. 11.3 Target diagrams summarizing the contrasting cognitive profiles of MC, NA, and ID across several cognitive domains. Cognitive impairment (estimated from percentile scores) is represented by the retreat of colour in each segment into the centre of the circle.

was very poor on both the VOSP test of spatial perception and the visuoconstructional task of figure copying. She was unable to place the numbers or hands correctly on a clock face and could not copy interlocking pentagons. In contrast, executive function was strikingly robust. Processing speed on a test that was not reliant on visual processing was normal. She scored in the mild range for both depression and anxiety on the Hospital Anxiety and Depression Scale (HADS), most likely underestimating somewhat low mood.

Interpretation

Although possibly exacerbated by mood, the profile is clearly organic. This was evident because of the relative specificity of her deficits; the nature of the difficulties she had with visual tasks which would not be seen in a functional disorder; and in her good scores on effortful verbal tests which indicated that level of effort was not at issue. Here, the profile was quite focal. Poor visuospatial function was the principal feature, with other aspects of cognition relatively intact apart from memory, which is usually but not always relatively spared in posterior cortical atrophy. This profile was confirmed on magnetic resonance imaging (MRI) which showed focal symmetrical volume loss in the parietal region bilaterally, in addition to some hippocampal atrophy which was also symmetrical.

2. Case NA: Semantic dementia

NA was a 71-year-old, right-handed professional woman who presented with a three- to four-year history of progressive difficulty thinking of words, especially nouns. She reported difficulty reading or following what she was watching on television. She had forgotten how to cook. Spontaneous speech was marked by word-finding difficulty and insertion of general substitutions (e.g. 'thingy') and semantic paraphasias (e.g. 'knife' for 'scissors'). Articulation and prosody were both preserved.

On formal examination, her score on the NART reading test suggested an estimated optimal premorbid IQ in the low-average range, clearly an underestimate given her education and employment history (see Table 11.2 and Fig. 11.3). The nature of her errors—trying to read the words by their spelling producing what are called 'regularization' errors—is a classic sign of semantic dementia.

In striking contrast to the previous patient, NA showed exactly the reverse finding on the verbal and performance IQs of the WAIS-III: here, the patient scored in the impaired range on the

verbal scale and in the high-average range on the non-verbal scale of the battery. The discrepancy points to very specific verbal deficits particular in relation to the vocabulary (production of definitions to words) and similarities (generation of abstract concepts which link two words) subtests. By the same token, recognition memory for words was impaired while recognition memory for faces remained intact. Unsurprisingly, object naming was profoundly impaired. Given the very prominent language impairment, additional language testing showed that single word comprehension was impaired (British Picture Vocabulary Test 22/32 correct) while repetition of both words and sentences was intact. Both visuoperceptual and visuospatial processing remained intact while executive function and processing speed were both reduced.

Interpretation

The profile was consistent with a diagnosis of semantic dementia, with the MRI showing selective, severe atrophy of the cortex and white matter of the anterior, medial, and inferior aspects of the *left* temporal lobe against a background of generalized atrophy.

3. Case ID: Functional cognitive symptoms

This 44-year-old man presented with complaints of forgetfulness in daily life dating back over the previous three to four years, possibly more noticeable in the months preceding the assessment. He had no other cognitive complaints although he did report a single conversational lapse while drinking with friends. Estimated optimal level of function based on NART and on his education and employment history was thought to be in the average range (see Table 11.3 and Fig. 11.3). Both verbal and performance IQ were in this range, indicating robust general intellectual function.

Recognition memory for words was quite robust (75–90th percentile) while recognition memory for faces was a little weaker, although still within normal limits (10–25th percentile). Both immediate and delayed recall of a short story were rather more impoverished than expected (both 10–25th percentile), with retention also a little weak (10–25th percentile). In contrast, both immediate and delayed recall of a complex figure were quite adequate (both 25–50th percentile) and here, retention after a delay was actually better than immediate recall (retention > 75th percentile)! Inconsistencies amongst memory tests pointed to attentional fluctuations and lapses that were most marked in response to complex

Table 11.2 Neuropsychology scores for patient NA

Test	Result
Estimated Premorbid Functioning	
NART FSIQ	85*
Current Intellectual Functioning	
WAIS–III	
Verbal IQ	69
Vocabulary	Borderline
Similarities	Impaired
Arithmetic	Low-average
Digit Span	Low-average
Performance IQ	111
Picture completion	High-average
Block design	High-average
Picture arrangement	Average
Memory	
WRMT—words	**<5th %ile**
WRMT—faces	50th %ile
D&P verbal recall	
Immediate	<10th %ile
Delayed	10th %ile
D&P visual recall	
Immediate	10–25th %ile
Delayed	25th %ile
Language	
Graded naming test	**<1st %ile**
Semantic fluency ('animals')	**<10th %ile**
Visuoperceptual Skills	
VOSP inc. letters	>5th %ile cut-off
Visuospatial Skills	
Doors and people copy	No errors
Executive Function	
Fluency—'S'	**<1st %ile**
Weigl sorting	½ categories
Processing Speed	
Letter cancellation	**4th %ile**

Table 11.3 Neuropsychology scores for patient ID

Test	Result
Estimated Premorbid Functioning	
NART FSIQ	108
Current Intellectual Functioning	
WAIS–III	
Verbal IQ	108
Vocabulary	High-average
Similarities	High-average
Arithmetic	Average
Digit span	Average
Performance IQ	95
Picture completion	Average
Block design	Average
Picture arrangement	Average
Memory	
WRMT—words	75–90th %ile
WRMT—faces	10–25th %ile
AMIPB story recall	
Immediate	10–25th %ile
Delayed	10–25th %ile
AMIPB figure recall	
Immediate	25–50th %ile
Delayed	25–50th %ile
Language	
Graded naming test	25–50th %ile
Semantic fluency ('animals')	25–50th %ile
Visuoperceptual Skills	
VOSP object decision	>5th %ile cut-off
Visuospatial Skills	
AMIPB figure copy	No errors
Executive Function	
Fluency—'S'	11th %ile
Stroop test	**2–4th %ile**
Processing Speed	
SDMT	47th %ile

auditory verbal material. However, conversational speech was fluent with no lapses and no word-finding difficulties.

Object naming was intact. There was no evidence of visuoperceptual or visuospatial impairment. Performance on executive tasks was a little poorer than expected. He was slow to complete the incongruent condition of the Stroop colour–word test, although he made only one error (2nd–4th percentile). Letter fluency was reduced (S: 11th percentile) in comparison with relatively intact category fluency (animals: 25–50th percentile). He scored in the moderate average range on the Hayling sentence completion task. Processing speed was normal.

ID expressed considerable anxiety about what he perceived to be the changes in his memory. Although the problems occurred more prominently at work, he reported that his mood was inclined to be low when he was away from the workplace. On a formal mood inventory he scored in the normal range for both anxiety and depression. Although there were no overt features of low mood and although he was generally cooperative and responsive on testing, there were several occasions in the course of the assessment when he seemed to give up in the face of an attention-demanding task. The MRI scan of the brain was normal with no evidence for atrophy.

Interpretation

The neuropsychological profile is therefore one of erratic scores on memory tests together with some executive inefficiency in the context of otherwise normal cognition. The overall impression, from the inconsistencies amongst the test scores and from his behaviour on testing, was that these lower than expected scores are most unlikely to be neurogenic in origin.

Psychological impact

Cognitive deficits can have a profound impact on the psychological dynamics of a couple and a family, particularly in the context of dementia as the patient's cognitive, affective, and mnestic processes disintegrate. Specific cognitive problems impact on a person's ability to function in particular ways: poor day-to-day memory makes it difficult to plan, organize, or anticipate what is going to happen, or to participate in the give-and-take of very much day-to-day conversation; visuospatial deficits may make it difficult to navigate familiar environments, even at home, or to function effectively in terms of knowing where to find things; apraxia may make it difficult to dress or to use everyday equipment (pens, cutlery) or appliances (remote control devices, microwave).

Difficulty with such everyday activities—with concomitant reliance and dependence on others to negotiate even simple aspects of daily life—dramatically affects a person's sense of themselves in the world and in their relations with others. Such changes can be profoundly distressing as well as anxiety-provoking to the patient. On the other hand, in some cases—most notably behavioural variant frontotemporal dementia (bvFTD)—the patient's unawareness of deficit is itself pathognomic of the disease, posing the problem of dramatic changes for the carer and family but to which the patient appears indifferent. The neuropsychological assessment can therefore also be helpful in guiding the patient's and/or the patient's family's understanding of the deficits, the development of strategies to assist in management of deficits where possible, and the basis of supportive psychotherapy towards adaptation and adjustment to very changed relationship dynamics.

References

1. Hodges JR, Patterson K, Oxbury S, et al. Semantic dementia. Progressive fluent aphasia with temporal lobe atrophy. *Brain*. 1992;115:1783–806.
2. Neary D, Snowden JS, Northen B, et al. Dementia of frontal lobe type. *J Neurol Neurosur Ps*. 1988;51:353–61.
3. Snowden JS, Thompson JC, Stopford CL, et al. The clinical diagnosis of early-onset dementias: diagnostic accuracy and clinicopathological relationships. *Brain*. 2011;134:2478–92.
4. Buschke H. Cued recall in Amnesia. *J Clin Exp Neuropsyc*. 1984;6(4):433–40.
5. Grober E and Buschke H. Genuine memory deficits in dementia. *Dev Neuropsychol*. 1987;3:13–36.
6. Warrington EK. *Recognition Memory Test*. Windsor: NFER-Nelson Publishing Co Ltd, 1984.
7. Saxton J, McGonigle KL, Swihart AA, et al. *The Severe Impairment Battery*. Suffolk: Thames Valley Test Company, 1993.
8. Rosen WG, Mohs RC, and Davis KL. A new rating scale for Alzheimer's disease. *Am J Psychiatry*. 1984 Nov;141(11):1356–64.
9. Wechsler D. *Wechsler Memory Scale—Revised*. New York, NY: Harcourt Brace Jovanovich, 1987.
10. Wechsler D. *The Wechsler Adult Intelligence Scale—Revised*. New York, NY: Harcourt Brace Jovanovich, 1981.
11. Folstein MF, Folstein SE, and McHugh PR. Mini-mental state. A practical method for grading the cognitive state of patients for the clinician. *J Psychiat Res*. 1975;12(3):189–98.
12. Bird CM, Papadopoulou K, Ricciardelli P, et al. Test-retest reliability, practice effects and reliable change indices for the recognition memory test. *Br J Clin Psychol*. 2003 Nov;42(Pt 4):407–25.
13. Baxter DM and Warrington EK. Measuring dysgraphia: A graded-difficulty spelling test. *Behav Neurol*. 1994;7(3–4):107–16.
14. Nelson HE. *The National Adult Reading Test*. Windsor: NFER-Nelson Publishing Co. 1991.
15. Lezak MD, Howieson DB, and Loring DW. *Neuropsychological Assessment*, 4th edn. New York, NY: Oxford University Press, 2004.
16. Wechsler D. *Wechsler Adult Intelligence Scale*, 4th edn. San Antonio, TX: Pearson, 2008.
17. Wechsler D. *Wechsler Abbreviated Scale of Intelligence*, 2nd edn (WASI-II). San Antonio, TX: NCS Pearson, 2011.
18. Coughlan AK, Oddy M, and Crawford JR. *The BIRT Memory and Information Processing Battery (BMIPB)*. West Sussex: BIRT, 2009.
19. Baddeley A, Emslie H, and Nimmo-Smith I. *Doors and People Test: A test of visual and verbal recall and recognition*. Bury St Edmunds: Thames Valley Test Company, 1994.
20. Welsh KA, Butters N, Hughes JP, et al. Detection and Staging of Dementia in Alzheimer's Disease: Use of the Neuropsychological Measures Developed for the Consortium to Establish a Registry for Alzheimer's Disease. *Arch Neurol*. 1992;49(5):448–52.
21. Wechsler, D. *Wechsler Memory Scale*, 3rd edn. San Antonio, TX: The Psychological Corporation, 1997.
22. Rohrer JD, Knight WD, Warren JE, et al. Word-finding difficulty: a clinical analysis of the progressive aphasias. *Brain*. 2008 Jan;131(Pt 1):8–38.
23. McKenna P and Warrington EK. *Graded Naming Test*. Windsor: NFER-Nelson Publishing Co. 1983.
24. Lambon Ralph MA, Patterson K, and Hodges JR. The relationship between naming and semantic knowkedge for different categories in dementia of Alzheimer's type. *Neuropsychologia*. 1997;35(9):1251–60.
25. Dell GS, Schwartz, MF, Martin, N, et al. Lexical access in aphasic and nonaphasic speakers. *Psychol Rev*. 1997;104(4):801–38.
26. Baldo JV, Schwartz S, Wilkins D, et al. Role of frontal versus temporal cortex in verbal fluency as revealed by voxel-based lesion symptom mapping. *J Int Neuropsych Soc*. 2006;12: 896–900.
27. Benson DF, Davis RJ, and Snyder BD. Posterior Cortical Atrophy. *Arch Neurol*. 1988;45(7):789–93.
28. Crutch SJ. Seeing why they cannot see: Understanding the syndrome and causes of posterior cortical atrophy. *J Neuropsychol*. 2013. doi:10.1111/jnp.12011.
29. Warrington EK and James M. *Visual Object and Space Perception Battery*. Bury St Edmunds: Thames Valley Test Company, 1991.
30. Goldenberg G. Imitating gestures and manipulating a mannikin—The representation of the human body in ideomotor apraxia. *Neuropsychologia*. 1995;33(1):63–72.
31. Reitan RM. Validity of the Trail Making test as an indicator of organic brain damage. *Percept. Mot Skills*. 1958;8:271–76.
32. Nelson H. A modified card sorting test sensitive to frontal lobe defects. *Cortex*. 1976;12:313–24.
33. Delis DC, Kaplan E, and Kramer JH. *Delis-Kaplan Executive Function System (D-KEFS)*. San Antonio, TX: The Psychological Corporation, 2001.
34. Burgess P and Shallice T. The Hayling and Brixton Tests. Test manual. Bury St Edmunds, UK: Thames Valley Test Company, 1997.
35. McDonald S, Flanagan S, Rollins J, et al. TASIT: A New Clinical Tool for Assessing Social Perception after traumatic brain injury Journal of Head Trauma Rehabilitation. 2003;18:219–38.

36. Baron-Cohen S, Wheelwright S, Hill J, *et al.* The 'Reading the Mind in the Eyes' Test revised version: a study with normal adults, and adults with Asperger syndrome or high-functioning autism. *J Child Psychol Psychiatry.* 2001 Feb;42(2):241–51.

37. Beck AT, Steer RA, and Brown GK. *Manual for the Beck Depression Inventory–II.* San Antonio, TX: Psychological Corporation, 1996.

38. Sheikh JI and Yesavage JA. *Geriatric Depression Scale (GDS): Recent Evidence and Development of a Shorter Version. Clinical Gerontology: A Guide to Assessment and Intervention.* New York, NY: The Haworth Press, 1986.

39. Alexopolous GS, Abrams RC, Young RC, *et al.* Cornell Scale for Depression in Dementia. Biological Psychiatry. 1998;23:271–84.

CHAPTER 12

Acquired disorders of language and speech

Dalia Abou Zeki and Argye E. Hillis

Introduction

Although the words 'speech' and 'language' are often used interchangeably, each of these systems has a distinct function, relies on a distinct set of representations and processes, and engages a distinct neural network.

Language is a non-instinctive, culturally driven system of voluntarily produced symbols, comprising receptive and expressive abilities allowing comprehension and communication of information respectively. Understanding and processing sound, word, phrase, sentence, and conversation involves retrieving vocabulary, concepts, grammar, and, on a higher scale, processing abstract inferences, idioms, or verbal problem-solving. There are five linguistic domains that comprise language (see Box 12.1).

Speech consists of the highly coordinated rapid motor function responsible for the actual act of vocal expression of language. Regulation of speech occurs via basal ganglia, cerebellum, and cortical systems, with the corticobulbar tracts via the nuclei of the vagal, hypoglossal, facial and phrenic nerves maintaining control and coordination of the muscles involved in speaking. Those include laryngeal, pharyngeal, palatal, lingual, oral, and respiratory muscles. Typically, the utterance of 2 words per second by a normal speaker is equivalent to 14 linguistically distinct sounds (phonemes), each one requiring the contraction or relaxation of 100 muscles.[1] Speech entails the combination of phonation (voicing), resonance (nasality), and articulation. It is also often characterized by fluency and prosody (Box 12.2).

Box 12.1 Linguists refer to five domains that comprise the language system

1. **Phonology:** the sound system and linguistic rules of sound combinations, pronunciation, and perception.

2. **Morphology:** the linguistic rules of word structure and construction.

3. **Semantics:** the systematic meaning of words reflecting content and utterance intent.

4. **Syntax:** the linguistic rules of sentence-element relationship or grammar.

5. **Pragmatics:** the rules for maintaining a conversation in terms of responsiveness, relevance, and so on.

Box 12.2 Speech consists of the following overlaid functions

1. **Phonation:** production of vocal sounds in relation to the length and mass of the membranous parts of the vocal cords. The duration of opening or closing of the vocal folds to produce a voiced versus voiceless consonant is often briefer than 20 msec.[2] Intratracheal pressure must be held long enough so that the 'ballistic opening gesture' produces the desired consonant.[3]

2. **Articulation:** interruption of vocal sounds by pharyngeal, palatal, lingual, and oral muscle contractions. Phonemes, or speech sounds, like [m], [b], and [p] are labial; [l] and [t] are lingual. While consonants are produced by this mechanism, vowels are solely laryngeal in origin.

3. **Fluency:** speech fluency (unlike language fluency) often refers to the ability to speak effortlessly, and smoothly, without forward flow interruption. In some cases it refers to rate of speech. On average, a normal speaker utters 120 words per minute during a conversation; that is, 2 words per second.

4. **Variations in pitch, loudness, and duration of syllables in speech:** these can be used to convey meaning (e.g. sarcasm versus factual content), affect (angry versus happy feeling), or even whether an utterance is a statement or a question (e.g. you are coming?).

Language localization

The outward production of language is a reflection of neural activation in vast network of brain structures and regions in the cortex, basal ganglia, cerebellum, and brainstem. There is clinical and imaging evidence of overlap in that network or with other networks of specialization that is responsible for the wide symptom spectrum following an acquired lesion. One lesion in an area can result in multiple deficits; lesions from multiple different sites can produce similar deficits; and multiple lesions in elements of the same network can severely impact function.[4] One of the most surprising findings from functional neuroimaging studies is that the 'language network' is remarkably similar across language tasks and across individuals (Fig. 12.1).

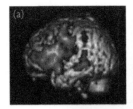
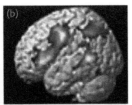
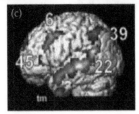

Fig. 12.1 The 'language network'—areas that are activated across a variety of language tasks across most healthy individuals. These areas include posterior inferior frontal cortex (Brodmann's area (BA) 44 and 45), a more dorsal posterior frontal area in BA 6, posterior middle/superior temporal cortex (in BA 22 and often BA 20/21), angular gyrus (BA 39), and posterior inferior temporal cortex (in BA 37). Panel (a) Areas activated during word generation.[131] Panel (b) Areas of activation throughout picture naming.[132] Panel (c) Areas of activation during passive watching and listening to video with language.

Yet, lesions to different nodes in the language tasks produce very different language impairments that are fairly predictable immediately after the lesion. However, the degree to which language will recover a year or more later is not predictable. Despite huge lesions that cover all of the 'language network', some individuals are able to recover language a year or so after stroke. These results allow two conclusions: (1) many areas that are recruited across all language tasks are not equally necessary for those tasks, and (2) it seems likely that there are no areas of the brain that are truly necessary for recovery of language at one year.

Certain manipulations in task paradigms allow functional magnetic resonance imaging (fMRI) or positron emission tomography (PET) to reveal areas more important for some language tasks than others. Lesion studies allow one to test what areas are normally 'necessary' for a task; that is, one assumes that when function on a task is impaired only when a particular area is damaged, that area is necessary for the task. However, lesion studies depend on identifying a sufficient number of people with lesions in all of the possible locations to test the hypotheses (or creating temporary lesions with transcranial magnetic stimulation, for example). Using a combination of these methods, some organization of the language network has been revealed. For example, ventral and dorsal language pathways have been proposed by some authors.[5,6] It has been suggested that the ventral temporal pathway might be critical for mapping sound to lexical representations and meanings of words, while the dorsal frontoparietal pathway has been proposed to be critical for syntactic and articulatory processes.

Using a variety of techniques, it has been established that core language functions are left-lateralized in the majority of both right-and left-handers (95 per cent and 75 per cent, respectively).[7] Only humans have this hemispheric specialization, most likely because of our reliance on language. While nearly all animal species communicate in some form, language is what sets us apart as a species. However, some aspects of language, such as conceptual semantics, may be broadly and even bilaterally distributed.

Disorders of language

Aphasia (in Greek ἀφασία, i.e. speechlessness) encompasses difficulty producing and/or understanding spoken language. Impairments in reading (alexia) and writing (agraphia) are often associated with aphasia. Much of our understanding of aphasia has come from the study of vascular cases, although the principles arising from such cases have often profitably been applied to other causes, including neurodegenerative disorders which are dealt with in detail elsewhere (see chapter 34).

Vascular aphasia syndromes have not typically corresponded to linguistic domains because lesions typically involve vascular territories, rather than being restricted to the 'dorsal frontoparietal language network' or the 'ventral temporal' language network, for example. The vascular syndromes refer to a collection of frequently co-occurring symptoms that are observed together because they represent functions that depend on tissue supplied by the same cerebral vessel (which can be occluded and cause a stroke), therefore each vascular aphasia syndrome is also associated with other neurological deficits (e.g. Broca's aphasia with right arm spastic monoplegia or right spastic hemiplegia).

Terminology for the vascular syndromes may vary. Broca's aphasia, for example, is also referred to as 'anterior', 'motor', or 'non-fluent' aphasia. Wernicke's aphasia, on the other hand, is sometimes termed, 'posterior', 'sensory', or 'fluent' aphasia. The classic Broca–Wernicke–Lichtheim–Geschwind model was the result of the efforts of Broca, Wernicke, and Lichtheim in the nineteenth century, with later modification by Geschwind in 1967. Broca proposed that part of the second or third convolutions of the left inferior frontal gyrus has a role in speech production, or what he, and Bouillaud before him, called the faculty of spoken language.[8,9] Wernicke observed that lesions in the posterior aspect of the superior temporal gyrus resulted in impaired comprehension and fluent but gibberish speech. He suggested this posterior superior temporal gyrus has a role in speech perception through its connections with other language areas.[10] Lichtheim synthesized the previous claims, adding an interfacing conceptual area.[11] Comprehension, language fluency (based on grammaticality, effortful articulation, prosody, and melody), repetition, naming, reading, and writing are the language domains that characterize the vascular aphasia syndromes described in the next section.

Vascular aphasia syndromes

Broca's aphasia

Broca's aphasia occurs after a lesion or dysfunction in the posterior inferior frontal cortex, the distribution of the superior division of the left middle cerebral artery, now known as Broca's area (see below). It is defined as arduous, non-fluent, telegraphic speech output, interrupted by word-finding pauses. Both speech and writing are characterized by agrammatic sentences, revealed by substitution and omission of function words (e.g. the, an) such as prepositions, inflexions, and auxiliary verbs. Three characteristics constitute the hallmark of this syndrome: (1) agrammatism, (2) verbal apraxia, and (3) preserved comprehension. Apraxia of speech is a disturbance in motor programming of speech articulation. Patients are aware of their problem and struggle to try and correct their misarticulation by trial-and-error, repetitively yet uneventfully. Groping articulatory movements are often produced instead.

It has long been recognized that infarction solely affecting Broca's area causes a brief deficit in motor speech ('apraxia of speech') that recovers very quickly.[12] Even lesions involving Broca's area and its immediate surrounding areas deep into the brain, cause mutism that is replaced by a rapidly improving dyspraxic and effortful articulation, but no significant disturbance in language function persists.[13] Lesions in this area typically cause deficits in action naming that are more severe than deficits in object naming. Infarctions that involve other structures beyond Broca's area in this vascular territory can cause the full-blown clinical syndrome of Broca's aphasia. The structures most commonly associated with this presentation are the rolandic operculum, capsulostriatal and periventricular areas. When the entire territory is involved there may be a persistence of some symptoms.

Transcortical motor aphasia

Transcortical motor aphasia, also known as adynamic or extrasylvian motor aphasia, occurs following an injury to a 'watershed area' between the left middle cerebral artery (MCA) and the left anterior cerebral artery (ACA), in the mesial frontal lobe, also referred to as the supplementary motor area (SMA),[14-16] This syndrome is characterized by poor spontaneous speech, with relatively good repetition and comprehension.

Wernicke's aphasia

Ten years after Paul Broca's description of the effect of motor area lesion on the proper speech output, Karl Wernicke proposed that the left superior posterior temporal lobe is an area critical for language comprehension and processing. More recently, it has been recognized that other areas are critical for language comprehension as well. Nevertheless, lesions in the inferior division of the left MCA, which supplies the posterior part of the temporal lobe and inferior parietal lobule, cause impairments in word meaning without disrupting fluency of speech articulation, resulting in meaningless jargon in both spontaneous speech and repetition, now termed Wernicke's aphasia. This syndrome consists of comprehension and repetition impairments, anomia, semantic paraphasias (semantically related word substitutions) and phonemic paraphasias (phonologically related word or nonword substitutions), and neologisms (jargon words). Alexia and agraphia are noted. These individuals, in contrast to those with Broca's aphasia, have poor insight regarding their deficits and seem unconcerned. Box 12.3 provides a case example of an individual with Wernicke's aphasia at onset of stroke.

Lastly and interestingly, cases of crossed Wernicke's aphasia in right-handed patients following lesions in the homologous area in the right hemisphere are reported.[17]

Transcortical sensory aphasia

This aphasia type is characterized by fluent, circumlocutory speech with semantic jargon and poor comprehension. The key feature that distinguishes it from Wernicke's aphasia is preserved repetition. It has been proposed that relatively spared repetition is due to preserved integrity of arcuate fasciculus,[16] but there is little direct evidence for this proposal. Others have proposed a right hemisphere contribution in language repetition given that transcortical sensory aphasia can occur post massive infarction involving the perisylvian

area.[18,19] Transcortical sensory aphasia is typically caused by posterior lesions involving the anterolateral thalamus, temporoparieto-occipital junction (watershed territory between the MCA and the posterior cerebral artery (PCA) territories), or second and third temporal gyri.[20] Semantic variant PPA, Alzheimer's disease, and Creutzfeldt–Jakob disease can cause a similar syndrome.

Transcortical mixed aphasia

Also known as isolation aphasia (or 'isolation of the speech area'), it combines features of both transcortical sensory and motor aphasia. Repetition is preserved but there is reduced spontaneous speech, echolalia, and palilalia, or even mutism, along with impaired comprehension, reading, and writing.[21-24]

Transcortical mixed aphasia, the term first coined by Goldstein,[14] follows lesions isolating the perisylvian language areas, thus the name 'syndrome of isolation of the speech area'.[25] Infarctions typically include the watershed territory between the left ACA and MCA in addition to the watershed territory between the left MCA and PCA. Lesions in the left thalamus, putamen, and periventricular white matter, and thalamo-mesancephalic infarcts have also been described.[24,26]

Prognosis is generally poor with persisting non-fluency and unrecovered comprehension.

Conduction aphasia

Three major characteristics comprise the vascular syndrome of conduction aphasia: a relatively fluent, though phonologically paraphasic speech; poor repetition, first described by Lichtheim;[11] and relatively spared comprehension.[14,27-32] Repetitive self-corrections, word-finding difficulties, and paraphrasing are attempts to approximate target phonemes, termed 'conduit d'approche'.

In 1874, Wernicke indicated that the symptoms in one of his patients might possibly be due to the disconnection between the superior temporal and the inferior frontal gyri.[10] This theory was later elaborated by Geschwind in 1968, giving rise to what is called the Wernicke–Geschwind model of aphasia.[25] He considered that

---

Box 12.3 A case of Wernicke's aphasia

Mr T awoke from cardiac surgery and seemed 'confused'. He was unable to follow even simple directions. His speech was fluent and well-articulated, but consisted only of jargon. When asked to state the month, he said, 'I haven't seen her (frip) (freep) around here, I know that.' He was not able to name any objects orally or in writing correctly although he gestured correctly their use. He called many of them 'another flap thing or something'. He was guessing on both spoken and written word/picture-matching tasks. His repetition was similar to his spontaneous speech: fluent, well-articulated English jargon, with occasional neologisms. MRI of the brain showed severe hypoperfusion of the left temporal cortex, including Wernicke's area. He was not a candidate for thrombolytics due to his recent surgery but underwent investigational therapy to increase perfusion. Repeat MRI on day 3 showed that he had a reperfused left temporal cortex (either a result of the intervention or due to spontaneous recanalization; Fig. 12.2). Repeat language testing on day 3 showed resolution of his language impairment, with good comprehension, repetition, naming, and spontaneous speech.

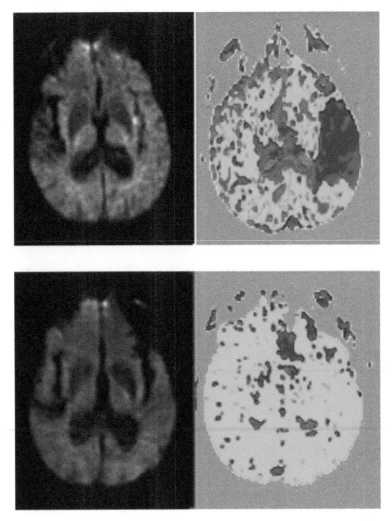

Fig. 12.2 Scans of individual with Wernicke's aphasia at day 1, which resolved by day 3. Top panel: Diffusion-weighted image (left) showing small acute infarct in left insula and perfusion-weighted image (right) at day 1, showing hypoperfusion of left temporal cortex, including Wernicke's area. Lower panel: Diffusion-weighted image (left) and perfusion-weighted image (right) at day 3, showing reperfusion of left temporal cortex.

lesions to the arcuate fasciculus, a large bundle of fibres connecting the frontal and posterior temporal cortex (and angular gyrus), caused the repetition impairments in this so-called disconnection syndrome.[33–35] However, most recent aphasiologists have ascribed the repetition impairment to limited working memory, and have found the associated lesions to be in areas critical for working memory: inferior parietal lobule (supramarginal and angular gyri), inferior frontal cortex, posterior temporal lobe, and/or their white matter connections. Box 12.4 describes a case of an individual with conduction aphasia.

On language testing, Mrs M's speech was well-articulated but she made some phonological errors that were self-corrected, and she had hesitations. Sentences were short and had simple syntax. She was accurate in following simple commands, but made errors on three-step commands. She understood simple, active sentences, but guessed at comprehension of passive sentences. Repetition of monosyllabic and bisyllabic words was accurate, but repetition of polysyllabic words and of sentences was completely incorrect. She often paraphrased the sentence rather than repeating it. (e.g. 'It's a sunny day in Baltimore' was repeated as 'it's nice out'.). Her forward digit span was three; her backward digit span was two. Her naming

---

Box 12.4 Case study of conduction aphasia

Mrs M is a 72-year-old woman who noted sudden difficulty in conversing on the telephone. Her friend mentioned the title of book they were going to read for book club, and she was unable to repeat it correctly or write down the name of the book. She reports that she was 'stuttering' and having trouble finding words. She looked up the phone number of her physician and could read it, but was not able to retain it long enough to correctly dial the number. She decided to wait until her husband got home from work. When he arrived four hours later her speech was unchanged so he called an ambulance. On arrival to the hospital, she was found to be in atrial fibrillation. An MRI showed an acute infarct (and comparable perfusion defect) in the left parietal cortex, including supramarginal gyrus, thought to be embolic (Fig. 12.3).

---

was mildly impaired. She had difficulty spelling and reading unfamiliar words (pseudowords) but correctly read and spelled words. She had language therapy five days per week for three weeks, and her language deficits resolved.

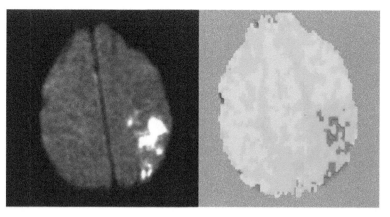

Fig. 12.3 Diffusion-weighted image (left) and perfusion-weighted image (right) at day 1 of individual with acute conduction aphasia.

Global aphasia

Destruction of anterior and posterior language areas causes reduction of all faculties of language, including comprehension and speech output.[27] Even though the most common cause behind this debilitating language disorder is a large left hemisphere ischaemic stroke due to carotid artery or middle cerebral artery stenosis or occlusion, cases following smaller haemorrhagic strokes are reported.[36] Global aphasia can be the initial presentation in a patient who later recovers into Broca's aphasia or transcortical motor aphasia. In this case, there is generally evidence of spared Wernicke's area.[37] Early comprehension recovery may result from reperfusion of Wernicke's area,[38] while later recovery of comprehension may result from reorganization of the language network such that another area of the brain assumes of the function of the damaged area.[39] Broca's and Wernicke's area may thus be hypoperfused in the acute period, such that the area is dysfunctional, causing global aphasia. When the area becomes reperfused through development of collateral blood flow or through treatment, the individual may show the vascular syndrome corresponding to the infarct rather than the initial vascular syndrome corresponding to the hypoperfused tissue (see Fig. 12.4).

Subcortical aphasia

Subcortical lesions have been reported to cause language deficits, ranging from anomia to global aphasia.[40–46] Fluctuating jargon aphasia with impaired fluency is often observed in patients with thalamic lesions.[47]

Two distinct mechanisms can account for subcortical aphasia. One is that plaques in the middle cerebral artery cut off blood supply to the lenticulostriate arteries, causing infarcts in the basal ganglia and subcortical white matter, but also cause hypoperfusion of the cortex, causing a variety of aphasia syndromes.[48] Aphasia due to cortical hypoperfusion has been demonstrated with single photon emission computed tomography (SPECT),[49] positron emission tomography (PET),[45,50,51] and perfusion-weighted imaging.[48,52] Improvement in cortical perfusion and metabolism corresponds to recovery of aphasia.[48,52–57] It has been also shown that recanalization of an occluded M1 branch of MCA in subjects with aphasia and a striatocapsular infarct can reverse the aphasic syndrome.[45]

Diaschisis, distant cortical hypometabolism caused by reduced input from the infarcted area, can account for aphasia due to thalamic lesions[54,58] and perhaps aphasia due to other subcortical lesions.[59–61]

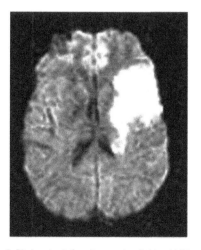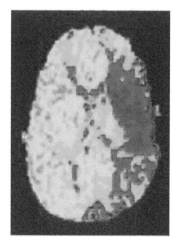

Fig. 12.4 Diffusion-weighted image (left) showing infarct in superior division MCA territory that included Broca's area, and perfusion-weighted image (right) showing larger area of hypoperfusion that included Wernicke's area in a patient who had global aphasia acutely. When he showed reperfusion of Wernicke's area, his comprehension improved, thus he had a Broca's aphasia.

Alexia and agraphia

Alexia is defined as the loss of reading ability following a brain insult while agraphia is impairment in writing ability following brain damage. Both these syndromes are discussed in more detail in the chapter concerning alexia and agraphia but are briefly considered here for sake of completeness within the framework of language disorders (chapter 18).

Pure alexia is at times referred to as visual alexia or word blindness, given that reading activates the left lateral occipitotemporal sulcus, mainly the so-called visual word form area (VWFA) area.[62] This area is reliably activated in reading tasks, but is also activated in spelling and other lexical tasks (see reference 63 for review of this controversial issue). Spelling dyslexia or surface dyslexia refers to a patient who tries to spell or sound each word and guess its meaning from the way it sounds. This presentation follows occipitotemporal damage.[64]

A neural model for reading and writing was first suggested by Dejerine in 1892[65] and supported in 1965 by Geschwind.[66] This model distinguishes between alexia without agraphia following occipital lobe lesions involving the splenium and its radiations, and alexia with the agraphia following a lesion to the angular gyrus. In the latter, other parietal signs are common on presentation (e.g. apraxia, anomia, and Gertsmann syndrome). Although Geschwind hypothesized that the angular gyrus is crucial for differentiating letters, Japanese researchers have argued that the neural circuit for this faculty is far more complicated. Ideographic (Kanji) and syllabic (Kana) reading and writing can be affected by various lesion areas, offering an additional emphasis on this extensive processing neuronal network. The latter was then specified as dual process, considering the angular gyrus as a the node for letter phonological processing and the posterior inferior temporal area as a node for letter semantic processing.[67]

Although ischaemia in the territory of the posterior cerebral artery is the most reported aetiology behind this reading impairment, compression to this artery by tentorial herniation or tumours is also reported.[68,69] Transitory alexia without agraphia was reported in an HIV-positive patient with toxoplasma encephalitis and another with neurocycticercosis.[70,71]

In agraphia, spelling can normally be accomplished via a direct lexical method of recalling a word's spelling or via a sublexical phonological method of sounding out its phonemes (speech sounds) and transforming them to graphemes (abstract letter identities). Retrieval of the learned spelling is likely to be important for the spelling of most familiar words and is critical for spelling irregular familiar words; while the computing plausible spellings of unfamiliar words (like proper names) and spelling of regular words may depend almost entirely on the sublexical phonological method of spelling. Either of these spelling mechanisms can be disrupted independently, indicating that the neural networks that support these cognitive processes are distinct.[72]

A common spelling impairment after stroke is a deficit in holding the string of graphemes in working memory ('the graphemic buffer') while the word is spelled. This spelling impairment equally affects regular and irregular words, and familiar and unfamiliar words, but affects longer words more than short words. It results in deletions, insertions, transpositions, and substitutions of graphemes.[73] Agraphia can be part of an aphasia syndrome, thus termed aphasic 'agraphia' where spelling and grammatical errors are defining features. Pure agraphia has also been reported.[63]

'Constructional agraphia' has been described, with disturbances in the perception of spatial relations resulting in wrongly arranged words or letters, either haphazardly, or diagonally, or superimposed. A right-to-left arrangement is also noted where only the right side of the page is used. In this case, researchers relate the writing disorder to left hemispatial neglect, affecting responsiveness to stimuli and space on the left side of the viewer. Right hemispatial neglect can also occur but tends to affect the right sides (final letters) of individual words, irrespective of the location with respect to the viewer. 'Apraxic agraphia' is reported after frontal and parietal lesions, due to impaired motor planning required to form the proper shapes of letters and words.

Pure word deafness

Pure word deafness refers to an inability to recognize spoken words in the absence of a peripheral deficit in auditory acuity or more general auditory discrimination impairment. In his 1884 memoir, Lichtheim mentioned the patient who produced no paraphasias or paragraphias and had no dyslexia, but had a repetition impairment and difficulty communicating using any means other than writing. When asked to write to dictation, though, the patient complained of an inability to hear. Pure word deafness, also known as 'auditory verbal agnosia', can occur after lesions in the left superior temporal gyrus and the superior temporal sulcus, both anterior. Bilateral temporal lesions can cause pure word deafness or a more general auditory discrimination deficit referred to as cortical deafness.[74]

Causes of aphasia

Any acute or transient insult or progressive pathologic process that affects the language network can cause aphasia. The most common lesion is ischaemic stroke,[75] and only ischaemic stroke typically causes the vascular syndromes described above. Haemorrhagic stroke, central nervous system infections,[76,77] tumours, and traumatic brain injury[78] are known aetiologies. Neurodegenerative diseases[79] and demyelinating diseases are reported also.[80,81] Transient ischaemic attacks, complicated migraines, and seizures cause transient aphasia. Primary progressive aphasia refers to three syndromes: the non-fluent, agrammatic variant is most commonly caused by a tauopathy such as frontotemporal degeneration-tau (FTLD-t), progressive supranuclear palsy, or corticobasal degeneration; the semantic variant is usually caused by frontotemporal degeneration-ubiquitin (FTLD-u); the logopenic variant is most commonly caused by Alzheimer's disease pathology.[82] Primary progressive aphasia is considered in detail in chapter 34.

Disorders of speech

Speech output is a highly organized task that requires coordination of respiratory musculature, larynx, pharynx, palate, tongue, and lips, via control by extrapyramidal structures, cerebellum, basal ganglia, and the corticobulbar tracts. Motor speech disorders are the result of an insult at any level of this system or multiple levels. Muscle weakness, paralysis, spasticity, and poor coordination are all reported findings.[83] A way to categorize this type of movement disorder is into the phenotypical presentation, as various dysarthrias or apraxia of speech.

The dysarthrias

Darley and colleagues classified the dysarthrias based on their effects on rate, range, tone, and timing of movement into the following categories: flaccid, spastic, mixed spastic and flaccid, ataxic, hypokinetic, hyperkinetic, and unilateral upper motor neuron dysarthrias.[83,84]

It was reported by the European Brain Council that about 20–30 per cent of people who have a stroke experience muscular disturbances impairing speech output.[85] More than 100 muscles are responsible for a proper articulation and phonation, important for the strength, speed, range, accuracy, steadiness, and tone of the speech.[86] In clinical practice, assessment of speech should be based on objective criteria about auditory–perceptual characteristics, repetition rate, oral mechanisms, and intelligibility testing. The last can be examined using the Assessment of Intelligibility in Dysarthric Speakers, for example.[87]

Flaccid dysarthria

Any impairment at the level of the cranial or spinal nerves innervating any of the muscles assisting speech output results in weakness of the corresponding muscles affecting several aspects of speech.[84] Lesions involving the motor nuclei in the medulla and lower pons can cause this disorder. Disorders of the neuromuscular junction can also cause flaccid dysarthria.

Because the insult involves a final common pathway, sole affected muscles can be observed. Although the presentation depends on the nerves affected, common features may be observed like hypernasality due to reduced velar movement and subsequent nasal emission.[86] Audible inspiration and hypophonia due to paralysis of unilateral or bilateral vocal folds in abducted position follows involvement of the vagal nerve. Pronunciation of lingual sounds becomes difficult following insults to the hypoglossal nerve.

Wallenberg's lateral medullary syndrome is the most common aetiology and occurs with a constellation of neurological symptoms (dizziness, nystagmus, crossed sensory loss, etc.), in addition to flaccid dysarthria.

Besides vascular causes, dysarthria has been described in muscular disorders, such as adult-onset myotonic dystrophy. Slowing down of relaxation of the muscles of the facial, jaw, and neck musculature after rest or activity are responsible for the dysarthria that is characterized by monotony, hypernasality, hoarseness, shorter stretches of speech, slow speech rate, and reduced intelligibility.[88] Warming-up phenomenon can be used for improving speech output.[89] Myasthenia gravis is the most common cause of flaccid dysarthria at the level of the neuromuscular junction. A bilateral insult to the vagal nerve, usually infectious in origin, can cause a nasal speech due to bilateral palatal paralysis. Bilateral insults to cranial nerve VII as seen in Guillain–Barre syndrome, Lyme disease, or sarcoidosis cause problems with consonant output, such as 'p' and 'b'.

Ataxic dysarthria

Ataxic dysarthria follows an insult to cerebellar structures, mainly the superior cerebellar peduncle or brachium conjunctivum.[90] Loss of motor organization and coordination of speech-responsible muscles is the key feature. The classic presentation is a 'drunken quality' of speech. The characteristic scanning speech is slurred, monotonous, with poor pitch control, and with unnatural separation of the syllables of words. Tremor of the laryngeal and respiratory muscles is common.[91] Breath may seem not enough for completing the utterance; a pause followed by explosive output is common. Intermittent hypo- and hypernasality is observed, suggesting an improper timing of the velar and articulatory gestures for consonants.[92] However, there is also abnormal variability in duration and intensity of vowel prolongation.

Common aetiologies of ataxic dysarthria include multiple sclerosis, spinocerebellar ataxia syndromes, paraneoplastic cerebellar degeneration, as well as stroke or tumour in the cerebellum.

Unilateral upper motor neuron dysarthria

There are several neurological disorders of speech that are due, in part, to unilateral damage to the pyramidal tracts.[93–95] Speech is mildly imprecise; phonation is harsh and low-pitched. This speech disturbance follows an insult to the upper motor neuron(s) that transmits the signal via cranial or spinal nerves to the articulation muscles.

Darley[86] and Melo[96] described this entity as impairment in articulation precision with 'incomplete pronunciation'. Added to this, Ropper[97] reported slowed speaking rates and monotonous voice as common features.

Pure dysarthria is generally observed with face and tongue weakness and is the result of 1 per cent of lacunar strokes involving the corona radiate or the internal capsule.[98,99] Genu of the internal capsule or hemispheric strokes that include the mouth area of the motor strip in the precentral gyrus are the most common lesion sites causing this type of dysarthria.

Spastic dysarthria

Damage to bilateral corticobulbar tracts by vascular, demyelinating, or motor neuron disease result in pseudobulbar palsy, the symptoms of which include 'spastic' dysarthria and pseudobulbar lability (laughter and crying).[84] Defining features are imprecision, monotony, hypernasality, 'strangled' breathy voice, pitch breaks, excess stress, and slow rate.[83]

Aetiologies include bilateral strokes, midbrain or upper pontine strokes, central pontine myelinolysis, bilateral inflammatory or infectious encephalitis, and progressive supranuclear palsy. Amyotrophic lateral sclerosis causes a mixed upper and lower motor neuron dysarthria, but the spastic component is often prominent.

Apraxia of speech

Apraxia of speech (AOS) is a motor speech disorder that can occur in the absence of aphasia or dysarthria. This disorder of speech has been the subject of continuous debate regarding its characteristics, corresponding anatomical lesions, and mechanism of deficits. It often occurs in the context of Broca's aphasia[84] but can occur in isolation.[100,101] While aphasic patients have a problem selecting the proper phonemes, apraxic individuals have a difficulty in the motor execution of this same phoneme.[102] They tend to have characteristically abnormal prosody[103] but are aware of their deficits, in contrast to the patients with conduction aphasia.[101] In contrast to dysarthria, which results in consistent and predictable errors, apraxia of speech results in inconsistent and non-predictable utterances.[84,86,88]

Briefly, though no single symptom has been solely attributed to AOS, Wertz[103] described five features of the disorder: (1) effortful trial and error with groping, (2) self correction of errors, (3) abnormal rhythm, stress, and intonation, (4) inconsistent articulation errors on repeated speech productions of the same utterance, and (5) difficulty initiating utterances.

Defining AOS in terms of anatomical lesions has been controversial. Broca's area has been found to be associated with AOS in acute and chronic stroke,[20,104] although other chronic lesion studies have found that failure to recover from AOS is associated with lesions in left temporoparital cortex,[101] the anterior superior insula,[105] and the basal ganglia.[84,106,106]

AOS is usually caused by stroke, due to a clot in the superior division of the left middle cerebral artery. However, any lesion that affects the left inferior frontal cortex, such as tumour, abscess, or focal atrophy can cause AOS. AOS is one of the two possible key features (along with agrammatic speech) of non-fluent agrammatic variant of primary progressive aphasia.[82]

Treatment of aphasia

Recovery of language function following vascular impairments has been the subject of extensive controversy. Knowing that this recovery still occurs with the persistence of the lesion,[108] the various factors predicting outcome remain controversial. Though transformation in aphasia types in the acute phase, mainly from non-fluent to fluent, not the opposite, and from severe to a milder form, is noted in 30–60per cent of aphasics,[109] the severity of the initial presentation predicts the final outcome.[110,111] The extent of spontaneous recovery in the first few months has been related to the lesion size and location,[112] age, and premorbid intelligence.[113] Moreover, systems or multivariate databases of combined clinical and functional imaging data have been introduced to provide individual outcome prediction post vascular aphasia.[114,115] It has been reported that all but severely aphasic patients improve by 70 per cent of their maximum potential by 90 days, as long as those who are aphasic receive at least some speech and language therapy.[116] However, controversy still exists concerning the efficacy of specific treatment modalities and the correlation between the intensity of the treatment and outcome.[117]

Nevertheless, there is strong evidence that recovery takes place by a number of different mechanisms, and can be augmented by speech and language therapy, as well as non-invasive brain stimulation techniques, such as transcranial magnetic stimulation (TMS), and transcranial direct current stimulation (tDCS).[118-125]

Pharmacotherapy with stimulants,[126] cholinesterase inhibitors, and dopamine agonists[127] has also been suggested for therapy augmentation. More clinical trials are needed for further proof of efficacy.

Treatment of dysarthria

Management strategies for patients with acquired dysarthria vary according to the severity and type of dysarthria. However, the overall cornerstone of therapy is enhancing orofacial muscle strength and mobility. Intelligibilty improvement with these techniques has been reported in single case or small group studies.[128,129] Post-stroke dysarthria is best managed by targeting respiratory, phonatory, articulatory, and resonatory systems for a more intelligible utterance,[130] Behavioural compensation through reduction of rate of speech,[131] provision of prosthetic devices, example palatal lift, or

training appliance to compensate for hypernasality,[132] and environmental listener training are used modalities. Computerized software to increase single function ability has also been implemented.

References

1. Lenneberg EH. *Biological Foundations of Language*. Oxford: Wiley, 1967.
2. Ludlow CL and Lou G. Observations on human laryngeal muscle control. In: N Fletcher and P Davis (eds). Controlling Complexity and Chaos: 9th vocal fold Physiology Symposium. San Diego, CA: Singular Press, 1996.
3. Borden GJ and Harris KS. *Speech Science Primer: Physiology, Acoustics, and Perception of Speech*, 2nd edn. Baltimore, MD: Williams and Wilkins, 1984.
4. Kertesz A. *The Western Aphasia Battery*. Philadelphia, PA: Gruyne & Stratton, 1982.
5. Poeppel D and Hickok G. Towards a new functional anatomy of language. *Cognition*. 2004 May–Jun;92(1–2):1–12.
6. Saur D, Kreher BW, Schnell S, *et al.* Ventral and dorsal pathways for language. *Proc Natl Acad Sci USA*. 2008 Nov 18; 105(46):18035–40.
7. Knecht S, Dräger B, Deppe M, *et al.* Handedness and hemispheric language dominance in healthy humans. *Brain*. 2000;Dec;123:Pt 12:2512–18.
8. Broca P. Perte de la parole. *Bulletins de la Societé Anthropologique de Paris*. 1861;2:235–8.
9. Bouillaud J. Recherches cliniques propres à démontrer que la perte de la parole correspond à la lésion des lobules antérieures du cerveau. *Archives Générales de Médecine*. 1825;8:25–45.
10. Wernicke C. *Der aphasische symptomen complex*. Breslau: Cohn and Weigert, 1874.
11. Lichtheim L. On aphasia. *Brain*. 1885;7:433–84.
12. Mohr J. Broca's area and Broca's aphasia. In: H Whitaker (ed.). *Studies in Neurolinguistics*, Vol 1. New York, NY: Academic Press, 1976, pp. 201–35.
13. Mohr J, Pessin M, Finkelstein S, *et al.* Broca's aphasia pathologic and clinical. *Neurology*. 1978 Apr;28(4):311–24.
14. Goldstein K. *Language and Language Disturbances: Aphasic Symptom Complexes and their Significance for Medicine and Theory of Language*. New York, NY: Grune & Stratton, 1948.
15. Kornyey E. Aphasie transcorticale et echolalie: Le probleme de l'initiative de la parole. *Cogn. Neuropsychol*. 1975;(3):291–308.
16. Rubens A. Aphasia with infarction in the territory of the anterior cerebral artery. *Cortex*. 1975 Sep;11(3):39–50.
17. Sweet EW, Panis W, and Levine DN. Crossed Wernicke's aphasia. *Neurology*. 1984 Apr;34(4):475–9.
18. Grossi D, Trojano L, and Soricelli A. Mixed transcortical aphasia: clinical features and neuroanatomical correlates. A possible role of the right hemisphere. *Eur Neurol*. 1991;31(4):204–11.
19. Turkeltaub PE, Messing S, Norise C, *et al.* Are networks for residual language function and recovery consistent across aphasic patients? *Neurology*. 2011 May 17;76 (20):1726–34.
20. Alexander M, Hiltbrubber B, and Fischer R. Distributed anatomy of transcortical sensory aphasia. *Arch Neurol*. 1989 Aug;46(8):885–92.
21. Maeshima S, Uematsu Y, and Terada T. Transcortical mixed aphasia with left frontoparietal lesions. *Neuroradiology*. 1996 May;38 Suppl 1:78–9.
22. Nagaratnam N, Grice D, and Kalouche H. Optic ataxia following unilateral stroke. *J Neurol Sci*. 1998 Mar 5;155(2):204–7.
23. Bougousslavsy J, Regli F, and Assal G (1985) Isolation of speech area from focal brain ischemia. *Stroke*. 1985;16(3):441–3.
24. Bogousslavsky J, Regli F, and Assal G. Acute transcortical mixed aphasia, a carotid occlusion syndrome with pial and watershed infarcts. *Brain*. 1988 Jun;111 (3):631–41.
25. Geschwind N, Quadfasel FA, and Sagarra JM. Isolation of the speech area. *Neuropsychologia*. 1968;6(4):327–40.

26. Rapcsak S, Krupp L, Rubens AB, *et al.* Mixed transcortical aphasia without anatomic isolation of the speech area. *Stroke.* 1990 Jun;21(6):953–6.

27. Kertesz A. *Aphasia and Associated Disorders.* New York, NY: Grune & Stratton, 1979.

28. Kertesz A. Aphasia. In: JA Frederiks (ed.). *Handbook of Clinical Neurology, Vol 45: Clinical Neuropsychology.* Amsterdam: Elsevier, 1985, pp. 287–332.

29. Kohn S. *Conduction Aphasia.* Mahwah, NJ: Erlbaum, 1992.

30. Benson D and Ardila A. Conduction aphasia: a syndrome of language network disruption. In: H Kirshner (ed.). *Handbook of Speech and Language Disorders.* 1994. New York, NY: Mercel Dekker, pp. 149–64.

31. Benson D and Ardila A. *Aphasia: A Clinical Perspective.* New York, NY: Oxford University Press, 1996.

32. Bartha L and Benke T. Acute conduction aphasia: an analysis of 20 cases. *Brain Lang.* 2003 Apr;85(1):93–108

33. Tanabe H, Sawada T, and Inoue N. Conduction aphasia and arcuate fasciculus. *Acta Neurol Scand.* 1987 Dec;76(6):422–7.

34. Geldmacher D, Quigg M, and Elias W. MR tractography depicting damage to the arcuate fasciculus in a patient with conduction aphasia. *Neurology.* 2007 Jul 17;69(3):321.

35. Yamada K, Nagakane Y, and Mizuno T. MR tractography depicting damage to the sarcuate fasciculus in a patient with conduction aphasia. *Neurology.* 2007 Mar 6;68(10):789.

36. Kumar R, Masih A, and Pard J. Global aphasia due to thalamic hemorrhage: A case report and review of the literature. *Arch Phys Med Rehabil.* 1996 Dec;77(12):1312–5.

37. Blumenfeld H. *Neuroanatomy through Clinical Cases*, 2nd edn. Sunderland, MA Sinauer Associates, 2010.

38. Hillis AE, Barker P, Beauchamp N, *et al.* Restoring blood pressure reperfused Wernicke's area and improved language, *Neurology.* 2001 Mar 13;56 (5):670–2.

39. Saur D, Lange R, Baumgaertner A, *et al.* Dynamics of language reorganization after stroke. *Brain.* 2006 Jun;129 (Pt 6):1371–84.

40. Damasio A, Damasio H, Rizzo M, *et al.* Aphasia with nonhemorrhagic lesions in the basal ganglia and internal capsule. *Arch Neurol.* 1982 Jan;39(1):15–24.

41. Naeser M, Alexander M, Helm-Estabrooks N, *et al.* Aphasia with predominantly subcortical lesion sites. Description of three capsular/putamenal aphasia syndromes. *Arch Neurol.* 1982 Jan;39(1):2–14.

42. Megens J, van Loon J, Goffin J, *et al.* Subcortical aphasia from a thalamic abscess. *J Neurol Neurosur Ps.* 1992;55:319–21.

43. Ferro JM and Kertesz A. Comparative classification of aphasic disorders. *J Clin Exp Neuropsychol.* 1987 Aug;9(4):365–75.

44. Weiller C, Ringlestein EB, Reiche W, *et al.* The large striatocapsular infarct: A clinical and pathophysiological entity. *Arch Neurol.* 1990 Oct;47(10):1085–91.

45. Weiller C, Willmes K, Reiche W, *et al.* The case of aphasia or neglect after striatocapsular infarction. *Brain.* 1993 Dec;116 (Pt6):1509–25.

46. Mazzocchi F and Vignolo L. Localisation of lesions in aphasia: Clinical-CT scan correlations in stroke patients. *Cortex.* 1979 Dec;15(4):627–53.

47. Mohr J, Walters W, and Duncan G. Thalamic hemorrhage and Aphasia. *Brain Lang.* 1975 Jan;2(1):3–17.

48. Hillis AE, Wityk RJ, Barker PB, *et al.* Subcortical aphasia and neglect in acute stroke: the role of cortical hypoperfusion. *Brain.* 2002 May;125(Pt 5):1094–104.

49. Skyhøj-Olsen T, Bruhn P, and Oberg RG. Cortical hypoperfusion as a possible cause of 'subcortical aphasia'. *Brain.* 1986 Jun;109(Pt3):393–410.

50. Nadeau SE and Crosson B. Subcortical Aphasia. *Brain Lang.* 1997 Jul;58(3):355–402.

51. Démonet J. Subcortical aphasia(s): a controversial and promising topic. *Brain Lang.* 1997 Jul;58(3):410–7.

52. Croquelois A, Wintermark M, Reichhart M, *et al.* Aphasia in hyperacute stroke: language follows brain penumbra dynamics. *Ann Neurol.* 2003 Sep;54(3):321–9.

53. Baron J, D'Antona R, Pantano P, *et al.* Effects of thalamic stroke on energy metabolism in the cerebral cortex. A Positron Tomography study in man. *Brain.* 1986 Dec;109 (Pt 6):1243–59.

54. Vallar G, Perani D, Cappa S, *et al.* Recovery from aphasia and neglect after subcortical stroke: neuropsychological and cerebral perfusion study. *J Neurol Neurosur Ps.* 1988 Oct;51(10):1269–76.

55. Hillis AE, Kane A, Tuffiash E, *et al.* Reperfusion of specific brain regions by raising blood pressure restores selective language functions in subacute stroke. *Brain Lang.* 2001;79(3):495–510.

56. Hillis AE, Ulatowski JA, Barker PB, *et al.* A pilot randomized trial of induced blood pressure elevation: effects on function and focal perfusion in acute and subacute stroke. *Cerebrovasc Dis.* 2003;16(3):236–46.

57. Hillis AE, Wityk RJ, Beauchamp NJ, *et al.* Perfusion-weighted MRI as a marker of response to treatment in acute and subacute stroke. *Neuroradiology.* 2004 Jan;46(1):31–9.

58. Perani D, Vallar G, Cappa S, *et al.* Aphasia and neglect after subcortical stroke. A clinical/cerebral perfusion correlation study. *Brain.* 1987 Oct;110(Pt 5):1211–29.

59. Metter E, Wasterlain C, Kuhl D, *et al.* FDG positron emission computed tomography in a study of aphasia. *Ann Neuro.* 1981 Aug;10(2):173–83.

60. Metter E. Neuroanatomy and physiology of aphasia: evidence from positron emission tomography. *Aphasiology.* 1987;1:3–33.

61. Wallesch C and Papagno C. Subcortical aphasia. In: F Rose, R Whurr, and M Wyke (eds). *Aphasia.* London: Whurr, 1988, pp. 256–87.

62. Dehaene S and Cohen L. The unique role of the visual word form area in reading. *Trends Cogn. Sci.* 2011 Jun;15(6):254–62.

63. Hillis AE. Neural correlates of the cognitive processes underlying reading: Evidence from Magnetic Resonance Perfusion Imaging. In: P Cornelissen, P Hansen, M Kringelbach, and K Pugh (eds). *The Neural Basis of Reading.* Oxford: Oxford University Press, 2010, pp. 264–80.

64. Bub D and Kertesz A. Deep agraphia. *Brain Lang.* 1982 Sep;17(1):146–65.

65. Dejerine J. Contribution a l'etude anatomo-pathologique et clinique des differentes varietes de cecites verbale. *Memoires de la Societe Biologique.* 1892;4:61–90.

66. Geschwind N. Disconnection syndromes in animals and man. *Brain.* 1965;88:237–94.

67. Iwata M. Kanji versus Kana. Neuropsychological correlates of the Japanese writing system. *Trends Neurosci.* 1982;7:290–3.

68. Caplan LR and Hedley-Whyte T. Cuing and memory dysfunction in alexia without agraphia. A case report. *Brain.* 1974 Jun;97(2):251–62.

69. Cohen D, Salanga V, Hully W, *et al* R. Alexia without agraphia. *Neurology.* 1976 May;26(5):455–9.

70. Luscher C and Horber FF. Transitory alexia without agraphia in HIV positive patient suffering from toxoplasma encephalitis: A case report. *Eur Neurol.* 1992;32(1):26.

71. Verma A, Singh N, and Misra S. Transitory alexia without agraphia: A disconnection syndrome due to neurocysticercosis. *Neurol India.* 2004 Sep;52(3):378–9.

72. Purcell JJ, Turkeltaub PE, Eden GF, *et al.* Examining the central and peripheral processes of written word production through meta-analysis. *Front Psychol.* 2011 Oct 11;2:239.

73. Cloutman LL, Newhart M, Davis CL, *et al.* Neuroanatomical correlates of oral reading in acute left hemispheric stroke. *Brain Lang.* 2011 Jan;116(1):14–21.

74. Kertesz A. Aphasia in clinical practice. *Can Fam Physician.* 1983 Jan;29:128–32.

75. Goodglass H. *Understanding Aphasia.* San Diego, CA: Academic Press, 1993.

76. Otero E, Cordova S, Diaz F, *et al.* Acquired epileptic aphasia (the Landau–Kleffner syndrome) due to neurocysticercosis. *Epilepsia.* 1989 Sep-Oct;30(5):569–72.

77. Senda J, Ito M, Atsuta N, *et al.* Paradoxical brain embolism induced by Mycoplasma pneumoniae infection with deep venous thrombus. *Intern Med.* 2010;49(18):2003–5.

78. Reeves RR and Panguluri RL. Neuropsychiatric complications of traumatic brain injury. *J Psychosoc Nurs Ment Health Serv.* 2011 Mar;49(3):42–50.

79. Rohrer J, Rossor M, and Warren J. Alzheimer's pathology in primary progressive aphasia. *Neurobiol Aging.* 2012 Apr;33(4):744–52.

80. Larner AJ and Lecky BR. Acute aphasia in MS revisited. *Int MS J.* 2007 Sep;14(3):76–7.

81. Staff N, Lucchinetti C, and Keegan B. Multiple sclerosis with predominant, severe cognitive impairment. *Arch Neurol.* 2009 Sep;66(9):1139–43.

82. Gorno-Tempini ML, Hillis AE, *et al.* Classification of primary progressive aphasia and its variants. *Neurology.* 2011 Mar 15;76(11):1006–14.

83. Darley F, Aronson A, and Brown J. Differential Diagnostic Patterns of Dysarthria. *J Speech Hear Res.* 1969;12(2):246–69 and 462–96.

84. Duffy J. *Motor Speech Disorders.* St. Louis, MO: Mosby, 1995.

85. Warlow C, Dennis M, and van Gijn J. *Stroke: A Practical Guide to Management*, 2nd edn. Oxford: Blackwell Scientific, 2000.

86. Darley F, Aronson A, and Brown J. *Motor Speech Disorders.* Philadelphia, PA: W.B. Saunders, 1975.

87. Yorkston K, Beukelman D, and Bell K. *Clinical Management of Dysarthric Speakers.* San Diego, CA: College-Hill Press, 1988.

88. de Swart BJ, van Engelen BG, van de Kerkhof JP, *et al* Myotonia and flaccid dysarthria in patients with adult onset myotonic dystrophy. *J Neurol Neurosur Ps.* 2004 Oct;75(10):1480–2.

89. de Swart B, van Engelen B, and Maassen B. Warming up improves speech production in patients with adult onset myotonic dystrophy. *J Commun Disord.* 2007 May–Jun;40(3):185–95.

90. Lechtenberg R and Gilman S. Speech disorders in cerebellar disease. *Ann Neurol.* 1978 Apr;3(4):285–90.

91. Ackermann H and Ziegler W. Articulatory deficits in Parkinsonian dysarthria: An acoustic analysis. *J Neurol Neurosur Ps.* 1991 Dec;54(12):1093–8.

92. Auzou P, Ozsancak C, Jan M, *et al.* Evaluation of motor speech function in the diagnosis of various forms of dysarthria. *Rev Neurol (Paris).* 2000 Jan;156(1):47–52.

93. Darley F, Brown J, and Goldstein N. Dysarthria in multiple sclerosis. *J Speech Hear Res.* 1972 Jun;15(2):229–45.

94. Fisher M. Lacunar strokes and infarcts: A review. *Neurology.* 1982;32;871–76.

95. Hartman DE and Abbs JH. Dysarthrias of movement disorders. *Adv Neurol.* 1988;49:289–306.

96. Melo T, Bocousslavsky J, Melle G, *et al.* Pure motor stroke: A reappraisal. *Neurology.* 1992 Apr;42(4) 789–95.

97. Ropper A. Severe dysarthria with right hemisphere stroke. *Neurology.* 1987 Jun;37(6):1061–3.

98. Ozaki I, Baba M, Narita S, *et al.* Pure dysarthria due to anterior internal capsule and/or corona radiata infarction: a report of five cases. *J Neurol Neurosur Ps.* 1986 Dec;49(12):1435–7.

99. Urban P, Wicht S, Hopf H, *et al* Isolated dysarthria due to extracerebellar lacunar stroke: a central monoparesis of the tongue. *J Neurol Neurosur Ps.* 1999 Apr;66(4):495–501.

100. Square-Storer P, Roy E, and Hogg S. The dissociation of aphasia from apraxia of speech, ideomotor limb and buccofacial apraxia. In: GR Hammond (ed.). *Cerebral Control of Speech and Limb Movements. Advances in Psychology.* Amsterdam: North-Holland, 1990, pp. 451–76.

101. Square P, Roy A, and Martin R. Apraxia of speech: Another form of praxis disruption. In: LJG Rothi and KM Heilman (eds). *Apraxia: The Neuropsychology of Action.* East Sussex: Psychology Press, 1997, pp. 173–206.

102. McNeil M, Pratt S, and Fossett T. The differential diagnosis of apraxia of speech. In: B Maassen. *Speech Motor Control in Normal and Disordered Speech.* New York, NY: Oxford University Press, 2004.

103. Wertz R, LaPointe L, and Rosenbek J. *Apraxia of Speech: The Disorder and its Management.* New York, NY: Grune & Stratton, 1984.

104. Hillis A, Work M, Barker P, *et al.* Re-examining the brain regions crucial for orchestrating speech articulation. *Brain.* 2004 Jul;127(Pt 7):1479–87.

105. Dronkers N. A new brain region for coordinating speech articulation. *Nature.* 1996 Nov 14;384(6605):159–61.

106. Square P, Martin R, Bose A. Nature and treatment of neuromotor speech disorders in aphasia. In: R Chapey. *Language Intervention Strategies in Aphasia and Related Neurogenic Communication Disorders*, 4th edn. Philadelphia, PA: Lippincott, Williams & Wilkins, 2001.

107. Peach R and Tonkovich J. Phonemic characteristics of apraxia of speech resulting from subcortical hemorrhage. *J Commun Disord.* 2004 Jan-Feb;37(1) 77–90.

108. Holland AL, Fromm DS, DeRuyter F, *et al.* Treatment efficacy: aphasia. *J Speech Hear Res.* 1996;Oct;39(5):S27–36.

109. Pashek GV and Holland AL. Evolution of aphasia in the first year post-onset. *Cortex.* 1988;Sep;24(3):411–23.

110. Kertesz A and McCabe P. Recovery patterns and prognosis in aphasia. *Brain.* 1977 Mar;100(1):1–18.

111. Pedersen PM, Vinter K, and Olsen TS. Aphasia after stroke: type, severity and prognosis. The Copenhagen aphasia study. *Cerebrovasc Dis.* 2004;17(1):35–43.

112. Plowman E, Hentz B, and Ellis C. Post-stroke aphasia prognosis: a review of patient-related and stroke-related factors. *J Eval Clin Pract.* 2012;Jun 18(3):689–94.

113. Lazar RM and Antoniello D. Variability in recovery from aphasia. *Curr Neurol Neurosci Rep.* 2008 Nov;8(6):497–502.

114. Price CJ, Seghier ML, and Leff AP. Predicting language outcome and recovery after stroke: the PLORAS system. *Nat Rev Neurol.* 2010 Apr;6(4):202–10.

115. Saur D, Ronneberger O, Kümmerer D, *et al.* Early functional magnetic resonance imaging activations predict language outcome after stroke. *Brain.* 2010 Apr;133(Pt 4):1252–64.

116. Lazar RM, Minzer B, Antoniello D, *et al.* Improvement in aphasia scores after stroke is well predicted by initial severity. *Stroke.* 2010 Jul;41(7):1485–8.

117. Bhogal SK, Teasell R, and Speechley M. Intensity of aphasia therapy, impact on recovery. *Stroke.* 2003 Apr;34(4):987–93.

118. Marsh EB and Hillis AE. Recovery from aphasia following brain injury: the role of reorganization. *Prog Brain Res.* 2006;157:143–56.

119. Sarasso S, Santhanam P, Määtta S, *et al.* Non-fluent aphasia and neural reorganization after speech therapy: insights from human sleep electrophysiology and functional magnetic resonance imaging. *Arch Ital Biol.* 2010 Sep;148(3):271–78.

120. Monti A, Cogiamanian F, Marceglia S, *et al.* Improved naming after transcranial direct current stimulation in aphasia. *J Neurol Neurosur Ps.* 2008 Apr;79(4) 451–53.

121. Baker JM, Rorden C, and Fridriksson J. Using transcranial direct-current stimulation to treat stroke participants with aphasia. *Stroke.* 2010 Jun;41:1229–36.

122. Kang EK, Kim YK, Sohn HM, *et al.* Improved picture naming in aphasia patients treated with cathodal tDCS to inhibit the right Broca's homologue area. *Restorative Neurol Neurosci.* 2011;29 (3):141–52.

123. Fridriksson J, Richardson JD, Baker JM, *et al.* Transcranial direct current stimulation improves naming reaction time in fluent aphasia: A double-blind, sham-controlled study. *Stroke.* 2011 Mar;42:819–21.

124. Martin PI, Naeser MA, Theoret H, *et al.* Transcranial magnetic stimulation as a complementary treatment for aphasia. *Semin Speech Lang.* 2004; 25:181–91.

125. Naeser M, Martin PI, Nicholas M, *et al.* Improved naming after TMS treatments in a chronic, global aphasia patient case report. *Neurocase.* 2005 Jun;11(3):182–93.

126. Walker-Batson D, Curtis S, Natarajan R, *et al.* A double-blind, placebo-controlled study of the use of amphetamine in the treatment of aphasia. *Stroke.* 2001 Sep;32(9):2093–8.

127. Klein RB and Albert ML. Can drug therapies improve language functions of individuals with aphasia? A review of the evidence. *Semin Speech Lang.* 2004 May;25(2):193–204.

128. Robertson S. The efficacy of oro-facial and articulation exercises in dysarthria following stroke. *Int J Lang Commun Disord.* 2001;36 Suppl:292–7.

129. Ray J. Orofacial myofunctional therapy in dysarthria: a study on speech intelligibility. *Int J Orofacial Myology.* 2002 Nov;28:39–48.

130. Freed DB. *Motor Speech Disorders.* San Diego, CA: Singular Thompson Learning, 2000.

131. Yorkston KM, Beukelman D, Strand EA, *et al. Management of Motor Speech Disorders in Children and Adults.* 2nd edn. Austin, TX: Pro-Ed, 1999.

132. Tudor C and Selley WG. A palatal training appliance and a visual aid for use in the treatment of hypernasal speech. A preliminary report. *Br J Disord Commun.* 1974 Oct;9(2):117–22.

CHAPTER 13

Memory disorders

Lara Harris, Kate Humphreys,
Ellen M. Migo, and Michael D. Kopelman

Theories of memory

Shortly after learning, we are temporarily able to access information over a period of seconds. After this, we can either recall this information in order to complete a task (short-term memory, STM), or the information may become consolidated into a longer-lasting memory (long-term memory, LTM). Memory takes various forms which can be defined separately, and different forms of memory are associated with different patterns of brain damage. Distinguishing types of memory is therefore important to develop theories of memory and also to understand the kinds of problems that different patients are likely to have.

LTM may be divided (Fig. 13.1) into *explicit, declarative memory*, which involves conscious recollection of facts and events, and *implicit, non-declarative memory*, where information is encoded without conscious memory of the learning event. Within explicit memory, there are episodic and semantic memory components. *Episodic memory* refers to memory for autobiographical events, often associated with contextual information (e.g. time and place), whereas *semantic memory* is defined as memory for factual information (e.g. meanings of words), which can be recalled without contextual information.

Episodic memories can be assessed through tests of recall and recognition. A recall memory test requires recollection of a target item or items perceived earlier. A recognition memory test involves identification of whether or not a given stimulus (or item) has been perceived before, either in a Yes/No format ('Yes–No recognition') or by selecting the item from one or more alternatives ('forced-choice recognition'). Both episodic and semantic memory have retrograde (memory for past events) and anterograde (memory for new events) components.

In contrast to explicit memory, implicit memory is where prior events support performance without conscious awareness of learning. Examples include priming, where subconscious awareness of previous information affects performance on future trials, and procedural memory, which supports acquisition of skills.

Traditionally, the role of the hippocampus was thought to be confined to LTM processes, grounded by early reports of dissociations between preserved STM and chronically impaired LTM in patients with hippocampal damage (e.g. patient HM).[9] However, more recent findings suggest the hippocampi are also involved in STM processes). In this section, we outline the main findings from neuropsychology, cognitive psychology, and neuroscience in the study of different types of memory, with particular reference to the role of the hippocampus.

Short-term and working memory

Within cognitive neuropsychology, STM is defined as the temporary storage of information over a period of around 20–30 seconds. The term 'working memory' refers to the storage and manipulation of information in order to complete a complex task.[10] The concept of working memory assumes that a limited capacity system temporarily maintains and stores information, and provides an interface between perception, LTM and action. Models of short-term memory can be divided into multi-store and unitary theories. Multi-component theories view STM and LTM as separate systems with distinct representations, whereas unitary models suggest that both STM and LTM use the same representations, differing only in terms of the level of activation of these representations and some of the processes that act upon them.[10]

The Baddeley and Hitch[8] model (Fig. 13.2), which has been the most highly influential account of working memory, comprises three functionally independent buffers: the phonological loop (responsible for information that can be rehearsed verbally), a visuospatial sketchpad (to maintain visual information), and an episodic buffer (for binding information from the other systems). Within this model, auditory information enters the phonological store directly and is then transferred to an output buffer, where the information may be either recalled or recycled through rehearsal. Remembering a list of words is easier when they form a meaningful sentence (e.g. 'chunking').[15] Within the Baddeley and Hitch model, this is because information from LTM supports the integration of words into sentences through the episodic buffer. According to their model, a supervisory system (or central executive) controls, coordinates, and regulates these systems, and is responsible for task shifting, retrieval strategies, selective attention, and inhibition.

There is support for neurologically and functionally distinct processes in STM and LTM. Patients with medial temporal lobe (MTL) damage present with preserved STM but impaired LTM,[12–16] while some patients, for example with parietal damage, show a profile of preserved STM despite disorders in LTM (e.g. patient KF).[15]

Support for the Baddeley and Hitch model[8] comes from neuropsychological double-dissociations in memory-impaired patients who show that visual and verbal STM can be independently impaired, following right and left hemisphere damage respectively.[16] Further support has come from dual-task experiments with healthy participants, where concurrent verbal tasks interfere with verbal STM and visual tasks with visual STM[17] (see section on classification of disorders of memory, this chapter, for a discussion of patients showing damage to component subsystems in STM). Evidence

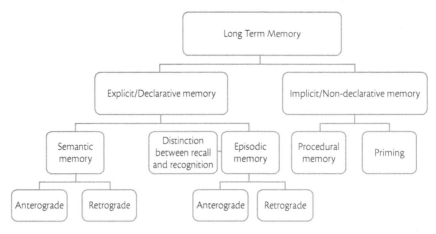

Fig. 13.1 An overview of long term memory (LTM).

Adapted from *Neurobiology of Learning and Memory.* 82(3), Squire LR, Memory systems of the brain: A brief history and current perspective, pp. 171–7, Copyright (2004), with permission from Elsevier.

from neuroimaging strongly suggests that verbal and visual STM processes may be neurologically distinct. Verbal STM is thought to be subserved by the left inferior frontal and parietal cortex, whereas spatial STM is made possible by the right posterior dorsal frontal and right parietal cortices and object/visual STM by the left inferior frontal and left parietal/left inferior temporal cortices.[18–22]

Perhaps the most influential unitary model of STM was described by Atkinson and Shiffrin.[21] Essentially, they proposed that STM consists of activated long-term representations, an idea that has been recently further developed.[22–27] Within their model, information is first submitted to sensory memory and is then transferred to a short-term store where information is fed into and out of long-term memory. Given this, STM consists of temporary activations of representations that may be associated with long-term memories, or information that was recently perceived. Crucially, representations that are more strongly activated (modulated by recency and frequency of occurrence) are more accessible. Oberauer[26] has suggested that four pieces (chunks) of information are available for access, but only one chunk of information can be the focus of attention at any one time.

Although the neural substrates of STM and LTM were traditionally assumed to be separate, there is some evidence that STM and LTM may share some neural processes. Patients with damage

to the MTL frequently perform well on standard STM tasks, but some amnesic patients have also shown impairment where STM tasks require the representation of novel materials,[28–32] and novel associations among stimuli, and between stimuli and context.[31,32] This finding has received strong support from neuroimaging.[33,34] The data suggest that MTL, and the hippocampus in particular, are employed in the encoding and retrieval of associative information during STM as well as in LTM. These findings challenge the simple STM/LTM dissociation that has been reported in classical lesion studies.

Long-term memory

Explicit/declarative memory

Explicit memory can be subdivided into episodic memory, defined as memory for a person's life events, and semantic memory, the memory for facts, concepts, and word meaning.[35] Crucially, episodic memory is described as *relational*, involving the representation of various associations between time, space, and the self, which is consistent with findings of hippocampal involvement in the short term, during associative memory tasks. Broadly, declarative memory is subserved by MTL structures: the hippocampal region (the dentate gyrus, the subicular complex, and the hippocampus itself; see chapter 4), midline diencephalic structures,[36] entorhinal cortex, perirhinal cortex, and parahippocampal cortex,[37–41] and the thalami, mammillary bodies, the mammillo-thalamic tract, retrosplenium, and the fornix. There may also be dorsolateral prefrontal cortex involvement.[42]

The hippocampus appears to have a specific role in the *binding* of information in memory. In a detailed case study of a patient with selective damage to the hippocampus (YR), Mayes and colleagues reported that associative memory for items of the same type (e.g. words) were preserved, while associative memory for different types of information (i.e. pictures and professions, faces and voices) was clearly impaired.[43] The authors suggest that different types of information processed in the neocortical regions is committed to the hippocampus for binding.[44,45] Further evidence supporting a specialized role of the hippocampus in associative memory has been found elsewhere (e.g. references 46, 47, see 48 for a review). It should be noted, though, that specialization of the hippocampus for relational memory has not always been found.[49–51]

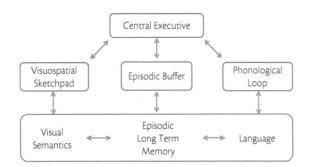

Fig. 13.2 The revised model of working memory, incorporating links with long-term memory (LTM) by way of both the subsystems and the episodic buffer.

Adapted from *Trends in Cognitive Sciences.* 4(11), Baddeley A, The episodic buffer: a new component of working memory? pp. 417–23, Copyright (2000), with permission from Elsevier.

Retrograde amnesia

Traditionally, it has been believed that in *retrograde amnesia* (RA), there is relative sparing of early memories, as is postulated by Ribot.[52] The two leading theories of remote declarative memory are consolidation theories[53–55] and multiple trace theory (MTT).[56–58] Consolidation theory suggests that encoded experiences are initially stored in the hippocampus and cortical regions (perirhinal cortex, parahippocampal cortex), and with repeated learning, this information is transferred to the neocortex for permanent storage (consolidated). MTT suggests instead that experiences form memory traces and older memories are associated with a greater number of memory traces acquired over time.

The perspectives differ in terms of the neural mechanisms assumed to subserve semantic memory and episodic memory; in particular, the effects of hippocampal or MTL damage on remote memory (retrograde amnesia). Consolidation theories state that hippocampal or MTL damage leads to an impairment in retrieval of remote episodic (event-based) and remote semantic (knowledge or fact-based) information, both with a temporal gradient (i.e. relative sparing of early memories compared to more recent ones). MTT, on the other hand, states that hippocampal or MTL damage leads to an extensive loss of remote episodic memories across all time periods, while remote semantic memories are spared.

Both theories agree that damage extending beyond the MTLs will affect remote episodic and semantic memories, but the MTT states that damage to the MTLs is sufficient to cause an extensive remote episodic memory loss (examples of cases showing disorders in LTM are described in section on classification of disorders of memory, this chapter). However, there is still considerable controversy over these issues.[59,04]

Topographical memory

Topographical memory involves relating information about landmarks and space from semantic and episodic memory for the purposes of navigation. In topographical amnesia, buildings and landmarks can frequently be recognized and recalled, but the memory for associations between them and how they relate to space is defective.[61–64]

Neuroimaging and neuropsychological evidence suggests that while the parahippocampus is implicated in relating visual and spatial information into a topographical representation, the hippocampus is involved in their *consolidation*. In an important study, Maguire and colleagues[65] took structural magnetic resonance imaging (MRI) scans of the brains of professional London taxi drivers, who undertake two to three years of training to learn the various spatial relations between destinations in the city. The authors reported that the taxi drivers had significantly larger posterior hippocampi, relative to a control group, concluding that the posterior hippocampus stores a map of spatial representations to enable navigation.

Topographical memory appears to be underpinned by a network including the medial parietal lobe, the posterior cingulate gyrus, occipitotemporal areas, the parahippocampal gyrus, and the right hippocampus.[65] This is consistent with neuropsychological reports of hippocampal patients who show impaired topographical memory in the context of better preserved memory for visual information.[66] On functional imaging, there is hippocampal activation during studies of navigation in virtual environments in PET[64,65] and activation of the right hippocampus during route-finding on fMRI.[67,68]

There is some suggestion that the role of the hippocampus in relating spatial representations may not be confined to LTM processes, as hippocampal damage impedes the memory for topographical information even over short delays.[69]

Implicit/non-declarative memory

While explicit memory processes are mediated by the MTL and diencephalic regions, the implicit (non-declarative) memory system is traditionally understood to be independent of the MTL, though the neural regions implicated in tests of implicit memory vary widely with the type of stimuli presented. Dissociations between implicit and explicit memory performance in amnesic patients[6] are consistent with theories positing separate neural systems for explicit and implicit memory.

More recent work has suggested that there may be some overlap between the neural mechanisms involved in implicit and explicit memory, which may indicate a unitary system. In particular, there is some evidence that MTL may be implicated in implicit memory where retrieval is of relational information rather than individual items. There is accumulating evidence from neuroimaging studies showing MTL activation during associative memory tasks (for reviews, see references 70, 71). Hippocampal activity during implicit relational memory encoding has been demonstrated in healthy participants,[47] and implicit relational memory effects were absent in hippocampal patients tested under the same conditions.[46]

Procedural memory

Procedural memory refers to the acquisition and retention of perceptuomotor skills. These memories are accessed and applied without the need for recalling information relating to the event where the skill was acquired. Procedural memory is less well understood than explicit memory, but it is likely to involve a network comprising frontal, basal ganglia, parietal, and cerebellar regions.[36,70,73] Unlike explicit memory, learning in the procedural memory system is gradual, and the automaticity with which procedural memory is applied is only achieved after repeated exposure and practice.

Skill acquisition has been tested experimentally using mirror-reading and pursuit rotor tasks. Mirror-reading tasks involve reading mirror-transformed words, and pursuit rotor tasks involve following a moving dot around a circle with a wand. Performance on these tasks should improve with practice. One study[74] compared the performance of patients with Huntington's disease with Korsokoff's syndrome patients and controls on mirror-reading and pursuit rotor tasks. Both Korsakoff's and control participants showed the expected pattern (increased speed of mirror-reversed words with increased exposure), whereas the performance of the Huntington's group was stable over incremental trials. Such lack of improvement with practice would be compatible with a special role of brain regions particularly affected in Huntington's in implicit memory (e.g. the basal ganglia).

Classification of disorders of memory

There are various types of memory disorders, each associated with different clinical characteristics and neuropsychological dissociations. In this section, we describe the most common memory disorders using vignettes of important neuropsychology cases from the literature.

Short-term memory

Much of the data on STM comes from memory *span tasks*, where lists of words, pictures, or numbers are presented and the participant is required to recall them in the order they were presented. Memory span is determined by the longest list of items reliably recalled in the correct order and is considerably reduced in patients with short-term memory disorders, relative to control norms.

Several STM-impaired patients have been described. Patients with phonological STM deficits are characterized by a marked impairment for verbally presented STM despite preserved visual STM. These patients are unaffected by phonological similarity or word length of the to-be-recalled items—effects commonly observed under STM conditions.[20,75–77] The first phonological STM patient to be described was patient KF[15,77] who, despite having a normal ability to articulate words and comprehend language, could recall sequences of only two auditorily presented items.[15,77] Strikingly though, KF performed within the normal range under conditions of visual presentation.

The authors attributed these results to avoidance of employing a defective phonological loop during STM tasks.[4,78] A similar patient (see Box 13.1) with a pure deficit for phonological information showed the same pattern of impaired auditory span, but with normal language comprehension with sentences comprised of simple structures (patient PV).[4] These dissociations strongly suggested selective impairment of an auditory short-term system, putatively localized in the left parietal or superior temporal regions[15,79] in a model with functionally separate short-term stores. Some other studies have also reported deficits of spatial span following lesions of the right parietal region.[80,81]

Box 13.1 Vignette: Patient PV

Patient PV[7] was a right-handed woman with 11 years of education, who suffered a large, left hemisphere CVA at the age of 23. Acutely, she had a right hemiparesis which cleared within a month, and some signs of aphasia, including phonemic paraphasias and word-finding difficulties, and sentence repetition was particularly impaired, though wider cognition was preserved.

Two years after her stroke, most of her language problems had resolved, though striking deficits in sentence repetition (for sentences containing more than eight syllables) and in comprehending complex language (e.g. using the Token test and Raven's progressive matrices) persisted. These difficulties were observed in the context of good repetition and comprehension of single words and short sentences suggesting that PV's problems were mnemonic in nature.

Her auditory span was severely restricted (to lists of two or three items) but she performed within the normal range with visual presentation. Her sentence repetition impairment was restricted to sentences of two to three words. Sentence comprehension was better and she experienced problems only with long, complex sentences. The absence of detrimental effects of phonological similarity and increased word length indicates subcomponents in STM, and suggests that a defective phonological loop[11] is the locus of PV's impairments in span, sentence repetition, and comprehension.

Box 13.2 Vignette: Patient HM

Patient HM[1,2] underwent a bilateral medial temporal lobe resection in 1953 at the age of 27, which included the hippocampus and most of the amygdaloid complex and entorhinal cortex, in order to control frequent and debilitating epileptic seizures. Surgery was partially successful in modifying his epilepsy but resulted in severe anterograde amnesia.

He failed to acquire new event-related, autobiographical memories (i.e. episodic memory, e.g. appointments, people he had just met) and memories for facts (i.e. semantic memory). HM famously reported that 'every day is alone in itself'.[1] In contrast, wider cognition, including perceptual abilities, short-term memory, procedural memory, and language skills were well-preserved.

The case of HM strongly influenced memory research, emphasizing the role of the medial temporal lobe structures in explicit, declarative memory, and demonstrating that the neural mechanisms responsible for memory can be dissociated from structures involved in other aspects of cognition.

As will be discussed below, MTL patients with impaired long-term memory and preserved STM have also been described.[2,14] These findings indicate that STM processes are broadly independent of MTL structures. Moreover, there is some evidence that while phonological (verbal) STM stores might be localized to posterior left hemisphere regions, visuospatial STM stores are in posterior right hemisphere areas.

Anterograde and retrograde amnesia

Anterograde amnesia is characterized by the failure to create new memories or acquire new information following the onset of a disease or brain injury. In contrast, retrograde amnesia refers to the loss of memories which occurred before the onset of a disease or head trauma. A highly influential case of anterograde amnesia following bilateral MTL lesions is patient H.M. (Box 13.2).

The association between anterograde amnesia and the MTL described in these original observations was subsequently replicated in several studies of amnesic patients with MTL damage (e.g. patient SS[82] and patient RB[83]; see also Box 13.3), and in experimental animals with tailored lesions to the MTL.[84] This work has sought to investigate the specific structures within the MTL involved in anterograde and retrograde amnesia.

Anterograde amnesia has been associated with bilateral loss of the pyramidal cells in the CA1 hippocampal area,[83] and damage to the anterior thalamus.[85–88] In herpes simplex encephalitis, the severity of anterograde amnesia is strongly modulated by the extent of pathology in the medial limbic regions, with bilateral damage typically predictive of very severe amnesia.[89–91]

In contrast, some studies have found that retrograde amnesia is associated with damage to the right temporal and frontal areas.[41,92–94] In a detailed case study, Levine and colleagues attributed retrograde amnesia in a traumatic brain injury patient to a focal right frontal lesion, and right frontotemporal disconnection.[95] Though some authors have described cases of disproportionate, 'isolated', or 'focal' retrograde amnesia,[87,96,97] many of these cases have in fact shown evidence of coexisting impairments in anterograde memory[98–102] (see reference 101 for a review).

Box 13.3 Vignette: Patient DJ

Patient DJ[10] suffered unilateral left temporal lobe damage due to herpes encephalitis in 1990, when he was aged 36. Initially, DJ was unable to remember events and could not read, speak, or comprehend spoken language. Recall of earlier memories was better preserved.

One year post-onset, his language abilities improved (though surface dyslexia persisted). Strikingly, he was still very unable to acquire new memories, though memory for remote news and autobiographical events was only moderately impaired. He made frequent confabulation errors when required to recall auditorily presented stories, both in immediate and delayed (20–30 minutes) recall conditions (logical memory, WMS–R).

Consistent with his left temporal lobe pathology, DJ's recognition memory was poor, though his memory for faces was better preserved than for words (using the Recognition Memory Test). Seven years post-onset, DJ was still severely amnesic and anomic, and showed on testing a pattern of poor verbal memory and preserved visual memory (WMS–R), though memory for recent episodic and semantic memory was much improved and he was able to name highly familiar items.

Box 13.5 Vignette: Patient IH

Patient IH[6] was diagnosed with semantic dementia aged 62. An MRI scan revealed marked atrophy of the left temporal lobe but crucially with better preservation of the left hippocampus and MTL, and minor atrophy in the right temporal lobe and neocortex.

He showed difficulties in word-finding, reading, naming, and language comprehension, despite good non-verbal reasoning, visual spatial processing, and day-to-day memory and orientation. This pattern of neuropsychological performance is characteristic of semantic dementia, though he was sometimes able to spontaneously recall events from his late teens.

IH showed a reversed temporal gradient (relative preservation of recent memories) in autobiographical memory using the Autobiographical Memory Interview, but not when recalling news events (semantic memory). However, IH's memory for early, remote events could be significantly improved with detailed cueing. The neuropsychological profile of IH suggests that lexical–semantic disturbances were the basis of his impaired retrieval from autobiographical memory, rather than deficiencies in autobiographical memory storage.

The partial dissociation of anterograde and retrograde amnesia has received support from studies of Korsokoff's syndrome patients, where the extent of retrograde amnesia is not well correlated with the severity of anterograde amnesia.[102–105]

Selective deficits in episodic memory?

Patients with impaired episodic memory show particular difficulties in remembering events with a specific spatial or temporal context in *both* anterograde and autobiographical memory. There are reports of patients who show dissociations between episodic and semantic memory (Box 13.4).

In a study of retrograde amnesia, Bright and colleagues[106] compared episodic and semantic memory performance in medial temporal, medial plus lateral temporal, and frontal lesion patients. MTL lesions were associated with impaired retrieval of recent episodic memories whereas patients with medial plus lateral temporal damage showed impaired recall of *both* recent and remote episodic memories (i.e. a flat temporal gradient).

Episodic memory disorder occurs in herpes simplex (HSV) encephalitis[107] and a similar pattern—though often to a lesser

extent—has been reported in limbic encephalitis.[108] In terms of neuroimaging findings, HSV encephalitis causes hyper-intense signal alteration on T2-weighted MRI scans and loss of volume in the MTL which is consistent with an association between episodic memory and the MTL.[89,109,110]

Selective deficits in semantic memory?

In the early stages, semantic dementia (SD) patients show frequent word-finding difficulties, and may demonstrate impaired reading of low-frequency, irregularly spelled words (surface dyslexia). In the later stages of the disease, speech becomes increasingly empty of meaning, though it remains fluent and grammatically sound (Box 13.5). Many semantic dementia patients have atrophy of the temporal pole, with relative preservation of MTL structures (see reference 111 for a review).

Under neuropsychological examination, these patients show impairments on tests of semantic knowledge (e.g. pyramids and palm trees).[112] Crucially, and as is consistent with preserved MTL regions on imaging, episodic memory in these patients is often relatively spared,[113–115] In a study comparing the memory performance of an MTL amnesic patient with a patient with semantic dementia, Westmacott and colleagues[116] showed that, unlike the amnesic patient, the semantic dementia patient EL had preserved episodic memory, at least on cueing, and a similar finding was made in patient IH (Box 13.5) by Moss and colleagues.[3] Further, EL's memory for semantic facts was significantly modulated by autobiographical significance, whereas this was not true of the amnesic patient KC, indicating that episodic memory may contribute to semantic memory in cases of SD. There is also evidence from a longitudinal study suggesting intact autobiographical memory in semantic dementia until the very late stages of the illness (patient AM).[117]

Semantic memory is also commonly affected in both Alzheimer's disease[118] and HSV encephalitis,[7,119] manifesting in surface dyslexia and difficulties on wider lexical semantic memory tasks. This impairment has been attributed to left inferolateral temporal lobe or temporal pole damage.[120]

Box 13.4 Vignette—Patient KC

Patient KC[3–5] is an amnesic patient with complete destruction of the left hippocampus, parahippocampal gyrus, entorhinal and perirhinal cortex following a road traffic accident.

He subsequently developed anterograde amnesia and a temporally graded retrograde amnesia for episodic information: he could not acquire new semantic or autobiographical memories, and could only reliably recall old semantic (fact-based) memories from his life prior to the accident. Notably, he could remember detailed factual information from his education but could not recall emotional details, such as those relating to his brother's death. KC was also unable to imagine himself in the future (autonoetic consciousness).

Box 13.6 Vignette: Patient Jon

Jon[8] is a developmental case of early onset amnesia. He was delivered prematurely and suffered two long-lasting convulsions at the age of four. Jon began to show evidence of memory problems a year-and-a-half later.

At the age of 19, Jon was assessed by Vargha-Khadem and colleagues.[8] On imaging, Jon showed abnormally small hippocampi bilaterally. Impressively, at this time he had an IQ of 120, could read successfully, and showed relatively preserved memory for factual information (semantic memory), even for information learned after his hippocampal damage. However, Jon was unable to find his way around familiar routes, was not well oriented in time, and could not acquire information about daily events (episodic memories).

Consistently, during assessment, he showed a striking impairment on the Rivermead Behavioural Memory Test, which includes tasks such as remembering a route, an appointment, and a message to be relayed. Despite his preserved ability to perceive and recognize objects, Jon's topographical memory was markedly impaired, as was his context-dependent episodic memory.

Topographical memory

Turriziani and colleagues[66] reported a patient with significant bilateral hippocampal atrophy and moderate cortical atrophy following cerebral hypoxia. Crucially, there was a chronic impairment in memory for spatial information that was significantly improved with visual cues, but a relatively well-preserved ability to learn verbal and visual information (including topographical information), which was only mildly impaired. The authors concluded that there was a (largely) preserved ability to form topographical representations (modulated by the preserved parahippocampus), but an impaired ability to consolidate them into LTM (owing to bilateral hippocampal damage). A developmental syndrome has also been described (Box 13.6).

The association between hippocampal damage and topographical memory has been observed even at very short delays. In a neuropsychological study of four focal hippocampal patients, Hartley and colleagues[69] found that two patients were impaired in both topographical perception and memory, but that two showed a selective impairment for topographical memory (i.e. despite preserved ability to perceive and process topographical representations), even at very brief (two-second) delays. This finding suggests the specific role of the hippocampus in topographical memory consolidation, and during specialized STM tasks tapping visualspatial information.

Implicit memory

A double dissociation between explicit and implicit memory in two neuropsychological cases, LH and HM, has been reported.[6] While HM was profoundly amnesic with severely impaired explicit memory and preserved performance on implicit memory tasks (perceptual identification, word completion, priming), LH demonstrated the reverse dissociation (Box 13.7).

Keane and colleagues[6] explained the difference in these patients' implicit memory performance in terms of occipital circuits that were intact in HM and damaged in LH. Ostergaard has contested the idea that there is complete preservation of implicit memory

---

Box 13.7 Vignette: Patient LH

Patient LH[9] was aged 18 when he was involved in a road traffic accident. He suffered a traumatic brain injury and underwent an extensive right temporal lobectomy and insertion of a shunt for hydrocephalus. MRI and SPECT conducted when he was aged 41 revealed damage to the right parietal and occipital lobes and a left hemisphere white matter lesion (extending from the inferior temporal gyrus to just below the occipital horn), but the diencephalic regions medial temporal lobe structures were spared.

LH's main complaint was an inability to recognize faces. He also showed other impairments in visuoperceptual skills. He showed an absent priming effect in perceptual identification of words and pseudowords and absent word completion priming in the context of normal (explicit) recognition memory.

---

in medial temporal amnesics, suggesting that implicit memory is often not preserved when studies are properly controlled with respect to baseline.[121]

Procedural memory is usually preserved in amnesia,[82,121–124] but can be impaired in Parkinson's and Huntington's disease.[74,125]

Recall and recognition memory

In both episodic and semantic memory, there are distinctions between recall and recognition tests. These tests ask participants to remember studied items in different ways. Recall tests are considered to be more difficult than recognition tests, requiring more effort, and patients often perform rather worse on them than in recognition tests. Performance on recall and recognition tests is usually interpreted in terms of the contributions of *recollection* and *familiarity*.[126,127] Recollection is where participants retrieve information beyond the represented stimulus, such as the context in which it was presented. Familiarity is simply the feeling that a stimulus has been encountered before.

Patients with apparently similar lesions of the hippocampi can show very different memory performance patterns.[128] A meta-analysis by Aggleton and Shaw[129] looked for associations between recognition performance and pathology in amnesic patients. They found that patients with more focal brain damage, particularly to the hippocampus, mamilliary bodies, and fornix, were more likely to show preserved recognition, despite profound impairments on recall tests. However, their meta-analysis was confounded by floor effects in some of their patients, and not all studies show disproportionate impairment on recall memory in hippocampal patients.[49] The reasons behind this inconsistency are not yet resolved.

Disproportionate recall over recognition deficits have also been reported in ageing[130] and a number of disorders, such as schizophrenia[131] and autism.[132] Damage to frontal brain regions has been shown to impair free recall performance more than cued recall, which in turn is more impaired than recognition, though recognition is commonly also affected in these patients.[133]

Testing memory

A wealth of standardized neuropsychological assessments of memory is available to the clinician to assist diagnosis. Some of the most well-known include the Wechsler Memory Scale,[134] the California Verbal Learning Test II,[135] and the Rey Complex Figure.[136] Most of these concentrate on episodic memory. However, specialist tests also exist for autobiographical memory (e.g. autobiographical memory interview),[137] prospective memory (e.g. Cambridge Prospective Memory Test),[138] and semantic memory (e.g. pyramids and palm trees).[112] Comprehensive critical reviews can be found in standard texts.[139,140] The reader is also referred to chapter 11. In this section, we outline practical considerations when testing for different types of memory disorder.

Diagnostic assessments

It is important to first establish the clinical history from both the patient and an informant relating to a memory complaint such as the time and nature of its onset and other related disease or psychiatric complaint, and then to assess whether there is objective evidence of a memory disorder on formal testing; that is, whether performance falls by at least 1.5 to 2 standard deviations based on estimated pre-morbid IQ (see chapter 11). Standardized tests of memory that give scores that can be compared directly against optimal IQ (i.e. that give age-scaled standardized scores) should be employed. Memory for both visual and verbal material should be tested as these can be impaired relatively independently,[141] and it is necessary to test free recall, ideally after a delay as well as immediately.

Recognition memory or cued recall should be assessed if performance on free recall is poor, as it may be that the information is being encoded but cannot be retrieved without a cue. Suitable test batteries for evaluating episodic memory include the Wechsler Memory Scale,[134] the doors and people test,[140] and the BIRT (Brain Injury Rehabilitation Trust) Memory and Information Processing Battery (BMIPB),[143] and the Recognition Memory Test 2007.[144] Performance on the Wechsler Adult Intelligence Scale[145] digit span subtest can be used as a measure of phonological STM and working memory either alone, or in combination with the arithmetic subtest with which it comprises the Wechsler Working Memory Index. Visuospatial STM and working memory can be evaluated using the symbol span subtest from the WMS–IV or the Corsi Block Tapping Test.[146]

If objective evidence of memory impairment is found, a second question is whether the pattern of impairment is more consistent with neurological or psychogenic causes (e.g. depression). In general, patients who are simply depressed will tend to make a large number of 'don't know' responses, to be reluctant to guess, and to show a pattern of generally poor performance. For these reasons, it is sometimes helpful to administer symptom validity tests such as the test of memory malingering,[147] the word memory test,[148] and the Camden Pictorial Memory Test.[149] Poor or below-chance performance on these tasks is strongly indicative of motivational factors rather than neurological disorder.

If the findings are more indicative of a neurological complaint, the question is whether the pattern of memory test scores has any lateralizing or localizing value or is consistent with a particular differential diagnosis. In general, difficulties remembering verbal material are associated with left hemisphere pathology while there is a less strong association between visual memory difficulties and pathology in the right hemisphere.[150]

Another important consideration in a diagnostic assessment is whether the memory difficulties are progressive or static in nature. This is particularly important in distinguishing between a cognitive impairment after a stable lesion and a dementia. Obviously this point can only be addressed by serial assessments. Memory batteries with parallel forms that increase slightly in difficulty, to counteract practice effects, are available (e.g. the BMIPB).[143]

Planning and monitoring rehabilitation

Results from memory assessments can inform memory rehabilitation programmes, which can be tailored to maximize the use of the individual's strengths and compensate for their areas of weakness. Findings from traditional standardized memory tests can be useful; for example, knowing that an individual scores at the 75th percentile on tests of verbal memory and only at the 5th percentile on tests of visual memory means that teaching verbal encoding strategies for visual material is likely to be of benefit. Furthermore, many clinicians find it more helpful to use so-called ecologically valid tests of memory to inform rehabilitation. These tests are designed to map on to real-life abilities in a much more direct way and aim to provide a measure of disability rather than impairment. Commonly used ecologically valid memory tests include the Rivermead Behavioural Memory Test[151] and the Cambridge Prospective Memory Test.[138]

Interpreting memory test scores in context

It is usually relatively meaningless to obtain memory test scores in isolation. First, poor performance on memory tests may be secondary to difficulties with other cognitive and perceptual domains such as processing speed, executive functions, language or visual cognition[152] rather than due to a primary 'memory deficit'. Thus, we would recommend at least screening these areas if difficulties are found on memory tests. Another reason to test more widely than just memory is that patients often report 'memory problems' when they mean that they experience word-finding difficulties or other cognitive problems.[139] Third, performance on memory tests must be considered relative to the individual's likely optimum level of functioning (see chapter 11); performance in the average range may constitute a strength for someone with an intellectual disability but a relative weakness for someone previously likely to have functioned in the superior range.

As well as the quantitative scores provided by memory tests, it is necessary to gather qualitative information regarding how the individual approached the task and the types of errors they made in order to aid interpretation of the results. For example, confabulation, intrusions, or perseverative responses, or an inability to initiate responses without frequent prompting and encouragement, can indicate fronto-executive dysfunction.

In addition to cognitive tests, it is desirable to administer a mood screen such as the Hospital Anxiety and Depression Scale[153] or the Beck Depression Inventory II[154] since depression and anxiety can affect performance on memory tests.[155] It is also good practice to administer a questionnaire asking about subjective memory difficulties, such as the Prospective and Retrospective Memory Questionnaire.[156]

Conclusion

Memory can be divided into various subtypes, and, while there are well-established findings (e.g. MTL involvement in episodic memory), there is still considerable controversy in some areas of the literature regarding the functional description and neural organization of memory processes. There is accumulating evidence attesting to the importance of hippocampi in representing novel items and associations both in the long- and (to some extent) the short-term, and in memory consolidation. Detailed neuropsychological case descriptions have contributed significantly to the evolution of memory theories. Standardized neuropsychological assessments are available that allow targeted evaluation of different types of memory (e.g. episodic and semantic), memory for different modalities of information (e.g. verbal and visual), and the underlying neurobiological process (e.g. static or progressive). However, when assessing memory-impaired patients, it is important to interpret evidence in the context of premorbid IQ and any wider cognitive or psychological disorders that may be causing impaired performance. Understanding memory disorders is of crucial importance for the clinician for making diagnoses and for planning rehabilitation. Moreover, neuropsychological descriptions of memory-impaired patients remain critically important for informing and evaluating memory theory.

References

1. Milner B, Corkin S, and Teuber HL. Further analysis of the hippocampal amnesic syndrome: 14-year follow-up study of H.M. *Neuropsychologia*. 1968;6(3):215–34.

2. Scoville WB and Milner B. Loss of recent memory after bilateral hippocampal lesions. 1957. *J Neuropsych Clin N*. 1957;12(1):103–13.

3. Moss HE, Kopelman MD, Cappelletti M, et al. Lost for words or loss of memories? Autobiographical memory in semantic dementia. *Cognitive Neuropsych*. 2003;20(8):703–32.

4. Vallar G and Baddeley AD. Fractionation of working memory: Neuropsychological evidence for a phonological short-term store. *Journal of Verbal Learning and Verbal Behavior*. 1984;23(2):151–61.

5. Vargha-Khadem F, Gadian DG, Watkins KE,et al. Differential Effects of Early Hippocampal Pathology on Episodic and Semantic Memory. *Science*. 1997;277(5324):376–80.

6. Keane MM, Gabrieli JDE, Mapstone HC, et al. Double dissociation of memory capacities after bilateral occipital-lobe or medial temporal-lobe lesions. *Brain*. 1995;118(5):1129–48.

7. Stanhope N and Kopelman MD. Art and memory: A 7-year follow-up of herpes encephalitis in a professional artist. *Neurocase*. 2000;6(2):99–110.

8. Baddeley A and Hitch GJ. Working memory. In: GA Bower (ed.). *Recent Advances in Learning and Motivation*. New York, NY: Academic Press, 1974, pp. 47–90.

9. Squire LR. The Legacy of Patient H.M. for Neuroscience. *Neuron*. 2009;61(1):6–9.

10. Baddeley A. Working memory: Looking back and looking forward. *Nat Rev Neurosci*. 2003;4(10):829–39.

11. Baddeley A. The episodic buffer: A new component of working memory? *Trends Cogn Sci*. 2000;4(11):417–23.

12. Squire LR. Memory and the hippocampus: A synthesis from findings with rats, monkeys, and humans. *Psychol Rev*. 1992;99(2):195–231.

13. Scoville WB and Milner B. Loss of recent memory after bilateral hippocampal lesions. *J Neurol Neurosur Ps*. 1957;20:11–21.

14. Baddeley AD and Warrington EK. Amnesia and the distinction between long- and short-term memory. *Journal of Verbal Learning and Verbal Behavior*. 1970;9(2):176–89.

15. Shallice T and Warrington EK. The dissociation between short term retention of meaningful sounds and verbal material. *Neuropsychologia*. 1974;12(4):553–5.

16. Wang PP and Bellugi U. Evidence from two genetic syndromes for a dissociation between verbal and visual-spatial short-term memory. *J Clin Exp Neuropsyc*. 1994;16(2):317–22.

17. Baddeley AD. *Working Memory*. Oxford: Oxford University Press, 1986.

18. Awh E, Jonides J, Smith EE, et al. Dissociation of Storage and Rehearsal in Verbal Working Memory: Evidence from Positron Emission Tomography. *Psychol Sci*. 1996;7(1):25–31.

19. Jonides J, Smith EE, Koeppe RA, et al. Spatial working memory in humans as revealed by PET. *Nature*. 1993;363(6430):623–5.

20. Warrington EK, Logue V, and Pratt RTC. The anatomical localisation of selective impairment of auditory verbal short-term memory. *Neuropsychologia*. 1971;9(4):377–87.

21. Atkinson RC and Shiffrin RM. Human Memory: A Proposed System and its Control Processes. In: WS Kenneth and JS Taylor (eds). *Psychology of Learning and Motivation*. New York, NY: Academic Press, 1968, pp. 89–195.

22. Anderson JR, Bothell D, Byrne MD, et al. An Integrated Theory of the Mind. Psychological Review. 2004;111(4):1036–60.

23. Cowan N. *Attention and Memory: An Integrated Framework*. Oxford: Oxford University Press, 1995.

24. Cowan N. The magical number 4 in short-term memory: A reconsideration of mental storage capacity. *Behav Brain Sci*. 2001;24(1):87–114; discussion 85.

25. McElree B. Working memory and focal attention. *J Exp Psychol Learn*. 2001;27(3):817–35.

26. Oberauer K. Access to information in working memory: Exploring the focus of attention. *J Exp Psychol Learn*. 2002;28(3):411–21.

27. Verhaeghen P, Cerella J, and Basak C. A Working Memory Workout: How to Expand the Focus of Serial Attention From One to Four Items in 10 Hours or Less. *J Exp Psychol Learn Mem Cogn*. 2004; 6:1322–37. doi:10.1037/0278-7393.30.6.1322.

28. Buffalo EA, Reber PJ, and Squire LR. The human perirhinal cortex and recognition memory. *Hippocampus*. 1998;8(4):330–9.

29. Holdstock JS, Shaw C, and Aggleton JP. The performance of amnesic subjects on tests of delayed matching-to-sample and delayed matching-to-position. *Neuropsychologia*. 1995;33(12):1583–96.

30. Olson I, Page K, Moore KS, et al. Working memory for conjunctions relies on the medial temporal lobe. *J Neurosci*. 2006;26(17):4596–601.

31. Hannula DE, Tranel D, and Cohen NJ. The long and the short of It: Relational memory impairments in amnesia, even at short lags. *J Neurosci*. 2006;26(32):8352–9.

32. Olson IR, Page K, Moore KS, et al. Working memory for conjunctions relies on the medial temporal lobe. *J Neurosci*. 2006;26(17):4596–601.

33. Miyashita Y and Chang HS. Neuronal correlate of pictorial short-term memory in the primate temporal cortex. *Nature*. 1988;331(6151):68–70.

34. Ranganath C and D'Esposito M. Medial temporal lobe activity associated with active maintenance of novel information. *Neuron*. 2001;31(5):865–73.

35. Tulving E. Episodic and semantic memory. In: E Tulving, W Donaldson (eds). *Organization of Memory*. New York, NY: Academic Press, 1972, pp. 381–402.

36. Squire LR and Zola SM. Structure and function of declarative and nondeclarative memory systems. *Proc Natl Acad Sci USA*.1996;93(24):13515–22.

37. Squire LR. Memory systems of the brain: A brief history and current perspective. *Neurobiol Learn Mem*. 2004;82(3):171–7.

38. Squire LR and Knowlton BJ. The Medial Temporal Lobe, the Hippocampus, and the Memory Systems of the Brain. In: MS Gazzaniga (ed.). *Memory*. Cambridge, MA: MIT Press, 2000, pp. 825–37.

39. Suzuki WA and Eichenbaum H. The neurophysiology of memory. *Annals of the New York Academy of Sciences*. 2000;911(1):175–91.

40. Kopelman MD, Stanhope N, and Kingsley D. Temporal and spatial context memory in patients with focal frontal, temporal lobe, and diencephalic lesions. *Neuropsychologia*. 1997;35(12):1533–45.

41. Kopelman MD, Stanhope N, and Kingsley D. Retrograde amnesia in patients with diencephalic,temporal lobe or frontal lesions. *Neuropsychologia*. 1999;37(8):939–58.

42. Prabhakaran V, Narayanan K, Zhao Z, et al. Integration of diverse information in working memory within the frontal lobe. *Nat Neurosci*. 2000;3(1):85–90.

43. Mayes AR, Holdstock JS, Isaac CL, et al. Associative recognition in a patient with selective hippocampal lesions and relatively normal item recognition. *Hippocampus*. 2004;14(6):763–84.

44. Mayes AR, Montaldi D, and Migo EM. Associative memory and the medial temporal lobes. *Trends Cogn Sci*. 2007;11(3):126–35.

45. Montaldi D and Mayes AR. The role of recollection and familiarity in the functional differentiation of the medial temporal lobes. *Hippocampus.* 2010;20(11):1291–314.

46. Hannula DE, Ryan JD, Tranel D, *et al.* Rapid Onset Relational Memory Effects Are Evident in Eye Movement Behavior, but Not in Hippocampal Amnesia. *J Cognitive Neurosci.* 2007;19(10):1690–705.

47. Hannula DE and Ranganath C. The Eyes Have It: Hippocampal Activity Predicts Expression of Memory in Eye Movements. *Neuron.* 2009;63(5):592–9.

48. Eichenbaum H. Hippocampus: Cognitive Processes and Neural Representations that Underlie Declarative Memory. *Neuron.* 2004;44(1):109–20.

49. Kopelman MD, Bright P, Buckman J, *et al.* Recall and recognition memory in amnesia: Patients with hippocampal, medial temporal, temporal lobe or frontal pathology. *Neuropsychologia.* 2007;45(6):1232–46.

50. Stark CE and Squire LR. Hippocampal damage equally impairs memory for single items and memory for conjunctions. *Hippocampus.* 2003;13(2):281–92.

51. Stark CEL, Bayley PJ, and Squire LR. Recognition memory for single items and for associations is similarly impaired following damage to the hippocampal region. *Learn Memory.* 2002;9(5):238.

52. Ribot TA. *The Diseases of Memory.* New York, NY: Appleton & Co., 1882.

53. Alvarez P and Squire LR. Memory Consolidation and the Medial Temporal Lobe: A Simple Network Model. *Proc Natl Acad Sci USA.* 1994;91(15):7041–5.

54. Squire LR. Lost forever or temporarily misplaced? The long debate about the nature of memory impairment. *Learn Memory.* 2006;13(5):522–9.

55. Squire LR, Stark CE, and Clark RE. The medial temporal lobe. *Annu Rev Neurosci.* 2004;27:279–306.

56. Moscovitch M, Nadel L, Winocur G, *et al.* The cognitive neuroscience of remote episodic, semantic and spatial memory. *Curr Opin Neurobiol.* 2006;16(2):179–90.

57. Nadel L and Moscovitch M. Memory consolidation, retrograde amnesia and the hippocampal complex. *Curr Opin Neurobiol.* 1997;7(2):217–27.

58. Winocur G and Moscovitch M. Memory Transformation and Systems Consolidation. *Journal of the International Neuropsychological Society.* 2011;17(05):766–80.

59. Kopelman MD and Bright P. On remembering and forgetting our autobiographical pasts: Retrograde amnesia and Andrew Mayes's contribution to neuropsychological method. *Neuropsychologia.* 2012;50(13):2961–72.

60. Kopelman MD and Stanhope N. Anterograde and retrograde amnesia following frontal lobe, temporal lobe, or diencephalic lesions In: LR Squire and D Schacter (eds). *Neuropsychology of Memory,* 3rd edn. New York, NY: Guilford Press, 2002, pp. 47–60.

61. Bottini G, Cappa S, Geminiani G, *et al.* Topographic disorientation—A case report. *Neuropsychologia.* 1990;28(3):309–12.

62. De Renzi E, Faglioni P, and Villa P. Topographical amnesia. *J Neurol Neurosur Ps.* 1977;40(5):498–505.

63. Habib M and Sirigu A. Pure Topographical Disorientation: A Definition and Anatomical Basis. *Cortex.* 1987;23(1):73–85.

64. Maguire EA, Burke T, Phillips J, *et al.* Topographical disorientation following unilateral temporal lobe lesions in humans. *Neuropsychologia.* 1996;34(10):993–1001.

65. Maguire EA, Frackowiak RSJ, and Frith CD. Recalling Routes around London: Activation of the Right Hippocampus in Taxi Drivers. *J Neurosci.* 1997;17(18):7103–10.

66. Turriziani P, Carlesimo GA, Perri R, *et al.* Loss of spatial learning in a patient with topographical disorientation in new environments. *J Neurol Neurosur Ps.*. 2003;74(1):61–9.

67. Gron G, Wunderlich AP, Spitzer M, *et al.* Brain activation during human navigation: Gender-different neural networks as substrate of performance. *Nat Neurosci.* 2000;3(4):404–8.

68. Hartley T, Maguire EA, Spiers HJ, *et al.* The Well-Worn Route and the Path Less Traveled: Distinct Neural Bases of Route Following and Wayfinding in Humans. *Neuron.* 2003;37(5):877–88.

69. Hartley T, Bird CM, Chan D, *et al.* The hippocampus is required for short-term topographical memory in humans. *Hippocampus.* 2007;17(1):34–48.

70. Cohen NJ, Ryan J, Hunt C, *et al.* Hippocampal system and declarative (relational) memory: Summarizing the data from functional neuroimaging studies. *Hippocampus.* 1999;9(1):83–98.

71. Davachi L. Item, context and relational episodic encoding in humans. *Curr Opin Neurobiol.* 2006;16(6):693–700.

72. Rizzolatti G, Fogassi L, and Gallese V. Cortical mechanisms subserving object grasping and action recognition: A new view on the cortical motor functions. In: MS Gazzaniga (ed.). *The New Cognitive Neurosciences.* Cambridge, MA: MIT Press, 2000, pp. 539–52.

73. Schacter D and Tulving E. *Memory Systems.* Cambridge, MA: MIT Press, 1994.

74. Martone M, Butters N, Payne M, *et al.* DIssociations between skill learning and verbal recognition in amnesia and dementia. *Arch Neurol-Chicago.* 1984;41(9):965–70.

75. Basso A, Spinnler H, Vallar G, *et al.* Left hemisphere damage and selective impairment of auditory verbal short-term memory. A case study. *Neuropsychologia.* 1982;20(3):263–74.

76. Saffran EM and Marin OSM. Immediate memory for word lists and sentences in a patient with deficient auditory short-term memory. *Brain Lang.* 1975;2(0):420–33.

77. Warrington EK and Shallice T. The Selective Impairment Of Auditory Verbal Short-Term Memory. *Brain.* 1969;92(4):885–96.

78. Vallar G and Shallice T. *Neuropsychological Impairments of Short-Term Memory.* Cambridge: Cambridge University Press, 1990.

79. Vallar G and Papagno C. Neuropsychological impairments of verbal short-term memory. In: A Baddeley, MD Kopelman, and BA Wilson (eds). *Handbook of Memory Disorders,* 2nd edn. Chichester: Wiley, 2002, pp. 249–70.

80. De Renzi E. *Disorders of Space Explanation and Cognition.* Chichester: John Wiley, 1982.

81. Hanley RJ, Pearson NA, and Young AW. Impaired Memory For New Visual Forms. *Brain.* 1990;113(4):1131–48.

82. Cermak LS and O'Connor M. The anterograde and retrograde retrieval ability of a patient with amnesia due to encephalitis. *Neuropsychologia.* 1983;21(3):213–34.

83. Zola-Morgan S, Squire LR, and Amaral DG. Human amnesia and the medial temporal region: Enduring memory impairment following a bilateral lesion limited to field CA1 of the hippocampus. *JNeurosci.*1986;6(10):2950–67.

84. Winocur G, McDonald RM, and Moscovitch M. Anterograde and retrograde amnesia in rats with large hippocampal lesions. *Hippocampus.* 2001;11(1):18–26.

85. Graff-Radford NR, Tranel D, *et al.* Diencephalic Amnesia. *Brain.* 1990;113(1):1–25.

86. Guinan EM, Lowy C, Stanhope N, *et al.* Cognitive effects of pituitary tumours and their treatments: Two case studies and an investigation of 90 patients. *J Neurol Neurosur Ps.* 1998;65(6):870–6.

87. Kapur N, Scholey K, Moore E, *et al.* Long-Term Retention Deficits in Two Cases of Disproportionate Retrograde Amnesia. *J Cognitive Neurosci.* 1996;8(5):416–34.

88. Parkin AJ and Hunkin NM. Impaired Temporal Context Memory on Anterograde But Not Retrograde Tests in the Absence of Frontal Pathology. *Cortex.* 1993;29(2):267–80.

89. Colchester A, Kingsley D, Lasserson D, *et al.* Structural MRI volumetric analysis in patients with organic amnesia, 1: Methods and comparative findings across diagnostic groups. *J Neurol Neurosur Ps.* 2001;71(1):13–22.

90. Kapur N, Barker S, Burrows EH, *et al.* Herpes simplex encephalitis: Long term magnetic resonance imaging and neuropsychological profile. *J Neurol Neurosur Ps.* 1994;57(11):1334–42.

91. Kopelman MD, Lasserson D, Kingsley D, *et al.* Structural MRI volumetric analysis in patients with organic amnesia, 2: Correlations with anterograde memory and executive tests in 40 patients. *J Neurol Neurosur Ps.* 2001;71(1):23–8.

92. Fink GR, Markowitsch HJ, Reinkemeier M, *et al.* Cerebral Representation of One's Own Past: Neural Networks Involved in Autobiographical Memory. *J Neurosci.* 1996;16(13):4275–82.

93. Kopelman MD, Lasserson D, Kingsley DR, *et al.* Retrograde amnesia and the volume of critical brain structures. *Hippocampus.* 2003;13(8):879–91.

94. Verfaellie M, Koseff P, and Alexander MP. Acquisition of novel semantic information in amnesia: Effects of lesion location. *Neuropsychologia.* 2000;38(4):484–92.

95. Levine B, Black SE, Cabeza R, *et al.* Episodic memory and the self in a case of isolated retrograde amnesia. *Brain.* 1998;121(10):1951–73.

96. Hodges JR and McCarthy RA. Loss of remote memory: A cognitive neuropsychological perspective. *Curr Opin Neurobiol.* 1995;5(2):178–83.

97. Kapur N. Focal Retrograde Amnesia in Neurological Disease: A Critical Review. *Cortex.* 1993;29(2):217–34.

98. Brown JW and Chobor KL. Severe retrograde amnesia. *Aphasiology.* 1995;9(2):163–70.

99. Markowitsch HJ, Calabrese P, Haupts M, *et al.* Searching for the anatomical basis of retrograde amnesia. *J Clin Exp Neuropsyc.* 1993;15(6):947–67.

100. O'Connor M, Butters N, Miliotis P, *et al.* The dissociation of anterograde and retrograde amnesia in a patient with herpes encephalitis. *J Clin Exp Neuropsyc.* 1992;14(2):159–78.

101. Kopelman, MD. *Focal Retrograde Amnesia and the Attribution of Causality: An Exceptionally Critical Review.* Abingdon: Taylor & Francis, 2000.

102. Kopelman MD. Remote and autobiographical memory, temporal context memory and frontal atrophy in Korsakoff and Alzheimer patients. *Neuropsychologia.* 1989;27(4):437–60.

103. Mayes AR, Downes JJ, McDonald C, *et al.* Two tests for assessing remote public knowledge: A tool for assessing retrograde amnesia. *Memory.*1994;2(2):183–210.

104. Parkin AJ. Recent advances in the neuropsychology of memory. In: J Weinman and J Hunter (eds). *Memory: Neurochemical and Abnormal Perspectives.* London: Harwood Academic, 1991, pp. 141–62.

105. Shimamura AP. Priming effects in amnesia: Evidence for a dissociable memory function. *Q J Exp Psychol–A.* 1986;38(4-A):619–44.

106. Bright P, Buckman J, Fradera A, *et al.* Retrograde amnesia in patients with hippocampal, medial temporal, temporal lobe, or frontal pathology. *Learn Memory.* 2006;13(5):545–57.

107. Reed LJ, Lasserson D, Marsden P, *et al.* Correlations of regional cerebral metabolism with memory performance and executive function in patients with herpes encephalitis or frontal lobe lesions. *Neuropsychology.* 2005;19(5):555–65.

108. Vincent A, Buckley C, Schott JM, *et al.* Potassium channel antibody-associated encephalopathy: A potentially immunotherapy-responsive form of limbic encephalitis. *Brain.* 2004;127(3):701–12.

109. Holmes EJ, Butters N, Jacobson S, *et al.* An examination of the effects of mammillary-body lesions on reversal learning sets in monkeys. *Physiol Psychol.* 1983;11(3):159–65.

110. Murray EA, Davidson M, Gaffan D, *et al.* Effects of fornix transection and cingulate cortical ablation on spatial memory in rhesus monkeys. *Exp Brain Res.* 1989;74(1):173–86.

111. Hodges JR and Patterson K. Semantic dementia: A unique clinico-pathological syndrome. *Lancet Neurol.* 2007;6(11):1004–14.

112. Howard D and Patterson K. *The Pyramids and Palm Trees Test.* Bury St. Edmunds: Thames Valley Test Company, 1992.

113. Hodges Jr, Patterson K, Oxbury S, *et al.* Semantic Dementia: Progressive Fluent Aphasia with Temporal Lobe Atrophy. *Brain.* 1992;115(6):1783–806.

114. Murre JMJ, Graham KS, and Hodges JR. Semantic dementia: Relevance to connectionist models of long-term memory. *Brain.* 2001;124(4):647–75.

115. Snowden JS, Goulding PJ, and Neary D. Semantic dementia: A form of circumscribed cerebral atrophy. *Behav Neurol.* 1989;2(3):167–82.

116. Westmacott R, Leach L, Freedman M, *et al.* Different Patterns of Autobiographical Memory Loss in Semantic Dementia and Medial Temporal Lobe Amnesia: A Challenge to Consolidation Theory. *Neurocase.* 2001;7(1):37–55.

117. Maguire EA, Kumaran D, Hassabis D, *et al.* Autobiographical memory in semantic dementia: A longitudinal fMRI study. *Neuropsychologia.* 2010;48(1):123–36.

118. Hodges JR, Salmon DP, and Butters N. Semantic memory impairment in Alzheimer's disease: Failure of access or degraded knowledge? *Neuropsychologia.* 1992;30(4):301–14.

119. Hokkanen L, Salonen O, and Launes J. AMnesia in acute herpetic and nonherpetic encephalitis. *Arch Neurol–Chicago.* 1996;53(10):972–8.

120. Binney RJ, Embleton KV, Jefferies E, *et al.* The Ventral and Inferolateral Aspects of the Anterior Temporal Lobe Are Crucial in Semantic Memory: Evidence from a Novel Direct Comparison of Distortion-Corrected fMRI, rTMS, and Semantic Dementia. *Cerebral Cortex.* 2010;20(11):2728–38.

121. Ostergaard AL. Priming deficits in amnesia: Now you see them, now you don't. *Journal of the International Neuropsychological Society.* 1999;5:175–90.

122. Corkin S, Amaral DG, Gonzalez RG, *et al.* H.M.'s medial temporal lobe lesion: Findings from magnetic resonance imaging. *J Neurosci.*1997;17(10):3964–79.

123. Moscovitch M. Multiple dissociations of function in amnesia. In: LS Cermak (ed.). *Human Memory and Amnesia.* Hillsdale, NJ: Lawrence Erlbaum, 1982, pp. 337–70.

124. Wilson BA and Wearing D. Prisoner of consciousness: A state of just awakening following herpes simplex encephalitis. In: R Campbell and MA Conway (eds). *Broken Memories.* Oxford: Blackwell, 1985, pp. 14–30.

125. Reber PJ and Squire LR. Intact learning of artificial grammars and intact category learning by patients with Parkinson's disease. *Behav Neurosci.* 1999;113(2):235–42.

126. Migo EM, Mayes AR, and Montaldi D. Measuring recollection and familiarity: Improving the remember/know procedure. *Conscious Cogn.* 2012;21(3):1435–55.

127. Yonelinas AP. The Nature of Recollection and Familiarity: A Review of 30 Years of Research. *J Mem Lang.* 2002;46(3):441–517.

128. Holdstock JS, Parslow DM, Morris RG, *et al.* Two case studies illustrating how relatively selective hippocampal lesions in humans can have quite different effects on memory. *Hippocampus.* 2008;18(7):679–91.

129. Aggleton JP and Shaw C. Amnesia and recognition memory: A re-analysis of psychometric data. *Neuropsychologia.* 1996;34(1):51–62.

130. Craik FIM and McDowd JM. Age Differences in Recall and Recognition. *J Exp Psychol Learn.* 1987;13(3):474–9.

131. Aleman A, Hijman R, de Haan EH, *et al.* Memory impairment in schizophrenia: A meta-analysis. *Am J Psychiat.* 1999;156(9):1358–66.

132. Bennetto L, Pennington BF, and Rogers SJ. Intact and Impaired Memory Functions in Autism. *Child Development.* 1996;67(4):1816–35.

133. Wheeler MA, Stuss DT, and Tulving E. Frontal lobe damage produces episodic memory impairment. *Journal of the International Neuropsychological Society.* 1995;1(06):525–36.

134. Wechsler, D. (2009). Wechsler Memory Scale—Fourth Edition (WMS-IV) technical and interpretive manual. San Antonio, TX: Pearson, 2009.

135. Delis DC, Kramer JH, Kaplan E, *et al.* The California Verbal Learning Test II. San Antonio, TX: Psychological Corporation, 2000.

136. Oserrieth PA. The test of copying a complex figure: A contribution to the study of perception and memory. *Archives de Psychologie.* 1944;30:286–356.

137. Kopelman MD, Wilson B, and Baddeley A. *Autobiographical Memory Interview.* Oxford: Pearson Assessments, 1990.

138. Shiel A, Wilson BA, Emslie H, *et al. Prospective Memory Test.* Cambridge: Pearson, 2005.

139. Lezak MD, Howieson DB, Bigler ED, *et al. Neuropsychological Assessment,* 5th edn. Oxford: Oxford University Press, 2012.

140. Strauss E, Sherman EMS, and Spreen O. *A Compendium of Neuropsychological Tests.* Oxord: Oxford University Press, 2006.

141. Saling MM. Verbal memory in mesial temporal lobe epilepsy: Beyond material specificity. *Brain*. 2009;132(3):570–82.

142. Baddeley AD, Emslie H, and Nimmo-Smith I. *Doors and People*. London: Pearson Assessment, 2006.

143. Oddy M, Coughlan A, and Crawford J. *BIRT Memory & Information Processing Battery*. Horsham: Brain Injury Research Trust, 2007.

144. Warrington E. *Recognition Memory Test Manual*. Windsor: Nfer-Nelson, 1984.

145. Wechsler D. *Wechsler Adult Intelligence Scale*, 4th edn. San Antonio, TX: Pearson, 2008.

146. Corsi PM. *Human Memory and the Medial Temporal Region of the Brain*. PhD thesis, McGill University, 1972.

147. Tombaugh TN. *Test of Memory Malingering*. Toronto: Multi-Health Systems, 1996.

148. Green P. *Green's Word Memory Test for Microsoft Windows: User's Manual*. Edmonton, Canada: Green's Publishing Inc., 2003.

149. Warrington EK. *Camden Pictorial Recognition Memory Test*. Windsor: Infernelson, 1996.

150. McConley R, Martin R, Palmer CA, *et al*. Rey Osterrieth complex figure test spatial and figural scoring: Relations to seizure focus and hippocampal pathology in patients with temporal lobe epilepsy. *Epilepsy & Behavior*. 2008;13(1):174–7.

151. Wilson BA, Greenfield E, Clare L, *et al*. *Rivermead Behavioural Memory Test*. London: Pearson, 2008.

152. Davidson PSR, Troyer AK, and Moscovitch M. Frontal lobe contributions to recognition and recall: Linking basic research with clinical evaluation and remediation. *Journal of the International Neuropsychological Society*. 2006;12(02):210–23.

153. Zigmond AS and Snaith RP. The Hospital Anxiety and Depression Scale. *Acta Psychiat Scand*. 1983;67(6):361–70.

154. Beck AT, Steer RA, Ball R, *et al*. Comparison of Beck Depression Inventories-IA and-II in Psychiatric Outpatients. *J Pers Assess*. 1996;67(3):588–97.

155. Kizilbash AH, Vanderploeg RD, and Curtiss G. The effects of depression and anxiety on memory performance. *Arch Clin Neuropsych*. 2002;17(1):57–67.

156. Smith G, Del Sala S, Logie RH, *et al*. Prospective and retrospective memory in normal ageing and dementia: A questionnaire study. *Memory*. 2000;8(5):311–21.

CHAPTER 14

Vision and visual processing deficits

Anna Katharina Schaadt and Georg Kerkhoff

Introduction

Visual disorders are frequent function losses after brain damage and occur in about 20–50 per cent of the patients with cerebrovascular disorders[1] and some 50 per cent of patients with traumatic brain injury (TBI).[2] In stroke patients > 65 years the incidence rises to 40–60 per cent.[3] In Alzheimer's disease (AD), visual impairments (low-level and high-level) occur in some 40 per cent of patients.[4] They are core features of posterior cortical atrophy (PCA). Consequently, routine screening of the various types of visual deficits is necessary both for diagnosis and rehabilitation planning. Patients with intact awareness can easily be questioned with a simple questionnaire (see Table 14.1), responses to which prove clinically useful in 95 per cent of cases.[5,6]

Visual acuity impairments

Visual acuity refers to the spatial resolution of the visual processing system[7] and is usually tested using high-contrast acuity plates (Fig. 14.1a). It is important to appreciate that impairments of visual acuity and spatial contrast sensitivity (see below) will often lead to difficulties for patients in performing higher-level neuropsychological tests, thus it is essential to test basic visual function before interpreting deficits on cognitive visual tests.[8]

Concerning deficits of visual acuity, primary and secondary causes have to be distinguished in patients with brain damage before initiating treatment.

Primary causes

Bilateral postchiasmatic lesions[9] which may cause partial up to total loss of visual acuity in both eyes which cannot be corrected by lenses. This is often associated with bilateral homonymous visual field defects.[10]

Secondary causes

Disturbed visual exploration, fixation difficulties due to Bálint–Holmes syndrome, impaired contrast sensitivity, eccentric fixation due to cerebral hypoxia, or nystagmus. Impairments in acuity for moving targets (dynamic acuity) are caused by deficient smooth pursuit eye movements,[11] due to cerebellar or parietal lesions.

Recovery is frequent in patients with secondary, but rare in those with primary causes of disturbed visual acuity. As impaired acuity affects all subsequent visual activities as well as neuropsychological testing, treatment of the secondary causes should be started immediately.

Treatment

The following short recommendations may be helpful, primarily for patients with non-progressive disorders (cf reference 2):

Bilateral postchiasmatic lesion: Use magnification software (for PCs) or screen-reading machines for permanent enlargement of printed text, pictures, and letters.

Visual exploration deficit: Improve visual search by providing the patient with a systematic (horizontally or vertically) saccadic search strategy. Acuity will improve when visual search is more systematic, quicker, and when omissions are reduced.

Nystagmus: Reduce nystagmus with orthoptic (prisms) or pharmacological means.[12]

Spasmodic fixation (Bálint–Holmes syndrome): Test acuity with *single* letter charts, as acuity for single letters should be normal as long as the patient can fixate the single target. Furthermore, improving simultaneous perception by repetitive treatment enlarges the useful field of view[13] and improves visual activities of daily living.

Dynamic visual acuity: Treat smooth pursuit eye movements in the horizontal domain (left, right) for different velocities. The recognition of moving objects is important for vocational tasks[14] and mobility in the environment. It improves in parallel with the increase of the smooth pursuit gain (relation of target velocity to eye–movement velocity).

Spatial contrast sensitivity (CS) impairments

Spatial CS denotes the ability to discriminate between striped patterns (gratings) of differing luminance (contrast) and stripe width (spatial frequency). It is often impaired in acute vascular posterior brain lesions (80 per cent).[15] In the majority of patients, recovery is rapid, although permanent deficits persist in about 20 per cent. An example for the assessment of CS is illustrated in Fig. 14.1b. CS also diminishes in AD.[16,17]

Treatment

CS can be trained effectively in normal subjects but this has rarely been tried in brain-damaged patients. In those 20 per cent with permanent deficits, the use of additional, indirect lighting is helpful because it improves contrast. Light-filtering lenses may increase contrast sensitivity.[18]

Table 14.1 Schema for the anamnesis of visual disorders after acquired brain lesions. Indent the questions in the table into the following phrase: 'Did you experience … since your brain lesion?'

Question	Purpose of Question, Underlying Disorder
1. any changes in vision?	◆ Awareness of deficits? Information about case history
2. diplopia? transiently/permanently?	◆ Type of gaze palsy? If transient: fusional disorder?
3. reading problems? syllables/words missing, change of line, reduced reading span?	◆ Hemianopic alexia? Differential diagnosis of neglect dyslexia, aphasic alexia, or pure alexia
4. problems in estimating depth on a staircase? reaching with your unimpaired hand for a cup, hand, door handle?	◆ Depth perception? Optic ataxia?
5. bumping into obstacles? failure to notice persons? at which side?	◆ Visual exploration deficits in homonymous visual field disorders?
6. blinding after exposure to bright light?	◆ Foveal photopic adaptation?
7. dark vision? that you need more light for reading?	◆ Foveal scotopic adaptation?
8. blurred vision? transiently/permanently?	◆ Contrast sensitivity? Acuity? Fusion?
9. that colours look darker, paler, less saturated?	◆ Colour hue discrimination? Impaired contrast sensitivity?
10. that faces look darker, paler, unfamiliar?	◆ Face discrimination/recognition disorders?
11. problems in recognizing objects?	◆ Object discrimination/recognition disorders?
12. problems in finding your way in familiar/unfamiliar environments?	◆ Topographic orientation deficits?
13. visual hallucinations (stars, dots, lines, fog, faces, objects) or illusions (distorted objects, faces)?	◆ Simple or complex visual hallucinations, illusions? Awareness about illusory character?

Adapted from *Neurorehabilitation & Neural Repair.* Neumann G, Schaadt A-K, Reinhart S, and Kerkhoff G, Clinical and psychometric evaluations of the Cerebral Vision Screening Questionnaire in 461 non-aphasic individuals post-stroke, Copyright (2016), with permission from SAGE Publications.

Disorders of foveal photopic or scotopic adaptation

Foveal photopic adaptation means the continuous adapting to a brighter illumination than the current one, scotopic adaptation the adaptation to a darker illumination than the present one. Both processes are dissociable and impaired in some 20 per cent of patients with posterior cerebral artery infarctions or cerebral hypoxia.[19] A questionnaire for the assessment of the most frequent subjective complaints

in these patients can be found at: http://tinyurl.com/SADQ-Kerkhoff. The case report in Box 14.1 illustrates the subjective visual impairments associated with a foveal photopic adaptation deficit. Concerning recovery, there is no evidence (even after years) that such deficits recover.[19]

Treatment

Photopic adapation

Avoid direct lighting, use a dimmer to adjust light individually; avoid flickering neon lights; use sunglasses outside buildings; avoid

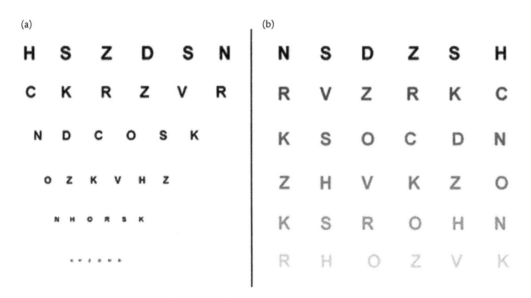

Fig. 14.1 Examples for assessing visual acuity (a) and spatial contrast sensitivity (b). For assessing visual acuity, size but not spatial contrast of the symbols diminishes; for assessing spatial contrast, sensitivity size of the characters is constant whereas spatial contrast diminishes.

Box 14.1 Foveal photopic adaptation

Case study

Since his stroke (right posterior cerebral artery infarction with associated left homonymous hemianopia), this patient has been unable to stay longer than 10 minutes in bright environments without feeling highly uncomfortable and getting severe headache. The adaptation deficit is subjectively more disturbing to him than the visual field loss. At work, for example, he would always darken the room he is sitting in. When colleagues come to his office, they would always complain about the darkness and turn on the lights. In the examiner's office, the patient considered the luminance as comfortable when the room was nearly fully darkened (50 lux).

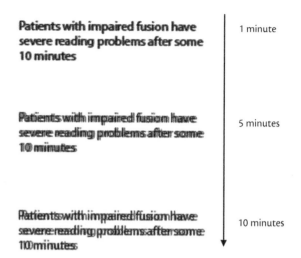

Fig. 14.2 Schematic illustration of the development of diplopic images in patients with fusion disorders as a function of time. Black and gray traces refer to the optic image of the left/right eye. Note blurring and finally diplopia after sustained binocular vision.

continuously adapting sunglasses (Varilux) because they are too slow in readapting inside a building. Driving at night ('blinding') is not advisable. If there is photophobia, light-filtering lenses can also reduce this sensation.[18]

Scotopic adaptation

Increase indirect lighting by additional light bulbs; use also portable dimmer to adjust lighting individually.

Disorders of convergent fusion and stereopsis

Stereopsis refers to the perception of spatial depth based on binocular integration. Convergent fusion is a prerequisite of stereopsis and means the fusion of the left and right eye's image into one combined (fused) picture of the world.[20] Fusion and stereopsis (local, global) are reduced in patients with vascular occipital, parietal, or temporal brain lesions,[21] and impair manual activities in near space (reaching and grasping, technical work, depth perception), which is also relevant for vocational rehabilitation. Astereopsis is also caused by TBI.[22] Fusion is impaired in some 20 per cent of patients with posterior vascular lesions and about one-third of TBI patients.[2] Those patients have severe reading problems after some 10 minutes (see Fig. 14.2). They rapidly develop diplopia and are impaired in all near-work activities.

The percentage of patients showing recovery is unknown in astereopsis. In TBI patients with fusional disorders, three-quarters have persistent impairments for years after their injury.[23]

Treatment

Fusion and stereopsis can be trained together using simple orthoptic or binocular devices.[24-26] First, determine from the history whether there are asthenopic symptoms (sensation of eye pressure, fatigue in reading or with PC work), blurred vision, problems in near-work activities, and how long the patient can read before blurred vision or diplopia emerges. Improvement of fusion and stereopsis can occur with repetitive display of dichoptic images with increasing disparity angle; 8–20 sessions advisable.[24-26] The outcome is favourable in 80 per cent of patients, with improvements in reading duration, stereopsis, and fusional range; relief from asthenopia; and better function in vocational life. However, this therapy is contra-indicated in patients with premorbid deficits in binocular integration or those with permanent diplopia of exophoria > 15°.

Visual discomfort

Looking at homogeneous, regular patterns like lines, written text, flagstones, or stripes of a certain spatial frequency (three to four cycles per degree visual angle)[27] may elicit unpleasant sensations (termed 'visual discomfort'; see Fig. 14.3a, b), blurred vision, and headaches in some healthy people, but much more so in patients with cerebral visual disorders. Visual discomfort in brain-lesioned patients may reduce sustained visual activities considerably and lead to asthenopic symptoms. There is no evidence so far that such symptoms recover naturally.

Treatment

In reading, visual discomfort can be eliminated by using a simple mask that covers all lines except the one that is currently read (see Fig. 14.3c).

Homonymous visual field disorders

Visual field disorders (VFDs) are present in 20–50 per cent of all neurological patients with stroke[1] and may also be present in patients with PCA. Visual field sparing is < 5° for the affected visual hemifield in 70 per cent of stroke cases with VFDs who receive specific neurovisual treatment in neurorehabilitation centres.[7,10] In acute neurology settings, visual field sparing on the blind side may be more variable. Fig. 14.4 demonstrates the most frequent types of VFD, although in patients with PCA such classical patterns are not usually present, or may vary, sometimes leading to the erroneous conclusion that the patient is psychogenic. Patients may present three types of associated deficits: visual exploration deficits, reading disorders, and visuospatial deficits.

Visual exploration deficit

Time-consuming, inefficient visual search due to loss of overview and unsystematic search strategies; numerous, small-amplitude staircase-saccades in the blind hemifield; omissions of targets in the blind field.[28-31]

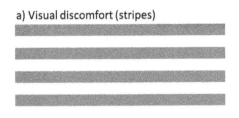

a) Visual discomfort (stripes)

b) Visual discomfort (text)

Looking at homogeneous written text
may elicit unpleasant sensations, blurred vision and headaches in some
healthy subjects, but much more so
in patients with cerebral visual disorders

c) Visual discomfort (cover template)

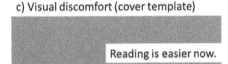

Reading is easier now.

Fig. 14.3 Illustration of the visual discomfort phenomenon with stripes (a), text (b), as well as its removal with a cover template (c).
Reproduced from Habermann C and Kolster F, *Ergotherapie im Arbeitsfeld Neurologie*, Copyright (2008), with permission from Thieme Medical Publishers.

Hemianopic reading disorder

For reading, the central visual field (+/–5° around the fovea) is crucial because only here visual acuity and form recognition are sufficient for letter recognition ('perceptual reading window'). Slow reading with errors is evident in patients with field sparing < 5°, as well as those with paracentral scotomas and quadrantanopia; however, reading of short, single words is normal (no aphasia or alexia).[32–34] Fig. 14.5 illustrates the impairment in reading depending on the type of VFD (see also chapter 18).

Visuospatial deficits

The patient's feeling of the subjective visual straight ahead in space or his subjective midline in bisecting horizontal lines and objects is shifted *towards* the blind field (horizontally in left/right VFDs, vertically in altitudinal VFDs, oblique in quadrantic VFDs) in 90 per cent of the patients.[35–38] This spatial shift is also evident in pointing[29] and in daily life (walking through doorways, sitting in front of a table). Line bisection can be used for the differential diagnosis of hemianopia versus visual neglect (see chapter 15). While the subjective midline in homonymous hemianopia is shifted *towards* the blind field (contralesional), it is ipsilesionally displaced away from the neglected side, in patients with visual neglect (see Fig. 14.6).[36,40,41] The line bisection error is not due to eccentric fixation[42] and attentional cueing does not change it.[43] A recent study identified lesions in Brodmann area 18 (lingual gyrus) as crucial.[44] Patients with homonymous quadrantanopia show a related, oblique shift of their subjective visual straight ahead towards the scotoma (see Fig. 14.6b).[37]

Field recovery is present in the first two to three months postlesion in up to 40 per cent of the patients with a stable aetiology such as stroke.[45] After six months post-lesion, spontaneous recovery is extremely unlikely.[45,46]

Treatment

Field recovery is very limited, and therefore restorative field training is appropriate only in a very small group of patients, detailed below. For the majority of VFD patients (95 per cent) compensatory visual field treatment of the associated disorders in reading and visual scanning is advocated as the standard treatment for patients with VFDs (see Table 14.2). While restorative visual field training induces only very small or no visual field increases (~1°) and improves visual search or reading only minimally,[47] hemianopic reading training and visual exploration training induce significant, lasting, and functionally relevant improvements in these treated domains. Thus, these treatments improve 'visual' activities of daily living and increase functional independence of the patient.[2,7,10,34,48] Cross-modal (visual-auditory) training has also

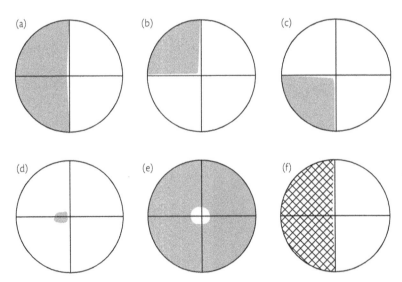

Fig. 14.4 Most frequent types of homonymous visual field defects: (a) left hemianopia, (b) left superior quadrantanopia, (c) left inferior quadrantanopia, (d) left paracentral scotoma, (e) tunnel vision, (f) left hemiamblyopia (loss of colour and form vision along with relatively intact light perception).
Reproduced from Habermann C and Kolster F, *Ergotherapie im Arbeitsfeld Neurologie*, Copyright (2008), with permission from Thieme Medical Publishers.

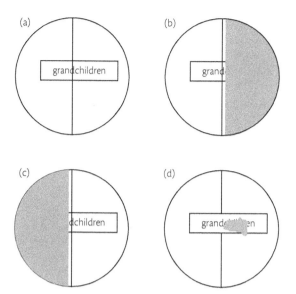

Fig. 14.5 Importance of the central visual field for reading ('perceptual reading window'). In healthy people with Western reading habits, the reading window is larger in the right paramacular hemifield so that right hemianopia (b) or a right paracentral scotoma (d) affect a bigger part of the reading window. In contrast, left hemianopia only affects a smaller part of the reading window (c), resulting in less marked reading impairment.

Reproduced from Habermann C and Kolster F, *Ergotherapie im Arbeitsfeld Neurologie*, Copyright (2008), with permission from Thieme Medical Publishers.

been used for improvement of reading and scanning in hemianopia.[49,50] Visual and auditory targets are presented time-locked in locations of the visual field, and the patient has to saccade to them. This training induces similar improvements as conventional visual scanning training but requires additional technical facilities.

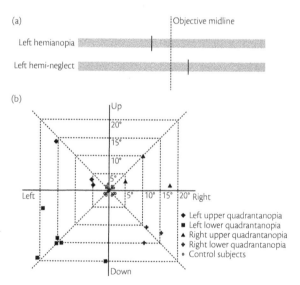

Fig. 14.6 Illustration of the horizontal line bisection error: (a) In left hemianopia, the subjective midpoint is shifted towards the blind hemifield, in left hemineglect it is biased towards the ipsilesional hemifield. (b) Oblique shifts of the subjective visual straight ahead direction towards the scotoma in different types of homonymous quarantanopia, without visual neglect.

Adapted from *Neuropsychologia*. 48(11), Kuhn C, Heywood C, Kerkhoff G. Oblique spatial shifts of subjective visual straight ahead orientation in quadrantic visual field defects, pp. 3205–10, Copyright (2010), with permission from Elsevier.

Table 14.2 Summary of restorative (visual field training) and compensatory approaches (hemianopic reading and visual exploration training) in patients with postchiasmatic scotomata

Restorative visual field training:

(1) *Anamnesis:* visual perimetry, tachistoscopic tests: identification of amblyopic transition zones which are most likely candidates for field recovery

(2) *Type of treatment:* improvement of saccadic localization at field border or in amblyopic transition zone; discourage head movements to target; recognition of colour, form, orientation, or luminance of the target; amount of treatment: 30–500 sessions (hours)

(3) *Transfer: very small* improvements in reading and subjective awareness of visual problems; minimal improvement in visual search

(4) *Outcome and follow-up: small or no visual* field increase; partial field recovery in exceptional patients with incomplete lesions

Hemianopic reading training:

(1) *Anamnesis:* problems with change of line, types of errors (omissions, substitutions, problems with long words or numbers), maximum reading duration, asthenopic disorders (eye strain)

(2) *Type of treatment:* improvement of oculomotor reading strategies (i.e. optokinetic reading therapy) substituting the lost parafoveal visual field; tachistoscopic reading of single words, moving window technique, floating words, search for words in a text, scanning reading technique, reading of numbers with embedded zeros: variation of physical and linguistic parameters: word length and frequency, position on screen (left, centre, right), number of words, presentation time, complexity of text, variation of instruction (read versus scan text), verbal working memory training

(3) *Transfer:* reading of newspaper, book, own manuscripts; text editing on a PC, increase of maximal reading duration

(4) *Outcome and follow-up:* increase in reading speed; reduction in reading errors; small field recovery in one-third of patients; improvements in reading eye movements

Visual exploration training:

(1) *Anamnesis:* limited overview, bumping into persons and obstacles, defective orientation in visual space, i.e. crowded situations, traffic

(2) *Type of treatment:* increasing amplitude of saccadic eye movements towards scotoma: variation of size, increase of velocity of saccade, reduction of saccadic reaction time, reduction of head movements; systematic, spatially organized visual search on wide-field displays: organized search strategy (horizontal or vertical); start search in blind field; visual displays requiring serial and parallel search

(3) *Transfer:* orientation in clinic, own urban district, new environments, management of visual activities of daily living: find objects on table or in room, find therapist's room, find objects in supermarket, cross street, use public traffic, find way home

(4) *Outcome and follow-up:* reduction of omissions and search time; improved eye- movements; significant improvements in functional visual tasks (e.g. find objects on table); subjective improvements in patient's functional independence in daily life

Compensatory versus restorative visual field training

In recent years, restorative visual field training has been revived after publication of advantageous results following new training procedures.[51] However, numerous replication studies have failed to find significant visual field enlargements[30,52–54] or found only minimal visual field increases as described above. In our view, restorative field training is only promising when lesions are incomplete and a high degree of residual visual capacities (light, motion, form, or colour perception) is preserved in specific regions of the scotoma.[2,48] Moreover, compensatory field training leads to a much quicker reduction of visual impairments and needs fewer treatment sessions. Recently, home-based treatments of visual search and reading have been successfully tested in VFDs.[30,55,56] These approaches are cost-effective, but require regular advice by the therapist (i.e. by telephone or visit).

Ineffective or disadvantageous therapies

Most hemianopic patients get confused when using prisms to substitute the visual field loss. However, small prisms fitted to a spectacle can be useful in some cases.[57] Compensatory head shifts towards the scotoma (either spontaneously adopted by the patient or to instruction) are of *no use* in the rehabilitation of VFDs because they lead to visual exploration deficits in the ipsilesional visual field, strain of the neck muscles, and delay treatment progress in visual scanning training.[58] Training of 'blindsight' (the ability of rare cases of cortical blindness which respond to stimuli in their visual field, e.g. by pointing to them, even if they are not able to consciously perceive them) is probably not useful for the majority of the patients[59] because it does not lead to improved functioning in daily life.

Anton's syndrome

Unawareness of visual field defects is not an unfrequent phenomenon, with up to one-third of the patients showing a denial of their impairment (Anton's syndrome).[7,60,61] One the other hand, there has been the reverse condition reported in which patients with spared vision after visual field loss deny any visual sensation in the intact parts of their visual field.[62] Insufficient awareness is negatively associated with development and use of compensatory strategies and rehabilitation outcome.[63] Consequently, detailed assessment and education of the patient are inevitable to assure compliance and the conditions for a good outcome.

Positive visual phenomena (visual hallucinations)

Whereas the previously described disorders refer to function losses (i.e. negative visual phenomena), visual hallucinations are positive symptoms in the absence of an external stimulus.[64] Simple formed visual hallucinations (light dots, bars, lines, stars, fog, coloured sensations, etc.)[65] are frequently reported by patients—although only when questioned systematically—with posterior, vascular lesions, most often after occipital lesions. More complex visual hallucinations and illusions are rare in structural lesions and most often associated with temporal lobe lesions; see Fig. 14.7).[66,67,68] Recovery is rapid and complete in 95 per cent of the patients with stroke aetiology, so that at six weeks post-lesion the occurrence is quite rare.[66,67] Positive visual phenomena have also been described in AD,[69] and well-formed visual hallucinations, typically non-threatening and of silent animals or people, are core diagnostic features of dementia with Lewy bodies (DLB),[128] and very common in Parkinson's disease with dementia. Visual hallucinations are not uncommon in prion diseases, and in particular those patients presenting with visual impairment—the so-called Heidenhain variant.[70]

Treatment

As hallucinations and illusions are irritating but—in the case of structural lesions—mostly transient phenomena, informing and reassuring the patient is important.

Complex visual scenes have a higher reality character than simple hallucinations and are therefore more frightening to the patient. These patients may be reluctant to talk about their experience for fear of being misdiagnosed as a psychogenic. Note that psychiatric patients much more often have *auditory* than *visual* hallucinations, while the opposite holds true for patients with organic visual hallucinations after posterior brain lesions. Further, brain-damaged patients very rarely report 'hearing voices'. The complex well formed halluciantions of DLB and Parkinson's disease with dementia may respond very well to treatment with cholinesterase inhibitors.

Persistent visual hallucinations

Check if there is an epileptic focus (EEG), the possibility of a new infarction developing, or a psychiatric disease. Lasting visual hallucinations that interfere with visual recognition have been reported in Parkinson's disease.[71,72]

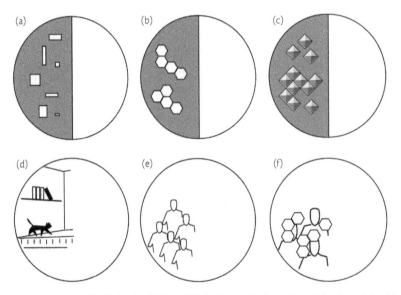

Fig. 14.7 Examples for positive visual phenomena (visual hallucinations); (a) and (b): simple visual hallucinations, (c): coloured visual hallucinations, (d), (e), (f) complex visual hallucinations.

Colour perception deficits

Colour perception can be impaired within a scotoma after a postchiasmatic VFD or within central vision caused by bilateral postchiasmatic lesions of various aetiologies.[73–75] The deficit is most apparent in central vision and may manifest as a subtle impairment in hue discrimination. Such disorders are often found after unilateral occipitotemporal lesions of vascular origin as well as after mild cerebral hypoxia or in Alzheimer's disease.[76,77] Total achromatopsia is much more rarely found, usually associated with bilateral occipitotemporal or diffuse lesions (see case study in Box 14.2).[78] Recovery of colour and form vision within a scotoma is often observed in patients with partial visual field recovery.[79] As a rule, the progression of visual recovery (if there is one) in VFDs is as follows: light detection → light localization → brightness discrimination → form discrimination → colour perception. In those patients with colour vision deficits in central vision no recovery has been reported over six years in one study.[80]

Treatment

Defective colour vision in visual field regions

In patients with residual colour perception in a scotoma and *incomplete* lesions, there is some evidence that improvement of colour discrimination can be trained by displaying coloured targets at the field border and having the patient saccade to them and discriminate the colour.

Defective colour perception in central vision

Forced discrimination of differently coloured forms is partially effective in cerebral anoxia, however with limited transfer to

---

Box 14.2 Cerebral achromatopsia

Case study

A 66-year-old man was washing his red car in a green meadow. Suddenly, he began to feel sick and noticed that his just-cleaned car appeared dirty, rusty brown, while the surrounding meadow looked more grey than green. The patient later reported that it seemed to him as if someone had switched off the colour TV into black-and-white mode. Furthermore, he described that although he had initially been able to recognize his car and house; later on he was not able anymore to see things in his upper field of vision. As illustrated below, the patient showed severe impairments in a colour-matching task. In contrast, discrimination of grey shades (not shown) as well as colour imagery were unimpaired. His symptoms were due to bilateral basal, temporo-occipital infarctions, associated with bilateral damage of lingual and fusiform gyri.

Examiner's arrangement of colours   Patient's attempt to match colours

     Original   *Patient's copy*

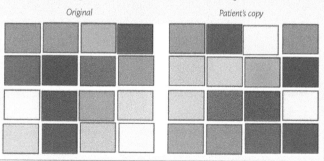

---

non-trained colours.[80] Often, patients can learn to base their colour judgments on other cues such as the brightness or saturation despite permanently impaired hue discrimination.

Visual form, object, and face perception deficits (visual agnosias)

The inability to recognize visual stimuli despite sufficiently intact elementary visual functions (e.g. visual acuity, spatial contrast sensitivity) as well as unaffected language processing and intact recognition in other modalities is defined as visual agnosia.[7] Depending on the severity and specifity of the visual recognition deficit, several types of agnosia can be distinguished.

Visual object agnosia refers to impairments in recognizing complex objects or pictures. Traditionally, a distinction has been made between apperceptive agnosia and associative agnosia. The former indicates a deficit in perception which leads to impaired object discrimination; the latter implies loss of semantic knowledge or understanding what the object is, despite patients seemingly having intact perceptual abilities. Thus while apperceptive agnosic patients have difficulty in copying objects or matching objects from different views (see Fig. 14.8a), patients with pure associative agnosia may copy and perform perceptual match tasks well but still not be able to say what an object is for—sometimes referred to as 'perception stripped of meaning',[81,82] a core feature of the semantic dementia subtype of frontotemporal dementia. Such behaviour needs to be distinguished from anomia where patients may not be able to name an object but nevertheless can describe what it is or how it might be used. Hence, patients with associative agnosia cannot even match objects by semantic properties as illustrated in Fig. 14.8c. Visual form agnosia refers to a severe type of apperceptive visual object agnosia, characterized by an inability to discriminate even simple forms like rectangles or squares (see Fig. 14.8b). Prosopagnosia corresponds to a selective deficit in recognizing faces.[7]

Visual agnosias are commonly described as rare conditions (less than 3 per cent of all neurological patients),[7,59,83] previously considered to occur most frequently after bilateral occipitotemporal lesions of vascular, traumatic, or anoxic origin.[81] However, recent evidence indicates that visual agnostic deficits might be more frequent than previously assumed when every patient with posterior brain lesions is quantitatively tested (e.g. Martinaud and colleagues[84] reporting a frequency of 65 per cent following posterior cerebral artery infarction). Moreover, with greater recognition of neurodegenerative conditions it is becoming evident that these too may lead to visual agnosia. Impairments in object processing have also been reported for neurodegenerative diseases like AD associated with or without PCA,[85–88] DLB,[85] corticobasal syndrome (CBS),[89] or Huntington's disease (HD) (e.g. recognition of overlapping figures).[90]

Standardized diagnostic is available with the Birmingham Object Recognition Battery (BORB),[91] or the Visual Object and Space Perception Battery (VOSP).[92]

Detailed case reports about recovery are rare. Partial recovery concerning object or face recognition of real-life objects has been occasionally noted, while recognition of photographs of objects or faces rarely improves. Recovery is particularly unlikely in anoxic brain damage, probably due to the widespread diffuse lesions and the additional cognitive impairment impeding the acquisition of compensatory strategies.[93] Partial recovery is more likely in

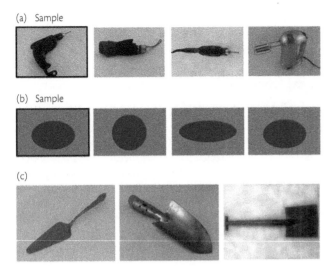

Fig. 14.8 Illustration of matching tasks in which agnostic patients depending on type of agnosia typically show deficits. (a) View-matching task: The patient has to match the sample to the target picture that is presented in a different view. Patients with apperceptive agnosia fail in such tasks as they are not able to form a coherent visual perception of an object. (b) Form-matching task (Efron shapes). Form agnostic patients typically have deficits in comparing and matching simple forms. (c) Function-match task: The subject has to match those two pictures that share a common function. Deficits in this task are characteristic for associative agnostic patients.

traumatic or vascular lesions and in those few cases with unilateral right sided lesions showing face agnosia.[81] A case of transient postoperative prosopagnosia that spontaneously recovered after six to seven days has been described,[94] demonstrating that recovery is in principle possible, but this may depend on lesion size.

Treatment

Visual form recognition can be improved in some cases by repetitive discrimination training for simple geometric forms equated for total luminance. Verbal or computerized feedback is essential with progressive increase in the similarity of the stimuli to be discriminated. Treatment can be accomplished either with self-constructed paper-made stimuli, or using computerized devices (e.g. Efron shapes) which give detailed quantitative feedback and allow variations of colours, sizes, and forms (cf. Kerkhoff & Marquardt).[95] Controlled treatment studies are rare for complex object- and face-recognition deficits. Improvements have been reported using errorless-learning paradigms focusing on specific search for key features of objects or faces.[7,59] In general, the use of context information (knowledge about objects and faces and the relevant social situation) and non-visual cues is advisable and may be helpful for some patients.[7]

Visuospatial disorders

Visuospatial disorders are frequent impairments following stroke affecting extrastriate cortical and subcortical brain areas (30–50 per cent after left, 50–70 per cent after right hemisphere stroke).[96] Moreover, poor visuospatial skills are often observed in conditions such as AD, PCA, DLB, and CBS.[85,97,98] Since intact visuospatial abilities are relevant for many activities of daily living (e.g. dressing, transfers, reading the clock), they are important predictors for rehabilitation outcome, particularly after right-hemisphere brain

damage.[99] Four categories of visuospatial disorders have been proposed that are compatible with the neuroanatomical conception of a dorsal and ventral visual pathway proposed by Ungerleider and Mishkin (see also individual chapters 3, 4, and 5).[100]

Perceptive visuospatial disorders

This group of impairments occurs after distinct lesions of (especially right-sided) parieto-occipital brain areas. More posterior lesions of these brain regions lead to deficits in estimation or discrimination of length, distance, or form. In contrast, more anterior (parieto-temporal) lesions are related to difficulties in estimating position or orientation as well as perceiving the subjective visual vertical/horizontal in the frontal and saggital plane; see Fig. 14.9a).[101,102]

Transformational visuospatial disorders

Some visuospatial tasks require spatial operations (rotation, mirroring, scale transformation). Deficits in perspective change or mental rotation tasks are related to parietal and parietooccipital lesions of both hemispheres; see Fig. 14.9b).[102]

Constructive visuospatial disorders

These deficits refer to a heterogenous group of functional deficits, manifest as impairments in the ability of patients to manually construct or copy a figure comprising simpler elements (e.g. drawing or copying a geometric figure in two or three dimensions, see Fig. 14.10a & b). 'Constructional apraxia' is the term often given to these deficits (not to be confused with limb apraxia). Despite their clinical and daily relevance as well as frequent co-occurrence with perceptive visuospatial, dysexecutive, and working memory deficits as well as neglect,[103] the core mechanisms of constructive visuospatial symptoms are still unknown.[102] Some authors have provided evidence for defective spatial remapping of locations across eye movements when information in retinal coordinates has to be transformed to locations in the external world.[104]

Topographic visuospatial disorders

Topographic visuospatial disorders refer to orientation deficits in the real as well as imagined three-dimensional space and are related

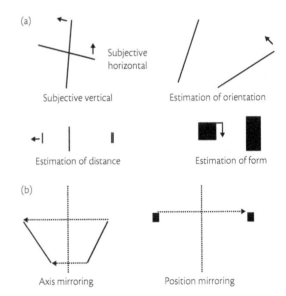

Fig. 14.9 (a) Examples for perceptual visuospatial tasks: subjective visual horizontal/vertical, estimation of orientation/distance/form. (b) Examples for cognitive visuospatial tasks: axis/position mirroring.

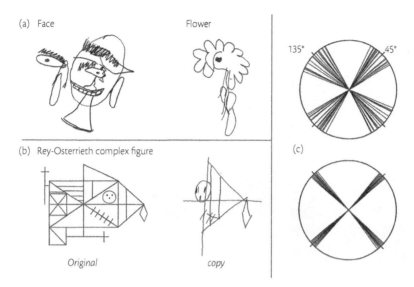

Fig. 14.10 (a) Performance of two patients with a constructive visuospatial disorder when requested to draw a flower respectively a face from memory. (b) Copying performance of a patient with constructive visuospatial disorder in the Rey–Osterrieth complex figure test. Note also neglect of left-sided elements. (c) Illustration of visual line-orientation-estimation performance before (above) and after systematic training for two oblique orientations (45° and 135°; following).

to parahippocampal lesions or can occur as secondary deficits in neglect or Bálint–Holmes syndrome.[102,105]

Treatment

Successful therapeutic approaches are feedback-based training of perceptual visuospatial abilities, visual background movement, constructive visuospatial training, reaction-chaining methods for topographic visuospatial disorders as well as ADL (activities of daily living) therapy.[106] These approaches including their therapeutic principles are summarized in Table 14.3. Concerning feedback-based training of visuospatial abilities, Funk and colleagues[107] have reported rapid and long-lasting improvements in visual line-orientation discrimination after systematic training along with transfer to other spatial domains such as visuoconstructive performance, clock reading, and horizontal writing (see Fig. 14.10c). In addition, non-invasive galvanic vestibular stimulation has been shown to improve subjective visual vertical judgements in patients suffering from right-sided stroke.[108] Treatments are, however, unlikely to help patients with progressive neurodegenerative disorders.

Visual motion perception deficits

Complete loss of movement perception (akinetopsia)[109] due to bilateral cerebral lesions is rather an unusual phenomenon.[78] More incomplete impairments of visual motion perception may occur with a frequency of 13 per cent after focal lesions of motion-sensitive regions, including area V5/MT in the occipito-parieto-temporal cortex, but permanent deficits are probably rare.[110] However, many brain-damaged patients report subjectively problems in estimating the velocity and position changes of moving vehicles in traffic situations as a pedestrian or when driving in a car. This may result either from impaired motion perception, possibly of impaired optic flow detection (radial patterns emerging when a subject moves),[111] disturbed visuospatial perception, smooth pursuit eye movements, or a combination of these factors. Moreover, deficits in motion perception have also been reported for patients

with AD, and particularly the PCA variant. While processing of linear moving patterns seems to be preserved, perception of optic flow is impaired in more than one-third of AD patients.[112,113]

Little is known about recovery. In those rare patients with bilateral lesions, no recovery has been reported,[114] while those with unilateral lesions may show recovery. Even the motion-blind patient reported by Zihl and colleagues re-adapted to moving stimuli in daily life by certain compensatory techniques, despite her permanent motion deficit under laboratory conditions.[114] Again, there are no realistic prospects for recovery in neurodegenerative cases.

Treatment

Due to the rarity of severe impairments in visual motion processing and probably the multiplicity of cortical and subcortical areas involved in motion perception, treatment approaches have not been developed. However, the treatment of an associated ability (i.e. smooth pursuit eye movements when tracking a moving target) is useful to improve visual scanning on computer screens and visual orientation in daily life.[14] This can be accomplished by use of a large PC screen, where the patient follows a moving target in different directions with a stabilized head. In addition, training for situations in daily life where motion is important (crossing a street, using an escalator) may improve orientation and reduce the likelihood of accidents due to reduced motion perception.

Optic ataxia

Optic ataxia refers to a visuomotor disorder characterized by an impairment in visually guided reaching that is not attributable to other primary motor or visual disorders.[115] At the bedside, this is assessed by asking the patient to fixate on the examiner's nose while the examiner's finger is presented as a target for a reach in either the left or right visual hemifield. Typically, healthy individuals can reach accurately even to a peripheral target while maintaining central fixation, but patients with optic ataxia misreach under such conditions.

Table 14.3 Therapeutic approaches for visuospatial disorders

Therapeutic approach	Therapeutic principle
Feedback-based training of perceptual visuospatial abilities	Improvement of spatial perception by graded training with verbal or visual feedback; basic concept: recalibration of spatial perception
Visual background movement to improve perceptual visuospatial deficits	Improvement of attention for spatial expansion and orientation (subjective visual vertical/horizontal) through repetitive stimulation; use of the attention-improving effect of optokinetic stimulation
Constructive visuospatial training	Improvement of perceptual, cognitive, and constructive visuospatial abilities as well as planning performance by graded practice with constructive material (e.g. Tangram, block design training)
ADL therapy	Direct practice of problematic 'spatial' daily procedures (e.g. wheelchair navigation, getting dressed)
Reaction-chaining and memory strategies for learning routes in the environment	Parsing longer routes into shorter distances, practicing them by conditioning and later 'chaining' or linking them together; eventually additional use of mnestic strategies

Adapted from *Der Nervenarzt*. 78(4), Kerkhoff G, Oppenländer K, Finke K, *et al.* Therapy of cerebral visual perception disturbances (German), pp. 457–70, Copyright (2007), with permission from Springer.

Beside the severe impairment in reaching, many patients also demonstrate a problem in grasping peripherally presented visual objects. By contrast, reaching to the patient's own body parts seems to be largely preserved,[116] although reaching to auditory targets is also impaired.[117] Furthermore, the accuracy of reaching can be improved by delaying the patient´s movement initiation after stimulus presentation.[118,119] Optic ataxia is associated with lesions in the parieto-occipital junction and the superior parietal lobule[120] and can occur both after unilateral or bilateral brain damage and as a result of neurodegenerative diseases including AD. Due to the neuroanatomical overlap, optic ataxia can co-occur with neglect after right parietal lesions (see chapter 5). For differential diagnosis, it is therefore important to note that neglect patients usually can reach and grasp accurately to visually presented objects in the neglected hemifield if they notice them.[116]

Treatment

Controlled treatment studies are rare. Since optic ataxia is less severe in the foveal than the affected peripheral visual hemifield,[120] prior fixation of the target *before* reaching or grasping usually improves reaching accuracy.

Bálint–Holmes syndrome, ocular motor apraxia

Bálint–Holmes syndrome designates a cluster of symptoms[121] including:

1. *Simultanagnosia*: Impaired simultaneous perception of more than one object[123]

2. *Optic ataxia*: see earlier in the chapter

3. *Visual neglect and visuospatial disorders* such as impaired retention of distance, orientation, and position[122]

4. *Oculomotor disorders*: severe and impaired fixation of gaze (sticky fixation) as well as problems in generating saccades voluntarily or on demand (oculomotor apraxia)[7,123]

Furthermore, patients show severe reading problems, while reading of short real words (four to six letters) is better than reading of non-words.[124]

Due to the bilateral or diffuse disseminated occipitoparietal lesions, recovery is limited in these severely and chronically disabled patients. It is estimated that some 30 per cent of patients with degenerative dementias might show aspects of Bálint–Holmes syndrome,[125,126] although rarely the complete syndrome, and this is much more common in PCA; the incidence in non-dementing, neurological disease is probably <0.5 per cent (Kerkhoff, unpublished results).

Treatment

Research on effective rehabilitation techniques is sparse (for review see references 13 and 127). It is likely that the disorder is often overlooked or misdiagnosed. Eye blinking may eliminate confusing visual images or the patient's subjective feeling of seeing the same object at multiple locations in space.[2,7] Zihl[59] noted some recovery of visual exploration and fixation after systematic training in three patients with Bálint–Holmes syndrome, but no recovery of the spatial disorder. Despite these occasional experiences effective treatment strategies are poorly developed and evaluated.

References

1. Rowe F, Brand D, Jackson C, *et al.* Visual impairment following stroke: do stroke patients require vision assessment? *Age Ageing.* 2009;38(2):188–93.
2. Kerkhoff G. Neurovisual rehabilitation, recent developments and future directions. *J Neurol Neurosur Ps.* 2000;68:691–706.
3. Suchoff IB, Kappor N, Ciuffreda KJ, *et al.* The frequency of occurrence, types, and characteristics of visual field defects in acquired brain injury: A retrospective analysis. *Optometry.* 2008;79:259–65.
4. Mendez MF, Mendez MA, Martin R, *et al.* Complex visual disturbances in Alzheimer's disease. *Neurology.* 1990;40(3): 439–43.
5. Kerkhoff G, Schaub J, and Zihl J. The anamnesis of cerebral visual disorders after brain damage (German). *Der Nervenarzt.* 1990;61:711–18.
6. Neumann G, Schaadt A-K, Reinhart S, *et al.* Clinical and psychometric evaluations of the Cerebral Vision Screening Questionnaire in 461 non-aphasic individuals post-stroke. *Neurorehabilitation and Neural Repair.* 30(3):187–98.
7. Zihl J. *Rehabilitation of Visual Disorders after Brain Injury,* 2nd edn. New York, NY: Psychology Press, 2011.
8. Skeel RL, Schutte C, Van Voorst W, *et al.* The relationship between visual contrast sensitivity and neuropsychological performance in a healthy elderly sample. *J Clin Exp Neuropsyc.* 2–6;28(5):696–705.
9. Frisén L. The neurology of visual acuity. *Brain.* 1980;103:639–70.
10. Kerkhoff G. Restorative and compensatory therapy approaches in cerebral blindness—a review. *Restorative Neurology and Neuroscience.* 1999;15:255–71.
11. Haarmeier T and Thier P. Impaired analysis of moving objects due to deficient smooth pursuit eye movements. *Brain.* 1999;122:1495–505.
12. Straube A and Kennard C. Ocular Motor Disorders. In: T Brandt, LR Caplan, J Dichgans, *et al.* (eds). *Neurological Disorders. Course and Treatment.* San Diego, CA: Academic Press, 1996, pp. 101–11.

13. Perez FM, Tunkel RS, Lachmann EA, *et al.* Bálints-Syndrome arising from bilateral posterior cortical atrophy or infarction—rehabilitation strategies and their limitation. *Disability and Rehabilitation.* 1995;18:300–4.

14. Gur S and Ron S. Training in oculomotor tracking, occupational health aspects. *Israel J Med Sci.* 1992;28:622–8.

15. Bulens C, Meerwaldt JD, van der Wildt GJ, *et al.* Spatial contrast sensitivity in unilateral cerebral ischaemic lesions involving the posterior visual pathway. *Brain.* 1989;112:507–20.

16. Corkin S, Nissen MJ, Buonanno FS, *et al.* Spatial vision in Alzheimer's disease. General findings and a case report. *Arch Neurol–Chicago.* 1985;42:667–71.

17. Cronin-Golomb A, Corkin S, and Growdon JH. Visual dysfunction predicts deficits in Alzheimer's disease. *Optometry Vision Sci.* 1995;72(3):168–76.

18. Jackowski MM, Sturr JF, Taub HA, *et al.* Photophobia in patients with traumatic brain injury: uses of light-filtering lenses to enhance contrast sensitivity and reading rate. *Neurorehabilitation.* 1996;6:193–201.

19. Zihl J and Kerkhoff G. Foveal photopic and scotopic adaptation in patients with brain damage. *Clin Vision Sci.* 1990;2:185–95.

20. Rizzo M. Astereopsis. In: F Boller and J Grafman (eds). *Handbook of Neuropsychology.* Amsterdam: Elsevier, 1989, pp. 415–27.

21. Koh SB, Kim BJ, Lee J, *et al.* Stereopsis and colour vision impairment in patients with right extrastriate cerebral lesions. *European Neurology.* 2008;60:174–8.

22. Miller LJ, Mittenberg S, Carrey VM, *et al.* Astereosis caused by traumatic brain injury. *Arch Clin Neuropsy.* 1999;14:537–43.

23. Hart CT. Disturbances of fusion following head injuries. *Proceedings of the Royal Society of Medicine.* 1969;62:704–6.

24. Schaadt A-K, Schmidt L, Kuhn C, *et al.* Perceptual re-learning of binocular fusion after hypoxic brain damage—four controlled single case treatment studies. *Neuropsychology.* 2014;28(3):382–87.

25. Schaadt A-K, Schmidt L, Reinhart S, *et al.* Perceptual relearning of binocular fusion and stereoacuity after brain Injury. *Neurorehabilitation and Neural Repair.* 2014;28(5):462–71.

26. Schaadt A-K, Brandt SA, Kraft A, *et al.* Holmes and Horrax (1919) revisited: Impaired binocular fusion as a cause of 'flat vision' after right parietal brain damage—A case study. *Neuropsychologia.* 2015;69:31–8.

27. Wilkins A. What is visual discomfort? *Trends Neurosci.* 1986;9:343–6.

28. Zihl J. Visual scanning behavior in patients with homonymous hemianopia. *Neuropsychologia.* 1995;33:287–303.

29. Pambakian A, Wooding D, Patel N, *et al.* Scanning the visual world: a study of patients with homonymous hemianopia. *J Neurol Neurosur Ps.* 2000;69(6):751–59.

30. Pambakian AL, Mannan SK, Hodgson TL, *et al.* Saccadic visual search training: a treatment for patients with homonymous hemianopia. *J Neurol Neurosur Ps.* 2004;75:1443–8.

31. Machner B, Sprenger A, Sander T, *et al.* Visual Search Disorders in Acute and Chronic Homonymous Hemianopia. *Ann NY Acad Sci.* 2009;116(4):419–26.

32. Zihl J. Eye movement patterns in hemianopic dyslexia. *Brain.* 1995;118:891–912.

33. Leff A, Scott S, Crewes H, *et al.* Impaired reading in patients with right hemianopia. *Ann Neurol.* 2000;47(2):171–8.

34. Spitzyna GA, Wise RJS, McDonald SA, *et al.* Optokinetic therapy improves text reading in patients with hemianopic alexia. A controlled trial. *Neurology.* 2007;68:1922–30.

35. Kerkhoff G. Displacement of the egocentric visual midline in altitudinal postchiasmatic scotomata. *Neuropsychologia.* 1993;31:261–5.

36. Barton JJS and Black S. Line bisection in hemianopia. *J Neurol Neurosur Ps.* 1998;64:660–62.

37. Kuhn C, Heywood C, and Kerkhoff G. Oblique spatial shifts of subjective visual straight ahead orientation in quadrantic visual field defects. *Neuropsychologia.* 2010;48:3205–10.

38. Kerkhoff G and Schenk T. Line bisection in homonymous visual field defects—recent findings and future directions. *Cortex.* 2011;47:53–58.

39. Hesse C, Lane A, Aimola L, *et al.* Pathways involved in human conscious vision contribute to obstacle-avoidance behaviour. *European Journal of Neuroscience.* 2012;36(3):2383–90.

40. Husain M. Hemispatial neglect. In: G Goldenberg and BV Miller (eds). *Handbook of Clinical Neurology.* Amsterdam: Elsevier, 2008, pp. 359–72.

41. Kerkhoff G and Bucher L. Line bisection as an early method to assess homonymous hemianopia. *Cortex.* 2008;44(2):200–5.

42. Kuhn C, Bublak P, Jobst S, *et al.* Contralesional spatial bias in chronic hemianopia: The role of (ec)centric fixation, spatial cueing and visual search. *Neuroscience.* 2012;210:118–27.

43. Kuhn C, Bublak P, Grotemeyer KH, *et al.* Does spatial cueing affect line bisection in chronic homonymous hemianopia? *Neuropsychologia.* 2012;50:1656–62.

44. Baier B, Mueller N, Fechir M, *et al.* Line bisection error and its anatomic correlate. *Stroke.* 2010;41(7):1561–3.

45. Zhang X, Kedar S, Lynn JJ, *et al.* Natural history of homonymous hemianopia. *Neurology.* 2006;66:901–5.

46. Zihl J and von Cramon D. Recovery of visual field in patients with postgeniculate damage. In: K Poeck, HJ Freund, H Gänshirt (eds). *Neurology.* Heidelberg: Springer, 1986, pp. 188–94.

47. Mödden C, Behrens M, Damke I, *et al.* A randomized controlled trial comparing 2 interventions for visual field loss with standard occupational therapy during inpatient stroke rehabilitation. *Neurorehabilitation and Neural Repair.* 2012;26(5):463–9.

48. Bouwmeester L, Heutink J, and Lucas C. The effect of visual training for patients with visual field defects due to brain damage: a systematic review. *J Neurol Neurosur Ps.* 2007;78:555–64.

49. Bolognini N, Rasi F, Coccia M, *et al.* Visual search improvement in hemianopic patients after audio-visual stimulation. *Brain.* 2005;128:2830–42.

50. Keller I and Lefin-Rank G. Improvement of visual search after audio-visual exploration training in hemianopic patients. *Neurorehabilitation and Neural Repair.* 2010;24(7):666–73.

51. Kasten E, Wüst S, Behrens-Baumann W, *et al.* Computer-based training for the treatment of partial blindness. *Nature Med.* 1998;4:1083–7.

52. Nelles G, Esser J, Eckstein A, *et al.* Compensatory visual field training for patients with hemianopia after stroke. *Neuroscience Letters.* 2001;306:189–92.

53. Reinhard J, Schreiber A, Schiefer U, *et al.* Does visual restitution training change absolute homonymous visual field defects? A fundus controlled study. *B J Ophthalmol.* 2005;89:30–35.

54. Roth TT, Sokolov AN, Messias AA, *et al.* Comparing explorative saccade and flicker training in hemianopia: A randomized controlled study. *Neurology.* 2009;72(4):324–31.

55. Lane AR, Smith DT, Ellison A, *et al.* Visual Exploration Training Is No Better than Attention Training for Treating Hemianopia. *Brain.* 2010;133(6):1717–28.

56. Aimola L, Lasne AR, Smith DT, *et al.* (submitted). Efficacy and feasibility of a home-based computer training for individuals with homonymous visual field defects. *Neurorehabilitation and Neural Repair.* 2014; 28(3):207–18.

57. Bowers A, Keeney K, and Peli E. Community-based trial of a peripheral prism visual field expansion device for hemianopia. *Arch Ophthalmol-Chic.* 2008;126(5):657–64.

58. Kerkhoff G, Münssinger U, Haaf E, *et al.* Rehabilitation of homonymous scotomata in patients with postgeniculate damage of the visual system: saccadic compensation training. *Restorative Neurology And Neuroscience.* 1992;4(4):245–54.

59. Zihl J and Kennard C. Disorders of higher visual functions. In: T Brandt, LR Caplan, J Dichgans, *et al.* (eds). *Neurological Disorders. Course and Treatment.* San Diego, CA: Academic Press, 1996, pp. 201–12.

60. Anton G. Ueber die Selbstwahrnehmung der Herderkrankungen des Gehirns durch den Kranken bei Rindenblindheit und Rindentaubheit. *Archiv für Psychiatrie und Nervenkrankheiten.* 1899;32:86–127.

61. Zihl J. Zerebrale Sehstörungen. In H -O. Karnath, W Hartje, and W Ziegler (eds). *Kognitive Neurologie.* Stuttgart: Thieme, 2006, pp. 1–18.

62. Hartmann J, Wolz W, Roeltgen D, *et al*. Denial of visual perception. *Brain Cognition*. 1991;16(1):29–40.

63. Kortte K, Wegener ST, and Chwalisz K. Anosognosia and denial: Their relationship to coping and depression in acquired brain injury. *Rehabilitation Psychology*. 2004;48(3):131–6.

64. Zihl J. Visuelle Reizerscheinungen. In H -O Karnath and P Thier (eds). *Neuropsychologie*. Heidelberg: Springer, 2006, pp. 84–7.

65. Lance JW. Simple formed hallucinations confined to the area of a specific visual field defect. *Brain*. 1976;99:719–34.

66. Kölmel HW. Coloured patterns in hemianopic fields. *Brain*. 1984;107:155–67.

67. Kölmel HW. Complex visual hallucinations in the hemianopic field. *J Neurol Neurosur Ps*. 1985;47:29–38.

68. Baier B, de Haan B, Mueller N, *et al*. Anatomical correlate of positive spontaneous visual phenomena: a voxelwise lesion study. *Neurology*. 2010;74(3):218–22.

69. Holroyd S, Shepherd ML, and Downs J. Occipital atrophy is associated with visual hallucinations in Alzheimer's disease. *J Neuropsych Clin N*. 2000;12(1):25–8.

70. Kropp S, Schulz-Schaeffer W, Finkenstaedt M, *et al*. The Heidenhain variant of Creutzfeldt–Jakob disease. *Arch Neurol*. 1999;56(1), 55–61.

71. Goetz C, Leurgans S, Pappert E, *et al*. Prospective longitudinal assessment of hallucinations in Parkinson's disease. *Neurology*. 2001;57(11):2078–82.

72. Meppelink A, de Jong B, Renken R, *et al*. Impaired visual processing preceding image recognition in Parkinson's disease patients with visual hallucinations. *Brain*.2009;132:2980–93.

73. Meadows JC. Disturbed perception of colours associated with localized cerebral lesions. *Brain*. 1974;97:615–32.

74. Zeki S. A century of cerebral achromatopsia. *Brain*. 1990;113:1721–77.

75. Bouvier SE and Engel SA. Behavioral deficits and cortical damage loci in cerebral achromatopsia. *Cerebral Cortex* 2006;16(2):183–91.

76. Vingrys A and Garner L. The effect of a moderate level of hypoxia on human color vision. *Documenta Ophthalmologica*. 1987;2:171–85.

77. Cronin-Golomb A, Sugiura R, Corkin S, *et al*. Incomplete achromatopsia in Alzheimer's disease. *Neurobiol Aging*. 1993;14(5):471–7.

78. Rizzo M and Barton JJS. Central disorders of visual function. In: NR Miller, NJ Newman, V Biousse, and JB Kerrison (eds). *Walsh and Hoyt's Clinical Neuro-Ophthalmology: The Essentials*. Philadelphia, PA: Lippincott Williams and Wilkins, 2008, pp. 263–84.

79. Zihl J and von Cramon D. Visual field recovery from scotoma in patients with postgeniculate damage. *Brain*. 1985;108:335–65.

80. Merrill MK and Kewman DG. Training of colour and form identification in cortical blindness, a case study. *Arch Phys Med Rehab*. 1986;67:479–83.

81. Farah M. *Visual Agnosia*. Cambridge, MA: MIT Press, 1990.

82. Riddoch MJ and Humphreys GW. Object recognition. In B. Rapp (ed.). *The Handbook of Cognitive Neuropsychology*. New York, NY: Psychology Press, 2001, pp. 45–74.

83. Zihl J and Nelles G. Rehabilitation von zerebralen Sehstörungen. In: G Nelles (ed.). *Neurologische Rehabilitation*. Stuttgart: Thieme, 2004, pp. 129–41.

84. Martinaud O, Pouliquen D, Gérardin E, *et al*. Visual agnosia and posterior cerebral artery infarcts: An anatomical-clinical study. *PLoS One*. 2012;7(1):1–14.

85. Mosimann UP, Mather GG, Wesnes KA, *et al*. Visual perception in Parkinson disease dementia and dementia with Lewy bodies. *Neurology*. 2004;63(11):2091–96.

86. Done D and Hajilou B. Loss of high-level perceptual knowledge of object structure in DAT. *Neuropsychologia*. 2005;43(1):60–8.

87. Caterini FF, Sala S, Spinnler HH, *et al*. Object recognition and object orientation in Alzheimer's disease. *Neuropsychology*. 2002;16(2):146–55.

88. Adlington RL, Laws KR, and Gale TM. Visual processing in Alzheimer's disease: Surface detail and colour fail to aid object identification. *Neuropsychologia*. 2009;47(12):2574–83.

89. Mori E, Shimomura T, Fujimori M, *et al*. Visuoperceptual impairment in dementia with Lewy bodies. *Arch Neurol*. 2000;57(4):489–93.

90. Finke K, Schneider WX, Redel P, *et al*. The capacity of attention and simultaneous perception of objects: A group study of Huntington's disease patients. *Neuropsychologia*. 2007;45(14):3272–84.

91. Riddoch MJ and Humphreys GW. *Birmingham Object Recognition Battery*. Hove: Lawrence Erlbaum Associates, 1993.

92. Warrington EK and James M. *The visual object and space perception battery*. Bury St Edmunds: Thames Valley Test Company, 1991.

93. Sparr SA, Jay M, Drislane FW, *et al*. A historic case of visual agnosia revisited after 40 years. *Brain*. 1991;114:789–800.

94. Mesad S, Laff R, and Devinsky O. Transient postoperative prosopagnosia. *Epilepsy and Behavior* 2003;4(5):567–70.

95. Kerkhoff G and Marquardt C. Standardised analysis of visuospatial perception after brain damage. *Neuropsychological Rehabilitation*. 1998;8:171–89.

96. Jesshope HJ, Clark MS, and Smith DS. The Rivermead Perceptual Assessment Battery: its application to stroke patients and relationship with function. *Clinical Rehabilitation*. 1991;5:115–22.

97. Tang-Wai D, Josephs K, Boeve B, *et al*. Pathologically confirmed corticobasal degeneration presenting with visuospatial dysfunction. *Neurology*.2003;61(8):1134–5.

98. Graham N, Bak T, and Hodges J. Corticobasal degeneration as a cognitive disorder. *Movement Disorders*. 2003;18(11):1224–32.

99. Kaplan J and Hier DB. Visuospatial deficits after right hemisphere stroke. *Am J Occup Ther*. 1982;36(5):314–21.

100. Ungerleider LG and Mishkin M. Two cortical visual systems. In: D Ingle and MA Goodale (eds). *Analysis of Visual Behavior*. Cambridge, MA: The MIT Press, 1982, pp. 549–85.

101. Utz KS, Keller II, Artinger FF, *et al*. Multimodal and multispatial deficits of verticality perception in hemispatial neglect. *Neuroscience*. 2011;188:68–79.

102. Kerkhoff G. Störungen der visuellen Raumorientierung. In: H -O Karnath and P Thier (eds). *Kognitive Neurowissenschaften*. Berlin: Springer, 2012, pp. 241–9.

103. Marshall RS, Lazar RM, Binder JR, *et al*. Intrahemispheric localization of drawing dysfunction. *Neuropsychologia*. 1994;32(4):493–501.

104. Russell C, Deidda C, Malhotra P, *et al* A deficit of spatial remapping in constructional apraxia after right-hemisphere stroke. *Brain*. 2010;133:1239–51.

105. Aguirre GK and D'Esposito M. Topographical disorientation: A synthesis and taxonomy. *Brain*. 199;122(9):1613–28.

106. Kerkhoff G, Oppenländer K, Finke K, *et al*. Therapy of cerebral visual perception disturbances (German). *Der Nervenarzt*. 2007;78(4):457–70.

107. Funk J, Finke K, Reinhart S, *et al*. (in press). Effects of feedback-based visual line-orientation discrimination training for visuospatial disorders after stroke. *Neurorehabilitation and Neural Repair*. 2013;27(2):142–52.

108. Oppenländer K, Utz KS, Reinhart S, *et al*. Subliminal galvanic-vestibular stimulation recalibrates the distorted visual and tactile subjective vertical in right-sided stroke. *Neuropsychologia*. doi:10.1016/j.neuropsychologia.2015. 03.004.

109. Zeki S. Cerebral akinetopsia (visual motion blindness). A review. *Brain*. 1991;114:811–24.

110. Schenk T and Zihl J. Visual motion perception after brain damage, I. Deficits in global motion perception. *Neuropsychologia*. 1997;35:1289–97.

111. Gibson JJ. *The Perception of the Visual World*. Boston: Houghton Mifflin, 1950.

112. Tetewsky S and Duffy CJ. Visual loss and getting lost in Alzheimer's disease. *Neurology*. 1999;52:958–65.

113. O'Brien H, Tetewsky S, Avery L, *et al*. Visual mechanisms of spatial disorientation in Alzheimer's disease. *Cerebral Cortex*. 2001;11(11):1083–92.

114. Zihl J, von Cramon D, Mai N, and Schmid C. Disturbance of movement vision after bilateral posterior brain damage. Further evidence and follow up observations. *Brain*. 1991;114:2235–51.

115. Perenin M and Vighetto A. Optic ataxia: a specific disruption in visuo-motor mechanisms. I. Different aspects of the deficit in reaching for objects. *Brain*. 1988;111:643–74.

116. Goldenberg G. The neuropsychological assessment and treatment of disorders of voluntary movement. In JM Gurd, U Kischka, and JC Marshall (eds). *The Handbook of Clinical Neuropsychology*. Oxford: Oxford University Press, 2010, pp. 387–400.

117. Phan M, Schendel K, Recanzone G, *et al.* Auditory and visual spatial localization deficits following bilateral parietal lobe lesions in a patient with Balint's syndrome. *J Cognitive Neurosci*. 2000;12(4):583–600.

118. Milner A, Dijkerman H, McIntosh R, *et al.* Delayed reaching and grasping in patients with optic ataxia. *Progress in Brain Research*. 2003;142:225–42.

119. Rossetti YY, Revol PP, McIntosh RR, *et al.* Visually guided reaching: Bilateral posterior parietal lesions cause a switch from fast visuomotor to slow cognitive control. *Neuropsychologia*. 2005;43(2):162–77.

120. Karnath H and Perenin M. Cortical control of visually guided reaching: Evidence from patients with optic ataxia. *Cerebral Cortex*. 2005;15(10):1561–9.

121. Rafal RD. Bálint syndrome. In: TE Feinberg and MJ Farah (eds). *Behavioral Neurology and Neuropsychology*. Boston: McGraw-Hill, 1997, pp. 337–56.

122. Moreaud O. Bálint syndrome. *Arch Neurol*. 2003;60(9):1329–31.

123. Zee DS and Newman-Toker D. Supranuclear and internuclear ocular motility disorders. In: NR Miller, NJ Newman, V Biousse, *et al.* (eds). *Walsh and Hoyt's Clinical Neuro-Ophthalmology: The Essentials*. Philadelphia, PA: Lippincott Williams & Wilkins, 2005, pp. 344–76.

124. Baylis GC, Driver J, Baylis LL, *et al.* Reading of letters and words in a patient with Balint's syndrome. *Neuropsychologia*. 1994;32(10): 1273–86.

125. Mendez M, Tomsak R, and Remler B. Disorders of the visual system in Alzheimer's disease. *J Clin Neuro-Ophthal*. 1990;10(1): 62–9.

126. Rizzo M. 'Bálint's syndrome' and associated visuospatial disorders. *Baillière's Clinical Neurology*. 1993;2(2):415–37.

127. Kerkhoff G and Heldmann B. Balint syndrome and associated disorders. Anamnesis—diagnosis—approaches to treatment (german). *Der Nervenarzt*. 1999;70(10):859–69.

128. Uchiyama M, Nishio Y, Yokoi K, Hirayama K, Imamura T, Shimomura T, and Mori E. Pareidolias: Complex visual illusions in dementia with Lewy bodies. *Brain*. 2012;135(8):2458–69.

CHAPTER 15

Disorders of attentional processes

Paolo Bartolomeo and Raffaella Migliaccio

Introduction

The term 'attention' refers to a heterogeneous set of cognitive processes which allow an organism to successfully cope with a continuously changing external and internal environment, while maintaining its goals.[1] This flexibility calls for mechanisms that (a) allow for the processing of novel, unexpected events, that could be either advantageous or dangerous, in order to respond appropriately with either approaching or avoidance behaviour; (b) allow for the maintenance of finalized behaviour despite distracting events.[2] To behave in a coherent and goal-driven way, we need to select stimuli appropriate to our goals while ignoring other less important objects. Thus, in a sense, objects in the world compete for recruiting our attention in order to be the focus of our subsequent behaviour, because of the obvious capacity limitations in our ability of dealing with multiple objects. Neural mechanisms of attention resolve this competition by taking into account both the agent's goals and the salience of the sensorial stimuli.[3] Neurological damage may impair these mechanisms and produce various sorts of attention disorders.[4]

The present chapter will focus on some of these disorders, such as the inability to process several visual objects at a time (simultagnosia), the unawareness of an object when presented in competition to another one (extinction), or when occurring on one side of space (visual neglect). Other disorders may affect the general ability to respond to external stimuli and to sustain attention over time,[5] or to plan and coordinate different activities and inhibit inappropriate responses (monitoring/executive control).[6,7]

With ageing, people often report a growing number of cognitive difficulties. In some cases, elderly persons complain of 'loss of efficiency', for example, forgetting where objects are placed, having the impression of being unsafe when driving, experiencing trouble when in new places or navigating new routes. Neurological conditions, on the other hand, can lead to severe impairments in different types of attention. These problems often occur in patients with acute vascular strokes (ischaemic or haemorrhagic), but they can also be observed in other neurological conditions, such as head trauma, brain tumours, or neurodegeneration. In several neurodegenerative conditions (e.g. corticobasal syndrome, CBS; Alzheimer's disease, AD; parkinsonian syndromes such as dementia with Lewy bodies, DLB), attention deficits can appear as part of more complex cognitive impairment profile. In others, such as in posterior cortical atrophy (PCA), they may constitute the central core of the syndrome.[8] Because we know far more about visual attention than any other sensory modality, in this chapter we focus on examples of visual inattention, although many of the conditions we discuss can also extend to other modalities.

Cortical networks for visuospatial attention and visual recognition

There is now considerable information on the functional anatomy, dynamics and pathological dysfunction of brain networks that subserve the spatial orienting of gaze and attention in the human brain. Important components of these networks include the dorsolateral prefrontal cortex (PFC) and the posterior parietal cortex (PPC). Physiological studies indicate that these two structures show interdependence of neural activity. In the rhesus monkey, analogous PPC and PFC areas show coordinated activity when the animal selects a visual stimulus as the goal of attention by, for example, moving their gaze to it.[9]

Functional MRI (fMRI) studies in healthy human participants (reviewed in reference 2 at p.1167) indicate the existence of frontoparietal networks for spatial attention (Fig. 15.1, right panel). A dorsal attentional network (DAN), composed of the intraparietal sulcus/superior parietal lobule and the frontal eye field/dorsolateral PFC, shows increased blood oxygenation level-dependent (BOLD) responses during the spatial orienting period. A more ventral attentional network (VAN), which includes the inferior parietal lobule (IPL) and the ventral PFC (inferior and middle frontal gyri) demonstrates increased BOLD responses when participants have to respond to targets presented at unexpected locations. Thus, the VAN is considered important for detecting salient, unexpected but behaviourally relevant events. Others have also argued for a role of the VAN in vigilance or sustaining attention over time.[11] Importantly, the VAN is considered to be strongly lateralized to the right hemisphere,[10] whereas the DAN appears to be more bilateral and symmetric (but see references 12 and 13 for possible asymmetries favouring the DAN in the right hemisphere).

Not surprisingly, PFC and PPC are directly and extensively interconnected. In particular, studies in the monkey brain have identified three distinct frontoparietal long-range pathways(see Fig 15.1, left panel).[14,15] Recent evidence from advanced *in vivo* tractography techniques and postmortem dissections suggests that a similar architecture exists in the human brain (Fig. 15.1, middle panel).[16] In humans, the most dorsal branch (SLF I) originates from BA (Brodmann's area) 5 and 7 and projects to BA 8, 9, and 32. The middle pathway (SLF II) originates in BA 39 and 40 within the IPL and

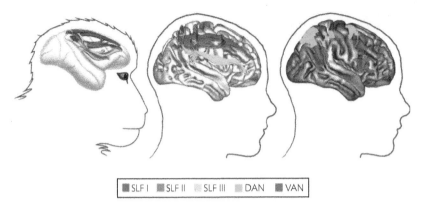

☐ SLF I   ■ SLF II   ▨ SLF III   ▨ DAN   ■ VAN

Fig. 15.1 Fronto-parietal networks in the monkey (left, from reference 15) and in the human right hemisphere (middle, from reference 16). Right: attentional networks in the right hemisphere according to Corbetta and Shulman.[104]
Reproduced from *Front Hum Neurosci.* 6(110), Bartolomeo P, Thiebaut de Schotten M, and Chica AB, Brain networks of visuospatial attention and their disruption in visual neglect, Copyright (2012), with permission from Frontiers Media S.A, reproduced under the Creative Commons CC BY-NC 3.0 License.

reaches prefrontal BA 8 and 9. The most ventral pathway (SLF III) originates in BA 40 and terminates in BA 44, 45, and 47.

These results are consistent with the fMRI evidence on attentional networks reviewed above. In particular, the SLF III connects the cortical nodes of the VAN, whereas the DAN is connected by the human homologue of SLF I. The SLF II connects the parietal component of the VAN to the prefrontal component of the DAN, thus allowing direct communication between ventral and dorsal attentional networks. Importantly, in good agreement with asymmetries of BOLD response during fMRI—with larger right-hemisphere response for the VAN and more symmetrical activity for the DAN[10]—the SLF III (connecting the VAN) is anatomically larger in the right hemisphere than in the left hemisphere, whereas the SLF I (connecting the DAN) is more symmetrically organized.[16] The lateralization of the SLF II is instead strongly correlated to behavioural signs of right-hemisphere specialization for visuospatial attention such as pseudo-neglect in line bisection (i.e. small leftwards deviations of the subjective midline observed in healthy individuals),[17–19] and asymmetries in the speed of detection of events presented in the right or in the left hemifield.[16]

These frontoparietal *attentional* systems are often considered important for spatially-based visual abilities (but see reference 20 for nonspatial functions of the IPL). They are to be distinguished from the dorsal and ventral *visual* streams which originate from the occipital cortex.[21,22]

Deficits of high-level visual abilities

The occipitoparietal cortical visual stream—or 'dorsal visual stream'—processes information about objects and their locations in a moment-to-moment manner, and mediates the visual control of skilled actions. More ventral, occipitotemporal networks are instead critical for other visual abilities, such as visual recognition[21,22] (see chapter 14). They appear to carry information about perceptual features, allowing the building of long-term representations necessary to identify and recognize objects.

Damage to the occipitotemporal cortical visual stream impairs the perceptual recognition of visual items such as objects, faces, colours, and written words, whereas more dorsal, occipitoparietal deficits concern the processing of spatial location (spatial

awareness and reaching movements) (see Box 15.1, cases 1 and 2). Anatomically, the ventral stream is composed of the occipitotemporal cortices and the white matter bundles running between these regions, which include the inferior longitudinal fasciculus and portions of the inferior fronto-occipital fasciculus.[23,24]

Visuospatial deficits in neurodegenerative conditions often develop and progress along these two main cortico-cortical axes. In particular, the distribution of neuropathology in neurodegeneration seems to follow specific trajectories for each syndrome, targeting specific cerebral networks.[25] For example, the pattern of network change in PCA is different to that in CBS, both of which can present with attention deficits, together with other features that might help distinguish between them. Within this framework, the anatomical definition of ventral and dorsal variants can assist clinicians in localization, and allow them to define the distribution of pathology by bedside testing.[26] Given these correspondences between disease, anatomically damaged patterns, and related cognitive impairment, the interpretation of neuropsychological tests of visuospatial cognition has important implications both for differential diagnosis and to monitor disease progression (see Box 15.1 and Fig. 15.3).

Visual neglect

Vascular, traumatic, neoplastic, or degenerative damage to frontoparietal networks in the right hemisphere is frequently associated with a disabling condition known as visual neglect.[27–29] About half of the patients with a lesion in the right hemisphere suffer from neglect for the contralesional, left side of space.[30] They are unaware of items to their left. Neglect patients may not eat from the left part of their dish, they often bump their wheelchair into obstacles situated on their left, and have a tendency to look to right-sided details in a visual scene, as if their attention were 'magnetically' attracted by these details.[31] Many of them are also inattentive to auditory or somatosensory stimuli to the left. Neglect patients are usually unaware of their deficits (anosognosia), and often obstinately deny being hemiplegic. Individuals with left brain damage may also show signs of contralesional, right-sided neglect, albeit more rarely and usually in a less severe form.[32,33]

Neglect is a substantial source of handicap and disability for patients, and entails a poor functional outcome. Diagnosis is important, because effective rehabilitation strategies are becoming

Box 15.1 Ventral/dorsal PCA (posterior cortical atrophy) variants

On the basis of the schematic dichotomy between dorsal (occipito-parieto-frontal) and ventral (occipito-temporal and occipito-frontal) cortical visual networks, here we present three patients affected by PCA, but showing a different pattern of white matter damage along these two main axes.[26]

Patient 1 was a 62-year-old woman who had been experiencing isolated difficulties in reading and writing for about seven years. At the time of the study, she complained of episodes of topographical disorientation, and her neuropsychological profile was dominated by a severe visual impairment. She was unable to copy the Rey complex figure. She was impaired in object and space perception and in face recognition tests. She performed poorly on reading words and pseudo-words. Despite her marked visual and gnosic difficulties, she had excellent episodic memory for recent events, and no difficulty in remembering appointments. She had a normal verbal working memory as measured by backwards digit span. Her speech was fluent and syntactically well formed. She performed normally on tests of word fluency tasks, as well as on tests of comprehension. Insight was preserved. The tractography study of this patient demonstrated white matter damage along all the components of the ventral cortical visual stream (namely, the inferior longitudinal and the fronto-occipital fasciculi) (Fig. 15.2a).

Patient 2 (Fig. 15.2b) was a 62-year-old lady. She had been experiencing episodes of misplacing of objects for the past two-and-a-half years, along with reading problems, prosopagnosia, left-right disorientation, and anomia. She was poorly oriented at the time of testing, with a severe visual agnosia. She also experienced deficits in working memory, visuospatial and verbal episodic memory. At the time of MRI, she had a severe optic ataxia, mild visuospatial neglect, and exhibited irritability and loss of interests. She had both dorsal and ventral dysfunction.[26] In contrast, another PCA patient, with selectively impaired 'ventral' abilities (object recognition deficits, reading difficulties, and impaired face recognition) had spared SLF (Fig. 15.2c).

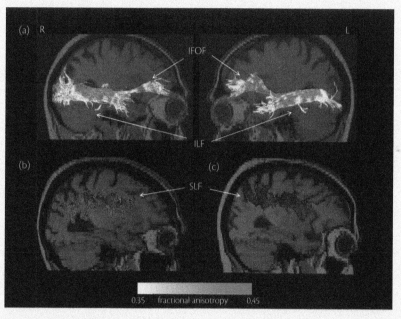

Fig. 15.2 An illustrative reconstruction of the ventral (inferior longitudinal fasciculus, ILF and the inferior fronto-occipital fasciculus, IFOF) and dorsal (fronto-parietal superior longitudinal fasciculus, SLF, branches II and III) stream pathways. Long-range white matter tracts of patients are rendered as maps of fractional anisotropy (FA, index of microstructural white matter integrity) and displayed on the native T1-weighted MRI. FA values range from 0.40 (yellow) to 0.50 (dark red). The lower the value, the greater the damage. (a) PCA patient 1 had a long clinical history of isolated deficits in reading and writing, followed by an impairment in object and space perception and face recognition, and showed a bilateral ventral white matter damage. (b) PCA patient 2, with optic ataxia and signs of mild left neglect two-and-a-half years after disease onset, had a diffusely damaged frontoparietal SLF (mean FA = 0.39). (c) Another PCA patient with preserved SLF (mean FA = 0.44). See Box 15.1 for more clinical details.

Reproduced from *Neurobiology of Aging*. 33(11), Migliaccio R, Agosta F, Scola E, *et al*. Ventral and dorsal visual streams in posterior cortical atrophy: A DT MRI study, pp. 2572–84, Copyright (2012), with permission from Elsevier.

available,[34] and there are promising possibilities for pharmacological treatments.[35] Furthermore, in many cases the nature of neglect deficits (impaired active exploration of a part of space) renders the diagnosis difficult or impossible if signs of neglect are not sought.

Neglect is especially frequent after focal vascular lesions of the right hemisphere, but signs of neglect have been described in AD.[36–39] More recently, signs of visual neglect have also been described in PCA. Out of 24 PCA patients, signs of neglect on at least one paper-and-pencil test were present in 16 patients, and

14 also had visual extinction or hemianopia.[40] In one patient with PCA and left-sided neglect as a presenting sign, MRI-based DTI tractography demonstrated damage to frontoparietal white matter bundles relatively selective to right-hemisphere pathways (reference 41 p. 4752) (see patient 3, Box 15.2).

Diagnostic tests

Patients' performance on paper-and-pencil tasks can easily demonstrate the presence and the extent of visual neglect. Here we

Pt #3

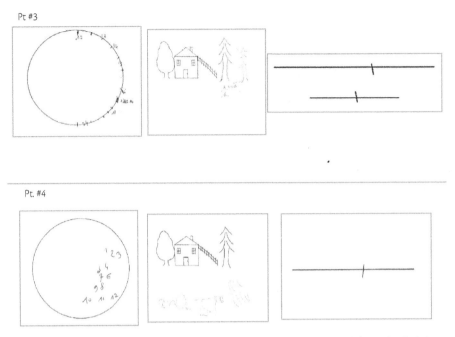

Pt. #4

Fig. 15.3 Performance on paper-and-pencil tests of PCA-AD patient 3 (see Box 15.2) and PCA-CBS patient 4. From left to right: clock-drawing test, copy of a drawing, line bisection. Note that patient 3, when copying the landscape, omitted the whole left part of the scene (scene-based pattern). Patient 4, on the other hand, tended to omit the left part of each element of the scene (object-based pattern); she also showed some spatial disorganization in placing the numbers during the clock drawing test.

Reproduced from *Cortex*. 48(10), Migliaccio R, Agosta F, Toba MN, *et al*. Brain networks in posterior cortical atrophy: a single case tractography study and literature review, pp. 1298–309, Copyright (2012), with permission from Elsevier.

briefly describe three visuomotor procedures simple enough as to be administered at the bedside (for other tests, see reference 4, p. 5198; reference 30, p. 1425; reference 42; reference 43, p. 4380). Care should be taken in the proper positioning of the test sheet; in the usual clinical conditions, the midline of the sheet should correspond to the trunk midline of the patient. Performance on these tasks is described by taking into account neglect for the left side of space, which is more common, severe, and durable than right-sided neglect in vascular patients.[32] The relative frequency of left and right neglect in neurodegenerative conditions is currently unknown. In some studies right-sided neglect was observed with an unexpected, relatively high frequency in neurodegenerative diseases as compared to vascular patients (reference 40, p. 4310; see also reference 37, p. 515 for discussion of possible mechanisms), whereas other studies found the usual predominance of left-sided neglect to be present also in degenerative patients.[44]

Importantly, patients who perform normally on these paper-and-pencil tests may nevertheless show spatial or nonspatial deficits on more demanding tests of visuospatial attention, such as speeded response time tests. It is important to be aware of the possibility of these seemingly 'subclinical' deficits, which might well have clinical implications, for example in taking decisions about the patient's ability to drive. In neurodegenerative conditions, such deficits of spatial attention have been described in patients with Alzheimer's disease.[45–47] Parkinson's disease,[48,49] Huntington's disease,[50,51] and progressive supranuclear palsy.[52]

Drawing tasks

When drawing figures, whether from memory or by copying them, neglect patients omit or distort the details on the left side (Fig. 15.3).[52] When copying patterns composed of several elements aligned horizontally, some patients neglect the whole left part of the model, while others copy all the items but leave unfinished the left part of each (Fig. 15.3 and 15.4).[53,54]

These distinct patterns of performance have been referred to, respectively, as scene- (or viewer-) based neglect and object-based neglect.[55]

Cancellation tasks

In cancellation tasks, patients are requested to search for and cross out items scattered on a paper sheet, such as lines,[56] letters,[57] or shapes.[58,59] Patients with right hemisphere damage typically begin to scan the sheet from the right side, unlike normal participants or patients with left brain damage, who start from the left side.[60] Patients with left neglect may omit a variable number of left-sided targets; some patients may continue to cancel the same right-sided items over and over again. Fig. 15.5 shows the performance on a shape cancellation test of a patient with PCA and mild signs of left neglect.

Line bisection

In line bisection tasks, patients have to mark the midpoint of a horizontal line; neglect patients deviate the subjective midpoint to the right of the true centre of the line (see Fig. 15.3).[61] The amount of deviation depends on several factors. The longer the line, the more rightward the bisection point; for the shortest lines there may be a paradoxical leftward deviation (the 'crossover effect').[62] The location in space of the line with respect to the patient's trunk midline also influences performance; rightward deviation increases when lines are located in the left hemispace and decreases when they are in the right hemispace.[61,63] Although patients' performance on line bisection may dissociate from their performance on other tasks, such as cancellation tests,[64] it remains a very useful test

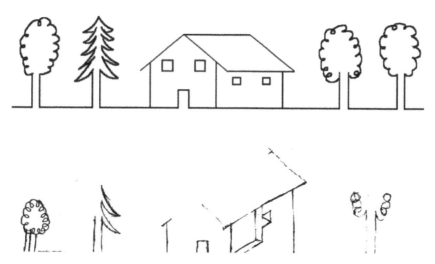

Fig. 15.4 Performance of a patient with probable AD on the copy of a landscape. Note the signs of left object-based neglect, similar to Patient 4 in Fig. 15.3.

particularly in situations, such as PCA, where simultagnosia may sometimes render difficult or impossible the completion of cancellation tests.[65]

Extinction

Sensory extinction refers to the failure of brain-damaged patients to report the stimulus contralateral to their lesion when stimulated on both sides, despite being able to report a single stimulus presented on either side. Extinction can occur in different sensory modalities: visual,[66] somatosensory,[67] acoustic,[68] olfactory,[69] and even cross-modally.[70] Accounts of extinction typically emphasize either a sensory problem not severe enough to impair perception of single stimuli,[71] or an attentional disorder favouring ipsilateral over contralateral stimuli,[72] or both.[73] Although visual extinction usually occurs after vascular strokes in the territory of medial cerebral artery, it has also been observed in neurodegenerative conditions such as PCA.[40]

Diagnostic tests

In clinical practice, the presence of extinction is traditionally investigated using various sorts of *double simultaneous stimulation*. The confrontation method is a common test of visual extinction. The examiner asks the patient to fixate the examiner's nose and then briefly moves his/her fingers either in one hemifield or in both hemifields simultaneously. For example, six single unilateral stimuli and six double simultaneous stimuli can be presented in pseudorandom order.[40] In practice, patients can be considered to show visual extinction when they fail at least twice to report a contralateral stimulus during bilateral simultaneous presentation, while accurately detecting all unilateral stimuli.[31] When the patient fails to report all stimuli on one side (whether single or double), homonymous hemianopia is a likely diagnosis which, however, requires confirmation with more detailed testing of the visual field in each eye at the bedside or with formal visual perimetry. Three patients out of the 24 PCA patients examined by Andrade and colleagues[40]

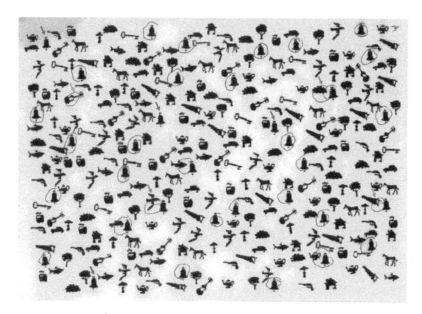

Fig. 15.5 Performance of a PCA patient on the Bells test.[58] The patient omitted three targets on the left side and one on the right side (red arrows). Note the false recognition on the left (green arrow) and the misreachings (blue arrows), perhaps depending on optic ataxia.

missed all the left-sided stimuli, thus suggesting the presence of left homonymous hemianopia, which is a rare occurrence in neurodegenerative diseases.[74] Of the remaining patients, eight had left extinction and three showed mild right extinction.

Somatosensory extinction can be tested by asking the patient to close the eyes and report light touches given by the examiner on the patient's limbs or face. To examine acoustic extinction, the examiner may lightly snap his/her fingers making a clicking sound near the patient's ears.

In typical amnesic Alzheimer's disease, general attentional deficits can occur early along with memory deficits. Later in the course of the disease, neglect signs may appear.[37,39] In some cases attentional deficits can precede the typical amnesic syndrome,[75] especially in the early-onset variant occurring before the age of 65.[76] More specifically, visuospatial attention deficits can have a central role in the impairment of higher-level cognitive processes concerning visual and spatial memory. As already mentioned, visuospatial neglect can represent the core symptom of clinical profile of patients affected by PCA (see Box 15.2, case 3). Even if less frequently, patients with CBS can also show signs of visuospatial neglect (see Box 15.3, case 4).[44]

Among the variety of tests used in clinical practice, line bisection might be more apt than target cancellation to demonstrate neglect in patients with neurodegenerative dementia, such as PCA,[40] because performance on isolated horizontal lines is less prone to be influenced by other concomitant deficits such as simultagnosia. In comparison with controls, PCA patients with signs of left-sided and right-sided neglect presented prominent hypoperfusion in right and left frontoparietal cortical networks, respectively.[77] In another recent study, rightward bias (sign of left-sided neglect) in line bisection test was strongly correlated with atrophy and hypoperfusion in a large-scale frontoparietal network in the right hemisphere, involving the parietotemporal cortex, the middle frontal gyrus, and in the postcentral region (Fig. 15.8).[65]

Thus, in these studies signs of neglect seemed to correlate with dysfunction in large-scale frontoparietal networks, beyond the sites of parietal atrophy ((see reference 41, p. 4755 and p. 4752), consistent with evidence from patients with vascular lesions.[28,78]

Similar results on the task of line bisection were reported also in patients with classic AD.[38] Obviously, in neurodegenerative patients, other aspects of the disease, such as simultagnosia and object recognition deficits, can interfere with patients' performance on visual search tasks, such as target cancellation.

Simultagnosia

Simultagnosia is a rare neuropsychological condition characterized by impaired spatial awareness of more than one object at time[79] which can occur in patients with posterior brain damage of vascular or degenerative origin. Wolpert[80] described simultagnosia as an inability to interpret a complex visual scene (processing multiple items and the relations between them), despite preservation of the ability to apprehend individual items. Simultagnosia can occur in isolation, or in association with other elements of Bálint's syndrome (see below), that is, oculomotor apraxia and optic ataxia. Simultagnosia has been reported in patients with bilateral parietal and occipital damage.[79] There have also been some documented cases following either left or right unilateral parietal brain damage, but at least in some of these unilateral cases[81,82] the lesions included damage to the corpus callosum. White matter tractography studies revealed associations with bilateral damage to major pathways within the visuospatial attention network, including the superior longitudinal fasciculus, the inferior fronto-occipital fasciculus, and the inferior longitudinal fasciculus.[83] Thus, simultagnosia typically occurs after bilateral damage to parieto-occipital regions, often associated with bilateral white matter disconnections.

Diagnostic tests

In clinical practice, simultanagnosia is assessed by the description of complex visual scenes, such as the cookie theft test.[84] The tests consists of a complex image displaying a mother cleaning

---

Box 15.2 Patient 3: Unilateral spatial neglect and PCA-early onset AD variant (PCA-AD)

Patient 3 is a 58-year-old, right-handed medical doctor, who came to our observation after about a year-and-a-half from disease onset, characterized by multiple minor car accidents against left-sided obstacles.

Clinical and neuropsychological examination revealed signs of severe left visual neglect (see Fig. 15.3), along with optic ataxia and ocular apraxia, as well as left ideomotor apraxia. There was a moderate rightward deviation (19 per cent) on line bisection; her performance was pathological on the landscape drawing copy and on the clock-drawing test. She showed no auditory extinction, although she had some difficulty to identify auditory stimuli presented on the left side. There were rare left tactile extinctions on double stimulation. Mild memory impairment, especially with visuospatial material, and a very mild *simultanagnosia* were also present. Executive functions and calculation were relatively spared. Rare difficulties in word finding and occasional phonologic paraphasias occurred.

Cerebrospinal fluid analysis revealed positive AD biomarkers (raised tau and phosphorylated tau proteins, and reduced amyloid β peptide). High-resolution MRI demonstrated bilateral cortical atrophy mainly located in the parietal lobes, confirmed by a detailed analysis performed by using voxel-based morphometry (VBM) (Fig. 15.6a). In agreement with current clinical criteria (see reference 103) a diagnosis of PCA was made.

During a two-year follow-up, the neuropsychological profile remained highly asymmetric with language and verbal memory largely preserved, while left visual neglect continued to represent the most severe symptom, and remained a substantial source of handicap in her everyday life.

A detailed anatomical study was conducted in order to study the grey and white matter status. VBM confirmed the bilateral posterior grey matter atrophy, including occipitotemporal and parietal cortices (Fig. 15.6a). Importantly, the tractography study of long-range white matter fibres demonstrated white matter damage largely restricted to the right hemisphere, including the superior and inferior longitudinal fasciculi and the inferior fronto-occipital fasciculus, while the homologous left-hemisphere tracts were spared (Fig. 15.6b). These data suggest that visuospatial deficits typical of PCA (such as neglect) may not result from cortical damage alone, but by a network-level dysfunction including white matter damage along the major large-scale pathways. The sparing of all the explored fasciculi in the left hemisphere, despite the cortical involvement of the occipital and parietal lobes, is consistent with the patient's cognitive profile, characterized by relatively intact language and calculation abilities.[41]

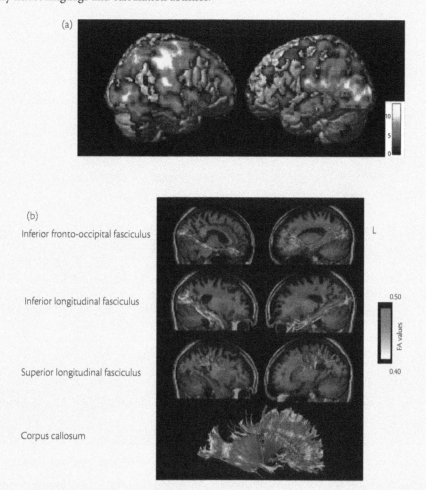

Fig. 15.6 PCA-AD patient 3. (a) Voxel-based morphometry as compared with a group of healthy controls. Regions of grey matter atrophy are shown in a colour code indicating the degree of atrophy, ranging from red (lower) to yellow (greater). Atrophy is displayed on the three-dimensional rendering of the Montreal Neurological Institute standard brain. (b) Long-range white matter tracts in the same patient, rendered as maps of fractional anisotropy (FA, an index of microstructural white matter integrity) displayed on the native T1-weighted MRI for both hemispheres. FA values range from 0.40 (yellow, greater damage) to 0.50 (red, lesser damage). In comparison to a group of healthy controls, maximum damage was found in the right frontoparietal superior longitudinal fasciculus. Inferior longitudinal fasciculus and inferior fronto-occipital fasciculus were also affected in the right hemisphere. There was also fibres loss in the posterior part of corpus callosum. Left hemisphere tracts did not differ from controls. See Box 15.2 for more clinical details.

Reproduced from *Cortex*, 48(10), Migliaccio R, Agosta F, Toba MN, et al., Brain networks in posterior cortical atrophy: a single case tractography study and literature review, pp. 1298–309, Copyright (2012), with permission from Elsevier.

dishes in a kitchen, and not noticing that the sink is overflowing and that a boy is about to fall while attempting to steal cookies behind her back. Patients with simultagnosia typically focus on one or two details of the scene, without being able to describe the others.

In the overlapping figures test,[31,85] multiple drawn objects are shown superimposed on each other. Patients are asked to name or indicate in a multiple-choice display all the objects seen, but may fail to identify most of them in case of simultagnosia.

Bálint syndrome

Bálint syndrome is a rare neurovisual disorder characterized by three elements: optic ataxia, oculomotor apraxia, and simultagnosia.[79] In 1909, Rezső Bálint described with the name of 'psychic paralysis of gaze' the case of a patient who had lost the ability to voluntarily move his gaze from one point to fixation to a new stimulus presented in the visual periphery.[86] This disorder is also known under the name of oculomotor apraxia. Patients cannot take

Box 15.3 Patient 4: Unilateral spatial neglect in PCA-CBD

Patient 4 is a 55-year-old woman, right-handed, was evaluated at about three years from clinical onset. She had a similar clinical history to patient 3; however, she deteriorated very rapidly in the visuospatial domain, while retaining almost normal performance in other cognitive domains. She mainly complained of visual deficit; her caregiver reported deficits occurring in everyday life and clearly resulting from visuospatial neglect.

Clinical and cognitive evaluation demonstrated signs of left visual neglect (see Fig. 15.3, lower panel, and Fig. 15.5), consisting in a moderate (17 per cent) rightward deviation on visual line bisection, and pathological scores on landscape drawing copy and clock drawing test, with an object-based pattern of omissions. Optic ataxia, visual and auditory left extinctions, along with alexia, and elements of Gerstmann syndrome (dysgraphia, finger agnosia, acalculia) were also present. She presented also constructional, ideomotor, and mielokinetic apraxia, with greater impairment for the execution of bimanual tasks and for the accurate movements and configurations involving the fingers. Memory and language were relatively preserved. Executive functions were slightly impaired. At neurological examination she was hypomimic and with a mild right-lateralized rigidity. CSF analysis was negative for AD biomarkers (tau and phosphorylated tau proteins, and amyloid β peptide levels were within normal range). MRI showed greater brain atrophy located in the posterior regions bilaterally, and in the frontal areas (with right predominance) (Fig. 15.7). Based on clinical features, such as hypomimia and rigidity, as well as the presence of limb apraxia, a clinical diagnosis of corticobasal syndrome was proposed. A presynaptic dopamine transporter (DAT)-scan study demonstrated an asymmetric decrease of the uptake, with right side predominance, corresponding to the rigidity. This finding confirmed the *in vivo* diagnosis of corticobasal syndrome.

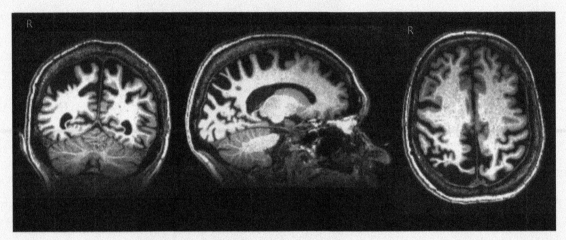

Fig. 15.7 Native high-resolution structural MRI of PCA-CBS patient 4. Note the bilateral posterior brain atrophy. There was also mild right frontal atrophy (data not shown). See Box 15.3 for more clinical details.

their eyes off fixed object (Holmes[87] called this disorder 'spasm of fixation'), in order to produce saccades towards other objects. Slow tracking movements may instead be preserved. The other two elements of Bálint syndrome are simultanagnosia (described in the previous paragraph) and optic ataxia—the inability to produce a correct movement of the hand to reach an object, typically presented in the periphery of visual field, under visual guidance. Similar to simultanagnosia, the typical lesion locations in Bálint syndrome are parietal or parieto-occipital bilateral. The most common cause is vascular (watershed strokes between middle and posterior cerebral arteries territories), tumour metastasis, or neurodegeneration (e.g. PCA, CBD; see also Boxes 15.2 and 15.3). Regarding optic ataxia, lesions of the superior parietal lobule and to its connections with frontal areas (supplementary motor area and frontal eye fields) appear to play a key role.[88]

Diagnostic tests

Clinically, oculomotor apraxia can be assessed asking the patient, who is seated in front of the examiner, to move the eyes towards

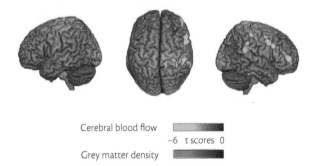

Cerebral blood flow

−6 t scores 0

Grey matter density

Fig. 15.8 Statistical parametric mapping results obtained in a sample of 15 patients with PCA, who underwent structural MRI and single photon emission computed tomography. The figure represents the regions of significant correlation between grey matter atrophy (red), regional brain hypoperfusion (green) and rightwards deviations on the bisection of 20-cm long horizontal lines.

Reproduced from *J Neurol Neurosur Ps.* 83(9), Andrade K, Kas A, Valabrègue R, *et al.*, Visuospatial deficits in posterior cortical atrophy: structural and functional correlates, pp. 860–3, Copyright (2012), with permission from BMJ Publishing Group Ltd.

a moving target after having fixated the examiner's nose. The four visual quadrants are evaluated.[89]

To assess optic ataxia, the examiner asks the patient to fixate his or her nose, then to use a designated hand (left or right) to reach a moving target (e.g. a pen) without losing fixation. The examiner moves the target across the four visual quadrants.[89]

Attention and monitoring deficits in vascular stroke and neurodegeneration

Focusing attention in space and sustaining it in time, as well as monitoring behaviour, are often considered to be mediated by cortical and subcortical frontal structures[90–92] and by their connections with parietotemporal regions.[4,11,16] Two principal neurodegenerative diseases can show deficits in these cognitive domains: AD and frontotemporal dementia (FTD, particularly behavioural-variant FTD).

Many clinical and cognitive studies have compared attention and monitoring in AD and FTD. Based on different patterns of neurodegeneration, peculiar general clinical and cognitive profiles have been described. Early memory impairment and following language, praxis, and visuospatial deficits are typically described in AD. In AD, the trajectory of the damage includes the hippocampal and perihippocampal regions, where the neurodegeneration originates causing memory failure, to the more posterior associative temporoparietal areas. Conversely, early changes in social conduct, insight, affective behaviour, along with impaired initiative, verbal fluency, attention, planning, set-shifting, problem-solving, and working memory depend on pathological changes in the orbitofrontal and dorsolateral prefrontal cortex, characteristically affected in patients with FTD.[93]

Notwithstanding their profound biological, anatomical, and cognitive differences, AD and FTD can have similar consequences in executive function. Executive deficits reflect an impaired integration of the frontal lobes with different brain areas, and in particular with more posterior brain regions. These functional and anatomical connections are damaged in both AD and FTD, thus perhaps accounting for their similarity in this specific domain. For this reason, it might prove difficult to differentiate, on the basis of these functions, patients with FTD and AD, particularly when AD patients are younger and atypical.

From the functional point of view, several large-scale brain networks, described as being dysfunctional in AD and FTD, are implicated in attention and monitoring behaviour, such as networks implicated in salience processing,[94] executive processes,[95] attention/working memory processes,[96] as well as the dorsal attentional network.[97] These functional networks are mainly impaired in FTD[98] and may represent a pathophysiological signature of this disease.

Little is known on the potential occurrence of visuospatial attention deficits in FTD, although patients with vascular stroke in the frontal lobes can sometimes demonstrate signs of spatial neglect.[99] Note, however, that frontal lobe neglect is typically observed after lateral frontal damage,[100] (i.e. in the prefrontal nodes of the attentional networks see Fig. 15.1), whereas in the behavioural variant of FTD, the atrophy affects first and foremost the frontomedian brain regions, the anterior insula, and the thalamus.[101]

Patients with DLB can show much more substantial deficits of attention. They can demonstrate a combination of severe attentional deficits and visuospatial dysfunction that can help to differentiate DLB from AD. DLB patients usually suffer from deficits in selective, sustained, and divided attention more severe than those found in AD patients. As a consequence, DLB patients typically perform better than AD patients on tests of verbal memory but worse on visuospatial performance tasks. Fluctuations in cognitive function—which may vary over minutes, hours, or days—occur in 50–75 per cent of patients and are associated with shifting degrees of attention and alertness.[102]

Conclusion

Disorders of attention are common in neurodegenerative conditions. These disorders often go undetected by the clinician, but can have a severe impact on patients' well-being and autonomy. These patients who are not able to explore their visual environment thoroughly can be far more handicapped in their daily life than patients with sensory deficits affecting perception directly, but leaving attention unimpaired, such as impaired visual acuity or homonymous hemianopia. Thus, the clinician should be aware of the variety of attention disorders which can occur in different neurodegenerative conditions, and of the (often very easy) diagnostic tests that can be used to detect them.

Acknowledgements

The authors received funding from the Fondation 'France Alzheimer', Fondation 'Philippe Chatrier' and from the programme 'Investissements d'Avenir' ANR-10-IAIHU-06.

References

1. Di Ferdinando A, Parisi D, and Bartolomeo P. Modeling orienting behavior and its disorders with 'ecological' neural networks. *J Cognitive Neurosc.* 2007;19(6):1033–49.
2. Allport DA. Visual attention. In: Posner MI, editor. *Foundations of Cognitive Science.* Cambridge, MA: MIT Press, 1989, pp. 631–87.
3. Desimone R and Duncan J. Neural mechanisms of selective visual attention. *Annu Rev Neurosci.* 1995;18:193–222.
4. Bartolomeo P. *Attention Disorders after Right Brain Damage: Living in Halved Worlds.* London: Springer-Verlag, 2014.
5. Robertson IH and Garavan H. Vigilant Attention. In: Gazzaniga MS (ed.). *The Cognitive Neurosciences*, 3rd edn. Cambirdge, MA:MIT Press, 2004, pp. 563–78.
6. Silvetti M, Seurinck R, and Verguts T. Value and prediction error in medial frontal cortex: integrating the single-unit and systems levels of analysis. *Front Hum Neurosci.* 2011;5:75.
7. Brown JW. Beyond conflict monitoring: cognitive control and the neural basis of thinking before you Act. *Current Directions in Psychological Science.* 2013 June 1, 2013;22(3):179–85.
8. Possin KL. Visual spatial cognition in neurodegenerative disease. *Neurocase.* 2010 Dec;16(6):466–87.
9. Buschman TJ and Miller EK. Top-down versus bottom-up control of attention in the prefrontal and posterior parietal cortices. *Science.* 2007 March 30, 2007;315(5820):1860–2.
10. Corbetta M and Shulman GL. Control of goal-directed and stimulus-driven attention in the brain. *Nature Neurosci.* 2002;3(3):201–15.
11. Singh-Curry V and Husain M. The functional role of the inferior parietal lobe in the dorsal and ventral stream dichotomy. *Neuropsychologia.* 2009 May;47(6):1434–48.
12. Nobre AC, Sebestyen GN, Gitelman DR, *et al.* Functional localization of the system for visuospatial attention using positron emission tomography. *Brain.* 1997;120:515–33.
13. Bourgeois A, Chica AB, Valero-Cabré A, *et al.* Cortical control of inhibition of return: Exploring the causal contributions of the left parietal cortex. *Cortex.* 2013.

14. Petrides M and Pandya DN. Projections to the frontal cortex from the posterior parietal region in the rhesus monkey. *J Comp Neurol.* 1984 Sep 1;228(1):105–16.

15. Schmahmann JD and Pandya DN. *Fiber Pathways of the Brain.* New York, NY: Oxford University Press, 2006.

16. Thiebaut de Schotten M, Dell'Acqua F, et al. A lateralized brain network for visuospatial attention. *Nature Neurosci.* 2011 Sep 18;14(10):1245–6.

17. Bowers D and Heilman KM. Pseudoneglect: Effects of hemispace on a tactile line bisection task. *Neuropsychologia.* 1980;18:491–8.

18. Jewell G and McCourt ME. Pseudoneglect: a review and meta-analysis of performance factors in line bisection tasks. *Neuropsychologia.* 2000;38(1):93–110.

19. Toba MN, Cavanagh P, and Bartolomeo P. Attention biases the perceived midpoint of horizontal lines. *Neuropsychologia.* 2011;49(2):238–346.

20. Husain M and Nachev P. Space and the parietal cortex. *Trends Cognit Sci.* 2007 Jan;11(1):30–66.

21. Mishkin M, Ungerleider LG, and Macko KA. Object vision and spatial vision: Two cortical pathways. *Trends Neurosci.* 1983;6:414–7.

22. Goodale MA and Milner AD. Separate visual pathways for perception and action. *Trends Neurosci.* 1992 Jan;15(1):20–5.

23. Catani M, Jones DK, Donato R, et al. Occipito-temporal connections in the human brain. *Brain.* 2003 Sep;126(Pt 9):2093–107.

24. ffytche DH and Blom JD, Catani M. Disorders of visual perception. *J Neurol Neurosur Ps.* 2010 Oct 22;81(11):1280–7.

25. Seeley WW, Crawford RK, Zhou J, et al. Neurodegenerative diseases target large-scale human brain networks. *Neuron.* 2009 Apr 16;62(1):42–52.

26. Migliaccio R, Agosta F, Scola E, Magnani G, Cappa SF, Pagani E, et al. Ventral and dorsal visual streams in posterior cortical atrophy: a DT MRI study. *Neurobiol Aging.* 2012 Nov;33(11):2572–84.

27. Bartolomeo P. A parieto-frontal network for spatial awareness in the right hemisphere of the human brain. *Archives of Neurology.* 2006;63:1238–41.

28. Bartolomeo P, Thiebaut de Schotten M, et al. Left unilateral neglect as a disconnection syndrome. *Cereb Cortex.* 2007;45(14):3127–48.

29. Parton A, Malhotra P, and Husain M. Hemispatial neglect. *J Neurol Neurosur Ps.* 2004;75(1):13–21.

30. Azouvi P, Bartolomeo P, Beis J-M, et al. A battery of tests for the quantitative assessment of unilateral neglect. *Restorative Neurology and Neuroscience.* 2006;24(4–6):273–85.

31. Gainotti G, D'Erme P, and Bartolomeo P. Early orientation of attention toward the half space ipsilateral to the lesion in patients with unilateral brain damage. *J Neurol Neurosur Ps.* 1991;54:1082–9.

32. Beis JM, Keller C, Morin N, et al. Right spatial neglect after left hemisphere stroke: *Qualitative and Quantitative Study. Neurology.* 2004 11 9;63(9):1600–5.

33. Bartolomeo P, Chokron S, and Gainotti G. Laterally directed arm movements and right unilateral neglect after left hemisphere damage. *Neuropsychologia.* 2001;39(10):1013–21.

34. Luaute J, Halligan P, Rode G, et al. Visuo-spatial neglect: a systematic review of current interventions and their effectiveness. *Neurosci Biobehav Rev.* 2006;30(7):961–82.

35. Gorgoraptis N, Mah YH, Machner B, et al. The effects of the dopamine agonist rotigotine on hemispatial neglect following stroke. *Brain.* 2012 Jul 2.

36. Mendez MF, Cherrier MM, and Cymerman JS. Hemispatial neglect on visual search tasks in Alzheimer's disease. *Neuropsy Neuropsy Be.* 1997;10:203–8.

37. Bartolomeo P, Dalla Barba G, Boissé MT, et al. Right-side neglect in Alzheimer's disease. *Neurology.* 1998;51(4):1207–9.

38. Ishiai S, Koyama Y, Seki K, et al. Unilateral spatial neglect in AD: significance of line bisection performance. *Neurology.* 2000 Aug 8;55(3):364–70.

39. Venneri A, Pentore R, Cotticelli B, et al. Unilateral spatial neglect in the late stage of Alzheimer's disease. *Cortex.* 1998;34(5):743–52.

40. Andrade K, Samri D, Sarazin M, et al. Visual neglect in posterior cortical atrophy. *BMC Neurology.* 2010;10:68.

41. Migliaccio R, Agosta F, Toba MN, Sa et al. Brain networks in posterior cortical atrophy: A single case tractography study and literature review. *Cortex.* 2012 Nov;48(10):1298–309.

42. Bartolomeo P and Chokron S. Levels of impairment in unilateral neglect. In: F Boller and J Grafman J (eds). *Handbook of Neuropsychology.* 2nd edn. Amsterdam: Elsevier Science Publishers, 2001, pp. 67–98.

43. Halligan PW and Bartolomeo P. Visual neglect. In: Ramachandran V (ed.). *Encyclopedia of Human Behavior,* 2nd edn. 2012, pp. 652–64.

44. Silveri MC, Ciccarelli N, and Cappa A. Unilateral spatial neglect in degenerative brain pathology. *Neuropsychology.* 2011;25(5):554–66.

45. Parasuraman R, Greenwood PM, Haxby JV, et al. Visuospatial attention dementia of the Alzheimer type. *Brain.* 1992;115 (Pt 3):711–33.

46. Balota DA and Faust ME. Attention in dementia of the Alzheimer's type. In: F Boller and J Grafman (eds). *Handbook of Neuropsychology.* 2nd edn. Amsterdam: Elsevier Science Publishers, 2001, pp. 51–80.

47. Danckert J, Maruff P, Crowe S, et al. Inhibitory processes in covert orienting in patients with Alzheimer's disease. *Neuropsychology.* 1998;12:225–41.

48. Wright MJ, Burns RJ, Geffen GM, and Geffen LB. Covert orientation of visual attention in Parkinson's disease: an impairment in the maintenance of attention. *Neuropsychologia.* 1990;28(2):151–9.

49. Cristinzio C, Bononi M, Piacentini S, et al. Attentional networks in Parkinson's disease. *Behavioural Neurology.* 2013;27(4):495–500.

50. Couette M, Bachoud-Lévi AC, Brugières P, et al. Orienting of spatial attention in Huntington's Disease. *Neuropsychologia.* 2008;46(5):1391–400.

51. Georgiou-Karistianis N, Farrow M, Wilson-Ching M, et al. Deficits in selective attention in symptomatic Huntington disease: assessment using an attentional blink paradigm. *Cogn Behav Neurol.* 2012 Mar;25(1):1–6.

52. Rafal RD, Posner MI, Friedman JH, et al. Orienting of visual attention in progressive supranuclear palsy. *Brain.* 1988;111(Pt 2):267–80.

53. Gainotti G, Messerli P, and Tissot R. Qualitative analysis of unilateral spatial neglect in relation to the laterality of cerebral lesions. *J Neurol Neurosur Ps.* 1972;35:545–50.

54. Marshall JC and Halligan PW. Visuo-spatial neglect: a new copying test to assess perceptual parsing. *J Neurol.* 1993;240(1):37–40.

55. Walker R. Spatial and object-based neglect. *Neurocase.* 1995;1:371–83.

56. Albert ML. A simple test of visual neglect. *Neurology.* 1973;23:658–64.

57. Mesulam MM. Attention, confusional states and neglect. In: MM Mesulam (ed.). *Principles of Behavioral Neurology.* Philadelphia, PA: F.A. Davis, 1985, pp. 125–68.

58. Gauthier L, Dehaut F, and Joanette Y. The bells test: A quantitative and qualitative test for visual neglect. *Int J Clin Neuropsych.* 1989;11:49–53.

59. Halligan PW, Cockburn J, and Wilson B. The behavioural assessment of visual neglect. *Neuropsychological Rehabilitation.* 1991;1:5–32.

60. Bartolomeo P, D'Erme P, and Gainotti G. The relationship between visuospatial and representational neglect. *Neurology.* 1994;44:1710–4.

61. Schenkenberg T, Bradford DC, and Ajax ET. Line bisection and unilateral visual neglect in patients with neurologic impairment. *Neurology.* 1980;30:509–17.

62. Marshall JC and Halligan PW. When right goes left: An investigation of line bisection in a case of visual neglect. *Cortex.* 1989;25(3):503–15.

63. Heilman KM and Valenstein E. Mechanisms underlying hemispatial neglect. *Ann Neurol.* 1979;5:166–70.

64. Binder J, Marshall R, Lazar R, et al. Distinct syndromes of hemineglect. *Arch Neurol–Chicago.* 1992;49(11):1187–94.

65. Andrade K, Kas A, Valabrègue R, et al. Visuospatial deficits in posterior cortical atrophy: structural and functional correlates. *J Neurol Neurosur Ps.* 2012;83(9):860–3.

66. Vuilleumier PO and Rafal RD. A systematic study of visual extinction. Between- and within-field deficits of attention in hemispatial neglect. *Brain.* 2000 Jun;123 (Pt 6):1263–79.

67. Bartolomeo P, Perri R, and Gainotti G. The influence of limb crossing on left tactile extinction. *J Neurol Neurosur Ps.* 2004;75(1):49–55.

68. De Renzi E, Gentilini M, and Pattacini F. Auditory extinction following hemisphere damage. *Neuropsychologia.* 1984;22(6):733–44.

69. Bellas DN, Novelly RA, Eskenazi B, *et al*. The nature of unilateral neglect in the olfactory sensory system. *Neuropsychologia*. 1988;26(1):45–52.

70. Mattingley JB, Driver J, Beschin N, *et al*. Attentional competition between modalities: extinction between touch and vision after right hemisphere damage. *Neuropsychologia*. 1997;35(6):867–80.

71. Bender MB. *Disorders in Perception*. Springfield, Ill.: Thomas, 1952.

72. Critchley M. *The Parietal Lobes*. New York: Hafner, 1953.

73. Marzi CA, Girelli M, Natale E, *et al*. What exactly is extinguished in unilateral visual extinction? Neurophysiological evidence. *Neuropsychologia*. 2001;39(12):1354–66.

74. Oda H, Ohkawa S, and Maeda K. Hemispatial visual defect in Alzheimer's disease. *Neurocase*. 2008;14(2):141–6.

75. D'Erme P, Bartolomeo P, and Masullo C. Alzheimer's disease presenting with visuo-spatial disorders. *Ital J Neurol Sci*. 1991 (abstract);12:117.

76. Frisoni GB, Pievani M, Testa C, *et al*. The topography of grey matter involvement in early and late onset Alzheimer's disease. *Brain*. 2007;130(Pt 3):720–30.

77. Andrade K, Kas A, Samri D, *et al*. Visuospatial deficits and hemispheric perfusion asymmetries in posterior cortical atrophy. *Cortex*. 2013;49(4):940–7.

78. Doricchi F, Thiebaut de Schotten M, *et al*. White matter (dis)connections and gray matter (dys)functions in visual neglect: Gaining insights into the brain networks of spatial awareness. *Cortex*. 2008;44(8):983–95.

79. Rizzo M and Vecera SP. Psychoanatomical substrates of Balint's syndrome. *J Neurol Neurosur Ps*. 2002 Feb;72(2):162–78.

80. Wolpert I. Die Simultanagnosie: Störung der Gesamtauffassung. *Zeitschrift für die gesamte Neurologie und Psychiatrie*. 1924;93:397–415.

81. Clavagnier S, Fruhmann Berger M, Klockgether T, *et al*. Restricted ocular exploration does not seem to explain simultanagnosia. *Neuropsychologia*. 2006;44(12):2330–6.

82. Naccache L, Slachevsky A, Levy R, *et al*. Simultanagnosia in a patient with right brain lesions. *J Neurol*. 2000;247(8):650–1.

83. Chechlacz M, Rotshtein P, Hansen PC, *et al* The neural underpinings of simultanagnosia: disconnecting the visuospatial attention network. *J Cogn Neurosci*. 2012;24(3):718–35.

84. Goodglass H and Kaplan E. *The Assessment of Aphasia and Related Disorders*. Philadelphia: Lea & Febiger, 1983.

85. Poppelreuter W. *Die psychischen Schädigungen durch Kopfschuss im Kriege 1914-1916*. Leipzig: Voss, 1917.

86. Husain M and Stein J. Rezsö Bálint and his most celebrated case. *Arch Neurol*. 1988;45(1):89–93.

87. Holmes G. Spasm of fixation. *Trans Ophthalmol Soc UK*. 1930;50:253–62.

88. Pisella L, Ota H, Vighetto A, *et al*. Optic ataxia and Bálint's syndrome: neuropsychological and neurophysiological prospects. In: PJ Vinken and GW Bruyn (eds). *Handbook of Clinical Neurology*. Amsterdam: Elsevier, 2008, pp. 393–415.

89. Kas A, de Souza LC, Samri D, *et al*. Neural correlates of cognitive impairment in posterior cortical atrophy. *Brain*. 2011;134(Pt 5):1464–78.

90. Duncan J. The structure of cognition: attentional episodes in mind and brain. *Neuron*. 2013;80(1):35–50.

91. Fuster JM. *The Prefrontal Cortex: Anatomy, Physiology and Neuropsychology of the Frontal Lobe*. 3rd edn. Philadelphia, PA: Lippincott-Raven, 1997.

92. Miller EK. The prefrontal cortex and cognitive control. *Nature Neurosci*. 2000;1(1):59.

93. Rosen HJ, Gorno-Tempini ML, Goldman WP, *et al*. Patterns of brain atrophy in frontotemporal dementia and semantic dementia. *Neurology*. 2002 Jan 22;58(2):198–208.

94. Seeley WW, Menon V, Schatzberg AF, *et al*. Dissociable intrinsic connectivity networks for salience processing and executive control. *J Neurosci*. 2007 Feb 28;27(9):2349–56.

95. Seeley WW, Crawford R, Rascovsky K, *et al*. Frontal paralimbic network atrophy in very mild behavioral variant frontotemporal dementia. *Arch Neurol*. 2008 Feb;65(2):249–55.

96. Damoiseaux JS, Rombouts SA, Barkhof F, *et al*. Consistent resting-state networks across healthy subjects. *Proc Natl Acad Sci USA*. 2006 Sep 12;103(37):13848–53.

97. Fox MD, Corbetta M, Snyder AZ, *et al*. Spontaneous neuronal activity distinguishes human dorsal and ventral attention systems. *Proc Natl Acad Sci USA*. 2006 June 27, 2006;103(26):10046–51.

98. Filippi M, Agosta F, Scola E, *et al*. Functional network connectivity in the behavioral variant of frontotemporal dementia. *Cortex*. 2012 Oct 24.

99. Husain M and Kennard C. Visual neglect associated with frontal lobe infarction. *J Neurol*. 1996 Sep;243(9):652–7.

100. Vallar G. Extrapersonal visual unilateral spatial neglect and its neuroanatomy. *Neuroimage*. 2001;14(1 Pt 2):S52–S8.

101. Schroeter ML, Raczka K, Neumann J, *et al*. Neural networks in frontotemporal dementia—A meta-analysis. *Neurobiol Aging*. 2008;29(3):418–26.

102. McKeith I, Mintzer J, Aarsland D, *et al*. Dementia with Lewy bodies. *Lancet Neurol*. 2004;3(1):19–28.

103. Migliaccio R, Agosta F, Rascovsky K, *et al*. Clinical syndromes associated with posterior atrophy: early age at onset AD spectrum. *Neurology*. 2009 Nov 10;73(19):1571–8.

104. Corbetta M, Kincade JM, and Shulman GL. Neural systems for visual orienting and their relationships to spatial working memory. *J Cogn Neurosci*. 2002 Apr 1;14(3):508–23.

CHAPTER 16

Apraxia

Georg Goldenberg

Concepts and classification of apraxia

Definition of apraxia

The term apraxia refers to 'higher-level' disorders of motor control. There is, however, no general agreement as to what counts as a high or a low level of motor control. Most agree though that apraxia should not be used to describe difficulties that might be attributed entirely to weakness, or loss of sensation, rigidity, tremor, or dystonia. However, this would be a diagnosis of exclusion. Moreover, in many neurological conditions apraxia can occur in the context of one or more of these deficits. Consequently, the history of apraxia has brought forward a wide variety of diverging definitions and classifications (Box 16.1).

The most influential of them was proposed some hundred years ago by the German psychiatrist Hugo Liepmann.[1,2] He distinguished two consecutive phases of voluntary motor action. The first is the creation of mental images of the intended actions, and the second their transduction into appropriate motor commands. Liepmann named disturbances of the first phase 'ideational' and that of the second phase 'ideo-kinetic' apraxia, which later authors re-baptized as *ideomotor* apraxia,[2,3] a distinction that still remains in widespread use (but see Box 16.1 for discussion of the utility of this distinction).

Although 'apraxia' has been applied to disturbances of widely different actions (e.g. lid closure, gait, gestures, or even spatial constructions), there is a core of clinical manifestations affecting limb function which have been the focus of the concept. They include:

- imitation of gestures
- communicative gestures on command and pantomime of tool use
- use of tools and objects

Deficits in all of these occur predominantly after left brain lesions and are frequently, though not invariably, associated with aphasia. In contrast to 'low-level' motor symptoms associated with unilateral hemispheric damage, they affect not only the contralesional limb (on the side of the body opposite to the cerebral lesion) but also the ipsilesional limb. In sections below, we examine each of these domains and how to examine for deficits in patients. In addition, we consider a particular aspect of tool and object use that involves:

- Multi-step actions involving several tools and objects

Box 16.1 Development of concepts of apraxia

Based on the associationist model of brain function prevalent at that time, Liepmann assumed that mental images emerge from revival of memory traces of previous sensations. He speculated that their translation into motor commands was accomplished by fibres that connect posterior sensory brain regions to the motor cortex in the anterior part of the brain. These fibres pass below the parietal cortex. Parietal lesions interrupt them and to cause 'ideo-kinetic' (now known as *ideo-motor*) apraxia.[4,5]

In the middle of the twentiehth century, when the localizing approach to mental function gave way to more functional and holistic theories, Liepmann's anatomical distinction between ideational and ideomotor apraxia fell into disfavour and was replaced by other systems of classification. Noteworthy, all of them retained some kind of dichotomy between high and low levels of motor controls. Thus, for example, they considered as opposites: autonomous action versus. environmental dependency; coping with novelty versus routine action, and abstract symbolic gestures versus material interactions with concrete objects (see references 6, 7, 8, and reference 9 for extensive historical review).

In the last third of the twentieth century, the renaissance of cerebral localization of mental function revamped Liepmann's ideas, which have strongly influenced modern accounts of apraxia and its cerebral localization.[10–14]

Ideomotor and ideational apraxia

Liepmann reasoned that in actual tool use, the interaction between the moving hand and external objects can compensate for an inability to direct movements that might arise because of a failure to transduce mental images into appropriate motor commands. In such cases, the deficit should be conspicuously apparent when actions have to be made without external counterpart. According to this reasoning *ideomotor apraxia* should affect *imitation* and the demonstration of *communicative gestures* but spare actual use of tools and objects.[1] Most modern authors who respect the traditional classification of apraxia adhere to this suggestion and apply the label 'ideomotor' to defective imitation as well as defective demonstration of communicative gestures, or compute compound scores from both for a diagnosis of ideomotor apraxia.[15–22]

However, the unity of imitation and demonstration of communicative gestures has been challenged by double dissociations between them. There are patients who are unable to correctly demonstrate communicative gestures but imitate flawlessly.[23] and others who have no problems with the demonstration of communicative gestures but commit many errors on imitation.[24–27] Their common classification as 'ideomotor' apraxia is misleading because it veils fundamental differences.

Most authors agree to apply the term *'ideational apraxia'* for *faulty use of tools and objects* but there is disagreement about the scope and nature of these errors. Liepmann had adopted the description of this variant of apraxia from the Prague psychiatrist, Arnold Pick.[28] who had reported gross errors in everyday *multi-step actions* like dressing or preparing a pipe by patients with dementia. Pick argued that most errors could be referred to perseveration and to neglect of the overarching goal of the multi-step sequence, rather than betraying problems that are specific for tool use. Liepmann agreed that ideational apraxia is the expression of a 'mental insufficiency which manifests itself in the domain of action but has its roots in deficits which are not specific for action'.[29]

By contrast, an alternative tradition originating with a seminal thesis of the French neurologist, Joseph Morlaas,[30] postulates that ideational apraxia can occur in patients without dementia and that it affects also the isolated use of *single tools*. Morlaas suggested the term *'agnosia of utilization'* to characterize the selective inability to recognize the way an object has to be used.[30,31]

In sum, the distinction between 'ideational' and 'ideomotor' does not correspond well with the clinical boundaries between different manifestations of apraxia and is confusing. It seems more productive to abandon it and to divide apraxia according to the affected *domain of action*. There are four of them: imitation of gestures, production of communicative gestures, use of single tools, and multi-step actions involving several tools and objects. Their autonomy is underlined by differences between the localizations of lesions interfering with each of them (Fig. 16.1).

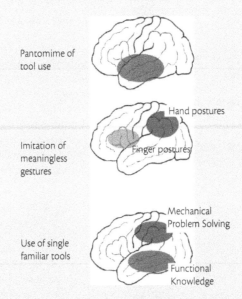

Fig. 16.1 Putative intra-hemispheric localization of left-sided lesions causing different manifestations of apraxia. Imitation of meaningless hand postures and mechanical problem solving depend on integrity of parietal region. By contrast, pantomime of tool use and retrieval of functional knowledge are vulnerable to temporal lesions. Imitation of finger configuration as well as performance of multi-step actions with multiple tools and objects are less strictly localized and can be impaired also by right hemisphere lesions.
Adapted from Goldenberg G. *Neuropsychologie—Grundlagen, Klinik, Rehabilitation,* Copyright (2007), with permission from Elsevier GmbH, Urban & Fischer, Munich.

Imitation of gestures

Success or failure of imitation of gestures may depend on the kind of gestures that are examined. A major distinction is that between meaningless and meaningful gestures (the meaning of meaningful gestures can be understood by other persons, thus they are, by definition, communicative, and I use the terms 'communicative' and 'meaningful' interchangeably).[23,32–34] This distinction derives from the fact that meaningful gestures have representations in semantic memory that associate their shapes with defined meanings. Their imitation may be accomplished by recognition of that meaning and reproduction of the corresponding shape. By contrast, the imitation of meaningless gestures requires reproduction of the shape of the gesture without support from semantic memory. Another factor influencing the success of imitation is whether *single static postures* or *movement sequences* are examined. Generally, sequences are more sensitive to brain damage but also less specific for its localization.[35–37] Here, we concentrate on the imitation of static meaningless gestures (Fig. 16.2).

Clinical diagnosis

Defective imitation will rarely be conspicuous in spontaneous behaviour but can easily be demonstrated on clinical examination. Even patients with severe aphasia mostly understand the instruction to imitate the examiner's actions. As with all manifestations of apraxia, the limb ipsilateral to the lesion should be tested to exclude contamination of results by the effects of hemiparesis. Many

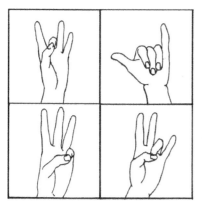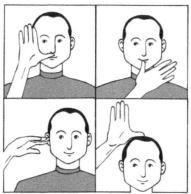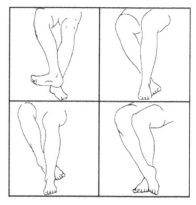

Fig. 16.2 Examples of hand, finger, and foot postures that show different sensitivity to left and right brain damage and within the left hemisphere to parietal and inferior frontal lesions. Scoring sheets for 10 hand and 10 finger postures with normative data are published as supplementary material to reference 53 and can also be obtained from the author.

Adapted from *Neurology*. 59(6), Goldenberg G and Strauss E, Hemisphere asymmetries for imitation of novel gestures, pp. 893–97, Copyright (2002), with permission from Wolters Kluwer Health, Inc.

clinicians ask patients to start their imitation only immediately *after* they have demonstrated the gesture. This brief delay introduces a working memory load that probably contributes to uncovering mild impairments. But patients with severe apraxia will show deficits even if the examiner's posture is still visible to them. The most reliable sign for the diagnosis of apraxia are spatially wrong final positions. Frequently, the movement path leading to the final position is hesitating with searching and self-correction, but there are apraxic patients who reach wrong final postures with swift and secure movements.[38]

Localization of lesions

The typical locations of lesions causing defective imitation depend on the body part performing it. Fig. 16.2 displays static postures of the finger, the hand, and the foot that have been used for assessing this body-part specificity.[39–41] Whereas defective imitation of hand postures is nearly exclusively bound to left hemisphere lesions, imitation of finger and foot postures is also susceptible to right hemisphere lesions.[39,42–44] Within the left hemisphere, defective imitation of hand postures is strongly linked to parietal lobe damage whereas defective imitation of finger postures can also be caused by frontal and subcortical lesions.[40,41,45–47]

Theoretical implications

The route from perception to imitation of meaningless gestures is direct in that it bypasses reference to semantic memory storage of conventional shapes of familiar gestures.[14] However, there are reasons to doubt that it is direct also in that it connects perception and execution of gestures without any interpolated cognitive processing. Thus patients who show apraxia for imitation of meaningless hand postures are also impaired when asked to replicate hand postures on a manikin[48] or to match pictures of meaningless gestures demonstrated by different persons under different angles of view,[49] although the motor actions of manipulating a manikin of pointing to pictures are very different from those of imitating the target posture on the own body. Findings such as these suggest that there is an intermediate stage—between perception and action—where a more abstract representation of the gesture is created that can serve not only for motor replication of the gesture but also for matching gestures or for their replication on a manikin.

It has been suggested that creation of this abstract representation relies on '*body-part coding*' that enables reduction of gestures to simple spatial relationships between a limited number of defined body parts.[40,48,49] The body-part specificity of the neural substrates of defective imitation can be accounted for by the assumption that body-part coding is bound to integrity of left parietal regions, but that frontal, subcortical, and right hemisphere regions are required when gestures pose high demands on the distribution of spatial attention or on selection between perceptually highly confusable items. Differential demands of hand, finger, and footpostures on body-part coding, attention, and selection might explain why different regions are crucial for their successful imitation.[39,44,50,51] The discrepancy between the associations of responsible brain lesions with body parts and the somatotopic organization of motor cortex further underlines the independence of apraxia from the anatomy of 'low-level' motor control.

Communicative gestures and pantomime of tool use

The clinical examination of communicative gestures probes gestures that have a habitual shape and meaning, allowing unambiguous assessment of their correctness. Gestures that fulfil this condition are either 'emblems' that have a conventional meaning like thumb up for 'OK', or pantomimes of tool use that indicate objects by miming their use. Usually, diagnosis and research on apraxia concentrates on pantomime of tool use. A practical reason for this preference is that aphasic patients may not understand the verbal label of emblems, whereas comprehension of the name of a tool whose use they should demonstrate can be facilitated by showing the tool or a picture of it.

Clinical diagnosis

In clinical practice, a patient is asked by the examiner to demonstrate how he would make a common gesture ('emblem') or use a common tool. Comprehension of the instruction may pose problems when examining patients with severe aphasia, even if the tool whose use should be pantomimed is pointed to or shown on a photo. Failure of comprehension is rather obvious when patients grasp for the demonstrated object, try to name or describe it,[52] or outline with the finger a more or less recognizable shape on the table.

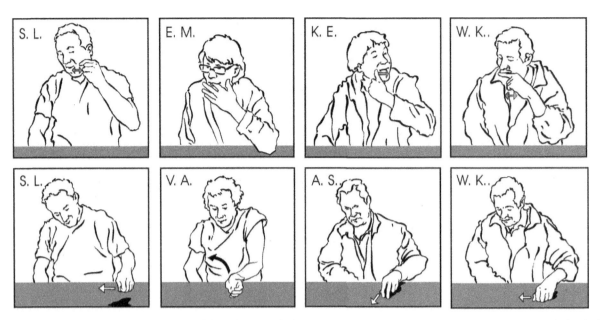

Fig. 16.3 Pantomimes of tool use made by patients with left brain damage and aphasia. Top row: Brushing teeth. S. L. makes a correct pantomime: The hand is formed to a precision grip, the distance between the hand and the mound corresponds to the approximate length of a toothbrush, and the hand is moved parallel to the mouth. E. M. only points to the mouth. K. E. moves the hand parallel to the mouth but neither the shape of the hand nor its distance to the mouth consider the imaginary toothbrush. W. K. shows 'body part as object' and moves the index as if it were the toothbrush. Bottom row: Ironing. Again, S. L. shows a correct pantomime. The hand is shaped as if it would rest on the handle of the flat iron, the distance to the table corresponds to the height of the iron, and it is moved in parallel to the table. V. A. demonstrates the approximate shape of the flat iron rather than pantomiming its use. A. S. slides the hand across the table as if it were the flat iron. W. K. shows the correct grip and the correct movement but disregards the distance between the hand and the table.

Adapted from Goldenberg G. *Neuropsychologie—Grundlagen, Klinik, Rehabilitation*, Copyright (2007), with permission from Elsevier GmbH, Urban & Fischer, Munich.

Exclusion of insufficient comprehension is more difficult, however, when patients outline the shape where the object would be used (e.g. a pipe in front of the mouth), or when they use the hand for symbolizing the object (using a body part as object, e.g. opening and closing index and middle finger for scissors). Even healthy people use such strategies and frequently prefer them to pure pantomime when communicating their needs to someone whose language they do not speak. They can switch to pure pantomime when explicitly asked to do so, but when patients with aphasia persist, it remains arguable whether they understood the request to switch to the less efficient strategy.

Independence of apraxic errors from language comprehension becomes obvious when patients make searching movements for the correct grip or movement or when their pantomime displays some but not all distinctive features of the intended pantomime (e.g. pantomiming drinking from a glass with a narrow grip not accommodated to the width of the pretended glass). Fig. 16.3 shows examples of apraxic errors for pantomimes of toothbrushing and ironing.

Qualitative assessment of a small number of pantomimes usually suffices for a clinical diagnosis of apraxia. Quantification of its severity requires standardized instruments. Reliable quantification can be accomplished by crediting points for the presence of predefined features for each pantomime. Table 16.1 shows such features for the pantomimes displayed in Fig. 16.3.[53]

Localization of lesions

In right-handers with typical laterality of cerebral functions, disturbance of pantomime is bound to left hemisphere lesions and virtually always associated with aphasia.[23,33,41,54–56] There are,

however, single case reports of left-handed patients with right-sided lesions who had apraxia for communicative gestures but no aphasia.[57–60] Contrary to widespread belief, there is no tight link between disturbed pantomime and parietal lesions. Independence of pantomime from integrity of the parietal lobe is demonstrated by single case reports of patients with parietal lesions who cannot imitate meaningless gestures but can produce pantomimes flawlessly,[24,27] and has been confirmed by group studies analysing lesions of patients with defective pantomime.[45,53,61,62] A growing number of systematic lesion symptom mapping studies indicate indicate inferior frontal and temporal regions as crucial for pantomime. If there is extension into parietal regions at all it is confined to the parietotemporal junction in the angular and supramarginal gyrus.[33,41,53,63,64]

Table 16.1 Examples from scoring sheet for pantomime of tool use. One point is credited for each of the features listed in the middle and right column

Command: Show me how you would	Grip	Movement and/or Position
brush teeth with a toothbrush	lateral or narrow cylindrical	repetitive small amplitude movements in frontal plane
		close to mouth but touching neither mouth nor face
iron with a flat iron	narrow cylindrical with axis of grip parallel to table	movement in horizontal plane
		distance to table appropriate for iron

Theoretical implications

A popular account of defective pantomime of tool use holds that patients have lost stored motor programmes required to direct the manual action of tool use,[10,65,66] but there are several arguments why this view might be too simplistic and does not cover all possible sources of error. Patients who fail pantomiming the use of tools have not necessarily lost the motor programmes of real use; indeed, a majority of them can use the same tools correctly.[67,68] Conversely, normal subjects can pantomime the use of objects which they are unable to manipulate in reality. For example, most persons can pantomime playing the violin or a trumpet but only a minority master the motor programmes for their actual use. Nor does normal pantomime faithfully replicate the motor acts of actual use. For example, when pantomiming taking up a glass for drinking, most people open their hand to the approximate width of the glass, transport the hand to its mimed location, stop there and move the hand to mouth without changing grip aperture. By contrast, for real grasping, the hand is initially opened wider than the glass and scaling is achieved by closing it around the glass in flight.

Such dissociations between pantomime and real use support the alternative suggestion that the manual action of pantomime is primarily intended *to communicate* the nature of the tool and its use.[53,56,69] Details of the manual actions that are not necessary for comprehension may not be expressed, whereas details that illustrate distinctive features of the object or its use may be exaggerated. Thus, for the pantomime of grasping a glass, the width of the hand aperture demonstrates the width of the glass, and stopping the transport of the hand suffices for indicating the grasp. According to this view, the problems of apraxic patient concern retrieval, selection, and demonstration of distinctive features of objects and their use, rather than replication of motor programmes for real use. Semantic knowledge about the tool and its use are necessary prerequisites for the selection of distinctive features whereas motor experience with actual use is not mandatory, as exemplified by the possibility of pantomiming actions for which one has no motor competence.

The idea that failure in pantomime is mainly due to insufficient retrieval and demonstration of semantic knowledge fits well with the predominant location of responsible lesions in left inferior frontal and temporal lobes as these regions do have a central role for semantic memory also beyond tool use.[70-72]

Use of single tools

Misuse of everyday tools and objects was the subject of the first printed use of the term 'apraxia'.[73] It remains an impressive symptom that may evoke a suspicion of general dementia. Patients may try to cut paper with closed scissors, eat soup with a fork, press the knife into the loaf without moving it to and fro, press the hammer upon the nail without hitting, and close the paper punch on top of the sheet without inserting the sheet.[51,50,74-76] Apparently, they have lost their knowledge of how to use these highly familiar tools.

Clinical diagnosis

For clinical diagnosis one presents to the patient a familiar tool and, if the tool is not used upon their own body (e.g. a comb), also the object—or 'recipient'—on which the tool acts (e.g. scissors and a sheet of paper, screwdriver and screw). Since many afflicted patients are hemiplegic, tool and object must be prepared for one-handed use (e.g. the sheet of paper kept in place by the examiner or the screw already partly placed into an unmovable support). Patients with right hemiparesis must perform with their non-dominant left hand, but their deviations from normal use surpass unmistakably the ineptness of a healthy person's left hand.

Localization of lesions

In patients with unilateral brain damage, defective use of single familiar tools and objects is bound to left hemisphere damage and associated with aphasia.[77,78] A group study of lesion symptom mapping pointed to a crucial role for left parietal lesions, but clinical experience suggests that at least for lasting impairment of single tool use the lesions must be quite extensive and frequently encroach also on temporal and frontal regions.[79]

The association with left brain damage applies also to deficits on tests that assess the putative components of knowledge about how to use single tools (see below) but indicate that they depend on different regions within the left hemisphere. Whereas retrieval of *functional knowledge* depends on integrity of the temporal lobes, *mechanical problem-solving* is disturbed mainly by parietal lesions.[79-81]

Theoretical implications

The gross misuse of familiar tools and objects evokes the impression that patients have lost their knowledge about how to use them. There are two possible sources of such knowledge. One of them is *functional knowledge* stored in semantic memory. It associates types of tools with their purpose, their 'recipient', and the action of their use. For example, a screwdriver serves for connecting or disconnecting parts, the recipient of its action is a screw, and the action is rotation. Retrieval of such functional knowledge can be probed without requiring the actual use of tools by asking subjects to match pictures of tools with pictures of other tools serving the same purpose or with pictures of the typical recipient of their action.[81-84]

An alternative source of knowledge about tool use is provided by *mechanical problem-solving* based on the direct inference of possible functions from structure.[78,81,84-87] The elements of mechanical problem-solving are not the prototypical functions of entire tools but the functional compatibilities of their parts.[88] Tools and objects are segmented into functionally significant parts and properties, and combinations of these parts and properties with parts and properties of other tools and objects are used for construction of mechanical chains. Mechanical problem-solving has been probed by confronting patients with novel tools and asking them to find out how to manipulate them or by presenting objects together with an array of tools but without the tool usually employed, and asking them to complete the task by using the tools in non-prototypical ways.[78,79,81,84,87,89]

There is controversy as to which of these two sources is more important for supporting correct tool use.[90,91] Probably both of them must be occluded to cause lasting deficits of single tool use in patients with patients with unilateral left-sided lesions.[78]

Multi-step actions involving several tools and objects

In daily living, one rarely encounters a situation as in testing for use of single tools where one is handed a tool and asked to perform the associated action on an adequately prepared 'recipient' of tool use. Typically, the use of single tools is embedded in a *chain of actions* involving several tools and objects and aiming at a superordinate goal. The need to keep track of completed and outstanding steps of actions, to avoid possible interferences between sequential action steps, and to maintain the superordinate goal against digressions create more opportunities for error than the isolated use of single tools. Whereas single tool use by healthy persons is virtually error-less, slips of actions in multi-step tasks are a common experience of everyday life, but they rarely attain the severity of errors that are committed by some patients with brain damage.

Clinical diagnosis

Assessment of multi-step actions with multiple objects trans-gresses the possibilities of routine clinical examination. In rehabilitation settings it is usually made by occupational thera-pists and concentrates on tasks that are important for everyday life like dressing or the preparation of meals and beverages.[75,92–98] Error rates increase when patients are required to coordinate two tasks; for example, when preparing two courses of a meal in par-allel,[99] or when they are confronted with unfamiliar and technical equipment.[96] Rating of success is quite straightforward when the number of completed steps of actions is evaluated but becomes intricate and less reliable when qualitative classifications of error types are attempted.[95,100]

Localization of lesions

In contrast to the tight link between left hemisphere damage and misuse of single tools, performance of multi-step actions with several tools and objects is about equally defective in patients with left-sided, right-sided, or diffuse brain damage.[96,99,100] Comparison between studies testing patients with frontal and with posterior lesions does not confirm the intuitive expectation that problems should be par-ticularly severe in patients with frontal lobe damage.[100,101]

Theoretical implications

The observation that execution of multi-step actions with sev-eral objects is vulnerable to brain damage in both hemispheres does not necessarily imply that the causes of failure are the same. Attempts to distinguish the types of errors committed by left and right brain-damaged patients did not yield convincing differ-ences,[99,100] but analysis of correlations with other symptoms of unilateral brain damage support the existence of different causal mechanisms.

In patients with left brain damage, the severity of difficulties on multi-step actions correlates with the errors on single tool use, with impairment of functional knowledge, and with severity of aphasia.[31,96] Since patients with right brain damage do not have these additional symptoms, the correlations cannot apply to their errors on multi-step actions. In patients with right brain dam-age, success on multi-step actions is correlated with the severity of hemi-neglect although errors are not necessarily confined to the left side of the working area.[96,99] Since neglect is generally absent or mild in patients with left brain damage, it cannot—conversely—be a prominent cause for their difficulties with multi-step actions.

A possible interpretation of these differential correlations could be that problems of patients with left brain damage concern retrieval of 'scripts' specifying the sequence and nature of action

Box 16.2 Bedside diagnosis of apraxia

Apraxia is not a unitary disorder. Failure on one test of apraxia does not necessarily predict similar impairment on another. For example, pantomime of tool use may be deficient but imitation preserved or vice versa. Separate assessment of all possible vari-ants of apraxia certainly exceeds the temporal limits of bedside testing. One possible reaction to this restriction is the assess-ment of sum scores. For example, communicative gestures may be probed both on verbal command and on imitation,[16,132,133] or imitation may be probed both for meaningful and meaning-less gestures,[18] and their results are added up. Such sum scores permit a reliable decision whether the general level of a patient's performance is within the range of healthy people, but they do not help to disentangle *individual patterns* of deficiencies and resources. Arguably, however, these individual differences are important not only for the theory of apraxia but also for clinical decisions concerning possible therapies of apraxia.

A practical solution to these difficulties is separate evaluation of a few clinically relevant domains of actions. I recommend testing imitation of meaningless static hand and finger postures, of pantomime of tool use and of use of single familiar tools. Observations of multi-step actions with multiple objects are usually beyond the limits of a clinical bedside examination, but can be made by prolonged assessment in daily life, and is often noted by nurses, occupational therapists, or the family. Hence, it is important to question carers and healthcare staff about their observations of patients' actions.

steps, whereas those of patients with right brain damage stem from insufficient maintenance of attention across the sequence of mul-tiple action steps and across the multiplicity of tools and objects involved in that sequence. This interpretation does not, however, exclude an additional contribution of less clearly lateralized apti-tudes like memory or problem-solving that are affected by lesions on either side of the brain.

The heterogeneity of apraxia makes a complete examination of all possible manifestations a cumbersome endeavour that can hardly be fulfilled within a routine neurological check-up. However, with some knowledge about the typical localization and clinical constellations underlying different manifestations it is possible to obtain relevant information within acceptable time limits and without a need for expensive technical equipment (see Box 16.2).

Apraxia in degenerative dementias

The overwhelming majority of studies on apraxia and hence of the evidence discussed in this chapter derive from patients with circum-scribed, mostly vascular, brain lesions. However, the decompos-ition of different components of apraxia allows speculations about their vulnerability to different variants of degenerative dementias, and the available empirical evidence allows some estimate of their plausibility.

Alzheimer's disease

Alzheimer's disease (AD) is characterized by widespread expan-sion of neuronal degeneration resulting in a combination of impairments of multiple cognitive functions, consequently one would expect that the neural substrates underlying all aspects of apraxia can be affected. Empirical studies have indeed revealed disturbances of imitation,[102–108] communicative gestures,[102,104–106,109–112] use of single tools,[102,113] and multi-step actions.[97,114] The disturbance of single tool use is likely to affect retrieval of functional knowledge as well as mechanical problem-solving.[113,115] Nonetheless, it has repeatedly been found to be less severe than that of pantomiming tool use.[109,110] In contrast to this relative preservation of single tool use, slips of actions and errors in daily life multi-step actions with multiple tools and objects are frequently among the earliest symptoms of AD reported by patients and their relatives.

Semantic dementia

Semantic dementia is a variant of frontotemporal dementia that affects left- more than right-sided inferior and anterior temporal regions but spares parietal cortex.[116] Comparison of this predilection with the lesions sites causing different manifestations of apraxia in patients with circumscribed brain damage (Fig. 16.1) leads to the expectation that retrieval of *functional knowledge* should be more severely affected than mechanical problem solving and imitation of meaningless gestures. Indeed, it has been convincingly demonstrated that imitation of meaningless hand postures can be intact, with preserved mechanical problem-solving but defective functional knowledge.[117,118] Preservation of mechanical problem-solving possibly explains why real object use can be preserved in spite of loss of any semantic knowledge about the used objects.[91,119–121]

Corticobasal degeneration

Apraxia in corticobasal degeneration has been held to be the opposite of apraxia in semantic dementia by sparing temporal but affecting parietal components.[118] However, the clinical picture is more intricate. Its analysis is complicated by the additional occurrence of prominent disturbances of motor control that have been labelled 'limb kinetic apraxia'[122] but do not fulfil the criteria for 'high-level' apraxia. They do not affect both sides of the body equally and they interfere with any motor actions of the afflicted limb regardless of their cognitive demands.[123–125] The belief that corticobasal degeneration selectively affects parietal regions is also weakened by its overlap with progressive supranuclear palsy, frontotemporal dementia, and AD.[116,126,127] There is nonetheless good evidence for particularly severe impairments of mechanical problem-solving and imitation, but the sparing of other components of apraxia is much less regular.[85,128]

Posterior cortical atrophy

Posterior cortical atrophy is often found on pathological diagnosis to be a variant of AD. It begins with selective degeneration of parieto-occipital cortex and may present with very severe deficits of visual and spatial perception.[129,130] Evaluation of apraxia is complicated by the deleterious influence of visuoperceptual problems on tool use and imitation, but the few studies that looked for it have reported normal performance of communicative gestures including pantomime on command.[129–131] In view of the severe damage to all established functions of the parietal cortex, this sparing is a strong argument against a crucial role of parietal regions for pantomime of tool use.

References

1. Liepmann H. *Drei Aufsätze aus dem Apraxiegebiet*. Berlin: Karger, 1908.
2. Goldenberg G. Apraxia and beyond—life and works of Hugo Karl Liepmann. *Cortex*. 2003;39:509–25.
3. Foix C. Contribution a l'étude de l'apraxie ideomotrice. *Rev Neurol*. 1916;29:283–98.
4. Goldenberg G. Apraxia and the parietal lobes. *Neuropsychologia*. 2009;47:1449–59.
5. Catani M and Ffytche DH. The rises and falls of disconnection syndromes. *Brain*. 2005;128:2224–39.
6. Denny Brown D. The nature of apraxia. *J Nerv Ment Dis*. 1958;126:9–32.
7. De Ajuriaguerra J and Tissot R. The apraxias. In: PJ Vinken and GW Bruyn (eds). *Handbook of Clinical Neurology* Vol 4. Amsterdam: North Holland, 1969, pp. 48–66.
8. Goldstein K. *Language and Language Disturbances*. New York, NY: Grune and Stratton, 1948.
9. Goldenberg G. Apraxia—*The Cognitive Side of Motor Control*. Oxford: Oxford University Press, 2013.
10. Geschwind N. The apraxias: Neural mechanisms of disorders of learned movements. *American Scientist*. 1975;63:188–95.
11. Heilman KM, Rothi LJG. Apraxia. In: KM Heilman and E Valenstein (eds). *Clinical Neuropsychology*. Oxford: Oxford University Press, 1993, pp. 141–64.
12. Roy EA and Hall C. Limb Apraxia: A Process Approach. In: L Proteau and D Elliott (eds). *Vision and Motor Control*. Amsterdam: Elsevier, 1992, pp. 261–82.
13. De Renzi E. Apraxia. In: F Boller and J Grafman (eds). Handbook of Clinical Neuropsychology, Vol 2. Oxford: Elsevier, 1990, pp. 245–63.
14. Rothi LJG, Ochipa C, and Heilman KM. A cognitive neuropsychological model of limb praxis and apraxia. In: LJG Rothi and KM Heilman (eds). Apraxia—*The Neuropsychology of Action*. Hove: Psychology Press, 1997, pp. 29–50.
15. Buxbaum LJ. Ideomotor apraxia: a call to action. *Neurocase*. 2001;7:445–58.
16. Alexander MP, Baker E, Naeser MA, *et al*. Neuropsychological and neuroanatomic dimensions of ideomotor apraxia. *Brain*. 1992;115:87–107.
17. Basso A, Luzzatti C, and Spinnler H. Is ideomotor apraxia the outcome of damage to well defined regions of the left hemisphere? *J Neurol Neurosur Ps*. 1980;43:118–26.
18. De Renzi E, Motti F, and Nichelli P. Imitating gestures—A quantitative approach to ideomotor apraxia. *Arch Neurol*. 1980;37:6–10.
19. Haaland KY, Harrington DL, and Knight RT. Spatial deficits in ideomotor limb apraxia—a kinematic analysis of aiming movements. *Brain*. 1999;122:1169–82.
20. Heilman KM, Rothie LJ, and Valenstein E. Two forms of ideomotor apraxia. *Neurology*. 1982;32:342–46.
21. Schnider A, Hanlon RE, Alexander DN, *et al*. Ideomotor apraxia: Behavioral dimensions and neuroanatomical basis. *Brain Lang*. 1997;58:125–36.
22. Lehmkuhl G, Poeck K, and Willmes K. Ideomotor apraxia and aphasia: An examination of types and manifestations of apraxic symptoms. *Neuropsychologia*. 1983;21:199–212.
23. Barbieri C and De Renzi E. The executive and ideational components of apraxia. *Cortex*. 1988;24:535–44.
24. Goldenberg G and Hagmann S. The meaning of meaningless gestures: A study of visuo-imitative apraxia. *Neuropsychologia*. 1997;35:333–41.
25. Mehler MF. Visuo-imitative apraxia. *Neurology*. 1987;37,Suppl 1:129.
26. Cubelli R, Marchetti C, Boscolo G, *et al*. Cognition in action: testing a model of limb apraxia. *Brain Cognit*. 2000;44:144–65.
27. Peigneux P, Van der Linden M, Andres-Benito P, *et al*. Exploration neuropsychologique et par imagerie fonctionelle cérébrale d'une apraxie visuo-imitative. *Rev Neurol*. 2000;156:459–72.
28. Pick A. Studien zur motorischen Apraxie und ihr nahe stehenden Erscheinungen;ihre Bedeutung in der Symptomatologie psychopathischer Symptomenkomplexe. Leipzig und Wien: Franz Deuticke, 1905.

29. Liepmann H. Klinische und psychologische Untersuchung und anatomischer Befund bei einem Fall von Dyspraxie und Agraphie [posthumos publication]. *Monatschr Psychiat Neurol.* 1929;71:169–214.

30. Morlaas J. *Contribution à l'étude de l'apraxie.* Paris: Amédée Legrand, 1928.

31. De Renzi E and Lucchelli F. Ideational apraxia. *Brain.* 1988;111:1173–85.

32. Tessari A, Canessa N, Ukmar M, *et al.* Neuropsychological evidence for a strategic control of multiple routes in imitation. *Brain.* 2007;130:1111–26.

33. Mengotti P, Corradi-Dell'Aqua C, Negri GAL, *et al.* Selective imitation impairments differentially interact with language processing. *Brain.* 2013;136:2602–18.

34. Buxbaum LJ, Shapiro AD, and Coslett HB. Critical brain regions for tool related and imitative actions: A componential analysis. *Brain.* 2014;137:1971–85.

35. Canavan AGM, Passingham RE, Marsden CD, *et al.* Sequencing ability in Parkinsonians, patients with frontal lobe lesions and patients who have undergone unilateral temporal lobectomies. *Neuropsychologia.* 1989;27:787–98.

36. Kolb B and Milner B. Performance of complex arm and facial movements after focal brain lesions. *Neuropsychologia.* 1981;19:491–503.

37. Luria AR. *Higher Cortical Functions in Man*, 2nd edn. New York, NY: Basic Books, 1980.

38. Hermsdörfer J, Mai N, Spatt J, *et al.* Kinematic analysis of movement imitation in apraxia. *Brain.* 1996;119:1575–86.

39. Goldenberg G, Strauss S. Hemisphere asymmetries for imitation of novel gestures. *Neurology.* 2002;59:893–97.

40. Goldenberg G and Karnath HO. The neural basis of imitation is body-part specific. *J Neurosci.* 2006;26:6282–87.

41. Goldenberg G and Randerath J. Shared neural substrates of aphasia and apraxia. *Neuropsychologia.* 2015;75:40–49.

42. Della Sala S, Faglioni P, Motto C, *et al.* Hemisphere asymmetry for imitation of hand and finger movements, Goldenberg's hypothesis reworked. *Neuropsychologia.* 2006;44:1496–1500.

43. Bekkering H, Brass M, Woschina S, *et al.* Goal-directed imitation in patients with ideomotor apraxia. *Cognit Neuropsychol.* 2005;22:419–32.

44. Goldenberg G. Defective imitation of gestures in patients with damage in the left or right hemisphere. *J Neurol Neurosur Ps.* 1996;61:176–80.

45. Dovern A, Fink G, Saliger J, *et al.* Apraxia impairs intentional retrieval of incidentally acquired motor knowledge. *J Neurosci.* 2011;31:8102–8.

46. Haaland KY, Harrington DL, and Knight RT. Neural representations of skilled movement. *Brain.* 2000;123:2306–13.

47. Hoeren M, Kümmerer D, Bormann T, *et al.* Neural bases of imitation and pantomime in acute stroke patients: distinct streams for praxis. *Brain.* 2014;137:2796–2810.

48. Goldenberg G. Imitating gestures and manipulating a mannikin—the representation of the human body in ideomotor apraxia. *Neuropsychologia.* 1995;33:63–72.

49. Goldenberg G. Matching and imitation of hand and finger postures in patients with damage in the left or right hemisphere. *Neuropsychologia.* 1999;37:559–66.

50. Goldenberg G. Apraxia. In: G Goldenberg and B Miller (eds). *Handbook of Clinical Neurology*, 3rd Series, Vol 88: Neuropsychology and Behavioral Neurology. Edinburgh: Elsevier, 2008, pp. 323–38.

51. Goldenberg G, Münsinger U, and Karnath HO. Severity of neglect predicts accuracy of imitation in patients with right hemisphere lesions. *Neuropsychologia.* 2009;47:2948–52.

52. Goodglass H and Kaplan E. Disturbance of gesture and pantomime in aphasia. *Brain.* 1963;86:703–20.

53. Goldenberg G, Hermsdörfer J, Glindemann R, *et al.* Pantomime of tool use depends on integrity of left inferior frontal cortex. *Cerebral Cortex.* 2007;17:2769–76.

54. Roy EA, Black SE, Blair N, *et al* Analysis of deficits in gestural pantomime. *J Clinic Experim Neuropsychol.* 1998;20:628–43.

55. Roy EA, Heath M, Westwood D, *et al.* Task demands in limb apraxia and stroke. *Brain Cognit.* 2000;44:253–79.

56. Goldenberg G, Hartmann K, and Schlott I. Defective pantomime of object use in left brain damage: apraxia or asymbolia? *Neuropsychologia.* 2003;41:1565–73.

57. Heilman KM, Coyle JM, Gonyea EF, *et al.* Apraxia and agraphia in a left-hander. *Brain.* 1973;96:21–28.

58. Valenstein E and Heilman KM. Apraxic agraphia with neglect-induced paragraphia. *Arch Neurol.* 1979;36:506–508.

59. Margolin DI. Right hemisphere dominance for praxis and left hemisphere dominance for speech in a left-hander. *Neuropsychologia.* 1980;18:715–19.

60. Goldenberg G. Apraxia in left-handers. *Brain.* 2013;136:2592–2601.

61. Manuel A, Radman N, Mesot D, *et al.* Inter-and intra-hemispheric dissociations in ideomotor apraxia: a large-scale lesion-symptom mapping study in subacute brain-damaged patients. *Cerebral Cortex.* 2013;23:2781–89.

62. Bohlhalter S, Vanbellingen T, Bertschi M, *et al.* Interference with gesture production by theta burst stimulation over left inferior frontal cortex. *Clinical Neurophysiology.* 2011;122:1197–202.

63. Buxbaum LJ, Shapiro A, and Coslett HB. Critical brain regions for tool related and imitative actions: A componential analysis. *Brain.* 2014;137:1971–85.

64. Weiss PH, Ubben SD, Kaesberg S, *et al.* Where language meets meaningful action: a combined behavior and lesion analysis of aphasia and apraxia. *Brain Structure and Function.* 2014;1–14. doi 10.1007/s00429-014-0925-3.

65. Poizner H, Mack L, Verfaellie M, *et al.* Three-dimensional computer-graphic analysis of apraxia. *Brain.* 1990;113:85–101.

66. Daprati E and Sirigu A. How we interact with objects: learning from brain lesions. *Trends Cogn Sci.* 2006;10:265–70.

67. Goldenberg G, Hentze S, and Hermsdörfer J. The effect of tactile feedback on pantomime of object use in apraxia. *Neurology.* 2004;63:1863–67.

68. De Renzi E, Faglioni P, and Sorgato P. Modality-specific and supramodal mechanisms of apraxia. *Brain.* 1982;105:301–12.

69. Duffy RJ and Duffy JR. Three studies of deficits in pantomimic expression and pantomimic recognition in aphasia. *J Speech Hear Res.* 1981;14:70–84.

70. Binder JR and Desai RH. The neurobiology of semantic memory. *Trends Cogn Sci.* 2011;15:527–36.

71. Jefferies E. The neural basis of semantic cognition: Converging evidence from neuropsychology, neuroimaging and TMS. *Cortex.* 2013;49:611–25.

72. Kemmerer D, Rudrauf D, Manzel K, *et al.* Behavioral patterns and lesion sites associated with impaired processing of lexical and conceptual knowledge of actions. *Cortex.* 2012;48:826–48.

73. Steinthal H. *Abriss der Sprachwissenschaft.* Berlin: Ferd.Dümmlers Verlagsbuchhandlung Harrwitz und Gossmann, 1871.

74. Rumiati RI, Zanini S, Vorano L, *et al.* A form of ideatonal apraxia as a selective deficit of contention scheduling. *Cognit Neuropsychol.* 2001;18:617–42.

75. Foundas AL, Macauley BL, Raymer AM, Maher LM, Heilman KM, and Rothi LJG. Ecological implications of limb apraxia: Evidence from mealtime behaviour. *J Intern Neuropsychol Soc.* 1995;1:62–66.

76. Poeck K. Ideatorische Apraxie. *J Neurol.* 1983;230:1–5.

77. De Renzi E, Pieczuro A, and Vignolo LA. Ideational apraxia: a quantitative study. *Neuropsychologia.* 1968;6:41–55.

78. Goldenberg G and Hagmann S. Tool use and mechanical problem solving in apraxia. *Neuropsychologia.* 1998;36:581–89.

79. Goldenberg G and Spatt J. The neural basis of tool use. *Brain.* 2009;132:1645–55.

80. Osiurak F, Aubin G, Allain P, *et al.* Object utilization and object usage. A single-case study. *Neurocase.* 2008;14:169–83.

81. Hodges JR, Bozeat S, Lambon Ralph MA, *et al.* The role of conceptual knowledge in object use—evidence from semantic dementia. *Brain.* 2000;123:1913–25.

82. Canessa N, Borgo F, Cappa SF, *et al.* The different neural correlates of action and functional knowledge in semantic memory: An fMRI study. *Cerebral Cortex.* 2008;18:740–51.

83. Boronat CB, Buxbaum LJ, Coslett HB, , *et al*. Distinctions between manipulation and function knowledge of objects: evidence from functional magnetic resonance imaging. *Cognit Brain Res*. 2005;23:361–73.

84. Kalénine S, Shapiro AD, and Buxbaum LJ. Dissociations of action means and outcomes processing in left hemisphere stroke. *Neuropsychologia*. 2013;51:1224–33.

85. Spatt J, Bak T, Bozeat S, Patterson K, *et al*. Apraxia, mechanical problem solving and semantic knowledge—Contributions to object usage in corticobasal degeneration. *J Neurol*. 2002;249:601–608.

86. Osiurak F, Jarry C, Aubin G, Allain P, *et al*. Unusual use of objects after unilateral brain damage. The technical reasoning model. *Cortex*. 2009;45:769–83.

87. Osiurak F, Jarry C, Lesourd M, *et al*. Mechanical problem—solving strategies in left—brain damaged patients and apraxia of tool use. *Neuropsychologia*. 2013;51:1964–72.

88. Vaina LM and Jaulent MC. Object structure and action requirements: A compatibility model for functional recognition. *Intern J Intell Syst*. 1991;6:313–36.

89. Heilman KM, Maher LM, Greenwald ML, *et al*. Conceptual apraxia from lateralized lesions. *Neurology*. 1997;49:457–64.

90. Osiurak F, Jarry C, and Le Gall D. Re-examining the gesture engram hypothesis. New perspectives on apraxia of tool use. *Neuropsychologia*. 2011;49:299–312.

91. Silveri MC and Ciccarelli N. Semantic memory in object use. *Neuropsychologia*. 2009;47:2634–41.

92. Walker CM, Sunderland A, Sharma J, *et al*. The impact of cognitive impairment on upper body dressing difficulties after stroke: a video analysis of patterns of recovery. *J Neurol Neurosur Ps*. 2004;75:43–48.

93. Humphreys GW and Forde EME. Disordered action schema and action disorganisation syndrome. *Cognit Neuropsychol*. 1998;15:771–812.

94. Schwartz MF, Segal M, Veramonti T, *et al*. The naturalistic action test: a standardised assessment for everyday action impairment. *Neuropsychol Rehab*. 2002;12:311–39.

95. Goldenberg G, Daumüller M, and Hagmann S. Assessment and therapy of complex ADL in apraxia. *Neuropsychol Rehab*. 2001;11:147–68.

96. Hartmann K, Goldenberg G, Daumüller M, *et al*. It takes the whole brain to make a cup of coffee: The neuropsychology of naturalistic actions involving technical devices. *Neuropsychologia*. 2005;43:625–37.

97. Feyereisen P, Gendron M, and Seron X. Disorders of everyday actions in subjects suffering from senile dementia of the Alzheimer's type: An analysis of dressing performance. *Neuropsychol Rehab*. 1999;9:169–88.

98. van Heugten CM, Dekker J, Deelman BG, *et al*. Measuring disabilities in stroke patients with apraxia: A validation study of an observational method. *Neuropsychol Rehab*. 2000;10:401–14.

99. Schwartz MF, Buxbaum LJ, Montgomery MW, *et al*. Naturalistic action production following right hemisphere stroke. *Neuropsychologia*. 1999;37:51–66.

100. Schwartz MF, Lee SS, Coslett HB, *et al*. Naturalistic action impairment in closed head injury. *Neuropsychology*. 1998;12:13–28.

101. Goldenberg G, Hartmann-Schmid K, Sürer F, *et al*. The impact of dysexecutive syndrome on use of tools and technical equipment. *Cortex*. 2007;43:424–35.

102. Benke T. Two forms of apraxia in Alzheimer's disease. Cortex. 1993;29:715–26.

103. Della Sala S, Lucchelli F, and Spinnler H. Ideomotor apraxia in patients with dementia of Alzheimer type. *J Neurol*. 1987;234:91–93.

104. Derouesné C, Lagha-Pierucci S, Thibault S, *et al*. Apraxic disturbances in patients with mild to moderate Alzheimer's disease. *Neuropsychologia*. 2000;38:1760–69.

105. Holl AK, Ille R, Wilkinson L, *et al*. Impaired ideomotor limb apraxia in cortical and subcortical dementia: A comparison of Alzheimer's and Hintington's disease. *Neurodegenerative Diseases*. 2011;8:208–15.

106. Rousseaux M, Rénier J, Anicet L, *et al*. Gesture comprehension, knowledge and production in Alzheimer's disease. Europ *J Neurol*. 2012;19:1037–44.

107. Lesourd M and Le Gall D. Apraxia and Alzheimer's disease: review and perspectives. *Neuropsycological Reviews*. 2013;23:234–56.

108. Nagahama Y, Okina T, and Suzuki N. Impaired imitation of gestures in mild dementia: comparison of dementia with Lewy bodies, Alzheimer's disease nd vascular dementia. *J Neurol Neurosur Ps*. In press.

109. Chainay H, Louarn GF, and Humphreys GW. Ideational action impairments in Alzheimer's disease. *Brain Cognit*. 2006;62:198–205.

110. Dumont C, Ska B, and Joanette Y. Conceptual apraxia and semantic memory deficit in Alzheimer's disease: Two sides of the same coin? *J Intern Neuropsychol Soc*. 2000;6:693–703.

111. Glosser G, Wiley MJ, and Barnoski EJ. Gestural communication in Alzheimer's disease. *J Clinic Experim Neuropsychol*. 1998;20:1–13.

112. Schwartz RL, Adair JC, Raymer AM, *et al*. Conceptual apraxia in probable Alzheimer's disease as demonstrated by the Florida Action Recall Test. *J Intern Neuropsychol Soc*. 2000;6:265–70.

113. Ochipa C, Rothi LFG, and Heilman KM. Conceptual apraxia in Alzheimer's disease. *Brain*. 1992;115:1061–71.

114. Giovannetti T, Libon DJ, Buxbaum LJ, *et al*. Naturalistic action impairment in dementia. *Neuropsychologia*. 2002;40:1220–32.

115. Falchook AD, Mosquerra DM, Finney GR, *et al*. The relationship between semantic knowledge and conceptual apraxia in Alzheimer Disease. *Cognitive and Behavioral Neurology*. 2012;25:167–74.

116. Kipps CM, Knibb JA, Patterson K, *et al*. Neuropsychology of frontotemporal dementia. In: G Goldenberg and B Miller B (eds). *Handbook of Clinical Neurology*, Vol 88 (3rd series) Neuropsychology and Behavioral Neurology. Amsterdam: Elsevier, 2008, pp. 527–48.

117. Bozeat S, Patterson K, and Hodges JR. When objects loose their meaning: What happens to their use? *Cognitive, Affective & Behavioral Neuroscience*. 2002;2:236–51.

118. Hodges JR, Spatt J, and Patterson K. 'What' and 'how': Evidence for the dissociation of object knowledge and mechanical problem-solving skills in the human brain. *Proc Natl Acad Sci USA*. 1999;96:9444–48.

119. Coccia M, Bartolini M, Luzzi S, *et al*. Semantic memory is an amodal, dynamic system: Evidence from the interaction of naming and object use in semantic dementia. *Cognit Neuropsychol*. 2004;21:513–27.

120. Lauro-Grotto R, Piccini C, and Shallice T. Modality-specific operations in dementia. *Cortex*. 1997;33:593–622.

121. Negri GA, Lunardelli A, Reverberi C, *et al*. Degraded semantic knowledge and accurate object use. *Cortex*. 2007;43:376–88.

122. Kleist K. Ueber Apraxie. *Monatschr Psychiat Neurol*. 1906;19:269–90.

123. Blasi V, Labruna L, Soricelli A, *et al*. Limb-kinetic apraxia: a neuropsychological description. *Neurocase*. 1999;5:201–11.

124. Moreaud O, Naegele B, and Pellat J. The nature of apraxia in corticobasal degeneration. *Neuropsychiatry, Neuropsychology, and Behavioural Neurology*. 1997;9:288–92.

125. Soliveri P, Piacentini M, and Girotti F. Limb apraxia in corticobasal degeneration and progressive supranuclear palsy. *Neurology*. 2005;64:448–53.

126. Boeve BF, Lang AE, and Litvan I. Corticobasal degeneration and its relationship to progressive supranuclear palsy and frontotemporal dementia. *Ann Neurol*. 2003;54:S15–19.

127. Shelley BP, Hodges JR, Kipps CM, *et al*. Is the pathology of corticobasal syndrome predictable in life? *Movement Disorders*. 2009;11:1593–99.

128. Peigneux P, Salmon E, Garraux G, Laureys S, Willems S, Dujardin K, *et al*. Neural and cognitive bases of upper limb apraxia in corticobasal degeneration. *Neurology*. 2001;57:1259–68.

129. Mendez MF, Gharajarania M, and Peru A. Posterior cortical atrophy: Clinical characteristics and differences compared to Alzheimer's disease. *Dementia and Geriatric Cognitive Disorders*. 2002;14:33–40.

130. Benson DF, Davis RJ, and Snyder BD. Posterior cortical atrophy. *Arch Neurol*. 1988;45:789–93.

131. De Renzi E. Slowly progressive visual agnosia or apraxia without dementia. *Cortex*. 1986;22:171–80.

132. Rothi LJG, Raymer AM, and Heilman KM. Limb praxis assessment. In: LJG Rothi and KM Heilman KM (eds). *Apraxia—The Neuropsychology of Action*. Hove: Psychology Press, 1997, pp. 61–74.

133. Vanbellingen T, Kersten B, Van de Winckel A, *et al*. A new bedside test of gestures in stroke: the apraxia screen of TULIA. *J Neurol Neurosurg. Psychiat*. 2011;82:389–92.

CHAPTER 17

Acquired calculation disorders

Marinella Cappelletti

The basic components of number and calculation processing

Number comprehension and production

Number comprehension is the ability to generate a semantic representation of numbers. The most common of such representations refers to the quantity associated with numbers, for instance '21' indicates the numerosity of 21, that is, that there are 21 items. The quantity expressed by numbers is often processed when comparing numbers, for instance when deciding which of two products is the most expensive. In doing so, we are usually faster and more accurate the more further apart two numbers are from each other; for example, £1.20 and £2.55, relative to £1.20 and £1.15. This phenomenon is referred to as 'distance effect'.[1] Besides quantities, number comprehension may, of course, also concern numbers used as verbal labels, for instance '21' could refer to a bus number or the age of consent.[2,3]

Number production is the process of converting numerals' semantic representation—for example, the numerosity of 21 items—onto an output format, most commonly the Arabic format, for example, the two-digit number '21' and the verbal format, for example, 'twenty-one'. The transformation of numbers from one format to another is also referred to as '*transcoding*'.[4–6]

Calculation

Oral and written arithmetical operations require a set of specific and independent processes to be performed. These include:

(i) Processing of arithmetical symbols, i.e. +, ×, −, ÷

(ii) Retrieval of arithmetical facts, such as '3 + 3 = 6' or '3 × 3 = 9'.

(iii) Execution of calculation procedures, which consist of the specific algorithms required to solve multi-digit calculation; for example, in written multi-digit multiplications the rightmost digit of the lower number is multiplied by the upper number starting from the rightmost digit;[7–9] other rules can be carrying (e.g. in '23 + 19') and borrowing (e.g. in '23 − 19').

(iv) Arithmetical conceptual knowledge, namely the understanding of the principles underlying arithmetical facts and procedures, like the principle of commutativity (e.g. 'a + b' = 'b + a').

Localization of brain lesions in number and calculation disorders

An overview of both group studies and single-case studies has suggested that the majority of patients with number production and/or number comprehension impairments had left posterior lesions almost always involving the parietal lobe.[10,11] Likewise, most patients with arithmetical fact retrieval impairments had lesions mainly implicating the left parietal lobe.

The neuropsychological evidence suggesting the involvement of the parietal lobe in numerical processing has been corroborated by neuroimaging studies showing that these brain regions are the most strongly activated in tasks requiring number processing.[12–15] However, it is important to observe that not all parietal lesions result in numerical impairments.[10,16] For instance, only about 20 per cent of patients with left parietal lesions show numerical deficits,[17] possibly because other brain regions are able to compensate when the parietal lobes or other number areas are damaged.[18]

Number impairments can also occur following lesions to brain areas different from parietal. For example, damage to the frontal lobes often leads to impaired calculation skills,[7,19,20–23] as well as disorders in quantity processing.[24–26] Similarly, damage to subcortical areas, especially the basal ganglia, can lead to impairment in quantity processing, arithmetical fact retrieval, and conceptual knowledge.[27–30,32,33]

Selective impairment of number processing and calculation

Patients may present with specific impairment in either the processing of numbers, or in calculation, or both. Table 17.1 provides an overview of the whole range of potential deficits that can be observed in acalculic patients.

Here the most commonly occurring number impairments are briefly described, specifically affecting: (1) number transcoding; (2) quantity processing; (3) calculation, which in turn may concern the processing of arithmetical signs, simple facts, procedures, or arithmetical conceptual knowledge.

Impairments of number transcoding

Several studies have reported patients with disorders in *reading and writing numbers*.[5,6,34,35] The analysis of the errors made by patients when reading or writing numbers has allowed the identification of two major cognitive processes within number transcoding. One of these—syntactic—involves the specification of the relationship among the elements of a number or number class; for instance, to read number '600', the correct number class (hundred) needs to be retrieved. Syntactic errors consist of selecting the wrong number class; for example, number '600' read as 'sixty' (see reference 33 for a clear description of patient SF making syntactic errors).

Table 17.1 Overview of the potential disorders of (A) number processing and (B) calculation

A. Disorders of number processing	
Disorders of number production	Disorders of lexical processing
	Disorders of syntactical processing
Disorders of number comprehension	Disorders of cardinal number meaning
	Disorders of sequence number meaning

B. Disorders of calculation	
	Disorders of arithmetical symbol processing
	Disorders of arithmetical fact retrieval
	Disorders of calculation procedures
	Disorders of conceptual knowledge

The other type of process—lexical—involves manipulation of individual elements in the number; for example, to read number '600', the correct class (hundred) and the unit (6) have to be retrieved. Lexical errors consist of the incorrect production of one or more of the individual elements in a number, such as number '600' read as 'seven hundred' (see reference 8 for a clear description of patient HY making lexical errors).

Another frequent type of error in writing numbers to dictation or from a written input has been referred to as 'intrusion errors' and observed both in patients with dementia of Alzheimer type as well as with focal brain lesions.[35,36] These errors consist of reproducing part of the input code into the output one; for instance, the Arabic number '75' written as 'SEVENTY5' or 'seventy' as '7ty'. Some authors explained these errors in terms of the combination of an impaired transcoding mechanism and impaired inhibitory processes,[36] or impairment in selective attention capacities.[37]

Impairments of quantity processing

A few studies have reported patients with a basic failure in understanding and processing the *quantity* indicated by numbers.[24–28,38–45] For example, patient NR with Alzheimer's disease could no longer understand Arabic numerals, was unable to point to the larger of two Arabic numerals (e.g. '34 vs 78' or '26 vs 23'), and had lost the ability to match spoken number names to the corresponding Arabic numeral.[43]

Another very profound acalculic patient with a left parietal lesion due to a stroke (CG) retained the ability to process abstract quantities, but completely lost the meaning of all numbers above four. For example, she was unable to say how many days there were in a week or whether 7 or 10 was the bigger number.[40] Her deficit was so pervasive that it seriously limited her activities of daily living such that, for instance, she could no longer deal with money or check her change, make phone calls, use a calendar, or read the time, although her intellectual skills, language, memory, and visuospatial abilities were largely preserved.[40]

A few case studies have recently focused on quantity processing in hemispatial neglect patients,[47–51] often testing whether neglect may affect the mental 'number line', a metaphor used to represent numbers as oriented from the smaller to the larger.[52] A way to test the integrity of the mental number line is with a bisection task, which consists of orally presenting two numbers (e.g. '1' and '5') and asking which number falls in the middle. Left-sided neglect patients with right hemisphere lesions typically select a number which is shifted towards the right relative to the correct middle one; for instance, they state that '4'—and not '3'—is mid-way between '1' and '5'.[48–51] This performance mirrors the classical bias that neglect patients show when bisecting physical lines, although their performance in number bisection also depends on working memory resources[49] and on the orientation of the physical and number lines.[48]

Impairments of calculation

Each of the different cognitive processes involved in calculation (arithmetic symbols, facts, procedures, and conceptual knowledge) is functionally independent and differentially susceptible to brain damage. Examples of selective impairments in these components of calculation are discussed below.

Disorders of arithmetical symbol processing

Very few cases with a selective impairment in processing arithmetical symbols have been reported.[53,54] For example, Laiacona and Lunghi[54] investigated a patient who misnamed and misidentified the arithmetical signs and performed written arithmetical operations according to their misidentification; for example, the patient systematically added the times (see Fig. 17.1a).

Disorders of arithmetical fact retrieval

Several patients have been documented with a selective impairment of arithmetic fact retrieval. Typically, these patients have severe difficulties in performing very simple single-digit addition, subtraction, multiplication, or division problems. They may produce errors such as '5 + 7' = '13 roughly', and their response times tend to be abnormally slow (e.g. >2 seconds).[8,28,55,56] Their errors can be classified as: *operand*, if the incorrect answer is correct for a problem that shares one of the operands (e.g. 6 × 5 = 25); *operation*, if the incorrect answer is correct for a problem involving the same operands but a different operation (e.g. 3 + 4 = 12); *table*, if the incorrect answer is the product of two other single digit numbers (e.g. 4 × 4 = 25); and *non-table*, if the incorrect answer is not an operand, table, or operation error (e.g. 9 × 8 = 52).[57,58] Patients who make these errors often show intact knowledge of arithmetical principles and procedures; they are usually able to retrieve and apply the appropriate arithmetical steps to solve complex arithmetical problems and they can define arithmetical operations adequately.[8,28,56] For these patients, everyday activities such as checking their change or bank statement pose great difficulties.

Disorders of calculation procedures

A few cases of selective impairments of calculation procedures show that patients may for example use unflexible procedures when solving problems. For instance, patient MT with a left frontoparietal lesion due to a stroke systematically subtracted the smaller number from the larger one, irrespective of whether the larger digit was at the top or on the bottom line (see Fig. 17.1b).[21]

Other impairments in the use of calculation procedures may consist of misaligning the digit in multi-digit operations, of errors using carrying procedures in addition problems, or of not applying problem-specific steps in the correct order.

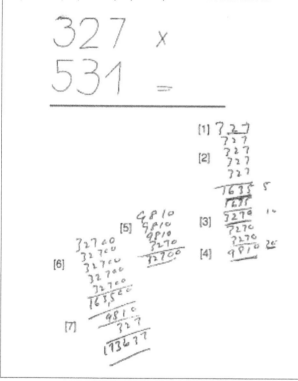

a) Performance of patient EB, with a selective impairment in arithmetical symbol processing such that he systematically plussed the times.[54]

```
   48        59
 × 67      × 29
  115        88
```

b) Performance of patient MT with a calculation procedure impairment such that he consistently subtracted the smaller from the larger number.[21]

```
  923       171
 − 644      − 48
  321       127
```

c) Performance of patient BE with impaired arithmetical fact retrieval but preserved conceptual knowledge. When asked to perform arithmetical problems such as 8 × 6, he adopted the strategy below.[30]

$$8 \times 10 = 80;\ 80 \div 2 = 40;\ 40 + 8 = 48$$

d) An example of a semantic dementia patient's (IH) performance in solving a multi-digit multiplication operation.[59] The patient spontaneously developed a series of procedures: first, number '531' was decomposed into the subparts '500', '30', and '1'; the following steps were then used, indicated by numbers in squared brackets. Step [1] is '27 × 1'. Steps [2] to [4] show how '327 × 30' was obtained. Step [2] is '327 × 5'; [3] is '327 × 10', and [4] is '327 × 30'; [5] is '327 × 100' obtained through multiple additions; [6] is '327 × 500', again obtained through multiple additions. Finally, [7] is (327 × 500) + (327 × 30) + (327 × 1). The final result is correct.

Fig. 17.1 Examples of specific impairments or preservations of calculation skills. (a) Adapted from *Neuropsychologia*. 35(3), Laiacona M and Lunghi A. A case of concomitant impairment of operational signs and punctuation marks, pp. 325–32, Copyright (1997), with permission from Elsevier; (b) Adapted from *Cortex*, 32(3), Girelli L and Delazer M. Subtraction bugs in an acalculic patient, pp. 547–55, Copyright (1996), with permission from Elsevier; (c) Source data from *Brain*. 117(4), Hittmair-Delazer M, Semenza C, and Denes G. Concepts and facts in calculation, pp. 715–28, Copyright (1994), Oxford University Press; (d) Adapted from *Cognitive Neuropsychology*. 22(7), Cappelletti M, Morton J, Kopelman M, and Butterworth B, The progressive loss of numerical knowledge in a semantic dementia patient: A follow-up study, pp. 771–93, Copyright (2005), with permission from Taylor & Francis.

Disorders of arithmetical conceptual knowledge

Delazer and Benke[28] described a patient (JG) with a left parietal lesion who had lost arithmetical conceptual knowledge, defined as 'an understanding of arithmetical operations and laws pertaining to these operations' (reference 30 at p. 117). Hence, JC could correctly retrieve the result of operations such as '3 × 9' from memory but was unable to recognize that the same multiplication problem could be transformed in repeated additions (i.e. 3 × 9 also equals 9 + 9 + 9), and she could not use basic principles such as commutativity in multiplication (i.e. 4 × 12 = 12 × 4).[28]

The opposite side of the dissociation—intact conceptual knowledge and impaired fact retrieval—has been reported in a few single-case studies.[30,31] For example, a patient who suffered from a left basal ganglia infarct could not solve from memory problems such as '8 × 6' but he could adopt the following strategy: 8 × 10 = 80; 80 ÷ 2 = 40; 40 + 8 = 48 (see Fig. 17.1c).[15,23,30] Similarly, a semantic dementia patient with left temporal lobe degeneration showed well-preserved understanding of arithmetical concepts despite the severe loss of arithmetical facts (see Fig. 17.1d).[59]

Selective preservation of number processing and calculation

It is now well established that numerical and calculation abilities can be largely independent from other cognitive abilities, such as general intellectual skills,[60] language,[61,62] short-term memory,[63] and semantic knowledge.[59,64–70] One of the most striking dissociations is observed in patients with semantic dementia who typically present with severe impairment in understanding the meaning of words and the use of objects, but with good understanding of numerical concepts and arithmetical operations.[59,64–70]

Assessment of acalculia

A list of the main numerical and calculation tasks that can be used for the diagnosis of acalculia is provided in Table 17.2. The diagnosis of acalculia relies on establishing with appropriate tools the presence of a number processing and/or calculation impairment in a patient who premorbidly had acquired normal numeracy skills. The diagnosis of acalculia can be made only when one can exclude that the deficit in numeracy skills is not a secondary consequence of other cognitive deficits, such as generalized impairments in language, attention, visuospatial functions, or other cognitive skills are not underpinning the failure of number processing and calculation.

A formal assessment of a patient's numeracy skills can be based on number reading, writing to dictation, and repetition tasks, with numerical stimuli presented as either Arabic numerals (8), written (*eight*), or spoken number names ('eight'). Patients can be simply asked to read, write, or repeat the numeral presented. Comprehension of number quantity is usually assessed with a magnitude comparison task, where patients are asked to indicate the larger of two numbers (e.g. 6 vs 9) while response times are recorded. Another test of number comprehension is the 'number composition task' whereby subjects have to compose the value of a given number using poker chips ranging in value from 1 to 500 (e.g. number '52' made of tokens 20, 20, 10, 2).

Calculation skills can be assessed by tests exploring knowledge of: arithmetical signs, for example by asking patients to read, point

Table 17.2 Suggested numerical and calculation tasks for the diagnosis of acalculia

Function	Task	How?
Sequence	Counting	◆ Reciting numbers forwards or backwards by 1 or 2 from 1 to 20 or 20 to 1
		◆ 'What comes next'? Given a number what comes before or after it
Transcoding	Writing	◆ Numbers to dictation (e.g. from spoken 'two' to written TWO or 2)
		◆ Numbers from Arabic (2) into alphabetic format (TWO) or vice-versa
	Reading	◆ Numbers from Arabic (2) or alphabetic (TWO) format
Quantity	Number comparison	◆ 'Which is bigger: 6 or 9'? Both accuracy and RTs to be collected
	Comparison of non-symbolic discrete quantity	◆ 'Which display contains more dots'? To be presented with either few fleshed dots or with many for unlimited time to test enumeration and counting respectively
	Comparison of non-symbolic continuous quantity	◆ Space or 'amount' discrimination (e.g. which line is longer or which container has more liquid?)
	Number composition task	◆ Composing the value of a number using poker chips ranging in value from 1 to 500
Calculation	Arithmetical signs	◆ Read, point, and write the arithmetical signs
	Simple facts	◆ Solve single-digit arithmetical problems mentally (e.g. 4 + 2, 3 × 4, or 5 − 2)
	Procedures	◆ Solve multi-digit calculation (e.g. 294 + 12 = 306), either in written form or orally

and write signs; arithmetical facts, by asking patients to solve orally presented single-digit arithmetical problems (e.g. 4 + 2, 3 × 4, or 5 − 2); and arithmetical procedures, by asking them to perform multi-digit calculation, such as 294 + 12 = 306, either in written form or orally.

A few test batteries that evaluate numerical skills in detail are available. One of these is the EC301 composite battery or its shorter form (EC301R),[71–73] and a more recent set of numerical and calculation tasks have been developed for which normative data have also been provided.[74] Standardized tests that evaluates mental calculation are the Graded Difficulty Arithmetic (GDA) test, which comprises 24 multi-digit addition and subtraction problems.[17] and the arithmetic subtest of the WAIS-R.[75]

Error analyses in reading and writing numerals (lexical or syntactical), and in retrieving arithmetical facts (operand, operation, table, and non-table errors) are usually not included in standardized tests but can be very useful additions to the assessment, in so far as they can provide information about the nature of the impairment.

Conclusion

Acalculia is a heterogeneous set of disorders consisting of impairments in processing numbers, in calculation or both. Specific components of number and calculation have been presented in this chapter in the context of both normal functioning and impaired performance following cerebral damage. This includes disorders in transcoding processing, quantity processing, in calculation, or in their sub-components. A few cases of selective preservation of number processing have also been briefly outlined. A short description of lesion localization in number and calculation disorders was provided, which indicates that parietal areas are the most relevant brain regions for numeracy impairments. Finally, some guidelines for the assessment of acalculia have been proposed.

Acknowledgements

This work was supported by a Royal Society Dorothy Hodgkin Fellowship.

References

1. Moyer RS and Landauer TK. Time required for judgements of numerical inequality. *Nature*. 1967;215:1519–20.
2. Butterworth B. *The Mathematical Brain*. London: Macmillan, 1999.
3. Dehaene S. *The Number Sense: How the Mind Creates Mathematics*. New York, NY: Oxford University Press, 1997.
4. Dehaene S and Cohen L. Towards an anatomical and functional model of number processing. *Mathematical Cognition*. 1995;1:83–120.
5. Deloche G and Seron X. From one to 1: An analysis of a transcoding process by means of neuropsychological data. *Cognition*. 1982;12:119–49.
6. McCloskey M, Sokol SM, and Goodman RA. Cognitive processes in verbal-number production: Inferences from the performance of brain-damaged subjects. *J Exp Psychol*. 1986;115(4):307–30.
7. Granà A, Hofer R, and Semenza C. Acalculia from a right hemisphere lesion Dealing with 'where' in multiplication procedures. *Neuropsychologia*. 2006;44:2972–86.
8. Sokol SM, McCloskey M, Cohen NJ, *et al.* Cognitive representations and processes in arithmetic: Inferences from the performance of brain-damaged subjects. *J Exp Psychol Learn*. 1991;17(3):355–76.
9. Sokol SM and McCloskey M. Levels of representation in verbal number production. *Applied Psycholinguistics*. 1988;9:267–81.
10. Cappelletti M and Cipolotti L. The neuropsychological assessment and treatment of calculation disorders. In: Halligan, U Kischka, and JC Marshall (eds). *Handbook of Clinical Neuropsychology*. Oxford: Oxford University Press, 2010.
11. Cipolotti L and van Harskamp NJ. Disturbances of number processing and calculation. In: F Boller and J Grafman (eds). *Handbook of Neuropsychology* New York, NY: Elsevier, 2001, pp. 305–31.
12. Cohen Kadosh R, Lammertyn J, and Izard V. Are numbers special? An overview of chronometric, neuroimaging, developmental and comparative studies of magnitude representation. *Prog Neurobiol*. 2008;84:132–47.
13. Dehaene S, Spelke E, Pinel P, *et al.* Sources of mathematical thinking: Behavioral and brain-imaging evidence. *Science*. 1999;284:970–74.
14. Dehaene S, Piazza M, Pinel P, *et al.* Three parietal circuits for number processing. *Cognitive Neuropsychology*. 2003;20:487–506.
15. Pesenti M, Thioux M, Seron X, *et al.* Neuroanatomical substrates of Arabic number processing, numerical comparison, and simple addition: A PET study. *J Cognitive Neurosci*. 2000;12(3):461–79.

16. Cappelletti M, Butterworth B, and Kopelman M. Numerical abilities in patients with focal and progressive neurological disorders: A neuropsychological study. *Neuropsychology.* 2012;26:1–19.

17. Jackson M and Warrington EK. Arithmetic skills in patients with unilateral cerebral lesions. *Cortex.* 1986;22:611–20.

18. Cappelletti M, Leff A, and Price C. How number processing survives left occipito-temporal damage, *Neurocase.* 2012;10.1080/13554794.2011.588179.

19. Basso A and Beschin N. Number transcoding and number word spelling in a left-brain-damaged non-aphasic acalculic patient. *Neurocase.* 2008;6:129–39.

20. Cohen L and Dehaene S. Calculating without reading: Unsuspected residual abilities in pure alexia. *Cognitive Neuropsycol.* 2000;17:563–83.

21. Girelli L and Delazer M. Subtraction bugs in an acalculic patient. *Cortex.* 1996;32:547–55.

22. Lucchelli F and De Renzi E. Primary dyscalculia after a medial frontal lesion of the left hemisphere. *J Neurol, Neurosur, Ps.* 1993;56:304–307.

23. Venneri A and Semenza C. On the dependency of division on multiplication: Selective loss for conceptual knowledge of multiplication. *Neuropsychologia.* 2011;49: 629–35.

24. Delazer M and Butterworth B. A dissociation of number meanings. *Cognitive Neuropsychol.* 1997;14:613–36.

25. Delazer M, Benke T, Trieb T, *et al.* Isolated numerical skills in posterior cortical atrophy–an fMRI study. *Neuropsychologia.* 2006;4:1909–13.

26. Polk T, Reed C, Keenan J, *et al.* A dissociation between symbolic number knowledge and analogue magnitude information. *Brain Cognition.* 2001;47:545–563.

27. Dehaene S and Cohen L. Cerebral pathways for calculation: double dissociation between rote verbal and quantitative knowledge of arithmetic. *Cortex.* 1997;33:219–50.

28. Delazer M and Benke T. Arithmetic facts without meaning. *Cortex.* 1997;33:697–710.

29. Delazer M, Domahs F, Lochy A, *et al.* Number processing and basal ganglia dysfunction: a single case study. *Neuropsychologia.* 2004;42:1050–1062.

30. Hittmair-Delazer M, Semenza C, and Denes G. Concepts and facts in calculation. *Brain.* 1994;117:715–28.

31. Hittmair-Delazer M, Sailer U, and Benke T. Impaired arithmetic facts but intact conceptual knowledge—A single case study of dyscalculia. *Cortex.* 1995;31:139–48.

32. Koss S, Clark R, Vesely L, *et al.* Numerosity impairment in corticobasal syndrome. *Neuropsychology.* 2010;24:476–92.

33. Lampl Y, Eshel Y, Gilad R, *et al.* Selective acalculia with sparing of the subtraction process in a patient with left parieto-temporal haemorrhage. *Neurology.* 1994;44:1759–61.

34. Cipolotti L, Warrington E, and Butterworth B. Selective impairment in manipulating Arabic numerals. *Cortex.* 1995;31:73–86.

35. McCloskey M, Sokol SM, Goodman-Schulman RA, *et al.* Cognitive representations and processes in number production: Evidence from cases of acquired dyscalculia. In: A Caramazza (ed.). *Advances in Cognitive Neuropsychology and Neurolinguistics.* Hillsdale, NJ: Lawrence Erlbaum, 1990, pp. 1–32.

36. Della Sala S, Gentileschi V, Gray C, *et al.* Intrusion errors in numerical transcoding by Alzheimer patients. *Neuropsychologia.* 2000;38:768–77.

37. Thioux M, Ivanoiu A, Turconi E, *et al.* Intrusion of the verbal code during the production of Arabic numerals: A single-case study in patient with probable Alzheimer Disease. *Cognitive Neuropsych.* 1999;16:749–73.

38. Macoir J, Audet T, Lecomte S, *et al.* From 'Cinquante-Six' to '5quante-Six': The origin of intrusion errors in a patient with probable Alzheimer disease. *Cognitive Neuropsych.* 2002;19:579–601.

39. Ashkenazi S, Henik A, Ifergane G, *et al.* Basic numerical processing in left intraparietal sulcus (IPS) acalculia. *Cortex.* 2008;44:439–48.

40. Cipolotti L, Butterworth B, and Denes G. A specific deficit for numbers in case of dense acalculia. *Brain.* 1991;114:2619–37.

41. Halpern CH, Clark R, Moore P, *et al.* Too much to count on: Impaired very small numbers in corticobasal degeneration *Brain Cognition.* 2007;64:44–149.

42. Lemer C, Dehaene S, Spelke E, *et al.* Approximate quantities and exact number words: Dissociable systems. *Neuropsychologia.* 2003;41:L1942–58.

43. Noël MP and Seron X. Arabic number reading deficit: A single case study. *Cognitive Neuropsych.* 1993;10:317–39.

44. Revkin SK, Piazza M, Izard V, *et al.* Verbal numerosity estimation deficit in the context of spared semantic representation of numbers: a neuropsychological study of a patient with frontal lesions. *Neuropsychologia.* 2008;46:2463–2475.

45. Rosselli M and Ardila A. Calculation deficits in patients with right and left hemisphere damage. *Neuropsychologia.* 1989;27:607–17.

46. Woods AJ, Mennemeier M, Garcia-Rill E, *et al.* Bias in magnitude estimation following left hemisphere injury. *Neuropsychologia.* 2006;44:1406–1412.

47. Cappelletti M and Cipolotti L. Unconscious processing of Arabic numerals in unilateral neglect. *Neuropsychologia.* 2006;44(10):1999–2006.

48. Cappelletti M, Freeman ED, and Cipolotti L. The middle house or the middle floor: bisecting horizontal and vertical mental number lines in neglect, *Neuropsychologia.* 2007;45:2989–3000.

49. Doricchi F, Guariglia P, Gasparini M, *et al.* Dissociation between physical and mental number line bisection in right hemisphere brain damage. *Nature Neurosci.* 2005;8(12):1663–66.

50. Vuilleumier P, Ortigue S, and Brugger P. The number space and neglect. *Cortex.* 2004;40:399–410.

51. Zorzi M, Priftis K, and Umilta' C. (Brain damage: neglect disrupts the mental number line. *Nature.* 2002417:138–9.

52. Dehaene S, Bossini S, and Giraux P. The mental representation of parity and number magnitude. *J Exp Psychol Human.* 1993;21:314–26.

53. Ferro JM and Botelho MAS. Alexia for arithmetical signs: a cause of disturbed calculation. *Cortex.* 1980;16:175–80.

54. Laiacona M and Lunghi A. A case of concomitant impairment of operational signs and punctuation marks. *Neuropsychologia.* 1997;35:325–32.

55. Dehaene S and Cohen L. Two mental calculation systems: A case study of severe acalculia with preserved approximation. *Neuropsychologia.* 1991;29:1045–74.

56. Warrington EK. The fractionation of arithmetical skills: A single study. *Q J Exp Psychol.* 1982;34:31–51.

57. McCloskey M, Aliminosa D, and Sokol SM. Facts, rules and procedures in normal calculation: Evidence from multiple single-patient studies of impaired arithmetic fact retrieval. *Brain Cognition.* 1991;17:154–203.

58. McCloskey M, Harley W, and Sokol SM. Models of arithmetic fact retrieval: An evaluation in light of findings from normal and brain-damaged subjects. *J Exp Psychol Learn.* 1991;17:377–97.

59. Cappelletti M, Morton J, Kopelman M, *et al.* The progressive loss of numerical knowledge in a semantic dementia patient: A follow-up study. *Cognitive Neuropsychology.* 2005;22:771–793.

60. Remond-Besuchet C, Noël MP, Seron X, *et al.* Selective preservation of exceptional arithmetical knowledge in a demented patient. *Mathematical Cognition.* 1999;5(1):41–63.

61. Rossor MN, Warrington EK, and Cipolotti L. The isolation of calculation skills. *J Neurol.* 1995;242:78–81.

62. Thioux M, Pillon A, Samson D, *et al.* The isolation of numerals at the semantic level. *Neurocase.* 1998;4:371–89.

63. Butterworth B, Cipolotti L, and Warrington EK. Short-term memory impairments and arithmetical ability. *Q J Exp Psychol.* 1995;49A:251–62.

64. Cappelletti M, Butterworth B, and Kopelman M. (2001). Spared numerical abilities in a case of semantic dementia. *Neuropsychologia.* 2001;39:1224–39.

65. Crutch SJ and Warrington EK. Preserved calculation skills in a case of semantic dementia. *Cortex.* 2002;38:389–99.

66. Halpern CH, Glosser G, Clark R, *et al*. Dissociation of numbers and objects in corticobasal degeneration and semantic dementia. *Neurology*. 2003;62:1163–69.

67. Jefferies E, Patterson K, Jones RW, *et al*. A category-specific advantage for numbers in verbal short-term memory: Evidence from semantic dementia. *Neuropsychologia*. 2004;42:639–660.

68. Jefferies E, Bateman D, and Lambon-Ralph MA. The role of the temporal lobe semantic system in number knowledge: Evidence from late-stage semantic dementia. *Neuropsychologia*. 2005;43:887–905.

69. Julien CL, Neary D, and Snowden JS. Personal experience and arithmetic meaning in semantic dementia. *Neuropsychologia*. 2010; 48:278–87.

70. Julien CL, Thompson JC, Neary D, *et al*. Arithmetic knowledge in semantic dementia: is it invariably preserved? *Neuropsychologia*. 2008;46:2732–44.

71. Deloche G, Seron X, Larroque C, *et al*. Calculation and number processing: Assessment battery; role of demographic factors. *J Clin Exp Neuropsyc. J Clin Exp Neuropsyc*. 1994;16:195–208.

72. Deloche G, Hannequin D, Carlomagno S, *et al*. Calculation and number processing in mild Alzheimer's disease. *J Clin Exp Neuropsyc*. 1995;7:634–39.

73. Deloche G, Dellatolas G, Vendrell J, *et al*. Calculation and number processing: Neuropsychological assessment and daily life difficulties. *Journal of the International Neuropsychological Society*. 1996;2:177–80.

74. Delazer M, Girelli L, Grana A, *et al*. Number processing and calculation-Normative data from healthy adults. *Clin Neuropsychol*. 2003;17(3):331–50.

75. Wechsler D. Wechsler Adult Intelligence Scale–Revised. The Psychological Corporation, 1981.

CHAPTER 18

Disorders of reading and writing

Alexander P. Leff

Introduction

Reading and writing are often not tested in clinical practice, with speaking and listening much higher up the clinician's bedside language-testing algorithm. However, perhaps because reading and writing develop later in life and seem to require more effortful practice to master, they quite often break down earlier than speaking or listening do and thus can be more sensitive markers of disease, especially in the dementias. Disorders of reading and writing have also shaped how we think about normal brain function. Perhaps more than in any other cognitive domain, the models of how the normal reading system works have been built upon a mass of single cases and case series, all delineating the differential ways reading breaks down in acquired brain injury.

Classification of acquired alexia

First we must distinguish the acquired alexias (the subject of this chapter) from the more common developmental dyslexias. We also note that the terms alexia and dyslexia have come to be used interchangeably, although it is perhaps preferable to use 'alexia' for acquired causes (where the normally developing language system has become damaged by an acquired disorder such as stroke or dementia) and 'dyslexia' for the developmental disorder, where, for reasons still not fully understood, reading fails to become normally instantiated. The two cannot be completely dissociated as people with developmental dyslexia are in no way protected from the usual causes of acquired alexia. In such cases it can be harder to classify patients behaviourally as the standard clinical tests of reading assume normal pre-existing reading behaviour. Those interested in developmental dyslexia may wish to refer to the following works.[1,2]

The central alexias

Central alexia is an acquired reading impairment in the context of a generalized language disorder. Dejerine used the short-hand 'alexia with agraphia'[3] to differentiate from cases of acquired alexia where only reading ability is affected—'alexia without agraphia'.[4] The lesion site for Dejerine's first case (left MCA territory infarct with involvement of the angular gyrus) turned out to be prescient as the vast majority of aphasic, and thus central alexic, patients have lesions affecting this vascular territory.

The neurological classification has not moved on much from Dejerine's time. However, in the late 1970s neuropsychologists were developing different models to explain normal reading behaviour by seeing how the process breaks down in patients with focal damage. In their simplest form, all of these models propose two ways that the reading brain can get from the written to the spoken word.[5] The first is a 'lexical' route where each word is recognized as a whole

and can be mapped directly onto a lexicon of how that word sounds and thus what sounds are required to produce a spoken form of the word. This is also called the 'direct' route, as the reader moves straight from the visual word form to the spoken word form without any intervening analysis; for example, breaking the word down into components such as syllables. Whether this route interacts with the semantic system in a serial or parallel manner is still debated. When this route is damaged patients have problems with 'exception words' such as [pint], misreading it to rhyme with [mint]. This is called *surface dyslexia*.[6]

The second route is called the '*nonlexical*' or '*sublexical*' route, whereby words are read by breaking down the written form into its constituent parts (graphemes) and applying learned rules as to how these elements sound. These sounds are assembled in order, and the word is read out. This route is also referred to as 'indirect' because the word form has to be dissembled before it can be read aloud. This route allows one to read novel words, and this is tested in adult readers by asking them to read non-words like [mune]. Patients with damage to this route have *phonological dyslexia* and cannot read non-words normally.[7] There is a more severe form of dyslexia called *deep dyslexia* which can be thought of as phonological dyslexia with added impairments.[8] Table 18.1 depicts the three canonical types of central alexia and the common error types when reading test words aloud.

We will now deal with each of the three main types of central alexia.

Surface dyslexia

This condition was defined by Marshall and Newcombe in a landmark paper as a, 'partial failure of grapheme-phoneme correspondence rules'.[6] They discussed two cases with surface dyslexia, giving examples of errors such as [lace] read as 'lass' and [island] read as 'izland'. The concept of surface alexia has been shaped primarily by patients with degenerative disorders as opposed to those with focal injury such as stroke. Indeed stroke patients with 'pure' surface alexia are rare. There appears to be pathological gradient: dementia > head injury > stroke associated with the condition, which perhaps suggests that multifocal damage is usually required to cause it. We will now consider in chronological order the key reports on this topic, and the related issue of semantic dementia, which have influenced our understanding.

In a famous paper in which she described three patients with semantic dementia (SD), Elizabeth Warrington argued they all had a selective impairment of semantic memory.[9] She used Tulving's definition of semantic memory, 'that system which processes, stores and retrieves information about the meaning of words, concepts

Table 18.1 The canonical three types of central alexia (rows) are characterized by the lexical types of words (also known as part of speech) patients make errors on (first three columns). Functors are a special class of word (such as a preposition, article, auxiliary, or pronoun) that chiefly expresses grammatical relationships, and have little semantic content of their own. The errors themselves (last four columns) are also considered diagnostic. Patients with *surface dyslexia* regularize irregular words [pint] read to thyme with [mint]. Patients with *deep dyslexia* often make semantic errors, for example, [little] read as 'small'. Morphological errors are formed by the deletion, addition, or substitution of an affix, for example, [govern] read as 'governor'. Visual errors usually occur when a letter or two has been misperceived, for example, [spy] misread as 'shy'

Subtype	Part of speech/Lexical class effects			Error types: reading aloud			
	Irregular	Non-words	Functors	Semantic	Morphological	Visual	Regularization
Surface	Errors*	OK	OK	No	Yes	No	Yes*
Phonological	OK	Errors*	OK	No	Yes	No	No
Deep	Variable^a	Errors	Errors*	Yes*	Yes	Yes	No

* = key element; a = deep dyslexics often show concreteness effects so highly imageable words are read best, then abstract words, then functors and lastly non-words. Irregular words can be of high or low imageability.

and facts',[10] which is differentiated from episodic memory because it is, 'a common pool of knowledge not unique to the individual'. Of course semantic memory is built up through experiential memory, but once established, it appears to be largely anatomically dissociable from structures supporting episodic memory.

The main thrust of Warrington's paper was on amodal semantic deficits, that is, regardless of whether the stimuli were visual or auditory in nature the patients had great trouble saying what they were (both naming and description), in the absence of a low-level perceptual impairment. Although not directly compared, Warrington noted that spoken and written word were equally affected in terms of accessing meaning. The patients could correctly read aloud written words, just not say what they meant, 'the mechanical aspects of reading were remarkably well preserved; words which were meaningless to the patients could be correctly read and written' (reference 9, p. 654).

Beyond this she also highlighted that irregular words presented a particular problem for these SD cases: 'That words which are spelt in a bizarre manner presented difficulty for these patients is consistent with the notion that the direct graphemic route was inoperative. That phonetically spelt words could be read with relatively little difficulty indicates that reading by the phonetic route alone can be quite effective.'[9] The suggestion being that these patients can 'read' aloud words they cannot understand by applying grapheme to phoneme rules. Read is in inverted commas because although sounding correct, the words frequently were meaningless to the patients, and the aim of reading is to comprehend the writer's message.

Is it possible that only a single class of words is affected in SD? It seems not, as Patterson and Hodges reported a series of six patients with SD and demonstrated an interaction between irregularity and frequency, with low frequency exception words being considerably harder to read,[11] suggesting that the patients were able to correctly read such words if they had been exposed to them enough prior to the onset of their illness. They ended their paper by speculating over the more common syndrome of Alzheimer's disease (AD), noting that reading errors seem more variable in this group. As if to answer this call, Arsland et al. published a paper that contained data from 16 patients with AD and an average disease duration of 3.4 years.[12] They tested the lexical (direct) and non-lexical (indirect) routes and showed that AD patients were significantly worse than controls for both routes in terms of both accuracy and reaction time. Moreover, reading performance correlated with severity of dementia as judged by mini-mental state examination (MMSE)[13] scores.

What about reading in progressive non-fluent aphasia (PNFA), a form of primary progressive aphasia (PPA)? A group study was published in 1997 on an impressive 112 cases.[14] They reported that reading was only mildly affected, with deficits rarely occurring before the 4th or 5th year post-presentation and 80 per cent of patients showing no deficit at all; although they employed clinical reading tests that may be insensitive to early impairments. More recently, Hodges and colleagues compared the neuropsychological profile of patients with AD, SD and the progressive non-fluent form of PPA with 19 cases in each group and patients were matched for age.[15] Reading was only assessed with the National Adult Reading Test (NART) which comprises 50 irregular words of varying difficulty.[16] As expected, SD patients were significantly worse than the other two groups on this test, who in turn were not significantly worse than controls. Unfortunately, no other reading tests were included, so this study adds little on the reading front to what was already known.

As an aside the NART is commonly used to provide an estimate of premorbid IQ following brain damage or disease, as the ability to read exception words correlates highly with intelligence measures (also in non-injured individuals). This means, of course, that the ability to read low frequency irregular words varies significantly in the normal population, a factor that is very important to take into account when assessing single patients.

The standard explanation for surface dyslexia is that regularizations suggest a lack of semantic knowledge, which begs the question: are surface dyslexia and semantic impairments inextricably linked? Yes, according to the largest study to date on reading in patients with SD (100 datasets on 51 patients), which was published in 2007.[17] They took longitudinal behavioral measures of reading ability and semantic knowledge and found strong correlations between performance on semantic tests and overall reading ability as well as regularization errors on irregular words. Interestingly, the patients were impaired on non-word reading too, even the relatively mildly impaired cases, although these scores did not correlate significantly with semantic knowledge. The relationship between composite semantic score and low-frequency exception word reading accuracy are impressive with $R^2 = 0.5$ (Fig. 18.1). They found the results so compelling that they dubbed the association between semantic dementia and surface dyslexia 'SD-squared'.

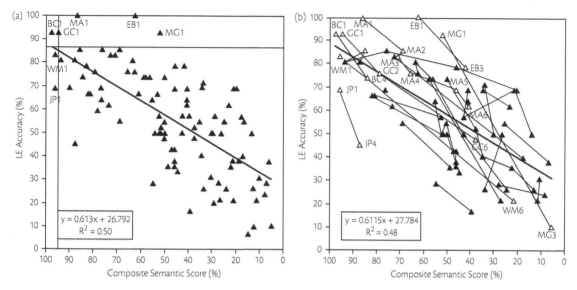

Fig. 18.1 (a) Overall accuracy results for 100 observations of reading performance from 51 semantic dementia patients for low-frequency exception (LE) words according to level of semantic knowledge. The horizontal line represents two standard deviations below control performance on LE words; the vertical line represents two standard deviations below control performance on the composite semantic score. (b) Overall accuracy results for 75 observations of reading performance from 27 semantic dementia patients for low-frequency exception words according to level of semantic knowledge. Repeated observations for each patient are connected by lines to indicate progression over time.

Reproduced from *Psychological Review.* 114(2), Woollams AM, Ralph MAL, Plaut DC, *et al.* SD-squared: On the association between semantic dementia and surface dyslexia, pp. 316–39, Copyright (2007), with permission from the American Psychological Association.

Phonological dyslexia

Phonological dyslexia—in its Platonic form—serves as a counterpoint to surface dyslexia. The syndrome was comprehensively described in 1983 in a patient who suffered a large left MCA stroke.[18] The patient was anomic and had a severe impairment of phonological memory (a digit span of only one) with auditory comprehension of speech also affected. His single word reading was affected, but with most grammatical classes of words equally affected (nouns, adjectives, verbs and functors (a word that chiefly expresses grammatical relationships and has little semantic content of its own) all read between 86–93 per cent correct). There was no effect of regularity. He was especially poor on non-words, unable to read any (0/20) of the four or five letter examples correctly. His errors were mainly close phonological non-words, but he did attempt to turn a few into real words (e.g. [sweal] read as 'sweat').

He was able to read suffixed words as well as the other classes of words, but could not read the suffixes alone (e.g. [ly] read as 'why'). This, combined with his ability to read functors, differentiated his reading behavior from that of patients with deep dyslexia (Table 18.1). In its purest form (an inability to read non-words only) phonological dyslexia looks like a neurological curiosity that should have little, if any, impact on normal reading. However, it means that new words will be hard to acquire and if there is any 'bleed' into other classes of word being affected, then these may be difficult to re-learn.

An important and as yet still unresolved issue is what is the root cause of phonological dyslexia. Is it in fact caused by a generalized phonological impairment? The most illuminating study to have examined this question used data from 31 stroke patients.[19] A key analysis investigated the relationship between phonological processing (here derived as a composite score taken from six tests taken from the PALPA or Psyhcolinguistics Assessments of Language Processing in Aphasia battery)[20] and scores on real and non-word

reading and writing (spelling to dictation). They found strong correlations between the phonological composite score (PC in Fig. 18.2) and non-word reading and writing (r = 0.66 and 0.69 respectively) and even stronger correlations with real word reading and writing (r = 0.80 and 0.78 respectively). Overall, the phonological composite scores proved to be powerful predictors of written language performance, accounting for 67 per cent of the variance in reading accuracy and 61 per cent of the variance in spelling accuracy. See Fig. 18.2.

A more recent study reported 16 patients with progressive non-fluent aphasia (PNFA).[21] Similar methodology was used to the SD squared paper mentioned above: namely, correlating phonological impairment (defined a little unusually by error rates on spoken word picture naming, rather than on tests of phonological perception) with real and non-word reading ability. All the patients had a central alexia of a pattern in which both low-frequency exception word and non-word reading were comparably compromised. They found that their phonological error rate significantly correlated with reading performance. The strength of this relationship was similar for low-frequency exception words and non-words, suggesting that reading deficits for these two types of items in this disorder shared a common cause: a progressive impairment of phonological processing. Thus the majority of the evidence in the literature points towards a 'central' phonological deficit in phonological alexia.

Lastly, a nice imaging study in 26 patients with PPA, clearly highlights the two different reading streams.[22] This was a voxel-based morphometry study which means that reading behaviour (as a continuous variable) was correlated with grey matter density (as a continuous variable). In this case the correlation was a positive one, that is, the better the patients were on a given reading task, the greater their grey matter density. Exception word reading (irregular words, read via the direct or lexical route) correlated with greater

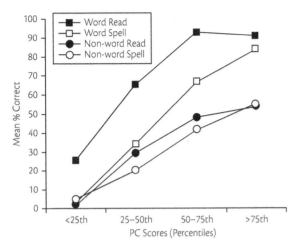

Fig. 18.2 Reading and spelling performance for subgroups of patients with peri-sylvian lesions falling into different quartiles based on the distribution of phonological composite (PC) scores for the peri-sylvian cohort (x-axis), plotted against reading and spelling performance (y-axis) across words and non-words. These graphs can be conceived of as a set of performance/resource curves with the x-axis reflecting the amount of phonological resources available to the different patient subgroups.

Reproduced from *Cortex.* 45(5), Rapcsak SZ, Beeson PM, Henry ML, *et al. Phonological dyslexia and dysgraphia: cognitive mechanisms and neural substrates*, pp. 575–91, Copyright (2009), with permission from Elsevier.

(more normal) grey matter values in the anterior and lateral temporal lobe, while non-word reading performance (read via the indirect or sub-lexical route) correlated with greater (more normal) grey matter values in the inferior parietal regions (Fig. 18.3).

Deep dyslexia

Deep dyslexia is related to phonological dyslexia but in its canonical form is clearly different. Patients make semantic errors when reading real words which are striking when they occur. From a 1930 account, the patient was shown the word [Cat] and, after each error, was asked to try again, 'Mice … Dog … Rat …'.[23] Deep dyslexic patients also have particular problems with function words, either being unable to read them at all, making a regularization error, [off] read as 'ov', or producing a different functor e.g. 'on'. The usual pattern of increasing difficulty that patients with deep dyslexia have, in terms of part-of-speech is: concrete > abstract > functors > non-words. These phenomena all suggest a problem with the way that the semantic system supports reading in these patients. Despite incorrect oral reading, are these patients able to extract the correct meaning from misread words? The answer appears to be 'Yes'.[8]

The majority of studies on deep dyslexia have focused on the semantic system, but such patients often make morphological errors too, e.g. [swimmer] misread as 'swim'. It has been proposed that this is actually a type of visual error driven by the target word's low concreteness or frequency.[24] So at their extremes, while there is overlap in terms of impaired non-word reading, phonological and deep dyslexia appear separable with deep dyslexics making semantic errors on word reading, being significantly worse at functors, and making morphological errors on genuinely suffixed words. Or are we seeing the effects of publication bias where cases that represent two ends of a clinical spectrum get reported, while those 'messy' cases that form a possible middle ground are missed out? In other words, do phonological dyslexia and deep dyslexia exist on a continuum?

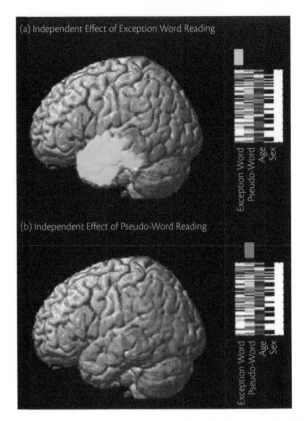

Fig. 18.3 Brain areas showing (a) independent effect of exception word reading; (b) independent effect of pseudo-word reading. Maps of significant correlation are superimposed the 3D rendering of the Montreal Neurological Institute standard brain.

Reproduced from *Neuropsychologia.* 47(8–9), Brambati SM, Ogar J, Neuhaus J, *et al. Reading disorders in primary progressive aphasia: A behavioral and neuroimaging study*, pp. 1893–900, Copyright (2009), with permission from Elsevier.

In almost all of the stroke patients that have been reported in papers discussed in this sub-section, there is little regard paid to where they were in terms of any potential recovery curve at the time of testing. Almost all were in the chronic phase (> 6 months post-stroke). The underlying assumption seems to be that little change is to be expected in their impairment profile, but this is unlikely to be the case. Friedman pointed this out when she described five patients whose reading evolved from deep to phonological.[25] Crisp and Lambon Ralph examined 12 cases recruited from a local speech and language therapy service. The patients had all suffered a stroke and were recruited on the basis of demonstrating the following when reading aloud: (a) a lexicality effect, (b) an imageability effect, or (c) production of semantic paralexias. The first 12 fulfilling these criteria were studied with a large battery (over ten) of psycholinguistic tests, mainly from the PALPA. In short, they could find no clear cut-offs between phonological and deep dyslexia. They proposed a two-dimensional space in which acquired dyslexic patients might be found (Fig. 18.4).[26] This suggests continua between all the main groups.

The peripheral alexias

Hemianopic alexia

Hemianopic alexia is the most peripheral of the peripheral alexias. It is also the commonest. In its most simplistic form, it can be thought

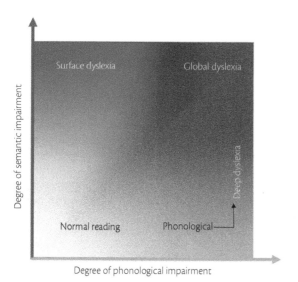

Fig. 18.4 The positioning of the acquired dyslexias within a phonological–semantic space.
Courtesy of Professor Matt Lambon Ralph.

of as a purely visual impairment that impacts upon text reading performance because the visuo-motor system requires visual information away from the point of fixation in order to plan efficient reading eye movements. Patients with homonymous, hemifield defects that encroach within five degrees of fixation, which the majority do,[27] can be expected to have some form of hemianopic alexia; although those with left-sided hemianopias are less likely to be impaired than those with right-sided hemianopias when reading languages that are written (and thus read) from left-to-right. The amount of visual sparing is important as there is a clear, monotonic relationship between this and reading speed.[28]

Therapy for this form of alexia has the strongest evidence base of all acquired alexias. Unlike all the others, visual word form and linguistic processes are preserved, so the various therapies are all based around retraining eye movements. There are at least five examples of these with effect sizes ranging from 0.2–1.[28–32] Both voluntary and involuntary (optokinetic nystagmus) saccades appear to work, with the latter available on a free-to-use website <http://www.read-right.ucl.ac.uk> that has been shown to be clinically effective.[33]

Pure alexia

Pure alexia is a selective disorder of reading, caused by damage to occipito-temporal structures in the dominant hemisphere. The disorder is selective in the sense that other language functions, including writing, are intact. However, subtle visual deficits have been reported to accompany pure alexia in many patients.[34–36] For a diagnosis of pure alexia to be made, a reading deficit evident in single word reading should be present, while writing and other language functions (speech production and comprehension) should be intact. Typically, patients read slowly, but can identify most letters, words, and nonwords correctly. In the more severe condition of global alexia, word reading and letter identification is very impaired, and most words and nonwords cannot be identified. Reaction times in reading are slower than normal even for short words, and many authors also use the presence of a word length effect (WLE: a linear increase in RT with the number of letters in a word) as a diagnostic criteria.

Pure alexia is in many ways a simple syndrome: it is the result of focal brain injury, affects only one function (word recognition), and commonly patients have residual function so that reading is not abolished but merely deficient. It would seem, then, that pure alexia should be an easy target for rehabilitation efforts. Unfortunately, it has proven rather difficult to help patients with pure alexia read better. Of course, many patients spontaneously use a letter by letter (LBL) strategy to compensate for their deficit, but this strategy does not allow them to read fluently, and many patients report that they do not read for pleasure, even years after their injury, as it is too demanding. There are a whole host of therapeutic approaches that have been tried with varying success.[37] Because the condition is rare, few groups studies have been published, although one cross-modal therapy (using audition to boost visual word form recognition) demonstrated small but significant (11 per cent) improvements in reading speed.[38]

Pure alexia, and indeed all the alexias discussed in this chapter result from damage to the left ('dominant') hemisphere. There are, however, two forms of acquired reading disorders that may result from lesions to the non-dominant hemisphere, or bilateral damage: neglect alexia and attentional alexia. As the names imply, these deficits are thought to reflect attentional dysfunctions, rather than being core reading deficits. The reason for mentioning them here, is that these two forms of alexia are not necessarily accompanied by writing deficits, and could thus be included under the heading 'alexia without agraphia'. They are, however, diagnostics entities in their own right.

Neglect alexia is seen in patients with damage to occipito-parietal areas, most commonly in the right hemisphere. The core symptom of these patients is that they ignore the contralesional (left) side of words and/or text. Neglect alexia is commonly seen in the context of more generalised unilateral neglect syndrome (inattention to contralesional space), but may in some instances be seen as an isolated symptom.[39]

Patients with attentional alexia have quite a curious deficit in reading: they may be relatively unimpaired in reading words, but unable to identify the constituent letters,[40] quite the opposite of what is seen in pure alexia, where each letter in a word is identified, before the word can be read. The core symptom of attentional alexia, migration errors, is almost never observed in pure alexia e.g. the words [win—fed] may be read 'fin—fed' or even 'fin—wed'. The majority of patients have bilateral parietal damage.[41]

Posterior cortical atrophy

Patients with posterior cortical atrophy (PCA) often present with reading problems, but they differ from patients with semantic dementia as their cortical atrophy starts posteriorly in the occipital lobes rather than ventrally in the temporal lobes. Posterior cortical atrophy is usually caused by Alzheimer's disease pathology but tends to present earlier than classical AD, in the 6th decade, with relative preservation of episodic memory.[42] Presenting symptoms are usually visual in nature and can affect any type of stimulus but reading makes such demands on the visual system that it is no great surprise that it is commonly affected. Initially, errors tend to be visual in nature with crowding effects, but as the disease process moves anteriorly, the ventral visual stream can be affected leading to pure alexia-like errors (letter confusability).[43] But this rarely progresses to a central alexia, as by that point, patients are so visually disorientated as to preclude reading at all.

Very occasionally, reading ability can be preferentially preserved in the face of quite impaired visuoperceptual and visuospatial function (but central acuity must be spared), presumably via strong top-down influences.[44] If the process moves dorsally, as it often does, then the parietal lobes become affected, and this causes an extra set of problems with text reading because the patients suffer from visuospatial disorientation and cannot plan reading eye movements.[45] Patients sometimes have a hemianopia as well (due to the occipital damage).[46] These multiple hits to posterior cortical regions explain why reading is often the presenting symptom.

Acquired dysgraphia

The debate over whether writing is carried out using dissociable brain region(s), and thus whether 'pure' agraphia can exist after focal brain damage, very much mirrors the debate over pure reading disorders with the same sorts of evidence brought to bear e.g. how can phylogenetically recent skills such as reading and writing become instantiated in designated neuronal networks? The answer, if there is one, is via practice and Cohen and Dehaene have written extensively on their 'neuronal recycling' hypothesis which they use to explain this phenomenon for reading and writing. In brief, they propose a form of short-term exaptation[47] whereby cultural inventions invade evolutionarily older brain circuits and inherit many of their structural constraints.[48]

The clinical data from stroke patients suggests that acquired dysgraphias are most commonly seen in the context of a generalized language (aphasic) disorder.[49] There are only a few functional imaging studies of writing in the normal population, and a representative study found much overlap in the cortical networks that support reading and writing.[50] The main candidate region for a specific writing area is named after the person to first describe it, Sigmund Exner (1849–1926). Exner's area is above (dorsal to) Broca's area in the middle frontal gyrus. Small ischemic lesions of this region have been reported as causing acute, seemingly pure, dysgraphia.[51] Interestingly, a recent review of Exner's original writing showed that the evidence put forward for a specific 'writing' centre of the brain in Exner's book was rather slim.[52] Only four of the 167 case reports in his seminal book 'Studies on the localisation of functions in the cerebral cortex of humans' explicitly mention agraphia.[53]

As with the acquired alexia literature, there are a few cases that claim to demonstrate pure agraphia, that is, only writing affected with reading and other linguistic skills left unharmed. But one could argue that as well as being linguistically pure, the syndrome must also be differentiated from a general motor output disorder affecting the dominant hand (a patient with a recently fractured dominant hand will be partially agraphic, but not in any clinically meaningful way). With this in mind, the most useful classification is to borrow that from acquired alexia and think about central dysgraphias, where linguistic functions are impaired, (such as phoneme-to-grapheme conversion); and peripheral dysgraphias, where the stages of letter selection and the planning and implementation of the motor movements break down.[54] These latter conditions are akin to the disorders that affect speech (but not language) such as speech apraxia and the various dysarthrias.

The central dysgraphias

Central dysgraphias are more common than peripheral dysgraphias and are usually seen in association with other language impairments. Their classification mirrors that for reading and depends on both part-of-speech effects (which classes of words are more or less affected), and error types so a patient with phonological dysgraphia will be more likely to make errors on low frequency words or abstract words. If they also make written semantic errors e.g. writing [wine] for 'beer' then they would have deep dysgraphia. One has to be particularly careful in enquiring about premorbid spelling ability before reading too much into mild written errors, as there is good evidence to suggest that writing errors may show up sooner than speaking errors in degenerative disorders. Homophone spelling appears to be a particularly sensitive test of mild Alzheimer's disease with patients making errors confusing [knit] and [nit] when asked to spell one of the words in context.[55] Treatment of central dyslexias is somewhat ad-hoc and depends on the patient's residual capacities; a variety of approaches have been championed.[54]

The peripheral dysgraphias

When the stages of letter selection or the planning and implementation of the motor movements involved in writing break down in isolation, then the patient is said to have an isolated peripheral alexia. Some patients have well formed letters but these are produced in the wrong order, have extra elements or transpositions, e.g. [flowrer] produced for 'flower', [winow] for 'window' or [chiar] for 'chair'. It has been argued that these rare patients have a problem with their graphemic buffer, so should be better at short words, even very irregular ones.[54] Oral spelling should be normal in cases of 'pure' agraphia.

The more common peripheral dysgraphias affect letter form generation and are analogous to dysarthria or dysphonia in speech where the rate, rhythm, force, or amplitude of the writing movements are affected. Neurological diseases of the pyramidal, extrapyramidal or cerebellar systems can all cause this type of peripheral dysgraphia.

Case History I

Peripheral alexia: Hemianopic alexia

This case demonstrates, in a single subject, how text reading speed depends on the degree of visual sparing there is to the right of fixation in left-to-right readers. The patient, a 48 year old right-handed male, was found to have a right-sided visual field defect. Subsequently, a cystic lesion was demonstrated on MRI, located between the left optic tract and lateral geniculate nucleus (LGN). He had a macular splitting hemianopia in his (dominant) right eye, and a macular sparing hemianopia (with 3-4° of foveal/parafoveal sparing) in his left eye (Fig. 18.5a). This type of field loss (non-identical defects in both eyes, also known as an incongruous hemianopia) happens because full segregation of the visual fields does not occur until fibres have synapsed in the LGN. His visual acuity was N6 corrected in both eyes.

He read a 32 word news paragraph spread over 8 lines of text with each eye (Fig. 18.5b). He was ~30 per cent faster when reading with his left eye.

Time is depicted on the x-axis, with the bars indicating 240 ms. Distance is on the y-axis with the left of the stimulus at top and right at bottom. Fixations (horizontal portions of the trace) lasting between 150 and 350 ms are interrupted by saccades (vertical portions) lasting ~20 ms. The start of the first fixation onto the first

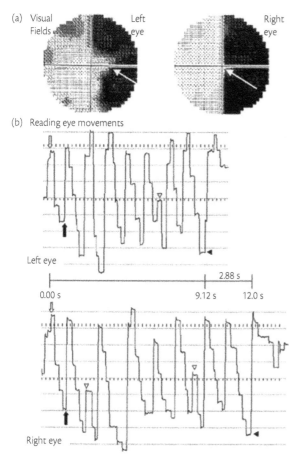

(a) Visual Fields   Left eye   Right eye

(b) Reading eye movements

Left eye

2.88 s

0.00 s   9.12 s   12.0 s

Right eye

Fig. 18.5 Peripheral alexia: hemianopic alexia.

Reproduced from *J Neurol Neurosur Ps.* 74(10), Upton NJ, Hodgson TL, Plant GT, *et al.* 'Bottom-up' and 'top-down' effects on reading saccades: a case study, pp. 1423–28, Copyright (2003), with permission from BMJ Publishing Group Ltd.

word of the opening line, 'There is a significant', is shown as an open arrow, with the end of the final fixation marked by a closed arrow. Regressive saccades occur in both traces (open arrowheads) but the patient clearly takes longer (12 secs as opposed to 9.1 secs) to get to the last word of the 8th line (closed arrowhead), when reading with his right eye.

References

1. Pugh K, and McCardle PD. *How Children Learn to Read: Current Issues and New Directions in the Integration of Cognition, Neurobiology and Genetics of Reading and Dyslexia Research and Practice.* New York, NY: Psychology Press, 2009.
2. Snowling MJ and Hulme C. *The Science of Reading: A Handbook.* Malden, MA: Blackwell, 2005.
3. Dejerine J. Sur un cas de cécité verbale avec agraphie, suivi d'autopsie. *CR Société du Biologie.* 1891;43:197–201.
4. Dejerine J. Contribution a l'étude anatomo-pathologique et clinique des différentes variétés de cécité-verbale. *Memoires Societé Biologique.* 1892;4:61–90.
5. Coltheart M, Rastle K, Perry C, *et al* DRC: A dual route cascaded model of visual word recognition and reading aloud. *Psychological Review.* 2001;108(1):204–56. doi:10.1037//0033-295x.108.1.204.
6. Marshall JC and Newcombe F. Patterns of paralexia: a psycholinguistic approach. *J Psycholinguist Res.* 1973;2(3):175–99.
7. Beauvois M -F and Derouesne J. Phonological alexia: three dissociations. *J Neurol Neurosur Ps.* 1979;42:1115–24.

8. Patterson KE. What is right with deep dyslexic patients. *Brain Lang.* 1979;8(1):111–29. doi:10.1016/0093-934x(79)90044-0.
9. Warrington EK. The selective impairment of semantic memory. *Q J Exp Psychol.* 1975;27:635–57.
10. Tulving G. Episodic and semantic memory. In: G Tulving and W Donaldson (eds). *Organization of Memory.* New York, NY: Academic Press, 1972, pp. 381–402.
11. Patterson K and Hodges JR. Deterioration of word meaning: implications for reading. *Neuropsychologia.* 1992;30(12):1025–40.
12. Arsland D, Larsen JP, and Hoien T. Alexia in dementia of the Alzheimer's type. *Acta Neurol Scand.* 1993;88(6):434–39.
13. Folstein MF, Folstein SE, and Mchugh PR. Mini-Mental State—Practical Method for Grading Cognitive State of Patients for Clinician. *Journal of Psychiatric Research.* 1975;12(3):189–198. doi:10.1016/0022-3956(75)90026-6.
14. Westbury C and Bub D. Primary progressive aphasia: A review of 112 cases. *Brain Lang.* 1997;60(3):381–406. doi:10.1006/brln.1997.1840.
15. Hodges JR, Patterson K, Ward R, *et al.* The differentiation of semantic dementia and frontal lobe dementia (temporal and frontal variants of frontotemporal dementia) from early Alzheimer's disease: a comparative neuropsychological study. *Neuropsychology,* 13(1999;13(1):31–40.
16. Nelson HE and Willison J. *The National Adult Reading Test (NART:2): Test Manual.* Windsor: NFER-Nelson, 1991.
17. Woollams AM, Ralph MAL, *et al.* SD-squared: On the association between semantic dementia and surface dyslexia. *Psychological Review.* 2007;114(2):316–39. doi:10.1037/0033-295x.114.2.316.
18. Funnell E. Phonological Processes in Reading—New Evidence from Acquired Dyslexia. *B J Psychol.* 1983;74(May):159–80.
19. Rapcsak SZ, Beeson PM, Henry ML, *et al.* Phonological dyslexia and dysgraphia: cognitive mechanisms and neural substrates. *Cortex.* 2009;45(5):575–91. doi: S0010-9452(08)00133-0 [pii] 10.1016/j.cortex.2008.04.006.
20. Kay J, Lesser R, and Coltheart M. *Psycholinguistic Assessments of Language Processing in Aphasia (PALPA): Reading and Spelling.* Hove: Lawrence Erlbaum Associates, 1992.
21. Woollams AM and Patterson K. The consequences of progressive phonological impairment for reading aloud. *Neuropsychologia.* 2012;50(14):3469–77. doi:10.1016/j.neuropsychologia.2012.09.020.
22. Brambati SM, Ogar J, Neuhaus J, *et al.* Reading disorders in primary progressive aphasia: A behavioral and neuroimaging study. *Neuropsychologia.* 2009;47(8–9):1893–900. doi:10.1016/j.neuropsychologia.2009.02.033.
23. Franz SI. The Relations of Aphasia. *J Gen Psychol.* 1930;3(3):401–11.
24. Funnell E. Morphological Errors in Acquired Dyslexia—a Case of Mistaken Identity. *Q J Exp Psychol–A.* 1987;39(3):497–539.
25. Friedman RB. Recovery from deep alexia to phonological alexia: Points on a continuum. *Brain Lang.* 1996;52(1):114–28. doi:10.1006/brln.1996.0006.
26. Crisp J and Ralph MAL. Unlocking the nature of the phonological-deep dyslexia continuum: The keys to reading aloud are in phonology and semantics. *J Cognitive Neurosci.* 2006;18(3):348–62. doi:10.1162/089892906775990543.
27. Zhang X, Kedar S, Lynn MJ, *et al.* Homonymous hemianopias: clinical-anatomic correlations in 904 cases. *Neurology.* 2006;66(6):906–910.
28. Zihl J. Eye movement patterns in hemianopic dyslexia. *Brain.* 1995:891–912.
29. Kerkhoff G, Munsinger U, Eberle-Strauss G, *et al.* Rehabilitation of hemianopic alexia in patients with postgeniculate visual field disorders. *Neuropsychological Rehabilitation.* 1992;2(1):21–41.
30. Schuett S, Heywood CA, Kentridge RW, *et al.* Rehabilitation of hemianopic dyslexia: are words necessary for re-learning oculomotor control? *Brain.* 2008;131(Pt 12):3156–68. doi: awn285 [pii] 10.1093/brain/awn285.
31. Schuett S, Kentridge RW, Zihl J, *et al.* Adaptation of eye-movements to simulated hemianopia in reading and visual exploration: Transfer or specificity? *Neuropsychologia.* 2009;47(7):1712–20. doi: S0028-3932(09)00079-7 [pii] 10.1016/j.neuropsychologia.2009.02.010.

32. Spitzyna GA, Wise RJ, McDonald SA, *et al.* Optokinetic therapy improves text reading in patients with hemianopic alexia: a controlled trial. *Neurology.* 2007;68(22):1922–30.

33. Ong YH, Brown MM, Robinson P, *et al.* Read-Right: a 'web app' that improves reading speeds in patients with hemianopia. *J Neurol.* 2012. doi:10.1007/s00415-012-6549-8.

34. Behrmann M, Nelson J, and Sekuler EB. Visual complexity in letter-by-letter reading: 'pure' alexia is not pure. *Neuropsychologia.* 1998;(11):1115–32.

35. Starrfelt R and Behrmann M. Number reading in pure alexia—a review. *Neuropsychologia.* 2011;49(9):2283–98. doi: S0028-3932(11)00228-4 [pii] 10.1016/j.neuropsychologia.2011.04.028.

36. Starrfelt R, Habekost T, and Leff AP. Too Little, Too Late: Reduced Visual Span and Speed Characterize Pure Alexia. *Cereb Cortex.* 2009. doi: bhp059 [pii] 10.1093/cercor/bhp059.

37. Starrfelt R, Olafsdottir RR, and Arendt IM. Rehabilitation of pure alexia: A review. *Neuropsychol Rehabil.* 2013;23(5):755–9. doi: 10.1080/09602011.2013.809661.

38. Woodhead ZV, Penny W, Barnes GR, *et al.* Reading therapy strengthens top-down connectivity in patients with pure alexia. *Brain.* 2013;(Pt 8):2579–91. doi: awt186 [pii] 10.1093/brain/awt186.

39. Haywood M and Coltheart M. Neglect dyslexia with a stimulus-centred deficit and without visuospatial neglect. *Cogn Neuropsychol.* 2001;18(7):577–615. doi: 713751919 [pii] 10.1080/02643290042000251.

40. Davis C and Coltheart M. Paying attention to reading errors in acquired dyslexia. *Trends Cogn Sci.* 2002;6(9):359. doi: S1364661302019502 [pii].

41. Shalev L, Mevorach C, and Humphreys GW. Letter position coding in attentional dyslexia. *Neuropsychologia.* 2008;46(8):2145–51. doi: S0028-3932(08)00088-2 [pii] 10.1016/j.neuropsychologia.2008.02.022.

42. McMonagle P, Deering F, Berliner Y, *et al.* The cognitive profile of posterior cortical atrophy. *Neurology,* 66(2006;66(3):331–38. doi:10.1212/01.wnl.0000196477.78548.db.

43. Crutch SJ and Warrington EK. The relationship between visual crowding and letter confusability: Towards an understanding of dyslexia in posterior cortical atrophy. *Cognitive Neuropsychology.* 2009;26(5):471–98. doi:10.1080/02643290903465819.

44. Yong KX, Warren JD, Warrington EK, *et al.* Intact reading in patients with profound early visual dysfunction. *Cortex.* 2013. doi: S0010-9452(13)00012-9 [pii] 10.1016/j.cortex.2013.01.009.

45. Crutch SJ. Seeing why they cannot see: Understanding the syndrome and causes of posterior cortical atrophy. *J Neuropsychol.* 2013. doi:10.1111/jnp.12011.

46. Formaglio M, Krolak-Salmon P, Tilikete C, *et al.* Homonymous hemianopia and posterior cortical atrophy. *Revue neurologique.* 2009;165(3):256–62. doi:10.1016/j.neurol.2008.10.010.

47. Gould SJ and Vrba ES. Exaptation—a Missing Term in the Science of Form. *Paleobiology.* 1982;8(1):4–15.

48. Dehaene S and Cohen L. Cultural recycling of cortical maps. *Neuron.* 2007;56(2):384–98. doi:10.1016/j.neuron.2007.10.004.

49. Swinburn K, Porter G, and Howard D. *Comprehensive Aphasia Test.* Hove and New York: Psychology Press, Taylor & Francis Group, 2004.

50. Purcell JJ, Napoliello EM, and Eden GF. A combined fMRI study of typed spelling and reading. *Neuroimage.* 2011;55(2):750–62. doi: S1053-8119(10)01520-X [pii] 10.1016/j.neuroimage.2010.11.042.

51. Keller C and Meister IG. Agraphia caused by an infarction in Exner's area. *J Clin Neurosci.* 2013. doi: S0967-5868(13)00159-8 [pii]. 10.1016/j.jocn.2013.01.014.

52. Roux FE, Draper L, Kopke B, *et al.* Who actually read Exner? Returning to the source of the frontal 'writing centre' hypothesis. *Cortex.* 2010;46(9):1204–10. doi: S0010-9452(10)00102-4 [pii] 10.1016/j.cortex.2010.03.001.

53. Exner S. *Untersuchungen über die Lokalisation der Functionen in der Grosshirnrinde des Menschen.* Wien: Wilhelm Braunmuller, 1881.

54. Beeson PM. Remediation of written language. *Top Stroke Rehabil.* 2004;11(1):37–48.

55. Neils J, Roeltgen DP, and Constantinidou F. Decline in homophone spelling associated with loss of semantic influence on spelling in Alzheimer's disease. *Brain Lang.* 1995;49(1):27–49. doi:S0093-934X(85)71020-6 [pii] 10.1006/brln.1995.1020.

CHAPTER 19

Neuropsychiatric aspects of cognitive impairment

Dylan Wint and Jeffrey L. Cummings

Emotional and behavioural dysfunction frequently accompany cognitive impairment[1-3] and dementia.[4,5] The study of these neuropsychiatric disturbances is critical because behavioural problems adversely affect quality of life, neurologic outcomes, caregiver burden, and cost of care for patients with cognitive disorders (Fig. 19.1).[6-10]

Neuropsychiatric profiles can also be used to distinguish between cognitive disorders while providing insights into anatomic, physiologic, and pathologic correlates of brain function and dysfunction (Table 19.1).[10-13] Unfortunately, medical providers continue to underestimate how common neuropsychiatric problems are and the extent to which they impact on patients' lives. Recognizing neuropsychiatric syndromes requires particular patience and thoughtfulness in cognitively disturbed patients, who may be less able to help identify symptoms.

Almost all individuals with Alzheimer's disease (AD)—the most common and most-studied acquired cognitive disorder—develop neuropsychiatric symptoms at some point during the course of illness. The large number of people with AD (more than 5 million in the United States alone) and the high prevalence of neuropsychiatric disturbances in this population make it one of the most common causes of mental illness.[10] Accordingly, dementia-associated neuropsychiatric symptoms have been best characterized in AD. However, there remain deficits even in the field of AD-associated neuropsychiatric symptoms. Among them are:

- Paucity and inconsistency of studies of neuropsychiatric phenomena other than depression[14]

- A lack of consensus definitions for many neuropsychiatric syndromes

- Few studies that have found safe and effective treatments for the neuropsychiatric aspects of cognitive impairment

The Neuropsychiatric Inventory (NPI)[15,16] is the most often-used tool for quantifying psychopathology associated with cognitive dysfunction. Its scoring system rates the frequency and severity of 12 neuropsychiatric abnormalities that can be grouped into clusters of co-occurring symptoms (Table 19.2).[17,18] This classification of neuropsychiatric disturbances provides a convenient scaffold upon which to build this chapter's discussion of selected mental disturbances that occur in cognitive diseases.

Agitation/aggression (hyperactive cluster)

Clinical phenomenology and importance

Of the hyperactive symptoms, agitation and aggression are the most serious and the most likely to require clinical attention. In part, this is because other hyperactive symptoms may go unreported unless they are accompanied by agitation or aggression. In addition, agitation and aggression are almost always accompanied by one or more of the other hyperactive symptoms. Agitation is an inappropriate and disruptive increase in activity, and may manifest as motoric (pacing, fidgeting, picking), verbal/vocal (shouting, cursing, grunting), or affective (anger, laughing, crying) symptoms. The judgment of someone as 'agitated' is necessarily subjective— the phrase 'inappropriate and disruptive' is open to interpretation. Nevertheless, assessment of agitation by clinicians and caregivers has demonstrated intra- and inter-test reliability.[15,19-21] Cognitive disorders reduce the patient's ability to communicate distress. Therefore, a cognitively impaired individual who appears agitated must be assessed for underlying causes, which may be physical (e.g. moaning because of pain), psychiatric (anxious fidgeting), or iatrogenic (pacing because of akathisia).

Although a careful evaluation will sometimes reveal a secondary cause for these behaviours, agitation can be a primary symptom of cognitive disease. It is now recognized that even individuals with mild cognitive impairment (MCI)—cognitive dysfunction not severe enough to cause dementia—exhibit elevated rates of agitation in comparison to cognitively intact peers.[22] Agitation occurs in more than 20 per cent of patients with AD.[23] There are also high prevalences of agitation in frontotemporal dementia (FTD),[24] vascular dementia (VaD),[25] and dementia with Lewy bodies (DLB).[26] Agitation seems to be generally less problematic in progressive supranuclear palsy (PSP)[27] but this is not a universal finding.[28] In addition to determining the likelihood of agitation, the underlying disorder also affects the longitudinal course of agitation. For example, agitation in AD is increasingly likely as the disease progresses,[29,30] while patients with FTD demonstrate increasing agitation into the middle stages of disease but lower levels of agitation in advanced illness.[24] Compared to patients with AD, those with DLB experience earlier occurrence of agitation but less worsening over time.[31]

Aggression refers to verbal or physical actions that if carried to completion would result in harm. This may include promised, threatened, or actual physical assault, property damage, or unwanted sexual activity. Self-mutilation and suicidality are forms of self-targeted aggression. Unlike agitation, therefore, aggression always implies violence. Among dementia patients, aggressive behaviours have been associated with depressive symptoms, male gender, and worse cognition.[30,32-34] On the other hand, Aarsland and colleagues found that aggression was not correlated with dementia severity or depression, but was highly correlated with

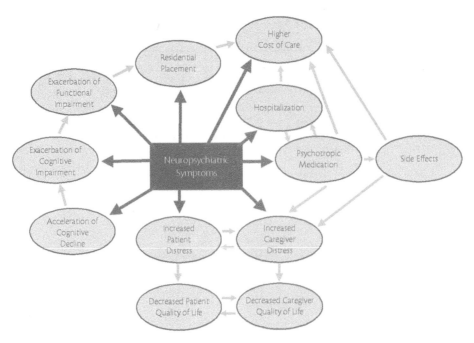

Fig. 19.1 The impact of neuropsychiatric symptoms.

psychotic symptoms.[35] Studies generally agree that verbal aggression is more common than physical aggression and that physical actions are generally preceded by verbal indications.[33,35–37] The number and type of verbal or motor actions that could signal aggressive intent are limitless, but it is important not to impute aggressive intent to benign actions.

Neurobiology

The neurobiology of agitation and aggression in dementia is not well understood. There are probably multiple underlying causes for these behaviours, further influenced by disease type and stage, underlying psychiatric history, psychosocial circumstances, and other variables. In general, studies have focused on roles of the neurotransmitters acetylcholine (Ach), serotonin (5-hydroxytryptamine, 5HT), noradrenaline (NA), and dopamine (DA) in modulating aggression in humans.

Many studies have demonstrated that the major metabolite of serotonin, 5-HIAA, is reduced in the cerebrospinal fluid

Table 19.1 Typical neuropsychiatric symptoms of major dementia syndromes

Dementia syndrome	Typical neuropsychiatric symptoms
Alzheimer disease	Apathy, irritability, depression, delusions
Dementia with Lewy bodies	Visual hallucinations, aberrant motor behaviour, depression
Vascular dementia	Depression, apathy, agitation/aggression
Frontotemporal dementia	Disinhibition, aberrant motor behaviour apathy, disinhibition
Parkinson's disease with dementia	Hallucinations, depression, agitation

(suggesting lower central 5HT activity) of individuals who have committed aggressive acts against themselves,[38] others,[39] or property.[40] These and other studies indicate that 5HT abnormalities are specifically associated with *impulsive* aggression.[41,42] However, these findings are subject to reasonable criticism and more study is needed.[43] Furthermore, relationships between neurobiology and behaviour in the cognitively intact brain may not be directly applicable to brains with abnormalities in cognitive processing.

Nevertheless, several lines of evidence suggest that 5HT dysregulation may be involved in aggressiveness of cognitively impaired individuals as well. In samples of temporal cortex from patients with AD, 5HT-1A receptor density was inversely correlated with aggression, suggesting that reduced ability to bind 5HT might mediate aggressive behaviour in AD.[44] Temporal 5HT-6 receptor density has also been correlated with both agitation and aggression, as measured by the Present Behavioural Examination.[45] Low 5HT levels in frontal cortex are associated with overactivity in AD.[46] Another study found a correlation between HVA (metabolite of DA)/5-HIAA ratio in CSF and aggression in FTD, but not in AD.[47] Studies investigating 5HT-related genetic predispositions toward AD-associated agitation and aggression have mixed results.[48–50]

The noradrenergic system has also been a target of investigation as a factor in dementia-related agitation and aggression. The noradrenergic locus coeruleus undergoes significant cell loss in AD and DLB,[51] although not in VaD.[52] The magnitude of noradrenergic cell loss is correlated with AD-related aggression.[53] This seems counterintuitive, as high levels of NA stimulation would be expected to promote agitated and aggressive behaviours, and behavioural hypersensitivity to NA stimulation has been demonstrated in AD patients.[54] However, there is evidence that locus coeruleus neuronal loss is compensated (possibly over-compensated) by increased NE production in remaining locus coeruleus neurons and postsynaptic NE receptor up-regulation in both AD51,[55–58] and DLB.[51]

Table 19.2 Neuropsychiatric inventory

Symptom cluster	NPI subscale	Representative questions
Hyperactivity	Agitation/Aggression	Is the patient stubborn, having to have things his/her way?
		Does the patient get upset with those trying to care for him/her or resist activities such as bathing or changing clothes?
		Does the patient shout or curse angrily?
	Elation/Euphoria	Does the patient find humour and laugh at things that others do not find funny?
		Does the patient tell jokes or make remarks that have little humour for others but seem funny to him/her?
		Does he/she play childish pranks such as pinching or playing 'keep away' for the fun of it?
	Irritability/Lability	Does the patient have sudden flashes of anger?
		Is the patient impatient, having trouble coping with delays or waiting for planned activities?
		Is the patient argumentative and difficult to get along with?
	Aberrant Motor	Does the patient pace around the house without apparent purpose?
		Does the patient rummage around opening and unpacking drawers or closets?
		Does the patient fidget excessively, seem unable to sit still, or bounce his/her feet or tap his/her fingers a lot?
	Disinhibition	Does the patient act impulsively without appearing to consider the consequences?
		Does the patient talk to total strangers as if he/she knew them?
		Does the patient take liberties or touch or hug others in a way that is out of character for him/her?
Mood/Apathy	Depression/Dysphoria	Does the patient put him/herself down or say that he/she feels like a failure?
		Does the patient express a wish for death or talk about killing him/herself?
		Does the patient seem very discouraged or say that he/she has no future?
	Apathy/Indifference	Does the patient seem less spontaneous and less active than usual?
		Does the patient seem less interested in the activities and plans of others?
		Does the patient show any other signs that he/she doesn't care about doing new things?
	Sleep	Does the patient have difficulty falling asleep?
		Does the patient wander, pace, or get involved in inappropriate activities at night?
		Does the patient awaken at night, dress, and plan to go out thinking that it is morning and time to start the day?
	Appetite / eating	Has he/she had a loss of appetite?
		Has he/she had an increase in appetite?
		Has he/she had a change in the kind of food he/she likes such as eating too many sweets or other specific types of food?
Psychosis	Delusions	Does the patient believe that others are stealing from him/her?
		Does the patient believe that unwelcome guests are living in his/her house?
		Does the patient believe that his/her spouse is having an affair?
	Hallucinations	Does the patient describe hearing voices or act as if he/she hears voices?
		Does the patient talk to people who are not there?
		Does the patient report smelling odours not smelled by others?
	Anxiety	Does the patient say that he/she is worried about planned events?
		Does the patient have periods of (or complain of) shortness of breath, gasping, or sighing for no apparent reason other than nervousness?
		Does the patient become nervous and upset when separated from your (or his/her caregiver)?

Furthermore, alpha-1 adrenoceptor density in post-mortem brain samples is correlated with aggressive behaviour of patients with AD.[59] More intriguing evidence for NA overactivity—despite locus coeruleus cell loss—in dementia-associated agitation/aggression is also suggested by treatment studies, which are described below.

Much of the evidence supporting a relationship between dopaminergic overactivity and agitation/aggression in the cognitively impaired is derived from animal data and DA's demonstrated role in aggression in cognitively healthy individuals.[60] However, DA may be only secondarily related to agitation and aggression, because heightened levels of DA activity are also associated with reward-seeking and motivational aspects of behaviour.[61] There are no studies that directly link DA activity with agitation or aggression,[62] although one older study found levels of the DA metabolite HVA in spinal fluid were lower in impulsive aggressors than in non-impulsive aggressors.[63] This seems to conflict with the finding that HVA/5-HIAA ratio in CSF is positively correlated with agitation and aggression in FTD.[47,64] In the cognitively impaired, non-significant associations between DA receptor and transporter genotypes and aggression have been detected.[65,66]

Low levels of acetylcholine and choline acetyltransferase activity in postmortem frontal and temporal cortex are correlated with overactivity in AD patients.[46,67] Other neurotransmitters such as GABA, glutamate, and acetylcholine are even less studied as mediators of agitation and aggression, especially in cognitively impaired humans. As with NA and DA, clinical responses to medications that modify these systems suggest a role for these less-studied transmitters.

Treatment

There are few controlled studies of treatments specifically for agitation/aggression in dementia, and these treatments have been largely unsuccessful.[68] There is increasing evidence that the treatments that help non-demented patients are not as likely to achieve measurable therapeutic responses in dementia.[69,70]

Cholinesterase inhibitors, which are often used to treat cognitive deterioration, have not shown marked benefit for agitation/aggression.[71] However, the glutamate antagonist memantine probably reduces irritability and agitation/aggression in dementia patients.[72] Memantine may be a particularly attractive option because its side-effect burden is relatively low and it can provide cognitive stabilization in addition to its neuropsychiatric benefits.[71]

Selective serotonin reuptake inhibitor (SSRI) antidepressants, which are taken by about one-third of patients with cognitive impairment,[73] have not shown robust efficacy for treating agitation or aggression. A large controlled study of citalopram 30 mg daily demonstrated an advantage over placebo in reducing some measures of agitation and caregiver distress at nine weeks.[74] However, subjects on citalopram exhibited more cognitive decline (1 point on MMSE) over the same period. In this study and others, citalopram treatment also appeared to confer a risk of QT$_c$ prolongation greater than that of other SSRI antidepressants.[75] Sertraline[76,77] may reduce restlessness and psychomotor agitation in AD patients. The heterocyclic antidepressant trazodone demonstrated effectiveness in reducing agitation in FTD.[78] Comprehensive reviews and meta-analyses of the relevant literature suggest that specific improvements in agitation/aggression with antidepressants are minimal,[79] although these drugs may help to improve general neuropsychiatric status.[80]

Anti-adrenergic agents may also be useful tools for addressing the problem of agitation/aggression in cognitive disorders. The non-selective beta-adrenergic antagonist propranolol reduced violent behaviours in a series of patients with chronic brain damage,[81] and it was significantly better than placebo at ameliorating NPI agitation/aggression in nursing home patients with possible and probable AD.[82] Prazosin, a selective alpha-1 adrenergic antagonist, reduced overall NPI scores in AD patients with agitation/aggression, but the sample was too small to allow for an analysis of its effects on specific NPI items.[83] The rate of adverse effects in studies of anti-adrenergic agents is fairly low, but close monitoring of blood pressure and heart rate is advised when using anti-adrenergic therapies in these often elderly patients.

The anti-epilepsy medications carbamazepine and valproate may help to reduce agitation/aggression, but valproate is associated with more rapid cerebral atrophy and cognitive decline, and several studies show no benefit of valproate over placebo.[84–86] Antipsychotic medications have also been studied for the treatment of dementia-associated agitation/aggression. Because many of these studies included patients with psychotic symptoms, specific details about the use of antipsychotics are discussed in the section on management of psychotic symptoms, below.

Depression and apathy (mood cluster)

Clinical phenomenology and importance

Most studies estimate the prevalence of major depression episodes in dementia to be between 20 per cent and 40 per cent, rates twice as high as those seen in the cognitively intact population, with even more patients suffering minor or subsyndromal depression,[23,87–89] rates twice as high as those seen in the cognitively intact population. Within the dementing disorders, the highest and lowest prevalences of depression have been reported in corticobasal syndrome (CBS) and PSP respectively, but findings have been quite varied.[11,27,90,91] Depression is associated with greater cognitive impairment in dementia and other neurological diseases,[92–94] but depression does not necessarily increase in prevalence or intensity as dementia progresses.[88] There is a rapidly enlarging body of evidence implicating depression as a risk factor for developing late-life cognitive disorders.[95–98] It may be that depressive episodes make limbic and cognitive circuits more vulnerable to damage by dementia-associated neuropathology. Alternately, mood symptoms could be the first signs of intrusions of dementia pathology that will later produce impaired cognition. The underpinnings of the relationship between depression and dementia—like most of what we have learned about each of these illnesses—are likely to be complex.[99]

Diagnosing depression in dementia is not straightforward. Patients with dementia usually have some degradation of recognition, recollection, and/or communication of emotional states and neurovegetative symptoms (see Box 19.1, case 1).[100] Informant reports, mental status examination, and clinical intuition must play the primary roles in gathering history about mood problems in this population. Specifics about depressive symptoms should be sought whenever possible. For example, the patient who reports her levels of interest and energy are 'good' should be asked to describe how she spends a typical day. The patient who claims he sleeps well should be asked what time he falls asleep, when he gets up for the day, and whether he feels refreshed in the mornings. Caregivers should be asked about their observations. In addition, agitation,

Box 19.1 Case 1

The family of a 72-year-old woman with moderate Alzheimer dementia was concerned that the patient might be depressed. In addition to sad mood, behavioural changes included insomnia, poor appetite, depressed affect (including tearfulness during the examination), disinterest in spending time with her family, and lack of energy. The family noted that she had stopped going for daily walks and did not want to attend her weekly card game. She was diagnosed with major depressive disorder and antidepressant medication was prescribed. Her cognitive impairments made psychotherapy unsuitable.

When the patient returned three months later, her family reported partial resolution of the depression symptoms. Appetite and sleep had returned to normal. She now appeared happy when her grandchildren visited. However, she still was not going on walks or playing cards. She spent most of her time in her bedroom. When asked whether she was still somewhat sad, she replied 'I'm the happiest I've ever been'. On a more specific review of the evolution of her depression, the family reported that the patient's activity level had declined 12 to 18 months before her sleep, appetite, and mood changed. At the time, the family attributed her waning activity level to 'normal slowing down' because of ageing. The medical provider educated the family and patient about dementia-related apathy, which all agreed was likely affecting this patient.

The provider offered a trial of stimulant medication. The patient and family declined, citing their reluctance to change the treatment regimen in the face of her recent improvement. They decided instead to pursue behavioural management—making a daily schedule of activities for the patient to follow, suggesting that she participate in activities (as opposed to asking whether she wanted to do them), visiting more frequently, and moving recreational supplies (television, bookshelf, radio) from her bedroom to the living room. They reported that although the patient still did not generate her own ideas about how to spend her day, her level of activity increased considerably over the next few months.

disinhibition, anxiety, irritability, aggression, and psychosis should be taken into account because they occur as atypical depressive symptoms in individuals with dementia.[101,102]

Apathy, a lack of directed thoughts and behaviour, is one of the most common neuropsychiatric disturbances in cognitive disorders, including PDD, FTD, DLB, and particularly AD.[103,104] Apathy contributes significantly to caregiver distress,[105,106] loss of independence,[107] and cognitive dysfunction.[108] Lack of consensus criteria and imprecise use of terms have sometimes led to conflation of depression (mainly anhedonia) and apathy. However, they are neither indistinguishable nor mutually exclusive.[109–112] Whereas anhedonia is a diminished response to agreeable stimulation, apathy is a lack of interest, drive, and persistence perhaps best conceptualized as an 'absence of will'.[113,114] The distinction has important therapeutic implications, as apathy is generally persistent[115] and unresponsive to antidepressants, while anhedonia is more likely to be a component of a potentially treatable depression.

Anxiety frequently accompanies depression but can also be present in non-depressed individuals. Like depression, anxiety impacts negatively on quality of life and creates caregiver distress, even at early stages of cognitive disturbance.[116]

Neurobiology

Although it is becoming clear that monoamines are not the only neurotransmitters that influence mood, a long-standing line of evidence links depression to dysfunction in monoamine transmitter systems.[117] As noted previously, adrenergic, serotonergic, and dopaminergic disruptions are also seen in AD, FTD, and DLB. However, there is much less evidence supporting differences in monamine activity between depressed and non-depressed dementia patients. Neuropathological examination has demonstrated greater loss of locus coeruleus (NA) and dorsal raphe (5HT) neurons in AD patients with depression than those without.[118] Lower levels of NA were also seen in cortical areas of depressed AD patients when compared to their non-depressed peers, but the same study showed no consistent or significant difference in 5HT or DA levels.[119] PET-measured densities of 5HT transporters (a surrogate for 5HT projections) in midbrain, caudate, and putamen were lower in depressed than non-depressed AD patients.[120] Limited studies have implicated the cholinergic system in mood and motivation abnormalities.[121] Further study of the relationships between monoaminergic state and mood in AD and other dementias is needed.

Anatomic changes may also be correlated with depression in dementia. Like AD, depression is associated with atrophy of the hippocampus and other regions that are important in cognitive processing.[122–124] Patients with MCI and depression had more frontal, temporal, and parietal white matter atrophy during two years of observation than did patients with no psychiatric symptoms. The same study did not detect accelerated atrophy in a group of MCI patients with non-depressive psychiatric symptoms, suggesting a specific neuroanatomical effect of depression.[125] There seems to be a relationship between the burden of AD-specific pathology (neurofibrillary tangles and neuritic plaques) and the presence of depression in individuals with AD, but not in elderly people with normal cognition.[126–128]

Apathy is associated neuroanatomical and neurochemical changes in the frontal cortex and regions with which it is extensively networked.[129] Several studies have demonstrated reduced cerebral perfusion in anterior temporal,[130] prefrontal,[130,131] and anterior cingulate[131,132] regions in dementia patients with apathy. The latter is also associated with apathy in non-demented patients.[132] Patients with apathy are under-responsive to amphetamine challenge, implicating DA and NA systems in its pathogenesis.[133] The early onset and persistence of apathy in AD, along with treatment studies using cholinesterase inhibitors, strongly suggest that cholinergic deficits also contribute to apathy.[134]

Treatment

Although they are widely used by clinicians, the evidence in favour of SSRI drugs for treating dementia-related depression is inconsistent at best.[135–138] Studies differ in definitions of depression, rating scales used to measure depression, and the severity of cognitive disturbance in the studied populations.[139] Furthermore, depression may be a time-limited phenomenon in patients with Alzheimer dementia, resulting in high rates of placebo response. Nevertheless, experts generally recommend use of SSRI antidepressant medication when a depressive episode is identified.[140] Although these drugs are generally considered quite safe, low starting doses and slow titration should be the overriding principles to reduce the risks of side-effects. A full therapeutic trial of at least eight weeks is necessary to determine an antidepressant's effectiveness.[141] Clinicians are particularly cautioned regarding antidepressants that have anticholinergic, antiadrenergic, and/or antihistaminic properties. These are more likely to cause side-effects in demented patients, and should be used for dementia-related depression only after failures of less problematic drugs, if at all.[142,143]

Electroconvulsive therapy (ECT) may also be of benefit, but it should be administered by an expert in treating the cognitively impaired population, because of specific and substantial cognitive risks.[144] Standardized evaluation of cognition and depression symptoms are recommended throughout the ECT course.[145] Individuals with better baseline cognition and those who are taking antidementia medications have better cognitive outcomes after a course of electroconvulsive therapy.[146] In addition to the assessment prior to starting the course of ECT, each individual stimulus should be preceded by a thorough risk/benefit analysis. In the authors' experience, patients who suffer significant cognitive decline during a course of ECT benefit from increased recovery time between treatments.

The results of studies evaluating treatments for apathy have been inadequate,[129,147] as most have measured apathy as a secondary or post hoc outcome. This evidence, from trials in a large number of patients, supports the use of cholinesterase inhibitors at typical treatment doses. The strongest evidence exists for donepezil in AD,[148,149] rivastigmine in DLB[150] and mixed AD/VaD,[151] and galantamine in mixed AD/VaD.[152] Ginkgo biloba extract EGb 761 240 mg daily was well tolerated, and superior to placebo in reducing apathy and other neuropsychiatric symptoms in AD, VaD, and mixed dementia.[153] In a study of non-depressed patients with AD and apathy, methylphenidate 20 mg daily was superior to placebo in two of three primary endpoints, with a low rate of adverse effects.[154] There is mixed evidence for the effectiveness of memantine, and no evidence favouring use of antidepressants or antipsychotics for AD- and VaD-associated apathy.[129] Apathy in FTD has proven even more resistant to treatment, with cholinesterase inhibitors,[155] memantine,[156] and antidepressants[157] showing no appreciable effect. However, it should be noted that treatment of apathy has not been studied nearly as well in FTD as in the more common dementias.

Delusions and hallucinations

Clinical phenomenology and importance

Psychosis—a disruption of one's connection to reality—is not as common as other neuropsychiatric symptoms, but is extremely disruptive to the lives of patients and caregivers (see Box 19.2, case 2). The overt manifestations of psychosis are hallucinations (aberrant sensory experiences), delusions (fixed false beliefs), and ideations (false beliefs not completely fixed). Psychosis may also include less obvious symptoms such as internal preoccupation and illogical/nonsensical patterns of thinking.[158]

Hallucinations in dementia, unlike those in schizophrenia or mood disorders, tend to be visual. Some types of delusions are more characteristic of dementias than primary psychiatric disorders. Among these are:

+ Infidelity: the patient's romantic partner has been unfaithful

+ Theft: someone has stolen important items from the patient

Box 19.2 Case 2

An 80-year-old woman with mild Alzheimer dementia complained that a small animal, the likes of which she had never seen before, was living in her house. She had only seen the animal once, when it 'snuck into my house' while a suspicious neighbor was moving out a few months ago. It had a body like a very small dog (about the size of a squirrel), with a head that resembled a cat's, except for long, hanging ears. Although she did not see it again, she knew it was in her house because she could hear it 'scratching around and knocking things over' as she tried to go to sleep each night. She also woke each morning with 'bite marks' on her skin, which she attributed to the animal's need to suck her blood. She attempted to demonstrate these marks to the examiner, who was unable to see the lesions to which she referred.

She was unable to sleep at night (because 'I don't know what it's gonna do next'). Her appetite was unchanged. She was still reading avidly and her mood was 'pretty good'. The patient's daughter said the patient appeared to be as sociable, happy, and energetic as before. However, she had stopped gardening and attending a twice-weekly senior breakfast because she spent much of the day catching up on sleep. Two thorough inspections of the patient's home, one by a rodent exterminator, found no evidence of infestation, although the patient pointed out a number of innocuous findings that signified to her that the animal was living there.

The patient did not see her concern about the animal as a medical problem, and did not want antipsychotic medication to reduce her preoccupation and anxiety about the animal. The daughter (who was the medical decision-maker) felt that the patient's symptoms were not severe enough to risk the serious potential side-effects of antipsychotics. They accepted trazodone, which did help the patient sleep better at night, but she discontinued it because of excessive daytime drowsiness.

Over the next eight months, the patient's worry about the animal slowly diminished, although she was convinced it was still roaming her house at night. Eventually the animal stopped biting her, 'or at least, not hard enough that I notice'. She attributed this to her new habit of leaving out a small bowl of milk each night, of which the animal drank 'just the tiniest bit, but you can tell'. Her sleep and daytime activities eventually returned to normal, and she continued putting out milk for the animal.

+ Misidentification: a loved one has been replaced by an identical-appearing impostor (Capgras syndrome), or a persecutor is disguising him/herself as other people (Fregoli syndrome)

+ Reduplicative paramnesia: a setting such as the patient's home has been relocated or duplicated in some other location

+ Phantom boarder: an unseen, sometimes unwanted, guest is living in the patient's home[158]

Rates of specific psychotic symptoms differ among the dementias. For example, although delusions and hallucinations are commonly seen in both AD and DLB,[12] DLB has much higher rates of hallucinations than the other dementias, and includes psychotic symptoms among its diagnostic features.[12,159] Studies of the prevalence of psychosis in VaD have varied results. Psychotic symptoms are more likely in very old patients and appear more frequently in multi-infarct dementia than in Binswanger disease.[160–163] Although PSP, CBD, and FTD are by no means immune to psychotic symptoms, they occur at lower rates in these disorders than in AD, DLB, and VaD.[11,12,27,90,164]

In addition to appearing as a consequence of the primary disease, psychotic symptoms can also result from delirium superimposed on dementia. Therefore, the sudden appearance or exacerbation of psychotic features should prompt a search for a new acute medical condition, such as infection or stroke. In addition, sensory deprivation such as impaired visual acuity or deafness can worsen psychotic symptoms in dementia patients.[165,166] Although it is not clear whether improving sensory deficits eliminates the psychotic phenomena, there are manifold reasons to improve sensory performance when possible.

Neurobiology

A core biological feature of both AD and DLB is loss of cholinergic activity in the brain. The high prevalence of psychosis in AD and DLB suggests that acetylcholine deficit may play a role in the pathogenesis of dementia-related hallucinations.[167,168] Indeed, cholinergic mechanisms are implicated by research observations. Psychotic symptoms are associated with cholinergic deficiency in frontal and temporal cortex in AD,[46,169] and in temporal and parietal cortex in DLB.[168] As with other forms of psychosis, limbic DA hyperactivity is also posited to play a role in dementia-related psychosis. Patients with DLB often experience worsening of psychotic symptoms when exposed to dopaminergic agents.[170] SPECT imaging has demonstrated a high correlation between severity of hallucinations and loss of striatal DA transporters (i.e. DAergic nerve terminals) in DLB patients.[171] PET imaging in a group of relatively early-stage AD patients showed increased striatal DA_2 and/or DA_3 receptor availability in patients with delusions; the study technique was not able to resolve whether this finding was due to decreased endogenous DA binding (which seems paradoxical) or increased DA receptor density in the patients with delusions.[172] There are sometimes contradictory implications about the contributions of glutamate, 5HT, and GABA dysregulation to psychosis in dementia.[173]

Studies of cerebral perfusion in AD patients with psychosis have found abnormally reduced or asymmetric blood flow in several regions, including striatum and thalamus, and frontal, temporal, and parietal cortex, as compared to cognitively healthy controls and AD patients without psychosis.[174-176] Parietotemporal hyper- and hypometabolism have both been seen with psychosis in AD.[177,178] Delusional misidentification syndromes are associated with reduced metabolism (FDG–PET) in orbitofrontal, mesial temporal, and cingulate regions,[177] and right temporal atrophy.[179] Neuropathological studies suggest that patients with AD and psychotic symptoms actually have greater neuronal preservation in parahippocampus, but higher levels of plaques, tangles, and dystrophic neurites throughout the rest of the cerebral cortex.[173,180] Conversely, visual hallucinations and delusions in DLB were associated with *less* neurofibrillary tangles and more Lewy bodies.[181]

Treatment

The issue of treatment of dementia-related psychotic phenomena is not straightforward. Psychotic symptoms are usually uncomfortable for patients and/or their caregivers, but the individual nature and circumstances of psychotic symptoms should always be taken into account when considering treatment. For example, if a patient has hallucinations of deceased loved ones but they do not bother

him, the most appropriate steps might be education, counselling, and support for a frustrated caregiver.[182] On the other hand, if similar hallucinations interfered with the patient's sleep and eating, then treatment to reduce the intensity or salience of the hallucinations could be in order.

Cholinesterase inhibitors demonstrate modest effectiveness in reducing dementia-related psychotic symptoms.[183] Because patients with AD, DLB, PDD, and VaD can benefit cognitively from cholinesterase inhibitors,[184-186] these medications are reasonable first-line agents for treating dementia-related psychosis. Antidepressant medicines may have some utility as well, with some studies demonstrating equal efficacy with lower side-effects when compared to antipsychotics.[79]

In the dementia population, antipsychotics have usually been studied in populations of patients who exhibit both psychosis and hyperactivity. The lessons learned from these studies can therefore be applied to both syndrome clusters. Meta-analytic studies of newer 'atypical' (combined 5HT and DA blockade) antipsychotics in dementia patients with agitation/aggression estimate small but significant benefits for using risperidone (1–2 mg daily), but poor support for aripiprazole, olanzapine, or quetiapine. Clinicians generally agree that psychotic symptoms are most effectively treated by antipsychotic medications, but benefits and risks can be difficult to balance in demented patients.

All current antipsychotics cause some level of postsynaptic DA blockade, which accounts for their class-specific side-effects—extrapyramidal syndromes (akathisia, dystonia, and parkinsonism), neuroleptic malignant syndrome, and tardive dyskinesia. The pharmacodynamic profiles of antipsychotics also predict potential antiadrenergic, antihistaminic, and anticholinergic side-effects.[187] These risks occur in all patient populations but the elderly are more sensitive. Importantly, antipsychotics have additional class-specific risks for the elderly and cognitively impaired. Antipsychotic medications are associated with clinically significant increases in short- and long-term rates of cognitive decline, stroke, sudden death, and acute hospitalization.[70,188,189] The authors recommend starting with low doses and titrating slowly, as antipsychotics can take some time to show their full therapeutic benefit. As with all pharmacotherapy, regular assessments of the need for continued medication are necessary. However, it should be noted that relapse rates after discontinuation are high, particularly in patients with severe symptoms.[190,191] Furthermore, as discussed above, other treatments for psychosis have low rates of effectiveness.

Pimavanserin, a selective 5HT-2A inverse agonist, is being investigated for the treatment of PD-related psychosis. Its effectiveness has been demonstrated in a placebo-controlled randomized trial.[192] This and other trials seemed to bear out the expectation that pimavanserin's pharmacodynamic selectivity would yield minimal motor (anti-DA), cognitive (anti-Ach), and sedative (antihistamine) side-effects.[193,194] Hopefully, pimavanserin will also be effective in treating psychosis associated with PDD and other dementias.[195]

Conclusion

Our understanding of cognitive disorders has been enhanced by study of the behavioural disturbances that so often accompany them. Although an impressive body of data has been accumulated about these symptoms, any clinician with experience in managing cognitive disorders will recognize that there is a pressing need for much more study. Increased attention to neuropsychiatric syndromes, better diagnostic criteria, and improvements in technology will produce a better understanding of their epidemiology, neurobiology, and—most importantly—the best ways to treat them.

References

1. Hwang TJ, Masterman DL, Ortiz F, et al. Mild cognitive impairment is associated with characteristic neuropsychiatric symptoms. *Alzheimer Dis Assoc Disord.* 2004 Jan–Mar;18(1):17–21.
2. Geda YE, Roberts RO, Knopman DS, et al. Prevalence of neuropsychiatric symptoms in mild cognitive impairment and normal cognitive aging: Population-based study. *Arch Gen Psychiatr.* 2008 Oct;65(10):1193–8.
3. Van der Mussele S, Le Bastard N, Vermeiren Y, et al. Behavioral symptoms in mild cognitive impairment as compared with Alzheimer's disease and healthy older adults. *Int J Geriatr Psychiatry.* 2012 Apr 30.
4. Lyketsos CG, Carrillo MC, Ryan JM, et al. Neuropsychiatric symptoms in Alzheimer's disease. *Alzheimer's and Dementia.* 2011 Sep;7(5):532–9.
5. Meeks TW, Ropacki SA, and Jeste DV. The neurobiology of neuropsychiatric syndromes in dementia. *Curr Opin Psychiatr.* 2006 Nov;19(6):581–6.
6. Phillips VL and Diwan S. The incremental effect of dementia-related problem behaviors on the time to nursing home placement in poor, frail, demented older people. *J Am Geriatr Soc.* 2003 Feb;51(2):188–93.
7. Murman DL, Chen Q, Powell MC, et al. The incremental direct costs associated with behavioral symptoms in ad. *Neurology.* 2002 Dec 10;59(11):1721–9.
8. Allegri RF, Sarasola D, Serrano CM, et al. Neuropsychiatric symptoms as a predictor of caregiver burden in Alzheimer's disease. *Neuropsychiatric Disease and Treatment.* 2006 Mar;2(1):105–10.
9. Somme JH, Fernandez-Martinez M, Molano A, et al. Neuropsychiatric symptoms in amnestic mild cognitive impairment: Increased risk and faster progression to dementia. *Current Alzheimer Research.* 2012 Sep 19.
10. Cummings JL, Vinters HV, and Felix J. *The Neuropsychiatry of Alzheimer's Disease and Other Dementias.* London Florence, KY: Martin Dunitz, 2003.
11. Levy ML, Miller BL, Cummings JL, et al. Alzheimer disease and frontotemporal dementias. Behavioral distinctions. *Arch Neurol–Chicago.* 1996 Jul;53(7):687–90.
12. Hirono N, Mori E, Tanimukai S, et al. Distinctive neurobehavioral features among neurodegenerative dementias. *J Neuropsychiatry Clin Neurosci.* 1999 Fall;11(4):498–503.
13. Konstantinopoulou E, Aretouli E, Ioannidis P, et al. Behavioral disturbances differentiate frontotemporal lobar degeneration subtypes and Alzheimer's disease: Evidence from the frontal behavioral inventory. *Int J Geriatr Psychiatry.* 2012 Nov 7:939–46.
14. van der Linde RM, Stephan BC, Savva GM, et al. Systematic reviews on behavioural and psychological symptoms in the older or demented population. *Alzheimer's Research & Therapy.* 2012 Jul 11;4(4):28.
15. Cummings JL, Mega M, Gray K, et al. The neuropsychiatric inventory: Comprehensive assessment of psychopathology in dementia. *Neurology.* 1994 Dec;44(12):2308–14.
16. Cummings JL. The neuropsychiatric inventory: Assessing psychopathology in dementia patients. *Neurology.* 1997 May;48(5 Suppl 6):S10–6.
17. Aalten P, de Vugt ME, Lousberg R, et al. Behavioral problems in dementia: A factor analysis of the neuropsychiatric inventory. *Dementia and Geriatric Cognitive Disorders.* 2003;15(2):99–105.
18. Lee WJ, Tsai CF, Gauthier S, et al. The association between cognitive impairment and neuropsychiatric symptoms in patients with Parkinson's disease dementia. *International Psychogeriatrics.* 2012 Dec;24(12):1980–7.
19. Finkel SI, Lyons JS, and Anderson RL. A brief agitation rating scale (bars) for nursing home elderly. *J Am Geriatr Soc.* 1993 Jan;41(1):50–2.
20. Shah A, Evans H, and Parkash N. Evaluation of three aggression/agitation behaviour rating scales for use on an acute admission and assessment psychogeriatric ward. *Int J Geriatr Psychiatry.* 1998 Jun;13(6):415–20.
21. Koss E, Weiner M, Ernesto C, et al. Assessing patterns of agitation in Alzheimer's disease patients with the cohen-mansfield agitation inventory. The Alzheimer's disease cooperative study. *Alzheimer Dis Assoc Disord.* 1997;11 Suppl 2:S45–50.
22. Brodaty H, Heffernan M, Draper B, et al. Neuropsychiatric symptoms in older people with and without cognitive impairment. *Journal of Alzheimer's Disease.* 2012;31(2):411–20.
23. Lyketsos CG, Steinberg M, Tschanz JT, et al. Mental and behavioral disturbances in dementia: Findings from the cache county study on memory in aging. *Am J Psychiat.* 2000 May;157(5):708–14.
24. Chow TW, Fridhandler JD, Binns MA, et al. Trajectories of behavioral disturbance in dementia. *Journal of Alzheimer's Disease.* 2012;31(1):143–9.
25. Echavarri C, Burgmans S, Uylings H, et al. Neuropsychiatric symptoms in Alzheimer's disease and vascular dementia. *Journal of Alzheimer's Disease.* 2012 Sep 21.
26. Borroni B, Agosti C, and Padovani A. Behavioral and psychological symptoms in dementia with Lewy-bodies (dlb): Frequency and relationship with disease severity and motor impairment. *Arch Geront Geriat.* 2008 Jan–Feb;46(1):101–6.
27. Litvan I, Mega MS, Cummings JL, et al. Neuropsychiatric aspects of progressive supranuclear palsy. *Neurology.* 1996 Nov;47(5):1184–9.
28. Han HJ, Kim H, Park JH, et al. Behavioral changes as the earliest clinical manifestation of progressive supranuclear palsy. *J Clin Neurol.* 2010 Sep;6(3):148–51.
29. Wetzels R, Zuidema S, Jansen I, et al. Course of neuropsychiatric symptoms in residents with dementia in long-term care institutions: A systematic review. *International Psychogeriatrics.* 2010 Nov;22(7):1040–53.
30. Majic T, Pluta JP, Mell T, et al. Correlates of agitation and depression in nursing home residents with dementia. *International Psychogeriatrics.* 2012 Nov;24(11):1779–89.
31. Stavitsky K, Brickman AM, Scarmeas N, et al. The progression of cognition, psychiatric symptoms, and functional abilities in dementia with Lewy bodies and Alzheimer disease. *Arch Neurol–Chicago.* 2006 Oct;63(10):1450–6.
32. Margari F, Sicolo M, Spinelli L, et al. Aggressive behavior, cognitive impairment, and depressive symptoms in elderly subjects. *Neuropsychiatric Disease and Treatment.* 2012;8:347–53.
33. Eastley R and Wilcock GK. Prevalence and correlates of aggressive behaviours occurring in patients with Alzheimer's disease. *Int J Geriatr Psychiatry.* 1997 Apr;12(4):484–7.
34. Isaksson U, Graneheim UH, Astrom S, et al. Physically violent behaviour in dementia care: Characteristics of residents and management of violent situations. *Aging Ment Health.* 2011 Jul 1;15(5):573–9.
35. Aarsland D, Cummings JL, Yenner G, et al. Relationship of aggressive behavior to other neuropsychiatric symptoms in patients with Alzheimer's disease. *Am J Psychiat.* 1996 Feb;153(2):243–7.
36. Brodaty H, Luscombe G, Anstey KJ, et al. Neuropsychological performance and dementia in depressed patients after 25-year follow-up: A controlled study. *Psychological Medicine.* 2003 Oct;33(7):1263–75.
37. Brodaty H, Draper B, Saab D, et al. Psychosis, depression and behavioural disturbances in Sydney nursing home residents: Prevalence and predictors. *Int J Geriatr Psychiatry.* 2001 May;16(5):504–12.
38. Asberg M, Traskman L, and Thoren P. 5-HIAA in the cerebrospinal fluid. A biochemical suicide predictor? *Arch Gen Psychiat.* 1976 Oct;33(10):1193–7.
39. Brown GL, Goodwin FK, Ballenger JC, et al. Aggression in humans correlates with cerebrospinal fluid amine metabolites. *Psychiatry Res.* 1979 Oct;1(2):131–9.
40. Virkkunen M, Nuutila A, Goodwin FK, et al. Cerebrospinal fluid monoamine metabolite levels in male arsonists. *Arch Gen Psychiat.* 1987 Mar;44(3):241–7.

41. Linnoila M, Virkkunen M, Scheinin M, *et al.* Low cerebrospinal fluid 5-hydroxyindoleacetic acid concentration differentiates impulsive from nonimpulsive violent behavior. *Life Sciences.* 1983 Dec 26;33(26):2609–14.

42. Brown CS, Kent TA, Bryant SG, *et al.* Blood platelet uptake of serotonin in episodic aggression. *Psychiatry Res.* 1989 Jan;27(1):5–12.

43. Roggenbach J, Muller-Oerlinghausen B, and Franke L. Suicidality, impulsivity and aggression—is there a link to 5-HIAA concentration in the cerebrospinal fluid? *Psychiatry Res.* 2002 Dec 15;113(1–2):193–206.

44. Lai MK, Tsang SW, Francis PT, *et al.* Reduced serotonin 5-HT1A receptor binding in the temporal cortex correlates with aggressive behavior in Alzheimer disease. *Brain Res.* 2003 Jun 6;974(1–2):82–7.

45. Garcia-Alloza M, Hirst WD, Chen CP, *et al.* Differential involvement of 5-HT(1b/1d) and 5-HT6 receptors in cognitive and non-cognitive symptoms in Alzheimer's disease. *Neuropsychopharmacology.* 2004 Feb;29(2):410–6.

46. Garcia-Alloza M, Gil-Bea FJ, Diez-Ariza M, *et al.* Cholinergic-serotonergic imbalance contributes to cognitive and behavioral symptoms in Alzheimer's disease. *Neuropsychologia.* 2005;43(3):442–9.

47. Engelborghs S, Vloeberghs E, Maertens K, *et al.* Evidence for an association between the CSF HVA: 5–HIAA ratio and aggressiveness in frontotemporal dementia but not in Alzheimer's disease. *J Neurol Neurosur Ps.* 2004 Jul;75(7):1080.

48. Sukonick DL, Pollock BG, Sweet RA, *et al.* The 5-HTTPR*S/*L polymorphism and aggressive behavior in Alzheimer disease. *Archives of neurology.* 2001 Sep;58(9):1425–8.

49. Pritchard AL, Pritchard CW, Bentham P, *et al.* Role of serotonin transporter polymorphisms in the behavioural and psychological symptoms in probable Alzheimer disease patients. *Dementia and geriatric cognitive disorders.* 2007;24(3):201–6.

50. Assal F, Alarcon M, Solomon EC, *et al.* Association of the serotonin transporter and receptor gene polymorphisms in neuropsychiatric symptoms in Alzheimer disease. *Archives of Neurology.* 2004 Aug;61(8):1249–53.

51. Szot P, White SS, Greenup JL, *et al.* Compensatory changes in the noradrenergic nervous system in the locus ceruleus and hippocampus of postmortem subjects with Alzheimer's disease and dementia with Lewy bodies. *J Neurosci.* 2006 Jan 11;26(2):467–78.

52. Mann DM, Yates PO, and Hawkes J. The noradrenergic system in Alzheimer and multi-infarct dementias. *J Neurol Neurosur Ps.* 1982 Feb;45(2):113–9.

53. Matthews KL, Chen CP, Esiri MM, *et al.* Noradrenergic changes, aggressive behavior, and cognition in patients with dementia. *Biol Psychiat.* 2002 Mar 1;51(5):407–16.

54. Peskind ER, Wingerson D, Murray S, *et al.* Effects of Alzheimer's disease and normal aging on cerebrospinal fluid norepinephrine responses to yohimbine and clonidine. *Archives of general psychiatry.* 1995 Sep;52(9):774–82.

55. Elrod R, Peskind ER, DiGiacomo L, *et al.* Effects of Alzheimer's disease severity on cerebrospinal fluid norepinephrine concentration. *Am J Psychiat.* 1997 Jan;154(1):25–30.

56. Szot P, White SS, Greenup JL, *et al.* Changes in adrenoreceptors in the prefrontal cortex of subjects with dementia: Evidence of compensatory changes. *Neuroscience.* 2007 Apr 25;146(1):471–80.

57. Hoogendijk WJ, Feenstra MG, Botterblom MH, *et al.* Increased activity of surviving locus ceruleus neurons in Alzheimer's disease. *Annals of neurology.* 1999 Jan;45(1):82–91.

58. Raskind MA, Peskind ER, Holmes C, *et al* Patterns of cerebrospinal fluid catechols support increased central noradrenergic responsiveness in aging and Alzheimer's disease. *Biol Psychiat.* 1999 Sep 15;46(6):756–65.

59. Sharp SI, Ballard CG, Chen CP, *et al.* Aggressive behavior and neuroleptic medication are associated with increased number of alpha1-adrenoceptors in patients with Alzheimer disease. *Am J Geriat Psychiat.* 2007 May;15(5):435–7.

60. Lindenmayer JP. The pathophysiology of agitation. *J Clin Psychiatry.* 2000;61 Suppl 14:5–10.

61. de Almeida RMM, Ferrari PF, Parmigiani S, *et al.* Escalated aggressive behavior: Dopamine, serotonin and gaba. *Eur J Pharmacol.* 2005 Dec 5;526(1–3):51–64.

62. Comai S, Tau M, and Gobbi G. The psychopharmacology of aggressive behavior: A translational approach part 1: Neurobiology. *J Clin Psychopharm.* 2012 Feb;32(1):83–94.

63. Linnoila M, Virkkunen M, Scheinin M, *et al.* Low cerebrospinal-fluid 5-hydroxyindoleacetic acid concentration differentiates impulsive from nonimpulsive violent behavior. *Life Sciences.* 1983;33(26):2609–14.

64. Engelborghs S, Vloeberghs E, Le Bastard N, *et al.* The dopaminergic neurotransmitter system is associated with aggression and agitation in frontotemporal dementia. *Neurochemistry International.* 2008 May;52(6):1052–60.

65. Pritchard AL, Ratcliffe L, Sorour E, *et al.* Investigation of dopamine receptors in susceptibility to behavioural and psychological symptoms in Alzheimer's disease. *Int J Geriatr Psych.* 2009 Sep;24(9):1020–5.

66. Pritchard AL, Pritchard CW, Bentham P, *et al.* Investigation of the role of the dopamine transporter in susceptibility to behavioural and psychological symptoms of patients with probable Alzheimer's disease. *Dementia and Geriatric Cognitive Disorders.* 2008;26(3):257–60.

67. Minger SL, Esiri MM, McDonald B, *et al.* Cholinergic deficits contribute to behavioral disturbance in patients with dementia. *Neurology.* 2000 Nov 28;55(10):1460–7.

68. Sink KM, Holden KF, and Yaffe K. Pharmacological treatment of neuropsychiatric symptoms of dementia: A review of the evidence. *JAMA.* 2005 Feb 2;293(5):596–608.

69. Schneider LS, Tariot PN, Dagerman KS, *et al.* Effectiveness of atypical antipsychotic drugs in patients with Alzheimer's disease. *New Engl J Med.* 2006 Oct 12;355(15):1525–38.

70. Schneider LS, Dagerman K, and Insel PS. Efficacy and adverse effects of atypical antipsychotics for dementia: Meta-analysis of randomized, placebo-controlled trials. *Am J Psychiat.* 2006 Mar;14(3):191–210.

71. Ballard CG, Gauthier S, Cummings JL, *et al.* Management of agitation and aggression associated with Alzheimer disease. Nature reviews Neurology. 2009 May;5(5):245–55.

72. Cummings JL, Schneider E, Tariot PN, *et al.* Behavioral effects of memantine in Alzheimer disease patients receiving donepezil treatment. *Neurology.* 2006 Jul 11;67(1):57–63.

73. Pitkala KH, Laurila JV, Strandberg TE, *et al.* Behavioral symptoms and the administration of psychotropic drugs to aged patients with dementia in nursing homes and in acute geriatric wards. *International Psychogeriatrics.* 2004 Mar;16(1):61–74.

74. Porsteinsson AP, Drye LT, Pollock BG, *et al.* Effect of citalopram on agitation in Alzheimer disease: The CITAD randomized clinical trial. *JAMA.* 2014 Feb 19;311(7):682–91.

75. Funk KA and Bostwick JR. A comparison of the risk of QT prolongation among SSRIs. *Ann Pharmacother.* 2013 Oct;47(10):1330–41.

76. Finkel SI, Mintzer JE, Dysken M, *et al.* A randomized, placebo-controlled study of the efficacy and safety of sertraline in the treatment of the behavioral manifestations of Alzheimer's disease in outpatients treated with donepezil. *Int J Geriatr Psychiatry.* 2004 Jan;19(1):9–18.

77. Gaber S, Ronzoni S, Bruno A, *et al.* Sertraline versus small doses of haloperidol in the treatment of agitated behavior in patients with dementia. *Arch Gerontol Geriat.* 2001:159–62.

78. Lebert F, Stekke W, Hasenbroekx C, *et al.* Frontotemporal dementia: A randomised, controlled trial with trazodone. *Dementia and Geriatric Cognitive Disorders.* 2004;17(4):355–9.

79. Seitz DP, Adunuri N, Gill SS, *et al.* Antidepressants for agitation and psychosis in dementia. *Cochrane Database Syst Rev.* 2011(2):CD008191.

80. Henry G, Williamson D, and Tampi RR. Efficacy and tolerability of antidepressants in the treatment of behavioral and psychological symptoms of dementia, a literature review of evidence. *Am J Alzheimers Dis.* 2011 May;26(3):169–83.

81. Yudofsky S, Williams D, and Gorman J. Propranolol in the treatment of rage and violent behavior in patients with chronic brain syndromes. *Am J Psychiat.* 1981 Feb;138(2):218–20.

82. Peskind ER, Tsuang DW, Bonner LT, *et al.* Propranolol for disruptive behaviors in nursing home residents with probable or possible Alzheimer disease: A placebo-controlled study. *Alzheimer Dis Assoc Disord.* 2005 Jan-Mar;19(1):23–8.

83. Wang LY, Shofer JB, Rohde K, *et al.* Prazosin for the treatment of behavioral symptoms in patients with Alzheimer disease with agitation and aggression. *American Journal of Geriatric Psychiatry.* 2009 Sep;17(9):744–51.

84. Tariot PN, Schneider LS, Cummings J, *et al.* Chronic divalproex sodium to attenuate agitation and clinical progression of Alzheimer disease. *Arch Gen Psychiat.* 2011 Aug;68(8):853–61.

85. Fleisher AS, Truran D, Mai JT, *et al.* Chronic divalproex sodium use and brain atrophy in Alzheimer disease. *Neurology.* 2011 Sep 27;77(13):1263–71.

86. Tariot PN, Erb R, Leibovici A, *et al.* Carbamazepine treatment of agitation in nursing home patients with dementia: A preliminary study. *J Am Geriatr Soc.* 1994 Nov;42(11):1160–6.

87. Di Iulio F, Palmer K, Blundo C, *et al.* Occurrence of neuropsychiatric symptoms and psychiatric disorders in mild Alzheimer's disease and mild cognitive impairment subtypes. *International Psychogeriatrics.* 2010 Jun;22(4):629–40.

88. Spalletta G, Musicco M, Padovani A, *et al.* Neuropsychiatric symptoms and syndromes in a large cohort of newly diagnosed, untreated patients with Alzheimer disease. *American Journal of Geriatric Psychiatry.* 2010 Nov;18(11):1026–35.

89. Chen P, Ganguli M, Mulsant BH, *et al.* The temporal relationship between depressive symptoms and dementia: A community-based prospective study. *Arch Gen Psychiat.* 1999 Mar;56(3):261–6.

90. Litvan I, Cummings JL, and Mega M. Neuropsychiatric features of corticobasal degeneration. *J Neurol Neurosur Ps.* 1998 Nov;65(5):717–21.

91. Schrag A, Sheikh S, Quinn NP, *et al.* A comparison of depression, anxiety, and health status in patients with progressive supranuclear palsy and multiple system atrophy. *Movement Disord.* 2010 Jun 15;25(8):1077–81.

92. Paradiso S, Hermann BP, Blumer D, *et al.* Impact of depressed mood on neuropsychological status in temporal lobe epilepsy. *J Neurol Neurosur Ps.* 2001 Feb;70(2):180–5.

93. Devanand DP, Sano M, Tang MX, *et al.* Depressed mood and the incidence of Alzheimer's disease in the elderly living in the community. *Arch Gen Psychiat.* 1996 Feb;53(2):175–82.

94. Starkstein SE, Mayberg HS, Leiguarda R, *et al.* A prospective longitudinal study of depression, cognitive decline, and physical impairments in patients with Parkinson's disease. *J Neurol Neurosur Ps.* 1992 May;55(5):377–82.

95. Saczynski JS, Beiser A, Seshadri S, *et al.* Depressive symptoms and risk of dementia: The Framingham heart study. *Neurology.* 2010 Jul 6;75(1):35–41.

96. Wilson RS, Barnes LL, Mendes de Leon CF, *et al.* Depressive symptoms, cognitive decline, and risk of AD in older persons. *Neurology.* 2002 Aug 13;59(3):364–70.

97. Bassuk SS, Berkman LF, and Wypij D. Depressive symptomatology and incident cognitive decline in an elderly community sample. *Arch Gen Psychiat.* 1998 Dec;55(12):1073–81.

98. Gao Y, Huang C, Zhao K, *et al.* Depression as a risk factor for dementia and mild cognitive impairment: A meta-analysis of longitudinal studies. *Int J Geriatr Psychiatry.* 2012 Jul 19.

99. Jorm AF. Is depression a risk factor for dementia or cognitive decline? A review. *Gerontology.* 2000 Jul–Aug;46(4):219–27.

100. Chemerinski E, Petracca G, Sabe L, *et al.* The specificity of depressive symptoms in patients with Alzheimer's disease. *Am J Psychiat.* 2001 Jan;158(1):68–72.

101. Prado-Jean A, Couratier P, Druet-Cabanac M, *et al.* Specific psychological and behavioral symptoms of depression in patients with dementia. *Int J Geriatr Psychiatry.* 2010 Oct;25(10):1065–72.

102. Volicer L, Van der Steen JT, and Frijters DH. Modifiable factors related to abusive behaviors in nursing home residents with dementia. *Journal of the American Medical Directors Association.* 2009 Nov;10(9):617–22.

103. Starkstein SE and Leentjens AF. The nosological position of apathy in clinical practice. *J Neurol Neurosur Ps.* 2008 Oct;79(10):1088–92.

104. Mega MS, Cummings JL, Fiorello T, *et al.* The spectrum of behavioral changes in Alzheimer's disease. *Neurology.* 1996 Jan;46(1):130–5.

105. Teri L. Behavior and caregiver burden: Behavioral problems in patients with Alzheimer disease and its association with caregiver distress. *Alzheimer Dis Assoc Disord.* 1997;11 Suppl 4:S35–8.

106. Kaufer DI, Cummings JL, Christine D, *et al.* Assessing the impact of neuropsychiatric symptoms in Alzheimer's disease: The neuropsychiatric inventory caregiver distress scale. *J Am Geriatr Soc.* 1998 Feb;46(2):210–5.

107. Boyle PA, Malloy PF, Salloway S, *et al.* Executive dysfunction and apathy predict functional impairment in Alzheimer disease. *Am J Geriat Psychiat.* 2003 Mar–Apr;11(2):214–21.

108. Starkstein SE, Jorge R, Mizrahi R, *et al.* A prospective longitudinal study of apathy in Alzheimer's disease. *J Neurol Neurosur Ps.* 2006 Jan;77(1):8–11.

109. Starkstein SE, Petracca G, Chemerinski E, *et al.* Syndromic validity of apathy in Alzheimer's disease. *Am J Psychiat.* 2001 Jun;158(6):872–7.

110. Levy ML, Cummings JL, Fairbanks LA, *et al.* Apathy is not depression. *J Neuropsychiatry Clin Neurosci.* 1998 Summer;10(3):314–9.

111. Pluck GC and Brown RG. Apathy in Parkinson's disease. *J Neurol Neurosur Ps.* 2002 Dec;73(6):636–42.

112. Starkstein SE, Mayberg HS, Preziosi TJ, *et al.* Reliability, validity, and clinical correlates of apathy in Parkinson's disease. *J Neuropsychiatry Clin Neurosci.* 1992 Spring;4(2):134–9.

113. Robert P, Onyike CU, Leentjens AF, *et al.* Proposed diagnostic criteria for apathy in Alzheimer's disease and other neuropsychiatric disorders. *European Psychiatry.* 2009 Mar;24(2):98–104.

114. Berrios GE and Gili M. Abulia and impulsiveness revisited: A conceptual history. *Acta Psychiat Scand.* 1995 Sep;92(3):161–7.

115. Hart DJ, Craig D, Compton SA, *et al.* A retrospective study of the behavioural and psychological symptoms of mid and late phase Alzheimer's disease. *Int J Geriatr Psychiatry.* 2003 Nov;18(11):1037–42.

116. Hynninen MJ, Breitve MH, Rongve A, *et al.* The frequency and correlates of anxiety in patients with first-time diagnosed mild dementia. *International Psychogeriatrics.* 2012 Nov;24(11):1771–8.

117. Schildkraut JJ. The catecholamine hypothesis of affective disorders: A review of supporting evidence. *Am J Psychiat.* 1965 Nov;122(5):509–22.

118. Zweig RM, Ross CA, Hedreen JC, *et al.* The neuropathology of aminergic nuclei in Alzheimer's disease. *Ann Neurol.* 1988 Aug;24(2):233–42.

119. Zubenko GS, Moossy J, and Kopp U. Neurochemical correlates of major depression in primary dementia. *Arch Neurol.* 1990 Feb;47(2):209–14.

120. Ouchi Y, Yoshikawa E, Futatsubashi M, *et al.* Altered brain serotonin transporter and associated glucose metabolism in Alzheimer disease. *J Nucl Med.* 2009 Aug;50(8):1260–6.

121. Francis PT, Pangalos MN, Stephens PH, *et al.* Antemortem measurements of neurotransmission: Possible implications for pharmacotherapy of Alzheimer's disease and depression. *J Neurol Neurosur Ps.* 1993 Jan;56(1):80–4.

122. Du MY, Wu QZ, Yue Q, *et al.* Voxelwise meta-analysis of gray matter reduction in major depressive disorder. *Prog Neuro-Psychoph.* 2012 Jan 10;36(1):11–6.

123. Sheline YI, Wang PW, Gado MH, *et al.* Hippocampal atrophy in recurrent major depression. *Proc Natl Acad Sci USA.* 1996 Apr 30;93(9):3908–13.

124. Sawyer K, Corsentino E, Sachs-Ericsson N, *et al.* Depression, hippocampal volume changes, and cognitive decline in a clinical sample of older depressed outpatients and non-depressed controls. *Aging Ment Health.* 2012;16(6):753–62.

125. Lee GJ, Lu PH, Hua X, *et al.* Depressive symptoms in mild cognitive impairment predict greater atrophy in Alzheimer's disease-related regions. *Biol Psychiat.* 2012 May 1;71(9):814–21.

126. Tsopelas C, Stewart R, Savva GM, *et al.* Neuropathological correlates of late-life depression in older people. *Brit J Psychiat.* 2011 Feb;198(2):109–14.

127. Rapp MA, Schnaider-Beeri M, Purohit DP, *et al.* Increased neurofibrillary tangles in patients with Alzheimer disease with comorbid depression. *Am J Geriat Psychiat.* 2008 Feb;16(2):168–74.

128. Rapp MA, Schnaider-Beeri M, Grossman HT, *et al.* Increased hippocampal plaques and tangles in patients with Alzheimer disease with a lifetime history of major depression. *Arch Gen Psychiat.* 2006 Feb;63(2):161–7.

129. Berman K, Brodaty H, Withall A, *et al.* Pharmacologic treatment of apathy in dementia. *Am J Geriat Psychiat.* 2012 Feb;20(2):104–22.

130. Craig AH, Cummings JL, Fairbanks L, *et al.* Cerebral blood flow correlates of apathy in Alzheimer disease. *Arch Neurol.* 1996 Nov;53(11):1116–20.

131. Lanctot KL, Moosa S, Herrmann N, *et al.* A SPECT study of apathy in Alzheimer's disease. *Dementia and Geriatric Cognitive Disorders.* 2007;24(1):65–72.

132. Migneco O, Benoit M, Koulibaly PM, *et al.* Perfusion brain spect and statistical parametric mapping analysis indicate that apathy is a cingulate syndrome: A study in Alzheimer's disease and nondemented patients. *Neuroimage.* 2001 May;13(5):896–902.

133. Lanctot KL, Herrmann N, Black SE, *et al.* Apathy associated with Alzheimer disease: Use of dextroamphetamine challenge. *Am J Geriat Psychiat.* 2008 Jul;16(7):551–7.

134. Cummings JL and Back C. The cholinergic hypothesis of neuropsychiatric symptoms in Alzheimer's disease. *Am J Geriat Psychiat.* 1998 Spring;6(2 Suppl 1):S64–78.

135. Weintraub D, Rosenberg PB, Drye LT, *et al.* Sertraline for the treatment of depression in Alzheimer disease: Week-24 outcomes. *Am J Geriat Psychiat.* 2010 Apr;18(4):332–40.

136. Rosenberg PB, Drye LT, Martin BK, *et al.* Sertraline for the treatment of depression in Alzheimer disease. *Am J Geriat Psychiat.* 2010 Feb;18(2):136–45.

137. Bains J, Birks JS, and Dening TR. The efficacy of antidepressants in the treatment of depression in dementia. *Cochrane Database Syst Rev.* 2002(4):CD003944.

138. Modrego PJ. Depression in Alzheimer's disease. Pathophysiology, diagnosis, and treatment. *Journal of Alzheimer's Disease.* 2010;21(4):1077–87.

139. Lee HB and Lyketsos CG. Depression in Alzheimer's disease: Heterogeneity and related issues. *Biol Psychiat.* 2003 Aug 1;54(3):353–62.

140. Alexopoulos GS, Jeste DV, Chung H, *et al.* The expert consensus guideline series. Treatment of dementia and its behavioral disturbances. Introduction: Methods, commentary, and summary. *Postgraduate Medicine.* 2005 Jan;Spec No:6–22.

141. Trivedi MH, Rush AJ, Wisniewski SR, *et al.* Evaluation of outcomes with citalopram for depression using measurement-based care in STAR*D: Implications for clinical practice. *Am J Psychiat.* 2006 Jan;163(1):28–40.

142. Richelson E. The clinical relevance of antidepressant interaction with neurotransmitter transporters and receptors. *Psychopharmacology Bulletin.* 2002 Autumn;36(4):133–50.

143. Richelson E. Interactions of antidepressants with neurotransmitter transporters and receptors and their clinical relevance. *J Clin Psychiatry.* 2003;64 Suppl 13:5–12.

144. Rao V and Lyketsos CG. The benefits and risks of ect for patients with primary dementia who also suffer from depression. *Int J Geriatr Psychiatry.* 2000 Aug;15(8):729–35.

145. Gardner BK and O'Connor DW. A review of the cognitive effects of electroconvulsive therapy in older adults. *Journal of ECT.* 2008 Mar;24(1):68–80.

146. Hausner L, Damian M, Sartorius A, *et al.* Efficacy and cognitive side effects of electroconvulsive therapy (ect) in depressed elderly inpatients with coexisting mild cognitive impairment or dementia. *J Clin Psychiatry.* 2011 Jan;72(1):91–7.

147. Drijgers RL, Aalten P, Winogrodzka A, *et al.* Pharmacological treatment of apathy in neurodegenerative diseases: A systematic review. *Dementia and Geriatric Cognitive Disorders.* 2009;28(1):13–22.

148. Gauthier S, Feldman H, Hecker J, *et al.* Efficacy of donepezil on behavioral symptoms in patients with moderate to severe Alzheimer's disease. *International Psychogeriatrics.* 2002 Dec;14(4):389–404.

149. Holmes C, Wilkinson D, Dean C, *et al.* The efficacy of donepezil in the treatment of neuropsychiatric symptoms in Alzheimer disease. *Neurology.* 2004 Jul 27;63(2):214–9.

150. McKeith I, Del Ser T, Spano P, *et al.* Efficacy of rivastigmine in dementia with Lewy bodies: A randomised, double-blind, placebo-controlled international study. *Lancet.* 2000 Dec 16;356(9247):2031–6.

151. Potkin SG, Alva G, Gunay I, *et al.* A pilot study evaluating the efficacy and safety of rivastigmine in patients with mixed dementia. *Drugs & Aging.* 2006;23(3):241–9.

152. Erkinjuntti T, Kurz A, Gauthier S, *et al.* Efficacy of galantamine in probable vascular dementia and Alzheimer's disease combined with cerebrovascular disease: A randomised trial. *Lancet.* 2002 Apr 13;359(9314):1283–90.

153. Scripnikov A, Khomenko A, Napryeyenko O, *et al.* Effects of ginkgo biloba extract EGb 761 on neuropsychiatric symptoms of dementia: Findings from a randomised controlled trial. *Wiener medizinische Wochenschrift.* 2007;157(13–14):295–300.

154. Rosenberg PB, Lanctot KL, Drye LT, *et al.* Safety and efficacy of methylphenidate for apathy in Alzheimer's disease: A randomized, placebo-controlled trial. *J Clin Psychiat.* 2013 Aug;74(8):810–6.

155. Moretti R, Torre P, Antonello RM, *et al.* Rivastigmine in frontotemporal dementia: An open-label study. *Drugs & Aging.* 2004;21(14):931–7.

156. Diehl-Schmid J, Forstl H, Perneczky R, *et al.* A 6-month, open-label study of memantine in patients with frontotemporal dementia. *Int J Geriatr Psychiatry.* 2008 Jul;23(7):754–9.

157. Lebert F and Pasquier F. Trazodone in the treatment of behaviour in frontotemporal dementia. *Hum Psychopharm Clin.* 1999 Jun;14(4):279–81.

158. Burns A, Jacoby R, and Levy R. Psychiatric phenomena in Alzheimer's disease. I: Disorders of thought content. *Brit J Psychiat.* 1990 Jul;157:72–6, 92–4.

159. McKeith IG, Galasko D, Kosaka K, *et al.* Consensus guidelines for the clinical and pathologic diagnosis of dementia with Lewy bodies (DLB): Report of the consortium on DLB international workshop. *Neurology.* 1996 Nov;47(5):1113–24.

160. Moretti R, Torre P, Antonello RM, *et al.* Different responses to rivastigmine in subcortical vascular dementia and multi-infarct dementia. *American Journal of Alzheimer's Disease and Other Dementias.* 2008 Apr–May;23(2):167–76.

161. Ostling S, Gustafson D, Blennow K, *et al.* Psychotic symptoms in a population-based sample of 85-year-old individuals with dementia. *J Geriatr Psych Neur.* 2011 Mar;24(1):3–8.

162. Cummings JL, Miller B, Hill MA, *et al.* Neuropsychiatric aspects of multi-infarct dementia and dementia of the Alzheimer type. *Arch Neurol.* 1987 Apr;44(4):389–93.

163. Binetti G, Bianchetti A, Padovani A, *et al.* Delusions in Alzheimer's disease and multi-infarct dementia. *Acta Neurol Scand.* 1993 Jul;88(1):5–9.

164. Engelborghs S, Maertens K, Nagels G, *et al.* Neuropsychiatric symptoms of dementia: Cross-sectional analysis from a prospective, longitudinal Belgian study. *Int J Geriatr Psychiatry.* 2005 Nov;20(11):1028–37.

165. Ballard C, Bannister C, Graham C, *et al.* Associations of psychotic symptoms in dementia sufferers. *Brit J Psychiat.* 1995 Oct;167(4):537–40.

166. Murgatroyd C and Prettyman R. An investigation of visual hallucinosis and visual sensory status in dementia. *Int J Geriatr Psychiatry.* 2001 Jul;16(7):709–13.

167. Cummings JL and Kaufer D. Neuropsychiatric aspects of Alzheimer's disease: The cholinergic hypothesis revisited. *Neurology.* 1996 Oct;47(4):876–83.

168. Perry EK, Irving D, Kerwin JM, *et al.* Cholinergic transmitter and neurotrophic activities in Lewy body dementia: Similarity to Parkinson's and distinction from Alzheimer disease. *Alzheimer Dis Assoc Disord.* 1993 Summer;7(2):69–79.

169. Lai MK, Lai OF, Keene J, *et al.* Psychosis of Alzheimer's disease is associated with elevated muscarinic M2 binding in the cortex. *Neurology.* 2001 Sep 11;57(5):805–11.

170. Goldman JG, Goetz CG, Brandabur M, *et al.* Effects of dopaminergic medications on psychosis and motor function in dementia with Lewy bodies. *Mov Disord* . 2008 Nov 15;23(15):2248–50.

171. Roselli F, Pisciotta NM, Perneczky R, *et al.* Severity of neuropsychiatric symptoms and dopamine transporter levels in dementia with Lewy bodies: A 123I-FP-CIT SPECT study. *Mov Disord.* 2009 Oct 30;24(14):2097–103.

172. Reeves S, Brown R, Howard R, *et al.* Increased striatal dopamine (d2/d3) receptor availability and delusions in Alzheimer disease. *Neurology.* 2009 Feb 10;72(6):528–34.

173. Zubenko GS, Moossy J, Martinez AJ, *et al.* Neuropathologic and neurochemical correlates of psychosis in primary dementia. *Arch Neurol.* 1991 Jun;48(6):619–24.

174. Kotrla KJ, Chacko RC, Harper RG, *et al.* Spect findings on psychosis in Alzheimer's disease. *Am J Psychiat.* 1995 Oct;152(10):1470–5.

175. Mega MS, Lee L, Dinov ID, *et al.* Cerebral correlates of psychotic symptoms in Alzheimer's disease. *J Neurol Neurosur Ps.* 2000 Aug;69(2):167–71.

176. Starkstein SE, Vazquez S, Petracca G, *et al.* A spect study of delusions in Alzheimer's disease. *Neurology.* 1994 Nov;44(11):2055–9.

177. Mentis MJ, Weinstein EA, Horwitz B, *et al.* Abnormal brain glucose metabolism in the delusional misidentification syndromes: A positron emission tomography study in Alzheimer disease. *Biol Psychiat.* 1995 Oct 1;38(7):438–49.

178. Grady CL, Haxby JV, Schapiro MB, *et al.* Subgroups in dementia of the Alzheimer type identified using positron emission tomography. *J Neuropsychiatry Clin Neurosci.* 1990 Fall;2(4):373–84.

179. Serra L, Perri R, Cercignani M, *et al.* Are the behavioral symptoms of Alzheimer's disease directly associated with neurodegeneration? *Journal of Alzheimer's disease.* 2010;21(2):627–39.

180. Forstl H, Burns A, Levy R, *et al.* Neuropathological correlates of psychotic phenomena in confirmed Alzheimer's disease. *Brit J Psychiat.* 1994 Jul;165(2):53–9.

181. Ballard CG, Jacoby R, Del Ser T, *et al.* Neuropathological substrates of psychiatric symptoms in prospectively studied patients with autopsy-confirmed dementia with Lewy bodies. *Am J Psychiat.* 2004 May;161(5):843–9.

182. Maci T, Pira FL, Quattrocchi G, *et al.* Physical and cognitive stimulation in Alzheimer disease. The Gaia project: A pilot study. *American Journal of Alzheimer's disease and Other Dementias.* 2012 Mar;27(2):107–13.

183. Rozzini L, Chilovi BV, Bertoletti E, *et al.* Cognitive and psychopathologic response to rivastigmine in dementia with Lewy bodies compared to Alzheimer's disease: A case control study. *American Journal of Alzheimer's disease and Other Dementias.* 2007 Feb–Mar;22(1):42–7.

184. Passmore AP, Bayer AJ, and Steinhagen-Thiessen E. Cognitive, global, and functional benefits of donepezil in Alzheimer's disease and vascular dementia: Results from large-scale clinical trials. *Journal of the Neurological Sciences.* 2005 Mar 15;229–230:141–6.

185. Mori E, Ikeda M, Kosaka K, *et al.* Donepezil for dementia with Lewy bodies: A randomized, placebo-controlled trial. *Ann Neurol.* 2012 Jul;72(1):41–52.

186. Rolinski M, Fox C, Maidment I, *et al.* Cholinesterase inhibitors for dementia with Lewy bodies, Parkinson's disease dementia and cognitive impairment in Parkinson's disease. *Cochrane Database Syst Rev.* 2012;3:CD006504.

187. Burns MJ. The pharmacology and toxicology of atypical antipsychotic agents. *J Toxicol–Clin Toxic.* 2001;39(1):1–14.

188. Schneider LS, Dagerman KS, and Insel P. Risk of death with atypical antipsychotic drug treatment for dementia—meta-analysis of randomized placebo-controlled trials. *JAMA.* 2005 Oct 19;294(15):1934–43.

189. Rochon PA, Normand SL, Gomes T, *et al.* Antipsychotic therapy and short-term serious events in older adults with dementia. *Arch Intern Med.* 2008 May 26;168(10):1090–6.

190. Devanand DP, Mintzer J, Schultz SK, *et al.* Relapse risk after discontinuation of risperidone in Alzheimer's disease. *New Engl J Med.* 2012 Oct 18;367(16):1497–507.

191. Ballard CG, Thomas A, Fossey J, *et al.* A 3-month, randomized, placebo-controlled, neuroleptic discontinuation study in 100 people with dementia: The neuropsychiatric inventory median cutoff is a predictor of clinical outcome. *J Clin Psychiatry.* 2004 Jan;65(1):114–9.

192. Cummings J, Isaacson S, Mills R, *et al.* Pimavanserin for patients with Parkinson's disease psychosis: A randomised, placebo-controlled phase 3 trial. *Lancet.* 2014 Feb 8;383(9916):533–40.

193. Meltzer HY, Mills R, Revell S, *et al.* Pimavanserin, a serotonin(2a) receptor inverse agonist, for the treatment of Parkinson's disease psychosis. *Neuropsychopharmacology.* 2010 Mar;35(4):881–92.

194. Friedman JH. Pimavanserin for the treatment of Parkinson's disease psychosis. Expert Opin Pharmacother. [Review]. 2013 Oct;14(14):1969–75.

195. Price DL, Bonhaus DW, and McFarland K. Pimavanserin, a 5-HT2A receptor inverse agonist, reverses psychosis-like behaviors in a rodent model of Alzheimer's disease. *Behav Pharmacol.* 2012 Aug;23(4):426–33.

SECTION 3

Cognitive impairment and dementia

CHAPTER 20

Epidemiology of dementia

Thais Minett and Carol Brayne

Demographic changes, the ageing population, and future projections costs

Demographic ageing is a major consequence of our success in extending life over the last century. People now live longer than at any other time in history. This is a worldwide process resulting from the extraordinary reductions in mortality and fertility rates. As population ages, the proportion of the older population (those aged 60 years or over) is growing faster than any other age segments. At the same time, the reductions in the proportion of children (persons under age 15) at the world level means that the balance between proportions of the young and the old is expected to shift for the first time in 2045, when the absolute number of old persons will exceed the number of children.[1]

The absolute number of older people has tripled over the last 50 years and will more than triple again over the next 50 years. In 1950, according to the United Nations (UN), there were 205 million people aged 60 or more worldwide. Only 59 years later, in 2009, this number rocketed to 737 million. It is predicted that in 2050 there will be just fewer than 2 billion people aged 60 or over. This phenomenon was first experienced by high-income countries (HIC) though it has recently become apparent in many of the low and medium-income countries (LAMIC). By 2050, six countries are forecast to have 55 per cent of all those people aged 80 or over in the world. Each of them will have more than 10 million people in this age group: China (101 million), India (43 million), United Sates of America (32 million), Japan (16 million), Brazil (14 million), and Indonesia (12 million).[1]

Fertility rates are now well below 2.1 children per woman, the level considered necessary to ensure the replacement of generations. Total fertility rate in the HIC has dropped from 2.8 children per woman in the period 1950–55 to 1.6 children per woman in 2005–10. Although this decline in the LAMIC has started later, it has progressed faster: from 6.0 children per woman in the period 1950–55 to 2.7 in 2005–10.[1]

Life expectancy at birth has shown a global increase of 21 years from 1990–95 to 2005–10.[1] This improvement is a by-product of epidemiological transition, where pandemics of infection are replaced by degenerative, neoplastic and 'lifestyle' driven diseases. This is a fact in the HIC as well as in the LAMIC, where this epidemiologic transition is underway.

In the current panorama, chronic diseases have become the primary causes of not only mortality but also morbidity. As a consequence, preventive measures are less effective, investigations and treatments are more complex and expensive, and life-long interventions may be required. The costs associated with these disorders are increasingly less affordable not only for LAMIC but also for HIC.

While longevity is widely seen as positive and is welcomed, the increase in the older population segment, which is typically more vulnerable to frailty and chronic conditions such as heart disease, dementia, arthritis, and stroke, will prompt a dramatic rise in medical and care costs in the years to come, posing financial risks for governments as well as pension and health providers.

Under the demographic trends expected by the United Nations, the aggregate pension costs incurred by the older population will roughly double over the period 2010–50.[2] Accounting for the likely increases in health and long-term care costs will yet further increase the financial burden associated with ageing.

The impact of population ageing on society means healthcare, retirement, and pensions will extend for longer, as there are increased numbers of potential beneficiaries of healthcare and pensions entitlements. On the other hand, there will be relatively less economically active contributors, aged 15–64, to support this growing segment of the population.

The ratio of those more likely to be economically productive (aged 16–64) and those more likely to be dependants (aged 65 or over) is termed the potential support ratio (PSR). In 2009, the PSR was 4.2 in Europe, under 3.5 in Japan, but considerably higher at 16.5, 10.2, and 9.6 in Africa, Asia, and Latin America respectively. Over the next four decades, the PSR is projected to drop substantially in Asia, Latin America, and the Caribbean as in those areas the demographic transition is rapidly taking place. By 2050, there will be about two people aged 16–64 per person aged 65 or over in Europe, about three in Latin America and the Caribbean, Northern America, and Oceania; in Japan, it is expected to drop below 1.5.[1] The financial impact of these changes will be particularly felt by the working-age population, who are already seeing retirement ages rise, their pensions under threat, and the requirement to pay more and higher taxes.

It is not difficult to see that these demographic trends will have adverse effects on economic growth and may lead to intergenerational conflicts. However, some factors may mitigate this scenario. It is forecast that although the older population labour force has been falling for men, labour force will increase by 1 per cent from 1980 to 2020 as the participation of older woman is expected to increase from 9 per cent to 17 per cent.[1]

Current impact of dementia: Numbers, costs, geographical distribution

Mortality

Cause of death statistics derived from civil registration systems are an important source of data for continuous and comprehensive monitoring of public health programmes over time. Yet, despite their central role in health development, their usefulness has been restricted because of many systemic difficulties ranging from systems that do not generate data at all, to malfunctioning systems that produce poor-quality data.

Country reports to the WHO (World Health Organzation Statistical Information Systems, WHOSIS) are the major source of international cause of death statistics from civil registration systems.[3]

According to WHO and based on analysis of latest available national information on levels of mortality and cause distributions as at late 2003, neurological disorders constitute 12 per cent of total deaths globally. Within these groups of diseases, Alzheimer's disease (AD) and other dementias were responsible for 6.3 per cent of the deaths in 2005, a number that is projected to rise to 7.5 per cent by 2030.[4]

Survival after estimated onset of dementia among participants aged 65 years or older in the UK's Medical Research Council's Cognitive Function and Ageing Study (MRC CFAS) was 4.6 years for women and 4.1 years for men. Those who were functionally impaired, older, and male had predicted shorter survival.[5]

Aguero-Torres and colleagues calculated a mean survival time of 3.0 years among 75-year-old patients with incident cases of dementia in contrast to a mean survival time of 4.2 years for persons without dementia.[6] Helmer and colleagues reported a mean survival time in incident cases of 4.5 years among 65-year-olds and a relative risk of 1.8 (95 per cent CI = 1.8, 2.7).[7]

In 2005, AD and other dementias contributed 6 per cent of the mortality within the neurological disorders. This figure is expected to be 8 per cent in 2030, being overridden only by the cerebrovascular diseases (85 per cent and 87 per cent, respectively).[4]

However, when taking into account the estimates for 2030 of years of healthy life lost (YLL) as a result of disability, AD and other dementias are forecast to have higher impact than cerebrovascular diseases, contributing to 18 per cent of the YLL among the neurological disorders in relation to 16 per cent represented by cerebrovascular diseases.

It is important to note that these estimates are based on all age groups. As dementia mainly affects older people with only 2 per cent of cases starting before the age of 65 years, dementia is one of the major causes of disability in later life. According to the World Health Organization,[8] dementia contributed 11 per cent of all years lived with disability among older people, more than stroke (9 per cent) and all forms of cancer (2 per cent).

Morbidity

The Global Burden of Disease (GBD) framework summarizes the disease burden across diagnostic categories of the International Classification of Diseases (ICD), and by adopting the concept of disability-adjusted life years (DALY),[9] many conditions which are highly incapacitating but have low mortality are aggregated to provide a single measure of overall population health. This is especially the case of the neuropsychiatric disorders. The DALY provides a measure of years expected to be lived in full health lost as a result of a disease that caused either disability or premature mortality.

This methodology uses vital statistics and epidemiological data, which allows for international comparisons as these now exist for many countries including LAMIC.

DALY is calculated as the sum of the years of life lost due to premature mortality (YLL) in the population and the years lost due to disability (YLD) for incident cases of the health condition (DALY = YLL + YLD).

According to the WHO, in 2005 AD and other dementias contributed for 12 per cent of the DALYs for neurological disorders, with projection suggesting a 66 per cent rise by 2030, that is, to account for 18 per cent of the DALY's for neurological disorders. This contribution is only surpassed by cerebrovascular diseases, which was 55 per cent in 2005 and is expected to be 59 per cent in 2030.[4]

Geographical distribution

In 2004, Alzheimer's Disease International convened an international group of experts to review all available epidemiological data and generate up-to-date evidence-based estimates for the prevalence of dementia for every WHO world region.[10] As evidence from well-conducted, representative epidemiological surveys was lacking in many regions, the panel used the Delphi consensus method to allow inferences in such regions by deriving quantitative estimates through the qualitative assessment of evidence. They estimated that globally 24 million people had dementia in 2005, with 4.6 million incident cases annually. They concluded that the prevalence would double every 20 years and that most people with dementia live in developing countries (60 per cent in 2001 rising to 71 per cent by 2040). Seven regions with the largest number of people with dementia in 2001 were: China (5.0 million), the European Union (5.0 million), US (2.9 million), India (1.5 million), Japan (1.1 million), Russia (1.1 million), and Indonesia (1.0 million).

As very little work had been done on evaluating prevalence and incidence of dementia in LAMIC, the 10/66 Dementia Research Group (http://www.alz.co.uk/1066/), as part of Alzheimer's Disease International, was formed to carry out population-based research into dementia, non-communicable diseases, and ageing in LAMIC. The name 10/66 refers to the two-thirds (66 per cent) of people with dementia living in LAMIC contrasting to less than 10 per cent of population-based research in the same areas. The prevalence of dementia varied widely, from 0.3 per cent in rural India to 6.3 per cent in Cuba. After standardization for age and sex, taking Europe as a reference population, the prevalence in all studied regions was less than that reported in Europe: in urban Latin American sites the standardized prevalence was four-fifths less than in Europe, in China it was half, and in India and rural Latin America it was a quarter. The interpretation of the group was that according to the adopted methodology, dementia might be underestimated, especially in regions with low awareness of dementia.[11]

Since these estimates from the Delphi consensus were published, the global evidence base has expanded considerably. There have been new studies from European countries, US, and the above-mentioned 10/66 Dementia Research Group studies in the LAMIC. In the World Alzheimer Report from 2009, the leaders of the Delphi consensus revisited the literature to summarize the evidence on the prevalence of dementia by carrying out quantitative meta-analyses of the available data, and where data were not available the estimates from the Delphi consensus or from recent good quality studies were used.[12] The estimates are summarized in Table 20.1.

Prevalence of dementia across time

Increasing vascular risk factors such as physical inactivity, obesity, diabetes, population ageing, and social inequalities might raise the risk of dementia across time. On the other hand, successful primary

Table 20.1 Estimates for dementia prevalence

Region	Age group							Standardized prevalence for those aged 60 and over
	60–64	65–69	70–74	75–79	80–84	85–89	90+	
Australasia*	1.8	2.8	4.5	7.5	12.5	20.3	38.3	6.91
Asia Pacific, high income*	1.0	1.7	2.9	5.5	10.3	18.5	40.1	5.57
Asia, East*	0.7	1.2	3.1	4.0	7.4	13.3	28.7	4.19
Asia, South*	1.3	2.1	3.5	6.1	10.6	17.8	35.4	5.78
Asia, South-east*	1.6	2.6	4.2	6.9	11.6	18.7	35.4	6.38
Europe, Western*	1.6	2.6	4.3	7.4	12.9	21.7	43.1	6.92
North America (USA only)*	1.1	1.9	3.4	6.3	11.9	21.7	47.5	6.46
Latin America*	1.3	2.4	4.5	8.4	15.4	28.6	63.9	8.48
Asia, Central	0.9	1.3	3.2	5.8	12.1	24.7		5.75
Oceania	0.6	1.8	3.7	7.0	14.4	26.2		6.46
Europe, Central	0.9	1.3	3.3	5.8	12.2	24.7		5.78
Europe, Eastern	0.9	1.3	3.2	5.8	11.8	24.5		5.70
Caribbean	1.3	2.6	4.9	8.5	16.0	33.2		8.12
North Africa/Middle East	1.0	1.6	3.5	6.0	12.9	23.0		5.85
Sub-Saharan Africa, Central	0.5	0.9	1.8	3.5	6.4	13.8		3.25
Sub-Saharan Africa, East	0.6	1.2	2.3	4.3	8.2	16.3		4.00
Sub-Saharan Africa, Southern	0.5	1.0	1.9	3.8	7.0	14.9		3.51
Sub-Saharan Africa, West	0.3	0.9		2.7		9.6		2.07

*Regions included in the meta-analyses.

Reproduced from World Alzheimer Report, Copyright (2009), with permission from Alzheimer's Disease International.

prevention of heart diseases and longer early life education might reduce the prevalence of dementia.

In a systematic review designed to gather evidence for intergenerational changes regarding dementia prevalence, Matthews and colleagues[13] found that that in higher-income countries, the prevalence and inferred or measured incidence of dementia might have decreased over the years. Most of the studies included were subject to different diagnostic criteria over time. This, could potentially act in both directions, leading either to a decrease in the figures (with some being classified in the mild cognitive impairment categories) or an increase (as a result of investigations showing abnormalities, which in fact might be common in non-demented older people).

To study the changes in prevalence and incidence of dementia over time, the UK CFAS compared data from 2011 to those gathered in 1991.[13] CFAS, now in its second generation, follows almost identical design and method of its parent study, which is ideal for intergenerational comparisons. Both CFAS I and CFAS II drew on the UK system of primary care registration which provides the most robust population base for sampling by age group for epidemiological studies in the UK. Comparison of standardized prevalence across time showed a substantial decrease in prevalence of dementia in the older population over two decades (OR(CFAS II vs I) 0.7; 0.6, 0.9). This results in stable estimates for the number of people with dementia on the UK over the last 20 years rather than the anticipated substantial increase. The reduction identified was substantial and might be accounted for societal changes such as improvements in education and prevention and treatment strategies in recent decades. In the UK, substantial evidence exists for inequality in health, and these findings suggest that some areas will have benefited more than others from reduction in risk.

Economic impact of dementia

The economic impact of dementia is considerable and includes not only forma but also informal care costs.

Formal care costs refer to those related to the medical care system, such as costs of hospital care, medication, and visits to clinics, services provided outside of the medical care system including community services such as home care, food supply, and transport, and residential or nursing home care. Informal care costs relate to the care provided by unpaid caregivers, normally family members or close friends who, as a consequence, are prevented from earning their own income.

According to the Alzheimer's Disease International,[14] the total cost of dementia, estimated worldwide, was US$604 billion in 2010, with about 70 per cent of the costs coming from Western Europe and North America. These costs account for around 1 per cent of the world's gross domestic product. The cost per person with dementia is more than 50 times higher in the richest world regions (e.g. North America, US$48,605) than in the poorest (e.g. South Asia region, US$903).

In LAMIC, informal care costs predominate, accounting for 58 per cent of all costs in low-income and 65 per cent of all costs in lower-middle-income countries, compared with 40 per cent in

HIC. Conversely, in HIC, the direct costs of care account for the largest element of costs, as between one-third and one-half of all people with dementia live in resource- and cost-intensive residential or nursing home care facilities. It was estimated that in LAMIC only 6 per cent of people with dementia live in care homes. However, this sector is expanding rapidly, particularly in urban settings in middle-income countries, boosted by demographic and social changes that reduce the availability of family members to provide care.

The costs of dementia are estimated to increase by 85 per cent by 2030 worldwide, based only on predicted rise in numbers of people with dementia. Costs in LAMIC are likely to rise faster than in HIC, due to the shift from informal to formal care as a consequence of economic development, and because of the sharper increase in numbers of people with dementia in those regions.[14]

In 2010, Alzheimer's Research Trust (now ARUK), a research charity in Britain, commissioned a report focusing on the economic burden of dementia and other chronic diseases. They estimated that every patient with dementia cost the economy £27,647 per year, more than the UK median salary (£24,700 at the time). By contrast, patients with cancer cost £5,999, stroke £4,770, and heart disease £3,455 per year. The total cost of dementia to the UK was estimated to be £23 billion, which almost matched those of cancer (£12 billion), heart disease (£8 billion), and stroke (£5 billion) combined. At the time, government and charitable spending on dementia research was 12 times lower than on cancer research: £590 million is spent on cancer research each year, compared to just £50 million in dementia research. For every person with cancer, £295 is spent each year on research, compared to £61 for dementia.[15]

The key findings from the 10/66 Dementia research group in LAMIC on the economic impact on dementia care were that a high proportion of caregivers had to reduce their paid work to provide care. Governmental compensatory financial support was negligible. Families faced the additional expense of paid carers and health services, required in addition to public healthcare, presumably because the latter was insufficient or failed to meet their needs.[16]

Limitations and problems: Diagnostic accuracy, ascertainment

Prevalence, incidence, and derived measures are heavily influenced by the methodological differences of studies and have restricted worldwide comparisons.

At the most basic level, case definition is not a straightforward process. Diagnosing exactly when an individual with cognitive impairment crosses over to dementia is, as discussed in other chapters, to some extent subjective, particularly in the older population where medical comorbidity, which may independently or concurrently interfere with normal functioning, is common.

Attempts have been made to address case definition through development of multiple classifications. However, depending on the system of diagnostic classification used, individuals can be identified as being a case according to one system, but not according to the other.[17]

Llibre Rodriguez and colleagues[11] conducted a study to verify the prevalence of dementia in LAMIC according to two definitions of dementia. The first was based on an algorithm derived from three measures:[18] the Geriatric Mental State Examination/Automated Geriatric Examination Computer Assisted Taxonomy (GMS/

AGECAT),[19] Community Screening Instrument for Dementia, and the modified Consortium to Establish a Registry of Alzheimer's Disease (CERAD) ten-word list-learning task.[20] The second definition used was derived from the diagnostic and statistic manual of mental disorders (DSM-IV).[21]

Across 10/66 regions dementia prevalence varied between 5.6 per cent and 11.7 per cent using the 10/66 dementia algorithm, and 0.4 per cent and 6.4 per cent when using the DSM-IV criteria. Prevalence determined by the DSM-IV criteria was generally half of that estimated by the 10/66 algorithm at every site.[11] When Erkinjuntti and colleagues[17] examined the effects of six different classification schemes for diagnosing dementia in the same population, they found that the frequency of dementia varied depending on the scheme adopted: 3.1 per cent using the international classification of diseases (ICD-10), 4.9 per cent with Cambridge mental disorders of the older population examination (CAMDEX), 5.0 per cent with ICD-9, 13.7 per cent with DSM-IV, 17.3 per cent with DSM-III-R, 20.9 per cent according to the Canadian Study of Health and Aging (CSHA) clinical-consensus method,[22] and 29.1 per cent with the DSM-III criteria.

Changes in diagnostic criteria over time also challenge diagnosis ascertainment, especially when defining dementia subtypes. Criteria for frontotemporal dementia, vascular cognitive impairment and dementia, dementia with Lewy bodies and AD have changed and continue to change with the advent of new neuroimaging techniques and biomarkers.

Some studies base the diagnosis of dementia on a consensus approach, where a multidisciplinary panel of expert clinicians meet to review detailed information on various aspects of an individual such as clinical examination, informant reports of cognition, behaviour, functional impairment, and neuropsychological diagnosis.[23] However, in such cases, the diagnosis process is inevitably influenced by the clinicians' philosophy, personality, discipline, and inherent biases. By standardizing data collection, the influence of between-clinician variability is attenuated, which assists study diagnostic reliability and, potentially, validity.[24]

Representativeness is also an important issue. Few studies can be considered as truly representative of the whole population (Box 20.1). Studies based on referral of patients can cause population bias affecting the results of epidemiological studies.[25] It is well known that referral is influenced not only by the condition itself but may vary according to burden of symptoms, recognition of problems in a given family, access to healthcare, how much attention the media are giving to the condition, and the presence of specialized centres nearby.[26] Furthermore, convenience or clinical studies may have strict selection criteria; for example, excluding individuals with common comorbidities. Similarly, many studies exclude individuals who live in institutions, potentially leading to underestimation of dementia prevalence, rates of cognitive decline, and mortality.

Studies based on performance on cognitive tests may be influenced by factors other than cognition. Educational background, cultural experiences, prior testing experience, emotional and physical states, testing environment, use of medicines, and measurement error are hard to control even when the same cognitive test is used.[27,28]

Another methodological source of bias is missing data. Missing values can be due to non-response at baseline or death or dropout during the study. Longitudinal and multi-stage studies are

Box 20.1 Main studies on the epidemiology of dementias (chronological order)

Longitudinal studies

- Lundby Study[59]
- Iceland birth cohort[60]
- Reykjavik Study[61]
- Gothenburg Study[62]
- Cambridge City over-75s Cohort Study (CC75C)[63]
- Framingham[64]
- Established Populations for Epidemiologic Studies of the Elderly (EPESE)[78]
- Gospel Oak study[65]
- Cognitive Function and Ageing Study (CFAS)[66]
- Rotterdam Study[67]
- Vantaa 85+[68]
- Personnes âgées QUID (Paquid)[69]
- Italian Longitudinal Study of Ageing (ILSA)[70]
- The Three-City study (3C)[71]
- The English Longitudinal Study of Ageing (ELSA)[72]
- Newcastle 85+ study[73]
- Epidemiological Clinicopathological Studies in Europe (EClipSE)[74]

Combined studies

- The EURODEM initiative[75]
- The 10/66 Dementia Research Group[76]

Synthesis of literature

- Delphi consensus study[10]
- Meta-analysis of dementia incidence[77]
- World Alzheimer Report 2009[12]

The causes of dementia in different age groups

Not only does dementia have different incidence and prevalence according to age but also the subtypes of dementia differ in terms of incidence and prevalence in different age groups.

Regardless of all these methodological issues, the most prevalent clinically diagnosed dementia subtypes are the neurodegenerative disorders, Alzheimer's disease (AD), vascular cognitive impairment/dementia (VaD), frontotemporal dementia (FTD), and dementia with Lewy bodies (DLB). In this chapter, other types of dementia such as metabolic, due to sleep apnoea, head trauma, dementia plus syndromes, etc., will not be covered.

Although it is generally agreed that AD is the commonest cause of dementia, studies show less agreement regarding the ordering of the other causes. In order to compare such studies, it is relevant to consider the changing pathological/clinical conceptual framework in which these disorders have been diagnosed over the years. Thus, for many years following Alois Alzheimer's 1907 seminal description,[30] linking the presence of neurofibrillary tangles and senile plaques with dementia AD was considered a presenile dementia. It was only in the 1960s that Blessed and colleagues[31] showed that the brains of patients derived from with senile dementia were associated with this same neuropathology, leading to the broader concept of AD across the age spectrum. Similarly, the presenile dementia with lobar brain atrophy described by Pick[32] and named in his honour by Alzheimer is now classified clinically within the FTD spectrum.

A further complexity is that although the neuropathological substrates of DLB and FTD were first described at the beginning of the twentieth century, the techniques which are currently used to identify them are relatively recent and are more sensitive than the originally used.[33,34] Therefore, these diseases have only recently[35,36] attracted more attention and have not been investigated in most population-based studies. FTD and DLB are also not fully supported by the DSM and ICD classification systems, with consensus guidelines used to define them changing over time. As a consequence, FTD and DLB have not been included in some population-driven studies of prevalence and incidence, perhaps leading to an overestimation of the incidence and prevalence of AD and VaD.

Two different perspectives have been looked at when creating diagnostic systems for dementia subtypes: the clinical manifestation and the underlying neuropathological features. Some classification criteria, such as the National Institute of Neurological and Communicative Disorders and Stroke and the Alzheimer's Disease and Related Disorders Association (NINCDS–ADRDA), rely on histopathological confirmation to diagnose AD as a definite condition.[37] Consequently, AD is structured as a neuropathological entity despite the diagnosis of AD in life being made based on clinical information.[38] Besides, the neuropathological diagnosis is far away from being gold standard as the neuropathological criteria for AD have changed several times over the past 30 years. In this context it is important to note that even in the well-established clinical centres when the diagnosis of AD is made during life, it is not unusual for it to be discordant with the pathological diagnosis. Beach and colleagues[39] reported a sensitivity for AD clinical diagnosis ranging from 71 per cent to 87 per cent, and specificity ranging from 44 per cent to 71 per cent, when non-demented patients were excluded. On the other hand, the Nun Study found substantial AD

especially prone to missing data due to death or dropout. However, in those cases, missing data cannot be assumed to be occurring at random as individuals with more severe cognitive impairment are more likely to dropout from a study. Missing data are even more common in retrospective studies when information is often gathered from medical records. There are no perfect solutions to the problem of missing data. Simply omitting variables or individuals who do not have complete data often affects final estimations. A number of statistical techniques based—so-called multiple imputation—where missing values are estimated from that individual's available data is increasingly used to handle missing data.[29] Following imputation, sensitivity analysis can be run to check for similarity in observed associations in the restricted (e.g. complete case analysis) compared to the imputation derived dataset. Many-study analysis and significance reporting do not fully take study design into account and this will increase the report of findings which are not fully robust.

lesions in brains of elderly subjects with normal cognition assessed shortly before death, creating the concept of status asymptomatic AD (ASYMAD).[40]

For extrapolation of results to the population to be valid, research must be conducted on a true population sample or on groups with well-characterized biases. However, paradoxically, the pathological criteria for the dementia subtypes rather than being based on the population, were derived from brains originated from highly selective clinical samples.[41] In truly population-based pathological samples, the neuropathological hallmarks of dementias often coexist, which makes determining dementia subtypes even more complex. Thus Xuereb JH and colleagues,[42] in the first truly population-based clinical neuropathological correlation study in dementia, demonstrated that participants with probable AD showed less severe AD pathology but more mixed pathologies. In a later publication when more brains were added to the sample,[43] these findings were confirmed: 22 per cent of the brains of participants with clinical dementia had mixed pathologies. The Honolulu–Asia Aging study[44] and the Hisayama study[45] also showed similar findings with respectively 16 per cent and 34 per cent of participants clinically diagnosed as having dementia having mixed pathologies, at post-mortem. The CFAS cohort has similarly reported both a high prevalence of vascular pathology and the co-occurrence of a mixture of AD and vascular pathology in populations with dementia.[46] Despite this evidence, most studies aiming to verify the distribution of dementia subtypes in the population disregard the possibility of mixed dementias, which is a particular problem in older age groups.

There is evidence not only that neuropathology is more heterogeneous than our clinical practice recognizes but also that the classic neuropathological features of AD, which are not pathognomonic of AD, can be seen in brains of people dying without dementia; this is true especially in the older age group. Studies that have included individuals in the oldest age groups consistently show that significant numbers of those who die in their 80s and 90s have pathological features of AD without a diagnosis of dementia during life.[46,47] Savva and colleagues[48] explored the effect of age on the relationship between the classical neuropathological features and clinical manifestation of dementia in a population-based cohort of older people. The burden of AD-type pathological lesions increased with age in individuals without dementia, in contrast to those with dementia where this burden was either constant or declined with age. This study indicated a convergence of AD-type pathological features in individuals with and without dementia at very advanced ages: the difference in the burden of AD neuropathology was more marked in the younger old with and without dementia than at older ages.

Besides, Boyle and colleagues[49] found that much of late life cognitive decline is not due to common neurodegenerative pathologies. When examining 856 brains of deceased participants from two longitudinal clinical-pathologic studies, the Rush Memory and Aging project and the Religious Orders Study, they found that although pathological indices of the common causes of dementia are important determinants of cognitive decline in old age, much of the variation in cognitive decline remains unexplained, suggesting that other important determinants of cognitive decline remain to be identified.

When studying the effect of age on dementia it is important to highlight that the other extreme of age, people younger than 65 years, are often left out of studies investigating dementia. AD can certainly manifest before this age, and some causes of dementia (e.g FTD) may be even more prevalent than in the very old.[50] The Lundby study,[51] which took into account participants of less than 65 years, found that among those who developed dementia from 1947 to 1972, 46 per cent had 'senile dementia of Alzheimer type' (SDAT) and the remaining 54 per cent, 'multi-infarct dementia' (MID). There was no mention of mixed dementias. The authors also did not look at FTD or DLB, probably because the collection of their sample pre-dated the formal identification of these entities.

The distribution of dementia subtypes according to the age groups is shown in Table 20.2.

More recent population-based studies have considered DLB and FTD diagnosis.

Stevens and colleagues[52] reported on the distribution of clinical dementia subtypes in a community-based study of people aged 65 years or over. They found that the prevalence of AD was 31 per cent, VaD 22 per cent, DLB 11 per cent, and FTD 8 per cent. When using the DSM-IV criteria, 57 per cent of patients diagnosed as having DLB according to the consensus criteria[53] were shifted to the AD category and 14 per cent to the VaD. Among the FTD patients (diagnosed according to the FTD consensus),[54] 50 per cent were re-classified as AD and 17 per cent as VaD.

Yamada and colleagues[55] studied the prevalence of dementing disorders in a rural town of Japan (Amino-cho). Of the 3715 individuals aged 65 years or older, the prevalence for all types of dementia was 4 per cent, and for the subtypes 2 per cent of AD, 1 per cent of VaD, and 0.1 per cent of DLB; no patients with FTD were identified. The distribution of dementia subtypes according to age is particularly relevant to those who see patients with young-onset dementia, where the subtypes prevalence and incidence differ from those in the older population.

Ratnavalli[56] estimated the prevalence of dementia subtypes in a population at 65 years of age or less, living in Cambridge city or east or south Cambridgeshire in the UK. Case ascertainment was by review of case records and inpatient admissions at a university hospital and checking with primary care. They identified 108 patients with early-onset dementia, with an overall prevalence of 81 per 100 000 in the 45–64 age-group. The prevalence of early-onset FTD and AD were the same (15.1 per 100 000) and for VaD 8.2 per 100 000. They identified no patients with DLB in that age group.

Similar results were found by Harvey and colleagues[50] when determining the prevalence of dementia in population of 65 years of age or less in three London boroughs, with diagnosis and age of onset established from all available health and social care records.

Table 20.2 Number of participants with first-time dementia diagnosis according to dementia subtype and age groups in the Lundby study from 1947–72

Age group	SDAT	MID
0–59	0	2
60–79	38	59
80+	27	33

Source data from *Neuroepidemiology.* 11(Suppl 1), Hagnell O, Ojesjo L, and Rorsman B, Incidence of dementia in the Lundby Study, pp. 61–6, Copyright (1992), S. Karger AG, Basel.

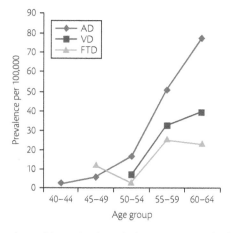

Fig. 20.1 Prevalence of dementia subtype in the younger in London boroughs of Kensington and Chelsea, Westminster, and Hillingdon, UK.
Adapted from *J Neurol Neurosur Ps.* 74(9), Harvey RJ, Skelton-Robinson M, and Rossor MN, The prevalence and causes of dementia in people under the age of 65 years, pp. 1206–9, Copyright (2003), with permission from BMJ Publishing Group Ltd.

They found that the prevalence of dementia in those aged 45–64 was 98.1 per 100 000. From the age of 35 onwards, the prevalence of dementia approximately doubled with each 5-year increase in age. In terms of dementia subtypes, the authors decided not to use mixed diagnoses but to make a 'highest confidence' single diagnosis in each case as follows: AD (34 per cent), VaD (34 per cent), FTD (12 per cent), and DLB (7 per cent). When prevalence of subtypes was assessed in relation to age, FTD was more common than AD or VaD in the younger age group, but this relationship was inverted in the older ages (Fig. 20.1).

In Japan, Ikejima and colleagues[57] found that the prevalence of dementia in 45–64 age-group was 83.3 per 100 000. They also found that in each five-year age group the prevalence of dementia almost doubles. VaD was the most frequent subtype of dementia (42 per cent), followed by AD (26 per cent), DLB and PD with

dementia (6 per cent), and FTD (3 per cent). Fig. 20.2 discloses the dementia subtypes by age groups, showing that for all, VaD was the most prevalent dementia subtype. Another interesting finding in this study was the high frequency of DLB. One possible explanation is that the authors amalgamated DLB patients with those with Parkinson's disease with dementia.

Studies such as these are, however, dependent on the accuracy of clinical diagnosis, consistent diagnostic criteria being used between studies and over time, and adequate ascertainment. In practice, these factors all prove difficult to identify, perhaps particularly in young-onset dementia where the differential diagnosis is often broad.[58]

Conclusion

The world population is ageing, a phenomenon which is true not only for HIC but also for LAMIC. With ageing, it is expected that the prevalence of dementias will increase considerably, causing huge social and economic impacts on society. Studies designed to verify the impact of dementia and its subtypes in the population have many methodological issues, especially regarding case ascertainment. In the population, dementia subtypes are often mixed, which is not often taken into account in most clinical studies. In the oldest old, the relationship between neuropathological burden and cognitive impairment is often less clear as many individuals without dementia have at least some, and sometimes marked, neuropathological hallmarks of neurodegenerative disease. In younger people, dementia is rarer and associated with a different distribution of causes compared to the older population.

References

1. Department of Economic and Social Affairs—Population Division. *World Population Ageing 2009.* New York, NY: United Nations, 2010.
2. International Monetary Fund. *Global Financial Stability Report.* Washington, DC: International Monetary Fund, Publications Services, 2012.
3. Mahapatra P, Shibuya K, Lopez AD, *et al.* Civil registration systems and vital statistics: Successes and missed opportunities. *Lancet.* 2007 Nov 10;370(9599):1653–63. PubMed PMID: 18029006. Epub 2007/11/22.
4. World Health Organization. *Neurological Disorders: Public Health Challenges.* Geneva: World Health Organization, 2006.
5. Xie J, Brayne C, and Matthews FE. Survival times in people with dementia: Analysis from population based cohort study with 14 year follow-up. *BMJ.* 2008 Feb 2;336(7638):258–62. PubMed PMID: 18187696. Pubmed Central PMCID: 2223023. Epub 2008/01/12.
6. Aguero-Torres H, Fratiglioni L, Guo Z, *et al.* Mortality from dementia in advanced age: A 5-year follow-up study of incident dementia cases. *J Clin Epidemiol.* 1999 Aug;52(8):737–43. PubMed PMID: 10465318. Epub 1999/08/28.
7. Helmer C, Joly P, Letenneur L, *et al.* Mortality with dementia: Results from a French prospective community-based cohort. *Am J Epidemiol.* 2001 Oct 1;154(7):642–8. PubMed PMID: 11581098. Epub 2001/10/03.
8. World Health Organization. *The World Health Report 2003: Shaping the Future.* Geneva: World Health Organization, 2003.
9. Murray CJ. Quantifying the burden of disease: The technical basis for disability-adjusted life years. *Bull World Health Organ.* 1994;72(3):429–45. PubMed PMID: 8062401. Pubmed Central PMCID: 2486718 Epub 1994/01/01.
10. Ferri CP, Prince M, Brayne C, *et al.* Global prevalence of dementia: A Delphi consensus study. *Lancet.* 2005 Dec 17;366(9503):2112–7.

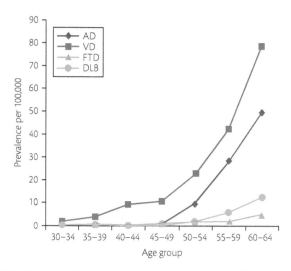

Fig. 20.2 Prevalence of dementia subtype in the younger in Ibaraki Prefecture, Japan.
Adapted from *Stroke.* 40(8), Ikejima C, Yasuno F, Mizukami K, *et al.* Prevalence and causes of early-onset dementia in Japan: a population-based study, pp. 2709–14, Copyright (2009), with permission from Wolters Kluwer Health, Inc.

PubMed PMID: 16360788. Pubmed Central PMCID: 2850264. Epub 2005/12/20.

11. Llibre Rodriguez JJ, Ferri CP, et al. Prevalence of dementia in Latin America, India, and China: A population-based cross-sectional survey. Lancet. 2008 Aug 9;372(9637):464–74. PubMed PMID: 18657855. Pubmed Central PMCID: 2854470. Epub 2008/07/29.

12. Alzheimer's Disease International. World Alzheimer Report 2009. London: Alzheimer's Disease International, 2009.

13. Matthews FE, Arthur A, Barnes LE, et al. A two-decade comparison of prevalence of dementia in individuals aged 65 years and older from three geographical areas of England: Results of the Cognitive Function and Ageing Study I and II. Lancet. 2013 Jul 17. PubMed PMID: 23871492.

14. Alzheimer's Disease International. World Alzheimer Report 2010: The Global Economic Impact of Dementia. London: Alzheimer's Disease International, 2010.

15. Luengo-Fernandez R, Leal J, and Gray A. Dementia 2010. The Economic Burden of Dementia and Associated Research Funding in the United Kingdom. Cambridge: Alzheimer's Research Trust, 2010.

16. Prince M. Care arrangements for people with dementia in developing countries. Int J Geriatr Psychiatry. 2004 Feb;19(2):170–7. PubMed PMID: 14758582. Epub 2004/02/06.

17. Erkinjuntti T, Ostbye T, Steenhuis R, et al. The effect of different diagnostic criteria on the prevalence of dementia. N Engl J Med. 1997 Dec 4;337(23):1667–74. PubMed PMID: 9385127. Epub 1997/12/04.

18. Prince M, Acosta D, Chiu H, et al. Dementia diagnosis in developing countries: A cross-cultural validation study. Lancet. 2003 Mar 15;361(9361):909–17. PubMed PMID: 12648969. Epub 2003/03/22.

19. Copeland JR, Dewey ME, and Griffiths-Jones HM. A computerized psychiatric diagnostic system and case nomenclature for elderly subjects: GMS and AGECAT. Psychol Med. 1986 Feb;16(1):89–99. PubMed PMID: 3515380. Epub 1986/02/01.

20. Mirra SS, Heyman A, McKeel D, et al. The Consortium to Establish a Registry for Alzheimer's Disease (CERAD). Part II. Standardization of the neuropathologic assessment of Alzheimer's disease. Neurology. 1991 Apr;41(4):479–86. PubMed PMID: 2011243. Epub 1991/04/01.

21. American Psychiatric Association. Diagnostic and Statistical Manual of Mental Disorders (DSM-IV).4th edn. Washington, DC: American Psychiatric Association, 1994.

22. Canadian Study of Health and Aging Working Group. Canadian study of health and aging: Study methods and prevalence of dementia. CMAJ. 1994 Mar 15;150(6):899–913. PubMed PMID: 8131123. Pubmed Central PMCID: 1486712. Epub 1994/03/15.

23. Weir DR, Wallace RB, Langa KM, et al. Reducing case ascertainment costs in U.S. population studies of Alzheimer's disease, dementia, and cognitive impairment-Part 1. Alzheimers Dement. 2011 Jan;7(1):94–109. PubMed PMID: 21255747. Pubmed Central PMCID: 3044596. Epub 2011/01/25.

24. Brayne C, Stephan BC, and Matthews FE. A European perspective on population studies of dementia. Alzheimers Dement. 2011 Jan;7(1):3–9. PubMed PMID: 21255739. Epub 2011/01/25.

25. Sackett DL. Bias in analytic research. J Chronic Dis. 1979;32(1–2):51–63. PubMed PMID: 447779. Epub 1979/01/01.

26. Brayne C. Research and Alzheimer's disease: An epidemiological perspective. Psychol Med. 1993 May;23(2):287–96. PubMed PMID: 8332643. Epub 1993/05/01.

27. Morris MC, Evans DA, Hebert LE, et al. Methodological issues in the study of cognitive decline. Am J Epidemiol. 1999 May 1;149(9):789–93. PubMed PMID: 10221314. Epub 1999/04/30.

28. The Medical Research Council Cognitive Function and Ageing Study (MRC CFAS). Cognitive function and dementia in six areas of England and Wales: The distribution of MMSE and prevalence of GMS organicity level in the MRC CFA Study. The Medical Research Council Cognitive Function and Ageing Study (MRC CFAS). Psychol Med. 1998 Mar;28(2):319–35. PubMed PMID: 9572090. Epub 1998/05/08.

29. Altman DG and Bland JM. Missing data. BMJ. 2007 Feb 24;334(7590):424. PubMed PMID: 17322261. Pubmed Central PMCID: 1804157. Epub 2007/02/27.

30. Alzheimer A, Stelzmann RA, Schnitzlein HN, et al. An English translation of Alzheimer's 1907 paper, 'Uber eine eigenartige Erkankung der Hirnrinde.' Clin Anat. 1995;8(6):429–31. PubMed PMID: 8713166. Epub 1995/01/01.

31. Blessed G, Tomlinson BE, and Roth M. The association between quantitative measures of dementia and of senile change in the cerebral grey matter of elderly subjects. Br J Psychiatry. 1968 Jul;114(512):797–811. PubMed PMID: 5662937. Epub 1968/07/01.

32. Pick A. Über die Beziehungen der senilen Hirnatrophie zur Aphasie. Prager Medizinische Wochenschrift. 1892;17:165–7.

33. Lennox G, Lowe J, Morrell K, et al. Anti-ubiquitin immunocytochemistry is more sensitive than conventional techniques in the detection of diffuse Lewy body disease. J Neurol Neurosur Ps. 1989 Jan;52(1):67–71. PubMed PMID: 2540286. Pubmed Central PMCID: 1032659. Epub 1989/01/01.

34. Love S, Saitoh T, Quijada S, et al. Alz-50, ubiquitin and tau immunoreactivity of neurofibrillary tangles, Pick bodies and Lewy bodies. J Neuropathol Exp Neurol. 1988 Jul;47(4):393–405. PubMed PMID: 2838588. Epub 1988/07/01.

35. Okazaki H, Lipkin LE, and Aronson SM. Diffuse intracytoplasmic ganglionic inclusions (Lewy type) associated with progressive dementia and quadriparesis in flexion. J Neuropathol Exp Neurol. 1961 Apr;20:237–44. PubMed PMID: 13730588. Epub 1961/04/01.

36. Brun A. Frontal lobe degeneration of non-Alzheimer type. I. Neuropathology. Arch Gerontol Geriatr. 1987 Sep;6(3):193–208. PubMed PMID: 3689053. Epub 1987/09/01.

37. McKhann G, Drachman D, Folstein M, et al. Clinical diagnosis of Alzheimer's disease: Report of the NINCDS-ADRDA Work Group under the auspices of Department of Health and Human Services Task Force on Alzheimer's Disease. Neurology. 1984 Jul;34(7):939–44. PubMed PMID: 6610841. Epub 1984/07/01.

38. Richards M and Brayne C. What do we mean by Alzheimer's disease? BMJ. 2010;341:c4670. PubMed PMID: 20940218. Epub 2010/10/14.

39. Beach TG, Monsell SE, Phillips LE, et al. Accuracy of the clinical diagnosis of Alzheimer disease at National Institute on Aging Alzheimer Disease Centers, 2005-2010. J Neuropathol Exp Neurol. 2012 Apr;71(4):266–73. PubMed PMID: 22437338. Pubmed Central PMCID: 3331862.

40. Iacono D, Markesbery WR, Gross M, et al. The Nun study: Clinically silent AD, neuronal hypertrophy, and linguistic skills in early life. Neurology. 2009 Sep 1;73(9):665–73. PubMed PMID: 19587326. Pubmed Central PMCID: 2734290. Epub 2009/07/10.

41. Zaccai J, Ince P, and Brayne C. Population-based neuropathological studies of dementia: Design, methods and areas of investigation—a systematic review. BMC Neurol. 2006;6:2. PubMed PMID: 16401346. Pubmed Central PMCID: 1397861. Epub 2006/01/13.

42. Xuereb JH, Brayne C, Dufouil C, et al. Neuropathological findings in the very old. Results from the first 101 brains of a population-based longitudinal study of dementing disorders. Ann NY Acad Sci. 2000 Apr;903:490–6. PubMed PMID: 10818543. Epub 2000/05/20.

43. Brayne C, Richardson K, Matthews FE, et al. Neuropathological correlates of dementia in over-80-year-old brain donors from the population-based Cambridge city over-75s cohort (CC75C) study. J Alzheimers Dis. 2009;18(3):645–58. PubMed PMID: 19661624. Epub 2009/08/08.

44. White L, Petrovitch H, Hardman J, et al. Cerebrovascular pathology and dementia in autopsied Honolulu–Asia Aging Study participants. Ann NY Acad Sci. 2002 Nov;977:9–23. PubMed PMID: 12480729. Epub 2002/12/14.

45. Noda K, Sasaki K, Fujimi K, et al. Quantitative analysis of neurofibrillary pathology in a general population to reappraise neuropathological criteria for senile dementia of the neurofibrillary tangle type (tangle-only dementia): The Hisayama Study. Neuropathology. 2006 Dec;26(6):508–18. PubMed PMID: 17203586. Epub 2007/01/06.

46. CFAS Neuropathology Group. Pathological correlates of late-onset dementia in a multicentre, community-based population in England and Wales. Neuropathology Group of the Medical Research Council

Cognitive Function and Ageing Study (MRC CFAS). *Lancet.* 2001 Jan 20;357(9251):169–75. PubMed PMID: 11213093. Epub 2001/02/24.

47. Katzman R, Terry R, DeTeresa R, *et al.* Clinical, pathological, and neurochemical changes in dementia: A subgroup with preserved mental status and numerous neocortical plaques. *Ann Neurol.* 1988 Feb;23(2):138–44. PubMed PMID: 2897823. Epub 1988/02/01.

48. Savva GM, Wharton SB, Ince PG, *et al.* Age, neuropathology, and dementia. *N Engl J Med.* 2009 May 28;360(22):2302–9. PubMed PMID: 19474427. Epub 2009/05/29.

49. Boyle PA, Wilson RS, Yu L, *et al.* Much of late life cognitive decline is not due to common neurodegenerative pathologies. *Ann Neurol.* 2013 Jun 24. PubMed PMID: 23798485.

50. Harvey RJ, Skelton-Robinson M, and Rossor MN. The prevalence and causes of dementia in people under the age of 65 years. *J Neurol Neurosur Ps.* 2003 Sep;74(9):1206–9. PubMed PMID: 12933919. Pubmed Central PMCID: 1738690. Epub 2003/08/23.

51. Hagnell O, Ojesjo L, and Rorsman B. Incidence of dementia in the Lundby Study. *Neuroepidemiology.* 1992;11 Suppl 1:61–6. PubMed PMID: 1603251. Epub 1992/01/01.

52. Stevens T, Livingston G, Kitchen G, *et al.* Islington study of dementia subtypes in the community. *Br J Psychiatry.* 2002 Mar;180:270–6. PubMed PMID: 11872521. Epub 2002/03/02.

53. McKeith IG, Galasko D, Kosaka K, *et al.* Consensus guidelines for the clinical and pathologic diagnosis of dementia with Lewy bodies (DLB): Report of the consortium on DLB international workshop. *Neurology.* 1996 Nov;47(5):1113–24. PubMed PMID: 8909416. Epub 1996/11/01.

54. Neary D, Snowden JS, Gustafson L, *et al.* Frontotemporal lobar degeneration: A consensus on clinical diagnostic criteria. *Neurology.* 1998 Dec;51(6):1546–54. PubMed PMID: 9855500. Epub 1998/12/17.

55. Yamada T, Hattori H, Miura A, *et al.* Prevalence of Alzheimer's disease, vascular dementia and dementia with Lewy bodies in a Japanese population. *Psychiatry Clin Neurosci.* 2001 Feb;55(1):21–5. PubMed PMID: 11235852. Epub 2001/03/10.

56. Ratnavalli E, Brayne C, Dawson K, *et al.* The prevalence of frontotemporal dementia. *Neurology.* 2002 Jun 11;58(11):1615–21. PubMed PMID: 12058088. Epub 2002/06/12.

57. Ikejima C, Yasuno F, Mizukami K, *et al.* Prevalence and causes of early-onset dementia in Japan: A population-based study. *Stroke.* 2009 Aug;40(8):2709–14. PubMed PMID: 19478230. Epub 2009/05/30.

58. Rossor MN, Fox NC, Mummery CJ, *et al.* The diagnosis of young-onset dementia. *Lancet Neurol.* 2010 Aug;9(8):793–806. PubMed PMID: 20650401. Pubmed Central PMCID: 2947856. Epub 2010/07/24.

59. Esson-Moller E, Larsson H, Uddenberg CE, *et al.* Individual traits and morbidity in a Swedish rural population. *Acta Psychiatr Neurol Scand Suppl.* 1956;100:1–160. PubMed PMID: 13326503. Epub 1956/01/01.

60. Helgason T. Epidemiology of Mental Disorders in Iceland. A Psychiatric and Demographic Investigation of 5395 Icelanders. *Acta Psychiatr Scand.* 1964;40:SUPPL 173:1+. PubMed PMID: 14154723. Epub 1964/01/01.

61. Harris TB, Launer LJ, Eiriksdottir G, *et al.* Age, Gene/Environment Susceptibility-Reykjavik Study: Multidisciplinary applied phenomics. *Am J Epidemiol.* 2007 May 1;165(9):1076–87. PubMed PMID: 17351290. Pubmed Central PMCID: 2723948. Epub 2007/03/14.

62. Rinder L, Roupe S, Steen B, *et al.* Seventy-year-old people in Gothenburg. A population study in an industrialized Swedish city. *Acta Med Scand.* 1975 Nov;198(5):397–407. PubMed PMID: 1081814. Epub 1975/11/01.

63. O'Connor DW, Pollitt PA, Hyde JB, *et al.* The prevalence of dementia as measured by the Cambridge Mental Disorders of the Elderly Examination. *Acta Psychiatr Scand.* 1989 Feb;79(2):190–8. PubMed PMID: 2923012. Epub 1989/02/01.

64. Linn RT, Wolf PA, Bachman DL, *et al.* The 'preclinical phase' of probable Alzheimer's disease. A 13-year prospective study of the Framingham cohort. *Arch Neurol.* 1995 May;52(5):485–90. PubMed PMID: 7733843. Epub 1995/05/01.

65. Livingston G, Hawkins A, Graham N, *et al.* The Gospel Oak Study: Prevalence rates of dementia, depression and activity limitation among elderly residents in inner London. *Psychol Med.* 1990 Feb;20(1):137–46. PubMed PMID: 2138793. Epub 1990/02/01.

66. Chadwick C. The MRC Multicentre Study of Cognitive Function and Ageing: A EURODEM incidence study in progress. *Neuroepidemiology.* 1992;11 Suppl 1:37–43. PubMed PMID: 1603246. Epub 1992/01/01.

67. Ott A, Breteler MM, van Harskamp F, *et al.* Incidence and risk of dementia. The Rotterdam Study. *Am J Epidemiol.* 1998 Mar 15;147(6):574–80. PubMed PMID: 9521184. Epub 1998/04/01.

68. Polvikoski T, Sulkava R, Haltia M, *et al.* Apolipoprotein E, dementia, and cortical deposition of beta-amyloid protein. *N Engl J Med.* 1995 Nov 9;333(19):1242–7. PubMed PMID: 7566000. Epub 1995/11/09.

69. Letenneur L, Jacqmin H, Commenges D, *et al.* Cerebral and functional aging: First results on prevalence and incidence of the Paquid cohort. *Methods Inf Med.* 1993 Apr;32(3):249–51. PubMed PMID: 8341161. Epub 1993/04/01.

70. Maggi S, Zucchetto M, Grigoletto F, *et al.* The Italian Longitudinal Study on Aging (ILSA): Design and methods. *Aging (Milano).* 1994 Dec;6(6):464–73. PubMed PMID: 7748921. Epub 1994/12/01.

71. Alperovitch A, Amouyel P, Dartigues JF, *et al.* Les études epidemiologiques sur le vieillissement en France: De l'étude Paquid a l'étude des Trois Cites. *C R Biol.* 2002 Jun;325(6):665–72. PubMed PMID: 12360853. Epub 2002/10/04.

72. Llewellyn DJ, Lang IA, Xie J, *et al.* Framingham Stroke Risk Profile and poor cognitive function: A population-based study. *BMC Neurol.* 2008;8:12. PubMed PMID: 18430227. Pubmed Central PMCID: 2386808. Epub 2008/04/24.

73. Collerton J, Davies K, Jagger C, *et al.* Health and disease in 85 year olds: Baseline findings from the Newcastle 85+ cohort study. *BMJ.* 2009;339:b4904. PubMed PMID: 20028777. Pubmed Central PMCID: 2797051. Epub 2009/12/24.

74. EClipSE Collaborative Members. Cohort profile: Epidemiological Clinicopathological studies in Europe (EClipSE). *J Alzheimers Dis.* 2009;18(3):659–63. PubMed PMID: 19661630. Epub 2009/08/08.

75. Hofman A, Rocca WA, Brayne C, *et al.* The prevalence of dementia in Europe: A collaborative study of 1980-1990 findings. Eurodem Prevalence Research Group. *Int J Epidemiol.* 1991 Sep;20(3):736–48. PubMed PMID: 1955260. Epub 1991/09/01.

76. Prince M, Ferri CP, Acosta D, *et al.* The protocols for the 10/66 dementia research group population-based research programme. *BMC Public Health.* 2007;7:165. PubMed PMID: 17659078. Pubmed Central PMCID: 1965476. Epub 2007/07/31.

77. Jorm AF and Jolley D. The incidence of dementia: A meta-analysis. *Neurology.* 1998 Sep;51(3):728–33. PubMed PMID: 9748017. Epub 1998/09/25.

78. Heyman A, Fillenbaum G, Prosnitz B, *et al.* Estimated prevalence of dementia among elderly black and white community residents. *Archives of Neurology.* 1991;48(6):594–98.

CHAPTER 21

Assessment and investigation of the cognitively impaired adult

Jonathan M. Schott, Nick C. Fox, and Martin N. Rossor

Introduction

Confronted by a patient with symptoms suggestive of cognitive impairment, the clinician has a number of key questions to address:

(1) Is there evidence of cognitive impairment representing a decline from previous levels of functioning?

(2) What is the cause of the cognitive impairment?

(3) How and to what extent are any impairments impacting on the individual's ability to function normally, and affecting those around them?

(4) What strategies—be they pharmacological or non-pharmacological—may be helpful both to improve the situation for the individual in question and those living with or caring for them?

The assessment of a patient in this setting requires a systematic approach: detailed history-taking remains the mainstay of the diagnostic process, complemented by a focused cognitive assessment and physical examination. A number of 'routine' investigations should be undertaken, supplemented by additional tests depending on the specific scenario. Once a diagnosis has been reached, appropriate management recommendations can then be made.

In this chapter, we provide an overview of this diagnostic process, with particular reference to the importance of establishing the time course over which impairments have occurred; which cognitive domains are affected and what cognitive deficits result; and how, taken together with the examination and investigation findings, a specific dementia syndrome and the probable underlying disease process can be diagnosed. Whilst for the primary neurodegenerative dementias, the cognitive history and examination are often the most important clues to diagnosis, in other, rarer cases, cognitive impairment may occur in the context of a range of other non-cognitive, often neurological or general features—so called dementia plus.[1] In these cases, the non-cognitive features may be more diagnostically pertinent.

A note on definitions

According to criteria dating from 1994, a diagnosis of 'dementia' requires an individual to have impairments of cognition, involving memory and at least one other cognitive domain *sufficient to interfere with activities of normal living*. This definition, whilst being recommended for use by the American Academy of Neurology Guidelines[2] does, however, have a number of problems: heavily weighted towards memory impairment and thus Alzheimer's disease, it may be less relevant to patients with other focal cognitive syndromes, where memory impairment is not the leading syndrome and indeed may not be present. A diagnosis of dementia says nothing about the *cause* of the cognitive impairment, and there may be some overlaps with delirium in certain conditions. Finally, the requirement for multiple domain impairments that impact on activities of daily living effectively precludes patients with early or isolated symptoms (see also chapter 32).

A number of other terms have been introduced to describe individuals with isolated or milder forms of cognitive impairment, the most commonly used of which is *mild cognitive impairment* (MCI), sometimes further divided into amnestic, non-amnestic, or multi-domain MCI.[3] New criteria for DSM–V include new definitions for delirium but also two new syndromes. *Major neurocognitive disorder*, including what is currently referred to as dementia, and *minor cognitive disorder*, for individuals with mild cognitive deficits in one or more domains but who are still able to function independently [Table 21.1]. Recognition of a cognitive problem is, however, not an end in itself, and as well as these broad syndromic definitions, more specific criteria for individual disorders have been proposed, discussed in detail in other chapters.

History-taking

Establishing as detailed a history as possible is a prerequisite for reaching an accurate diagnosis. The cognitively impaired individual may not be in a position to provide a detailed history of their current problems alone, and for this reason, and with the patient's permission, a collateral history should be taken from an *informant*—ideally interviewed alone—wherever possible.

The patient's *age* is clearly relevant to the likely diagnosis: in general, sporadic neurodegenerative dementias are diseases of the elderly although they can occur in mid-life, whereas metabolic and genetically inherited dementias are more likely to present earlier. *Handedness* should always be recorded, having potential bearing on the interpretation of cognitive testing. Ascertaining an individual's *prior level of functioning*, for example from educational achievement and employment history, provides useful information about previous level of cognitive functioning which might be crucial for interpretation of some cognitive test results.

Table 21.1 Criteria for dementia and cognitive impairment

Dementia (DSM–IV)	◆ Short- and long-term memory impairment ◆ Impairment in abstract thinking, judgment, other higher cortical function or personality change ◆ Cognitive disturbance interferes significantly with work, social activities, or relationships ◆ Cognitive changes do not occur exclusively in the setting of delirium
Mild Cognitive Impairment (MCI)	**Amnestic MCI** ◆ Cognitive complaints from patient ◆ History suggestive of decline from previous level of functioning ◆ Objective memory impairment for age ◆ Preserved functional abilities ◆ Not demented ◆ Memory alone affected; or memory + other cognitive domains (multi-domain amnestic MCI) **Non-amnestic MCI** ◆ Cognitive complaints from patient ◆ History suggestive of decline from previous level of functioning ◆ Evidence for impairment on testing ◆ Preserved functional abilities ◆ Not demented ◆ Single or multiple (multi-domain non-amnestic MCI) non-memory domains affected
Neurocognitive Disorder (DSM–V)	**Major Neurocognitive Disorder** Significant cognitive decline from a previous level of performance in one or more of the following: ◆ Complex attention ◆ Executive ability ◆ Learning and memory ◆ Language (expressive, receptive, naming) ◆ Visuoconstructional-perceptual ability ◆ Social cognition Based on: 1. Reports by the patient or caregiver of clear decline; and 2. Clear deficits (typically <2SDs or <2.5th %-ile) on objective testing Cognitive deficits are: ◆ Sufficient to interfere with independence ◆ Not exclusively in the context of delirium ◆ Not wholly or partially attributable to major psychiatric disease **Minor Neurocognitive Disorder** Minor cognitive decline from a previous level of performance in one or domains above, based on: 1. Reports by patient/caregiver (e.g. greater difficulty; using compensatory strategies) 2. Mild deficits (e.g. 1–2SDs below mean or 2.5–16th %-ile) on objective testing or a significant decline (e.g. 0.5SD) on serial testing; Cognitive deficits are: ◆ Not sufficient to interfere with independence (but greater effort/compensation required) ◆ Not exclusively in the context of delirium ◆ Not wholly or partially attributable to major psychiatric disease

Source data from American Psychiatric Association, Diagnostic and Statistical Manual of Mental Disorders Fourth Edition (DSM–IV), Copyright (2000), and Fifth Edition (DSM–5), Copyright (2013), American Psychiatric Association; Adapted from *J Int Med*. 256(3), Petersen RC, *et al*. Mild cognitive impairment as a diagnostic entity, pp. 183–94, Copyright (2004), with permission from John Wiley and Sons.

Timing and clinical course

The *timing* of development of any impairments has direct relevance to the diagnosis: whilst there may be considerable overlap in individual cases, most neurodegenerative dementias and metabolic diseases slowly progress over years, whilst prion disease, and infective and inflammatory conditions typically progress much more rapidly. Acute confusional states are more likely to reflect delirium than dementia and a different range of aetiologies, but of course delirium can also occur in the context of dementia. It is therefore helpful to ask the patient and informant to try and identify the timing of the earliest possible symptoms relating to the current problems. The *pattern* of progression should also be noted: abrupt onset or decline may suggest a vascular cause, although many cases of vascular cognitive impairment do not have the step-wise progression previously considered a core feature;[4] fluctuations are commonly seen in cortical Lewy body disease,[5] but may also suggest metabolic problems or seizures.

Determining the cognitive domains affected

The next stage in the history is to determine both the patient and informant's reports of the specific cognitive problems. When so doing, it is important to try to determine whether there has been objective decline from a previous level of functioning—a distinction that is important for the diagnosis of a dementia or major/minor neurocognitive disorder—and thus establishing concrete examples of change and its impact at home and work is important. An initial question to be addressed is which cognitive domains are involved. 'Memory impairment' is often used as a surrogate for cognitive impairment in more general terms, but for some patients presenting at cognitive disorders clinics, memory impairment may not be present, or may not be the major problem.

Where memory is the major issue, the commonest problem encountered will be the insidious erosion of event or episodic memory as seen in the majority of patients with Alzheimer's disease with, for example, difficulties remembering recent events, telephone conversations, or appointments, reflecting medial temporal lobe compromise. This, however, should be distinguished from other forms of memory impairment including those for names of common objects (semantic memory) and faces/routes, which suggest different anatomical localization (left and right temporal lobe respectively).

Symptoms referable to other cognitive domains should be sought: these include problems with spelling, numeracy, or object use (apraxia) that suggest dominant (left) parietal lobe dysfunction; problems related to vision including visual perception and location of objects in space, as seen in non-dominant (right) parietal lobe or occipital lobe dysfunction; or behavioural change, including apathy, socially inappropriate behaviour, impulsivity, loss of sympathy/empathy, ritualistic behaviour or dietary changes, that reflect dysfunction of the frontal lobe or its connections. Very prominent cognitive slowing may suggest subcortical involvement. Where possible, documenting specific examples of any impairment is often particularly helpful. In this way, the clinician should aim to build up a picture both of the extent of any cognitive problems and the impact they have on the individual and those around him/her, but also which anatomical brain regions are either involved or spared.

Neurological history

It is important to consider a relevant review of a number of neurological symptoms, whose presence or absence may both give clues to an underlying diagnosis—particularly in unusual dementia syndromes—and have bearing on management. Visual disturbance may reflect cortically based problems with visual processing (e.g. optic ataxia, ocular apraxia, simultagnosia) but may also be seen in cranial nerve dysfunction, in which case the differential diagnosis is very different. The presence or absence of speech and swallowing problems is important both diagnostically and may also have practical management issues. Focal weakness, ataxia, extrapyramidal involvement (particularly the emergence of parkinsonian features or hyperkinetic movements), sensory disturbance, symptoms suggestive of denervation (muscular thinning, weakness, cramps), falls, or gait impairments disturbance can all narrow the differential diagnosis considerably (Table 21.2).

Psychiatric history

The presence of depression or anxiety may be sufficient to lead to cognitive complaints per se but may also complicate established dementia and occur as early manifestations of neurodegenerative disease. Early behavioural change is a cardinal feature of frontotemporal dementia but can also accompany vascular cognitive impairment and a range of other dementing disorders. Delusions and hallucinations may reflect a primary psychiatric disorder, particularly when long standing. However, the development of these symptoms later in life should serve as a 'red flag' for the possibility of an emerging dementia. In particular, the emergence of well-formed visual hallucinations, particularly in the presence of motor parkinsonism is very suggestive of dementia with Lewy bodies; and psychosis can be seen in some forms of frontotemporal dementia (e.g. due to mutations in the *c9orf72* gene).[6]

Past medical history and medications

The presence of significant vascular risk factors (hypertension, smoking, diabetes, hypercholesterolaemia, and atrial fibrillation) may alert the clinician to the possibility of vascular cognitive impairment (VCI); conversely, their absence should prompt a reappraisal of this diagnosis. A history of frank epilepsy or symptoms suggestive of seizures, psychiatric disorders, autoimmunity, significant head trauma, cranial surgery, obstructive sleep apnoea, rapid-eye-movement sleep behaviour disturbance (shouting during sleep, acting-out dreams, and vivid dreams), metabolic disturbance, multiple sclerosis, vascular events, or prior malignancy may all be relevant. Similarly, current and past medication use may both cause cognitive impairment or influence phenotype. Commonly encountered problems in this context include the interpretation of extrapyramidal signs in patients who have been exposed to neuroleptics, the cognitive blunting that can accompany sedative or opiate use, and confusion associated with the use of anticholinergic drugs.

Family history

In all patients presenting with a cognitive disorder, detailed family history-taking is mandatory. A family history suggestive of autosomal dominant inheritance of a similar disorder, particularly but not exclusively at young age, may suggest an underlying single gene disorder (Fig. 21.1). This has implications for both how an individual may be diagnosed, but potentially also for other family members. Particular care should be taken in the presence of a censored or unknown family history; an absence of family history does not entirely exclude an autosomal dominant dementia due to mis-paternity. The possibility of an autosomal recessive inheritance should also not be discounted: whilst none of the principle neurodegenerative forms of dementia have yet been shown to be inherited in this way, a number of disorders within the 'dementia plus' spectrum may be.

Social history

The patient's social circumstances should be explored, including whom they may live with and what level of support is available at home. In many patients, including those who present with subjective memory complaints but do not have a diagnosis of dementia, discussing the social network of the individual and stressors

Table 21.2 Causes of dementia plus

Dementia plus ...	Differential diagnosis
Ataxia	Spinocerebellar ataxia, paraneoplastic diseases, prion diseases, DRPLA, fragile x-associated tremor ataxia syndrome, familial British and Danish dementias, mitochondrial disorders, superficial siderosis, neuronal ceroid lipofuscinosis, Niemann–Pick disease type C, multiple system atrophy, Alexander's disease, and multiple sclerosis
Pyramidal signs	Multiple sclerosis, frontotemporal lobar degeneration with motor neuron disease, Alzheimer's disease (some presenilin mutations), spinocerebellar ataxias, phenylketonuria, familial British and Danish dementias, some forms of hereditary spastic paraparesis, adrenoleukodystrophy, vanishing white matter disease, polyglucosan body disease, polycystic lipomembranous sclerosing leukoencephalopathy (Nasu–Hakola disease)
Dystonia/chorea	Huntington's disease (and related disorders), Kuf's disease, Wilson's disease, neuroacanthocytosis, neurodegeneration with brain iron accumulation, Lesch–Nyhan syndrome, DRPLA, corticobasal degeneration, neuroferritinopathy, anti-NMDA receptor-mediated limbic encephalitis, variant CJD
Bucco-lingual mutilation	Neuroacanthocytosis, Lesch–Nyhan syndrome
Akinetic-rigid syndrome	Lewy body disease, progressive supranuclear palsy, multiple system atrophy Huntington's disease, corticobasal degeneration, dementia pugilistica, Wilson's disease, neurodegeneration with brain iron accumulation, frontotemporal lobar degeneration with parkinsonism-17, Alzheimer's disease (usually advanced)
Peripheral neuropathy	Neuroacanthocytosis, cerebrotendinous xanthomatosis, HIV infection, giant axonal neuropathy, alcohol-related diseases, metachromatic leukodystrophy, porphyria, adrenoleukodystrophy, GM2 gangliosidosis, polyglucosan body disease, Krabbe's disease, sialidosis, Fabry's disease, mitochondrial disorders, spinocerebellar ataxias (particularly type 3)
Myoclonus/early seizures	Prion disease, Alzheimer's disease, Lewy body disease, DRPLA, mitochondrial disorders, Gaucher's disease, GM2 gangliosidosis, neuroserpinopathy, polycystic lipomembranous sclerosing leukoencephalopathy, subacute sclerosing panencephalitis, progressive myoclonic epilepsy syndromes, Kuf's disease, Lafora body disease, sialidosis
Gaze palsy	Niemann–Pick disease type C, Gaucher's disease, progressive supranuclear palsy, mitochondrial disorders, spinocerebellar ataxias (particularly type 2), paraneoplastic disorders, Whipple's disease
Deafness	Superficial siderosis, mitochondrial disorders, familial Danish dementia, alpha mannosidosis, sialidosis
Dysautonomia	Lewy body disease, multiple system atrophy, prion disease, porphyria, adrenoleukodystrophy, anti-NMDA receptor-mediated limbic encephalitis
Cataracts	Myotonic dystrophy, cerebrotendinous xanthomatosis, mitochondrial disorders, familial Danish dementia
Splenomegaly	Niemann–Pick disease type C, Gaucher's disease
Tendon xanthomas	Cerebrotendinous xanthomatosis
Bone cysts	Polycystic lipomembranous sclerosing leucoencephalopathy
Paget's disease/Inclusion body myositis	Valosin-associated frontotemporal lobar degeneration
Renal impairment	Fabry's disease, Lesch–Nyhan syndrome, mitochondrial disorders
Liver dysfunction	Wilson's disease, Gaucher's disease, mitochondrial disorder
Respiratory failure	Frontotemporal lobar degeneration and motor neuron disease, Perry syndrome, mitochondrial disease (e.g. POLG), anti-NMDA receptor-mediated limbic encephalitis
Gastrointestinal dysfunction	Coeliac disease, Whipple's disease, porphyria
Anaemia	Vitamin B12 deficiency, neuroacanthocytosis (McLeod's syndrome), Wilson's disease, Gaucher's disease
Skin lesions	Behcet's disease, systemic vasculitides and connective tissue disease, Fabry's disease
Metabolic/infectious crises	Vanishing white matter disease, Alexander's disease, ornithine transcarbamylase deficiency, alpha mannosidosis, porphyria
Hyponatraemia	Lgl1 antibody associated encephalitis

Adapted from *Lancet Neurol*. 9(8), Rossor MN, Fox NC, Mummery CJ, Schott JM, and Warren JD, The diagnosis of young-onset dementia, pp. 793–806, Copyright (2010), with permission from Elsevier.

at home and work provides crucial insights into potential factors that might be exacerbating cognitive symptoms. Some patients with cognitive impairment may be very vulnerable, and poor judgment or memory can result in significant financial problems. Ascertaining what the individual in question is able to do around the house, whether they are safe or need supervision, and in the younger population, whether they are still able to work, has implications for management. Estimating current and past alcohol use is also important, as is obtaining a smoking history. It is often important to establish whether the patient is driving, and if so, whether there is any evidence to suspect that this is being influenced by their cognitive problems.

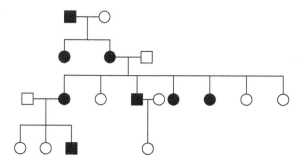

Fig. 21.1 Family tree in family Alzheimer's disease due to a presenilin1 mutation. Squares = male; Circles = female; Black centre = gene positive; White centre = gene negative.

Overview

Having taken the history, the clinician should aim to answer a number of key questions:

(1) Is there clear evidence for cognitive decline from a higher baseline?

(2) Which cognitive domains appear to be affected?

(3) Does the pattern and progression of cognitive impairment combined with the other clinical features suggest a specific diagnosis?

With these questions in mind, the examination and investigations, whilst needing to be comprehensive, can be focused towards confirming or refuting the putative diagnosis reached at this stage.

Examination

Cognitive examination

The bedside cognitive examination is discussed in detail in chapter 10. In brief, such an assessment generally starts with a broad screening tool to establish the level of any cognitive impairment, with the caveat that no single screening tool can reliably assess severity across all dementia syndromes. The assessment then should focus on establishing—in the same way as was done during history-taking—which cognitive domains are affected or spared, through the use of tests which probe specific cognitive domains; for example, implicating dysfunction within one or more lobes of the brain, or where possible more fine-grained neuroanatomical description. In general, it is important to observe the patient's behaviour and interaction with the environment and those around them. Patients with Alzheimer's disease usually maintain a preserved social façade at least in the early stages of the disease, but may turn to their partner/carer when questioned, and become withdrawn and tentative. By contrast, patients with dysexecutive syndromes may be overfamiliar, withdrawn, or inappropriate, sometimes showing utilization behaviour (inappropriately using objects with specific functions, e.g. seeing a pen, picking it up, and writing unasked during a consultation[7]). Note should be made about whether a patient engages when tested, and whether their performance is in keeping with their functioning in everyday life.

Physical examination

Patients evaluated for a cognitive problem should have a physical examination. Whilst for most patients with Alzheimer's disease this will be normal, there are important physical findings that can guide a diagnosis for many other forms of dementia. Particularly in the case of young-onset, unusual or rapid dementias, where unlike many of the cortical dementias, the pattern of cognitive impairment may not give major clues to the underlying diagnosis, the allied physical (neurological and/or non-neurological) symptoms and signs can provide vital clues to narrow the differential diagnosis (Table 21.2).

General examination

The general examination should include a cardiovascular assessment (pulse, blood pressure, and the heart sounds), all of which may be very relevant to helping establish a diagnosis of (or contribution from) vascular cognitive impairment, and in some instances can help define much rarer causes such as endocarditis or arteritis. A note should be made of significant weight loss or cachexia: examination of the chest and abdomen may be particularly pertinent in patients who smoke and drink respectively. In the case of patients with young onset or more complex dementia syndromes, a detailed systems review and examination may narrow diagnosis considerably (Table 21.2).

Neurological examination

In many of the primary neurodegenerative dementias, the neurological examination will be unremarkable. However, where present, neurological signs may help significantly narrow the differential diagnosis. Examination of the eye movements is often very rewarding, allowing for the assessment of cerebellar dysfunction, ocular apraxia (suggestive of parietal lobe dysfunction), or either a nuclear or supranuclar gaze palsy. Speech will have been assessed as part of the cognitive assessment, but it may be relevant to assess the swallow, alongside fundal appearances and visual fields. The presence of a brisk jaw jerk and myotatic facial reflexes (elicited by gently tapping around the mouth) provides evidence for upper motor neurone lesions at brainstem level or above, as does the presence of a pout. By contrast, movement of the lips towards an approaching target or reaction to gentle stroking around the mouth is a frontal release sign.[7] Observing the facial appearances may also be very revealing: facial hypomimia is suggestive of extrapyramidal disease; staring facies with frontalis overactivity and decreased blink rate are features of progressive supranuclear palsy;[8] facial weakness or asymmetry may be suggestive of prior stroke.

Examination of the limbs may reveal signs of parkinsonism, suggestive of dementia with Lewy bodies, or in the case of an existing diagnosis of Parkinson's disease, Parkinson's disease dementia, or a number of other disorders including progressive supranuclar palsy, and the corticobasal syndrome classically but by no means invariably accompanied by asymmetric dystonia, myoclonus, and cortical sensory impairment. The presence of chorea focuses the differential diagnosis considerably (Table 21.2). The presence of a cerebellar syndrome is unusual in most of the cortical dementias, raising the possibility of alcohol, vascular cerebellar/brainstem lesions, or a range of genetic or metabolic disorders depending on the clinical context. Focal upper motor neuron weakness is most commonly due to vascular lesions, although this has a large differential diagnosis, including inflammatory disorders such as multiple sclerosis or neurodegenerative disorders such as amyotrophic lateral sclerosis. A potentially useful observation is that in vascular cognitive impairment, the reflexes including jaw jerk are often brisk, but the plantars flexor. Particularly in unusual dementia syndromes, the presence of a peripheral neuropathy may provide clues to diagnosis, although in the elderly, comorbidities are common, and a mild peripheral neuropathy is not uncommon. Examination of the gait may provide useful clues to a parkinsonian syndrome or cerebellar disorder, the effects of cerebrovascular disease, or possibly hydrocephalus. The presence of prominent retropulsion is often seen in parkinsonian disorders, and perhaps particularly progressive supranuclear palsy.

Investigation

Following clinical evaluation, the clinician should have narrowed the differential diagnosis and can use investigations to try to secure the diagnosis as far as possible. For all patients with cognitive impairment, a number of investigations including a panel of blood tests and structural brain imaging are recommended. Where possible, all patients with a possible dementing illness should have a formal neuropsychometric assessment to provide quantifiable measures of cognitive performance against age-related norms both globally and in specific domains. This is discussed in detail in chapter 21. A range of other investigations may be appropriate depending on the clinical context.

How far to investigate patients in whom primary problems with mood or anxiety are thought to underpin the cognitive complaints will depend on the specific circumstance and the individual patient. Where possible, obtaining baseline neuropsychometric, blood, and imaging data may help support the hypothesis that there is not a significant organic component, provide reassurance to the patient, and act as a baseline against which subsequent testing can be compared objectively. Where investigation is either not feasible or wanted by the patient, reassessment after an interval is often very helpful in determining whether there is a significant and progressive cognitive problem.

Blood testing

All patients with possible cognitive impairment should have a range of blood investigations, including a full blood count, blood sugar, liver function, electrolytes, thyroid function, B12, folate, and at least some inflammatory indices (e.g. ESR and/or C-reactive protein).[2,9] Whilst principally designed to exclude 'treatable' causes of cognitive impairments, in practice, at least in our experiences it is rare for any of these conditions in isolation to be sufficient to cause cognitive impairment. However, anaemia, liver and renal failure, recurrent and significant hypoglycaemia, vitamin B12 deficiency, and thyroid dysfunction can certainly all cause cognitive impairment and as significant comorbidities, worsen other causes of dementia. Abnormalities in any of these parameters should be investigated and treated as appropriate.

Depending on the clinical setting, a large range of other blood tests may be appropriate. Outlines for the screening of potential metabolic problems are given in chapter 24; for infections in chapter 23; and for autoimmune causes of cognitive impairment in chapter 28. HIV testing may be appropriate both as a treatable cause for dementia in itself[10] but in addition, it raises the possibility of other opportunistic infections. In atypical parkinsonism, testing copper, caeruloplasmin, and ferritin, and excluding the presence of acanthocytes on a blood film may all be appropriate.

Brain imaging

Brain imaging can be usefully divided into structural, functional, and metabolic imaging.

Structural imaging

Structural imaging, with magnetic resonance imaging (MRI) or computed tomography (CT), is recommended for *all* patients being investigated for dementia.[2,9] MRI is the modality of choice, providing high white/grey matter contrast without exposure to ionizing radiation. Modern MRI scanning provides very detailed visualization of brain structure, allowing for an assessment of atrophy, and of signal change typically reflecting the presence of vascular disease or demyelination. A standard dementia sequence including a T1-weighted, T2-weighted/FLAIR (fluid-attenuated inversion recovery) sequence complemented where necessary by susceptibility-weighted imaging (sensitive to iron, and thus blood products) and diffusion-weighted imaging (for recent infarcts or spongiosis), and can be performed within half an hour.[11] Whilst traditionally undertaken to exclude 'treatable' causes (i.e. mass lesions such as tumours), MRI is increasingly being used to aid in the differential diagnosis of the different dementias and is being incorporated into new diagnostic criteria.[12]

We recommend that examination of MRI images be done in a structured manner.[13] T2/FLAIR images should be reviewed for evidence of white matter lesions. In the elderly patient, the most likely explanation for these will be on the basis of vascular disease. It is, however, important not to over-interpret the presence of a few small lesions, which is common with advancing age. However, the presence of multiple and particularly confluent vascular lesions, may be sufficient, in the correct clinical context, to support a diagnosis of either vascular cognitive impairment, or in the presence of medial temporal atrophy, mixed (e.g. VCI and Alzheimer's disease) pathology. Small focal lesions involving thalamocortical circuitry can be sufficient alone to cause memory or other cognitive impairments.[14] Similarly, the presence of focal large infarcts demonstrating prior large vessel stroke would be expected to produce neuropsychological deficits in the regions affected. White matter change, however, does not always implicate vascular disease, and in the correct clinical context, may be compatible with the effects of multiple sclerosis and inherited or genetically determined metabolic diseases. Susceptibility-weighted imaging can be very useful in detecting microbleeds which, when present in the brainstem and basal ganglia, typically reflect hypertensive changes, with cortical lesions being more commonly associated with the effects of amyloid angiopathy (Fig. 21.2, panel f).[15]

T1-weighted volumetric imaging, particularly viewed in the coronal plane with angulations through medial temporal lobe structures, can provide valuable evidence for *focal atrophy*, which has predictive value for different dementia syndromes (Fig. 21.2).[16] Alzheimer's disease is typically associated with bilateral symmetrical hippocampal atrophy in excess to that seen elsewhere in the cortex (Fig. 21.2, panel a). Involvement of parietal lobe structures and the cingulate gyrus is very common, with the general pattern usually being of a posterior greater than anterior gradient.[17] In some patients with Alzheimer's disease—the posterior cortical atrophy variant—atrophy may be restricted to the occipitoparietal lobes with sparing of the hippocampi (Fig. 21.2, panel b).[18]

Dementia with Lewy bodies tends to produce relatively less hippocampal atrophy than is seen in Alzheimer's disease,[5] although

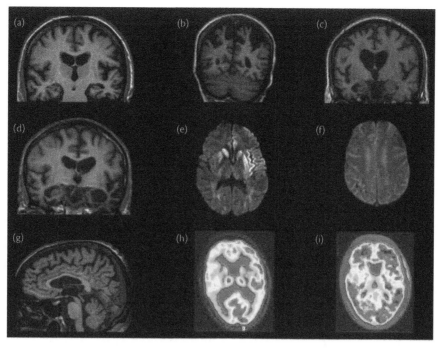

Fig. 21.2 Imaging in the investigation of dementia. (a) Coronal MRI scan showing selective hippocampal volume loss in postmortem (PM) confirmed Alzheimer's disease. (b) Coronal MRI scan showing prominent parietal lobe atrophy in PM confirmed posterior cortical atrophy (due to Alzheimer's disease). (c) Coronal MRI scan showing right temporal lobe atrophy and right lateral ventricle prominance in PM confirmed frontotemporal dementia. (d) Coronal MRI scan showing very asymmetric left temporal lobe atrophy involving the hippocampus and fusiform gyrus in PM confirmed semantic dementia. (e) Diffusion-weighted MRI showing basal ganglia and cortical signal change in sporadic Creutzfeldt–Jakob disease. (f) T2* MRI showing multiple cortical microbleeds in cerebral amyloid angiopathy. (g) Sagittal MRI scan shows pontine atrophy (the 'Hummingbird sign') in PM-proven progressive supranuclear palsy. (h) FDG-PET scan shows marked parietal hypometabolism in Alzheimer's disease. (i) Amyloid PET imaging shows widespread cortical fibrillar amyloid deposits in Alzheimer's disease.

this may not necessarily be helpful on an individual basis. Patients with frontotemporal lobar degeneration often have striking atrophy patterns, with prominent asymmetrical frontal and/or temporal atrophy in some cases of behavioural variant FTD (Fig. 21.2, panel c), focal dominant temporal lobe atrophy particularly involving the temporal pole and fusiform gyrus in semantic dementia (Fig. 21.2, panel d), widening of the dominant Sylvian fissure in progressive non-fluent aphasia, marked hemispheric atrophy in patients with progranulin mutations, and symmetrical very focal atrophy of the anterior medial temporal lobes in certain tau mutations.[19]

Assessments of brainstem and subcortical structures may be helpful in certain parkinsonian conditions; for example, progressive supranuclear palsy (Fig. 21.2, panel g). Asymmetric hippocampal and medial temporal lobe atrophy particularly with signal change may be suggestive of autoimmune limbic encephalitis. Numerous other rare conditions are associated with often fairly specific patterns of imaging abnormality. These are reviewed in detail in reference 20.

Prion diseases are often associated with specific patterns of restricted diffusion on diffusion-weighted imaging, which has revolutionized the diagnosis of sporadic Creutzfeldt–Jakob disease (CJD) (Fig. 21.2, panel e). Variant CJD typically shows high signal on diffusion-weighted or FLAIR imaging within the thalamus, showing higher signal than that seen within the basal ganglia. Inherited prion diseases can be associated with focal cerebellar atrophy.[21]

Metabolic and molecular imaging

Imaging using either 18F-fluoro-deoxyglucose (FDG) positron emission tomography (PET) or single photon computed

tomography (SPECT) allows for *in vivo* assessment of brain metabolism, and both are licensed for the investigation of dementia in both the UK and the US. The pattern of hypometabolism (e.g. in temporoparietal regions) has positive predictive value for a diagnosis of Alzheimer's disease (Fig. 21.2, panel h).[22] Conversely, hypometabolism in frontotemporal regions can be very useful in the diagnosis of frontotemporal dementia, particularly in patients with behavioural symptoms in whom a non-degenerative syndrome is possible.[23]

In patients where dementia with Lewy bodies is suspected, dopamine transporter (DAT) imaging, which allows for demonstration of dopamine uptake *in vivo*, can be very useful, demonstrating central dopamine depletion.[24] A normal DAT scan does not, however, help to distinguish between DLB and Parkinson disease dementia (PDD), and is also often abnormal in other typical parkinsonian syndromes. It may be particularly valuable in differentiating central dopaminergic depletion from the effects of neuroleptics (where the scan would typically be normal) in patients with combinations of cognitive impairment, movement disorders, and psychiatric disease.[25]

The development of the amyloid PET binding radiotracer ^{11}C-Pittsburg compound (PIB) allowed for fibrillar amyloid plaques to be visualized during life for the first time.[26]. In recent years, the development of 18F-based amyloid tracers has allowed for the commercialization of this approach. At the time of writing, three compounds, florbetapir (Amyvid), flutemetamol (Vizamyl), and florbetaben (Neuraceq) have been licensed for use in both Europe and the US to rule in or out the presence of fibrillar amyloid in the brain. The clinical context in which this new technology should best be applied has yet to be fully defined, but it is potentially extremely valuable in differentiating Alzheimer from non-Alzheimer's dementias in patients with established cognitive impairment (Fig. 21.2, panel i).

Cerebrospinal fluid

Examination of the CSF, at least in the UK and the US, has traditionally been used to exclude infection or inflammation as the cause of cognitive decline in young-onset cases.[2] This remains very important for patients with an unusual 'dementia plus' or rapidly progressive cognitive syndrome. The ability to quantify neuronal specific proteins in the CSF, however, means that lumbar puncture can now be used to increase the certainty of a diagnosis of AD during life. In established AD, concentrations of Aβ1-42 are reduced, probably reflecting deposition of Aβ1-42 within the brain, and concentrations of tau and phosphorylated tau are increased.[27] A combination of low Aβ1-42 and elevation of tau and/or phospho tau (often expressed as a tau:Aβ1-42 ratio) has good sensitivity and specificity for a diagnosis of AD, and for predicting which patients with mild memory impairment will go onto develop dementia due to AD.[28]

These AD-specific biomarkers are now being incorporated into new criteria for AD.[12,29,30] As evidence suggests that they become abnormal prior to the development of symptoms, they may have utility in defining individuals with presymptomatic disease for clinical trials.[31] Performing CSF examination to aid in the diagnosis of dementia varies widely between countries, being very commonly used in some European countries, but less so in the US and the UK. Given the very valuable diagnostic information that can be provided and the ability in the correct clinical context to measure other CSF proteins within the CSF, our practice is increasingly to offer CSF testing to all patients with young-onset dementia, and to more elderly patients when the diagnosis is in doubt. In due course it is likely that CSF markers with high sensitivity/specificity for other neurodegenerative diseases will become available.

Genetic testing

Some conditions causing dementia, including Huntington's disease and a range of other conditions, occur exclusively on an autosomal dominant basis and genetic testing is necessary for definitive diagnosis. In the case of the common neurodegenerative dementias, a minority of cases of Alzheimer's occur secondary to mutations in either the APP (amyloid precursor protein), PSEN1 (presenilin 1), or PSEN2 genes; up to 40 per cent of patients with frontotemporal dementia have causative mutations, as will a proportion of patients with prion disease. The decision to undertake genetic testing should always be made in consultation with the patient and the family and should follow standard guidelines.[32] Predictive, as opposed to diagnostic, genetic testing should always be performed via a clinical genetics department. Request for genetic testing varies considerably between clinicians, perhaps reflecting differences in populations seen. Our practice is to offer genetic testing for patients with clear autosomal dominant family histories, particularly although not exclusively, occurring at young ages. As genetic techniques advance and more patients are tested, the phenotypic spectrum of autosomal dominant dementia syndromes is expanding. The arrival of next-generation genetic sequencing techniques allows for much wider and cheaper genetic testing,[33] undoubtedly increasing both the number of mutations positive individuals identified and the associated phenotypic diversity.

Other investigations

Depending on the clinical scenario, and particularly in the case of patients with young-onset disease, rapid progression, or 'dementia plus', it may be appropriate to undertake a very wide range of other tests in order to reach a definitive diagnosis,[1] including but not limited to body imaging using CT, FDG-PET, mammography, or ultrasonography with/without biopsy (e.g. for suspected paraneoplasia, systemic inflammation, or infection); bone marrow biopsy (e.g. for haematological malignancy); neuro-ophthalmological or otological assessment (e.g. for complex eye movements, or in the case of suspected inflammatory disease); neurophysiology, including electroencephalography (seizures) or (EMG) electromyogram/nerve conduction studies (myopathy or neuropathy); or sleep studies (e.g. for obstructive sleep apnoea or rapid-eye-movement (REM) sleep behaviour disorder). Ultimately, and particularly if an underlying inflammatory condition, particularly CNS vasculitis which is notoriously difficult to diagnose during life, is considered, it may be necessary to proceed to a brain biopsy. Where possible, a targeted biopsy from a clinically non-eloquent area should be taken. Failing this, a full thickness biopsy involving grey matter, white matter, and dura is usually taken from the non-dominant frontal lobe. Particularly in the case of rapidly progressive dementia, the possibility of prion disease should always be considered, and appropriate surgical procedures followed to prevent transmission. In our experience of over 130 cerebral biopsies for dementia, a treatable cause was determined in 10 per cent and an alternative diagnosis in around 60 per cent. There was some—transient—morbidity in around 10 per cent, but no deaths attributable to the procedure.[34]

Management

Management of the cognitively impaired patient will clearly depend on the specific diagnosis, with management issues and specific treatments for the different causes covered in their relevant chapters. Generic issues that should always be considered in patients diagnosed with significant cognitive impairment or dementia include: treatment of intercurrent mood or sleep problems and other comorbidites; control of vascular risk factors; and appropriate counselling and support for the patient and family. Referral to support services may be appropriate depending on the needs and wishes of the patient and carer, and again depending on the specific circumstance, the patient should be advised about driving. Accurate diagnosis may not only direct appropriate therapeutic strategies but also may provide useful prognostic information influencing future planning. Importantly however, individual treatments and care plans need to be directed on an individual-by-individual basis, taking into account matters specific to the disease and the cognitive domains affected, the individual's personal circumstances, and their and their carers' responses to their problems and diagnosis.

References

1. Rossor MN, Fox NC, Mummery CJ, et al. The diagnosis of young-onset dementia. *Lancet Neurol.* 2010 Aug;9(8):793–806.
2. Knopman DS, DeKosky ST, Cummings JL, et al. Practice parameter: diagnosis of dementia (an evidence-based review). Report of the Quality Standards Subcommittee of the American Academy of Neurology. *Neurology.* 2001. p. 1143–53.

3. Petersen RC. Clinical practice. Mild cognitive impairment. *N Engl J Med*. 2011 Jun 9;364(23):2227–34.

4. Bowler JV. Modern concept of vascular cognitive impairment. *Br Med Bull*. 2007;83:291–305.

5. McKeith IG, Dickson DW, Lowe J, et al. Diagnosis and management of dementia with Lewy bodies: third report of the DLB Consortium. *Neurology*. 2005. p. 1863–72.

6. Snowden JS, Rollinson S, Thompson JC, et al. Distinct clinical and pathological characteristics of frontotemporal dementia associated with C9ORF72 mutations. *Brain*. 2012 Mar;135(Pt 3):693–708.

7. Schott JM and Rossor MN. The grasp and other primitive reflexes. *J Neurol Neurosur Ps*. 2003 May;74(5):558–60.

8. Williams DR and Lees AJ. Progressive supranuclear palsy: clinico-pathological concepts and diagnostic challenges. *Lancet Neurol*. 2009 Mar;8(3):270–79.

9. Sorbi S, Hort J, Erkinjuntti T, et al. EFNS-ENS Guidelines on the diagnosis and management of disorders associated with dementia. *Eur J Neurol*. 2012. p. 1159–79.

10. Nightingale S, Michael BD, Defres S, et al. Test them all; an easily diagnosed and readily treatable cause of dementia with life-threatening consequences if missed. *Pract Neurol*. 2013 Dec;13(6):354–56.

11. Schott JM, Warren JD, Barkhof F, et al. Suspected early dementia. *BMJ*. 2011;343:d5568.

12. McKhann GM, Knopman DS, Chertkow H, et al. The diagnosis of dementia due to Alzheimer's disease: Recommendations from the National Institute on Aging–Alzheimer's Association workgroups on diagnostic guidelines for Alzheimer's disease. *Alzheimer's & Dementia*. 2011 May;7(3):263–69.

13. Harper L, Barkhof F, Scheltens P, et al. An algorithmic approach to structural imaging in dementia. *J Neurol Neurosur Ps*. 2013 Oct. 16.

14. Carrera E and Bogousslavsky J. The thalamus and behavior: effects of anatomically distinct strokes. *Neurology*. 2006 Jun. 27;66(12):1817–23.

15. Greenberg SM, Vernooij MW, Cordonnier C, et al. Cerebral microbleeds: a guide to detection and interpretation. *Lancet Neurol*. 2009 Feb;8(2):165–74.

16. Likeman M, Anderson VM, Stevens JM, et al. Visual assessment of atrophy on magnetic resonance imaging in the diagnosis of pathologically confirmed young-onset dementias. *Arch Neurol*. 2005 Sep;62(9):1410–15.

17. Frisoni GB, Fox NC, Jack CR, et al. The clinical use of structural MRI in Alzheimer disease. *Nat Rev Neurol*. 2010 Feb;6(2):67–77.

18. Crutch SJ, Lehmann M, Schott JM, et al. Posterior cortical atrophy. *Lancet Neurol*. 2012 Feb;11(2):170–78.

19. Warren JD, Rohrer JD, and Rossor MN. Clinical review. Frontotemporal dementia. *BMJ*. 2013;347:f4827.

20. Barkhof F, Fox NC, Bastos-Leite AJ, et al. *Neuroimaging in Dementia*. Berlin: Springer-Verlag, 2011.

21. Macfarlane RG, Wroe SJ, Collinge J, et al. Neuroimaging findings in human prion disease. *J Neurol Neurosur Ps*. 2007 Jul;78(7):664–70.

22. Foster NL, Heidebrink JL, Clark CM, et al. FDG-PET improves accuracy in distinguishing frontotemporal dementia and Alzheimer's disease. *Brain*. 2007 Oct;130(Pt 10):2616–35.

23. Kipps CM, Hodges JR, Fryer TD, et al. Combined magnetic resonance imaging and positron emission tomography brain imaging in behavioural variant frontotemporal degeneration: refining the clinical phenotype. *Brain*. 2009 Sep;132(Pt 9):2566–78.

24. McKeith I, O'Brien J, Walker Z, et al. Sensitivity and specificity of dopamine transporter imaging with 123I-FP-CIT SPECT in dementia with Lewy bodies: A phase III, multicentre study. *Lancet Neurol*. 2007 Apr;6(4):305–13.

25. Kägi G, Bhatia KP, and Tolosa E. The role of DAT-SPECT in movement disorders. *J Neurol Neurosur Ps*. 2010 Jan;81(1):5–12.

26. Klunk WE, Engler H, Nordberg A, et al. Imaging brain amyloid in Alzheimer's disease with Pittsburgh Compound-B. *Ann Neurol*. 2004;55(3):306–19.

27. Blennow K, Hampel H, Weiner M, et al. Cerebrospinal fluid and plasma biomarkers in Alzheimer disease. *Nat Rev Neurol*. 2010 Mar;6(3):131–44.

28. Mattsson N, Zetterberg H, Hansson O, et al. CSF biomarkers and incipient Alzheimer disease in patients with mild cognitive impairment. *JAMA*. 2009 Jul 22;302(4):385–93.

29. Albert MS, DeKosky ST, Dickson D, et al. The diagnosis of mild cognitive impairment due to Alzheimer's disease: Recommendations from the National Institute on Aging–Alzheimer's Association workgroups on diagnostic guidelines for Alzheimer's disease. *Alzheimer's & Dementia*. 2011 May;7(3):270–79.

30. Dubois B, Feldman HH, Jacova C, et al. Revising the definition of Alzheimer's disease: a new lexicon. *Lancet Neurol*. 2010 Nov;9(11):1118–27.

31. Sperling RA, Aisen PS, Beckett LA, et al. Toward defining the preclinical stages of Alzheimer's disease: Recommendations from the National Institute on Aging–Alzheimer's Association workgroups on diagnostic guidelines for Alzheimer's disease. *Alzheimers & Dementia*. 2011 May;7(3):280–92.

32. Burgunder J-M, Finsterer J, Szolnoki Z, et al. EFNS guidelines on the molecular diagnosis of channelopathies, epilepsies, migraine, stroke, and dementias. *Eur J Neurol*. 2010 May;17(5):641–48.

33. Beck J, Pittman A, Adamson G, et al. Validation of next-generation sequencing technologies in genetic diagnosis of dementia. *Neurobiol Aging*. 2014 Jan;35(1):261–65.

34. Schott JM, Reiniger L, Thom M, et al. Brain biopsy in dementia: clinical indications and diagnostic approach. *Acta Neuropathol*. 2010 Sep;120(3):327–41.

CHAPTER 22

Delirium, drugs, toxins

Barbara C. van Munster, Sophia E. de Rooij, and Sharon K. Inouye

History

The ancient Greeks described a mental disturbance associated with fever and other serious illnesses. They distinguished two different forms of this mental disturbance: an agitated phrenitis (frenzy) and a quiet lethargus (lethargy). Celsius was the first who introduced the concept delirium (*de lira*, off the path) in the first century, where it was used to distinguish this clinical entity from mania, depression, and hysteria. In sixteenth century Italy, Antonio Guainerio recognized the need for a comprehensive examination of the delirious patient, and in 1769, Morgagni replaced the concept of phrenitis by the term febrile delirium.[1] In 1959, Engel and Romano developed the concept of delirium as a 'syndrome of cerebral insufficiency',[2] but it was not until 1980, however, that delirium was standardized for the first time as a clinical entity in the American Psychiatric Association's (APA) Diagnostic and Statistical Manual, 3rd edition (DSM–III).

Epidemiology

Delirium is a frequently encountered syndrome with a prevalence of 0.4 per cent in the general population rising to 1 per cent in the population aged 55 years and older.[3] In hospital, delirium has been reported in 22 per cent of medical, 11–35 per cent of surgical, and 80 per cent of intensive care unit (ICU) patients.[4,5] In nursing homes the reported prevalence varies widely from 1 per cent[6] to 72 per cent, mainly explained by the poor reliability of the method used for diagnosis.[7] Terminal delirium is also a common symptom affecting up to 90 per cent in patients with cancer at end of life and is a major cause of distress for patients and their families.[8] Alcohol withdrawal delirium (AWD) is reported in 5 per cent of placebo-treated alcohol dependent patients entered into clinical trials of inpatient drug treatment for alcohol withdrawal.[9] The consequence of an ageing population (chapter 20) which is at greater risk for delirium is that the absolute number of patients with delirium and associated problems can be expected to rise.

There is a paucity of information about the incidence, prevalence, and severity of delirium in children, since well-validated instruments for diagnosing delirium in children have not been available; such scales are, however, currently being developed.[10]

Diagnosis

Numbers on prevalence and incidence vary greatly based on the different instruments used to diagnose delirium, and different diagnostic criteria for delirium.[11] The formal gold standard has been based on the diagnostic criteria of the Diagnostic and Statistical Manual of the APA (DSM version III to DSM–5) or the 9th and 10th edition of the International Classification of Diseases and Related Health Problems (ICD) (World Health Organization (WHO) 1992; American Psychiatric Association 1994).[12] The syndrome is defined by an acute disturbance in attention, a change in cognition, or a perceptual derangement (See Box 22.1| case history). In 2013, DSM–5, defined delirium more restrictively in comparison to the former DSM versions. The disturbance in consciousness (DSM–III to DSM–IV TR) has been replaced by a disturbance in attention, and the inattention or changes in cognition 'must not be occurring in the context of a severely reduced level of arousal such as coma'.

Box 22.1 Case history

Ms B, 92 years, was admitted to hospital because of dehydration and pneumonia. She lived at home independently and was not known to have previous cognitive impairment. On admission she was confused and could not tell the nurses where she lived. She was treated with antibiotics and stimulated to drink. During the evening she was restless and saw cats sitting on her bed, which made her fearful. Her son was encouraged to stay with her in hospital at night, in an attempt to avoid the need to treat her with antipsychotics with possible associated side-effects. Also, a calendar was placed on the wall and her son brought pictures to make her feel at home.

After a relatively good night's sleep, she felt better but the following day she was tired and fell asleep even during conversation. An activity programme was instigated to keep her awake during the day, and she fell asleep in the evening without restlessness or hallucinations. The following day she remembered having seen cats at some stage but could not recall anything of her day in hospital. Her son, having been concerned that his mother had developed dementia, reported that she was more or less back to normal. She was discharged home but temporarily needed some additional help at home because of reduced concentration.

Conclusion: Ms B experienced delirium, with mainly hyperactive symptoms during the first day and hypoactive elements during the second day. Non-medical management and treatment of the underlying condition resolved these problems. It can be expected that her attention level will return to baseline after a few months.

By definition, there is evidence from history, physical, or investigation that the symptoms are caused by direct physiological consequences of a general medical condition, or substance abuse, or withdrawal. To enable non-psychiatric clinicians to detect delirium quickly, the confusion assessment method (CAM) was developed (see Table 22.1). The CAM has become the most widely used instrument in recent years and it is translated and validated in many languages and in various specialty settings, including the adult and paediatric ICU.[10,13] To rate the assessment properly, brief instruments to test cognition such as the the Pfeiffer short portable mental status questionnaire (SPMSQ),[14] Mini-Cog,[15] or Montreal cognitive assessment (MOCA) test[16] are required.

Before delirium is present in its full form, some prodromal symptoms (e.g. memory impairments, vivid dreams, incoherence, disorientation, and symptoms of underlying acute illness) are often present.[17] If patients do not completely fullfil the criteria for delirium but experience changes in sleep–wake cycle, thought process, language, attention, orientation, and visuospatial processes, the non-DSM term 'subsyndromal delirium' is used.[18] Delirium in childhood typically has a more acute onset, less circadian variety in symptoms, and less sleep–wake cycle disturbances as compared to adults.[19] There are several scales both for screening, diagnosing, and assessing the severity and/or subtyping delirium (Table 22.2).

Three clinical subtypes of delirium (*hyperactive*, *hypoactive*, and *mixed* subtype) can be distinguished based on the predominant clinical symptoms.[21] Hyperactive patients are restless, agitated, and hyperalert, and often show hallucinations and delusions. Hypoactive delirium, which is particularly easy to miss in clinical practice, is characterized by sleepiness, lack of interest in activities, slow response to questions, and minimal spontaneous movements.[20] Mixed delirous patients can move between the two subtypes. Delirium recognition rates are low (12–43 per cent) and its management remains consequently inadequate in up to 80 per cent of the patients.[22] Apart from failure to recognize the symptoms, misdiagnosis is a considerable problem since depression and dementia (especially vascular dementia) are important differential diagnoses for hypoactive delirium. Hyperactive and mixed subtype of delirium may falsely be diagnosed as functional psychosis, dementia (especially Lewy body dementia), (hypo)mania, anxiety disorders, or akathisia.[23]

In the palliative care setting, it has been shown that subtypes often remain stable during a given episode.[24] Distinguishing the different delirium subtypes is important both to guide treatment

Table 22.2 Available scales for screening, diagnosis severity, and subtype of delirium

Test	Aim	Population
Clinical Assessment Confusion-A	Screening	Hospital ward
Confusion Rating Scale	Screening	Hospital ward
Delirium Observation Screening Scale	Screening	Hospital
Neelon/Champagne Confusion Scale	Screening	Hospital ward
Nursing Delirium Screening Scale	Screening	Hospital ward
Confusion Assessment Method (CAM)	Screening/Diagnosis	Hospital ward
CAM–ICU		Intensive care unit (ICU)
pCAM-ICU		Paediatric ICU
Nursing-Home CAM		Nursing home
Minimum Data Set CAM		Nursing home
Delirium Rating Scale–Revised-98	Diagnosis/Severity/Subtype	Hospital
Delirium Symptom Interview	Diagnosis/Subtype	Hospital ward
Memorial Delirium Assessment Scale	Diagnosis/Severity/Subtype	Hospital
Cogniteve Test for Delirium	Diagnosis	Hospital ward
RAI–MDS/RAI–LTCF	Diagnosis	Nursing home
Confusional State Evaluation	Severity	Hospital ward
Delirium Index	Severity	Hospital ward
Delirium Severity Scale	Severity	Hospital ward
Delirium motor subtype scale	Subtype	Palliative care
Dublin Delirium Assessment Scale	Subtype	Geriatric ward
Lipowski criteria	Subtype	Neuropsychiatric ward

Source data from *JAMA*. 304(7), Wong CL, Holroyd-Leduc J, Simel DL, *et al*. Does this patient have delirium?: value of bedside instruments, pp. 779–86, Copyright (2010), American Medical Association; *Int J Geriatr Psychiatry*. 20(7), de Rooij SE, Schuurmans MJ, van der Mast RC, *et al*. Clinical subtypes of delirium and their relevance for daily clinical practice: a systematic review, pp. 609–15, Copyright (2005), John Wiley and Sons; *Int Rev Psychiatry*, 21(1), Meagher D, Motor subtypes of delirium: past, present and future, pp. 59–73, Copyright (2009), Informa Healthcare.

Table 22.1 Confusion assessment method (CAM) algorithm

(1) acute onset and fluctuating course
-and-
(2) inattention
-and either-
(3) disorganized thinking
-or-
(4) altered level of consciousness

Reproduced from 2003 Hospital Elder Life Program, LLC with permission.

(see treatment section below) as well as for research purposes. Lack of a reproducible method to standardize classification for delirium subtypes has been an important limitation in the field.[20] Studies using actigraphy, devices that are capable of measuring the 24-hour motor activity patterns by measuring accelerations, have revealed psychomotoric differences between the subtypes, even in small samples of patients,[25] and when used together with a well-validated subtype scale, may yet prove useful in distinguishing the different subtypes. Currently, however, there is insufficient evidence linking specific phenomenology with aetiology, pathophysiology, management, course, and outcome.[26]

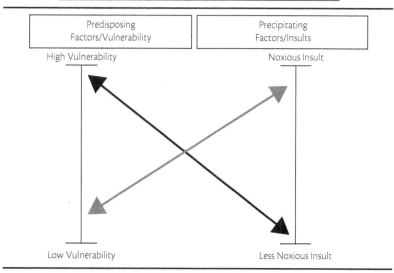

Fig. 22.1 Relationship between predisposing and precipitating factors.
Adapted from *JAMA*. 275(11), Inouye SK *et al*. Precipitating Factors for Delirium in Hospitalized Elderly Persons: Predictive Model and Interrelationship With Baseline Vulnerability, pp. 852–7, Copyright (1996), with permission from American Medical Association.

Predisposing and precipitating factors

Knowledge of the predisposing and precipitating factors is relevant for clinical practice and implementing appropriate prevention and treatment strategies. Fig. 22.1 describes the multiplicative relationship between predisposing and precipitating factors underlying the risk for delirium, as proposed by Inouye.[27,28] While a person with many predisposing factors will only need a minor trigger to develop delirium (e.g. an old patient with dementia experiencing a mild urinary tract infection), a person without predisposing factors requires a much more severe trigger (e.g. severe sepsis in a younger and otherwise fit patient).

This conceptual framework can be of assistance in guiding the search for one or more precipitating factors for the individual patient. Thus, in a relatively healthy person developing delirium, one relatively minor precipitating factor may not be sufficient explanation and other perhaps potentially more serious precipitants should be sought. Factors precipitating delirium can include any illness, medication, drug, or surgical procedure, but in a geriatric population infections, metabolic abnormalities, adverse drug effects, and cardiovascular events are the most common precipitants.[29] The exact underlying cause or trigger for delirium, however, often remains unknown and is multifactorial in over 50 per cent of cases.[30] Predisposing and precipitating factors overlap, and when investigated in a cross-sectional study design it may not be possible to distinguish causality from association.[31] Dehydration, for example, can be considered both a predisposing as well as a precipitating factor.

Recent literature tends to split risks for delirium into modifiable and non-modifiable factors, which makes sense from the point of view of prevention and (early) treatment. Risk factors identified in multiple studies include pre-existing cognitive impairment/dementia or functional impairment, increasing age, severity of disease, infection, fracture at admission, visual impairment, and the use of physical restraints.[31,32] With increasing age, the duration of delirium might be longer and the symptoms more severe.[31] Other

factors that are associated with a more serious course of delirium are ICU admission, change of rooms during hospitalization, and absence of help in orientation or provision of appropriate vision/hearing aids.[31] There are no indications that risk factors in nursing homes differ from those in hospitalized patients.[7]

With regard to medication, there are some indications that use of benzodiazepines and opioids lead to higher risk for delirium.[31] Controversy still exists about the exact role of benzodiazepines since they continue to be prescribed to sedate delirious patients, for instance in intensive care and palliative care.[8,33] Lorazepam and (to a lesser extent) midazolam have been shown to be associated with a slightly increased risk of delirium.[34] Diphenhydramine administration is associated with an increased risk of delirium with a dose-response relationship due to its anticholinergic activity.[35,36] All opiates can increase delirium risk, with meperidine a particularly high risk; conversely, the evidence implicating fentanyl, morphine and oxycodone is less strong.[34,36,37] Anticholinergic medications as a group are associated with a high risk of delirium.[38] Different scales to assess the anticholinergic burden of medication are available but the correlation between serum anticholinergic activity level and risk of delirium is uncertain.[39]

With respect to delirium in children, infection, use and withdrawal of medication, including anticholinergic agents and opioids, and young age are the most important risk factors.[40]

Pathophysiology

Despite a growing and widespread interest in delirium in elderly patients, relatively few research studies have attempted to elucidate the pathophysiology of delirium. This is likely to be a reflection of the specific methodological and ethical issues related to studies of the brain in a fluctuating neuropsychiatric disorder in persons with a (temporarily) impaired capacity to consent. Additionally, the underlying pathophysiological mechanisms may differ between the diverse subtypes of delirium and different aetiologies. Clinical observations in many different populations, biomarker studies in blood[41] as well as in cerebrospinal fluid (CSF)[42], and a recently developed rodent model[43] have resulted in several hypotheses being advanced to explain the processes.

Taking into account the multiple precipitating and predisposing factors, involvement of a number of interacting systems in the brain, leading to disturbance of a final common pathway, seems to be the most plausible explanation for the development of delirium.[44] The main candidates for this final common pathway are changes in the relative ratio of acetylcholine (decreased) and dopamine (increased). Thus, drugs or infections resulting in anticholinergic effects are well-recognized risk factors for delirium in elderly people; these effects may be also mediated via the lower anticholinergic activity associated with cognitive impairment (see chapters 32, 33, and 36) and higher age.[45,46]

Peripheral inflammation can influence the central nervous system (CNS) by a number of routes including the circumventricular organs (structures in the brain that are characterized by their extensive vasculature and lack of a normal blood–brain barrier), vagal afferents, and the brain endothelium forming the blood–brain barrier.[47] Activation of cerebral microglia is considered pivotal for mediation of the behavioural effects of systemic infections, and in this context delirium can be considered as an extreme form of sickness behaviour.[43,48–51] Sickness behaviour is a coordinated set of adaptive behavioural changes that develop in ill individuals during the course of an infection. Rodent studies have shown CNS inflammatory responses to acute inflammatory insults of peripheral origin are exaggerated both in the aged as in the neurodegenerative brain.[52,53] Decreasing cholinergic inhibition may cause normally protective microglial responses to become neurotoxic[46] and this may cause neuronal damage, reflected by biomarkers like (CSF) S100B.[54,55] This cascade could account for the strong association between delirium and its sequelae like long-term cognitive impairment, although associations between these markers and long-term outcomes are still lacking.

There is also growing evidence that dysregulation of the limbic–hypothalamic–pituitary–adrenal axis, with pathologically sustained high levels of cortisol occurring with acute stress, can play a mediating role.[51] Disruption of the sleep–wake cycle, another important characteristic of delirium, may be evoked by lower levels of tryptophan, serotonin, or melatonin, all hormones involved in the circadian rhythm,[56] which might be induced by a higher activity of indoleamine 2,3-dioxygenase.[57]

The two most important neurochemical systems involved in alcohol withdrawal are gamma-aminobutyric acid and glutamine. It is unknown whether both these neurosystems are involved in the pathophysiology of AWD as well, but it is notable that glutamine plays an important role in hepatic encephalopathy.[58]

Genetics

Information about heritability or predisposition to delirium is lacking. There are no known families with a high frequency of affected members nor in whom delirium occurs at younger age without serious precipitating factors. However, it is hypothesized that the heritability rate of delirium might be comparable to the estimated heritability of 30 per cent for the occurrence of any psychotic episode in late-onset Alzheimer's disease.[59] Genetic studies in delirium have been scarce until recently, due to the difficulties in establishing

the diagnosis and aetiology of the syndrome, and the pitfalls inherent in the design of genetic studies.[27,60] In AWD, positive associations were found in three different candidate genes involved in the dopamine transmission (dopamine receptor D3 (DRD3), the solute carrier family 6 (SLC6A3), and tyrosine hydroxylase); one gene involved in the glutamate pathway (glutamate receptor ionotropic kainate 3); one neuropeptide gene (brain-derived neurotrophic factor); and one cannabinoid gene (cannabinoid receptor 1).[61] In older patients with delirium, a meta-analysis suggested an association between delirium and possession of an APOE ε4 allele.[62] In independent cohorts, a variation in the SLC6A3 gene and possibly the DRD2 gene were found to be protective against delirium.[63] In one population, homozygous carriage of the BclI–TthIIII haplotype of the glucocorticoid receptor gene was associated with a reduced risk (92 per cent) of developing delirium.[64]

Treatment

Treatment of delirium and its symptoms can be classified in four parts, summarized in Table 22.3. The most important and first steps both for the prevention and treatment of delirium are well-proven *non-pharmacological* measures. These multidisciplinary, multicomponent interventions have been shown to reduce the incidence and duration of delirium in hospitalized patients and reduce functional decline in older patients.[65–69] Such interventions should focus on several domains, including addressing cognitive impairment or disorientation, sensory deprivation, sleep disturbance, limited mobility, dehydration, constipation, hypoxia, pain, poor nutrition, and medication use.[67,68,70] Optimal management requires implementation throughout the hospital on a 24/7 basis and actively promoting these interventions in patients at increased risk for delirium.[68,69]

The second step is to identify and treat the underlying disease or factors contributing to the delirium; for example, rectifying dehydration or commencing antibiotic therapy for a suspected infection.

Third, and only when patients are severely agitated or when they will not comply with steps one and two should antipsychotic medications be considered. When necessary, these should be started at the lowest possible dose. Evidence for their efficacy in the context of delirium, and specifically in the target group of vulnerable and often cognitively impaired patients in which it is most commonly used, is limited.[71] Haloperidol is still the first-choice medication for symptom reduction because it can be used orally, intramuscularly, and intravenously, and most experience both in research and in daily practice has been acquired with this antipsychotic. Antipsychotics have important side-effects such as extrapyramidal effects, sedation, increased risk of cerebrovascular accidents and mortality, and when used in high intravenous doses, *torsade des points* and other ventricular dysrhythmias have been decribed.[72–74] People with Lewy body dementia, Parkinson's disease, or parkinsonism should not be prescribed typical antipsychotic drugs because they are at particular risk of severe adverse reactions. Atypical antipsychotics have never been investigated for delirium, but clozapine has been shown to be effective for hallucinations in Parkinson's disease (NICE clinical guideline 35).

Whilst commonly used, the evidence to support the use of benzodiazepines in the treatment of non-alcohol withdrawal-related delirium among hospitalized patients is lacking, with some evidence of worsening or prolongation of delirium symptoms in HIV patients.[75,76] On the other hand, for AWD, benzodiazepines are the first choice of treatment as well as for prevention.[77] For delirium

Table 22.3 Work-up steps for delirium treatment (steps 1, 2, 3, and 4) and prevention in at-risk patients (primary step 1 and secondary step 4)

1. Non-medical measures*

- cognitive impairment or disorientation: appropriate lighting, clear signage, clock and calendar easily visible to the person, reorient verbally, introduce cognitively stimulating activities, facilitate visits from well-known persons
- dehydration: adequate fluid intake by encouraging patient to drink (by family)
- constipation: adequate fluid, dietary fibre, no opiates, laxatives
- hypoxia: optimize oxygen saturation
- limited mobility: mobilize soon as possible, if unable to walk carry out active range-of-motion exercises
- pain: look for (nonverbal) signs of pain, initiate and review appropriate pain management
- poor nutrition: adequate nutrition, ensure that dentures fit
- medication use: reduce anticholinergic medications
- sensory deprivation: resolve any reversible cause of the impairment, ensure hearing and visual aids are available and in good working order
- sleep disturbance: promote good sleep patterns and sleep hygiene

2. Identify and treat precipitating factors

- Medical history
- Medication review
- Physical examination (including neurological examination)
- Blood testing (as indicated by clinical judgement): renal function, glucose, infection parameters, haemoglobin
- Urinalysis

If not clarified by first screening, do a step-by-step more invasive diagnostic evaluation based on prior probability. Consider calcium, medication level, liver and thyroid function tests, culture, of urine, blood, sputum, EKG, chest X-ray, CT brain, etc.

3. Medical treatment

Only when patients are severely agitated or will interrupt essential medical therapies despite the first two steps:

antipsychotics (first choice haloperidol 0.25–0.50 mgs) in the lowest possible dose

4. Post-delirium treatment

- Evaluate impact of delirium episode for patient and family
- Perform cognitive tests for post-delirium cognitive impairment
- Critical medication review
- Limit risk factors as described in step 1

Source data from National Institute for Health and Care Excellence, Delirium: Diagnosis, prevention and management, Clinical Guideline 103, Copyright (2010), National Clinical Guideline Centre.

in the ICU, the evidence is even more limited both for pharmacological treatment and for pharmacological prevention.[78] Current evidence suggests that cholinesterase inhibitors may be contraindicated for prevention or treatment of delirium, at least in intensive care and surgical patients.[79,80]

Medication trials for the above populations did not discriminate in efficacy for the different subtypes. Experts doubt the benefit of antipsychotic medication for hypoactive delirium based on lack of evidence and the potential serious side-effects such as *torsades*.

Limited evidence is available for the prevention of (severe) delirium with antipsychotics or melatonin and they are not recommended at this time. There is no evidence that children with

delirium respond differently to antipsychotics compared to adults.[40] In palliative care, delirium is the most common indication for sedation.[81]

After delirium, patients should be followed intensively to counsel them about the episode, diagnose possible cognitive impairment, and limit risk factors for a new episode. A systematic intervention in elderly patients after a delirious state found that institutionalization could be delayed by using rehabilitation periods and case management.[82] Case management strives to provide proactive individualized care supported by a multidisciplinary team of providers of elderly care.

Prognosis

Adjusted for age, sex, comorbid illness or illness severity, and baseline dementia, delirium is associated with an increased risk of death compared with controls (hazard ratio (HR): 1.95 [95% confidence interval (CI), 1.51–2.52]).[83] Moreover, patients experiencing delirium are also at increased risk of institutionalization (odds ratio (OR): 2.41 [95% CI, 1.77–3.29]), or dementia (OR: 12.52 [95% CI, 1.86–84.21]),[28,83] and patients with Alzheimer's disease experiencing delirium have an increased rate of cognitive decline maintained for up to five years.[84,85]

Although patients usually recover after treatment of the precipitating factors, persistent delirium in older hospital patients is frequent (exact percentages are highly variable) especially in patients with pre-existing cognitive impairment. This persistence is associated with adverse outcomes and such individuals have a poor prognosis.[86]

Summary

Delirium is a serious neuropsychiatric syndrome caused by a variety of factors, with serious effects on overall outcome. Delirium and dementia overlap in many ways: the symptoms may overlap, delirium is a risk factor for developing dementia, and dementia increases the risk of delirium. Many avenues of future research exist in the delirium field.[87] From a pathophysiological perspective, the potential roles of inflammation and impaired cholinergic neurotransmission and the interactions between these two factors need further exploration and may provide opportunities for development of targeted preventive strategies. Determining the underlying pathophysiology and identifying specific biomarkers may explain the subtypes of delirium presentation and guide specific therapies. Current data support the use of nonpharmacological treatment protocols and in case of severe agitation antipsychotics. However, further randomized trials are required to evaluate other prevention and treatment strategies in populations stratified according to delirium risk, delirium subtype, or associated comorbid dementia, and to investigate whether or not pharmacologic treatments improve long-term outcomes following delirium.

References

1. Frederiks JA. Inflammation of the mind. On the 300th anniversary of Gerard van Swieten. *J Hist Neurosci.* 2000 Dec;9(3):307–10.
2. Engel GL and Romano J. Delirium, a syndrome of cerebral insufficiency. 1959. *J Neuropsychiatry Clin Neurosci.* 2004;16(4):526–38.
3. Folstein MF, Bassett SS, Romanoski AJ, et al. The epidemiology of delirium in the community: the Eastern Baltimore Mental Health Survey. *Int Psychogeriatr.* 1991;3(2):169–76.

4. Ely EW, Inouye SK, Bernard GR, *et al*. Delirium in mechanically ventilated patients: Validity and reliability of the confusion assessment method for the intensive care unit (CAM–ICU). *JAMA*. 2001 Dec 5;286(21):2703–10.

5. Young J, Murthy L, Westby M, *et al*. Diagnosis, prevention, and management of delirium: Summary of NICE guidance. *BMJ*. 2010;341:c3704.

6. Dosa D, Intrator O, McNicoll L, *et al*. Preliminary derivation of a Nursing Home Confusion Assessment Method based on data from the Minimum Data Set. *J Am Geriatr Soc*. 2007 Jul;55(7):1099–105.

7. Voyer P, Richard S, Doucet L, *et al*. Detection of delirium by nurses among long-term care residents with dementia. *BMC Nurs*. 2008;7:4.

8. Moyer DD. Review article: Terminal delirium in geriatric patients with cancer at end of life. *Am J Hosp Palliat Care*. 2011 Feb;28(1):44–51.

9. Mayo-Smith MF, Beecher LH, Fischer TL, *et al*. Management of alcohol withdrawal delirium. An evidence-based practice guideline. *Arch Intern Med*. 2004 Jul 12;164(13):1405–12.

10. Smith HA, Fuchs DC, Pandharipande PP, *et al*. Delirium: An emerging frontier in the management of critically ill children. *Anesthesiol Clin*. 2011 Dec;29(4):729–50.

11. Wong CL, Holroyd-Leduc J, Simel DL, *et al*. Does this patient have delirium? Value of bedside instruments. *JAMA*. 2010 Aug 18;304(7):779–86.

12. American Psychiatric Association. Diagnostic and Statistical Manual of Mental Disorders: DSM IV-TR. APA:Washington, DC, 2000.

13. Ely EW, Margolin R, Francis J, *et al*. Evaluation of delirium in critically ill patients: Validation of the Confusion Assessment Method for the Intensive Care Unit (CAM–ICU). *Crit Care Med*. 2001 Jul;29(7):1370–9.

14. Pfeiffer E. A short portable mental status questionnaire for the assessment of organic brain deficit in elderly patients. *J Am Geriatr Soc*. 1975 Oct;23(10):433–41.

15. Borson S, Scanlan JM, Chen P, *et al*. The Mini-Cog as a screen for dementia: Validation in a population-based sample. *J Am Geriatr Soc*. 2003 Oct;51(10):1451–4.

16. Nasreddine ZS, Phillips NA, Bedirian V, *et al*. The Montreal Cognitive Assessment, MoCA: A brief screening tool for mild cognitive impairment. *J Am Geriatr Soc*. 2005 Apr;53(4):695–9.

17. de Jonghe JF, Kalisvaart KJ, Dijkstra M, *et al*. Early symptoms in the prodromal phase of delirium: A prospective cohort study in elderly patients undergoing hip surgery. *Am J Geriatr Psychiatry*. 2007 Feb;15(2):112–21.

18. Trzepacz PT, Franco JG, Meagher DJ, *et al*. Phenotype of subsyndromal delirium using pooled multicultural Delirium Rating Scale—Revised-98 data. *J Psychosom Res*. 2012 Jul;73(1):10–7.

19. Turkel SB and Tavare CJ. Delirium in children and adolescents. *J Neuropsychiatry Clin Neurosci*. 2003;15(4):431–5.

20. de Rooij SE, Schuurmans MJ, van der Mast RC, *et al*. Clinical subtypes of delirium and their relevance for daily clinical practice: A systematic review. *Int J Geriatr Psychiatry*. 2005 Jul;20(7):609–15.

21. Meagher D. Motor subtypes of delirium: Past, present and future. *Int Rev Psychiatry*. 2009 Feb;21(1):59–73.

22. Michaud L, Bula C, Berney A, *et al*. Delirium: Guidelines for general hospitals. *J Psychosom Res*. 2007 Mar;62(3):371–83.

23. Meagher DJ and Trzepacz PT. Motoric subtypes of delirium. Semin Clin *Neuropsychiatry*. 2000 Apr;5(2):75–85.

24. Meagher DJ, Leonard M, Donnelly S, *et al*. A longitudinal study of motor subtypes in delirium: Relationship with other phenomenology, etiology, medication exposure and prognosis. *J Psychosom Res*. 2011 Dec;71(6):395–403.

25. van Uitert M, de Jonghe A, de Gijsel S, *et al*. Rest-activity patterns in patients with delirium. *Rejuvenation Res*. 2011 Oct;14(5):483–90.

26. Gupta N, de JJ, Schieveld J, Leonard M, *et al*. Delirium phenomenology: What can we learn from the symptoms of delirium? *J Psychosom Res*. 2008 Sep;65(3):215–22.

27. van Munster BC, de Rooij SE, and Korevaar JC. The role of genetics in delirium in the elderly patient. *Dement Geriatr Cogn Disord*. 2009;28(3):187–95.

28. Inouye SK. Delirium in older persons. *N Engl J Med*. 2006 Mar 16;354(11):1157–65.

29. Laurila JV, Laakkonen ML, Tilvis RS, *et al*. Predisposing and precipitating factors for delirium in a frail geriatric population. *J Psychosom Res*. 2008 Sep;65(3):249–54.

30. Webster R and Holroyd S. Prevalence of psychotic symptoms in delirium. *Psychosomatics*. 2000 Nov;41(6):519–22.

31. National Institute for Health and Clinical Excellence. DELIRIUM: Diagnosis, prevention and management. Clinical Guideline 103, 2010 Jul.

32. Korevaar JC, van Munster BC, and de Rooij SE. Risk factors for delirium in acutely admitted elderly patients: A prospective cohort study. *BMC Geriatr*. 2005 Apr 13;5(1):6.

33. Frontera JA. Delirium and sedation in the ICU. *Neurocrit Care*. 2011 Jun;14(3):463–74.

34. Pandharipande P and Ely EW. Sedative and analgesic medications: Risk factors for delirium and sleep disturbances in the critically ill. *Crit Care Clin*. 2006 Apr;22(2):313–27, vii.

35. Agostini JV, Leo-Summers LS, and Inouye SK. Cognitive and other adverse effects of diphenhydramine use in hospitalized older patients. *Arch Intern Med*. 2001 Sep 24;161(17):2091–7.

36. Marcantonio ER, Juarez G, Goldman L, *et al*. The relationship of postoperative delirium with psychoactive medications. *JAMA*. 1994 Nov 16;272(19):1518–22.

37. Morrison RS, Magaziner J, Gilbert M, *et al*. Relationship between pain and opioid analgesics on the development of delirium following hip fracture. *J Gerontol A Biol Sci Med Sci*. 2003 Jan;58(1):76–81.

38. Tune LE. Anticholinergic effects of medication in elderly patients. *J Clin Psychiatry*. 2001;62 Suppl 21:11–4.

39. Mangoni AA, van Munster BC, Woodman RJ, *et al*. Measures of Anticholinergic Drug Exposure, Serum Anticholinergic Activity, and All-cause Postdischarge Mortality in Older Hospitalized Patients With Hip Fractures. *Am J Geriatr Psychiatry*. 2012 May 28.

40. Creten C, Van Der Zwaan S, Blankespoor RJ, *et al*. Pediatric delirium in the pediatric intensive care unit: A systematic review and an update on key issues and research questions. *Minerva Anestesiol*. 2011 Nov;77(11):1099–107.

41. Marcantonio ER, Rudolph JL, Culley D, *et al*. Serum biomarkers for delirium. *J Gerontol A Biol Sci Med Sci*. 2006 Dec;61(12):1281–6.

42. Hall RJ, Shenkin SD, and Maclullich AM. A systematic literature review of cerebrospinal fluid biomarkers in delirium. *Dement Geriatr Cogn Disord*. 2011;32(2):79–93.

43. Cunningham C and Maclullich AM. At the extreme end of the psycho-neuroimmunological spectrum: Delirium as a maladaptive sickness behaviour response. *Brain Behav Immun*. 2012 Aug 3.

44. Trzepacz PT. Is there a final common neural pathway in delirium? Focus on acetylcholine and dopamine. *Semin Clin Neuropsychiatry*. 2000 Apr;5(2):132–48.

45. van Munster BC, Thomas C, Kreisel SH, *et al*. Longitudinal assessment of serum anticholinergic activity in delirium of the elderly. *J Psychiatr Res*. 2012 Oct;46(10):1339–45.

46. Van Gool WA, van de BD, and Eikelenboom P. Systemic infection and delirium: When cytokines and acetylcholine collide. *Lancet*. 2010 Feb 27;375(9716):773–5.

47. Dantzer R, O'Connor JC, Freund GG, *et al*. From inflammation to sickness and depression: When the immune system subjugates the brain. *Nat Neurosci*. 2008 Jan;9(1):46–56.

48. Munster BC, Aronica E, Zwinderman AH, E*et al*. Neuroinflammation in delirium: A postmortem case-control study. *Rejuvenation Res*. 2011 Dec;14(6):615–22.

49. Godbout JP, Chen J, Abraham J, *et al*. Exaggerated neuroinflammation and sickness behavior in aged mice following activation of the peripheral innate immune system. *FASEB*. J 2005 Aug;19(10):1329–31.

50. Cerejeira J, Firmino H, Vaz-Serra A, *et al*. The neuroinflammatory hypothesis of delirium. *Acta Neuropathol*. 2010 Jun;119(6):737–54.

51. Maclullich AM, Ferguson KJ, Miller T, *et al*. Unravelling the pathophysiology of delirium: A focus on the role of aberrant stress responses. *J Psychosom Res*. 2008 Sep;65(3):229–38.

52. Godbout JP and Johnson RW. Age and neuroinflammation: A lifetime of psychoneuroimmune consequences. *Immunol Allergy Clin North Am.* 2009 May;29(2):321–37.

53. Combrinck MI, Perry VH, and Cunningham C. Peripheral infection evokes exaggerated sickness behaviour in pre-clinical murine prion disease. *Neuroscience.* 2002;112(1):7–11.

54. van Munster BC, Bisschop PH, Zwinderman AH, *et al.* Cortisol, interleukins and S100B in delirium in the elderly. *Brain Cogn.* 2010 Oct;74(1):18–23.

55. van Munster BC, Korse CM, de Rooij SE, *et al.* Markers of cerebral damage during delirium in elderly patients with hip fracture. *BMC Neurol.* 2009;9:21.

56. de Jonghe A, Korevaar JC, van Munster BC, *et al.* Effectiveness of melatonin treatment on circadian rhythm disturbances in dementia. Are there implications for delirium? A systematic review. *Int J Geriatr Psychiatry.* 2010 Dec;25(12):1201–8.

57. de JA, van Munster BC, Fekkes D, *et al.* The tryptophan depletion theory in delirium: Not confirmed in elderly hip fracture patients. *Psychosomatics.* 2012 May;53(3):236–43.

58. Desjardins P, Du T, Jiang W, *et al.* Pathogenesis of hepatic encephalopathy and brain edema in acute liver failure: Role of glutamine redefined. *Neurochem Int.* 2012 Jun;60(7):690–6.

59. Bacanu SA, Devlin B, Chowdari KV, *et al.* Heritability of psychosis in Alzheimer disease. *Am J Geriatr Psychiatry.* 2005 Jul;13(7):624–7.

60. Adamis D, van Munster BC, and Macdonald AJ. The genetics of deliria. *Int Rev Psychiatry.* 2009 Feb;21(1):20–9.

61. van Munster BC, Korevaar JC, de Rooij SE, *et al.* Genetic polymorphisms related to delirium tremens: A systematic review. *Alcohol Clin Exp Res.* 2007 Feb;31(2):177–84.

62. van Munster BC, Korevaar JC, Zwinderman AH, *et al.* The association between delirium and the apolipoprotein E epsilon 4 allele: New study results and a meta-analysis. *Am J Geriatr Psychiatry.* 2009 Oct;17(10):856–62.

63. van Munster BC, de Rooij SE, Yazdanpanah M, *et al.* The association of the dopamine transporter gene and the dopamine receptor 2 gene with delirium, a meta-analysis. *Am J Med Genet B Neuropsychiatr Genet.* 2010 Mar 5;153B(2):648–55.

64. Manenschijn L, Van Rossum EF, Jetten AM, *et al.* Glucocorticoid receptor haplotype is associated with a decreased risk of delirium in the elderly. *Am J Med Genet B Neuropsychiatr Genet.* 2011 Jan 13.

65. Marcantonio ER, Flacker JM, Wright RJ, *et al.* Reducing delirium after hip fracture: a randomized trial. *J Am Geriatr Soc.* 2001 May;49(5):516–22.

66. Bo M, Martini B, Ruatta C, *et al.* Geriatric ward hospitalization reduced incidence delirium among older medical inpatients. *Am J Geriatr Psychiatry.* 2009 Sep;17(9):760–8.

67. Vidan MT, Sanchez E, Alonso M, *et al.* An intervention integrated into daily clinical practice reduces the incidence of delirium during hospitalization in elderly patients. *J Am Geriatr Soc.* 2009 Nov;57(11):2029–36.

68. Inouye SK, Bogardus ST, Jr, Charpentier PA, *et al.* A multicomponent intervention to prevent delirium in hospitalized older patients. *N Engl J Med.* 1999 Mar 4;340(9):669–76.

69. Inouye SK, Baker DI, Fugal P, *et al.* Dissemination of the hospital elder life program: Implementation, adaptation, and successes. *J Am Geriatr Soc.* 2006 Oct;54(10):1492–9.

70. O'Mahony R, Murthy L, Akunne A, *et al.* Synopsis of the National Institute for Health and Clinical Excellence guideline for prevention of delirium. *Ann Intern Med.* 2011 Jun 7;154(11):746–51.

71. Lonergan E, Britton AM, Luxenberg J, *et al.* Antipsychotics for delirium. *Cochrane Database Syst Rev.* 2007;(2):CD005594.

72. Recupero PR and Rainey SE. Managing risk when considering the use of atypical antipsychotics for elderly patients with dementia-related psychosis. *J Psychiatr Pract.* 2007 May;13(3):143–52.

73. Blom MT, Bardai A, van Munster BC, *et al.* Differential changes in QTc duration during in-hospital haloperidol use. *PLoS One.* 2011;6(9):e23728.

74. Mittal V, Kurup L, Williamson D, *et al.* Risk of cerebrovascular adverse events and death in elderly patients with dementia when treated with antipsychotic medications: A literature review of evidence. *Am J Alzheimers Dis Other Demen.* 2011 Feb;26(1):10–28.

75. Breitbart W, Marotta R, Platt MM, *et al.* A double-blind trial of haloperidol, chlorpromazine, and lorazepam in the treatment of delirium in hospitalized AIDS patients. *Am J Psychiatry.* 1996 Feb;153(2):231–7.

76. Lonergan E, Luxenberg J, Areosa SA, *et al.* Benzodiazepines for delirium. *Cochrane Database Syst Rev.* 2009;(1):CD006379.

77. Amato L, Minozzi S, Vecchi S, *et al.* Benzodiazepines for alcohol withdrawal. *Cochrane Database Syst Rev.* 2010;(3):CD005063.

78. Bledowski J and Trutia A. A review of pharmacologic management and prevention strategies for delirium in the intensive care unit. *Psychosomatics.* 2012 May;53(3):203–11.

79. van Eijk MM, Roes KC, Honing ML, *et al.* Effect of rivastigmine as an adjunct to usual care with haloperidol on duration of delirium and mortality in critically ill patients: A multicentre, double-blind, placebo-controlled randomised trial. *Lancet.* 2010 Nov 27;376(9755):1829–37.

80. Gamberini M, Bolliger D, Lurati Buse GA, *et al.* Rivastigmine for the prevention of postoperative delirium in elderly patients undergoing elective cardiac surgery—a randomized controlled trial. *Crit Care Med.* 2009 May;37(5):1762–8.

81. Maltoni M, Scarpi E, Rosati M, *et al.* Palliative sedation in end-of-life care and survival: a systematic review. *J Clin Oncol.* 2012 Apr 20;30(12):1378–83.

82. Rahkonen T, Eloniemi-Sulkava U, Paanila S, *et al.* Systematic intervention for supporting community care of elderly people after a delirium episode. *Int Psychogeriatr.* 2001 Mar;13(1):37–49.

83. Witlox J, Eurelings LS, de Jonghe JF, *et al.* Delirium in elderly patients and the risk of postdischarge mortality, institutionalization, and dementia: A meta-analysis. *JAMA.* 2010 Jul 28;304(4):443–51.

84. Weiner MF. Impact of Delirium on the Course of Alzheimer Disease. *Arch Neurol.* 2012 Sep 17;1–2.

85. Gross AL, Jones RN, Habtemariam D, *et al.* Delirium and Long-term Cognitive Trajectory Among Persons With Dementia. *Arch Intern Med.* 2012;In Press.

86. Cole MG, Ciampi A, Belzile E, *et al.* Persistent delirium in older hospital patients: A systematic review of frequency and prognosis. *Age Ageing.* 2009 Jan;38(1):19–26.

87. Fong TG, Tulebaev SR, and Inouye SK. Delirium in elderly adults: Diagnosis, prevention and treatment. *Nat Rev Neurol.* 2009 Apr;5(4):210–20.

CHAPTER 23

CNS infections

Sam Nightingale, Benedict Daniel Michael, and Tom Solomon

Acute central nervous system infection

Acute central nervous system (CNS) infections can be broadly divided into infections involving the meninges, 'meningitis', those affecting the brain parenchyma, 'encephalitis', and those with discrete space occupying lesions such as brain abscesses.[1] Meningitis and encephalitis are most frequently caused by viral and bacterial infection, but fungi and parasites can occasionally be responsible, particularly in the immunocompromised.[1,2] These pathogens have multiple acute clinical manifestations, often affecting various cognitive domains. In addition to acute CNS disorders, sequaelae of CNS damage sustained at the time of infection can lead to long-term cognitive dysfunction.

Epidemiology

Common viral infections causing meningitis, include enteroviruses, which are acquired by faeco-oral transmission, other viruses acquired by respiratory droplet spread, such as the influenza family, and those acquired sexually, such as herpes simplex virus (HSV) type 2, which may be recurrent. The most common viral cause of sporadic encephalitis is HSV type 1 reactivation, following acquisition early in childhood via droplet spread.[2] Globally, the most common cause of epidemic viral encephalitis is currently Japanese encephalitis virus despite ongoing vaccination programmes.[3]

Bacterial CNS infections are typically limited to the meninges, however there may be some para-meningeal parenchymal inflammation. In the developed world, these are typically caused by *Streptococcus pneumoniae* and *Haemophilus influenza* which often follow or co-present with an upper respiratory tract infection.[4] The other major bacterial cause of meningitis is *Neisseria meningitides*, which is a particularly common cause of meningitis across the 'meningitis belt' of Africa, from Senegal to Ethiopia.[88]

Clinical features

Classically, meningitis presents with an acute febrile illness associated with headache, nausea and vomiting, photophobia, rashes and signs of meningeal irritation, such as neck stiffness, Kernig's and Brudzinski's signs.[4] In contrast, on admission 10–15 per cent of patients with viral encephalitis will not be febrile, and in febrile cases the fever will be of a lower grade or intermittent.[2,3] In addition, patients typically have a headache, which may be severe; nausea and vomiting, and signs of meningeal irritation. Whilst there is clearly some clinical overlap, and indeed in some cases there is histological overlap too, clinical features reflecting parenchymal inflammation are more suggestive of encephalitis than meningitis. These include focal neurological signs and alterations in consciousness, cognition, personality, and/or behaviour.[2]

Acute cognitive presentations in patients with encephalitis due to HSV type 1 may reflect temporal lobe involvement such as dysphasia, or features reflecting frontal lobe involvement, such as aggressive and socially inappropriate behaviour (Fig. 23.1). In addition, features reflecting involvement of the limbic system such as impaired short-term memory and/or emotional lability may be seen in limbic encephalitis, which may be due to HSV, other viral infections or antibody-mediated disease.[2]

With the exception of the pathognomonic non-blanching, petechial rash of meningococcal septicaemia, there are no clinical features or specific cognitive syndromes which can definitively determine the aetiological agent in a patient with meningitis or encephalitis.

Investigation

Whilst there is no established gold-standard tool, initial bedside investigations should include assessment of cognition and consciousness. In many cases, even of encephalitis, the Glasgow Coma Score (GCS) may be normal and the clinician must instead actively look for changes in cognition, personality, and behaviour; consequently a collateral history is invaluable.[2] A travel history is vital as many infections have geographical limitations.[3]

Investigation involves prompt lumbar puncture with gram stain, culture, and polymerase chain reaction (PCR) of cerebrospinal fluid (CSF).[2] Neuroimaging may be helpful but should not delay lumbar puncture unless there are clear clinical contraindications, including focal neurological weakness, significant reduction in the GCS (<13 or fall of >2), seizures, immunocompromise, or signs of raised intracranial pressure (e.g. papilloedema, Cushing's reflex).[4] National UK guidelines recommend that all patients should be tested for human immunodeficiency virus (HIV) as both seroconversion and opportunistic infection can cause acute CNS infection.[5]

Management

Prompt treatment is essential to limit sequelae. Initial management involves stabilizing the patient; this may necessitate controlling seizures and/or airway management. Where possible, antimicrobial treatment should be postponed until the lumbar puncture (LP) has been performed. However, if there will be delays beyond 30 minutes from admission for antibiotics and beyond 6 hours for acyclovir,

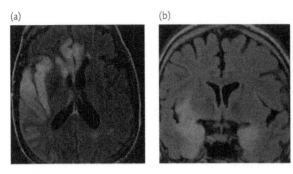

Fig. 23.1 (a) Sagittal FLAIR MRI of a patient with encephalitis due to herpes simplex virus 1 demonstrating oedema of the left temporal lobe and medial frontal lobes bilaterally with effacement of the sulci and compression of the lateral ventricles. (b) Coronal FLAIR MRI of a patient with encephalitis due to herpes simplex virus 1 demonstrating asymmetric oedema of both temporal lobes, greater on the right.
Courtesy of Dr Ian Turnbull.

then these treatments should be started before the LP.[2,6] Aciclovir has virostatic activity against HSV and, to a lesser extent, varicella zoster virus, and is therefore started empirically whilst the results of the virological investigations are awaited in patients with suspected encephalitis. Antibiotics should follow local protocols, but typically involve a third-generation cephalosporin, with the addition of amoxicillin in those aged >50 years, or who are pregnant or alcoholic, to cover *listeria monocytogenes*.[6]

Sequelae of infection

Bacterial meningitis continues to be associated with 15 per cent mortality. If there are delays or failure to start treatment in HSV encephalitis, the mortality can be >70 per cent and, whilst this can be reduced to <20–30 per cent if aciclovir is started early, at least 60 per cent of survivors will have significant neurological disability.[2] In addition to consequent epilepsy, the most common complaints following all causes of encephalitis are short-term memory problems, difficulty sustaining concentration, speech disturbance, and behavioural disorders.[7] Features most commonly reported in HSV encephalitis include cognitive impairments, such as receptive and/or expressive dysphasia, frontal lobe features, such as perseveration, impulsivity, and social disinhibition. If the limbic system is involved, there may be ongoing emotional liability and anterograde amnesia. However, encephalitis can result in any syndrome of cognitive impairment depending on both aetiology and the region of the brain affected. Notably, previously acquired skills such as musical ability may be retained, and interestingly there is evidence that some patients who otherwise have anterograde amnesia may be able to learn new music.[8] However, whilst others retain some of their premorbid skill sets, implicit long-term memory may not be coordinated with declarative memory and working memory for them to adjust their existent skills to new scenarios.[9]

There is some evidence that the certain markers of global cognitive performance may be more severe in patients with HSV encephalitis in comparison to those with other aetiologies.[10] There may be some association between post-encephalitis depression and some aspects of cognitive and interpersonal anxiety, and this may be greatest in those with impaired insight into their condition. In addition, some patients suffer with phobic anxiety and compulsive behaviours, which may be present in the absence of significant cognitive impairment.[11]

Impairments suffered during the acute insult may subsequently show improvements or may remain static. Children with encephalitis due to enterovirus infection may more frequently return to baseline levels.[12] Progression of symptoms following acute infectious encephalitis is unusual and should prompt investigation into other causes, such antibody-associated encephalitis, neoplastic processes, or a progressive post-infectious phenomena such as subacute sclerosing panencephalitis (discussed below).[13–15]

Subacute central nervous system infection

Cognitive impairment forms part of the presentation of several subacute CNS infections. In some cases, cognitive features may be the predominant symptoms at presentation. The most important causes are discussed below. In addition, many of the causes of acute CNS infection can present subacutely in patients with significant immunocompromise.[2]

Tuberculosis

Epidemiology

Approximately one-third of the world's population has been infected with *mycobacterium tuberculosis*.[16] The disease is endemic to many parts of the world, in particular in developing countries in Africa and Asia.

Pathogenesis

CNS infection occurs in 5–15 per cent of active tuberculosis cases. This is most commonly due to reactivation of latent infection in adults, but may occur as a complication of primary infection, particularly in children.[17]

Clinical features

Confusion, decreased consciousness, and impairment in a number of cognitive domains may occur in addition to the typical features of fever, headache, and meningism.[2] Presentation is highly variable and cognitive features may initially be the predominant feature; fever may only be present in approximately two-thirds of patients.[17]

Investigation

If tuberculosis is suspected larger volumes of CSF should be collected—ideally at least 6 ml—for there to be sufficient sensitivity of staining, extended culture, and PCR.[2] Some have also demonstrated the use of CSF lactate levels to distinguish TB meningitis from other causes of meningitis, and in distinguishing bacterial from viral infection, although this may not be routinely available.[89–91] In areas with limited available investigations, some have advocated the use of composite scores of clinical and laboratory features, such as the Thwaites criteria,[17] to guide management. Magnetic resonance imaging is more sensitive than computed tomography, and may identify meningeal gandolinium enhancement, with a predilection for the basal meninges, parenchymal tuberculomas, oedema, and hydrocephalus (Fig. 23.2).

Management

Decisions regarding appropriate antituberculous treatment should be made in conjunction with local microbiological and infectious disease teams, but a typical regime would include isoniazid,

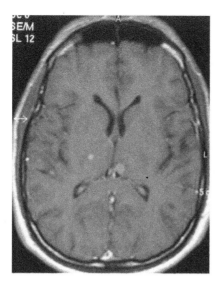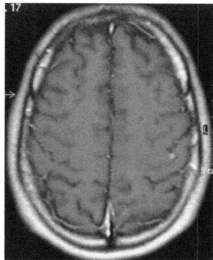

Fig. 23.2 Gadolinium enhanced T1 MRI of a patient with tuberculous meningitis showing leptomeningeal enhancement, and enhancing nodules in thalamus, basal ganglia, and sulci.

rifampicin, pyrazinamide, and streptomycin. The patient should be watched closely for signs of hydrocephalus, which may necessitate neurosurgical intervention, such as emergency extraventricular shunt insertion.[6] The prognosis is worse in those with delayed access to therapy and with comorbid conditions such as alcoholism and diabetes.[17] Dexomethasone is recommended in the acute phase for those with and without HIV co-infection, although the strongest evidence is in the latter group.[92]

Subacute sclerosing panencephalitis

Epidemiology

Subacute sclerosing panencephalitis (SSPE) is a rare, late complication of infection with the measles virus typically described in areas with poor vaccine uptake, with an incidence ranging between 0.01 cases per million in the United States (US) and 21 per million in India.[2,18] It is estimated that there are 4–11 cases of SSPE for every 100 000 cases of clinical measles infection. The highest incidence is in those who have the primary infection when aged under 5 years, and may be as high as 360 per 100 000 in those aged under 1 year at the time of primary infection.[18] There is also a higher risk of developing SSPE in males.

Pathogenesis

The pathophysiology remains poorly understood but is thought to involve an immune response to primary infection that is predominantly humoral rather than cellular, and results in latent viral infection in neurons and the development of highly mutated viruses.[18]

Clinical features

Patients usually present between 8–11 years old, approximately 6 years after primary infection. Symptoms initially begin with intellectual decline and consequent poor educational activity, associated with personality and behavioural changes. During this period, or sometimes in the preceding two years, there may be early visual symptoms, such as visuospatial disorientation. Within six months this progresses to include motor features which begin as repetitive and frequent myoclonic jerks, sometimes with abrupt-onset periodic dystonic myoclonus, and progress to extrapyramidal features,

including rigidity. During this period, focal and/or generalized seizures often develop and the patient progresses towards a state of akinetic mutism, autonomic failure, vegetative state, coma and death.[18] Nevertheless, approximately 10 per cent will present with a more accelerated phenotype with significant neurological deficit within three months and death within six months.

SSPE may also present in adults, usually around 20 years of age, with visual symptoms typically dominating for 2–5 years before motor involvement.

Investigation

The diagnosis requires the presence of an appropriate clinical phenotype with evidence of intrathecal anti-measles antibodies, although MRI and EEG findings may also be supportive. CSF-serum IgG ratios of anti-measles IgG range from 5–40:1. MRI may be normal in the early stages and does not correlate with the clinical stage but rather the duration of the disease. There may initially be cortical and subcortical hyperintensities on T2 images, progressing to involve the thalamus and basal ganglia, and then periventricular white matter lesions and cortical atrophy and the progressive atrophy of the brainstem and deep structures. Many EEG features have been described, with the most common being stereotyped bilateral synchronous, but asymmetrical, periodic complexes (Fig. 23.3). These are highly stereotyped within an individual but differ between patients. Background cerebral activity between complexes is normal initially, with increasing slow activity and then attenuation in later stages. In cases in which there is diagnostic uncertainty, a brain biopsy may be required for definitive diagnosis.

Management

SSPE is a severe progressive neurological infection resulting in death in 94–95 per cent of patients, with the remaining 5–6 per cent developing spontaneous remission, which is more common in adults. Combination therapy with intrathecal interferon alpha and oral isoprinosine is generally recommended, but well-standardized randomized controlled trials (RCTs) are still needed, as despite current therapy, most patients die within three years. The single

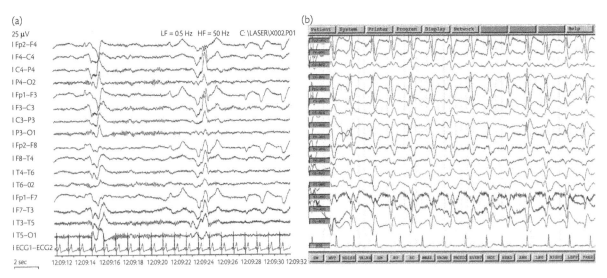

Fig. 23.3 (a) The characteristic electroencephalograph (EEG) picture in SSPE demonstrating stereotyped high-voltage periodic complexes, here at a frequency of 0.3 hertz. In contrast, EEG (b) shows complexes occurring at around 1 hertz in sporadic Creutzfeldt–Jakob disease.
Reproduced from *J Neurol Neurosur Ps.* 76(suppl.2), SJ Smith. EEG in the diagnosis, classification, and management of patients with epilepsy, pp. ii2–7, Copyright (2005), with permission from BMJ Publishing Group Ltd.

intervention with greatest impact to reduce the burden of SSPE is improving access to healthcare and comprehensive vaccination programmes.

Progressive multifocal leukoencephalopathy

Progressive multifocal leukoencephalopathy (PML) is a demyelinating condition due to John Cunningham (JC) virus infection in association with immunosuppression.

Epidemiology

Most cases of PML occur in HIV-positive individuals and PML is an AIDS-defining condition. Prior to antiretroviral therapy, PML occurred in around 5 per cent of people with HIV prior to death.[19] Incidence has decreased in areas where antiretroviral treatment is available, although prevalence has increased with improved survival. PML occurs disproportionately in HIV compared to other forms of immunosuppression,[20] but can occur in those with severe immunodeficiency such as transplant recipients,[21] and is becoming an increasingly common complication of monoclonal antibody treatment, and in particular of Natalizumab for multiple sclerosis.[22]

Pathogenesis

JC virus causes central demyelination through destruction of oligodendrocytes and myelin processes. Typically this process is characterized by lack of inflammation, although inflammatory forms do occur, particularly in association with immune reconstitution.[23]

Clinical features

Typically there is an insidious onset of focal neurological deficit without headache, fever, or meningism. Cognitive deficits occur in around one-third of cases, usually alongside focal neurology, but may be the sole presenting feature, particularly in those with bifrontal lesions. Seizures occur in 20 per cent.[19]

Investigation

Demonstration of JC viral DNA in the CSF in those with an appropriate clinical syndrome is highly specific for PML. Sensitivity of viral PCR is greater than 70 per cent; this increases with progression of disease so lumbar puncture should be repeated if initial tests are negative but clinical suspicion remains high.

MRI shows characteristic multifocal white matter lesions corresponding to the areas of clinical deficits (Fig. 23.4). Typically there is no mass effect or contrast enhancement. PML lesions can be distinguished from the white matter changes of HIV-associated dementia by the asymmetry, lack of atrophy, and involvement of the subcortical U-fibres.

Management

There is currently no specific treatment of PML.[22] A number of agents with *in vitro* effect against JC virus have not proved efficacious in clinical trials.[24]

Treatment involves correcting immunosuppression. Without this, PML is invariably fatal, usually within months of diagnosis. In those with PML secondary to HIV infection, antiretroviral treatment can stabilize disease, sometimes for months or years.[25] Cases of PML secondary to monoclonal antibody treatment should receive plasma exchange, and other causes of immunosuppression should be corrected if possible.[22] Rapid improvements in immune function may lead to a paradoxical worsening of clinical disease associated with inflammation and swelling of lesions. This is termed immune reconstitution inflammatory syndrome (IRIS) and can be managed with corticosteroids.

Neuroborreliosis

Epidemiology

Borrelia are zoonotic spirochetes transmitted by the bite of an infected tick. Several species causing Lyme disease are prevalent in woodland and heath areas across Europe, Russia, and parts of Asia and North America. Transmission occurs to a lesser degree in the UK, particularly in the New Forest of Hampshire and the Scottish highlands.

Clinical features

Initial infection produces the typical erythema migrans rash, although this is not invariably present and may have gone unnoticed

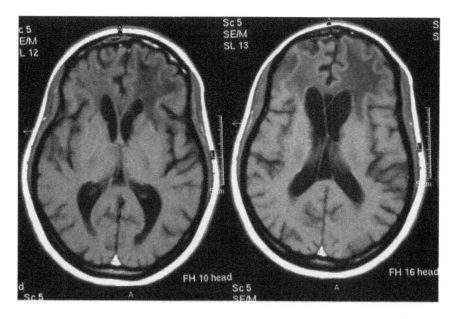

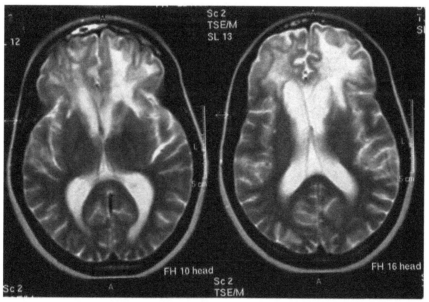

Fig. 23.4 T1- and T2-weighted MRI demonstrating extensive bifrontal demyelination due to progressive multifocal leukoencephalopathy secondary to immunosuppressive treatment post renal transplant.

by the patient. Neurological involvement occurs in around 35 per cent of European cases, but is less common in American strains of *Borrelia*. Neurological involvement is typically with subacute meningitis with or without facial palsy, painful radiculitis (Bannwarth's syndrome) or transverse myelitis in the weeks to months following initial infection. Myalgia, arthralgia, fatigue, and malaise are common. Acute encephalitis due to *Borellia* is uncommon but encephalopathy can occur, particularly in those in whom infection has persisted for long periods without treatment. Cognitive problems include deficits in processing speed, visual and verbal memory, and executive/attention functions.[26]

Investigation

The spirochete is rarely demonstrated in the CSF or other tissues and diagnosis is by the detection of specific antibodies to *Borrelia* in the CSF and serum. Relative levels of antibody between the CSF and serum can be used to calculate an antibody index; an index of over 1 suggests intrathecal synthesis of antibodies directed against spirochaetes.

Management

Treatment is with parenteral cephalosporin or oral doxycycline for 2–4 weeks.[27]

Neurobrucellosis

Epidemiology

Brucellosis is a highly contagious zoonosis endemic to many Mediterranean countries, South and Central America, Eastern Europe, Asia, Africa, the Caribbean, and the Middle East. It is the most common zoonosis in the world accounting for 500 000 human cases annually.[28] Transmission has been described in the UK but is rare and most human cases are acquired abroad. *Brucella* species are transmitted to humans by ingestion of unsterilized milk or cheese, or by close contact with infected animals.

Clinical features

Clinical features are diverse and include prolonged fever, cough, constitutional symptoms, arthritis, hepatosplenomegaly, and endocarditis. Neurological involvement occurs in 3–5 per cent of cases, usually after a period of untreated acute brucellosis.[29] The most common presentation is with diffuse encephalopathy or meningoencephalitis occurring in approximately 50 per cent of neurobrucellosis cases. Multiple cortical functions are affected with varying degrees of headache, meningism, and decreased conciousness. Seizures can occur. Other manifestations of neurobrucellosis include inflammatory transverse myelitis, polyradiculoneuritis, cranial nerve palsies, cerebral demyelination, and neuropsychiatric syndromes.[30]

Investigation

Brucella species are slow-growing fastidious organisms and culture of CSF or blood is rarely positive. Serological diagnosis is by ELISA or serum and CSF agglutination (STA) tests. IgM antibody titres rise during the first one to three weeks following infection and IgG after four weeks. Endemic areas have relatively high background positivity of *Brucella* IgG, and in such cases a fourfold rise or fall should be demonstrated.

Management

Treatment for neurological disease is typically with two to four weeks of doxycycline and rifampicin with or without streptomycin or a third-generation cephalosporin.

Chronic central nervous system infection

Some pathogens infect the CNS chronically to cause dementia syndromes. Pathogens such as HIV or *treponema pallidum* may have infected the CNS for a decade or more before presentation with cognitive impairment. However, it is important to note that although the CNS infection is chronic, presentation of the cognitive syndrome may have a relatively acute onset.

Human immunodeficiency virus

HIV-associated dementia describes a syndrome of marked cognitive impairment that occurs in advanced disease, usually at CD4 counts less than 200, and is an AIDS-defining illness. It is due to HIV infection itself rather than the effect of opportunistic infection. Since combination antiretroviral therapy has been widely available in the West the incidence of HAD has declined, however, more subtle neurocognitive impairments remain prevalent and are discussed separately.

HIV-associated dementia

Terminology

The terminology around HIV-associated dementia (HAD) can be confusing.

- HIV encephalopathy (HIVE) and AIDS dementia complex describe severe impairment and are synonymous with HAD.

- HIV encephalitis is the neuropathological correlate of HAD, but this term is also sometimes used to describe the syndrome.

- HIV can cause an acute meningoencephalitis at seroconversion which can be severe, leading to seizures and coma.[31] Confusingly, this is also sometimes referred to as 'HIV encephalitis' due to clinical similarities with acute viral encephalitis, but it is an entirely different syndrome.

In this chapter, we use HAD to describe severe impairment and HIV encephalitis for its neuropathological correlate. Specific discussion of HIV-meningoencephalitis at seroconversion is beyond the scope of this chapter.

Epidemiology

Approximately 34 million people are infected with human immunodeficiency virus (HIV) type 1 globally.[32] In the UK, over 90 000 people are infected, a quarter of whom are unaware of their diagnosis, and the number of new infections continues to rise.[33] Prior to antiretroviral therapy, dementia was common and affected up to 50 per cent prior to death.[34] HAD is now uncommon in those stable on antiretroviral treatment, but occurs in those failing treatment, or as the first presentation of HIV infection in advanced disease. Importantly, HIV frequently presents in its late stages as unexplained cognitive impairment in a young person, with or without obvious risk factors, and all such patients should be offered a HIV test as routine.[5]

Pathogenesis

HIV enters the brain early in infection via infected macrophages and monocytes. Pathologically, activated macrophages and astrocytes, sometimes with multinucleated giant cells, are seen in brain parenchyma (Fig. 23.5). Infection persists within the CNS in perivascular macrophages and microglia, although direct neuronal infection is rare.[35] Pro-inflammatory cytokines and toxic viral products cause blood–brain barrier breakdown, rarefaction of white matter, astrocyte apoptosis, dendritic simplification, and neuronal loss.[36] Subcortical structures such as basal ganglia and the hippocampus appear to be the most vulnerable.[37]

Clinical features

HAD is associated with a slowly progressive decline in cognition associated with motor slowing and spasticity. As it primarily affects the subcortical white matter, it classically has a subcortical dementia phenotype with a combination of cognitive and motor impairment. Features may include bradykinesia, pyramidal signs, predominant apathy, social withdrawal, and emotional blunting.

Early symptoms include forgetfulness and inability to concentrate, as well as personality changes such as apathy, diminished libido, emotional lability, and depression. Individuals may withdraw from social activities or have difficulty managing the financial and administrative aspects of their life. In moderate disease, motor abnormalities become more prominent, particularly slowing and impairment of fine movements (e.g. typing, buttoning up). Disturbance of gait, leg weakness, tremor, and ataxia may occur. Late features include psychiatric disturbances, mutism, paraplegia, seizures, incontinence, myoclonus and frontal release signs.

Differential diagnosis

HAD is a diagnosis of exclusion and multiple CNS pathologies may coexist. In HAD, symptoms typically develop slowly over the course of weeks or months. Rapidly developing symptoms should warrant investigation for a different aetiology, particularly if associated with impairment of consciousness, headache, or neck stiffness which are

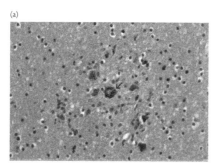
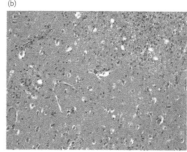

Fig. 23.5 (a) High-power microscopic view of a section of brain from a child with HIV encephalitis. A multinucleate giant cell is arrowed. (b) Parenchymal inflammatory infiltrates in a patient with encephalitis due to herpes simplex virus 1.

(a) Courtesy of the Wellcome Library, reproduced under the Creative Commons CC BY- NC 4.0 License. (b) Courtesy of Daniel Crooks.

not features of HAD. There should be a low threshold for lumbar puncture to exclude infections such as neurosyphilis, cryptococcal meningitis, tuberculous meningitis, Epstein–Barr virus related primary CNS lymphoma, or encephalitis due to varicella zoster, cytomegalovirus, or Epstein–Barr virus (see Table 23.1).

Marked generalized weakness and spasticity occurring before cognitive impairment is advanced is unusual and should also prompt investigation for other causes such as HIV-associated vacuolar myelopathy or human T-lymphotropic virus-1 (HTLV-1) infection causing tropical spastic paraparesis. Focal neurological signs do not occur in HAD and may be related to cerebral toxoplasmosis, primary CNS lymphoma, or progressive multifocal leucoencephalopathy.

Both antiretroviral medications and HIV infection itself can cause endothelial dysfunction and accelerated atherosclerosis. Stroke and vascular dementia are more common in HIV.[38] Subcortical arteriosclerotic encephalopathy can mimic HAD.

Metabolic, endocrine, and nutritional disorders may occur in HIV. Electrolytes, renal and hepatic function, blood count, B12/folate levels, and thyroid function should be routinely checked.

Mood should always be assessed in any HIV-positive individual presenting with cognitive symptoms. Depression and anxiety are common and may occur in over 50 per cent of those infected with HIV.[39] Substance misuse should also be excluded.

Investigation

Neuroimaging

MRI may show large, confluent periventricular lesions, hyperintense and relatively symmetrical in the white matter, with atrophy representing leukoencephalopathy. However, none of these findings are specific for HAD and the disease may be present with a normal MRI. Although there may be some faint symmetrical contrast enhancement symmetrically in the basal ganglia, oedema, space-occupying lesions and frank asymmetry of the white matter are not typical for HAD and should raise suspicion of other conditions (Fig. 23.6).

Lumbar puncture

CSF analysis is normal or shows a mild pleocytosis, rarely exceeding $50 \times 10^6/l$. Total protein and albumin concentrations may be slightly elevated due to blood–brain barrier disruption. Oligoclonal bands are often present, matched or unmatched in the serum; however, this is nonspecific and frequently found in the asymptomatic stages of HIV infection. In the pre-antiretroviral therapy era, greater levels of HIV RNA in the CSF was associated with HAD.[40,41]

Management

Many individuals with HAD improve when commenced on antiretroviral medications.[42,43] This response can be quite marked and some individuals return to independence following treatment; however, response is variable and some show only modest improvement. Several adjunctive anti-inflammatory treatments have been assessed but none has shown clinical benefit to date. Choice of antiretroviral treatment should be based on clinical factors, side-effects, efficacy, tolerability, and resistance profile of the virus. Some antiretroviral drugs achieve higher levels in CSF, however at present there is no strong evidence for benefit of these drugs in patients with HAD.[5,44] Opinion varies as to whether to prescribe antiretroviral treatment to patients with HAD on the basis of CNS penetration.[93]

Mild cognitive impairment in HIV

Milder forms of cognitive impairment that do not meet criteria for HAD occur in HIV infection. The full spectrum of cognitive impairment in HIV has been classified under the 'Frascati criteria' (Fig. 23.7).[45] Individuals falling at least one standard deviation from norms in at least two cognitive domains are classified as impaired. These patients are further divided into asymptomatic neurocognitive impairment (ANI) or mild neurocognitive impairment (MND), depending on whether it has a functional impact on daily activities. Along with HAD, these are referred to collectively as HIV-associated neurocognitive disorders (HANDs). ANI is currently a term used in research studies and the clinical consequences of ANI remain to be defined.

Epidemiology

Since effective antiretroviral therapy (ART) has been available, the incidence of HAD has dramatically decreased in countries with access to this treatment.[46] However, milder forms of cognitive impairment remain common despite treatment.[47] These milder forms of cognitive impairment may be very common. US and European cohort studies have suggested neurocognitive impairment may be present in 20–50 per cent of HIV-infected subjects, even those on stable antiretroviral therapy.[48–50] Although mild, these subtle impairments represent a significant clinical problem as they have been shown to affect basic daily activities such as driving, shopping, medication adherence, and financial management, as well as being associated with unemployment and a poorer quality of life.[51] As such, cognitive impairment in HIV is an increasingly concerning limitation of ART.

Table 23.1 Neurological infections causing cognitive impairment

Disease	Pathogen	Comments
Acute presentation		
Viral encephalitis	Herpes simplex virus type 1 or 2, varicella zoster virus, enteroviruses and others	Acute encephalitis with current or antecedent febrile illness with headache, seizures, and/or changes in behaviour, personality, cognition, or consciousness. Neurocognitive sequelae may follow
Bacterial menigitis	*Streptococcus pneumonae, Haemophillus influenza, Neisseria meningitides* and others	Acute meningitis with fever, neck stiffness, headache, vomiting, and photophobia. Neurocognitive sequelae may follow
Subacute or chronic presentation		
HIV-associated dementia and milder forms of cognitive impairment	Human immunodeficiency virus	HIV-associated dementia may be first presentation. Cognitive impairment remains prevelant despite antiretroviral therapy
Neurosyphilis	*Treponema pallidium*	CNS can be affected at any stage of infection. Dementia from general paresis is late complication
Tuberculous meningitis	*Mycobacterium tuberculosis*	Usually in the context of fever, meningism, and/or cranial neuropathy. Intracerebral lesions may coexist
Subacute sclerosing panencephalitis	Measles virus	Rare late complication of infection with the measles virus
Neuroborreliosis	*Borrellia species*	May be accompanied by constitutional symptoms, meningism, facial palsy, or painful radicultis
Neurobrucellosis	*Brucella species*	May be preceded by systemic features of acute brucellosis. Infection typically aquired outside of UK
Whipple's disease	*Tropheryma whipplei*	Usually accompanied by diarrhoea, weight loss, abdominal pain, and/or arthralgia.
In patients known to be HIV positive or otherwise immunocompromised		
Progressive multifocal leucoencephalopathy	JC virus	Nature of impairment dependant on site of lesions. Focal signs may be present
Cerebral toxoplasmosis	*Toxoplasma gondii*	Encephalitis can occur with or without focal signs from space occupying lesion
Fungal meningitis	*Cryptococcus neoformans*	Meningitic features may be minimal or absent. Often associated with raised intracranial pressure
Primary CNS lymphoma/encephalitis	Ebstein Barr virus	Signs related to space occupying lesion from primary CNS lymphoma. Less comonly a subacute encephalitis may occur
Ventricuoencephalitis	Cytomegalovirus	CMV has predeliction to infect ependyma of ventricles. There may be CMV related disease elsewhere such as retinitis or colitis
In patients with tropical foreign travel		
Cerebral malaria	*Plasmodium falciparum*	Fever and decreased concious level in returning traveller from endemic region
African sleeping sickness	*Trypanosoma species*	Confusion, disruption of sleep–wake cycle and lymphadenopathy in returning traveller from rural Africa, e.g. game reserves
Arboviral encephalitis	Japanese encephalitis, West Nile, chicungunya, dengue, and other arboviruses	Acute encephalitis and sequelae as described above. Pathogen is dependant on geographical location and exposure

Pathogenesis

Antiretroviral CNS penetration is poor, and in some cases CSF levels do not exceed the minimal inhibitory concentration for wild-type HIV, suggesting the virus may not be fully controlled in this compartment.[52] Other potential causes of CNS damage in those on antiretroviral treatment include low-grade immune reconstitution inflammatory syndrome (IRIS) directed at the CNS,[53] and neurotoxicity of antiretroviral drugs.[54] However, it remains unclear to what extent these phenomena lead to the high prevalence of HAND in treated populations as there are multiple other factors contributing to cognitive impairment, including hepatitis C coinfection,[55] substance misuse,[56] and the systemic effects of HIV on atherosclerosis and cerebrovascular disease.[57] Nadir (lowest ever) CD4 is associated with HAND;[47,50] this reflects the degree of CNS damage sustained before antiretroviral treatment was commenced, some of which will be irreversible, leaving a legacy effect.

Clinical features

MCI and ANI may be phenotypically different to HIV dementia rather than simply a milder form of the same syndrome. Some have

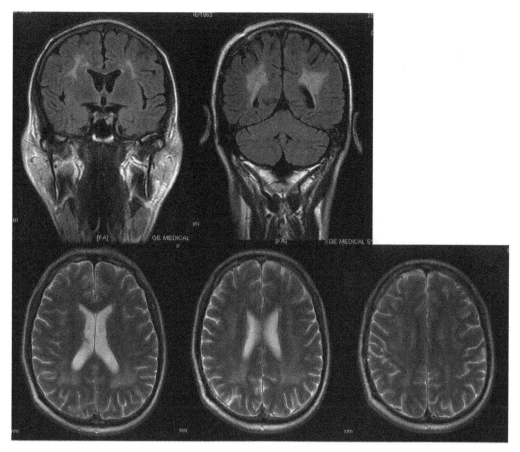

Fig. 23.6 Magnetic resonance imaging (MRI) appearance of HIV-associated dementia. White matter hyper-intensity on coronal fluid-attenuated inversion recovery (FLAIR) and sagittal T2-weighted MRI.

reported executive function to be worse in MND in contrast to the classical subcortical pattern in HAD. Motor features that are typical of HAD such as bradykinesia, spasticity, and weakness tend to be absent in ANI and MND.[58]

Investigation

HIV can be detected in the CSF of some patients who are on treatment with undetectable viral load in the plasma.[59] It is, however, unclear to what extent this phenomenon leads to mild cognitive impairment, and CSF HIV viral load has not been shown to consistently relate to neurocognitive outcomes.[60]

HIV isolated from within the CNS and from the plasma may have different viral characteristics in the same individual, suggesting that the CNS virus is partially independent from the haemato-lymphatic compartment and can evolve separately.[61,62] In cases of HAND with grossly discordant CSF and plasma HIV viral loads,

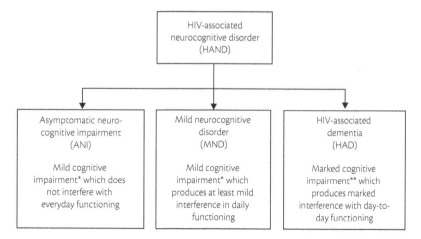

Fig. 23.7 Frascati criteria for HIV-associated neurocognitive disorders.

*Performance on neuropsychological tests of at least one standard deviation below the mean for norms in at least two cognitive domains.

**Performance on neuropsychological tests of at least two standard deviations below the mean for norms in at least two cognitive domains.

Adapted from *Clin Infect Dis.* 54(10), Mailles A, De Broucker T, Costanzo P, *et al.* Long-term outcome of patients presenting with acute infectious encephalitis of various causes in France, pp. 1455–64, Copyright (2012), with permission from Oxford University Press.

Table 23.2 Neurological complications of syphilis

	Description	Time to presentation	Proportion affected*
Neuroinvasion	*T pallidum* in CSF. Most clear infection from CNS spontaneously	days	?100%
Asymptomatic neurosyphilis	CSF abnormalities due to persistant asymptomatic meningitis	<12 months	13–20%
Meningeal disease			
Early meningeal syphilis	Meningism, fever, and cranial nerve palsys	<12 months	4%
Meningovascular syphilis	Menigitis with stroke	5–12 years	5–10%
Parenchymal disease			
Tabes dorsalis	Posterial column spinal cord disease	15–25 years	3–9%
General paresis	Dementia with personality change	15–20 years	5%
CNS gumma	Mass lession	late	rare
Acute encephalitis	Can mimic herpes simplex encephalitis	? early	rare

*natural progression, i.e. assumes untreated.

genotypic resistance testing can be performed on virus from the CSF.[44]

Management

Studies have attempted to determine a hierarchy of CNS penetration between different antiretrovirals agents; the CNS penetration effectiveness (CPE) score is based on drug chemical properties, CSF concentration, and effectiveness in clinical studies.[52] Antiretroviral drug combinations with higher composite CPE scores have been shown to have lower CSF HIV viral loads,[63,64] however, to date, no conclusive evidence has shown that higher CPE scores have any benefit on neurocognitive function. Use of this score does not form part of current UK or European guidelines.[5,44]

Hepatitis C virus co-infection

Hepatitis C virus (HCV) is neurotropic, and replicative forms of HCV have been found in autopsy brain tissue.[65] Chronic HCV infection is associated with neurocognitive dysfunction that does not correlate with the severity of liver disease and cannot be accounted for by hepatic encephalopathy or drug abuse.[66,67] The effect of HCV on cognition is compounded by HIV infection; HIV and HCV co-infected patients may be almost twice as likely to have neurocognitive impairment as HIV positive individuals without HCV infection.[55,68]

Neurosyphilis

Syphilis is due to infection with the spirochete bacterium *Treponema pallidum*. The CNS can be involved at any stage of infection (Table 23.2). Neurocognitive impairment and psychiatric manifestations occur as a late complication of untreated parenchymal neurosyphilis, known as general paralysis of the insane, or general paresis.[69]

Epidemiology

In the pre-antibiotic era, up to 10 per cent of the population in some urban areas were infected with syphilis, and the natural history of untreated disease is well described.[69] The incidence declined dramatically following the introduction of penicillin in the 1940s, however, since 2000 there has been an increase in new infections, mainly in homosexual men and those with HIV infection.[70]

Infection remains common in many parts of the developing world and approximately 12 million people are infected globally.[70]

Pathogenesis

Treponemes disseminate systemically early and CNS infection is common if not universal following primary infection.[71] CNS infection may then be cleared or can progress to an asymptomatic stage where CSF abnormalities can be demonstrated without evidence of CNS disease. In a minority of cases there is further progression to symptomatic neurosyphilis with meningeal or parenchymal manifestations. Those with HIV are less likely to clear spirochetes following initial neuroinvasion, and CNS disease is more common in this group.[72]

Clinical features

See Table 23.2.

Early meningeal syphilis

Acute syphilitic leptomeningitis occurs within 12 months of primary infection and is more common is association with HIV. Symptoms are of meningeal inflammation with headache, neck stiffness, nausea, and photophobia. Cranial nerve palsies may occur.

Meningovascular syphilis

Endarteritis of vessels results in thrombosis and infarction which is most common in the territory of the middle cerebral artery but can occur anywhere in the CNS. This manifestation tends to occur 5–12 years after primary infection.

Tabes dorsalis

Late disease, typically 20–25 years after infection, resulting from degeneration of the posterior column and roots of the spinal cord. Symptoms include ataxic gait, paresthesia, bladder dysfunction, and failing vision due to associated optic atrophy. Signs include impaired vibration sense and proprioception, Argyl Robertson pupils, Charcot's joints, and extensor plantar responses with absent tendon reflexes at the ankle.

CNS gumma

Syphilitic gummas can occur anywhere in the CNS, causing focal signs related to site of the space-occupying lesion. They are uncommon, occurring only rarely in large untreated cohorts from the pre-antibiotic era, but may occur in HIV co-infected patients.[73]

Acute encephalitis

An acute encephalitic syndrome mimicking herpes simplex encephalitis has been described secondary to neurosyphilis.[74,75] Patients are typically younger and present with seizures and altered conscious level in association with parenchymal abnormalities on neuroimaging. Most have a brief history of cognitive impairment leading up to presentation. Electroencephalogram typically demonstrates periodic lateralizing epileptiform discharges (PLEDS) or nonconvulsive status epilepticus.[76]

General paresis/General paralysis of the insane

General paresis is a neuropsychiatric disorder developing 15–20 years after infection. It occurs in approximately 5 per cent of patients infected with syphilis if untreated. There is widespread atrophy of the cerebral cortex, most severe in the frontal lobes and becoming less pronounced more posteriorly. Focal neurological signs can occur in the 'Lissauer' form of the disease, characterized by focal atrophy and seizures.

Although presentation follows long-term infection, the onset of disease may be relatively rapid. Early symptoms include irritability, forgetfulness, and personality changes. Progressive cognitive impairment follows with psychiatric manifestations which include depression, mania, delusions, hallucinations, and psychosis. In late stages there may be dysarthria, generalized weakness, and hypertonia. Argyl Robertson pupils may be seen but are more often present in tabes dorsalis. Optic atrophy and ocular muscle palsies are described.[69]

Investigation

It is not possible to culture treponemes; they can be visualized by dark field microscopy of lesions or infected lymph nodes, however this is not useful for the diagnosis of CNS disease. PCR tests have been developed but are not available in all centres. In most cases serological tests are used to confirm the diagnosis.

Serological tests

Serological tests are divided into treponemal specific and non-treponemal specific tests:

◆ Non-treponemal-specific
  • VDRL (venereal disease research laboratory)
  • RPR (rapid plasma reagin)

Non-treponemal tests are quantitative and titres indicate disease severity. Levels fall following successful treatment so they can be used to monitor response. Levels decrease over time even without treatment, and false negatives occur in around 30 per cent of those with late neurosyphilis.

◆ Treponemal-specific
  • FTA-Abs (fluorescent treponemal antibody-absorption)
  • TPHA (*treponema pallidum* haemaglutination assay)
  • TPPA (*treponema pallidum* particle agglutination)
  • TPI (*treponema pallidum* immobilization)

Treponemal-specific tests become positive early in infection and remain reactive indefinitely regardless of treatment. They are useful for diagnosing the late stages of neurosyphilis but cannot be used for monitoring response to treatment.

CSF tests

A positive VDRL in the CSF is considered diagnostic of neurosyphilis in the absence of heavy contamination with blood; however, false negatives may occur in up to 50 per cent of those with symptomatic disease.[77,78] In this situation, a CSF pleocytosis indicates neurosyphilis, although the level considered abnormal is higher in those with HIV infection particularly if not on antiretroviral treatment. Testing RPR is not recommended in CSF as the false negative rate is higher than with VDRL.[79] CSF treponemal specific tests are sensitive however passive transfer from blood causes specificity to be low. This can be improved by looking at the titre of the test or calculating the TPHA index. Although some guidelines suggest a negative treponemal specific test in CSF rules out neurosyphilis, this may not be the case when clinical suspicion is high (Fig. 23.8).[78]

All patients diagnosed with neurosyphilis should be tested for other sexually transmitted infections including HIV.

Management

Penicillin remains the mainstay of therapy to treat neurosyphilis. Longer duration of treatment and parenteral route of administration is required for syphilis involving the central nervous system. Current UK treatment guidelines can be found at <http://www.bashh.org/documents/1771>.[80]

Whipple's disease

Whipple's disease is a relapsing, slowly progressive systemic infectious disease caused by the bacterium *Tropheryma whipplei*. It is primarily a gastrointestinal disorder causing malabsorbtion but can affect multiple other parts of the body including the brain. Although rare, it is important to consider as it is fatal without antibiotic treatment.[81]

Epidemiology

Fewer than 1000 cases of Whipple's disease have been reported, of whom less than half have CNS involvement. This is likely to be an underestimation due to the low index of suspicion and difficulties making a diagnosis, however Whipple's disease remains an uncommon infectious cause of cognitive impairment.

Clinical features

Infection is systemic and Whipple's disease may affect almost any part of the body. The most common manifestations are diarrhoea, weight loss, abdominal pain, and arthralgia with low-grade fever and lymphadenopathy. These features may be absent and neurological symptoms can occur in isolation.[82,83]

Cognitive changes are the most common manifestation of CNS disease occurring in around 75 per cent of cases.[84] Around half have concomitant psychiatric features including depression, anxiety, hypomania, and psychosis. Oculomasticatory or oculofacial-skeletal myorhythmia is a pathognomonic sign of neuro-Whipple's.[83,85] It occurs in around 20 per cent of cases and is associated with supranuclear gaze palsy.[84] Other CNS features include seizures and symptoms related to hypothalamic dysfunction such as polydipsia, polyuria, hypogonadism, and hypersomnia.

Investigation

Early diagnosis can be difficult due to the variable clinical features and occasional absence of gastrointestinal symptoms. There is no

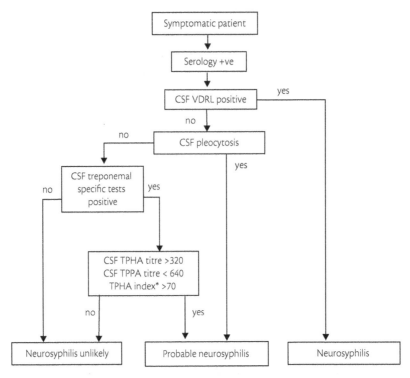

Fig. 23.8 Flowchart for the diagnosis of neurosyphilis in a symptomatic patient.
*TPHA index = CSF TPHA/albumin quotient (CSF albumin ×10³/serum albumin).

specific serologic test for *Tropheryma whipplei* and diagnosis is usually based on histopathogical appearances on small bowel biopsy. Patients with only CNS involvement may require stereotactic brain biopsy.[83] Characteristic changes of villous atrophy and periodic acid–Schiff–positive macrophages can be absent in up to 30 per cent; however, newer PCR techniques have a higher sensitivity.[86] PCR can also be performed on CSF.[86]

Management
For Whipple's disease involving the CNS initial treatment with parenteral streptomycin, benzylpenicillin or cephalosporins is followed by long-term trimethoprim-sulphamethoxazole with folate supplementation for up to two years.[87]

References

1. Beckham JD and Tyler KL. Neuro-intensive care of patients with acute CNS infections. *Neurotherapeutics*. 2012;9(1):124–38.
2. Solomon T, Michael BD, Smith PE, *et al*. Management of suspected viral encephalitis in adults—Association of British Neurologists and British Infection Association National Guidelines. *J Infect*. 2012;64(4):347–73.
3. Granerod J, Ambrose HE, Davies NW, *et al*. Causes of encephalitis and differences in their clinical presentations in England: a multicentre, population-based prospective study. *Lancet Infect Dis*. 2010;10(12):835–44.
4. Michael B, Menezes BF, Cunniffe J, *et al*. Effect of delayed lumbar punctures on the diagnosis of acute bacterial meningitis in adults. *Emerg Med J*. 2010;27(6):433–8.
5. Williams I, Churchill D, Anderson J, *et al*. British HIV Association guidelines for the treatment of HIV-1-positive adults with antiretroviral therapy 2012. *HIV Med*. 2012;13 Suppl 2:1–85.
6. Heyderman RS. Early management of suspected bacterial meningitis and meningococcal septicaemia in immunocompetent adults—second edition. *J Infect*. 2005;50(5):373–4.
7. Mailles A, De Broucker T, Costanzo P, *et al*. Long-term outcome of patients presenting with acute infectious encephalitis of various causes in France. *Clin Infect Dis*. 2012;54(10):1455–64.
8. Cavaco S, Feinstein JS, van Twillert H, *et al*. Musical memory in a patient with severe anterograde amnesia. *J Clin Exp Neuropsychol*. 2012;34(10):1089–100.
9. Geffen G, Isles R, Preece M, and Geffen L. Memory systems involved in professional skills: a case of dense amnesia due to herpes simplex viral encephalitis. *Neuropsychol Rehabil*. 2008;18(1):89–108.
10. Hahn K, Schildmann EK, Baumeister C, *et al*. Cognitive impairment after acute encephalitis: an ERP study. *Int J Neurosci*. 2012;122(11):630–6.
11. Pewter SM, Williams WH, Haslam C, *et al*. Neuropsychological and psychiatric profiles in acute encephalitis in adults. *Neuropsychol Rehabil*. 2007;17(4–5):478–505.
12. Huang MC, Wang SM, Hsu YW, *et al*. Long-term cognitive and motor deficits after enterovirus 71 brainstem encephalitis in children. *Pediatrics*. 2006;118(6):e1785–8.
13. Gustaw-Rothenberg K. Cognitive impairment after tick-borne encephalitis. *Dement Geriatr Cogn Disord*. 2008;26(2):165–8.
14. Deramecourt V, Bombois S, Debette S, *et al*. Bilateral temporal glioma presenting as a paraneoplastic limbic encephalitis with pure cognitive impairment. *Neurologist*. 2009;15(4):208–11.
15. Lebon S, Maeder P, Maeder-Ingvar M, *et al*. An initial MRI picture of limbic encephalitis in subacute sclerosing panencephalitis. *Eur J Paediatr Neurol*. 2011;15(6):544–6.
16. World Health Organization. Tuberculosis Fact sheet No. 104. Geneva: World Health Organization. 2015.
17. Pehlivanoglu F, Yasar KK, and Sengoz G. Tuberculous meningitis in adults: a review of 160 cases. *Scientific World Journal*. 2012;169028.
18. Gutierrez J, Issacson RS, and Koppel BS. Subacute sclerosing panencephalitis: an update. *Dev Med Child Neurol*. 2010;52(10):901–7.
19. Saribas AS, Ozdemir A, Lam C, *et al*. JC virus-induced Progressive Multifocal Leukoencephalopathy. *Future Virol*. 2010;5(3):313–23.
20. Berger JR. Progressive multifocal leukoencephalopathy in acquired immunodeficiency syndrome: explaining the high incidence and

disproportionate frequency of the illness relative to other immunosuppressive conditions. *J Neurovirol.* 2003;9 Suppl 1:38–41.

21. Mateen FJ, Muralidharan R, Carone M, et al. Progressive multifocal leukoencephalopathy in transplant recipients. *Ann Neurol.* 2011;70(2):305–22.

22. Yousry TA, Major EO, Ryschkewitsch C, et al. Evaluation of patients treated with natalizumab for progressive multifocal leukoencephalopathy. *N Engl J Med.* 2006;354(9):924–33.

23. Major EO, Amemiya K, Tornatore CS, et al. Pathogenesis and molecular biology of progressive multifocal leukoencephalopathy, the JC virus-induced demyelinating disease of the human brain. *Clin Microbiol Rev.* 1992;5(1):49–73.

24. Brew BJ, Davies NW, Cinque P, et al. Progressive multifocal leukoencephalopathy and other forms of JC virus disease. *Nat Rev Neurol.* 2010;6(12):667–79.

25. Antinori A, Cingolani A, Lorenzini P, et al. Clinical epidemiology and survival of progressive multifocal leukoencephalopathy in the era of highly active antiretroviral therapy: Data from the Italian Registry Investigative Neuro AIDS (IRINA). *J Neurovirol.* 2003;9 Suppl 1:47–53.

26. Eikeland R, Ljostad U, Mygland A, et al. European neuroborreliosis: Neuropsychological findings 30 months post-treatment. *Eur J Neurol.* 2012;19(3):480–7.

27. Pachner AR and Steiner I. Lyme neuroborreliosis: Infection, immunity, and inflammation. *Lancet Neurol.* 2007;6(6):544–52.

28. Pappas G, Papadimitriou P, Akritidis N, et al. The new global map of human brucellosis. *Lancet Infect Dis.* 2006;6(2):91–9.

29. Pappas G, Akritidis N, and Christou L. Treatment of neurobrucellosis: what is known and what remains to be answered. *Expert Rev Anti Infect Ther.* 2007;5(6):983–90.

30. Ceran N, Turkoglu R, Erdem I, et al. Neurobrucellosis: clinical, diagnostic, therapeutic features and outcome. Unusual clinical presentations in an endemic region. *Braz J Infect Dis.* 2011;15(1):52–9.

31. Meersseman W, Van Laethem K, Lagrou K, et al. Fatal brain necrosis in primary HIV infection. *Lancet.* 2005;366(9488):866.

32. WHO/UNAIDS/UNICEF. Global HIV/AIDS Response: Epidemic update and health sector progress towards Universal Access 2011. 2011, pp. 1–10. Accessed at www.who.int/hiv/pub/progress_report2011/en/.

33. Health Protection Agency. HIV in the United Kingdom: 2011 Report. In: *London: Health Protection Services C*, editor. London: November 2011. Accessed at www.gov.uk/government/statistics/hiv-in-the-united-kingdom.

34. Grant I, Atkinson JH, Hesselink JR, et al. Evidence for early central nervous system involvement in the acquired immunodeficiency syndrome (AIDS) and other human immunodeficiency virus (HIV) infections. Studies with neuropsychologic testing and magnetic resonance imaging. *Ann Intern Med.* 1987;107(6):828–36.

35. Budka H. Neuropathology of human immunodeficiency virus infection. *Brain Pathol.* 1991;1(3):163–75.

36. Navia BA, Cho ES, Petito CK, et al. The AIDS dementia complex: II. Neuropathology. *Ann Neurol.* 1986;19(6):525–35.

37. Wiley CA, Soontornniyomkij V, Radhakrishnan L, et al. Distribution of brain HIV load in AIDS. *Brain Pathol.* 1998;8(2):277–84.

38. Samaras K, Wand H, Law M, et al. Prevalence of metabolic syndrome in HIV-infected patients receiving highly active antiretroviral therapy using International Diabetes Foundation and Adult Treatment Panel III criteria: Associations with insulin resistance, disturbed body fat compartmentalization, elevated C-reactive protein, and [corrected] hypoadiponectinemia. *Diabetes Care.* 2007;30(1):113–9.

39. Myers HF and Durvasula RS. Psychiatric disorders in African American men and women living with HIV/AIDS. *Cultural Diversity and Ethnic Minority Psychology.* 1999;5(3):249–62.

40. Brew BJ, Pemberton L, Cunningham P, et al. Levels of human immunodeficiency virus type 1 RNA in cerebrospinal fluid correlate with AIDS dementia stage. *J Infect Dis.* 1997;175(4):963–6.

41. Sonnerborg AB, Ehrnst AC, Bergdahl SK, et al. HIV isolation from cerebrospinal fluid in relation to immunological deficiency and neurological symptoms. *AIDS.* 1988;2(2):89–93.

42. Cysique LA, Vaida F, Letendre S, et al. Dynamics of cognitive change in impaired HIV-positive patients initiating antiretroviral therapy. *Neurology.* 2009;73(5):342–8.

43. Tozzi V, Balestra P, Galgani S, et al. Positive and sustained effects of highly active antiretroviral therapy on HIV-1-associated neurocognitive impairment. *AIDS.* 1999;13(14):1889–97.

44. European AIDS Clinical Society Guidelines. Version 6.1 November 2012. <http://www.europeanaidsclinicalsociety.org/images/stories/EACS-Pdf/EACSGuidelines-v6.1-English-Nov2012.pdf>.

45. Antinori A, Arendt G, Becker JT, et al. Updated research nosology for HIV-associated neurocognitive disorders. *Neurology.* 2007;69(18):1789–99.

46. Maschke M, Kastrup O, Esser S, et al. Incidence and prevalence of neurological disorders associated with HIV since the introduction of highly active antiretroviral therapy (HAART). *J Neurol Neurosur Ps.* 2000;69(3):376–80.

47. Heaton RK, Clifford DB, Franklin DR, Jr, et al. HIV-associated neurocognitive disorders persist in the era of potent antiretroviral therapy: CHARTER Study. *Neurology.* 2010;75(23):2087–96.

48. Woods SP, Moore DJ, Weber E, et al. Cognitive neuropsychology of HIV-associated neurocognitive disorders. *Neuropsychol Rev.* 2009;19(2):152–68.

49. Cysique LA, Maruff P, and Brew BJ. Prevalence and pattern of neuropsychological impairment in human immunodeficiency virus-infected/acquired immunodeficiency syndrome (HIV/AIDS) patients across pre- and post-highly active antiretroviral therapy eras: A combined study of two cohorts. *J Neurovirol.* 2004;10(6):350–7.

50. Robertson KR, Smurzynski M, Parsons TD, et al. The prevalence and incidence of neurocognitive impairment in the HAART era. *AIDS.* 2007;21(14):1915–21.

51. Gorman AA, Foley JM, Ettenhofer ML, et al. Functional Consequences of HIV-Associated Neuropsychological Impairment. *Neuropsychol Rev.* 2009;19(2):186–203.

52. Letendre S, Ellis RJ, Deutsch R, et al. Correlates of Time-to-Loss-of-Viral-Response in CSF and Plasma in the CHARTER Cohort. Paper # 430. 17th Conference on Retroviruses and Opportunistic Infections (CROI 2010); San Fransisco, CA. 2010.

53. Robertson KR, Robertson WT, Ford S, et al. Highly active antiretroviral therapy improves neurocognitive functioning. *J Acquir Immune Defic Syndr.* 2004;36(1):562–6.

54. Liner J, Meeker R, and Robertson K. CNS Toxicity of Antiretroviral Drugs. Paper #435. 17th Conference on Retroviruses and Opportunistic Infections (CROI 2010) San Fransisco, CA. 2010.

55. Letendre SL, Cherner M, Ellis RJ, et al. The effects of hepatitis C, HIV, and methamphetamine dependence on neuropsychological performance: Biological correlates of disease. *AIDS.* 2005;19 Suppl 3:S72–8.

56. Rippeth JD, Heaton RK, Carey CL, et al. Methamphetamine dependence increases risk of neuropsychological impairment in HIV infected persons. *J Int Neuropsychol Soc.* 2004;10(1):1–14.

57. Wright EJ, Grund B, Robertson K, et al. Cardiovascular risk factors associated with lower baseline cognitive performance in HIV-positive persons. *Neurology.* 2010;75(10):864–73.

58. Dore GJ, McDonald A, Li Y, et al. Marked improvement in survival following AIDS dementia complex in the era of highly active antiretroviral therapy. *AIDS.* 2003;17(10):1539–45.

59. Eden A, Fuchs D, Hagberg L, et al. HIV-1 viral escape in cerebrospinal fluid of subjects on suppressive antiretroviral treatment. *J Infect Dis.* 2010;202(12):1819–25.

60. Brew BJ and Letendre SL. Biomarkers of HIV related central nervous system disease. *Int Rev Psychiatry.* 2008;20(1):73–88.

61. Soulie C, Fourati S, Lambert-Niclot S, et al. HIV genetic diversity between plasma and cerebrospinal fluid in patients with HIV encephalitis. *AIDS.* 2010;24(15):2412–4.

62. Cunningham PH, Smith DG, Satchell C, et al. Evidence for independent development of resistance to HIV-1 reverse transcriptase inhibitors in the cerebrospinal fluid. *AIDS.* 2000;14(13):1949–54.

63. Letendre S, Marquie-Beck J, Capparelli E, *et al.* Validation of the CNS Penetration-Effectiveness rank for quantifying antiretroviral penetration into the central nervous system. *Arch Neurol.* 2008;65(1):65–70.

64. Letendre S, Fitzsimons C, Ellis RJ, *et al.* Correlates of CSF Viral Loads in 1,221 Volunteers of the CHARTER Cohort. Paper #172. 17th Conference on Retroviruses and Opportunistic Infections (CROI 2010); San Fransisco, CA.2010.

65. Laskus T, Radkowski M, Adair DM, *et al.* Emerging evidence of hepatitis C virus neuroinvasion. *AIDS.*2005; 19 Suppl 3:S140–4.

66. Forton DM, Thomas HC, Murphy CA, *et al.* Hepatitis C and cognitive impairment in a cohort of patients with mild liver disease. *Hepatology.* 2002;35(2):433–9.

67. Richardson JL, Nowicki M, Danley K, *et al.* Neuropsychological functioning in a cohort of HIV- and hepatitis C virus-infected women. *AIDS.* 2005;19(15):1659–67.

68. Perry W, Carlson MD, Barakat F, *et al.* Neuropsychological test performance in patients co-infected with hepatitis C virus and HIV. *AIDS.* 2005;19 Suppl 3:S79–84.

69. Ghanem KG. Review: Neurosyphilis: A historical perspective and review. *CNS Neurosci Ther.* 2010;16(5):e157–68.

70. Stamm LV. Global challenge of antibiotic-resistant Treponema pallidum. *Antimicrob Agents Chemother.* 2010;54(2):583–9.

71. Collart P, Franceschini P, and Durel P. Experimental rabbit syphilis. *Br J Vener Dis.* 1971;47(6):389–400.

72. Taylor MM, Aynalem G, Olea LM, *et al.* A consequence of the syphilis epidemic among men who have sex with men (MSM): Neurosyphilis in Los Angeles, 2001–2004. *Sex Transm Dis.* 2008;35(5):430–4.

73. Weinert LS, Scheffel RS, Zoratto G, *et al.* Cerebral syphilitic gumma in HIV-infected patients: case report and review. *Int J STD AIDS.* 2008;19(1):62–4.

74. Szilak I, Marty F, Helft J, *et al.* Neurosyphilis presenting as herpes simplex encephalitis. *Clin Infect Dis.* 2001;32(7):1108–9.

75. Bash S, Hathout GM, and Cohen S. Mesiotemporal T2-weighted hyperintensity: neurosyphilis mimicking herpes encephalitis. *AJNR Am J Neuroradiol.* 2001;22(2):314–6.

76. Marra CM. Update on neurosyphilis. *Curr Infect Dis Rep.* 2009;11(2):127–34.

77. Brown ST, Zaidi A, Larsen SA, *et al.* Serological response to syphilis treatment. A new analysis of old data. *JAMA.* 1985;253(9):1296–9.

78. Harding AS and Ghanem KG. The performance of cerebrospinal fluid treponemal-specific antibody tests in neurosyphilis: A systematic review. *Sex Transm Dis.* 2012;39(4):291–7.

79. Marra CM, Tantalo LC, Maxwell CL, *et al.* The rapid plasma reagin test cannot replace the venereal disease research laboratory test for neurosyphilis diagnosis. *Sex Transm Dis.* 2012;39(6):453–7.

80. Kingston M, French P, Goh B, *et al.* UK National Guidelines on the Management of Syphilis 2008. *Int J STD AIDS.* 2008;19(11):729–40.

81. Ratnaike RN. Whipple's disease. *Postgrad Med J.* 2000;76(902):760–6.

82. Durand DV, Lecomte C, Cathebras P, *et al.* Whipple disease. Clinical review of 52 cases. The SNFMI Research Group on Whipple Disease. Societe Nationale Francaise de Medecine Interne. *Medicine (Baltimore).* 1997;76(3):170–84.

83. Mendel E, Khoo LT, Go JL, *et al.* Intracerebral Whipple's disease diagnosed by stereotactic biopsy: A case report and review of the literature. *Neurosurgery.* 1999;44(1):203–9.

84. Louis ED, Lynch T, Kaufmann P, *et al.* Diagnostic guidelines in central nervous system Whipple's disease. *Ann Neurol.* 1996;40(4):561–8.

85. Schwartz MA, Selhorst JB, Ochs AL, *et al.* Oculomasticatory myorhythmia: a unique movement disorder occurring in Whipple's disease. *Ann Neurol.* 1986;20(6):677–83.

86. Ramzan NN, Loftus E, Jr, Burgart LJ, *et al.* Diagnosis and monitoring of Whipple disease by polymerase chain reaction. *Ann Intern Med.* 1997;126(7):520–7.

87. Singer R. Diagnosis and treatment of Whipple's disease. *Drugs.* 1998;55(5):699–704.

88. http://www.who.int/gho/epidemic_diseases/meningitis/en/ (accessed 30th October 2013)

89. Thwaites GE, Chau TT, and Farrar JJ. Improving the bacteriological diagnosis of tuberculous meningitis. *J Clin Microbiol.* 2004 Jan;42(1):378–9.

90. Bailey EM, Domenico P, and Cunha BA. Bacterial or viral meningitis? Measuring lactate in CSF can help you know quickly. *Post-grad Med.* 1990;88:217e9. 223.

91. Cunha BA. Distinguishing bacterial from viral meningitis: The critical importance of the CSF lactic acid levels. *Intensive Care Med.* 2006;32:1272e3. author reply 1274.

92. Thwaites GE and Tran TH. Tuberculous meningitis: Many questions, too few answers. *Lancet Neurol.* 2005 Mar;4(3):160–70.

93. Nightingale S, Winston A, Letendre S, *et al.* Controversies in HIV-associated neurocognitive disorders. *Lancet Neurol.* 2014 Nov;13(11):1139–51. doi: 10.1016/S1474–4422(14)70137–1.

CHAPTER 24

Metabolic dementia

Nicholas J.C. Smith and Timothy M. Cox

Introduction

In clinical practice, 'metabolic dementias' are often considered as singular diagnostic entities, giving little attention to their complex manifestations and protean causes. Defined as progressive cognitive impairment sufficient to impair independent function, dementia induced by disorders of metabolism may be acquired or the result of inborn errors of cellular function (Table 24.1).

Clinical manifestations may arise from infancy to old age, with presenting features ranging from precipitant encephalopathy to indolent cognitive decline. Variation in clinical presentation is often explained by the time that cellular decompensation occurs in the brain and the neurodevelopmental stage and cognitive function that has been attained at that age. Indeed, normal development may at first mask degenerative pathology in childhood, and deterioration in an intellectually impaired patient might be overlooked. Conversely, onset *in utero* may be associated with profound disease that is declared in infancy, while delayed presentation of inborn metabolic errors is increasingly recognized. Relapsing–remitting patterns of dementing disease are also common; these are typically due to external influences on cellular homeostasis, including metabolic stressors (e.g. intercurrent illness and relative starvation), deficiencies of enzyme co-factors (e.g. vitamin and mineral deficiencies), or intoxication (e.g. excess protein load) [Fig. 24.1].

Given the importance of identifying genetic diseases in affected pedigrees, and as some conditions may be treatable, metabolic causes of, or contributions to, cognitive impairment should always be considered and specific diagnoses sought. Advances in biochemical genetics have greatly expanded the opportunities for effective treatments: these include replacement of cofactors, enzyme replacement and augmentation, removal of toxic substrates via scavenging chemical agents, or restriction of dietary substrates. While in some monogenic disorders gene transfer techniques show considerable promise.

Here we restrict discussion to a practical diagnostic framework for primary metabolic dementia: the contribution of disturbed cellular metabolism to the classically defined dementias and the effects of systemic metabolic conditions, such as accelerated cerebrovascular disease in patients with diabetes are discussed in relevant chapters; dementia resulting from mitochondrial disease is discussed in chapter 31 and is summarized only briefly herein.

Table 24.1 Metabolic disorders associated with adult-onset cognitive decline

Acquired
Nutritional deficiencies
Acid-base and electrolyte disturbances
Endocrinopathies
Visceral insufficiency
Hypoxia and hypercapnia
Toxins and medication

Inborn errors of metabolism
Disorders of carbohydrate metabolism
Disorders of mitochondrial energy metabolism
Disorders of amino acid metabolism and transport
Vitamin responsive disorders
Disorders of neurotransmitter metabolism and function
Disorders of purine and pyrimidine metabolism
Disorders of lipid and bile acid metabolism
Disorders of haem metabolism
Disorders of elemental co-factor transport and metalloprotein dysfunction
Other disorders of lysosomal macromolecule catabolism

Classification of the metabolic dementias

Many different ways of classifying the metabolic dementia have been proposed. From a practical perspective, an approach based on clinical phenotype is most relevant for clinicians, with the caveat that the clinical behaviour of some disorders may be confounded by the sheer diversity of potential manifestations—particularly when these come to light at different neurodevelopmental ages.

To simplify the diagnostic conspectus for practising clinicians rather than biochemists, here we present a working classification which first distinguishes acquired pathologies from inborn errors of metabolism and subclassifies the given entities on the basis of the principal metabolic pathways affected (Fig. 24.2). In making this pathophysiological distinction, the main presenting phenotypes are set out, with emphasis on conditions with onset in adult life. For these purposes, dementia is defined broadly as progressive cognitive impairment, without limitation to the classical dementias and includes acute encephalopathy.

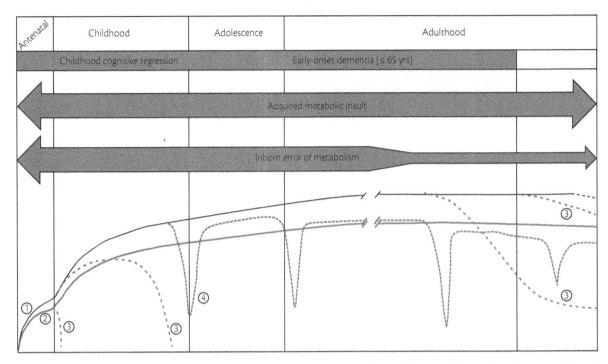

Fig. 24.1 Patterns of neurocognitive decline in metabolic dementia. Dementia due to inborn errors of metabolism is usually manifest in infancy or childhood, with adult-onset disease most commonly presenting as early-onset dementia (before 65 years of age). However, both inborn and acquired disease may declare at any age and proceed at variable velocities, dependent upon cause. This figure depicts: neurocognitive development in a healthy individual (solid line, black) with variable age-related cognitive decline (dashed line, black) (1); non-progressive intellectual impairment (solid line, red) (2); pathological neurocognitive decline (multiple dashed lines, red) (3); acute deterioration with a relapsing-remitting course and evident recovery (dotted line, red) (4).

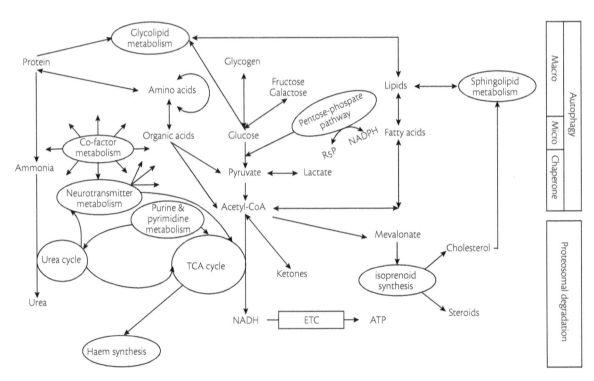

Fig. 24.2 Major pathways of cellular metabolism affected in metabolic neurocognitive decline. The principal substrate pathways for generating acetyl coenzyme A from carbohydrates, lipids, and proteins are shown; acetyl-CoA is the primary carbon donor to the tricarboxylic acid (TCA) cycle and adenosine triphosphate (ATP) is generated by mitochondrial oxidative phosphorylation. Critical pathways of intermediate and macromolecular metabolism are included: pathological disruption of each of these has been implicated in neurocognitive decline.

ETC: electron transport chain; NADH: reduced nicotinamide adenine dinucleotide; NADPH: reduced nicotinamide adenine dinucleotide phosphate; R5P: ribose-5-phosphate.

The scope of metabolic disorders with cognitive manifestations is vast, and with the increasing use of massive parallel DNA sequencing for diagnostic purposes, rare inherited variants of inborn errors of metabolism are emerging as causes of cognitive decline with onset in adult life. The advent of methods for systematic analysis of whole-exome and even individual genome sequences has enabled numerous ultra-rare disorders to be identified within the pool of previously undiagnosed neurodegenerative disorders. These exciting initiatives are improving diagnostic power; moreover, they offer the promise of new insights into potential therapy.

When to suspect metabolic dementia

While some clinical features are highly suggestive of a metabolic cause and, with experience, specific patterns can often be recognized, there can be few certainties. Nonetheless, several features in the clinical presentation should alert the physician to the possibility of a metabolic disorder in the dementing patient (Box 24.1).

Acquired disease may arise at any age; indeed, it may precipitate deterioration in those patients harboring metabolic conditions due to underlying genetic defects. However, early-onset dementia—generally accepted as presenting before 65 years of age[1]—should certainly prompt consideration of a metabolic cause, particularly with onset in adolescence or young adulthood, where suspicion of a metabolic dementia is at the forefront of diagnostic possibility.

Box 24.1 Features suggestive of metabolic dementia

- Early age of onset
- Precipitant onset
- Rapidly progressive dementia
- Global encephalopathy/impaired conscious state
- Episodic course
- Risk factors for acquired nutritional deficiency

   Malnutrition, malabsorption, alcoholism, metabolic consumption (pregnancy, cancer)

- Childhood neurocognitive impairment
- Family history
- Familial consanguinity
- Presence of associated features / comorbid pathology (dementia plus)

   Neurological: seizures, pyramidal, extrapyramidal, cerebellar, neuro-ophthalmological, peripheral neuropathic/neuronopathic, neuromuscular
   Psychiatric: affective spectrum, personality and behavioural changes, psychosis
   Somatic: ophthalmological, visceral, endocrinological, cutaneous, connective tissue, skeletal

---

In metabolic conditions the cognitive manifestations are usually more varied than in the primary dementias; they may range from developmental intellectual delay to late-onset delirium and progressive dementia. Moreover, global encephalopathy and impaired consciousness are more suggestive of a secondary dementing illness than one of the classic dementias.

Rapid decline, often at times of metabolic stress (e.g. starvation, inflammation, and surgery), increased catabolic load (e.g. high dietary protein), or following a closed head injury, strongly suggests an inborn metabolic error—particularly those affecting intermediate metabolism and cellular energy production. Episodic fluctuations (sometimes with near-complete recovery) are also common, reflecting interval restitution of metabolic homeostasis upon removal of precipitating factors. Of note, hyperemesis gravidarum places the pregnant woman under considerable metabolic stress, compounded by the risk of micronutrient deficiency; the postpartum period is also a vulnerable period for women with latent inborn errors of metabolism and it is important not to overlook such diagnoses when maternal neuropsychiatric disturbances have occurred. Subacute progressive forms of dementia are typical of disorders of macromolecular biosynthesis and degradation, such as the disorders of lipid breakdown and many of the elemental transport disorders; certain mitochondrial cytopathies may also present in this manner.

The presence of additional neurological features and concomitant systemic manifestations may also indicate a metabolic derangement; the presence of such features giving rise to the designation of 'dementia plus' disorders.[1] In the assessment of dementing patients, the pattern of these additional features may provide invaluable diagnostic clues (see chapter 21).

A premorbid history of childhood neurodevelopmental delay, presumed static intellectual impairment (often reflected in poor scholastic performance), or behavioural disorder might reflect early and previously unrecognized manifestations of disease. Indeed, early confirmation of indolent regressive disease is often difficult in the absence of formal neurocognitive assessments carried out serially, especially when slow regression is 'masked' by parallel neurodevelopmental gains in childhood. A transient illness in childhood may similarly provide clues to the cause neurodegenerative disease that comes to light later in life—a history of prolonged neonatal jaundice, for example, raises the possibility of disorders of bile acid and cholesterol metabolism[2] as is seen in Niemann–Pick disease type C.[3,4]

Familial occurrence of disease may suggest a genetic cause and the pattern of inheritance may clarify the differential diagnosis. However, the absence of disease in any known ancestor or family member cannot exclude an inborn metabolic disorder, particularly those inherited as autosomal recessive traits. Consanguinity (immediate, or more typically, in antecedents) often provides vital clues to inform diagnosis in cases presumed to be sporadic; often consanguinity may emerge from enquiring as to the geographic origin and birthplace of the parents of an index case. At the same time, the potential for de-novo mutation and confounding factors such as non-paternity (often withheld) are of critical diagnostic value. Phenotypic variability amongst family members with inborn errors of metabolism (e.g. childhood cerebral X-linked adrenoleukodystrophy and adult-onset adrenomyelneuropathy) may further confound the true genetic basis for the condition. Thus, a wider knowledge of familial medical history may prove informative; for example, a history of maternal miscarriage might suggest presentation of disease *in utero*.

As with all cases of dementia, a thorough review of medication is mandatory—also with consideration of the potential metabolic effects of prescribed and non-prescription drugs. The often dramatic triggering of acute porphyria by adverse exposure to drugs and metabolic stress, including surgical operations, is a paradigmatic example. Indeed, the temporal relationship of disease onset and exacerbation, especially in relation to use of medication, may lead to the diagnosis in the metabolic dementias.

Acquired nutritional deficiencies occur frequently in developing and displaced populations; although uncommon in Western populations, the possibility must be considered in the context of alcoholism and in situations of restricted intake as may occur in the chronically ill or anorexic patient, and pregnant women with hyperemesis gravidarum. Indeed, multiple nutritional deficiencies often coexist. Of note, specific deficiencies are increasingly evident in those adhering to specialist diets or after bariatric surgery.[5] Patients receiving total parenteral nutrition or cytotoxic chemotherapy are also at risk and careful attention should be given to the micronutrient and elemental composition of replacement nutrition.

Finally, in a dementing patient with a known inborn error of metabolism, where treatment is expected to attenuate disease the possibility of non-compliance should be considered, particularly given the strict dietary regulation that is often needed to maintain health in many inborn metabolic disorders. A review of the consequences of specific therapies must also be considered: acquired nutritional deficiencies may occur, as exemplified by symptomatic cobalamin deficiency in patients with phenylketonuria managed by dietary protein restriction,[6] and secondary zinc deficiency in patients with Wilson's disease receiving copper-chelation therapy without supplementation.[7]

An approach to the investigation of suspected metabolic dementia

Given their protean nature and heterogeneity, the approach to diagnosis of neurometabolic disease favours targeted investigation over protocol-driven screening. Investigations should be guided by clinical insight, with clear understanding as to their diagnostic value and priority given to the rapid identification of treatable pathology. While in certain cases the clinical phenotype is highly suggestive, such as Fabry disease presenting with an acute stroke in a young man with angiokeratoma and a history of acroparaesthesia, or hypothyroidism in a middle-aged woman with confusion and myxoedema, in most cases the clinical features are non-specific. Where aetiology is uncertain, initial consideration should be given to whether the features of the patient's condition fall within one or more broad 'functional' phenotypes (Table 24.2), at the same time recognizing such distinctions are not concrete. Finally, before deciding upon the likely conditions to investigate, in each case it is prudent to consider whether an acquired or inborn metabolic disorder is the more likely.

Clinical assessment should include detailed neurocognitive, systemic, cutaneous, and ophthalmological examinations; metabolic disorders rarely present as isolated cognitive decline, with adjunct central and peripheral neurological impairment ('dementia plus') common and often proving to be the presenting feature of the illness, while non-neurological features may also inform diagnosis. Attention to biochemical consequences of aberrant metabolism can assist diagnosis, such as dark-red to brown urine reflecting excess porphyrin excretion or the presence of malodorous biofluids (perspiration and urine) which may occur in the context of substrate accumulation, particularly the disorders of amino acid metabolism.

Formal neuropsychological assessment is helpful in defining the pattern of cognitive impairment and establishes a baseline level of function which facilitates determination of time-dependent reduction in performance, typical of many inborn errors of metabolism.

Routine haematological and biochemical assays may identify a primary metabolic defect (e.g. thyroid function tests) or provide indirect evidence of underlying pathology (e.g. megaloblastic anaemia in B_{12} deficiency or abnormal liver-related tests and acanthocytosis in Wilson's disease). However, these findings are of variable specificity and in many cases remain within healthy reference limits, particularly if decompensation is episodic.

Where clinical phenotype and routine laboratory investigations fail to suggest a specific cause, a general screening algorithm, intended to identify the more common consequences of metabolic disruption and several rare but potentially treatable causes of cognitive decline, may prove to be useful. Here, consideration is given to a more inclusive screen of cerebrospinal fluid (CSF) neurochemistry, rather than a stepwise approach, reflecting the more invasive nature of diagnostic lumbar puncture (Fig. 24.3). However, it must be noted that while stratagems of high diagnostic utility may become evident, sensitivity and specificity of these screening investigations are variable and care must be exercised when selecting and interpreting them. Furthermore, consideration to practical constraints of sample collection, transport, and processing is essential to avoid metabolite artefact in many cases.

Consideration must also be given to the wider consequences of investigations ordered, including the patient and their family members, in whom the genetic implications of inborn metabolic disorders may have profound implications; as with all genetic disorders, strict confidentiality and attentive pre- and post-test counselling are paramount.

Biochemical laboratory investigations

Generally, biochemical screening assays quantify major biological substrates and products of metabolism that accumulate *in vivo* or assess specific enzymatic activity by *in vitro* assay. While frankly disordered homeostasis is usually evident, diagnostic features may only be present at times of cellular metabolic stress or substrate load (particularly in many of the intermediate metabolism disorders); thus apparently normal results are often obtained when studies are carried out at times of greater or more compensated metabolic stability. Conversely, a negative result during such an episode has greater value in excluding an inborn metabolic error. Furthermore, in most inborn metabolic disorders, late-onset disease reflects an attenuated variant and the pathological biochemical changes may be barely notable, limiting detection, depending upon assay sensitivity. Care must be taken to ensure the appropriate sample is

Table 24.2 Functional classification of metabolic disease presenting with adult-onset neurocognitive decline

Intermediate metabolite ('small molecule') disorders

Disorders of cellular energy production	Examples
Disorders of cellular energy production reflect impaired production of ATP or its utilization, a process dependent upon several interacting metabolic pathways. Breakdown of complex carbohydrate to glucose and its glycolytic conversion to pyruvate provides the main substrate for mitochondrial generation of acetyl CoA, the main carbon donor to the tricarboxylic acid (TCA) cycle and oxidative phosphorylation pathway, from which the majority of cellular ATP is derived. In addition, products of protein (amino and organic acids), fatty acid, and ketone body metabolism also generate acetyl CoA and are critical in states of impaired carbohydrate availability or utilization. Inborn defects in energy production therefore include disorders of carbohydrate metabolism, including defects of glycolysis, gluconeogenesis, and glycogenolysis, primary disorders of pyruvate metabolism, and disorders affecting the TCA cycle and mitochondrial respiratory chain function. Aberrant organic and amino metabolism may also affect energy production via reduced substrate availability and secondary dysequilibrium of TCA cycle metabolites. Disordered β-oxidation of fatty acids also impairs acetyl-CoA synthesis and ATP production; fatty oxidation defects induce critical dependence on glycolysis and hence the supply of glucose units, especially in the brain where energy production adapts slowly to ketone bodies generated by the liver. Additionally, dysregulation of purine and pyrimidine metabolism impairs ATP synthesis and generation of TCA cycle intermediates. In the majority of cases, presentation is acute, precipitated by metabolic stress (e.g. fasting or illness), often with rapid cognitive decline typical of an encephalopathy; episodic exacerbation with complete or partial recovery and stroke-like episodes are common. However, chronic dementing disease is also recognized, typified by several syndromic mitochondrial cytopathies and characteristic of the cerebral glycogenosis (e.g. adult polyglucosan body disease). Additional neurological features are frequent, including cortical (e.g. seizures and myoclonus) and deep grey matter involvement (e.g. extrapyramidal disease), cerebellar dysfunction, dysautonomic features, and peripheral neuromuscular disease (including optic atrophy, extraocular paresis, polyneuropathy, and primary myopathic disease). Of note, white matter disease and spastic paresis are less common, with the exception of certain co-factor deficiencies (e.g. B12 and copper) and adult Polyglucosan body disease. Systemic disease is frequently present, particularly in the mitochondrial energy defects (e.g. cardiomyopathy, hepatic disease, gastrointestinal dysmotility, and diabetes mellitus), and reflects involvement of tissues outside the central nervous system with high energy requirements.	**Acquired disorder of metabolism** **Co-factor deficiencies:** e.g. B group vitamin deficiencies, copper deficiency **Inborn error of metabolism** **Disorders of carbohydrate metabolism** e.g. cerebral glycogenosis, glucose transporter deficiency **Disorders of mitochondrial energy metabolism** e.g. mitochondrial cytopathies, disorders of fatty acid β-oxidation **Vitamin responsive disorders** e.g. cobalamin C disease, cerebral folate deficiency, biotin-thiamine-responsive basal ganglia disease **Disorders of amino acid metabolism and transport*** e.g. phenylketonuria, organic acidaemias, urea cycle disorders

Disorders of metabolite intoxication	
Disorders of metabolite intoxication can be considered as a broad collective of disparate aetiology, characterized by acute or chronic accumulation of compounds which are toxic in excess—here we consider those resulting from an inherent defect of intermediate metabolism (choosing to exclude the inborn disorders of elemental co-factor metabolism which are categorized as a distinct group in this context). Typically a symptom-free period is observed before cognitive manifestations of intoxication arise—indeed first presentation may be well into adulthood; the intoxication is often acute, usually in the context of metabolic stress (e.g. fever or illness) or increased substrate load, such as hyperammonaemic encephalopathy after protein ingestion in acquired hepatic insufficiency or urea cycle disorders; more insidious cognitive impairment may occur in late-onset disorders of amino and organic acid metabolism. Interval recovery, between acute episodes of decompensation may occur, such as in the hepatic porphyrias, where psycocognitive impairment, sometimes resembling delirium or acute anxiety may be interpreted as a primary psychiatric illness or 'toxic confusional state'. Adjunctive neurological features are common, including cortical manifestations (e.g. seizures) and prominent white matter disease with a progressive leukoencephalomyelopathy seen in several aminoacidopathies (e.g. phenylketonuria and the homocysteine remethylation defects). Cerebellar impairment, extrapyramidal disease, and akinetic parkinsonian features may also arise. While less common, peripheral neuropathy is often recognized in the disorders of homocysteine metabolism and constitutes a dominant feature of acute hepatic porphyria, typically with exuberant autonomic features. Systemic manifestations in this group are less prominent than in the disorders of energy metabolism, although the presence of corneal clouding or cataract formation may suggest metabolite accumulation (e.g. galactosaemia). Features overlap with the disorders of cellular energy production and toxicity may give rise to the latter, exemplified by secondary impairment of TCA cycle metabolism in the context of many amino and organic acidopathies, as well as the hyperammonaemias.	**Acquired** **Exogenous toxins and medications** e.g. lead inhibition of aminolevulinate dehydratase **Visceral insufficiency** e.g. uraemic encephalopathy, hepatic encephalopathy **Inborn error of metabolism** **Select disorders of carbohydrate metabolism** e.g. Galactosaemia, hereditary fructose intolerance **Disorders of amino acid metabolism and transport** e.g. phenylketonuria, tyrosinaemia type 1, organic acidaemias, urea cycle disorders **Disorders of Haem metabolism** e.g. acute hepatic (neurovisceral) porphyrias

(continued)

Table 24.2 Continued

Intermediate metabolite ('small molecule') disorders	
Disorders of neurotransmitter metabolism	**Examples**
Monogenic disorders of monoamine, gamma aminobutyric acid, and glycine metabolism are typically recognized in infancy and childhood, although late-onset variants occur; however, with the exception of glycine encephalopathy (non-ketotic hyperglycinaemia), late-onset neurocognitive decline and dementia are not characteristic. While, disordered regulation of many neurotransmitters, particularly acetylcholine, are thought to underpin several psychocognitive diseases, the mechanisms by which homeostasis is disturbed are uncertain. Clinically, monoamine deficiencies reflect the primary neurotransmitters affected; dopamine (parkinsonism, dystonia, and autonomic features), noradrenalin (ptosis, myosis, and orthostatic hypotension), and serotonin (sleep disturbance, dysthymia, and behavioural change). Adult presentations of glycine encephalopathy more readily resemble intoxication states, with acute confusional encephalopathy precipitated by metabolic stress, often upon a background of intellectual delay and disturbed behaviour, although features are variable and have also included paroxysmal choreoform movement disorders and white matter disease. Also considered among 'acquired' disorders of neurotransmission are several of the autoimmune encephalopathies, where autoantibodies target the post-synaptic N-methyl-D-aspartate (NMDA) receptor; subacute cognitive decline is typically associated with headache, behavioural change, prominent neuropsychiatric symptoms, generalized seizures, or myoclonus.	**Acquired** **Exogenous toxins and medications** e.g. dopamine antagonists, anticholinergics **Co-factor deficiencies:** e.g. copper deficiency **Neurotransmitter receptor antibodies (autoimmune encephalitis)** e.g. autoimmune encephalopathy (anti-NMDA receptor antibodies)
	Inborn error of metabolism
	Inborn error of glycine metabolism e.g. glycine encephalopathy
Disorders of elemental co-factor transport and metalloprotein dysfunction	
Disorders of elemental co-factor transport and metalloprotein dysfunction are recognized causes of metabolic dementia and neuropsychiatric manifestations; in most cases the consequence of disordered metal trafficking and utilization, resultant tissue accumulation underlies end-organ pathology. Neurocognitive decline is typically subacute in presentation, often with dominant psychiatric features. Metal accumulation within the basal ganglia prompts diagnostic consideration when demonstrated by neuroimaging; extra-pyramidal manifestations including dystonia (often including orofacial dyskinesia), choreoathetosis, and parkinsonism are characteristic. Cerebellar dysfunction may be prominent. Visceral involvement, such as cirrhosis, cardiomyopathy, renal tubular disease, and endocrine pancreatic failure (diabetes mellitus), should also raise the possibility of elemental tissue deposition in this context and may arise independently from neurological disease.	**Acquired** **Metal intoxication** e.g. lead, copper, manganese **Elemental deficiency** e.g. copper, iron, iodine, zinc **Inborn error of metabolism** **Disorder of copper transport** e.g. Wilson's disease **Disorder of iron transport** e.g. aceruloplasminaemia, neuroferritinopathy
Disorders of endocrine function	
Endocrinopathy-associated cognitive decline represents a unique subgroup of acquired metabolic dementia; diagnosis is rarely mistaken when attention is given to the associated systemic features present.	**Acquired** **Endocrinopathies** e.g. hyperthyroid encephalopathy, Cushing's disease, diabetes mellitus
Macromolecule disorders	
Disorders of lipid metabolism and transport	
Disorders of lipid metabolism and transport are increasingly recognized amongst the late-onset metabolic dementias, encompassing a heterogeneous group of diseases which includes disorders of cholesterol and bile acid synthesis, disordered fatty acid catabolism, aberrant cholesterol trafficking, and the disorders of sphingolipid catabolism. While clinical features are disease-specific, general associations hold true; cognitive decline is typically of a slowly progressive nature and neuropsychiatric presentations are common, constituting the presenting feature in many cases. Dysmyelination and leukoencephalopathic disease is frequent and peripheral neuropathy is often a feature; cerebellar ataxia, choreoathetosis, seizures, and retinopathy also occur. Systemic pathology may also prove suggestive; splenomegaly suggesting a disorder of lipid storage, or features of cutaneous deposition such as xanthomata. A history of prolonged neonatal jaundice may suggest a disorder of cholesterol or bile acid metabolism.	**Acquired** **Acquired dyslipiaemias** e.g. metabolic syndrome **Malabsorption of fat-soluble vitamins** e.g. cystic fibrosis, pancreatitis, intestinal malabsorptive disease

Table 24.2 Continued

Disorders of lipid metabolism and transport	Examples
	Inborn error of metabolism
	Hereditary dyslipidaemias
	e.g. abetalipoproteinaemia
	Disorders of bile acid synthesis
	e.g. cerebrotendinosis xanthomatosis, 2-methylacyl-CoA racemase deficiency
	Disorders of sphingolipid metabolism
	e.g. Gaucher disease, GM1 gangliosidosis, GM2 gangliosidosis, metachromatic leukodystrophy
	Disorder of cholesterol transport
	e.g. Niemann–Pick disease type C
	Disorders of peroxisomal function
	e.g. X-linked adrenoleukodystrophy/adrenomyeloneuropathy
Other disorders of macromolecule catabolism and autophagy	
Representing a significant proportion of the inborn metabolic dementia spectrum, disorders of lysosomal function reflect anomalous macromolecule catabolism.	**Inborn error of metabolism**
Progressive cognitive decline and, at times, neuropsychiatric features, are typical of adult manifesting disease, while adjunct neurological involvement is more variable. Visceral disease may be present with enlargement of viscera and skeletal abnormalities and, in the mucopolysaccharidoses and oligosaccharidoses (glycoproteinoses), dysmorphism and coarsening of facial cutaneous tissues. Skeletal dysplasisa, cutaneous angiokeratoma, and peripheral neuropathy occur in the oligosaccharidoses and are near pathognomic when presenting a comorbid tetrad with central neurological disease. The numerous genetically distinct neuronal ceroid lipofuscinoses are characterized by a central neurological phenotype without systemic features; seizures, ataxia, and parkinsonism often accompany dementia, typically with progressive blindness due to retinal dystrophy and optic nerve atrophy.	**The mucopolysaccharidoses**
	e.g. Sanfilippo syndrome (MPSIII)
	The oligosaccharidosis (glycoproteinoses)
	e.g. mannosidosis, fucosidosis, sialidosis
	The neuronal ceroid lipofuscinoses
	e.g. adult-onset NCL (Kuf's disease), cathepsin D (CTSD) deficiency
Disordered cellular catabolism in the lysosomal compartment includes pathological disruption of autophagy and proteosomal degradation, a feature that appears to be associated with neurodegenerative disease, including the primary dementias. While the pathogenesis is not fully understood, it is of great interest that mutations affecting several proteins involved in lysosomal metabolism are implicated in parkinsonism—first noted to occur with increased frequency in patients with Gaucher disease who were homozygous for causal mutations in the GBA1 gene: Notably, heterozygotes for mutations causing Gaucher disease, Niemann–Pick C disease, and neuronal ceroid lipofuscinosis also demonstrate an increased risk of age-related parkinsonism.	

*Secondary impairment of TCA cycle metabolism and cellular energy production arise in a number of aminoacidopathies (e.g. organic acidurias and disorders of urea cycle metabolism)

obtained (blood, CSF, urine, or tissue); sample collection (timing and methodology), transport, and processing are also critical for avoiding artefactual errors, the details of which are within the territory of specialist biochemical advice and should be confirmed, if unfamiliar.

Magnetic resonance imaging

Magnetic resonance imaging (MRI) serves as an important diagnostic modality in the investigation of suspected neurometabolic disease. While stereotypic patterns may prove diagnostic, imaging features are often non-specific and, in many cases normal, particularly amongst attenuated late-onset disease variants. Standard T1 sequences permit regional delineation of structure, including atrophy (best determined with dedicated volumetric acquisitions), while T2 and fluid-attenuation inversion recovery (FLAIR) sequences reflect white matter integrity and may reveal a typically symmetrical leukodystrophic process, the pattern of which aids pathological discrimination in many

cases.[8–10] Indeed, two broad categories of inborn metabolic disease dominate the metabolic leukoencephalopathies: lipid storage disorders, in which involvement is typically restricted to tracts within the deep white matter, sparing the juxtacortical fibres (U-fibres), and disorders of amino acid metabolism, which usually extend to a juxtacortical distribution.[8] Regional involvement, including the presence of peripheral nerve involvement, may provide additional diagnostic clues.[9,10] Signal change within the basal ganglia should always precipitate consideration of acquired or inborn disorder of metabolic function, particularly, but not limited to, those impacting cellular energy production (typified by the mitochondrial cytopathies) and many of the toxic encephalopathies.[11,12] Additional sequences should include diffusion-weighted acquisitions (DWI/ADC), as restricted diffusion is a sensitive marker of cytotoxic oedema, a pathophysiological process present in a number of primary and secondary disorders of metabolism. While, susceptibility-weighted images (SWI) utilize flow-compensated gradient-echo imaging to exploit susceptibility variations between tissues, allowing definition of paramagnetic

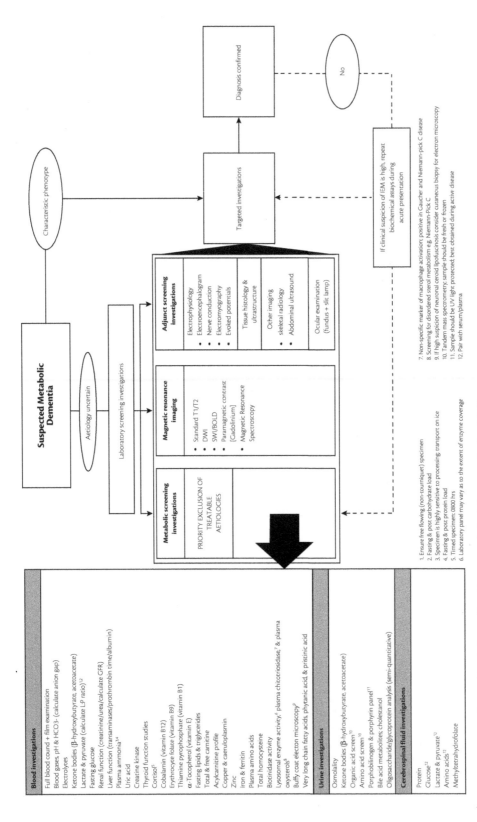

Blood investigations

Full blood count + film examination
Blood gases pH & HCO3- (calculate anion gap)
Electrolytes
Ketone bodies (β-hydroxybutyrate, acetoacetate)
Lactate & pyruvate (calculate L:P ratio)[12]
Fasting glucose
Renal function (creatinine/urea/calculate GFR)
Liver function (transaminases/prothrombin time/albumin)
Plasma ammonia[14]
Uric acid
Creatine kinase
Thyroid function studies
Cortisol[5]
Cobalamin (vitamin B12)
Erythrocyte folate (vitamin B9)
Thiamine pyrophosphate (vitamin B1)
α-Tocopherol (vitamin E)
Fasting lipids & triglycerides
Total & free carnitine
Acylcarnitine profile
Copper & caeruloplasmin
Zinc
Iron & ferritin
Plasma amino acids
Total homocysteine
Biotinidase activity
Lysosomal enzyme activity,[6] plasma chitotriosidase,[7] & plasma oxysterols[8]
Buffy coat electron microscopy[9]
Very long chain fatty acids, phytanic acid, & pristinic acid

Urine investigations

Osmolality
Ketone bodies (β-hydroxybutyrate, acetoacetate)
Organic acid screen[10]
Amino acid screen[10]
Porphobilinogen & porphyrin panel[11]
Bile acid metabolites; cholestanol
Oligosaccharide/glycoprotein analysis (semi-quantitative)

Cerebrospinal fluid investigations

Protein
Glucose[12]
Lactate & pyruvate[12]
Amino acids[12]
Methyltetrahydrofolate

1. Ensure free flowing (non-tourniquet) specimen
2. Fasting & post carbohydrate load
3. Specimen is highly sensitive to processing; transport on ice
4. Fasting & post protein load
5. Timed specimen: 0800 hrs
6. Laboratory panel may vary as as the extent of enzyme coverage

7. Non-specific marker of macrophage activation; positive in Gaucher and Niemann-pick C disease
8. Screening for disordered sterol metabolism e.g. Niemann-Pick C
9. If high suspicion of neuronal ceroid lipofuscinosis consider cutaneous biopsy for electron microscopy
10. Tandem mass spectrometry; sample should be fresh or frozen
11. Sample should be UV light protected; best obtained during active disease
12. Pair with serum/plasma

Fig. 24.3 Screening investigations for cognitive decline attributable to a metabolic defect presenting in adult life.

(e.g. deoxyhaemoglobin, ferritin, haemosiderin), diamagnetic (e.g. calcium), and ferromagnetic (e.g. iron and manganese-rich) molecules,[13] deposition of which is intrinsic to several neurodegenerative disorders.[14,15] Finally, T1 sequences following the administration of a paramagnetic contrast agent (e.g. gadolinium) should be considered, enabling definition of blood–brain barrier integrity and aiding diagnosis in some cases (e.g. the inflammatory margins typical of adenoleukodystrophy and patchy enhancement characteristic of Alexander's disease).[10] Imaging of the entire neuraxis may also be of valuable; pathologic changes in the spinal cord are present in numerous metabolic disorders, exemplified by subacute combined degeneration of cobalamin deficiency and peripheral findings might come to light (e.g. nerve root enhancement in Krabbe disease).[16] As well as providing positive evidence for a metabolic disorder, MRI may also suggest an alternate diagnosis (e.g. multiple sclerosis in a younger patient), or concurrent pathology (e.g. cerebrovascular disease).

Proton magnetic resonance spectroscopy (^{1}H-MRS)

Complementary to standard sequences, proton magnetic resonance spectroscopy (^{1}H-MRS) enables relative metabolite concentrations to be quantified within the target region of interest (single voxel spectroscopy) or averaged over multiple sampling regions (chemical shift imaging), in each case reflecting radiofrequency emissions from the proton nuclei of the present metabolites. These are expressed as parts per million, by convention relative to creatine.[17,18] However, in clinical practice, in vivo spectral resolution is limited to compounds present at minimum concentrations of 0.5–1.0 mM, permitting broad inference only. Pathognomic profiles are limited, including elevated N-acetyl aspartate in aspartoacylase deficiency[19] and the absence of creatine in disorders of creatine synthesis;[20] nevertheless, non-specific findings may prove informative and often preceed changes in standard sequences, such as the presence of a lactate doublet (an inverted peak at 1.3 ppm in long TE acquisitions), occurring in the context of a suspected mitochondrial cytopathy.[12] Moreover, advances in MRS technology, in part due to the availability of high field magnets are permitting greater spectral resolution and more definitive metabolite identification, with the promise of increased clinical utility.

Positron emission tomography

Positron emission tomography has limited utility in the screening assessment of neurometabolic disorders, although this more accurately reflects a current lack of data for this modality amongst the heterogeneous cohort of neurometabolic disorders—for the most part limited to individual case reports and small series.

Neurophysiology

While electrophysiological studies have limited utility in the adjunctive assessment of suspected metabolic cognitive decline, they are inexpensive, non-invasive, and may demonstrate functional aberrations not evident with neuroimaging. Electroencephalography is often normal, although background slowing consistent with an encephalopathic state is common and temporospatial changes may reflect transient cognitive impairment, a feature of many metabolic diseases. Characteristic findings may also provide diagnostic clues; triphasic waves are often considered to indicate a metabolic aetiology, most commonly present in hepatic and renal encephalopathy—although

non-metabolic causes are also recognized. Epileptiform features, while of limited discriminatory value, are present in several neurometabolic dementias, and in some cases, electrographic patterns suggest a specific aetiology (e.g. prominent occipital potentials and photoparoxysmal discharges in several of the neuronal ceroid lipofuscinoses).[21,22] Similarly, evoked potentials, nerve conduction studies, and electromyography may assist diagnosis.

Tissue biopsies

Histopathological, ultrastructural (electron microscopy), and tissue biochemical studies may prove informative in cases of suspected metabolic dementia. Tissue biopsies allow for histopathological analysis of substrate storage, as evident in the cerebral glycogenosis (e.g. adult polyglucosan body disease) and many of the lysosomal disorders, while transmission electron microscopy may identify disordered ultrastructural pathology (e.g. mitochondrial dysmorphology) or characteristic intracellular inclusions (e.g. neuronal ceroid lipofuscinoses), the latter often identified upon preparation of buffy coat leucocytes. Fibroblast culture is often useful, providing an enduring source of tissue for analysis of ubiquitously expressed enzymes, substrate loading studies (e.g. fillipin staining after incubation of Niemann–Pick C fibroblasts in the presence of cholesterol-loaded low-density lipoprotein), and extraction of genomic DNA for molecular analysis of causal genes, while metabolically active tissues such as skeletal muscle and liver are typically utilized for the biochemical analyses of respiratory chain complexes in fresh or snap-frozen samples. Of special note, specimens derived postmortem should always be considered in suspected cases of inborn metabolic disease where inherited pathology has relevance for remaining family members. Appropriate preservation of tissue samples is, of course, critical and advice regarding collection, processing, and storage of samples should be sought.

Acquired metabolic causes of cognitive decline

Nutritional deficiency

Critical to nervous system development and cellular biochemical function, nutritional deficiency of macronutrients and essential micronutrients (vitamins and trace elements) remains a dominant contributing factor to neurocognitive health globally, particularly in at-risk populations, where multiple deficiencies are common. Specific deficiencies, while comparatively rare, are more typical in micronutrient-replete Western diets, encountered in restrictive dietary regimens, psychiatric eating disorders, and, increasingly, after bariatric surgery.[5] However, multiple deficiencies in the context of self-neglect and the impact of illness upon nutritional state must also be considered, particularly in vulnerable persons such as the itinerant, elderly, and chronic alcohol abusers; pathological restriction of intake (e.g. malabsorptive disease), increased utilization (e.g. malignancy), and excessive losses (e.g. renal tubular disease) must not be forgotten. Iatrogenic deficiency (e.g. inappropriate parenteral nutrition) may also occur. It is noteworthy that many inborn errors of metabolism parallel acquired micronutrient deficiencies, emphasizing the importance of these compounds as co-factors for normal enzyme function.

Nutritional excesses are also recognized in the path genesis of cognitive impairment, either through accumulative consequences of dietary excess (the metabolic syndrome) or specific toxicities, as may occur in heavy metal exposure or alcohol.

Vitamin deficiency

Vitamin deficiencies dominate amongst the acquired causes of neurocognitive dysfunction.

B-group vitamin deficiencies[22-24] reflect their importance as specific enzyme co-factors, typically occurring in the context of malnutrition, pathological malabsorption, or states of increased metabolic demand (e.g. malignancy); alcoholism is a common association. Pharmacological interactions may impair bioavailability (eg. folate analogues, including trimethoprim) and dietary inhibitors can impact absorption. The neurocognitive consequences of B-vitamin deficiency are varied, in many cases reflecting compound losses, although isolated deficiencies with characteristic phenotypes do occur—commonly thiamine, cobalamin, and niacin deficiencies manifesting Wernicke–Korsakoff syndrome, combined degeneration of the spinal cord and pellagra respectively. Subacute cognitive impairment and psychiatric manifestations dominate, often associated with apathy. Systemic features are typically prominent, including anorexia, abdominal pain, glossitis, and a seborrheic-like dermatitis; cardiomyopathy is a feature of thiamine deficiency (wet beriberi). While a role for individual vitamin deficiencies in primary dementia and geriatric cognitive decline has been postulated (e.g. B_6, B_9, and B_{12}), a clear association remains unproven and the population benefit of widespread supplementation in the non-deficient population remains unsubstantiated.[25,26] Early treatment response is usual, although irreversible manifestations occur when replacement is delayed, emphasizing the importance of prompt recognition and diagnosis. Biochemical deficiency is readily confirmed via fasting assay in plasma or erythrocytes, although laboratory variability can be wide and acess to specialist assays may be limited. Indeed, clinical response to replacement is often sufficient to confirm a presumptive diagnosis, particularly when rapid intervention is indicated. Urinary organic acids may reveal excretion of characteristic metabolites such as methylmalonic acid in the presence of cobalamin deficiency, which must be excluded in any case where elevation is present. Rarely, functional enzyme studies are required to confirm increased activity following co-factor loading. Neurophysiological parameters are non-specific and may demonstrate an encephalopathic EEG, at times with epileptic features. Imaging is typically non-specific, with the exception of thiamine (see below) and cobalamin deficiencies, the later presenting subacute combined deficiency of the spinal cord.

Vitamins D and E (α-tocopherol) deficiency, while not primarily causing dementia, have also been implicated in neurocognitive decline; the latter, when severe, manifesting a phenotype of cerebellar and posterior column dysfunction, ophthalmoparesis (typically of upgaze) and axonal neuropathy resembling Friedreich ataxia. Each have been hypothesized to contribute to age-related cognitive decline and primary dementia,[27-29] although as with the B-group vitamins, benefits of replacement within the wider population remain inconclusive.

Example: Thiamine (vitamin B₁) deficiency

Thiamine (vitamin B_1), a heterocyclic carbine, serves as a critical co-factor in carbohydrate and amino acid metabolism; its active phosphorylated form (thiamine pyrophosphate) serves as a co-factor in the decarboxylation of α-keto acids—intermediaries in the generation of ATP via the tricarboxylic acid cycle—and transketolase in the formation of ribose and dexoyribose via the pentose monophosphate shunt. Within the central nervous system, thiamine is critical to the processes of myelin formation, axonal conduction, and the synthesis of specific neurotransmitters (e.g. acetylcholine).

Most commonly arising in states of nutritional deficiency, classically starvation and malabsorption, thiamine depletion may also reflect reduced bioavailability due to dietary antithiamine factors, and increased metabolic consumption; hepatic stores are limited and clinical manifestations can arise in as little as one to three months.

Cognitive manifestations reflect impairment of cellular energy production resulting in cytotoxic oedema and parenchymal injury. Disease features range from irritability and mild confusion, often with an apathetic quality, to frank encephalopathy and irreversible deficiencies of anterograde and retrograde amnesia (Korsakoff psychosis). Acutely, focal neurological deficits are common with the triad of ophthalmoparesis, cerebellar ataxia, and encephalopathy defining Wernicke's encephalopathy.

Clinical suspicion is often confirmed by treatment response; fasting plasma thiamine can be measured, although it is subject to protein binding, and quantification of erythrocyte thiamine pyrophosphate levels has largely replaced this assay. Urinary excretion of thiamine and its metabolites can be confirmed by HPLC, typically expressed as a spot ratio relative to creatinine, and organic acid profiles may demonstrate elevated levels of pyruvate, lactate, and α-ketoglutarate, reflecting impairment of thiamine-dependent enzymes. Erythrocyte transketolase activity, measured pre- and post-thiamine load, remains the most sensitive indicator, with an increase of enzyme activity in excess of 25 percent indicative of deficiency. Folate deficiency and hypomagnesaemia must also be excluded as both may exacerbate thiamine deficiency.

Neuroimaging lacks sensitivity and may prove normal; however, acute disease may demonstrate symmetrical T2/FLAIR signal hyperintensity, restricted diffusion, and gadolinium enhancement within the mamillary bodies, mediodorsal thalamus, tectal plate, and periaqueductal grey matter. In chronic disease, cerebral and cerebellar volume loss may additionally be seen. Proton spectroscopy may demonstrate increased lactate, reduced NAA, and reduced choline, the latter suggested to reflect reduced incorporation of lipids into myelin or disordered acetylcholine production. A length-dependent axonal polyneuropathy is often prominent in chronic deficiency, and non-neurological features, particularly cardiomyopathy, may result. Variability of clinical phenotype is well documented and polygenic influences have been suggested with variations in transketolase affinity and the thiamine transporter proteins implicated.[30,31]

Early recognition is critical as prompt thiamine replacement may effect symptom resolution, albeit permanent amnestic deficits are common (100 mg/day parenterally for 1 week followed by 10 mg/day orally until symptom resolution).

Elemental deficiency

Biologically present in trace amounts, many elements are absolutely required for life: although they are often fastidiously conserved in the body and recycled through various compartments, they must be obtained from the diet—usually in amounts < 1 mg/day. Trace elements are integral to the structure and function of many proteins (metalloproteins), and when deficient or found in excess, cognitive function is often impaired; indeed elemental deficiencies including copper, iron, selenium, and zinc, have been implicated in the causation of neuropsychiatric disease, non-specific cognitive decline and primary dementing illnesses, albeit definitive mechanisms remain poorly defined.[32–35]

With the exception of iodine, where one-third of the global population live in deficient regions,[36] isolated losses are rare, more typically occurring in the context of multiple nutritional insufficiency, the result of inadequate diet, intestinal malabsorption (copper, often follows gastric bypass surgery), and renal protein losses (e.g. nephrotic syndrome). Specific iatrogenic deficiencies may occur, as seen with chelating agents, particularly penicillamine which has wider medicinal indications, or other pharmaceutical actions such as urinary zinc losses secondary to thiazide diuretics. Chronic dialysis and dependence upon unsupplemented pareneteral nutrition are also a risk where strict monitoring is not observed; indeed, rare deficiencies of molybdenum, an essential co-factor of sulphite oxidase, xanthine oxidoreductase, and aldehyde oxidase, leading to irritability and coma have been reported in this context.[37]

Recognizable phenotypes may inform diagnosis. **Cuproproteins** serve important roles in cellular energy production, free-radical scavenging, neurotransmitter metabolism, phospholipid synthesis, and iron transport, deficiency of which may also contribute to disturbed cognition and adjunct features including sensory ataxia, proprioceptive loss, and spasticity, reflecting peripheral neuropathy and myelopathic disease. **Zinc** is an integral component of more than 300 metalloenzymes and transcription factors and serves multiple functions within the central nervous system including synthesis of coenzymes requisite in bioamine metabolism and the modulation of postsynaptic N-methyl-D-aspartate (NMDA) receptors, suggesting a role in the regulation of synaptic plasticity.[38] Neurological features range from impaired concentration and irritability to neuropsychiatric features and variable cognitive impairment; hypogeusia (decreased taste) may alert the treating physician, while the presence of a concomitant vesiculopustular dermatitis should prompt strong consideration. Secondary exacerbation of hepatic encephalopathy and hyperammonaemia, resulting from impaired ornithine transcarbamylase activity (OTC), akin to the inborn error of this enzyme, is also a recognized consequence of zinc deficiency.[39,40] The neurocognitive effects of severe **iodine** deficiency reflect impaired thyroid hormone synthesis; presenting at at any age, with features ranging from mild sequalae in adults to profound intellectual impairment in the context of congenital deficiency (cretinism). Adjunct neurological findings include sensorineural deafness and spasticity of a characteristic axial and proximal appendicular distribution. Only in severe iodine deficiency does hypothyroidism develop, accompanied by an elevated serum TSH value and decreased T3 and T4 levels.

In most cases neuroimaging is non-specific, although myelopathy with increased T2 signal in the dorsal columns is suggestive of copper deficiency.[41] Screening biochemical abnormalities may reflect enzyme dysfunction (e.g. reduced alkaline phosphatase level, a zinc-dependent enzyme); however, diagnosis relies upon quantification of elemental plasma and urinary levels (spot ratios relative to creatinine or 24-hour collection); activity assays of dependent enzymes may also inform diagnosis. In all cases, prompt replacement is warranted, as delayed correction may result in permanent neurological sequalae.

Marchiafava–Bignami disease

Marchiafava–Bignami disease (MBD) is an extremely rare condition characterized by dementia with axonal injury and demyelination within the corpus callosum, typically beginning in the corpus and extending to the genu and splenium; involvement of the centrum semiovale, brachium pontis, and other white matter tracts may also occur, although sparing of the internal capsule, corona radiata, and subcortical association fibres is usual. Gliosis in the frontotemporal regions, predominantly in the third cortical layer (Morel cortical laminar sclerosis), is often a feature. Commonly, but not absolutely described in patients with chronic alcoholism, aetiology has been attributed to non-specific nutritional deficiency and may reflect a reduction in multiple B-group compounds. A panethnic disease, cases are dominated by men, the majority arising after 45 years of age. Clinical symptoms vary; onset may be precipitous with lethargy, stupor, and rapid progression to coma, while subacute or chronic dementia, often with ideomotor apraxia and psychiatric disturbance, is also observed. Progressive corticospinal tract involvement, ataxia, and seizures evolve—with distinction from associated disease and comorbid pathology often difficult. Diagnosis is made upon clinical and neuroradiological grounds, characteristically manifesting a 'sandwich sign' wihin the corpus callosum on saggital T2/FLAIR series due to relative sparing of the ventral and dorsal fibres; restricted diffusion is evident within acute lesions, and cystic necrosis eventuates. Prognosis is poor, however early detection and supportive management including abstinence from alcohol and administration of B-complex vitamins has improved outcomes in contemporary practice.

Macronutrient deficiency and excess

Critical for normal neurodevelopmental outcomes, the cognitive effects of macronutrient insufficiency on the developed brain can be profound, albeit distinction from comorbid micronutrient deficiency is often difficult. Macronutrient excess is similarly linked to dementia, largely through secondary consequences of insulin resistance and chronic metabolic dysregulation.

Endocrinopathy-associated cognitive decline

Endocrinopathy-associated cognitive decline is well recognized as a primary consequence of the precipitant disorder (e.g. thyroid, parathyroid, and adrenal disease) or as sequalae of the disordered metabolic state that results—exemplified by diabetes mellitus, in which multiple factors contribute to cerebral pathology, including abnormal protein glucosylation, recurrent hypoglycaemic insult, and cerebrovascular disease. Patterns of neurocognitive dysfunction vary from acute encephalopathy and subacute cognitive decline to late-onset dementing disease and neuropsychiatric manifestations. Systemic features are often prominent in thyroid and adrenal disease, with recognizable phenotypes in many cases alerting the diagnosis. Biochemical confirmation is readily determined and early initiation of treatment with sustained endocrinological homeostasis the priority.

Whilst not a primary endocrinopathy, the consequence of recurrent non-diabetic hypoglycaemia should also be considered in the cognitively declining patient, particularly if stepwise deterioration is evident; plasma glucose is confirmatory during an acute episode; however, transient episodes may require pre- and post-prandial sampling to substantiate, with an observed fast (up to 72 hours) most sensitive. Once confirmed, diagnostic investigations must follow and the differential causes of hypoglycaemia investigated.

Visceral insufficiency and cognitive decline

Disordered metabolic homeostasis, as a result of visceral failure, frequently precipitates acute, recurrent encephalopathy; however, more indolent cognitive dysfunction may also occur. In each case, disease can be considered a consequence of neurotoxic metabolite accumulation—chiefly ammonia and manganese in hepatic disease and multiple renally cleared substrates (urea, phosphates, parathyroid hormone, and amino acids) in the presence of renal failure; iatrogenic neurocognitive decline in the context of long-term dialysis (dialysis dementia) has also been recognized—the result of aluminium toxicity, now rarely observed, with removal of this contaminant from dialysate.[42] The pathophysiological basis of pancreatic encephalopathy is more protean, implicating cytokine release and consequences of the acute inflammatory response, microcirculation abnormalities, and concomitant bacterial infection. Moreover, in all cases of visceral failure, comorbid electrolyte disturbance and micronutrient insufficiency are often present; indeed, co-morbid thiamine deficiency has been implicated in both hepatic- and pancreatic-associated encephalopathies.[43,44] The contribution of visceral pathology to other dementia subtypes (e.g. nephrogenic hypertension and multi-infarct dementia) should also be considered. In all cases acute management pertains to reduction of the accumulating toxins, through dietary, pharmacotherapeutic, and other means including dialysis, in addition to treatment of the underling systemic pathology. Attention to minimizing precipitants of metabolic decompensation (e.g. increased protein load in hepatic and renal disease) is critical to improving longer-term stability.

Inborn disorders of metabolic function causing cognitive decline in adulthood

Whilst the inborn errors of metabolism remain individually rare causes of adult-onset dementia, recognition is critical: effective therapeutic intervention is increasingly available and the genetic implications of inborn metabolic errors require consideration. Accurate epidemiological data are lacking—in part due to underdiagnosis—however it is notable that the greatest burden is within young adult presentations and amongst those with adjunct neurological and/or systemic disease.

A contemporary view of inborn metabolic diseases includes other genetic disorders affecting metabolic function, a premise which could be extended to almost all neurodegenerative processes. Nevertheless, here we focus on recognition of important classes of neurometabolic disease presenting with adult-onset cognitive dysfunction. Readers are refered to specialist resources for further detail.

Disorders of carbohydrate metabolism

As a primary substrate for energy production, inborn errors of carbohydrate metabolism include defects of glucose production and utilization (e.g. disorders of gluconeogenesis and glycolysis), disorders of transport (e.g. glucose transporter deficiency), and abnormalities of glucose storage and mobilization (e.g. the glycogenopathies). Neurons do not synthesize glycogen and rely upon mitochondrial oxidation of astrocyte-derived lactate, generated by glycogenolysis, to provide an alternative energy source during neuroglycopaenia. Cognitive involvement ranges from childhood intellectual impairment to acute encephalopathy, classic dementing disease, and episodic decline. Neuroglycopaenic-associated cognitive impairment and recurrent hypoglycaemic insult must also be considered in this context. Biochemical identification corresponds to the protocols for such diagnoses, excepting the glycogenoses. In several cases effective therapeutic intervention can be implemented, again emphasizing the need so far as possible to confirm diagnosis.

Example: The cerebral glycogenoses

Characterized by the intracellular accumulation of polyglucosan—an abnormal storage form of glycogen—the cerebral glycogenoses[45,46] are an important consideration in the dementing adult. Two subtypes dominate, adult polyglucosan body disease (APGBD), over-represented in the Ashkenazi Jewish population, is the consequence of an autosomal recessive mutation in the GBE1 gene, encoding the 1,4-α-glucan-branching enzyme-1; and Lafora body disease, primarily associated with autosomal recessive mutations in either of two genes: epilepsy, progressive myoclonus 2a and 2b (EPM2A and EPM2B) which encode the complicit glycogen regulatory proteins, laforin phosphatase and malin ubiquitin ligase, respectively. Disease reflects aberrant glycogen synthesis with deposition of periodic acid–Schiff (PAS) positive polyglucosan aggregations in neural tissues; the pathophysiological consequences of which remain poorly understood, however a secondary deficit of cellular energy production has been suggested, possibly related to inadequate reserves of normally compacted glycogen.[47,48]

Adult polyglucosan body disease typically presents after age 40 years, with progressive neurogenic bladder dysfunction, lower limb weakness, and spasticity of a mixed upper and lower motor neuron pattern; distal sensory deficit, cerebellar dysfunction, and cognitive difficulties also occur, typified by mild deficits in executive function. Lafora disease presents in adolescence (12–17 years), with progressive myoclonic epilepsy and mixed semiology seizures; occipital seizures presenting as visual hallucinations are often striking. Of note, a history of infantile seizures is common. Neurocognitive decline, with a frontal dementia pattern ensues with progression to myoclonic status, and death within 10 years of onset. Clinical diagnosis is supported by neuroimaging in APBD where progressive cerebral, cerebellar, and upper cervical spinal cord atrophy is typical, with non-enhancing white matter disease involving the subcortex (periventricular), brainstem, and cerebellum; imaging is normal or reveals non-specific cerebral atrophy in Lafora disease. Conversley, electroencephalography is non-specific in APBD, and typically epileptiform in Lafora disease, with photosensitivity an early feature and generalized, irregular spike-wave discharges of occipital predominance. Histological demonstration of periodic acid–Schiff (PAS) positive, diastase resistant, polyglucosan inclusions strongly suggests the diagnosis; confirmation is achieved by molecular analysis. In each case, targeted therapy remains unmet and management is symptomatic; while recent attempts to ameliorate the suspected deficit of cellular energy in APBD (using dietary supplementation of the 7-carbon triglyceride, triheptanoin), may afford some attenuation of clinical deterioration, functional recovery is not expected.[47]

Disorders of mitochondrial energy metabolism

The primary mitochondrial cytopathies and related disorders of pyruvate, tricarboxylic acid cycle, and respiratory chain metabolism are an important subclass of metabolic cognitive disease (see chapter 31). Childhood onset dominates but late-onset decline, often with specific deficits of visual construction, attention, and abstraction (in the absence of general intellectual deterioration) has been reported in mutations involving both the mitochondrial genome (e.g. MELAS, MERRF, MNGIE) as well nuclear-encoded mitochondrial proteins (e.g. POLG, DDP1). Searching for these mutations should be considered in work-up of early-onset dementing patients.[49]

Fatty acid oxidation disorders similarly reflect an end-deficit of mitochondrial energy failure; four subgroups are defined 1) carnitine cycle disorders, 2) fatty acid ß-oxidation disorders, 3) electron transfer disturbances (e.g. type II glutaric aciduria), and 4) anomalies of ketone body production—in each case resulting in disordered synthesis of acetyl CoA. These diseases typically occur in childhood, however, adult presenting disease is recognized, often during periods of metabolic stress, and in many cases preceeded by prolonged periods of normal health. Infantile presentations are dominated by non-ketotic hypoglycaemia and encephalopathy, accompanied by hepatomegaly and 'Reye-like' liver dysfunction. Cognitive involvement is rare in adult disease and hypertrophic cardiomyopathy and skeletal muscle involvement, often with rhabdomyolysis, dominate the clinical picture.

These disorders are briefly summarized.

Disorders of amino acid metabolism and transport

Disorders of amino acid metabolism and transport are a large group of intermediate metabolism defects, reflecting the importance of amino acids in cellular function. These diseases occur principally in infancy and childhood; however, adult-onset variants, typically of an attenuated phenotype, are increasingly recognized. Many of these prove amenable to therapeutic intervention, necessitating timely and accurate diagnosis. Disease is largely attributed to toxic accumulation of specific amino acids, their precursors, and derivatives, including secondary impairment of complicit metabolic pathways such as disruption of the tricarboxylic acid

cycle in many of the organic acidopathies and urea cycle disorders. Porphyria-like decompensation, characteristic of tyrosinemia type 1, is another example, reflecting inhibition of aminolevulinate dehydratase, an enzyme in haem biosynthesis, by pathogenic metabolites. Less frequently, disruption of cellular homeostasis is due to deficiency of exogenous amino acids, best exemplified in Hartnup disease, in which impairment of the neutral amino acid transporter, SLC6A19 results in renal and gastrointestinal losses of the niacin precursor tryptophan, giving rise to frank pellagra.

These are protean disorders, particularly amongst attenuated, late-onset variants: detailed summaries can be obtained from dedicated texts, nevertheless several common features may inform diagnosis. While dementia occurs, the neurocognitive decline is more often acute or subacute in nature, often preceded by a prolonged asymptomatic period or relapsing–remitting decompensation, usually in the context of interval metabolic stress (e.g. fever or illness) or increased protein loading. Dietary aversion to protein-rich diets may be discovered, particularly in phenylketonuria, the organic acidopathies, and urea cycle disorders, which may present following protein loading. Mutations in the transporter, citrin (citrullinaemia type 2) are a notable exception; here carbohydrate-rich diets trigger decompensation. Neurocognitive decline in the context of childhood intellectual impairment should also suggest an undiagnosed aminoacidopathy. Insidious cognitive impairment in the context of known diagnoses may also occur, prompting consideration of either lack of compliance or iatrogenic restriction of essential nutrients, as a result of inappropriate dietary therapy. In general, psychiatric and neurobehavioural manifestations are common and additional neurological and systemic features often occur. Progressive leukoencephalopathy revealed by MRI, extending to involve the subcortical fibres, necessitates exclusion of disordered amino acid metabolism. Stroke-like episodes may be identified, particularly in patients with branched chain aminoacidopathies and urea cycle disorders; while peripheral thromboembolism is a feature of homocystinuria—most commonly due to deficiency of the pyridoxine-dependent enzyme, cystathionine β-synthase, which causes disrupted methionine transsulfuration (classical homocystinuria). In this condition, unique amongst the aminoacidopathies, there is a prominent Marfanoid phenotype which is a distinguishing feature in hyperhomocysteinaemia. In the case of several aminoacidopathies, a characteristic body odour may be reported, reflecting accumulation of the odiferous compound.

Diagnosis relies upon quantification of pathological compounds and their derivatives in biological fluids—typically plasma and urine, including ammonia and the aminoacids—detection of the latter has been advanced through contemporary refinement of chromatographic techniques and mass spectrometry. In the case of the organic acidopathies, patterns of aberrant acylcarnitine conjugation may assist diagnosis. Secondary metabolic consequences may also provide supportive data (e.g. ketoacidosis in the organic acidemias). Caution should be exercised in the diagnosis of hyperammonaemia in this context, as the presentation of many organic acidemias may suggest a urea cycle anomaly, consequent to accumulation of CoA derivatives which inhibit the formation of N-acetylglutamate, the activator of hepatic carbamoyl phosphate synthetase. It is important to be aware of assay limitations, including factors which lead to artefactual results and, where possible, sampling should be performed during symptomatic states or under conditions of metabolic stress as this will improve detection of pathogenic metabolites, which may fall below levels of detection during asymptomatic periods. Given the potential for decompensation, timed collections under conditions of substrate load should only be performed under careful clinical observation; while occasionally required to confirm diagnoses, the advent of genetic analyses has rendered such tests increasingly unnecessary.

Many of the aminoacidopathies are treatable, however, particularly when neurological disease is advanced, not all sequalae are reversible. Interventions are subtype specific and focus upon removal of accumulated toxic compounds by substrate-restrictive diets (in most cases protein restriction), extracorporeal procedures or target specific 'cleansing' drugs such as carnitine, sodium benzoate or phenylacetate and betaine; and through supplementation of critical intermediates such as urea cycle metabolites (e.g. arginine, citrulline), essential co-factors (e.g. pyridoxine in homocystinaemia), and suppression of disordered biosynthesis, particularly during periods of metabolic stress.

Example: Phenylketonuria and disordered biopterin metabolism

Phenylketonuria is the most prevalent of the aminoacidopathies and is usually the result of an autosomal recessive deficiency of phenylalanine hydroxylase, which catalyses the conversion of phenylalanine (an essential amino acid) to tyrosine. Functional deficiency of the enzyme may also arise from disordered synthesis or recycling of its co-factor, tetrahydrobiopterin (BH4), although such disorders have only been described in childhood-onset disease. Central nervous system pathology ensues when excess phenylalanine accumulates and, while the exact mechanism of disease is uncertain, consequences include disruption of synaptogenesis and dendritic arborization, glial cell dysfuncton, and oligodendrocyte toxicity—the latter resulting in dysmyelination and white matter vacuolization. Aberrant equilibria of large neutral amino acids within the brain, as a result of competive transport across the blood-brain barrier and impaired synthesis of biogenic amines (e.g. dopamine and norepinephrine) due to a reduction in their precursor, tyrosine, also contribute.[50–52]

Classical disease presents with progressive neurocognitive impairment in infancy and childhood, typified by irreversible intellectual retardation and spasticity; seizures and parkinsonian features may result. However, rare instances of adult-onset disease have been reported, with progressive leukoencephalopathy, dementia, optic atrophy, and neuropsychiatric decline.[53–55] Moreover, asymptomatic cases are recognized. Hypopigmentation, the result of reduced melanin synthesis, and a musty odour, caused by excreted phenylacetic acid may be prominent. Increasingly patients are identified through newborn screening programmes, facilitating initiation of presymptomatic therapy and amelioriating consequences of chronic hyperphenylalaninaemia.

Hyperphenylalaninaemia is readily confirmed through quantification of plasma and urinary amino acids; urinary organic acid profiles may also demonstrate increased excretion of phenylpyruvic and phenylacetic acid. Cofactor deficiencies (disorders of biopterin synthesis or recycling) are excluded via urinary pterin analysis and quantification of dihydropteridine reductase activity within erythrocytes, while molecular confirmation is now widely available. Neuroimaging findings are non-specific, however a leukodystrophy, predominantly of an occipitoparietal (periventricular) distribution and including the subcortical fibres is typical (this may reverse with treatment); cerebral and cerebellar atrophy may also occur. An increased phenylalanine peak (7.4 ppm) may resolve on 1H-MRS, however it is not usually prominent on standard clinical spectra.

Management includes implementation of a phenylalanine-(protein) restricted diet and, in responsive cases, adjuvant therapy with tetrahydrobiopterin, which acts to stabilize and augment endogenous PAH activity.[56] Consideration must also be given to late-onset neuropsychiatric manifestations in patients, arising in the context of treatment non-compliance, although such outcomes are not absolute and some patients may tolerate a relaxation of phenylalanine restriction. Iatrogenic B_{12} deficiency may account for the dementing phenylketonuria patient—a consequence of low-protein diet without supplementation of this essential vitamin.[57,58]

Vitamin-responsive inborn errors of metabolism

The vitamin-responsive inborn errors of metabolism include homocysteine remethylation defects, and disorders of cobalamin transport and utilization, methylenetetrahydrofolate reductase deficiency, cerebral folate deficiency, and the disorders of biotin metabolism; familial vitamin E deficiency can also be considered in this context. In most of these conditions, disease resembles that seen in the respective acquired co-factor deficiencies. Clinical suspicion is reinforced by response to replacement therapy, while diagnostic screening relies on demonstration of specific cofactor deficiencies and their related biochemical consequences, such as elevated homocysteine in disorders of remethylation (cobalamin-C disease and methylenetetrahydrofolate reductase deficiency), in the case of cerebral folate deficiency necessitating cerebrospinal fluid analysis as plasma levels are normal. Functional studies of enzyme activity may also be required, for example in biotinidase deficiency where plasma biotin may fall within normal range, while in other cases, such as biotin–thiamine-responsive basal ganglia disease, biochemical parameters are typically normal and molecular diagnosis is required.

Example: Cobalamin C deficiency

The inborn disorders of cobalamin transport and utilization represent defects of intracellular cobalamin metabolism, defined by biochemical phenotype and genetic complementation analysis. The most common of these is cobalamin-C disease (cblC), which results in disordered homocysteine remethylation secondary to a deficiency of the cobalamin binding protein, Methylmalonic aciduria and homocystinuria type C (MMACHC), responsible for catalysing removal of ligands from alkylcobalamins and cyanocobalamin. Typically presenting during infancy, a small number of cblC patients present as late as the fourth decade of life with confusion, disorientation, dementia, and neuropsychiatric disease, often associated with subacute combined degeneration of the spinal cord; leukoencephalopathy may also emerge. Systemic features, including macrocytic anaemia, while suggestive, are not invariably present and do not preclude consideration of B_{12} deficiency in isolated neurological presentations.

Biochemical hallmarks of disease include increased plasma total homocysteine with low to normal plasma methionine; homocystinuria and methylmalonic aciduria. Treatment with parenteral hydroxycobalamin and oral betaine may normalize biochemical parameters, however disease reversal may prove incomplete, particularly if instigated late in the course of the illness.[59–61]

Disorders of neurotransmitter metabolism and function

Disorders of gamma aminobutyric acid, glycine, and monoamine metabolism (including disorders of biopterin synthesis) typically present in infancy and childhood, however in many cases survival to adulthood occurs. Late-onset neurocognitive decline and dementia are not characteristic, although adult presentation of non-ketotic hyperglycinaemia is recognized.[62,63] In this autosomal recessive disorder of glycine cleavage, accumulation of the excitatory neurotransmitter manifests as cognitive decline, which may be triggered by fever or prescription of sodium valproate (an inhibitor of glycine cleavage), often on a background of existing intellectual delay. Neurobehavioural lability, seizures, optic atrophy, and paroxysmal choreiform movements may occur, with eventual progression to a vacuolating leukoencephalopathy, typically sparing the subcortical U-fibres. Diagnosis requires demonstration of an isolated elevation in glycine and increased CSF:plasma ratio; confirmation of the molecular defect usually follows. Treatment response is at most partial; a restricted protein diet with additional sodium benzoate may reduce plasma concentration of glycine, while more recently, N-methyl D-aspartate (NMDA) receptor antagonists have been employed to minimize NMDA receptor activation.[64]

Disordered neurotransmitter homeostasis, particularly acetylcholine, is also implicated in a number of neuroocognitive diseases, including Alzheimer's disease and Lewy body dementias, the mechanisms of which are likely multifactorial. However quantification of CSF acetylcholine is technically limited and of little practical use.[65] Monoamine metabolites and pterin profiles are increasingly accessible in specialist laboratories, albeit these too have little utility in the context of adult-onset dementia. Nevertheless, the spectrum of neurotransmitter disease remains undefined and consideration to screening of the CSF biochemical profile may prove to be decisive.

Brief consideration should also be given to 'acquired' disorders of neurotransmission; autoantibodies targeting the post-synaptic N-methyl-D-aspartate (NMDA) receptor may contribute to the spectrum of autoimmune encephalitidies, often occurring in the context of an ovarian teratoma or other occult malignancy and manifesting after a prodromal 'influenza-like' illness, with behavioural change, prominent neuropsychiatric symptoms, and seizures. This important diagnosis is covered in detail in chapter 28.

Disorders of lipid and bile acid metabolism

Disorders of lipid metabolism and transport are very diverse, but they are increasingly recognized amongst the late-onset disorders of metabolism and prominently represented amongst the metabolic

dementias. Broadly these can be considered under several main categories:

1) Disorders of cholesterol and bile acid synthesis, cerebrotendinous xanthomatosis (sterol 27-hydroxylase deficiency) and α-methylacyl-CoA racemase (AMACR) deficiency, each reflecting disordered oxidation of cholesterol side chains.

2) X-linked adrenoleukodystrophy/adrenomyeloneuropathy.

3) Disorders of cholesterol trafficking, exemplified by Niemann–Pick disease type C.

4) The sphingolipidoses, each the result of a specific lysosomal hydrolase deficiency that impairs catabolism of complex sphingolipids with resultant accumulation leading to neuronal dysfunction.

While clinical features and diagnostic investigations tend to be disease-specific, several generalizations apply across to this cohort. Cognitive decline is typically slowly progressive and neuropsychiatric presentations are common, while leukoencephalopathic disease and peripheral neuropathy are frequently observed. Cerebellar dysfunction, extrapyramidal features, seizures, and retinopathy may also occur. Systemic pathology can inform diagnosis; splenomegaly might suggest a disorder of lipid storage, while tissue deposition of storage material, such as tendon xanthomata, may be evident. A history of prolonged neonatal jaundice in the dementing patient necessitates exclusion of disordered cholesterol metabolism, disordered bile acid metabolism or Niemann–Pick disease type C, a cholesterol-trafficking defect.

Example: Cerebrotendinosus xanthomatosis

Cerebrotendinosus xanthomatosis reflects a recessive defect in the mitochondrial enzyme, sterol 27-hydroxylase, required for the synthesis of bile acids from cholesterol; accumulation of cholesterol, bile acid precursors, and their metabolites (including cholestenol) results. A history of infantile cholestatic jaundice is common and should always raise suspicion in the dementing adult. Neurocognitive decline is usual and may occur as early as the first decade, however it appears more typically from adolescence and early adulthood, with concomitant neurobehavioural and psychiatric manifestations. Adjunct neurological features are prominent, including cerebellar dysfunction, spasticity and seizures; axonal neuropathy is frequent. Childhood-onset cataract is common and the presence of tendon xanthomas—evident from early to mid adulthood—are highly suggestive. Visceral xanthomata may also occur and focal neurological presentations in the context of cerebral lesions are recognized—most frequently within the cerebellar white matter. Neuroimaging demonstrates leukodystrophic changes within the cerebral and cerebellar white matter, with characteristic involvement of the dentate nuclei. Biochemical diagnosis is confirmed by demonstration of elevated plasma and urinary cholestanol in the context of a reduced plasma cholesterol and bile acids. Treatment with chenodeoxycholic acid effects a reduction in cholestanol synthesis and neurological improvement by suppression of cholesterol 7α-hydroxylase, the first enzyme within the predominant bile acid synthetic pathway. Adjunct strategies include the use of statins (3-hydroxy-3-methylglutaryl-coenzyme A (HMG-CoA) reductase inhibitors) and low-density lipoprotein apheresis.[66,67]

Example: Disorders of sphingolipid catabolism

The disorders of sphingolipid catabolism are lysosomal disorders characterized by the pathological accumulation of sphingolipids and their derivatives. The diseases result from deficient function of a given lysosomal hydrolase or a cognate activator protein. Panethnic in distribution, inheritance is autosomal recessive, with the exception of Andersen–Fabry disease which is X-linked. Individual disorders usually show a spectrum of neurovisceral disease, with attenuated, late-onset, cognitive decline in several (Gaucher disease, GM1 and GM2 gangliosidoses, and metachromatic leukodystrophy), generally of a slowly progressive nature and often with comorbid neuropsychiatric features, acute decompensation may, however, occur. Symmetrical leukoencephalopathy, sparing the subcortical U-fibres, suggests metachromatic leukodystrophy [Fig. 24.4], while cerebellar dysfunction, extrapyramidal disease, and seizures are common, although not invariably present. Systemic features are mostly seen in Gaucher disease (e.g. prominent visceromegaly) and GM1 gangliosidosis; these are not present in metachromatic leukodystrophy or the GM2 gangliosidoses (aside from mild visceral involvement in Sandhoff variant disease). With the exception of metachromatic leukodystrophy, neuroimaging is largely non-specific and diagnosis relies primarily on the demonstration of low residual enzyme activities – specific to each disease (typically performed in leucocytes or cultured fibroblasts); excepting rare cases of activator protein deficiency where *in vitro* activity assays are normal. Consequently, methods to identify pathogenic substrate accumulation via tandem mass spectrometry and molecular screening protocols are increasingly employed. In all cases, treatment of neurological disease remains limited, although attempts to effect central nervous system delivery of recombinant human enzyme, substrate reduction therapy and gene transfer approaches are in development.[66–72]

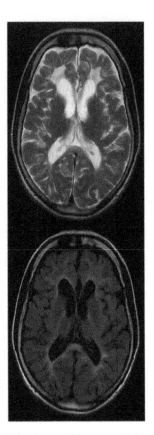

Fig. 24.4 Cerebral MRI in a 23-year-old woman with late-onset metachromatic leukodystrophy: T2 (above) and FLAIR axial images demonstrate frontally predominant white matter volume loss with symmetrically distributed signal hyperintensity and sparing of the subcortical U-fibres.
Reproduced from *Journal of Inherited Metabolic Disease*. 33(Suppl 3), Smith NJ, Marcus RE, Sahakian BJ, *et al.* Haematopoietic stem cell transplantation does not retard disease progression in the psycho-cognitive variant of late-onset metachromatic leukodystrophy, pp. 471–5, Copyright (2010), with permission from Springer.

Example: Nieman–Pick disease type C

One of the more common of the inborn metabolic dementias, Niemann–Pick type C disease shares many features with the disorders of sphingolipid catabolism. This defect of endocytosed cholesterol cellular trafficking, is due to mutations in either of two related proteins, NPC1 (≈ 95 percent) and NPC2 (≈ 5 percent). The disease is characterized by pathological accumulation of unesterified cholesterol and complex sphingolipids (including GM2 and GM3 ganglioside) within the endosomal–lysosomal system. The spectrum of clinical disease is widely variable, ranging from progressive neurovisceral disease in infancy (typically with prominent hepatosplenomegaly and infantile cholestasis) to more indolent adult-onset variants, the latter often presenting with progressive dystonia, cerebellar dysfunction, and variable cognitive impairmen; neuropsychiatric symptoms and dementia tend to be dominant and isolated psychiatric presentations are not uncommon. Movement disorders including myoclonus and action-induced dystonia are frequent and seizures may arise. Gelastic cataplexy and vertical supranuclear gaze palsy, with delayed saccadic initiation, are highly suggestive of the diagnosis, although less common in late-onset presentations. Similarly, visceral symptoms are less prominent in adult-onset disease. Neuroimaging is initially normal, with progressive cerebral and cerebellar atrophy (usually involving the cerebellar vermis), and thinning of the corpus callosum, with variable white matter hyperintensity, evident in some cases at late-stages of disease. Diagnostic confirmation is often complex; traditional demonstration of lipid storage within tissue samples (e.g. 'foamy', lipid-laden macrophages upon bone marrow biopsy) is rarely utilized in contemporary practice. Elevated serum chitotriosidase (a marker of macrophage activation) is non-specific; demonstration of reduced cholesterol esterification and its pathological accumulation after loading of cultured fibroblasts with exogenous cholesterol (using the fluorescent polyene macrolide, filipin) is often employed, however, reliable interpretation of this assay requires specialist expertise and is subject to normal variation. Molecular analysis is also incomplete, with mutations of the *NPC1* and *NPC2* genes in approximately 94 percent of cases. More recently, the demonstration of altered serum oxysterol profiles has proved an effective screening assay and is likely to replace filipin staining in this context. Disease is invariably progressive, and management remains largely symptomatic although inhibition of glycosphingolipid synthesis by the non-selective glucosylceramide synthase inhibitor, n-butyldeoxynojirimycin (miglustat) may, incompletely slow progression of late-onset disease.[3,4,73]

Disorders of haem metabolism

The hereditary porphyrias are a group of inborn metabolic errors of haem biosynthesis. Pathological accumulation of toxic pathway intermediates and their derivatives occurs, the majority of which are reduced porphyrins (porphyrinogens) which oxidize upon excretion from the intracellular environment to their corresponding porphyrins—these pigmented photoactive molecules fluoresce when exposed to visible light. Accumulation of the first committed precursor of haem biosynthesis in the liver, 5-aminolaevulinic acid, is associated with the acute neurovisceral effects of the disorder. Clinical features vary amongst subtypes, with neurovisceral disease largely restricted to the three acute hepatic porphyrias. Disease typically presents after puberty and may follow a prolonged period of clinical latency, with episodic decompensation often manifesting in the context of precipitants such as medication, illness or hormonal factors—especially progestogens formed during the luteal phase of the menstrual cycle—which increase demand for hepatic P450 synthesis and haem biosynthesis. While classic dementia is not usually a feature, neurocognitive symptoms include florid agitation and affective manifestations, often with features of sympathetic activation and, at their extreme, frank delirium, in many cases leading to an erroneous diagnosis of psychiatric disease. Visceral symptoms are prominent and include poorly characterized but often incapacitating abdominal pain, often with associated nausea or constipation; other effects such as tachycardia and arterial hypertension, reflect sympathetic overactivity. Additional features may include a mixed sensorimotor peripheral neuropathy (motor dominant), characteristically affecting the upper limbs and progressing to tetraparesis with ventilatory paralysis in some cases. While darkly pigmented urine is strongly suggestive, such findings are not acutely present in the hepatic porphyrias, due to the slow rate of colourless porphobilinogen oxidation to pigmented porphobilin; 5-aminoleavulinate excretion is also acutely elevated but this metabolite is colourless. Hyponatraemia is common, the result of electrolyte depletion and inappropriate antidiuretic hormone secretion; intractable seizures may result. Diagnosis relies upon detecting elevated urinary porphobilinogen and in some forms of acute porphyria, raised total porphyrin analyses during symptomatic episodes; while excretion patterns typically normalize upon recovery this is not always the case. Neuroimaging may demonstrate subcortical T2 signal intensity, without restricted diffusion, suggesting vasogenic oedema which resolves upon clinical recovery; a biooccipital pattern may be evident, resembling changes seen in posterior reversible (hypertensive) encephalopathy; differentiation of which is aided by the presence of contrast enhancement in porphyric lesions. Prompt treatment of acute decompensation is critical; identified triggers should be removed (care must be taken to avoid aggravating medications) and supportive measures including fluid resuscitation, electrolyte replacement, and analgesia initiated. Intravenous therapy with dextrose should be avoided in the face of rapidly progressive hyponatraenmia which characterizes the acute attack; intravenous haem arginate given daily for several days shortens duration of the acute attack. Long-term management centres upon the avoidance of triggering factors and consideration to hepatic transplantation in patients with frequently relapsing disease.[74–76]

Disorders of elemental co-factor transport and metalloprotein dysfunction

Disorders of elemental co-factor transport and metalloprotein dysfunction are well recognized causes of dementia and neuropsychiatric dysfunction, in most cases the consequence of disordered metal trafficking and utilization, with resultant tissue accumulation leading to toxic effects. Disrupted copper and iron metabolism dominate adult-onset presentations, with often striking clinicopathological similarities; typified by the autosomally recessive copper transport disorder, **Wilson** disease, and abnormalities of iron-binding proteins ferritin and careuloplasmin, giving rise to autosomally dominant **neuroferritinopathy** and recessive **acaeruloplasminaemia**. These conditions are members of the heterogeneous cohort of disorders classified as neurodegeneration with brain iron accumulation (NBIA), other members of which may also present in adulthood (e.g. pantothenate kinase-associated neurodegeneration).

In Wilson disease, copper accumulation reflects dysfunction of an ATPase copper transporter, encoded by the *ATP7B* gene, and responsible for excretion of copper and its incorporation into ceruloplasmin, a ferroxidase enzyme, critical to copper and iron transport. Resultant tissue accumulation of copper is responsible for local injury. By comparison, acaeruloplasminaemia results from a deficiency of caeruloplasmin's ferroxidase activity, required for iron export, while neuroferritinopathy stems from a mutation in a subunit of the iron storage protein, ferritin. Increasingly, other disorders of elemental metabolism are recognized, including the recent indentification of autosomal recessive hypermanganesaemia, in which a parkinsonian phenotype with hepatic cirrhosis and polycythaemia reflect dysfunction of the manganese transporter, SLC30A10.[77]

Most often presenting in late adolescence and throughout adulthood, metal accumulation within the basal ganglia is prominent across these heterogeneous disorders; extrapyramidal manifestations are characteristic—commonly dystonia, choreoathetosis, and parkinsonism. Tremor and a deterioration in handwriting are often an early feature of Wilson disease, while speech-induced, orofacial dystonia, and frontalis overactivity are common in neuroferritnopathy; striking asymmetry of limb dystonia may also feature. Cerebellar dysfunction is often prominent and isolated psychiatric presentations may arise with progressive neurodegeneration typical. Ocular pathlogy may inform diagnosis—retinal dysfunction suggests acaeruloplasminaemia (particularly if comorbid with diabetes mellitus), while cataracts are common in Wilson disease and the presence of copper deposition within Descemet's membrane (Kayser–Fleischer rings) near pathognomic, especially when present in association with neurological disease. Visceral involvement, such as cirrhosis, cardiomyopathy, renal tubular disease, and endocrine pancreatic failure (diabetes mellitus is near universal in acaeruloplasminaemia) should also raise the possibility of elemental tissue deposition and may arise independently. Clinical consequences of visceral disease are notably absent in both neuroferritinopathy and pantothenate kinase-associated neurodegeneration.

Screening investigations vary: neuroimaging often reveals signal change within the basal ganglia, secondary to metal deposition with cytotoxic oedema, often with a subregional pattern that is usually specific.[14,78] In late-stage disease, generalized cerebral and cerebellar atrophy occurs. Biochemical screening must include serum copper, iron and manganese levels, ferritin, and caeruloplasmin, with careful consideration towards artefactual confounding of ferritin and caeruloplasmin which are acute phase proteins. Wilson disease is characterized by low serum protein-bound copper and ceruloplasmin, with elevated unbound copper and increased urinary excretion (best quantified by accumulative 24-hour assay); molecular analysis of the *ATP7B* gene will usually confirm the diagnosis, although rarely, hepatic biopsy and confirmation of pathogenic copper storage is required. Acaeruloplasminaemia demonstrates low serum copper and iron, reflecting deficient caeruloplasmin function, typically with a marked reduction in ceruloplasmin concentration and plasma ceruloplasmin ferroxidase activity, and increased serum ferritin. Hepatic iron stores are increased, although, as with Wilson disease, biopsy is generally reserved for cases where molecular analysis of the caeruloplasmin gene (*CP*) is unavailing. Conversely, ferritin is decreased in neuroferritinopathy; clinical suspicion is confirmed through molecular analysis of the ferritin light chain (*FLT*) gene. Biochemical abnormalities are absent in pantothenate kinase-associated neurodegeneration, with diagnosis focusing upon neuroradiological features and molecular analysis; the presence of acanthocytosis on a peripheral blood film and low or absent plasma pre-beta lipoprotein fractions may be evident in certain subsets of this disease.

Treatment is directed to removal of excess metal via chelation therapy and restriction of dietary intake and intestinal absorption, an approach best employed early within the disease course. In Wilson disease, early recognition and aggressive copper reduction strategies greatly improve outcome; chelation typically employs penicillamine, although trientine has a more favourable side-effect profile and is increasingly the preferred option. Oral zinc supplementation is also used to induce metallothionein synthesis, a copper binding protein within the small intestinal enterocytes, effecting increased faecal excretion of copper. In those who fail medical therapy, orthotopic liver transplantation may be considered, although this has marginal effect upon established neuropathology. Similarly, reduction of iron load via regular venesection and the use of high affinity iron chelators (e.g. desferrioxamine) to reduce iron stores and zinc sulphate supplements, which reduce gastrointestinal absorption of ironmay ameliorate diabetes and improve hepatic and neurological symptoms in patients with acaeruloplasminaemia, although such approaches have had minimal effect in neuroferritinopathy to date. Trials of adjunct coenzyme Q10 and anti-oxidant therapy are also under investigation, although unlikely to confer significant clinical benefit in any of these disorders.[79–83]

Other inborn disorders of lysosomal macromolecule catabolism

In addition to its integral role in sphingolipid catabolism, the endosomal–lysosomal pathway is critical for the degradation and recycling of glycosaminoglycans and complex proteins, disruption of which gives rise to a further group of neurodegenerative disorders. Disease burden is greatest in childhood, however late-onset variants occur. Among these diseases are the adult neuronal ceroid lipofuscinosis and several of the oligosaccharidoses (glycoproteinoses).

The **neuronal ceroid lipofuscinoses** are 14 genetically distinct diaseases characterized by pathological accumulation of ceroid pigments (lipofuscin and other proteins such as cytochrome C and saposins) within neurons—inducing an autofluorescent aggregate of oxidized protein and lipid residues, with bound metals including iron, copper, and zinc—believed to interfere with cellular autophagy and sensitize cells to oxidative stress.[84] Wide molecular heterogeneity is observed and an increasing number of causative mutations, of both recessive (e.g. *CLN6* and *PPT1*) and dominant (e.g. *DNAJC5* and *CTSF*) inheritance identified, the majority involving proteins integral to endosomal-lysosomal processing, albeit, the pathogenic mechanisms remain incompletely understood. Adult-onset disease manifests from adolescence, most frequently in the third to fourth decades and progressing to death within 10 years of onset. Unlike other lysosomal disorders, ceroid neuronal lipofuschinoses are restricted to a central neurological phenotype; broadly, two overlapping subtypes are defined: type A, dominated by progressive myoclonic epilepsy, cerebellar disease, and cognitive decline, and type B by the absence of epilepsy, with prominent behavioural disturbance and dementia. Pyramidal and extrapyramidal disease often results; however, unlike childhood variants, retinal dysfunction is less commonly evident. Diagnosis of neuronal ceroid lipofuscinoses can be very challenging in the early phases of the illness; neuroimaging is often normal although parietal predominant cortical atrophy and attenuation of T2-signal within the putamen may be observed. Electroencephalography is typically nonspecific with both encephalopathic and epileptogenic features described; prominent photo-paroxysmal responses, as seen in childhood-onset disease, are uncommon, however, when present should raise the index of suspicion. Screening enzymatic assay (typically performed within leukocytes or cultured fibroblasts) is limited to palmitoyl-protein thioesterase 1 (PPT-1) and cathepsin D (CTSD) in adult-onset disease; thus, diagnostic confirmation relies largely upon molecular analysis of known genes. However, in many cases, no defect in DNA can be identified and the diagnosis is made on the basis of ultrastructural examination, demonstrating characteristic intracytoplasmic inclusions within leukocytes (buffy coat analysis) or skin biopsy specimens. Treatment remains, largely symptomatic although enzyme replacement for *CLN2* as well as gene transfer techniques are under investigation.[85–87]

The **oligosaccharidoses** also represent a heterogeneous group, with neurocognitive impairment in adulthood typically restricted to α mannosidosis, galactosialidosis and α-*N*-acetylgalactosaminidase deficiency, each the consequence of specific lysosomal hydrolase dysfunction causing disordered glycoprotein catabolism and accumulation of incompletely degraded oligosaccharides. Inherited in an autosomally recessive fashion, adult-onset variants typically manifest progressive cognitive decline, at times, prominent neuropsychiatric features and seizures—often myoclonic. Visceromegaly is typically prominent although by no means universal, while coarsening of facial cutaneous tissues and corneal clouding, reflecting substrate storage, should raise suspicion. In some cases (e.g. adult-onset galactosialidosis) fundoscopy reveals a macular cherry-red spot, reflecting retinal disease. Skeletal dysplasisa (dysostosis multiplex), cutaneous angiokeratoma, and peripheral neuropathy are suggestive of many oligosaccharidoses and are highly suggestive of the diagnosis in the context of central neurological disease. Late-onset cognitive decline in patents with childhood-onset disease also occurs and disease complicated by communicating hydrocephalus has been reported.[88] Diagnosis relies upon detection of urinary oligosaccharide excretion, with confirmation by specific enzyme activity assays and molecular analysis. As with many of the lysosomal disorders, treatment is symptomatic, although targeted approaches utilizing enzyme replacement therapies and gene transfer techniques are under investigation.[89–92]

Disordered endosomal–lysosomal function and dementia

While not strictly constituting a primary 'metabolic dementia', the pathogenic role of disordered endosomal–lysosomal function and other autophagic processes is increasingly implicated in the pathogenesis of primary dementias.[93] Moreover, heterozygous mutations in several genes encoding lysosomal proteins—homozygous mutations in which, give rise to recognized lysosomal diseases—have been identified amongst the known genetic risk factors for Parkinson disease and related Lewy body disorders.[94–96] While the pathogenic mechanisms remain poorly understood, common pathways of neurodegeneration are likely amongst these varied disorders and serve as strong motivation for further investigation.

Conclusion

In comparison to major neurodegenerative diseases, metabolic causes of dementia are rare. However, recognition is vital as, in many cases, specific treatments are available and there are often genetic implications for other family members. In addition, metabolic disorders, particularly those that are acquired, may complicate other causes of dementia and should not be overlooked as contributing factors. Whilst there are myriad metabolic causes of cognitive impairment, focused investigations based on clinical phenotype, with involvement of clinical biochemists and metabolic specialists as required, allows for a specific diagnosis to be reached in most cases.

References

1. Rossor MN, Fox NC, Mummery CJ. The diagnosis of young-onset dementia. *Lancet Neurol.* 2010;9:793–806.
2. Clayton PT, Verrips A, Sistermans E. Mutations in the sterol 27-hydroxylase gene (CYP27A) cause hepatitis of infancy as well as cerebrotendinous xanthomatosis. *J Inherit Metab Dis.* 2002; 25:501–13.
3. Vanier MT. Niemann–Pick disease type C. *Orphanet J Rare Dis.* 2010 Jun 3;5:16. doi: 10.1186/1750-1172-5-16.
4. Patterson M. Niemann–Pick Disease Type C. 2000 Jan 26 [Updated 18 Jul 2013]. In: RA Pagon, MP Adam, HH Ardinger, *et al.* (eds). GeneReviews® [Internet]. Seattle, WA: University of Washington, 1993–2015. Available at: <http://www.ncbi.nlm.nih.gov/books/NBK1296/>.
5. Berger JR and Singhal D. The neurologic complications of bariatric surgery. *Handb Clin Neurol.* 2014;120:587–94. doi: 10.1016/B978-0-7020-4087-0.00039-5. Review.
6. Robert M, Rocha JC, van Rijn M, *et al.* Micronutrient status in phenylketonuria. *Mol Genet Metab.* 2013;110 Suppl:S6–17. doi:10.1016/j.ymgme.2013.09.009. Epub 2013 Sep 19.
7. Van Caillie-Bertrand M, Degenhart HJ, Luijendijk I, *et al.* Wilson's disease: assessment of D-penicillamine treatment. *Arch Dis Child.* 1985 Jul;60(7):652–5.
8. Sedel F, Tourbah A, Fontaine B, *et al.* Leukoencephalopathies associated with Inborn Errors of Metabolism in adults: a diagnostic approach. *J Inherit Metab Dis.* 2008;31:295–307.
9. Schiffmann R and van der Knaap MS. An MRI-based approach to the diagnosis of white matter disorders. *Neurology.* 2009;72:750–9.
10. Ahmed RM, Murphy E, Davagnanam I, *et al.* A practical approach to diagnosing adult onset leukodystrophies. *J Neurol Neurosur Ps.* 2014 Jul;85(7):770–81. doi:10.1136/jnnp-2013-305888. Epub 2013 Dec 19.
11. Hegde AN, Mohan S, Lath N, *et al.* Differential diagnosis for bilateral abnormalities of the basal ganglia and thalamus. *Radiographics.* 2011 Jan–Feb;31(1):5–30. doi: 10.1148/rg.311105041.l.
12. Saneto RP, Friedman SD, and Shaw DW. Neuroimaging of mitochondrial disease. *Mitochondrion.* 2008 Dec;8(5–6):396–413. doi:10.1016/j.mito.2008.05.003. Epub 2008 May 23.
13. Roberts TP and Mikulis D. Neuro MR: Principles. *J Magn Reson Imaging.* 2007 Oct;26(4):823–37.
14. Hingwala DR, Kesavadas C, Thomas B, *et al.* Susceptibility weighted imaging in the evaluation of movement disorders. *Clin Radiol.* 2013 Jun;68(6):e338–48. doi:10.1016/j.crad.2012.12.003. Epub 2013 Mar 26.
15. McNeill A, Birchall D, Hayflick SJ, *et al.* T2* and FSE MRI distinguishes four subtypes of neurodegeneration with brain iron accumulation. *Neurology.* 2008 Apr 29;70(18):1614–9. doi:10.1212/01.wnl.0000310985.40011.d6.
16. Vasconcellos E and Smith M. MRI nerve root enhancement in Krabbe disease. *Pediatr Neurol.* 1998 Aug;19(2):151–2.
17. Rae CD. A guide to the metabolic pathways and function of metabolites observed in human brain 1H magnetic resonance spectra. *Neurochem Res.* 2014 Jan;39(1):1–36. doi: 10.1007/s11064-013-1199-5. Epub 2013 Nov 21.
18. Rossi A and Biancheri R. Magnetic resonance spectroscopy in metabolic disorders. *Neuroimaging Clin N Am.* 2013 Aug;23(3):425–48. doi:10.1016/j.nic.2012.12.013. Epub 2013 Feb 10.
19. Gordon N. Canavan disease: a review of recent developments. *Eur J Paediatr Neurol.* 2001;5(2):65–9.
20. Clark LN, Chan R, Cheng R, *et al.* Gene-wise association of variants in four lysosomal storage disorder genes in neuropathologically confirmed Lewy body disease. *PLoS One.* 2015 May 1;10(5):e0125204. doi:10.1371/journal.pone.0125204. eCollection 2015.
21. Guellerin J, Hamelin S, Sabourdy C, *et al.* Low-frequency photoparoxysmal response in adults: an early clue to diagnosis. *J Clin Neurophysiol.* 2012 Apr;29(2):160–4. doi: 10.1097/WNP.0b013e31824d949f.
22. Cook CC, Hallwood PM, and Thomson. B Vitamin deficiency and neuropsychiatric syndromes in alcohol misuse. *Alcohol Alcohol.* 1998 Jul–Aug;33(4):317–36.
23. Kumar N. Acute and subacute encephalopathies: Deficiency states (nutritional). *Semin Neurol.* 2011 Apr;31(2):169–83. doi:10.1055/s-0031-1277986. Epub 2011 May 17.
24. Pfeiffer RF. Neurologic manifestations of malabsorption syndromes. *Handb Clin Neurol.* 2014;120:621–32. doi:10.1016/B978-0-7020-4087-0.00042-5.
25. Morris MC, Schneider JA, and Tangney CC. Thoughts on B-vitamins and dementia. *J Alzheimers Dis.* 2006 Aug;9(4):429–33.
26. Morris MS. The role of B vitamins in preventing and treating cognitive impairment and decline. *Adv Nutr.* 2012 Nov 1;3(6):801–12. doi:10.3945/an.112.002535.
27. Kontush K and Schekatolina S. Vitamin E in neurodegenerative disorders: Alzheimer's disease. *Ann NY Acad Sci.* 2004 Dec;1031:249–62.
28. Rafnsson SB, Dilis V, and Trichopoulou A. Antioxidant nutrients and age-related cognitive decline: a systematic review of population-based cohort studies. *Eur J Nutr.* 2013 Sep;52(6):1553–67. doi:10.1007/s00394-013-0541-7. Epub 2013 Jun 7.
29. Toffanello ED, Coin A, Perissinotto E, *et al.* Vitamin D deficiency predicts cognitive decline in older men and women: The Pro.V.A. Study. *Neurology.* 2014 Dec 9;83(24):2292–8. doi:10.1212/WNL.0000000000001080. Epub 2014 Nov 5.

30. McCool BA, Plonk SG, Martin PR, *et al.* Cloning of human transketo-lase cDNAs and comparison of the nucleotide sequence of the coding region in Wernicke–Korsakoff and non-Wernicke–Korsakoff individuals. *J Biol Chem.* 1993 Jan 15;268(2):1397–404.

31. Guerrini I, Thomson AD, and Gurling HM. Molecular genetics of alcohol-related brain damage. *Alcohol Alcohol.* 2009 Mar-Apr;44(2):166–70. doi: 10.1093/alcalc/agn101. Epub 2008 Dec 18.

32. Yavuz BB, Cankurtaran M, Haznedaroglu IC, *et al.* Iron deficiency can cause cognitive impairment in geriatric patients. *J Nutr Health Aging.* 2012 Mar;16(3):220–4.

33. Berr C, Arnaud J, and Akbaraly TN. Selenium and cognitive impairment: a brief-review based on results from the EVA study. *Biofactors.* 2012 Mar–Apr;38(2):139–44. doi:10.1002/biof.1003. Epub 2012 Mar 15.

34. Brewer GJ, Kanzer SH, Zimmerman EA, *et al.* Subclinical zinc deficiency in Alzheimer's disease and Parkinson's disease. *Am J Alzheimers Dis Other Demen.* 2010 Nov;25(7):572–5. doi:10.1177/1533317510382283. Epub 2010 Sep 14.

35. Pajonk FG, Kessler H, Supprian T, *et al.* Cognitive decline correlates with low plasma concentrations of copper in patients with mild to moderate Alzheimer's disease. *J Alzheimers Dis.* 2005 Sep;8(1):23–7.

36. Pearce EN, Andersson M, and Zimmermann MB. Global iodine nutrition: Where do we stand in 2013? *Thyroid.* 2013 May. 23(5):523–8.

37. Abumrad NN, Schneider AJ, Steel D, *et al.* Amino acid intolerance during prolonged total parenteral nutrition reversed by molybdate therapy. *Am J Clin Nutr.* 1981 Nov;34(11):2551–9.

38. Amico-Ruvio SA, Murthy SE, Smith TP, *et al.* Zinc effects on NMDA receptor gating kinetics. *Biophys J.* 2011 Apr 20;100(8):1910–8. doi 10.1016/j.bpj.2011.02.042.

39. Reding P, Duchateau J, and Bataille C. Oral zinc supplementation improves hepatic encephalopathy. Results of a randomised controlled trial. *Lancet.* 1984 Sep 1;2(8401):493–5.

40. Riggio O, Merli M, Capocaccia L, *et al.* Zinc supplementation reduces blood ammonia and increases liver ornithine transcarbamylase activity in experimental cirrhosis. *Hepatology.* 1992 Sep;16(3):785–9.

41. Jaiser SR and Winston GP. Copper deficiency myelopathy. *J Neurol.* 2010 Jun;257(6):869–81. doi:10.1007/s00415-010-5511-x. Epub 2010 Mar 16.

42. Gault PM, Allen KR, and Newton KE. Plasma aluminium: a redundant test for patients on dialysis? *Ann Clin Biochem.* 2005 Jan;42(Pt 1):51–4.

43. Zhang XP and Tian H. Pathogenesis of pancreatic encephalopathy in severe acute pancreatitis. *Hepatobiliary Pancreat Dis Int.* 2007 Apr;6(2):134–40.

44. Butterworth RF. Thiamine deficiency-related brain dysfunction in chronic liver failure. *Metab Brain Dis.* 2009 Mar;24(1):189–96. doi:10.1007/s11011-008-9129-y. Epub 2008 Dec 6.

45. Klein CJ. Adult Polyglucosan Body Disease. 2009 Apr 2 [Updated 19 Dec 2013]. In: RA Pagon, MP Adam, HH Ardinger, *et al.* (eds). GeneReviews® [Internet]. Seattle, WA: University of Washington, Seattle, 1993–2015. Available at: <http://www.ncbi.nlm.nih.gov/books/NBK5300/>.

46. Jansen AC and Andermann E. Progressive Myoclonus Epilepsy, Lafora Type. 2007 Dec 28 [Updated 22 Jan 2015]. In: RA Pagon, MP Adam, HH Ardinger, *et al.* (eds). GeneReviews® [Internet]. Seattle, WA: University of Washington, Seattle, 1993–2015. Available at: <http://www.ncbi.nlm.nih.gov/books/NBK1389/>.

47. Roe CR and Mochel F. Anaplerotic diet therapy in inherited metabolic disease: therapeutic potential. *J Inherit Metab Dis.* 2006 Apr–Jun;29(2–3):332–40.

48. Benarroch EE. Glycogen metabolism. Metabolic coupling between astrocytes and neurons. *Neurology.* 2010;74:919–23.

49. Finsterer J. Cognitive decline as a manifestation of mitochondrial disorders (mitochondrial dementia). *J Neurol Sci.* 2008 Sep 15;272(1–2):20–33. doi:10.1016/j.jns.2008.05.011. Epub 2008 Jun 24.

50. Huttenlocher PR. The neuropathology of phenylketonuria: Human and animal studies. *Eur J Pediatr.* 2000 Oct;159 Suppl 2:S102–6.

51. Oberdoerster J, Guizzetti M, and Costa LG. Effect of phenylalanine and its metabolites on the proliferation and viability of neuronal and astroglial cells: Possible relevance in maternal phenylketonuria. *J Pharmacol Exp Ther.* 2000 Oct;295(1):295–301.

52. van Spronsen FJ, Hoeksma M, and Reijngoud DJ. Brain dysfunction in phenylketonuria: is phenylalanine toxicity the only possible cause? *J Inherit Metab Dis.* 2009 Feb;32(1):46–51. doi:10.1007/s10545-008-0946-2. Epub 2009 Jan 13.

53. Kasim S, Moo LR, Zschocke J, *et al.* Phenylketonuria presenting in adulthood as progressive spastic paraparesis with dementia. *J Neurol Neurosur Ps.* 2001 Dec;71(6):795–7.

54. Rosini F, Rufa A, Monti L, *et al.* Adult-onset phenylketonuria revealed by acute reversible dementia, prosopagnosia and parkinsonism. *J Neurol.* 2014 Dec;261(12):2446–8. doi:10.1007/s00415-014-7492-7. Epub 2014 Oct 31. No abstract available.

55. Seki M, Takizawa T, Suzuki S, *et al.* Adult phenylketonuria presenting with subacute severe neurologic symptoms. *J Clin Neurosci.* 2015 Aug;22(8):1361–3. doi:10.1016/j.jocn.2015.02.011. Epub 2015 Apr 23.

56. Erlandsen H, Pey AL, Gámez A, *et al.* Correction of kinetic and stability defects by tetrahydrobiopterin in phenylketonuria patients with certain phenylalanine hydroxylase mutations. *Proc Natl Acad Sci USA.* 2004;101:16903–8.

57. Robinson M, White FJ, Cleary MA, *et al.* Increased risk of vitamin B12 deficiency in patients with phenylketonuria on an unrestricted or relaxed diet. *J Pediatr.* 2000;136:545–7.

58. Mitchell JJ. Phenylalanine Hydroxylase Deficiency. 2000 Jan 10 [Updated 31 Jan 2013]. In: RA Pagon, MP Adam, HH Ardinger, *et al.* (eds). GeneReviews® [Internet]. Seattle, WA: University of Washington, Seattle, 1993–2015. Available at: <http://www.ncbi.nlm.nih.gov/books/NBK1504/>.

59. Bodamer OAF, Rosenblatt DS, Appel SH, *et al.* Adult-onset combined methylmalonic aciduria and homocystinuria (cblC). *Neurology* 2001;56:1113.

60. Thauvin-Robinet C, Roze E, Couvreur G, Horellou MH, Sedel F, Grabli D, *et al.* The adolescent and adult form of cobalamin C disease: Clinical and molecular spectrum. *J Neurol Neurosur Ps.* 2008 Jun;79(6):725–8. doi:10.1136/jnnp.2007.133025. Epub 2008 Feb 1.

61. Rahmandar MH, Bawcom A, Romano ME, *et al.* Cobalamin C deficiency in an adolescent with altered mental status and anorexia. *Pediatrics.* 2014 Dec;134(6):e1709–14. doi:10.1542/peds.2013-2711. Epub 2014 Nov 3.

62. Hasegawa T, Shiga Y, Matsumoto A, *et al.* Late-onset nonketotic hyperglycinemia: a case report]. *No To Shinkei.* 2002 Dec;54(12):1068–72. Review. Japanese.

63. Hall DA and Ringel SP. Adult nonketotic hyperglycinemia (NKH) crisis presenting as severe chorea and encephalopathy. *Mov Disord.* 2004;19:485–6.

64. Van Hove J, Coughlin C II, and Scharer G. Glycine Encephalopathy. 2002 Nov 14 [Updated 2013 Jul 11]. In: RA Pagon, MP Adam, HH Ardinger, *et al.* (eds). GeneReviews® [Internet]. Seattle, WA: University of Washington, Seattle, 1993–2015. Available at: <http://www.ncbi.nlm.nih.gov/books/NBK1357/>.

65. Yamada H, Otsuka M, Fujimoto K, *et al.* Determination of acetylcholine concentration in cerebrospinal fluid of patients with neurologic diseases. *Acta Neurol Scand.* 1996 Jan;93(1):76–8.

66. Federico A, Dotti MT, and Gallus GN. Cerebrotendinous Xanthomatosis. 2003 Jul 16 [Updated 1 Aug 2013]. In: RA Pagon, MP Adam, HH Ardinger, *et al.* (eds). GeneReviews® [Internet]. Seattle, WA: University of Washington, Seattle, 1993–2015. Available at: <http://www.ncbi.nlm.nih.gov/books/NBK1409/>.

67. Gallus GN1, Dotti MT, and Federico A. Clinical and molecular diagnosis of cerebrotendinous xanthomatosis with a review of the mutations in the CYP27A1 gene. *Neurol Sci.* 2006 Jun;27(2):143–9.

68. Fluharty AL. Arylsulfatase A Deficiency. 2006 May 30 [Updated 6 Feb 2014]. In: RA Pagon, MP Adam, HH Ardinger, *et al.* (eds). GeneReviews® [Internet]. Seattle, WA: University of Washington, Seattle, 1993–2015. Available at: <http://www.ncbi.nlm.nih.gov/books/NBK1130/>.

69. Kaback MM and Desnick RJ. Hexosaminidase A Deficiency. 1999 Mar 11 [Updated 11 Aug 2011]. In: RA Pagon, MP Adam, HH Ardinger, *et al.* (eds). GeneReviews® [Internet]. Seattle, WA: University of Washington, Seattle, 1993–2015. Available at: <http://www.ncbi.nlm.nih.gov/books/NBK1218/>.

70. Regier DS and Tifft CJ. GLB1-Related Disorders. 2013 Oct 17. In: RA Pagon, MP Adam, HH Ardinger, *et al.* (eds). GeneReviews® [Internet]. Seattle, WA: University of Washington, Seattle, 1993–2015. Available at: <http://www.ncbi.nlm.nih.gov/books/NBK164500/>.

71. Platt FM. Sphingolipid lysosomal storage disorders. *Nature*. 2014 Jun 5;510(7503):68–75. doi:10.1038/nature13476.

72. Pastores GM and Hughes DA. Gaucher Disease. 2000 Jul 27 [Updated 2015 Feb 26]. In: RA Pagon, MP Adam, HH Ardinger, *et al.* (eds). GeneReviews® [Internet]. Seattle, WA: University of Washington, Seattle, 1993–2015. Available at: <http://www.ncbi.nlm.nih.gov/books/NBK1269/>.

73. Mengel E, Klünemann HH, Lourenço CM, *et al.* Niemann–Pick disease type C symptomatology: an expert-based clinical description. *Orphanet J Rare Dis*. 2013 Oct 17;8:166. doi:10.1186/1750-1172-8-166.

74. Solinas C and Vajda FJ. Neurological complications of porphyria. *J Clin Neurosci*. 2008 Mar;15(3):263–8. doi:10.1016/j.jocn.2006.11.015. Epub 2008 Jan 9.

75. Whatley SD and Badminton MN. Acute Intermittent Porphyria. 2005 Sep 27 [Updated 7 Feb 2013]. In: RA Pagon, MP Adam, HH Ardinger, *et al.* (eds). GeneReviews® [Internet]. Seattle, WA: University of Washington, Seattle, 1993–2015. Available at: <http://www.ncbi.nlm.nih.gov/books/NBK1193/>.

76. Tracy JA and Dyck PJ. Porphyria and its neurologic manifestations. *Handb Clin Neurol*. 2014;120:839–49. doi:10.1016/B978-0-7020-4087-0.00056-5.

77. Stamelou M, Tuschl K, Chong WK, *et al.* Dystonia with brain manganese accumulation resulting from SLC30A10 mutations: a new treatable disorder. *Mov Disord*. 2012 Sep 1;27(10):1317–22. doi:10.1002/mds.25138. Epub 2012 Aug 23.

78. King AD, Walshe JM, Kendall BE, *et al.* Cranial MR imaging in Wilson's disease. *AJR Am J Roentgenol*. 1996 Dec;167(6):1579–84.

79. Chinnery PF. Neuroferritinopathy. 2005 Apr 25 [Updated 23 Dec 2010]. In: RA Pagon, MP Adam, HH Ardinger, *et al.* (eds). GeneReviews® [Internet]. Seattle, WA: University of Washington, Seattle, 1993–2015. Available at: <http://www.ncbi.nlm.nih.gov/books/NBK1141/>.

80. Gregory A and Hayflick SJ. Pantothenate Kinase-Associated Neurodegeneration. 2002 Aug 13 [Updated 31 Jan 2013]. In: RA Pagon, MP Adam, HH Ardinger, *et al.* (eds). GeneReviews® [Internet]. Seattle, WA: University of Washington, Seattle, 1993–2015. Available at: <http://www.ncbi.nlm.nih.gov/books/NBK1490/>.

81. Miyajima H. Aceruloplasminemia. 2003 Aug 12 [Updated 18 Apr 2013]. In: RA Pagon, MP Adam, HH Ardinger, *et al.* (eds). GeneReviews® [Internet]. Seattle, WA: University of Washington, Seattle, 1993–2015. Available at: <http://www.ncbi.nlm.nih.gov/books/NBK1493/>.

82. Weiss KH. Wilson Disease. 1999 Oct 22 [Updated 16 May 2013]. In: RA Pagon, MP Adam, HH Ardinger, *et al.* (eds). GeneReviews® [Internet]. Seattle, WA: University of Washington, Seattle, 1993–2015. Available at: <http://www.ncbi.nlm.nih.gov/books/NBK1512/>.

83. Bandmann O, Weiss KH2, and Kaler SG. Wilson's disease and other neurological copper disorders. *Lancet Neurol*. 2015 Jan;14(1):103–13. doi:10.1016/S1474-4422(14)70190-5.

84. Seehafer SS and Pearce DA. You say lipofuscin, we say ceroid: defining autofluorescent storage material. Neurobiol Aging. 2006 Apr;27(4):576–88. Epub 2006 Feb 7.

85. Mole SE and Williams RE. Neuronal Ceroid-Lipofuscinoses. 2001 Oct 10 [Updated 1 Aug 2013]. In: RA Pagon, MP Adam, HH Ardinger, *et al.* (eds). GeneReviews® [Internet]. Seattle, WA: University of Washington, Seattle, 1993–2015. Available at: <http://www.ncbi.nlm.nih.gov/books/NBK1428/>.

86. Cotman SL, Karaa A, Staropoli JF, *et al.* Neuronal ceroid lipofuscinosis: impact of recent genetic advances and expansion of the clinicopathologic spectrum. *Curr Neurol Neurosci Rep*. 2013 Aug;13(8):366. doi:10.1007/s11910-013-0366-z.

87. Mole SE and Cotman SL. Genetics of the neuronal ceroid lipofuscinoses (Batten disease). *Biochim Biophys Acta*. 2015 May 27. pii: S0925-4439(15)00154-4. doi:10.1016/j.bbadis.2015.05.011. [Epub ahead of print].

88. Halperin JJ, Landis DM, Weinstein LA, *et al.* Communicating hydrocephalus and lysosomal inclusions in mannosidosis. *Arch Neurol*. 1984 Jul;41(7):777–9.

89. Cantz M and Ulrich-Bott B. Disorders of glycoprotein degradation. *J Inherit Metab Dis*. 1990;13(4):523–37.

90. Okamura-Oho Y, Zhang S, and Callahan JW. The biochemistry and clinical features of galactosialidosis. *Biochim Biophys Acta*. 1994 Feb 22;1225(3):244–54.

91. Michalski JC and Klein A. Glycoprotein lysosomal storage disorders: alpha- and beta-mannosidosis, fucosidosis and alpha-N-acetylgalactosaminidase deficiency. *Biochim Biophys Acta*. 1999 Oct 8;1455(2–3):69–84.

92. Malm D and Nilssen Ø. Alpha-Mannosidosis. 2001 Oct 11 [Updated 3 May 2012]. In: RA Pagon, MP Adam, HH Ardinger, *et al.* (eds). GeneReviews® [Internet]. Seattle, WA: University of Washington, Seattle, 1993–2015. Available at: <http://www.ncbi.nlm.nih.gov/books/NBK1396/>.

93. Nixon RA. The role of autophagy in neurodegenerative disease. *Nat Med*. 2013 Aug;19(8):983–97. doi: 10.1038/nm.3232. Epub 2013 Aug 6.

94. Beavan MS and Schapira AH. Glucocerebrosidase mutations and the pathogenesis of Parkinson disease. *Ann Med*. 2013 Dec;45(8):511–21. doi:10.3109/07853890.2013.849003.

95. Murphy KE and Halliday GM. Glucocerebrosidase deficits in sporadic Parkinson disease. *Autophagy*. 2014 Jul;10(7):1350–1. doi: 10.4161/auto.29074. Epub 2014 May 15.

96. Deng H, Xiu X, and Jankovic J. Genetic convergence of Parkinson's disease and lysosomal storage disorders. *Mol Neurobiol*. 2015 Jun;51(3):1554–68. doi: 10.1007/s12035-014-8832-4. Epub 2014 Aug 7.

CHAPTER 25

Vascular cognitive impairment

Geert Jan Biessels and Philip Scheltens

Changing concepts: From vascular dementia to VCI

The difficulty in capturing the vascular burden in cognitive dysfunction in operational diagnostic criteria is reflected in the evolution such criteria over the past decades. The first diagnostic criteria that were proposed in the early 1990s focused on vascular dementia (VaD).[1,2] These criteria have been widely used, both in clinical practice and research, but have also been criticized. A key issue in the critique was the way in which dementia was defined. First, the definition of dementia was largely based on clinical features of Alzheimer's disease and required memory impairment, whereas cognitive impairment due to vascular disease involves multiple other cognitive domains. Second, by focusing on dementia, the diagnosis VaD did not apply to patients with cognitive impairment due to vascular disease with relatively preserved daily functioning. Therefore in the mid-1990s, the term vascular cognitive impairment (VCI) was introduced to refer to all forms of mild to severe cognitive impairment associated with and presumed to be caused by cerebrovascular disease.[3–5] The term covers the whole spectrum of cognitive dysfunction from mild cognitive impairments to severe impairments meeting criteria for dementia, with a presumed vascular aetiology, regardless of the pathogenesis (e.g. cardioembolic, atherosclerotic, ischaemic, haemorrhagic, or genetic).[4]

VCI is thus an umbrella term encompassing all forms of cognitive dysfunction associated with cerebrovascular disease. Just like other umbrella terms such as, for example, 'stroke' or 'dementia', it is not very well suited as a diagnostic label in individual patients due to lack of diagnostic specificity and clear leads for prognosis or treatment. Therefore, over the past years, there have been efforts to develop the concept of VCI into diagnostic criteria that are applicable in daily care. The criteria for vascular cognitive impairment from the American Heart Association/American Stroke Association (Table 25.1)[5] and the criteria for vascular cognitive disorders (VCD) from VAS COG[6] (Table 25.2) are the most recent and relevant examples. Just like the initial VaD criteria, these VCI (or VCD) criteria rely on three pillars: 1) demonstration of the presence of cognitive dysfunction, 2) demonstration of the presence of cerebrovascular disease, and 3) evidence that the two are causally linked. Although this may seem straightforward, it is unfortunately often not the case.

Let us first consider the first pillar: demonstration of 'cognitive dysfunction.' Only in a subset of patients with cerebrovascular disease cognitive dysfunction has an acute onset or stepwise progression. If this stepwise decline co-occurs with a cerebrovascular event cognitive dysfunction is often easily noted and the causal relationship with the vascular event readily established. However, in the majority of patients that fall under the concept of VCI, cognitive decline is insidious and can evolve over many years. Loss of cognitive function in such patients is a continuous process. Therefore, making a dichotomy between presence or absence of cognitive dysfunction in such cases can be difficult and is to some extent arbitrary. Nevertheless, for a patient to meet the VCI criteria, cognitive dysfunction must be present and confirmed by formal assessment and may not, by definition, include episodic memory impairment. Most often, the deficits include slowing of information processing, executive dysfunction, and memory retrieval impairment.

The second pillar, demonstration of cerebrovascular disease, can be based on a history of clinical stroke but is generally supported by demonstrating vascular lesions on brain imaging (Tables 25.1 and 25.2). Vascular lesions on imaging are heterogeneous and may include different manifestations of cerebral small vessel disease (SVD; i.e. white matter hyperintensities, lacunes, microbleeds), but also large infarcts, intracerebral haemorrhage, and subarachnoid haemorrhage. Several of these lesions, like a large cortical infarct, can be easily classified as 'abnormal.' For the different manifestations of SVD, however, it is more difficult to draw the line between normal and abnormal. White matter hyperintensities, for example, are extremely common in people over the age of 60, and also in people without any cognitive complaints. Moreover, in the general population lacunes and microbleeds can be observed in 20–30 per cent of people over the age of 75.[7,8] Let us consider two individuals, one 40 and one 80 years of age. Both have a similar burden of white matter hyperintensities on brain MRI, with bands around the ventricles and several punctate lesions in the deep white matter. This would be considered as perfectly normal in an 80 year old, but would definitely be classified as abnormal in a 40 year old. Hence, the context—patient-related factors—determine whether we classify these lesions as abnormal rather than the lesions themselves. This links to the third pillar: to establish causality between cognitive dysfunction and cerebrovascular disease in an individual patient. If the 40-year-old patient displayed slowed information processing and executive dysfunction on cognitive testing, the white matter hyperintensities would be readily accepted as a probable cause and this would prompt extensive investigations. If the 80-year-old man was a healthy volunteer in a research project, the same white matter hyperintensities would be considered as clinically irrelevant and prompt no further action. If this man presented at a memory clinic with progressive memory loss interfering with daily functioning, the clinical diagnosis would most probably be Alzheimer's disease and again, the white matter hyperintensities would not automatically be considered the cause of his cognitive dysfunction but most

Table 25.1 Criteria for vascular cognitive impairment: Statement from the American Heart Association/American Stroke Association (2011)

1. The term VCI characterizes all forms of cognitive deficits from vascular dementia (VaD) to MCI of vascular origin (VaMCI).

2. These criteria cannot be used for subjects who have an active diagnosis of drug or alcohol abuse/dependence. Subjects must be free of any type of substance for at least three months.

3. These criteria cannot be used for subjects with delirium.

Dementia

1. The diagnosis of dementia should be based on a decline in cognitive function from a prior baseline and a deficit in performance in two cognitive domains that are of sufficient severity to affect the subject's activities of daily living.

2. The diagnosis of dementia must be based on cognitive testing, and a minimum of four cognitive domains should be assessed: executive/attention, memory, language, and visuospatial functions.

3. The deficits in activities of daily living are independent of the motor/sensory sequelae of the vascular event.

Probable VaD

1. There is cognitive impairment and imaging evidence of cerebrovascular disease, and

   a. There is a clear temporal relationship between a vascular event (e.g. clinical stroke) and onset of cognitive deficits, or

   b. There is a clear relationship in the severity and pattern of cognitive impairment and the presence of diffuse, subcortical cerebrovascular disease pathology (e.g. as in CADASIL).

2. There is no history of gradually progressive cognitive deficits before or after the stroke that suggests the presence of a nonvascular neurodegenerative disorder.

Possible VaD

There is cognitive impairment and imaging evidence of cerebrovascular disease but

1. There is no clear relationship (temporal, severity, or cognitive pattern) between the vascular disease (e.g. silent infarcts, subcortical small-vessel disease) and the cognitive impairment.

2. There is insufficient information for the diagnosis of VaD (e.g. clinical symptoms suggest the presence of vascular disease, but no CT/MRI studies are available).

3. Severity of aphasia precludes proper cognitive assessment. However, patients with documented evidence of normal cognitive function (e.g. annual cognitive evaluations) before the clinical event that caused aphasia could be classified as having probable VaD.

4. There is evidence of other neurodegenerative diseases or conditions in addition to cerebrovascular disease that may affect cognition, such as:

   a. A history of other neurodegenerative disorders (e.g. Parkinson's disease, progressive supranuclear palsy, dementia with Lewy bodies);

   b. The presence of Alzheimer's disease biology is confirmed by biomarkers (e.g. CSF, PET amyloid ligands) or genetic studies (e.g. PS1 mutation); or

   c. A history of active cancer or psychiatric or metabolic disorders that may affect cognitive function.

VaMCI

1. VaMCI includes the four subtypes proposed for the classification of MCI: amnestic, amnestic plus other domains, nonamnestic single domain, and nonamnestic multiple domain.

2. The classification of VaMCI must be based on cognitive testing, and a minimum of four cognitive domains should be assessed: executive/attention, memory, language, and visuospatial functions. The classification should be based on an assumption of decline in cognitive function from a prior baseline and impairment in at least one cognitive domain.

3. Instrumental activities of daily living could be normal or mildly impaired, independent of the presence of motor/sensory symptoms.

Probable VaMCI

1. There is cognitive impairment and imaging evidence of cerebrovascular disease and

   a. There is a clear temporal relationship between a vascular event (e.g. clinical stroke) and onset of cognitive deficits, or

   b. There is a clear relationship in the severity and pattern of cognitive impairment and the presence of diffuse, subcortical cerebrovascular disease pathology (e.g. as in CADASIL).

2. There is no history of gradually progressive cognitive deficits before or after the stroke that suggests the presence of a nonvascular neurodegenerative disorder.

Possible VaMCI

There is cognitive impairment and imaging evidence of cerebrovascular disease but:

1. There is no clear relationship (temporal, severity, or cognitive pattern) between the vascular disease (e.g. silent infarcts, subcortical small-vessel disease) and onset of cognitive deficits.

2. There is insufficient information for the diagnosis of VaMCI (e.g. clinical symptoms suggest the presence of vascular disease, but no CT/MRI studies are available).

3. Severity of aphasia precludes proper cognitive assessment. However, patients with documented evidence of normal cognitive function (e.g. annual cognitive evaluations) before the clinical event that caused aphasia could be classified as having probable VaMCI.

4. There is evidence of other neurodegenerative diseases or conditions in addition to cerebrovascular disease that may affect cognition, such as:

   a. A history of other neurodegenerative disorders (e.g. Parkinson's disease, progressive supranuclear palsy, dementia with Lewy bodies);

   b. The presence of Alzheimer's disease biology is confirmed by biomarkers (e.g. PET, CSF, amyloid ligands) or genetic studies (e.g. PS1 mutation); or

   c. A history of active cancer or psychiatric or metabolic disorders that may affect cognitive function.

Unstable VaMCI

Subjects with the diagnosis of probable or possible VaMCI whose symptoms revert to normal should be classified as having 'unstable VaMCI'.

VCI, vascular cognitive impairment; VaD, vascular dementia; MCI, mild cognitive impairment; CADASIL, cerebral autosomal dominant arteriopathy with subcortical infarcts and leukoencephalopathy; CT/MRI, computed tomography/magnetic resonance imaging; PET, positron emission tomography; CSF, cerebrospinal fluid; and VaMCI, vascular mild cognitive impairment.

Reproduced from *Stroke*. 42(9). Gorelick PB, Scuteri A, Black SE, *et al.* Vascular Contributions to Cognitive Impairment and Dementia: A Statement for Healthcare Professionals from the American Heart Association/American Stroke Association, pp. 2672–713, Copyright (2011), with permission from Wolters Kluwer Health, Inc.

Table 25.2 Diagnostic criteria for vascular cognitive disorders: Statement from VASCOG (2014)

Proposed Criteria for Mild Cognitive Disorder and Dementia (or Major Cognitive Disorder)

Mild cognitive disorder

(A) Acquired decline from a documented or inferred previous level of performance in ≥ 1 cognitive domains as evidenced by the following:

    (a) Concerns of a patient, knowledgeable informant, or a clinician of mild levels of decline from a previous level of cognitive functioning. Typically, the reports will involve greater difficulty in performing the tasks, or the use of compensatory strategies; and

    (b) Evidence of modest deficits on objective cognitive assessment based on a validated measure of neurocognitive function (either formal neuropsychological testing or an equivalent clinical evaluation) in ≥ 1 cognitive domains. The test performance is typically in the range between one and two SDs below appropriate norms (or between the 3rd and 16th percentiles) when a formal neuropsychological assessment is available, or an equivalent level as judged by the clinician.

(B) The cognitive deficits are not sufficient to interfere with independence (i.e. instrumental activities of daily living are preserved), but greater effort, compensatory strategies, or accommodation may be required to maintain independence.

Dementia or major cognitive disorder

(A) Evidence of substantial cognitive decline from a documented or inferred previous level of performance in ≥ 1 cognitive domains. Evidence for decline is based on

    (a) Concerns of the patient, a knowledgeable informant, or the clinician, of significant decline in specific abilities; and

    (b) Clear and significant deficits in objective assessment based on a validated objective measure of neurocognitive function (either formal neuropsychological testing or equivalent clinical evaluation) in ≥ one cognitive domain. These typically fall ≥ two SDs below the mean (or below the 3rd percentile) of people of similar age, sex, education, and sociocultural background, when a formal neuropsychological assessment is available, or an equivalent level as judged by the clinician.

(B) The cognitive deficits are sufficient to interfere with independence (e.g. at a minimum requiring assistance with instrumental activities of daily living, i.e. more complex tasks such as managing finances or medications).

Evidence for Predominantly Vascular Aetiology of Cognitive Impairment

(A) One of the following clinical features

(1) The onset of the cognitive deficits is temporally related to ≥ 1 CVEs. (Onset is often abrupt with a stepwise or fluctuating course owing to multiple such events, with cognitive deficits persisting beyond three months after the event. However, subcortical ischaemic pathology may produce a picture of gradual onset and slowly progressive course, in which case A2 applies.) The evidence of CVEs is one of the following

    (a) Documented history of a stroke, with cognitive decline temporally associated with the event

    (b) Physical signs consistent with stroke (e.g. hemiparesis, lower facial weakness, Babinski sign, sensory deficit including visual field defect, pseudobulbar syndrome—supranuclear weakness of muscles of face, tongue, and pharynx, spastic dysarthria, swallowing difficulties, and emotional incontinence)

(2) Evidence for decline is prominent in speed of information processing, complex attention, and/or frontal-executive functioning in the absence of history of a stroke or transient ischaemic attack. One of the following features is additionally present

    (a) Early presence of a gait disturbance (small-step gait or marche petits pas, or magnetic, apraxic–ataxic, or parkinsonian gait); this may also manifest as unsteadiness and frequent, unprovoked falls

    (b) Early urinary frequency, urgency, and other urinary symptoms not explained by urologic disease

    (c) Personality and mood changes: abulia, depression, or emotional incontinence

(B) Presence of significant neuroimaging (MRI or CT) evidence of cerebrovascular disease (one of the following)

(1) One large vessel infarct is sufficient for mild VCD, and ≥ two large vessel infarcts are generally necessary for VaD (or major VCD)

(2) An extensive or strategically placed single infarct, typically in the thalamus or basal ganglia may be sufficient for VaD (or major VCD)

(3) Multiple lacunar infarcts (> two) outside the brainstem; one to two lacunes may be sufficient if strategically placed or in combination with extensive white matter lesions

(4) Extensive and confluent white matter lesions

(5) Strategically placed intracerebral haemorrhage, or ≥ two intracerebral haemorrhages

(6) Combination of the above

Exclusion criteria (for mild and major VCD)

(1) History

    (a) Early onset of memory deficit and progressive worsening of memory and other cognitive functions such as language (transcortical sensory aphasia), motor skills (apraxia), and perception (agnosia) in the absence of corresponding focal lesions on brain imaging or history of vascular events

    (b) Early and prominent parkinsonian features suggestive of Lewy body disease

    (c) History strongly suggestive of another primary neurological disorder such as multiple sclerosis, encephalitis, toxic, or metabolic disorder, etc. sufficient to explain the cognitive impairment

(2) Neuroimaging

    (a) Absent or minimal cerebrovascular lesions on CT or MRI

(3) Other medical disorders severe enough to account for memory and related symptoms

(4) *For research*: The presence of biomarkers for Alzheimer disease (cerebrospinal Ab and pTau levels or amyloid imaging at accepted thresholds) exclude diagnosis of probable VCD, and indicate AD with CVD

AD, Alzheimer disease; CT, computed tomography; CVD, cerebrovascular disease; CVE, cerebrovascular event; MRI, magnetic resonance imaging; VaD, vascular dementia; VCD, vascular cognitive disorder.

Reproduced from *Alzheimer Dis Assoc Disord*. 28(3), Sachdev P, Kalaria R, O'Brien J, *et al*. Diagnostic criteria for vascular cognitive disorders: A VASCOG statement, pp. 206–18, Copyright (2014), with permission from Wolters Kluwer Health, Inc.

likely be considered a comorbidity. The bottom line is that causality is easy to establish for clear-cut cognitive dysfunction that is linked to a specific vascular process or event but much more difficult in instances of subtle cognitive changes with multiple non-specific vascular lesions, or in the context of other coexistent disease processes, such as Alzheimer-type pathology. The majority of patients with VCI fall in the latter categories because the most common vascular lesions, in particular manifestations of SVD, are often not very strongly linked to cognitive functioning in individual patients, and co-occur with other pathologies, especially in older patients. Nevertheless, at the population level the burden of SVD is considerable and as such it is an important and potentially preventable contributor to dementia. The key importance of the concept VCI is that it highlights these latter aspects.

Neuropathology of VCI

The neuropathology of VCI is heterogeneous and can be expressed in the blood vessels themselves or in the parenchyma (see references 9–12 for comprehensive overviews). These pathologies are summarized in Table 25.3. Few patients have a single type of pathology and in most cases cerebrovascular pathology is accompanied by other pathologies, most often Alzheimer type. Pathological changes in the vessels can affect the whole arterial tree and, less commonly, also the veins.[9] Cerebrovascular disease can be grouped under large- and small-vessel domains. Large ischaemic parenchymal lesions can be due to emboli, from cardiac origin or from large-vessel disease, including atherosclerosis, plaque rupture, thrombotic occlusion and dissection, but can also result from haemodynamic events, causing borderzone or watershed lesions.[9] Although atherosclerotic changes in the large arteries supplying the brain are very common in old age, large parenchymal lesions occur only in a subset

of individuals. At the population level, these large parenchymal lesions are not a major contributor to VCI. By comparison, parenchymal lesions due to abnormalities in the smallest vessels (i.e. the small arteries, arterioles, venules, and capillaries of the brain) are much more common, some clearly linked to cognitive impairment (Table 25.3). Abnormalities in these vessels include arteriolosclerosis, lipohyalinosis, fibrinoid necrosis, microatheromas, and cerebral amyloid angiopathy (CAA). Parenchymal lesions that are associated with these vessel abnormalities include lacunes, diffuse white matter changes, and microinfarcts (Fig. 25.1).[9,12] Abnormalities in the smallest vessels and the parenchymal lesions which they cause are collectively referred to as cerebral SVD.[13] Age-related and hypertension-related SVD and cerebral amyloid angiopathy (see also chapter 26) are the most common forms.[13]

Neuroimaging features of VCI

Brain imaging is a cornerstone in the evaluation of VCI. The preferred imaging modality is magnetic resonance imaging (MRI). Computed tomography (CT) can be used as an alternative but it is much less sensitive to white matter hyperintensities and cannot detect microbleeds.

Vascular lesions on brain imaging can roughly be grouped under large- and small-vessel domains, along the same lines as has been described for neuropathology. Large vessel disease most commonly manifests itself in the form of ischaemic stroke. Cortical or cerebellar ischaemic lesions and brainstem or subcortical hemispheric infarcts larger than 1.5 cm in diameter on CT or MRI are generally considered to be of large-artery origin, mostly due to atherosclerosis, or to be due to an embolus from the heart.[14] For large spontaneous intracerebral haemorrhages the most common cause is SVD, due to arteriolosclerosis or CAA. Particularly for SVD, a major

Table 25.3 Types of vascular and parenchymal neuropathological changes in VCI

Pathological Feature	Predominant Location	Frequency	Association with CI
Atheromas	Carotid artery bifurcation and internal	High	Weak
Atheromatous and occlusive disease	Circle of Willis, proximal branches of MCA, ACA, PCA	High	Moderate
Complete infarctions (macroscopic), arterial territorial infarctions	Cortical and subcortical regions	Moderate	Weak
Lacunar infarcts	WM, basal ganglia, thalamus	Moderate	Moderate
Cystic infarcts	WM, basal ganglia, thalamus	Moderate	Unknown
Small or microinfarcts	Cortical and subcortical	High	Strong
Hyalinosis, lipohyalinosis, fibroid necrosis	WM, cortical and subcortical grey matter	Moderate	Unknown
Cribriform change, perivascular spacing	WM, basal ganglia, internal and external capsules	High	Strong
Demyelination and oligodendrocyte changes	WM	High	Strong
Gliosis: astrocytosis and microgliosis	WM, cortical and subcortical	Variable	Moderate
Cerebral amyloid angiopathy	Cortical	Moderate	Moderate
Intracerebral haemorrhages	Cortical, subcortical and lobar	Low	Moderate
Microspongiform change	Neocortical layer I–II	Moderate	Unknown
Laminar necrosis, gliosis	Neocortical ribbon	Low	Unknown
Hippocampal atrophy and sclerosis	CA1–CA4	Moderate	Strong
Alzheimer type of pathology (concomitant)	Hippocampus, neocortex	Low	Strong

VaD, vascular dementia; CI, cognitive impairment; MCA, middle cerebral artery; ACA, anterior cerebral artery; PCA, posterior cerebral artery; WM, white matter. Reproduced from Kalaria (9), based on a review of the neuropathological literature on VCI.

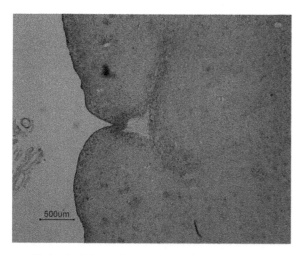

Fig. 25.1 Gliotic microinfarct in the upper layers of the cerebral cortex in an 83-year-old male with a neuropathologically confirmed diagnosis of vascular dementia. The microinfarct shows up on GFAP (glial fibrillary acidic protein) immunohistochemistry staining and has a cystic core.

Courtesy of SV Veluw and W Spliet, UMC Utrecht.

difference with neuropathology is that brain imaging does not depict the abnormalities in the small vessels themselves but rather the associated parenchymal lesions. Recently, an international working group has provided definitions and imaging standards for specific markers and consequences of SVD, the so-called STandards for ReportIng Vascular changes on nEuroimaging (STRIVE) criteria.[15] These standards were developed for use in research studies but use in the clinical setting should also be encouraged to standardize image interpretation, acquisition, and reporting. On brain imaging, the core manifestations of SVD include small subcortical infarcts, white matter MRI hyperintensities (WMH), prominent perivascular spaces (PVS), and cerebral microbleeds (CMBs) (Fig. 25.2) (15). Importantly, cerebral atrophy, which is often used as an indicator of neurodegeneration, can also be due to vascular disease[15]

Small subcortical infarcts

On imaging, small subcortical infarcts can be detected in the acute stage, but in the context of VCI these lesions are more commonly detected in the chronic stage. According to the STRIVE criteria acute lesions are termed 'recent small subcortical infarcts (SSI)'. These SSI,

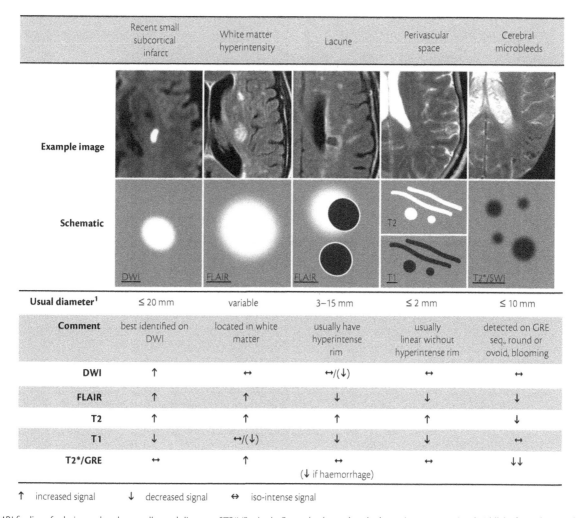

	Recent small subcortical infarct	White matter hyperintensity	Lacune	Perivascular space	Cerebral microbleeds
Example image					
Schematic	DWI	FLAIR	FLAIR	T1	T2*/SWI
Usual diameter¹	≤ 20 mm	variable	3–15 mm	≤ 2 mm	≤ 10 mm
Comment	best identified on DWI	located in white matter	usually have hyperintense rim	usually linear without hyperintense rim	detected on GRE seq., round or ovoid, blooming
DWI	↑	↔	↔/(↓)	↔	↔
FLAIR	↑	↑	↓	↓	↓
T2	↑	↑	↑	↑	↓
T1	↓	↔/(↓)	↓	↓	↔
T2*/GRE	↔	↑	↔ (↓ if haemorrhage)	↔	↓↓

↑ increased signal   ↓ decreased signal   ↔ iso-intense signal

Fig. 25.2 MRI findings for lesions related to small vessel disease—STRIVE criteria. Examples (upper) and schematic representation (middle) of MRI features for changes related to small vessel disease, with a summary of imaging characteristics (lower) for individual lesions. DWI = diffusion-weighted imaging. FLAIR = fluid-attenuated inversion recovery. SWI = susceptibility-weighted imaging. GRE = gradient-recalled echo.

Reproduced from *Lancet Neurol.* 12(8). Wardlaw JM, Smith EE, Biessels GJ, *et al.* Neuroimaging standards for research into small vessel disease and its contribution to ageing and neurodegeneration, pp. 822–38, Copyright (2013), with permission from Elsevier.

often referred to clinically as 'lacunar stroke' or 'lacunar syndrome,' represent about 25 per cent of all ischaemic strokes, but recent SSI are occasionally also found in patients without symptoms of acute stroke. A recent SSI is defined as 'imaging evidence of infarction in the territory of a single perforating arteriole with imaging features or correlating clinical symptoms consistent with a lesion occurring in the last few weeks'.[15] 'Recent' is derived from symptoms or imaging features—most commonly a diffusion weighted imaging lesion on MRI—suggesting that the SSI occurred within the last few weeks. 'Small' indicates a lesion that should generally be less than 20 mm maximum diameter in the axial plane. In the chronic stage, a small subcortical infarct can manifest itself on CT and MRI as a so-called lacune. A *lacune of presumed vascular origin* is defined as a round or ovoid, subcortical, fluid-filled (similar signal to CSF) cavity between 3 mm and 15 mm in diameter, compatible with a previous acute small deep brain infarct or haemorrhage in the territory of a single perforating arteriole.[15] On FLAIR, lacunes of presumed vascular origin usually have central hypointensity with a surrounding rim of hyperintensity. However, in some cases the central fluid may not be suppressed on FLAIR such that the entire lesion appears hyperintense, in which case it is often not possible to distinguish these lesions from WMH. Also, in some cases a rim of hyperintensity is not seen on FLAIR. Lacunes of presumed vascular origin should be distinguished from PVS. Although pathological studies show that there is no absolute cut-off, lesions < 3 mm in diameter are more likely to be PVS than lacunes.

White matter lesions

White matter lesions are a common finding on brain imaging, particularly in older individuals.[16] On CT, these white matter lesions appear as periventricular or subcortical areas of hypointensity. On MRI FLAIR and T2/proton density-weighted images these lesions are hyperintense (WMH). The term WMH of presumed vascular origin has been proposed to exclude white matter lesions from other diseases such as multiple sclerosis or leukodystrophies.[15] The shape, size, and distribution of white matter lesions provide clues to the differential diagnosis, but the most likely nature of the lesions is best derived from a combination of these imaging features, other lesions that may be present, and clinical data, including age, neurological, psychiatric, medical, and family history and medication use.[17] If WMH are found in older people, they are generally considered to be of vascular origin, even more so if other vascular lesions are also present. Below the age of 50, however, particularly if the shape and distribution of WMH are atypical, the differential diagnosis is long, including many non-vascular causes such as hereditary, inflammatory, infectious, and metabolic-toxic conditions.[17]

Postmortem studies show that WMH of presumed vascular origin reflect tissue abnormalities that range from slight disentanglement of the white matter structure to varying degrees of myelin and axonal loss.[18] The aetiology includes ischaemia, hypoperfusion, blood–brain barrier leakage, inflammation, degeneration, and amyloid angiopathy.[18]

MRI classifications of white matter changes usually distinguish between periventricular and deep/subcortical signal abnormalities.[16] Periventricular WMH typically include caps around the frontal horns of the lateral ventricles and pencil-thin lining or a smooth halo along the side of the lateral ventricles. Deep/subcortical WMH can occur as punctate changes or beginning confluent or

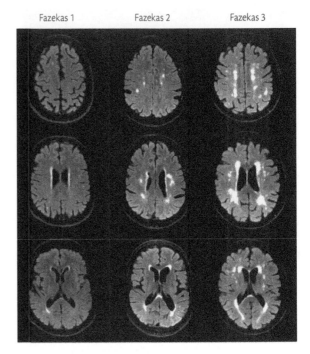

Fig. 25.3 Grading white matter hyperintensities (WMH). For clinical purposes, severity of WMH is generally assessed with ordinal visual rating scales. To this end, the Fazekas scale is widely used. Periventricular WMH are rated as 0: absent, 1: 'caps' or pencil-thin lining, 2: smooth 'halo', and 3: irregular periventricular hyperintensities extending into the deep white matter. Separate deep WMH are rated as 0: absent, 1: punctuate foci, 2: beginning confluence of foci, and 3: large confluent areas.

confluent abnormalities. For clinical purposes severity of WMH is generally assessed with ordinal visual-rating scales (Fig. 25.3). For research purposes (semi)automated volumetric methods are often used.[15]

Enlarged perivascular spaces

A perivascular space (PVS) is defined as a fluid-filled space, which follows the typical course of a vessel penetrating/traversing the brain through grey or white matter, with signal intensity similar to CSF on all sequences.[15] Their diameter commonly not exceeds 2 mm. PVS tend to be most prominent in the inferior basal ganglia and can also often be seen coursing centripetally through the hemispheric white matter. As PVSs are a normal anatomical structure, they are present in all individuals. However, due to their small diameter, normal PVSs are often below the detection limit of low-resolution MR or CT scans. They may, however, exhibit focal enlargement particularly enlarged (up to in the inferior basal ganglia, where it can sometimes be difficult to differentiate them from lacunes; see Fig. 25.2 for distinguishing features). Although the clinical significance of presence of numerous visible PVSs is still controversial, a generalized enlargement of PVS has been associated with other markers of SVD and cognitive dysfunction,[15] and may therefore be relevant to VCI.

Cerebral microbleeds

Microbleeds are visualized as small (usually 2–5 mm or sometimes 10 mm in size) areas of signal void with associated 'blooming' on T2* or other MR sequences sensitive to paramagnetic material.[15] Microbleeds are generally not visualized on CT or on FLAIR, T1w-, or T2w-MR sequences. They are well defined and regular, either round or oval, in shape. Neuropathological studies show that these MR lesions correspond to haemosiderin-laden macrophages consistent with vascular leakage of blood cells, that is, a small haemorrhage.[15,19] The underlying vascular pathology most commonly involves hypertensive vasculopathy or cerebral amyloid angiopathy.[18] Cerebral microbleeds are associated with other forms of SVD. Particularly lobar microbleeds are common in Alzheimer's disease and can be detected in 10–40 pe cent of patients, depending on the sensitivity of the MR protocol.[19,20] Lobar microbleeds are also linked to CAA and are incorporated into research criteria for this condition (see chapter 26).

Clinical evaluation of VCI

As has been noted earlier in this chapter, VCI is an umbrella term and as such is not very well suited as a diagnostic label in an individual patient because it lacks specificity and does not provide sufficiently clear leads for prognosis or treatment. Nevertheless, the umbrella term does offer guidance on some general principles in the evaluation and management of patients with cognitive dysfunction presumed to be caused by cerebrovascular disease (see references 5 and 21 for published recommendations). There are two main pillars in evaluation that jointly guide management. First, the nature and severity of cognitive, psychiatric, and behavioural symptoms should be assessed. Next, the vascular risk-factor profile should be evaluated and the nature of the vascular aetiology should be established as accurately as possible. In this respect it is important to note that simply labelling the aetiology as 'vascular' is too generic and therefore does not direct patient management. Based on the symptom profile, symptomatic treatment or support may be offered. Based on the most likely aetiology, vascular risk management may be optimized and the risk benefit ratio of, for example, antithrombotic treatment considered.

Cognitive and behavioural symptoms

In essence the clinical evaluation of cognitive and behavioural symptoms of patients suspected of VCI is based on the same principles as the evaluation of any other patient suspected of cognitive impairment as has been presented in earlier chapters of this book. It is important to note, however, that the cognitive profile of patients with VCI can be quite different from that of, for example, Alzheimer's disease. Cognitive deficits may involve any cognitive domain, but executive dysfunction, with slowed information processing and impairments in the ability to shift between tasks and to hold and manipulate information (i.e. working memory), is a relatively common manifestation of VCI.[21] Neuropsychological protocols should therefore be sensitive to these domains for reliable assessment of cognitive dysfunction due to vascular causes. To this end, different test protocols have been proposed, from five-minute protocols for screening purposes in, for example, primary care, to more extensive protocols that allow breakdown of functional deficits in the executive/activation, language, visuospatial, and memory domains.[21]

Behavioural changes that should be addressed include change in personality, apathy or disinhibition, and depressive symptoms. In addition, other symptoms of cerebovascular disease should be sought, including focal neurological deficits, gait and balance problems, and incontinence (see chapter 10).

Vascular risk profile

The history and physical examination should provide information about vascular risk factors and clinical manifestations of cardiovascular disease. Presence of and duration of exposure to hypertension, hyperlipidaemia, diabetes mellitus, and alcohol or tobacco use should be recorded, as well as physical activity and medications. A family history should be obtained, establishing if there are first-degree relatives (also record the total number of first-degree relatives) with a history of stroke, vascular disease, or dementia (record age at which these conditions occurred).

Vital signs should be collected, including height, weight, blood pressure (orthostatic), waist circumference, heart rate, vision, and hearing.[21]

Other clinical manifestations of cardiovascular disease are generally retrieved from medical history or records and include ischaemic heart disease, congestive heart failure, peripheral vascular disease, transient ischaemic attacks or strokes, and carotid endarterectomy.

Establishing the 'vascular cause'

When there is a clear link between an acute stroke and the onset of a cognitive deficit it is generally straightforward to establish causality. Still, brain imaging will be required to classify the causative vascular lesion as this will guide secondary prevention. In this context the so-called TOAST criteria, that classify acute ischaemic strokes into 1) large-artery atherosclerosis, 2) cardioembolism, 3) small-vessel occlusion, 4) stroke of other determined aetiology, and 5) stroke of undetermined aetiology, are still of use.[14] Also, for haemorrhagic stroke it is clear that the aetiological subtype provides essential information with regard to long-term prognosis and risk of stroke recurrence. In all cases, secondary prevention should proceed according to established guidelines for that particular stroke subtype, also taking into account the functional ability of the patient (e.g. other medical problems, independence, risk of falls).

As has been noted in an earlier section of this chapter, causality is more difficult to establish when a clear temporal relationship between a vascular event and the onset of cognitive decline is lacking. In such cases, evidence of a possible vascular cause will predominantly be derived from brain-imaging studies. While the relationship between the different neuroimaging features of VCI, as reviewed later in this chapter, and cognitive dysfunction at the population level is evident, establishing causality between a certain burden of vascular lesions and cognitive functioning is often not possible in an individual patient. In such cases, the vascular lesions can merely be considered as either incidental or contributing to the functional loss. Another issue is that vascular brain lesions on MRI have quite limited specificity for underlying aetiology. This issue is probably one of the key factors that hamper the development of treatment that targets specific aetiological processes in SVD. Hence, classification of the possible causative lesions therefore currently predominantly guides general vascular risk-factor management, which is nonetheless important.

Management of VCI

Due to its heterogeneous nature, there are few generalizable principles that apply to the treatment of all patients with VCI. As has been noted earlier, an individualized approach is required in which the symptom profile guides symptomatic treatment and supportive measures, and the aetiological diagnosis directs vascular risk management. In this final section we will highlight the treatment of two very common VCI subtypes, post-stroke cognitive dysfunction and mixed dementia (i.e. Alzheimer's disease with vascular lesions). The reader is also referred to other chapters in this book that provide guidance on the clinical management of cerebral amyloid angiopathy (see chapter 26) and rare genetic causes of VCI, in particular CADASIL (see chapters 30 and 31).

Post-stroke cognitive dysfunction

Cognitive dysfunction commonly occurs after stroke. In population-based studies, 5–10 per cent of patients experiencing a first-ever stroke, who were without dementia prior to stroke, develop dementia within a year after the event.[22] In hospital-based series, the post-stroke dementia rate in the first year is 10–14 per cent in those with first-ever stroke and 18–23 per cent if patients with recurrent strokes are also considered.[22] Even more patients experience cognitive dysfunction not meeting criteria for dementia, and these deficits may involve any cognitive domain, but most commonly involve visual perception and construction and executive functioning.[23] As with other, non-cognitive, symptoms of stroke, cognitive functioning may improve during the first months, but deficits persist in around one in three patients with acute (i.e. within the first weeks) post-stroke cognitive impairment.[23] There are also a substantial number of patients with persisting post-stroke cognitive complaints whose actual level of cognitive functioning does not even meet formal criteria for cognitive impairment (i.e. cognitive test scores do not fall below the 5th percentile of normative values) but who are still likely to have experienced a decline from pre-stroke level of performance (see Box 25.1 for case history).

Particularly in patients with a first stroke, without pre-stroke cognitive deficits, the acute lesion may be the only cause of cognitive dysfunction. In the large majority of such cases no further cognitive decline will occur in the following years, as long as recurrent strokes can be prevented. In many other patients, however, strokes occur in the context of pre-existent SVD or other pathologies, such as incipient Alzheimer's disease and the prognosis will be much less favourable.

Apart from acute stroke management and prevention of post-stroke complications, which is not the focus of this chapter, initiating adequate secondary prevention is essential. This may not only protect the patient against recurrent vascular events but may also help to preserve cognition. The selection of the right preventive measures again depends on the accurate aetiological subtyping of the stroke. Because post-stroke cognitive dysfunction is so common, high vigilance for its occurrence is warranted and cognitive functioning should be addressed in follow-up outpatient clinics after stroke. Even in patients who do return to their pre-stroke activities cognitive complaints may occur. In such patients, brief cognitive rehabilitation programmes that provide the patient with some insight into the source of the complaints and offer tips and tricks on how to deal with the deficits may be of use.

Mixed dementia: Alzheimer's disease with vascular lesions

Vascular lesions, in particular various manifestations of SVD, are an extremely common finding in patients who meet the diagnostic criteria for Alzheimer's disease. Data from epidemiological and

---

Box 25.1 Case history

A 57-year-old man developed an acute left-sided hemiparesis with dysartria. An initial CT showed no abnormalities, but the MRI three days later showed a small subcortical infarct at the lateral border of the right thalamus (Left image: FLAIR; middle image: diffusion-weighted image). He was treated with aspirin and dipyridamol, a statin, and an antihypertensive agent.

One year later he returned to the outpatient clinic because of cognitive complaints. Since the occurrence of the infarct he experienced problems with concentration and keeping oversight at his work as owner of a store for kitchen equipment. He could still perform most of his duties, albeit requiring a greater effort. His wife corroborated his history. On neuropsychological assessment his performance on the domains attention and executive functioning was around the 10th–15th percentile of normative values, whereas he performed above the 50th percentile on other domains. The MRI now showed cavitation of the infarct, which had evolved into a lacune (right image). The MRI did not show any other manifestations of small vessel disease except WMH with Fazekas grade 1 (see also Fig. 25.3).

His level of cognitive functioning did not meet formal criteria for cognitive impairment (i.e. cognitive test scores did not fall below the 5th percentile of normative values). He therefore does not meet the formal criteria for VCI (Tables 25.1 and 25.2). Nevertheless, the neuropsychological test profile clearly matches with his complaints and the temporal relation with the infarct—and its location in the thalamus—make the infarct a very likely cause of the cognitive decrements.

The test results were explained to the patient. Because all findings are indicative of a single aetiology (i.e. the infarct) no rapid cognitive decline is expected as long as no other strokes occur. The patient participated in a brief rehabilitation programme aimed to provide insight into his limitations and to acquire compensation strategies.

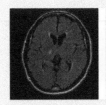 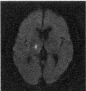 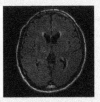

---

community-based pathology studies have indicated that many people with dementia have a combination of Alzheimer-type and vascular pathology, thereby challenging the conventional distinction between Alzheimer's disease and vascular dementia based on widely used clinical criteria.[24,25] Dementia in older people is mostly a heterogeneous condition in which different pathologies contribute to the clinical dementia syndrome.

When the burden of CVD is exceeding a presumed threshold, patients may be diagnosed with mixed dementia. There are no real fixed criteria for this threshold and thus clinicians use this label at their own discretion, resulting in a very heterogenous category, unsuitable for comparative research. It is probably better to state that SVD may be a contributor, to a greater or lesser extent, to the development of dementia in almost every patient with Alzheimer's disease who shows these lesions.

Studies in MCI patients have shown that vascular lesions are not predictive of progression to Alzheimer's disease but do contribute to the development of other dementia syndromes.[26-28] Apart from cognitive outcomes, vascular changes may affect mobility (i.e. balance and gait)[29] and are linked to mortality in memory clinic populations, as has been shown for microbleeds.[30,31] These data have fuelled the discussion on optimal management of patients with Alzheimer's disease and vascular lesions. In the EVA trial, a randomized controlled clinical trial in 123 subjects, intensive vascular care was compared with standard care in patients with Alzheimer disease with concomitant cerebrovascular lesions on MRI. Subjects receiving vascular care showed less WMH progression but the number of new lacunes or change in global cortical atrophy or medial temporal lobe atrophy did not differ between groups, nor was there any effect on clinical function between the intervention and control group.[32,33] Of note, treatment with aspirin in the vascular care group was associated with an increased risk of intracerebral haemorrhage. A subsequent pooled analysis of the EVA data with the Aspirin in Alzheimer's disease (AD2000) trial indicated that the pooled hazard ratio for an intracerebral haemorrhage in patients with Alzheimer's disease using aspirin is 7.6 (95% CI, 0.72 to 81; P = 0.09).[34] In our view, in light of the current evidence, vascular risk-factor management in patients with Alzheimer's disease and small vessel disease should therefore still be guided by general guidelines for cardiovascular risk management. In patients who have suffered a cardiovascular event, this event will dictate the type and intensity of treatment. In patients with cerebral small vessel disease who have not experienced a clinically manifest cardiovascular event, risk-factor management should follow guidelines for primary prevention of cardiovascular disease. In other words, demonstration of small vessel disease should not be regarded as a 'cardiovascular event' when deciding on the appropriate therapy. A final word of caution concerns the use of anticoagulants in patients with small vessel disease, in particular white matter hyperintensities and microbleeds. Judging the balance of risk and benefit of anticoagulant treatment in such patients can be very difficult. If there is an indication for anticoagulants to prevent occlusive vascular events this needs to be weighed against the increased risk of haemorrhage. Unfortunately, the available evidence to guide decisions is limited, and currently mainly relies on expert opinion.

References

1. Roman GC, Tatemichi TK, Erkinjuntti T, et al. Vascular dementia: diagnostic criteria for research studies. Report of the NINDS-AIREN International Workshop. Neurology. 1993;43(2):250–60.
2. Chui HC, Victoroff JI, Margolin D, et al. Criteria for the diagnosis of ischemic vascular dementia proposed by the State of California Alzheimer's Disease Diagnostic and Treatment Centers. Neurology. 1992;42(3 Pt 1):473–80.
3. Hachinski V. Vascular dementia: A radical redefinition. Dementia. 1994;5(3–4):130–2.
4. O'Brien JT, Erkinjuntti T, Reisberg B, et al. Vascular cognitive impairment. Lancet Neurol. 2003;2(2):89–98.
5. Gorelick PB, Scuteri A, Black SE, et al. Vascular Contributions to Cognitive Impairment and Dementia: A Statement for Healthcare Professionals from the American Heart Association/American Stroke Association. Stroke. 2011;42(9):2672–713.
6. Sachdev P, Kalaria R, O'Brien J, et al. Diagnostic criteria for vascular cognitive disorders: A VASCOG statement. Alzheimer Dis Assoc Disord. 2014;28(3):206–18.
7. Poels MM, Vernooij MW, Ikram MA, et al. Prevalence and risk factors of cerebral microbleeds: An update of the Rotterdam scan study. Stroke. 2010;41(10 Suppl):S103-S106.
8. Vermeer SE, Longstreth WT, Jr, and Koudstaal PJ. Silent brain infarcts: A systematic review. Lancet Neurol. 2007;6(7):611–9.
9. Kalaria RN. Cerebrovascular Disease and Mechanisms of Cognitive Impairment: Evidence from Clinicopathological Studies in Humans. Stroke. 2012.
10. Kalaria RN, Kenny RA, Ballard CG, et al. Towards defining the neuropathological substrates of vascular dementia. J Neurol Sci. 2004;226(1–2):75–80.
11. Deramecourt V, Slade JY, Oakley AE, et al. Staging and natural history of cerebrovascular pathology in dementia. Neurology. 2012;78(14):1043–50.
12. Jellinger KA. The enigma of vascular cognitive disorder and vascular dementia. Acta Neuropathol. 2007;113(4):349–88.
13. Pantoni L. Cerebral small vessel disease: from pathogenesis and clinical characteristics to therapeutic challenges. Lancet Neurol. 2010;9(7):689–701.
14. Adams HP, Jr, Bendixen BH, Kappelle LJ, et al. Classification of subtype of acute ischemic stroke. Definitions for use in a multicenter clinical trial. TOAST. Trial of Org 10172 in Acute Stroke Treatment. Stroke. 1993;24(1):35–41.
15. Wardlaw JM, Smith EE, Biessels GJ, et al. Neuroimaging standards for research into small vessel disease and its contribution to ageing and neurodegeneration. Lancet Neurol. 2013;12(8):822–38.
16. Schmidt R, Schmidt H, Haybaeck J, et al. Heterogeneity in age-related white matter changes. Acta Neuropathol. 2011;122(2):171–85.
17. Barkhof F and Scheltens P. Imaging of white matter lesions. Cerebrovasc Dis. 2002;13 Suppl 2:21–30.
18. Gouw AA, Seewann A, van der Flier WM, et al. Heterogeneity of small vessel disease: a systematic review of MRI and histopathology correlations. J Neurol Neurosur Ps. 2011;82(2):126–35.
19. Greenberg SM, Vernooij MW, Cordonnier C, et al. Cerebral microbleeds: a guide to detection and interpretation. Lancet Neurol. 2009;8(2):165–74.
20. Goos JD, van der Flier WM, Knol DL, et al. Clinical relevance of improved microbleed detection by susceptibility-weighted magnetic resonance imaging. Stroke. 2011;42(7):1894–900.
21. Hachinski V, Iadecola C, Petersen RC, et al. National Institute of Neurological Disorders and Stroke-Canadian Stroke Network vascular cognitive impairment harmonization standards. Stroke. 2006;37(9):2220–41.
22. Pendlebury ST and Rothwell PM. Prevalence, incidence, and factors associated with pre-stroke and post-stroke dementia: a systematic review and meta-analysis. Lancet Neurol. 2009;8(11):1006–18.
23. Nys GM, Van Zandvoort MJ, de Kort PL, et al. The prognostic value of domain-specific cognitive abilities in acute first-ever stroke. Neurology. 2005;64(5):821–7.
24. Pathological correlates of late-onset dementia in a multicentre, community-based population in England and Wales. Neuropathology Group of the Medical Research Council Cognitive Function and Ageing Study (MRC CFAS). Lancet. 2001;357(9251):169–75.
25. Schneider JA, Arvanitakis Z, Bang W, et al. Mixed brain pathologies account for most dementia cases in community-dwelling older persons. Neurology. 2007;69(24):2197–204.
26. Staekenborg SS, Koedam EL, Henneman WJ, et al. Progression of mild cognitive impairment to dementia: contribution of cerebrovascular disease compared with medial temporal lobe atrophy. Stroke. 2009;40(4):1269–74.
27. van de Pol LA, Korf ES, van der Flier WM, et al. Magnetic resonance imaging predictors of cognition in mild cognitive impairment. Arch Neurol. 2007;64(7):1023–8.
28. DeCarli C, Mungas D, Harvey D, et al. Memory impairment, but not cerebrovascular disease, predicts progression of MCI to dementia. Neurology. 2004;63(2):220–7.
29. Baezner H, Blahak C, Poggesi A, et al. Association of gait and balance disorders with age-related white matter changes: the LADIS study. Neurology. 2008;70(12):935–42.

30. van der Vlies AE, Goos JD, Barkhof F, *et al.* Microbleeds do not affect rate of cognitive decline in Alzheimer disease. *Neurology.* 2012;79(8):763–9.

31. Henneman WJ, Sluimer JD, Cordonnier C, *et al.* MRI biomarkers of vascular damage and atrophy predicting mortality in a memory clinic population. *Stroke.* 2009;40(2):492–8.

32. Richard E, Kuiper R, Dijkgraaf MG, *et al.* Vascular care in patients with Alzheimer's disease with cerebrovascular lesions-a randomized clinical trial. *J Am Geriatr Soc.* 2009;57(5):797–805.

33. Richard E, Gouw AA, Scheltens P, *et al.* Vascular Care in Patients With Alzheimer Disease With Cerebrovascular Lesions Slows Progression of White Matter Lesions on MRI. The Evaluation of Vascular Care in Alzheimer's Disease (EVA) Study. *Stroke.* 2010.

34. Thoonsen H, Richard E, Bentham P, *et al.* Aspirin in Alzheimer's Disease. Increased Risk of Intracerebral Hemorrhage: Cause for Concern? *Stroke.* 2010.

CHAPTER 26

Cerebral amyloid angiopathy and CNS vasculitis

Sergi Martinez-Ramirez, Steven M. Greenberg, and Anand Viswanathan

Cerebral amyloid angiopathy

Cerebral amyloid angiopathy (CAA) refers to a heterogeneous group of entities characterized by the deposit of amyloid proteins in the vessel walls of small-sized arteries and capillaries of leptomeninges and cerebral cortex.[1,2] CAA can be either occur in the more common sporadic form[3] or in more rare hereditary forms.[4] The accumulation of amyloid in brain vessels may compromise their self-regulation, narrow their lumen, and eventually compromise their structural integrity.[5,6] Sporadic CAA underlies most lobar intracerebral haemorrhages (ICH) in the elderly[7] but its clinical spectrum also includes cerebral ischaemia and cognitive decline.[8] Furthermore, all magnetic resonance imaging-based markers of small vessel disease are typically found in CAA, especially lobar microbleeds (MB) and white matter hyperintensities (WMH).[3] Estimates from autopsy studies suggest that CAA could be present in as many as 57 per cent of asymptomatic ageing subjects, and in up to 85 per cent when subjects with dementia are also included.[9,10]

Pathophysiology

In the sporadic form of CAA, it is thought that most of the accumulated $A\beta$ is neuronal in origin,[11] although a potential role of circulating plasma $A\beta$ is still under debate.[12,13] Neurons produce amyloid precursor protein (APP), which undergoes sequential proteolytic cleavage by secretase enzymes. As a consequence, two major amyloid species may be formed: $A\beta_{1-40}$ and $A\beta_{1-42}$. In normal conditions $A\beta$ is effectively removed, both through enzymatic degradation[14,15] and drainage along arterial perivascular spaces.[16,17] However, in pathologic conditions, an imbalance between production and clearance of $A\beta$ may occur, resulting in aggregation both in vascular and parenchymal tissue. The more soluble $A\beta_{1-40}$ mainly accumulates in the vessel walls (resulting in CAA) while the less soluble $A\beta_{1-42}$ polymerizes, aggregates, and forms insoluble complexes in the parenchyma. These latter complexes comprise senile plaques, a pathologic feature of Alzheimer's disease (AD).[18,19]

The exact relationship between CAA and AD remains unclear. As CAA shares a common pathogenic mechanism with AD, some degree of CAA is observed in virtually all AD brains.[20] However, only ~25 per cent of AD cases harbour advanced CAA, while the remaining show lesser degrees of vascular $A\beta$.[21] Similarly, AD pathology is identified in only ~50 per cent of patients who die of CAA-related haemorrhage.[20] These observations suggest that CAA and AD, whilst commonly seen together, can exist as distinct entities, and that this may relate to differences in $A\beta_{1-40}$:$A\beta_{1-42}$ ratio. As yet, the factors influencing the dominant $A\beta$ moieties produced and the associated clinical phenotype remain poorly understood.

Topographically, it has been shown that CAA largely affects superficial vessels, especially those in the temporal and occipital lobes.[21,22] This may be the consequence of age-related changes of vessel walls, resulting in reduced pulsatility of vessels running through the brain surface compared to those supplying deep regions due to their respective anatomical features.[11] As already mentioned, one of the main clearance pathways for $A\beta$ is its drainage along the arterial perivascular spaces.[23] Although the dynamics of interstitial fluid and solutes within perivascular spaces are still speculative, pulsations of the arterial walls seem to be the driving force;[24,25] thus, vessels with lower pulsatility would be more prone to stasis and accumulation of $A\beta$ along perivascular spaces. In support of this theory, it has been shown that arterial perivascular routes match with the topography of $A\beta$ deposits in CAA.[16]

Genetics

Hereditary forms of CAA manifest earlier in life and are typically more severe than sporadic CAA. Most of these familiar forms occur due to mutations affecting the APP gene,[4,26–29] although in some cases it is not $A\beta$ but other amyloid peptides that accumulate in the brain (i.e. amyloid forms of transthyretin[30] or cystatin C[31]). Hereditary $A\beta$-amyloidoses are restricted to the brain and may present with the classic picture of recurrent lobar haemorrhages, with or without accompanying cognitive decline, but they may also present with progressive cognitive decline alone, as seen in individuals harboring the Arctic (Icelandic) APP mutation.[28] Non-$A\beta$ amyloidoses tend to affect both the cerebral and systemic circulation and thus are associated with a range of extracerebral clinical manifestations.[32]

In the sporadic form of CAA, only ApoE ε2 and ε4 alleles have been identified as genetic risk factors of the disease.[33] ApoE co-localizes and interacts with $A\beta$ in experimental studies,[34] but its exact biological role in $A\beta$ accumulation is not clear. Clinical studies have shown that both ApoE ε2 and ε4 are associated with CAA-related ICH, but interestingly, these 2 alleles may act through different pathways: ε4 by promoting widespread vascular amyloid deposition, and ε2 by promoting vasculopathic changes on amyloid-laden vessels.[35]

Clinical-radiological manifestations

Weakening of vessel walls due to amyloid deposition may lead to their rupture and subsequent bleeding. Location of CAA-related haemorrhages is typically lobar, cortical, or juxta-cortical, and small foci of subarachnoid bleeding may also occur.[5,36] These topographies correlate with the anatomical distribution of amyloid deposits (cortex and leptomeninges).[37,38] Depending on the magnitude of the bleeding, haemorrhages may be small and subclinical (MB) or large and symptomatic (ICH) (Fig. 26.1).

Lobar ICH in the context of CAA is associated with high morbidity and mortality, particularly when recurrent,[39,40] and sporadic CAA is the most common cause of lobar ICH in the elderly.[3] The presence of lobar MB is also a common feature among CAA patients, and they may be detected in the presence or absence of lobar ICH. In fact, lobar MB are believed to be at least twice more frequent than large, symptomatic ICH, in CAA patients.[41] The clinical impact of MB has not been completely ascertained: in patients with lobar ICH, the number of both MB at baseline and incident MB at follow-up predicts a higher risk of ICH recurrence.[42] MB have been correlated with a higher mortality in CAA[42] and AD cohorts,[43,44] though this association seems not to be explained by speed of cognitive decline.[45] In population-based autopsy studies, CAA severity has been associated with increased risk of cognitive impairment during life and worse cognitive performance in patients with AD, controlling for the severity of AD pathology.[46,47] Indeed, a recent study on community-dwelling persons found the presence of CAA to be associated with impairment of selective cognitive domains (i.e. perceptual speed), separately from AD pathology.[10] Thus, even though MB may have a modest or marginal effect on cognition, this evidence suggests that CAA independently causes cognitive decline.

Loss of normal architecture of vessel walls may lead to impaired vascular reactivity in CAA patients.[48,49] This phenomenon, combined with progressive narrowing of the lumen, is finally responsible for severe hypoperfusion and brain ischaemia. White matter hyperintensities (WMH) are the most easily identifiable expression of chronic hypoperfusion of white matter on magnetic resonance imaging (MRI) studies, and are common among individuals with CAA.[3] Although previous studies had shown contradictory results, a recent work using automated detection of WMH centre of mass showed that WMH in CAA patients have a more posterior predominance (occipital > frontal) than in non-CAA cases, even in the absence of lobar haemorrhages, which is potentially helpful to differentiate white matter damage by CAA versus other forms of small-vessel disease. The clinical importance of WMH relies on their association with cognitive impairment, independently of the effects of ICH.[51] A further form of ischaemic injury attributable to CAA is cortical microinfarcts,[52,53] a reflection of capillary occlusion at a cortical level. To date, the clinical impact of cortical microinfarcts in CAA subjects is not well studied. In recent years, dilated perivascular spaces (DPVS) in the white matter have been postulated as potential markers of CAA, as opposed to DPVS in the basal ganglia, which are more associated to hypertension and other vascular risk factors.[54,55] It has been hypothesized that cortical vascular amyloid spreading into the surrounding perivascular spaces may lead to the blockage of the interstitial fluid circulating within, thus causing a retrograde dilation of perivascular spaces in the white matter.[56]

Finally, another part of the clinical spectrum of CAA refers to transient focal neurological deficits (TFND),[57,58] also called 'amyloid spells.' TFND may present as 'aura-like symptoms' (positive) or 'TIA-like symptoms' (negative). Subarachnoid blood in the convexity (cSAH) appears to be the most characteristic feature when comparing patients with TFND to those without.[59] Also, TFND may predict a high early risk of ICH in CAA patients.[59] Radiologically, cSAH may evolve into focal, lineal deposits of blood degradation products outlining the brain sulci. This feature, so-called superficial siderosis (SS), is also considered as another relatively specific marker of CAA.[60,61]

Diagnosis

Pathological diagnosis

The definitive diagnosis of CAA still requires the direct examination of the brain. On pathologic specimens, multiple effects of vascular

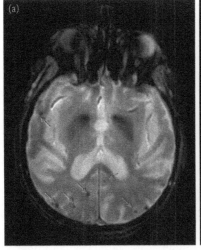
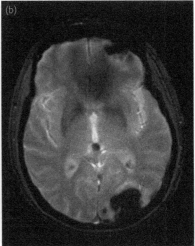

Fig. 26.1 Lobar hemorrhages in two pathologically-confirmed CAA cases: (a) with multiple microbleeds; (b) with a large intracerebral haemorrhage.

amyloid deposition may be observed, though the most characteristic feature is the loss of smooth muscle cells with replacement of the media layer by amyloid. Wall thickening, lumen narrowing, splitting of the vessel wall, microaneurysms, and perivascular haemorrhages are also frequently reported in CAA.[5,62] Amyloid proteins have been traditionally identified with Red Congo staining using polarized light.[63] Due to the low sensitivity of this method, complementary techniques are used to rule out small amounts of Aβ deposition; that is, immunohistochemistry with fluorescent antibodies against specific precursor proteins (Fig. 26.2).[64]

CAA is characteristically a patchy disease.[65,66] In practice, this means that pathologic evaluation should include as much brain tissue as possible. Autopsy studies, therefore, represent the best source of documentation of CAA. However, definitive histological diagnosis during life is sometimes required, especially when symptoms are rapidly evolving or atypical, and not infrequently when the clinical picture resembles the inflammatory form of CAA (see section on CNS vasculitis, following). *In-vivo* pathologic diagnosis of CAA requires surgical brain biopsy. Although its sensitivity is not 100 per cent, this is a highly reliable method for CAA detection when cortex is sampled appropriately and contains leptomeninges.[66] In terms of grading the severity of CAA, several scales have been proposed, such as the Vonsattel scale.[66]

The Boston criteria

The development of MRI sequences particularly susceptible to blood-degradation products including gradient-recalled echo (GRE) or susceptibility-weighted image (SWI) demonstrates that old haemorrhages, mainly MB, were already present in many patients suffering a first symptomatic lobar ICH.[67] The absence or presence of prior exclusively lobar haemorrhages forms the basis of the Boston criteria for CAA, which have been validated pathologically. The term 'possible CAA' referred to cases with a single symptomatic lobar ICH without the presence of old lobar haemorrhages on neuroimaging, while 'probable CAA' refers to the presence of old lobar haemorrhages in cases with symptomatic lobar ICH. The Boston criteria allow physicians to approach the diagnosis of CAA during life without the need to obtain brain tissue. Two histology-based diagnostic categories complete the Boston criteria: 'Probable CAA with supporting pathology' and 'Definite CAA' (Table 26.1). Validation studies have shown that the categories of 'possible CAA' and 'probable CAA' diagnoses predict pathologic evidence of CAA

in around 60 per cent and 100 per cent of cases, respectively.[7] The inclusion of additional CAA radiologic markers in the Boston Criteria, such as SS or DPVS in the white matter, has been shown to increase their sensitivity.[68,69]

The diagnostic value of lobar MB in the absence of lobar ICH has not yet been determined. Although the Boston criteria do not specifically refer to the size of lobar haemorrhages, these criteria are based on survivors of lobar ICH and may not apply to patients with asymptomatic haemorrhages. This point is of major importance, as many patients with CAA will not experience major haemorrhagic complications during life. From population-based studies, it is known that ~8–19 per cent of healthy subjects may harbor incidental, strictly lobar MB.[70,71] Although the presence of multiple, strictly lobar MB is highly suggestive of CAA, the significance of only one or a few MB may be more diagnostically challenging. Furthermore, there is some evidence to suggest the vessel pathology in underlying symptomatic ICH may be different from the vessel pathology underlying MB in patients with probable or possible CAA.[72] Therefore, radiological–pathological correlation studies on patients without lobar ICH are needed in order to ascertain the specific predictive value of lobar MB for CAA.

Other diagnostic approaches

In recent years, *in-vivo* positron emission tomography (PET) imaging using amyloid specific tracers, such as Pittsburgh Compound-B (PiB), has been an intensive field of research, mainly focused on patients with AD.[73] Vascular amyloid alone can be detected with PiB as one study has imaged vascular amyloid in a single patient with hereditary CAA.[74] Further studies using both MRI and PiB–PET have revealed that the location of lobar MB correlates with the highest concentrations of PiB retention in CAA,[37] and that PiB cortical retention positively correlates with WMH burden in subjects with CAA.[75] Although these novel imaging techniques are promising their clinical applications are still not defined and, consequently, their use remains confined to research purposes.

The analysis of the cerebrospinal fluid (CSF) has become another focus of interest in CAA as it has been shown to be sensitive and specific in distinguishing between AD and healthy controls.[76] CSF in AD patients is characterized by low levels of $A\beta_{1-42}$ and high levels of tau, whereas $A\beta_{1-40}$ is not particularly altered.[77] In contrast, CAA is associated with low levels of $A\beta_{1-42}$ but also $A\beta_{1-40}$, which is likely to reflect the depletion of this protein in the CSF

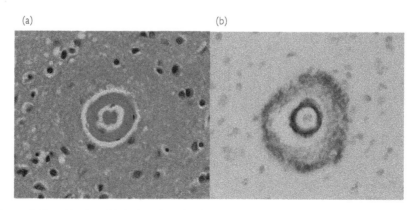

(a)   (b)

Fig. 26.2 Histological images of a vessel affected by CAA. (a) Thickened vessel walls staining by eosin (H&E, 40×). (b) Positivity for anti-Aβ antibodies (anti-Aβ immunohistochemistry, 40×).

Table 26.1 Boston Criteria for diagnosis of CAA-related haemorrhage*

1. Definite CAA

Full postmortem examination demonstrating:

◆ Lobar, cortical, or corticosubcortical haemorrhage

◆ Severe CAA with vasculopathy†

◆ Absence of other diagnostic lesion

2. Probable CAA with supporting pathology

Clinical data and pathologic tissue (evacuated haematoma or cortical biopsy) demonstrating:

◆ Lobar, cortical, or corticosubcortical haemorrhage

◆ Some degree of CAA in specimen

◆ Absence of other diagnostic lesion

3. Probable CAA

Clinical data and MRI or CT demonstrating:

◆ Multiple haemorrhages restricted to lobar, cortical, or corticosubcortical regions (cerebellar haemorrhage allowed)

◆ Age > 55 years

◆ Absence of other cause of haemorrhage‡

4. Possible CAA

Clinical data and MRI or CT demonstrating:

◆ Single lobar, cortical, or corticosubcortical haemorrhage

◆ Age > 55 years

◆ Absence of other cause of haemorrhage‡

*Criteria established by the Boston Cerebral Amyloid Angiopathy Group: Steven M Greenberg, MD, PhD, Daniel S Kanter, MD, Carlos S Kase, MD, and Michael S Pessin, MD.

†As defined in: Von sattel JP, Myers RH, Hedley–Whyte ET, Ropper AH, Bird ED, Richardson EP Jr. Cerebral amyloid angiopathy without and with cerebral hemorrhages: a comparative histological study. *Ann Neurol.* 1991;30:637–49.

‡Other causes of intracerebral haemorrhage: excessive warfarin (INR.3.0); antecedent head trauma or ischaemic stroke; CNS tumour, vascular malformation, or vasculitis; and blood dyscrasia or coagulopathy. (INR.3.0 or other nonspecific laboratory abnormalities permitted for diagnosis of possible CAA.)

Reproduced from *Neurology.* 56(4), Knudsen KA, Rosand J, Karluk D, *et al.* Clinical diagnosis of cerebral amyloid angiopathy: Validation of the Boston Criteria, pp. 537–9, Copyright (2001), with permission from Wolters Kluwer Health, Inc.

pool due to its extensive vascular accumulation.[78] Thus, $A\beta_{1-40}$ levels in CSF may be a good biological marker to differentiate between AD and CAA.

Management

No effective treatment currently exists for the acute phase of any kind of spontaneous ICH, including CAA-related lobar ICH. After lobar ICH, modelling studies have suggested that anticoagulants may place patients at an increased risk of recurrence. It is thus generally recommended to avoid these medications after lobar ICH.[79] In patients with MB but not ICH, the risk:benefit ratio of antithrombotic drugs is controversial. Although there is no formal contraindication, some studies have identified MB as an independent risk factor for warfarin-related ICH.[80] Even antiplatelet agents, traditionally safer than anticoagulants, have been associated with an increased risk of ICH, especially in subjects with a high number of MB.[81,82] Considering these findings, it seems reasonable to individualize decisions on antithrombotic therapy in patients with lobar MB only.

Regarding disease-modifying therapies for CAA, a phase-II multicentre, randomized, placebo-controlled clinical trial is currently testing the safety and efficacy of ponezumab, a monoclonal antibody targeting Aβ, on individuals with 'probable CAA' without cognitive impairment. This monoclonal antibody is expected to clear vascular amyloid from the blood vessels of patients with CAA. The primary outcome is the change in cerebrovascular reactivity as measured on functional functional MRI (fMRI), based on previous work by Dumas and colleagues;[48] the trial will test whether ponezumab can improve vascular reactivity in CAA with no significant adverse effects. Enrollment is expected to be completed by late 2015.

Vasculitis of the central nervous system

The term CNS vasculitis refers generically to the inflammation of cerebral blood vessels. A wide and heterogeneous group of diseases may cause CNS vascular inflammation, either primarily or secondarily. Primary CNS vasculitidies are rare but they deserve major attention for two main reasons. First, they are pure CNS vasculitis, implying particular pathophysiologic mechanisms and clinical features. Second, diagnosis is more challenging than in secondary CNS vasculitidies, as inflammation can only be demonstrated in the cerebral tissue. Primary CNS vasculitidies are largely represented by two entities: CAA-related inflammation (CAA-RI) and primary angiitis of the CNS (PACS). CAA-RI is particularly interesting as it establishes a unique link between a deposition disease (CAA) and a primary inflammatory process of the CNS. A summary of causes of CNS vasculitis can be found in Table 26.2.

Cerebral amyloid angiopathy-related inflammation

CAA-related inflammation (CAA-RI) is a vasculitic form of CAA that may occur spontaneously in a subset of patients. A report of meningoencephalitis cases from clinical trials testing active immunization against Aβ in AD patients[83] provided indirect evidence that vascular amyloid is likely to be responsible for triggering the inflammatory response observed in CAA-RI, but little is known about the factors contributing to it. Well-characterized series of patients with CAA-RI are very limited in the literature. However, available literature clearly shows that CAA-RI is clinically, pathologically, genetically, and radiographically differentiated from CAA; importantly, these particular characteristics translate into distinct and effective therapeutic approaches, which do not apply to the non-inflammatory form of CAA.[84]

The clinical presentation of CAA-RI also differs from other forms of CAA. The most commonly reported symptoms of CAA-RI are subacute cognitive decline/behavioural changes, seizures, and headache.[84–86] Focal neurological signs are also part of the clinical spectrum, but are seen less frequently. The presence of at least two of these four symptoms is present in almost 80 per cent of the patients described thus far. 'TIA-like symptoms', which may represent an acute form of presentation of the disease, have been observed only in a few cases.[87] In contrast to the non-inflammatory form of CAA, lobar ICH is a very rare presentation.

Brain imaging with MRI shows abnormalities in virtually all patients with CAA-RI. The finding of extensive and asymmetrical WMH on T2 and FLAIR sequences, which can be either patchy or confluent, is very common (Fig. 26.3). These WMH have characteristics of vasogenic oedema rather than ischaemia, including swelling and sometimes contrast enhancement. The oedema may be pronounced enough to generate mass effect, sometimes

Table 26.2 Vasculitides that affect the central nervous system

CAA-related inflammation
Primary angiitis of the CNS
Systemic necrotizing arteritis
    Polyarteritis nodosa
    Churg–Strauss syndrome
Hypersensitivity vasculitis
    Henoch–Schönlein purpura
    Hypocomplementemic vasculitis
    Cryoglobulinemia
Systemic granulomatous vasculitis
    Wegener granulomatosis
    Lymphomatoid granulomatosis
    Lethal midline granuloma
Giant cell arteritis
    Temporal arteritis
    Takayasu arteritis
Connective tissue disorders associated with vasculitis
    Systemic lupus erythematosus
    Scleroderma
    Rheumatoid arthritis
    Sjögren syndrome
    Mixed connective tissue disease
    Behçet disease
Vasculitis associated with infection
    Varicella zoster virus
    Spirochetes
      Treponema pallidum
      Borrelia burgdorferi
    Fungi
    Rickettsia
    Bacterial meningitis
    Mycobacterium tuberculosis
    HIV-1
Paraneoplastic vasculitis

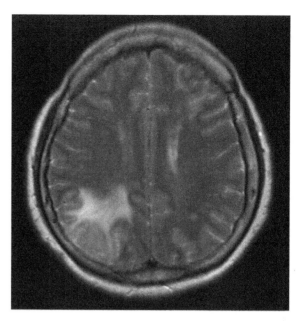

Fig. 26.3 Vasogenic oedema affecting white matter and cortex (FLAIR sequence) in a confirmed case of CAA-related inflammation. The MRI FLAIR sequence shown above is from a 72-year-old woman with subacute behavioural and cognitive changes.

sufficient to resemble a brain tumour. When hemosiderin-sensitive MRI sequences (e.g. GRE or SWI) are performed on patients with CAA-RI, lobar MB are a highly frequent finding, and even subarachnoid haemorrhage can be detected. Cerebral angiography is not routinely indicated when CAA-RI is strongly suspected, but when angiography is performed, typical findings of vasculitis (such as 'beading') may be found.[88]

Although blood tests typically lack diagnostic value in CAA-RI, the study of CSF may provide further proof of the autoimmune nature of the disease. In a recent small study,[89] patients with CAA-RI (n = 10) showed significantly higher levels of autologous anti-Aβ antibodies in the CSF compared to patients with the non-inflammatory form of CAA (controls, n = 7). Furthermore, CSF levels of $A\beta_{1-40}$ and $A\beta_{1-42}$, as well as markers of axonal injury (tau and P-181 tau), were found increased in CAA-RI. Interestingly, the levels of all these proteins decreased to control levels once the disease had resolved clinically and radiologically, and regardless of the use of immunosupressant agents. In the correct clinical context, genotyping of APOE may also provide

supportive evidence towards a diagnosis of CAA-RI. In a series of 14 confirmed CAA-RI cases, 10 out of 13 (76.9 per cent) were ApoE ε4 homozygotes.[84] In the same study it was reported that the frequency of ε4/ε4 in 39 confirmed cases of non-inflammatory CAA with available APoE genotype was only 5.1 per cent. The marked over-representation of the homozygous form in CAA-RI patients suggest that ε4 may play a role in the immunological response against vascular Aβ.

Pathological evidence of Aβ-related vascular inflammation is needed to confirm the diagnosis of CAA-RI. Although one case has been reported with proven increase of anti-Aβ antibodies in CSF,[90] brain biopsy is the only means of definitively diagnosing the disease during life.

Histological studies of CAA-RI cases have revealed that inflammatory infiltrates may be either perivascular (strictly a non-vasculitic form of CAA-RI) or transmural (a 'true' vasculitic form, often accompanied by the formation of granulomas)[88] (Fig. 26.4). Considering that surgical biopsy of the brain is an invasive, potentially dangerous exam, several authors have suggested a conservative approach in cases with clinical and neuroimaging findings highly suggestive of CAA-RI.[84,85] A set of diagnostic criteria for CAA-RI have been proposed, which include a 'probable CAA-RI' category for those cases without pathological study.[85] These criteria, however, still require validation.

Treatment of CAA-RI is not standardized, but typically high-dose corticosteroids are given as initial therapy.[84,85,91–95] Most treated patients will show some degree of improvement, both clinically and radiologically, within a few weeks of treatment onset.[84] Immunosuppressive agents, such as cyclophosphamide, may also be used as the initial treatment, or may be used if there is no rapid clinical improvement with corticosteroids. The duration of treatment is not well established and thus must be individualized. Three different patterns of response to treatment may be observed: improvement (persistent over time after treatment withdrawal); relapsing

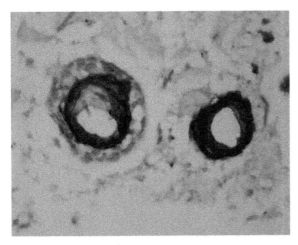

Fig. 26.4 CAA-related inflammation. Intracortical vessels have complete replacement of the vessel wall with Aβ, and the left-hand vessel demonstrates a lymphocytic reaction to the deposited Aβ (anti-Aβ immunohistochemistry, 40×).

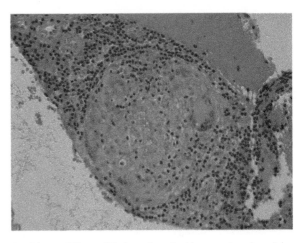

Fig. 26.5 Primary CNS vasculitis. A medium-sized leptomeningeal arteriole demonstrates inflammatory infiltrate throughout the vessel wall, with giant cells as well as a mixed lymphocytic population (H&E, 40×).

(initial improvement and relapse after treatment withdrawal), and stable/progressive (no response at all).[84]

Primary angiitis of the central nervous system (PACS)

PACS is a rare inflammatory condition of the cerebral blood vessels of unknown origin. PACS is traditionally considered a small-vessel vasculitis but reports of focal neurological signs are not uncommon, suggesting that major vessels may be involved as well.[96] Two major histological forms have been described: granulomatous and non-granulomatous, the latter being more frequent.[97] Untreated, PACS generally leads to progressive neurological dysfunction, with high morbidity and mortality. The inflammatory nature of the disease carries a favourable response to corticosteroids and/or cytotoxic drugs. However, diagnosis is often delayed, which may result in a poorer outcome.[96–98]

PACS mostly affects middle-aged men.[96,97,99] Headache and acute/subacute cognitive impairment or encephalopathy are the most common symptoms, and they present in an insidious, progressive way.[96] The insidious progression of the disorder combined with the often nebulous or nonspecific symptoms mean that the diagnosis is often very difficult to make in the earliest stages, the mean delay between symptoms onset and diagnosis of PACS being as long as six months.[98] Severe complications of PACS, such as TIA/stroke, seizures, and permanent neurologic deficits occur later in the course of the disease;[96,100] while they are not helpful to establish an early diagnosis, they can be prevented if treatment is initiated promptly. In contrast to many secondary vasculitidies with central nervous system involvement, fever, night sweats, and other systemic symptoms are not very prevalent in PACS (<20 per cent).[96,101]

In PACS, peripheral blood tests may occasionally show an increase in the erythrocyte sedimentation rate[96] but are often normal. CSF is abnormal in more than 80 per cent of cases,[96,102] typically showing protein elevation and/or a raised white cells count. MRI studies show abnormalities in almost 100 per cent of cases.[96,103] The most distinctive finding is the presence of bi-hemispheric infarcts affecting the subcortical white matter and even the overlying cortex.[96,104] Gadolinium enhancement is only observed in one-third of the patients, with leptomeningeal enhancement even more infrequent

(10–15 per cent). However, when leptomeningeal enhancement is present in the non-dominant hemisphere, it may serve as an ideal site for biopsy.[96] Cerebral angiography, may demonstrate morphologic signs frequently associated with vasculitis. 'Beading' (or multiple regions of narrowing in a given vessel, with interposed regions of ectasia or normal luminal architecture) is the most recognized angiographic abnormality.[105] Angiography, however, has some limitations that considerably limit its sensitivity and specificity for PACS: inability to detect abnormalities in vessels whose caliber is below the resolution of angiography, even when they are responsible for infarcts seen on MRI, and, more importantly, inability to provide a pathologic substrate for those morphologic alterations detected. Therefore cerebral biopsy, which remains the only way to confirm the diagnosis *in vivo*, is recommended in all patients with suspected PACS.[98] Biopsy may not only demonstrate vascular inflammation (Fig. 26.5) but also rule out other entities that mimic PACS. It should be noted that brain biopsy may result in false negatives, given that PACS may have a patchy distribution.[96]

No specific guidelines exist for a standardized treatment of PACS. However, expert consensus suggests treating patients with corticosteroids and a cytotoxic agent,[98] typically cyclophosphamide, However, given the high incidence of long-term adverse effects of cyclophosphamide,[106] switching to azathioprine is encouraged once remission is achieved. The cytotoxic agent should be continued for 2–3 years, while corticosteroid may be tapered off after 12 months of treatment. Given the powerful and broad immunosuppressant action of all these drugs, it is crucial to rule out other diagnosis (such as reversible vasoconstriction syndrome and CNS infections) prior to initiating treatment.

References

1. Biffi A and Greenberg SM. Cerebral amyloid angiopathy: a systematic review. *J Clin Neurol*. 2011;7:1–9.
2. Viswanathan A and Greenberg SM. Cerebral amyloid angiopathy in the elderly. *Ann Neurol*. 2011;70:871–80.
3. Smith EE and Greenberg SM. Beta-amyloid, blood vessels, and brain function. *Stroke*. 2009;40:2601–06.
4. Zhang-Nunes SX, Maat-Schieman ML, van Duinen SG, *et al*. The cerebral beta-amyloid angiopathies: Hereditary and sporadic. *Brain Pathol*. 2006;16:30–9.

5. Vinters HV. Cerebral amyloid angiopathy. A critical review. *Stroke.* 1987;18:311–24.

6. Vinters HV, Secor DL, Read SL, *et al.* Microvasculature in brain biopsy specimens from patients with Alzheimer's disease: an immunohisto-chemical and ultrastructural study. *Ultrastruct Pathol.* 1994;18:333–48.

7. Knudsen KA, Rosand J, Karluk D, *et al.* Clinical diagnosis of cerebral amyloid angiopathy: Validation of the Boston criteria. *Neurology.* 2001;56:537–39.

8. Greenberg SM, Gurol ME, Rosand J, *et al.* Amyloid angiopathy-related vascular cognitive impairment. *Stroke.* 2004;35:2616–19.

9. Coria F and Rubio I. Cerebral amyloid angiopathies. *Neuropathol Appl Neurobiol.* 1996;22:216–27.

10. Arvanitakis Z, Leurgans SE, Wang Z, *et al.* Cerebral amyloid angiopathy pathology and cognitive domains in older persons. *Ann Neurol.* 2011;69:320–27.

11. Herzig MC, Van Nostrand WE, and Jucker M. Mechanism of cerebral beta-amyloid angiopathy: murine and cellular models. *Brain Pathol.* 2006;16:40–54.

12. Eisele YS, Obermuller U, Heilbronner G, *et al.* Peripherally applied Abeta-containing inoculates induce cerebral beta-amyloidosis. *Science.* 2010;330:980–82.

13. Sutcliffe JG, Hedlund PB, Thomas EA, *et al.* Peripheral reduction of beta-amyloid is sufficient to reduce brain beta-amyloid: implications for Alzheimer's disease. *J Neurosci Res.* 2011;89:808–14.

14. Miners JS, Baig S, Palmer J, *et al.* Abeta-degrading enzymes in Alzheimer's disease. *Brain Pathol.* 2008;18:240–52.

15. Selkoe DJ. Clearing the brain's amyloid cobwebs. *Neuron.* 2001;32:177–80.

16. Weller RO, Massey A, Newman TA, *et al.* Cerebral amyloid angiopathy: amyloid beta accumulates in putative interstitial fluid drainage pathways in Alzheimer's disease. *Am J Pathol.* 1998;153:725–33.

17. Weller RO, Subash M, Preston SD, *et al.* Perivascular drainage of amyloid-beta peptides from the brain and its failure in cerebral amyloid angiopathy and Alzheimer's disease. *Brain Pathol.* 2008;18:253–66.

18. Ishii K, Tamaoka A, Mizusawa H, *et al.* Abeta1-40 but not Abeta1-42 levels in cortex correlate with apolipoprotein E epsilon4 allele dosage in sporadic Alzheimer's disease. *Brain Res.* 1997;748:250–52.

19. Harper JD, Lieber CM, and Lansbury PT, Jr. Atomic force microscopic imaging of seeded fibril formation and fibril branching by the Alzheimer's disease amyloid-beta protein. *Chem Biol.* 1997;4:951–59.

20. Jellinger KA. Alzheimer disease and cerebrovascular pathology: an update. *J Neural Transm.* 2002;109:813–36.

21. Ellis RJ, Olichney JM, Thal LJ, *et al.* Cerebral amyloid angiopathy in the brains of patients with Alzheimer's disease: the CERAD experience, Part XV. *Neurology.* 1996;46:1592–96.

22. Attems J, Jellinger KA, and Lintner F. Alzheimer's disease pathology influences severity and topographical distribution of cerebral amyloid angiopathy. *Acta Neuropathol.* 2005;110:222–31.

23. Hawkes CA, Hartig W, Kacza J, *et al.* Perivascular drainage of solutes is impaired in the ageing mouse brain and in the presence of cerebral amyloid angiopathy. *Acta Neuropathologica.* 2011;121:431–43.

24. Schley D, Carare-Nnadi R, Please CP, *et al.* Mechanisms to explain the reverse perivascular transport of solutes out of the brain. *J Theor Biol.* 2006;238:962–74.

25. Arbel-Ornath M, Hudry E, Eikermann-Haerter K, *et al.* Interstitial fluid drainage is impaired in ischemic stroke and Alzheimer's disease mouse models. *Acta Neuropathologica.* 2013;126:353–64.

26. Bornebroek M, De Jonghe C, Haan J, *et al.* Hereditary cerebral hemorrhage with amyloidosis Dutch type (AbetaPP 693): decreased plasma amyloid-beta 42 concentration. *Neurobiol Dis.* 2003;14:619–23.

27. De Jonghe C, Zehr C, Yager D, *et al.* Flemish and Dutch mutations in amyloid beta precursor protein have different effects on amyloid beta secretion. *Neurobiol Dis.* 1998;5:281–86.

28. Stenh C, Nilsberth C, Hammarback J, *et al* L. The Arctic mutation interferes with processing of the amyloid precursor protein. *Neuroreport.* 2002;13:1857–60.

29. Van Nostrand WE, Melchor JP, Cho HS, *et al.* Pathogenic effects of D23N Iowa mutant amyloid beta -protein. *J Biol Chem.* 2001;276:32860–66.

30. Ushiyama M, Ikeda S, and Yanagisawa N. Transthyretin-type cerebral amyloid angiopathy in type I familial amyloid polyneuropathy. *Acta Neuropathologica.* 1991;81:524–28.

31. Palsdottir A, Snorradottir AO, and Thorsteinsson L. Hereditary cystatin C amyloid angiopathy: genetic, clinical, and pathological aspects. *Brain Pathol.* 2006;16:55–9.

32. Falk RH, Comenzo RL, and Skinner M. The systemic amyloidoses. *N Engl J Med.* 1997;337:898–909.

33. Sudlow C, Martinez Gonzalez NA, Kim J, *et al.* Does apolipoprotein E genotype influence the risk of ischemic stroke, intracerebral hemorrhage, or subarachnoid hemorrhage? Systematic review and meta-analyses of 31 studies among 5961 cases and 17,965 controls. *Stroke.* 2006;37:364–70.

34. Strittmatter WJ, Saunders AM, Schmechel D, *et al.* Apolipoprotein E: high-avidity binding to beta-amyloid and increased frequency of type 4 allele in late-onset familial Alzheimer disease. *Proc Natl Acad Sci USA.* 1993;90:1977–81.

35. Greenberg SM, Vonsattel JP, Segal AZ, *et al.* Association of apolipoprotein E epsilon2 and vasculopathy in cerebral amyloid angiopathy. *Neurology.* 1998;50:961–65.

36. Linn J, Herms J, Dichgans M, *et al.* Subarachnoid hemosiderosis and superficial cortical hemosiderosis in cerebral amyloid angiopathy. *Am J Neuroradiol.* 2008;29:184–86.

37. Dierksen GA, Skehan ME, Khan MA, *et al.* Spatial relation between microbleeds and amyloid deposits in amyloid angiopathy. *Ann Neurol.* 2010;68:545–48.

38. Gurol ME, Dierksen G, Betensky R, *et al.* Predicting sites of new hemorrhage with amyloid imaging in cerebral amyloid angiopathy. *Neurology.* 2012;79:320–26.

39. Neau JP, Ingrand P, Couderq C, *et al.* Recurrent intracerebral hemorrhage. *Neurology.* 1997;49:106–13.

40. Passero S, Burgalassi L, D'Andrea P, *et al.* Recurrence of bleeding in patients with primary intracerebral hemorrhage. *Stroke.* 1995;26:1189–92.

41. Greenberg SM, O'Donnell HC, Schaefer PW, *et al.* MRI detection of new hemorrhages: potential marker of progression in cerebral amyloid angiopathy. *Neurology.* 1999;53:1135–38.

42. Greenberg SM, Eng JA, Ning M, *et al.* Hemorrhage burden predicts recurrent intracerebral hemorrhage after lobar hemorrhage. *Stroke.* 2004;35:1415–20.

43. Altmann-Schneider I, Trompet S, de Craen AJ, *et al.* Cerebral microbleeds are predictive of mortality in the elderly. *Stroke.* 2011;42:638–44.

44. Henneman WJ, Sluimer JD, Cordonnier C, *et al.* MRI biomarkers of vascular damage and atrophy predicting mortality in a memory clinic population. *Stroke.* 2009;40:492–98.

45. van der Vlies AE, Goos JD, Barkhof F, *et al.* Microbleeds do not affect rate of cognitive decline in Alzheimer disease. *Neurology.* 2012;79:763–69.

46. Neuropathology Group of the Medical Research Council Cognitive Function and Ageing Study (MRC CFAS). Pathological correlates of late-onset dementia in a multicentre, community-based population in England and Wales. *Lancet.* 2001;357:169–75.

47. Pfeifer LA, White LR, Ross GW, *et al.* Cerebral amyloid angiopathy and cognitive function: the HAAS autopsy study. *Neurology.* 2002;58:1629–34.

48. Dumas A, Dierksen GA, Gurol ME, *et al.* Functional magnetic resonance imaging detection of vascular reactivity in cerebral amyloid angiopathy. *Ann Neurol.* 2012;72:76–81.

49. Smith EE, Vijayappa M, Lima F, *et al.* Impaired visual evoked flow velocity response in cerebral amyloid angiopathy. *Neurology.* 2008;71:1424–30.

50. Thanprasertsuk S, Martinez-Ramirez S, Pontes-Neto OM, *et al.* Posterior white matter disease distribution as a predictor of amyloid angiopathy. Neurology. 2014;83:794–800.

51. Smith EE, Gurol ME, Eng JA, *et al.* White matter lesions, cognition, and recurrent hemorrhage in lobar intracerebral hemorrhage. *Neurology.* 2004;63:1606–12.

52. Haglund M, Passant U, Sjobeck M, *et al.* Cerebral amyloid angiopathy and cortical microinfarcts as putative substrates of vascular dementia. *Int J Geriatr Psychiatry.* 2006;21:681–87.

53. Soontornniyomkij V, Lynch MD, Mermash S, *et al.* Cerebral microinfarcts associated with severe cerebral beta-amyloid angiopathy. *Brain Pathol.* 2010;20:459–67.

54. Martinez-Ramirez S, Pontes-Neto OM, Dumas AP, *et al.* Topography of dilated perivascular spaces in subjects from a memory clinic cohort. *Neurology.* 2013;80:1551–56.

55. Charidimou A, Meegahage R, Fox Z, *et al.* Enlarged perivascular spaces as a marker of underlying arteriopathy in intracerebral haemorrhage: a multicentre MRI cohort study. *J Neurol Neurosur Ps.* 2013;84:624–29.

56. Roher AE, Kuo YM, Esh C, *et al.* Cortical and leptomeningeal cerebrovascular amyloid and white matter pathology in Alzheimer's disease. *Molecular Medicine.* 2003;9:112–22.

57. Greenberg SM, Vonsattel JP, Stakes JW, *et al.* The clinical spectrum of cerebral amyloid angiopathy: presentations without lobar hemorrhage. *Neurology.* 1993;43:2073–79.

58. Roch JA, Nighoghossian N, Hermier M, *et al.* Transient neurologic symptoms related to cerebral amyloid angiopathy: usefulness of T2*-weighted imaging. *Cerebrovasc Dis.* 2005;20:412–14.

59. Charidimou A, Peeters A, Fox Z, *et al.* Spectrum of transient focal neurological episodes in cerebral amyloid angiopathy: multicentre magnetic resonance imaging cohort study and meta-analysis. *Stroke.* 2012;43:2324–30.

60. Charidimou A, Jager RH, Fox Z, *et al.* Prevalence and mechanisms of cortical superficial siderosis in cerebral amyloid angiopathy. *Neurology.* 2013;81:626–32.

61. Shoamanesh A, Martinez-Ramirez S, Oliveira-Filho J, *et al.* Interrelationship of superficial siderosis and microbleeds in cerebral amyloid angiopathy. *Neurology.* 2014;83:1838–43.

62. Vonsattel JP, Myers RH, Hedley-Whyte ET, *et al.* Cerebral amyloid angiopathy without and with cerebral hemorrhages: a comparative histological study. *Ann Neurol.* 1991;30:637–49.

63. Puchtler H, Waldrop FS, and Meloan SN. A review of light, polarization and fluorescence microscopic methods for amyloid. *Appl Pathol.* 1985;3:5–17.

64. Yamaguchi H, Hirai S, Morimatsu M, *et al.* A variety of cerebral amyloid deposits in the brains of the Alzheimer-type dementia demonstrated by beta protein immunostaining. *Acta Neuropathologica.* 1988;76:541–49.

65. Vinters HV and Gilbert JJ. Cerebral amyloid angiopathy: incidence and complications in the aging brain. II. The distribution of amyloid vascular changes. *Stroke.* 1983;14:924–28.

66. Greenberg SM and Vonsattel JP. Diagnosis of cerebral amyloid angiopathy. Sensitivity and specificity of cortical biopsy. *Stroke.* 1997;28:1418–22.

67. Rosand J, Muzikansky A, Kumar A, *et al.* Spatial clustering of hemorrhages in probable cerebral amyloid angiopathy. *Ann Neurol.* 2005;58:459–62.

68. Linn J, Halpin A, Demaerel P, *et al.* Prevalence of superficial siderosis in patients with cerebral amyloid angiopathy. *Neurology.* 2010;74:1346–50.

69. Charidimou A, Jaunmuktane Z, Baron JC, *et al.* White matter perivascular spaces: an MRI marker in pathology-proven cerebral amyloid angiopathy? *Neurology.* 2014;82:57–62.

70. Vernooij MW, van der Lugt A, Ikram MA, *et al.* Prevalence and risk factors of cerebral microbleeds: the Rotterdam Scan Study. *Neurology.* 2008;70:1208–14.

71. Sveinbjornsdottir S, Sigurdsson S, Aspelund T, *et al.* Cerebral microbleeds in the population based AGES-Reykjavik study: prevalence and location. *J Neurol Neurosur Ps.* 2008;79:1002–1006.

72. Greenberg SM, Nandigam RN, Delgado P, *et al.* Microbleeds versus macrobleeds: evidence for distinct entities. *Stroke.* 2009;40:2382–86.

73. Klunk WE, Engler H, Nordberg A, *et al.* Imaging brain amyloid in Alzheimer's disease with Pittsburgh Compound-B. *Ann Neurol.* 2004;55:306–19.

74. Greenberg SM, Grabowski T, Gurol ME, *et al.* Detection of isolated cerebrovascular beta-amyloid with Pittsburgh compound B. *Ann Neurol.* 2008;64:587–91.

75. Gurol ME, Viswanathan A, Gidicsin C, *et al.* Cerebral amyloid angiopathy burden associated with leukoaraiosis: a positron emission tomography/magnetic resonance imaging study. *Ann Neurol.* 2013;73:529–36.

76. De Meyer G, Shapiro F, Vanderstichele H, *et al.* Diagnosis-independent Alzheimer disease biomarker signature in cognitively normal elderly people. *Arch Neurol.* 2010;67:949–56.

77. Sunderland T, Linker G, Mirza N, *et al.* Decreased beta-amyloid1-42 and increased tau levels in cerebrospinal fluid of patients with Alzheimer disease. *JAMA.* 2003;289:2094–103.

78. Verbeek MM, Kremer BP, Rikkert MO, *et al.* Cerebrospinal fluid amyloid beta(40) is decreased in cerebral amyloid angiopathy. *Ann Neurol.* 2009;66:245–49.

79. Eckman MH, Rosand J, Knudsen KA, *et al.* Can patients be anticoagulated after intracerebral hemorrhage? A decision analysis. *Stroke.* 2003;34:1710–16.

80. Lee SH, Ryu WS, and Roh JK. Cerebral microbleeds are a risk factor for warfarin-related intracerebral hemorrhage. *Neurology.* 2009;72:171–76.

81. Soo YO, Yang SR, Lam WW, *et al.* Risk vs benefit of anti-thrombotic therapy in ischaemic stroke patients with cerebral microbleeds. *J Neurol.* 2008;255:1679–86.

82. Biffi A, Halpin A, Towfighi A, *et al.* Aspirin and recurrent intracerebral hemorrhage in cerebral amyloid angiopathy. *Neurology.* 2010;75:693–98.

83. Orgogozo JM, Gilman S, Dartigues JF, *et al.* Subacute meningoencephalitis in a subset of patients with AD after Abeta42 immunization. *Neurology.* 2003;61:46–54.

84. Kinnecom C, Lev MH, Wendell L, *et al.* Course of cerebral amyloid angiopathy-related inflammation. *Neurology.* 2007;68:1411–16.

85. Chung KK, Anderson NE, Hutchinson D, *et al.* Cerebral amyloid angiopathy related inflammation: three case reports and a review. *J Neurol Neurosur Ps.* 2011;82:20–26.

86. Eng JA, Frosch MP, Choi K, *et al.* Clinical manifestations of cerebral amyloid angiopathy-related inflammation. *Ann Neurol.* 2004;55:250–56.

87. Amick A, Joseph J, Silvestri N, and Selim M. Amyloid-beta-related angiitis: a rare cause of recurrent transient neurological symptoms. *Nat Clin Pract Neurol.* 2008;4:279–83.

88. Scolding NJ, Joseph F, Kirby PA, *et al.* Abeta-related angiitis: primary angiitis of the central nervous system associated with cerebral amyloid angiopathy. *Brain.* 2005;128:500–15.

89. Piazza F, Greenberg SM, Savoiardo M, *et al.* Anti-amyloid beta autoantibodies in cerebral amyloid angiopathy-related inflammation: implications for amyloid-modifying therapies. *Ann Neurol.* 2013;73:449–58.

90. DiFrancesco JC, Brioschi M, Brighina L, *et al.* Anti-Abeta autoantibodies in the CSF of a patient with CAA-related inflammation: a case report. *Neurology.* 2011;76:842–44.

91. Fountain NB and Eberhard DA. Primary angiitis of the central nervous system associated with cerebral amyloid angiopathy: report of two cases and review of the literature. *Neurology.* 1996;46:190–97.

92. Ginsberg L, Geddes J, and Valentine A. Amyloid angiopathy and granulomatous angiitis of the central nervous system: a case responding to corticosteroid treatment. *J Neurol.* 1988;235:438–40.

93. Harkness KA, Coles A, Pohl U, *et al.* Rapidly reversible dementia in cerebral amyloid inflammatory vasculopathy. *Eur J Neurol.* 2004;11:59–62.

94. Marotti JD, Savitz SI, Kim WK, *et al.* Cerebral amyloid angiitis processing to generalized angiitis and leucoencephalitis. *Neuropathol Appl Neurobiol.* 2007;33:475–79.

95. Murphy MN and Sima AA. Cerebral amyloid angiopathy associated with giant cell arteritis: a case report. Stroke. 1985;16:514–17.

96. Salvarani C, Brown RD, Jr, Calamia KT, *et al.* Primary central nervous system vasculitis: analysis of 101 patients. *Ann Neurol.* 2007;62:442–51.

97. Lie JT. Primary (granulomatous) angiitis of the central nervous system: a clinicopathologic analysis of 15 new cases and a review of the literature. *Hum Pathol.* 1992;23:164–71.

98. Birnbaum J and Hellmann DB. Primary angiitis of the central nervous system. *Arch Neurol.* 2009;66:704–709.

99. Calabrese LH and Mallek JA. Primary angiitis of the central nervous system. Report of 8 new cases, review of the literature, and proposal for diagnostic criteria. *Medicine (Baltimore).* 1988;67:20–39.

100. Crane R, Kerr LD, and Spiera H. Clinical analysis of isolated angiitis of the central nervous system. A report of 11 cases. *Arch Intern Med.* 1991;151:2290–94.

101. Vollmer TL, Guarnaccia J, Harrington W, *et al.* Idiopathic granulomatous angiitis of the central nervous system. Diagnostic challenges. *Arch Neurol.* 1993;50:925–30.

102. Stone JH, Pomper MG, Roubenoff R, *et al.* Sensitivities of noninvasive tests for central nervous system vasculitis: A comparison of lumbar puncture, computed tomography, and magnetic resonance imaging. *J Rheumatol.* 1994;21:1277–82.

103. Woolfenden AR, Tong DC, Marks MP, *et al.* Angiographically defined primary angiitis of the CNS: Is it really benign? *Neurology.* 1998;51:183–88.

104. Pomper MG, Miller TJ, Stone JH, *et al.* CNS vasculitis in autoimmune disease: MR imaging findings and correlation with angiography. *AJNR Am J Neuroradiol.* 1999;20:75–85.

105. Alhalabi M and Moore PM. Serial angiography in isolated angiitis of the central nervous system. *Neurology.* 1994;44:1221–26.

106. Hoffman GS, Kerr GS, Leavitt RY, *et al.* Wegener granulomatosis: an analysis of 158 patients. *Ann Intern Med.* 1992;116:488–98.

CHAPTER 27

Cognition in multiple sclerosis

Maria A. Ron

Introduction

Multiple sclerosis (MS) is the commonest disabling neurological disease affecting young adults in the UK. MS is two to three times commoner in women. MS is also commoner in white populations and in northern latitudes.[1]

The cause of MS remains uncertain. The increased incidence in first-degree relatives and concordance rates in monozygotic twins (30 per cent) point to the relevance of genetic factors. Genome-wide association studies have identified more than 50 susceptibility loci, many of them closely mapped to immunological relevant genes.[2] Epstein–Barr virus infection, vitamin D deficiency, latitude, and smoking are possible environmental risk factors interacting with a genetic predisposition.

In 85 per cent of patients, MS has a relapse onset with an acute episode of neurological symptoms known as a clinically isolated syndrome or CIS. The course of MS after a CIS is variable. After the CIS, half of the patients continue to experience relapses and remissions (relapsing and remitting MS or RRMS). One-third of the patients follow a benign course with minimal disability. Permanent disability occurs when relapses fail to recover or when the course of the disease becomes progressive (secondary progressive MS or SPMS). Conversion to SPMS tends to occur 15–20 years after the initial CIS. Around 15 per cent of patients have a progressive course from the beginning (primary progressive MS or PPMS), although superimposed relapses may occur in up to 25 per cent.[1]

The diagnosis of MS can be made solely on clinical grounds, but magnetic resonance imaging (MRI) can help to demonstrate dissemination of typical lesions in time and space and allows for the diagnosis to be made in some patients presenting with a CIS.[3]

The neuropathology of MS is complex. Active focal inflammatory demyelinating white matter lesions are typical of acute relapses. These lesions occur preferentially in the optic nerve, periventricular white matter, corpus callosum, brainstem, cerebellar white matter, and cervical cord. In progressive forms of MS the acute inflammatory reaction is less marked and damage to the normal-appearing white matter with diffuse axonal injury, microglial activation, and cortical demyelination is more prominent.[4] The demyelination and transection of nerve fibres interferes with the smooth and rapid conduction of electrical impulses. Opinions vary as to whether the acute inflammatory lesions and the widespread neurodegenerative changes observed in progressive disease occur independently or whether the focal inflammatory lesion is the primary event. Demyelinating cortical lesions and cortical atrophy are now recognized as important elements of MS pathology and are known to be present in the early stages of the disease. Recent research[5] suggests that cortical lesions also have a marked inflammatory component and that they may be triggered by adjacent meningeal inflammation. Tissue damage in a particular cortical area also gives rise to anterograde or retrograde neurodegeneration in connected cortical regions.

Cognitive impairment in MS: Prevalence, pattern, and clinical correlates

Cognitive impairment occurs in 40–70 per cent of MS patients[6] and adds considerably to their disability, limiting independence, ability to work, adherence to treatment, driving safety, and successful rehabilitation. Cognitive impairment can be detected in about one-quarter of patients when they present with a CIS, but its prevalence increases with age and disease duration and it is more severe in those with a progressive disease course. Long-term follow-up studies have documented the accumulation of cognitive deficits over time.[7]

Impairment can be detected in a wide range of cognitive functions, but speed of information processing, complex attention, long-term memory, and executive functions (i.e. reasoning, planning, fluency, and organizational skills) are worst affected, while simple attention and essential verbal skills (word naming and comprehension) tend to be better preserved.[7] A decline in IQ from estimated premorbid levels has also been well documented.[8] Decrements in cognitive function tend to be moderate and frank dementia is rare. Decreased information-processing speed and visual memory impairment are the commonest deficits and often the first to be detected.[9] Slow information processing is often associated with impaired working and long-term memory, and tests tapping processing speed (e.g. paced auditory serial addition test or PASAT) are often used to screen for the presence of cognitive impairment and can predict later cognitive decline. Deficits in long-term memory can be detected in 40–60 per cent of MS patients, and impaired initial learning, rather than defective recall or recognition, is considered to responsible for the memory decline. The cognitive deficits detected in MS are closely interrelated and impaired initial learning may be explained, at least in part, by the slow information processing and defective working memory; while impaired learning may in turn result in poor decision-making. Cognitive reserve, as estimated by premorbid IQ and years of education,[10] appears to modulate the severity of cognitive impairment and may provide a partial explanation for the variability in the severity and pattern of cognitive impairment in a given patient.

Cognitive impairment in patients presenting with a CIS predicts conversion to MS and hence accumulation of physical disability.[11] In cross-sectional studies the correlation between the severity of cognitive impairment and physical disability is only modest, as the latter is often determined by spinal cord pathology, and in some patients cognitive and behavioural abnormalities are the most prominent symptoms in the absence of significant physical disability.[12] The pattern and the severity of cognitive impairment are similar in those with PPMS and SPMS.

Fatigue, depression, and cognitive performance

Cognitive performance may be influenced by fatigue and depression, both common features of MS. Fatigue is reported by about 90 per cent of patients and its relationship with cognitive performance is complex. Some studies, but not all, have reported that patients reporting fatigue performed worse in tests of attention[13] and information-processing speed.[14] More consistent decrements in cognitive performance have been reported in MS patients compared to healthy controls when cognitive fatigue is induced using tests that require sustained attention.[15]

Depression has a life-time prevalence of around 50 per cent in MS patients. The neuropathological substrate of depression in this context is unclear, but associations have been described with lesions located in medial inferior frontal regions and with left anterior temporal atrophy.[16] Cortico-subcortical disconnection caused by frontoparietal white matter lesions has been put forward as a possible mechanism.[17] Depression has been linked to poor performance on a variety of cognitive tasks, but the link is particularly strong for tasks that demand large cognitive processing capacity and in particular those that also involve working memory.[18]

Cognitive impairment and cerebral pathology as detected by MRI

Conventional MRI is best at detecting white matter lesions and providing measures of brain atrophy, but it is less sensitive for the detection of grey matter pathology or abnormalities in the normal-appearing white matter (NAWM). These limitations explain the modest correlations between clinical status, including cognition, and conventional MRI. New sequences such as double inversion recovery (DIR) and in particular phase-sensitive inversion recovery (PSIR) have improved the detection of grey matter lesions (Fig. 27.1),[19] while diffusion and magnetization transfer (MTI) and proton MR spectroscopy (^{1}H-MRS) are able to detect abnormalities in the normal appearing brain tissue.

Cognitive impairment in MS is thought to result from damage to cognitively relevant white matter tracts (e.g. cingulum, uncinate fasciculus, superior and middle cerebellar peduncles) leading to a multisystem cortico-subcortical disconnection syndrome.[20] Disruption of functional connectivity between different brain regions leads to cortical thinning,[21] although primary cortical pathology also plays a part.

Integrity of white matter tracts as indexed by the presence of lesions and by abnormalities in the NAWM correlate with global measures of cognitive performance.[22] Studies using diffusion-based tractography, a technique that allows the study of specific white matter tracts, have provided evidence of how pathology in different white matter tracts results in specific cognitive deficits. Thus damage to the corpus callosum and tracts connecting

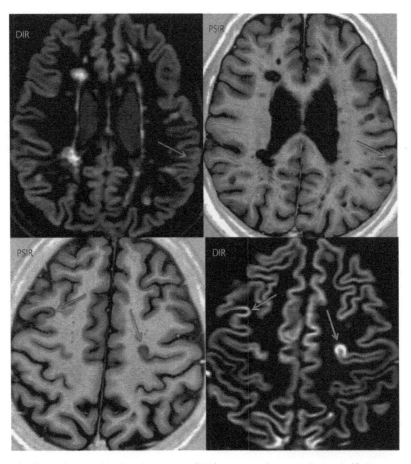

Fig. 27.1 Double inversion recovery (DIR) and phase-sensitive inversion recovery (PSIR) sequences demonstrating cortical lesions.

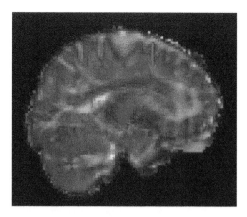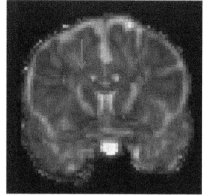

Fig. 27.2 Diffusion images showing white matter lesion in the corpus callosum that resulted in marked reduction of information processing speed.

prefrontal (Fig. 27.2) regions result in impaired processing speed, attention, and working memory, while damage to the uncinate fasciculus is related to memory impairment.[22] Measures of whole brain atrophy, indicative of irreversible neuroaxonal damage and reflecting cortico-subcortical disconnection, are associated with cognitive impairment.[23] Lesion metrics and atrophy detected early in the disease have also been found to predict future cognitive impairment.[8,10] This is in keeping with the findings of a recent study using resting state fMRI[24] that reported diffusely impaired functional connectivity involving many large-scale neuronal networks, including the salience, executive, and default mode networks. Changes in functional connectivity were correlated with disability, including poor cognitive performance and with the severity of MS-related pathology.

Changes in brain plasticity in patients with MS have been described using fMRI in conjunction with attention-[25] and memory-activation[26] paradigms. MS patients with preserved cognitive performance showed increased activation in the areas normally activated in healthy controls, and also extensive, usually bilateral, activation in areas commonly silent in normal subjects. The extent of increased activation was correlated with measures of pathology in the normal-appearing white and grey matter.[27] These findings have been interpreted as indicating compensatory neural activity early in the disease. Another fMRI study[28] has reported that patients with greater expression of the default mode network, an index of cognitive reserve, can withstand more severe brain pathology before manifesting cognitive impairment.

Approaches to treatment

Available *disease modifying therapies* (DMTs) target the inflammatory process of MS and there is good evidence that they reduce the number of relapses, but there is no clear indication that DMTs prevent or delay the onset of SPMS or long-term disability. Few studies have looked at the effect of DMTs on cognition. A systematic review of available trials[29] suggests that interferon β1a may slow down the rate of cognitive impairment and of brain atrophy. There is also some evidence that interferon β1b may also improve information-processing speed and memory in patients with RRMS and that it may protect against cognitive decline in patients with CIS.[30] No beneficial cognitive effects have been reported in association with glatiramer acetate. The effects of DMTs in patients with PPMS are uncertain, but recent evidence[31] suggests that interferon β1b may

have modest beneficial long-term effects on cognition and in slowing down the rate of atrophy. Short-term trials of the monoclonal antibody natalizumab have also reported cognitive improvement in patients with RRMS.[32]

Beneficial effects have also been reported when acetylcholinesterase inhibitors (AChE) donepezil and rivastigmine were administered in double-blind placebo-controlled trials. Donepezil was found to improve verbal learning and memory[33] and rivastigmine has been reported to alter functional connectivity, enhancing prefrontal function and limiting cognitive failure.[34] A recent study[35] has reported improvements in speed of information processing and memory in MS patients given lisdexanphetamine dimesylate (LDX) a medication used to treat attention deficit/hyperactivity disorder.

Neuroprotection in MS is still in its infancy, and the effect of neuroprotective drugs (e.g. glutamate antagonists, sodium channel blockers, and cannabinoids) on cognition remains to be determined.

Cognitive rehabilitation—a systematic review of the 16 available trials of cognitive rehabilitation that met required standards[36] found some evidence of success for memory rehabilitation techniques that use visual imagery and context. Improved memory performance was associated with increased fMRI activation in frontal, temporal, and parietal areas associated with memory, visual processing, and executive control (i.e. the areas subserving the mnemonic treatment strategies). It remains to be determined whether these effects are long-lasting.[37] Cognitive remediation appears to be more effective in patients with only mild brain atrophy. There is no evidence so far to suggest that rehabilitation aimed at attention or executive function is of value.

References

1. Cole A. The bare essentials. Multiple sclerosis. *Practical Neurology*. 2009;9: 118–26.
2. Lin R, Charlesworth J, and van der Mei I, *et al*. The Genetics of Multiple Sclerosis. *Practical Neurology*. 2012;12:279–88.
3. Swanton JK, Rovira A, Tintore M, *et al*. MRI criteria for multiple sclerosis in patients presenting with clinically isolated syndromes: a multicentre retrospective study. *Lancet Neurol*. 2007;8:677–86.
4. Kutzelnigg A, Lucchinetti CF, Stadelmann C, *et al*. Cortical demyelination and diffuse white matter injury in multiple sclerosis. *Brain*. 2005;128:2705–12.
5. Lassman H. Cortical lesions in multiple sclerosis: inflammation versus neurodegeneration. *Brain*. 2012;136:2904–5.

6. Chiaravalloti ND and DeLuca J. Cognitive impairment in multiple sclerosis. *Lancet Neurol.* 2008;12:1139–51.

7. Amato MP, Ponziani G, Siracusa G, *et al.* Cognitive dysfunction in early-onset multiple sclerosis: a reappraisal after 10 years. *Arch Neurol.* 2001;58:1602–6.

8. Summers M, Fisniku L, Anderson V, *et al.* Cognitive impairment in relapsing-remitting multiple sclerosis can be predicted by imaging performed several years earlier. *Mult Scler.* 2008 14:197–204.

9. Benedict RH, Cookfair D, Gavett R, *et al.* Validity of the minimal assessment of cognitive function in multiple sclerosis. J Int Neuropsychol Soc 2006; **12**: 549–58.

10. Summers M, Swanton J, Fernando K, *et al.* Cognitive impairment in multiple sclerosis can be predicted by imaging early in the disease. *J Neurol Neurosur Ps.* 2008; 79:955–8.

11. Zipoli V, Goretti B, Hakiki B, *et al.* Cognitive impairment predicts conversion to multiple sclerosis in clinically isolated syndromes. *Multiple Sclerosis.* 2010;16: 62–67.

12. Zarei M, Chandran S, Compston A, *et al.* Cognitive presentation of multiple sclerosis: evidence for a cortical variant. *J Neurol Neurosur Ps.* 2003;74:872–877.

13. Weinges-Evers N, Brandt AU, Bock M, *et al.* Correlation of self-assessed fatigue and alertness in multiple sclerosis. *Mult Scler.* 2010; 9:1134–40.

14. Andreasen AK, Spliid PE, Andersen H, *et al.* Fatigue and processing speed are related in multiple sclerosis. *Eur J Neurol.* 2010;17:212–8.

15. Schwid SR, Tyler CM, Scheid EA, *et al.* Cognitive fatigue during a test requiring sustained attention: a pilot study. *Mult Scler.* 2003;9:503–8.

16. Feinstein A, Roy P, Lobaugh N, *et al.* Structural brain abnormalities in multiple sclerosis patients with major depression. *Neurology.* 2004;62:586–90.

17. Bakshi R, Czarnecki D, Shaikh ZA, *et al.* Brain MRI lesions and atrophy are related to depression in multiple sclerosis. *Neuroreport.* 2000;11:1153–8.

18. Arnett PA, Higginson CI, Voss WD, *et al.* Depressed mood in multiple sclerosis: relationship to capacity-demanding memory and attentional functioning. Neuropsychology 1999; 13:434–446.

19. Sethi V, Yousry TA, Muhlert N, *et al.* Improved detection of cortical MS lesions with phase-sensitive inversion recovery MRI. *J Neurol Neurosur Ps.* 2012;83:877–82.

20. Mesaros S, Rocca MA, Kacar K, *et al.* Diffusion tensor MRI tractography and cognitive impairment in multiple sclerosis *Neurology.* 2012;78:969–975.

21. He Y, Dagher A, Chen Z, *et al.* Impaired small-world efficiency in structural cortical networks in multiple sclerosis associated with white matter lesion load. *Brain.* 2009;132:3366–79.

22. Filippi M, Rocca MA, Benedict RH, *et al.* The contribution of MRI in assessing cognitive impairment in multiple sclerosis. *Neurology.* 2010;75:2121–8.

23. Lanz M, Hahn HK, and Hildebrandt H. Brain atrophy and cognitive impairment in multiple sclerosis: A review. *J Neurol.* 2007;254 Suppl 2:II43–8.

24. Rocca MA, Valsasina P, Martinelli V, *et al.* Large-scale neuronal network dysfunction in relapsing-remitting multiple sclerosis. *Neurology.* 2012;79:1449–57.

25. Staffen W, Mair A, Zauner H, *et al.* Cognitive function and fMRI in patients with multiple sclerosis: evidence for compensatory cortical activation during an attention task. *Brain.* 2002; 125:1275–82.

26. Chiaravalloti N, Hillary F, Ricker J, *et al.* Cerebral activation patterns during working memory performance in multiple sclerosis using FMRI. *J Clin Exp Neuropsychol.* 2005; 27:33–54.

27. Audoin B, Au Duong MV, Malikova I, *et al.* Functional magnetic resonance imaging and cognition at the very early stage of MS. *J Neurol Sci.* 2006; 245:87–91.

28. Sumowski JF, Wylie GR, *et al.* Intellectual enrichment is linked to cerebral efficiency in multiple sclerosis: functional magnetic resonance imaging evidence for cognitive reserve. *Brain.* 2010;133:362–74.

29. Galetta SL, Markowitz C, and Lee AG. Immunomodulatory agents for the treatment of relapsing multiple sclerosis: a systematic review. *Arch Intern Med.* 2002;162:2161–9.

30. Patti F, Amato MP, Bastianello S, *et al.* Subcutaneous interferon beta-1a has a positive effect on cognitive performance in mildly disabled patients with relapsing-remitting multiple sclerosis: 2-year results from the cogimus study. *Ther Adv Neurol Disord.* 2009;2:67–77.

31. Tur C, Montalban X, Tintore M, *et al.* Interferon beta-1b for the treatment of primary progressive multiple sclerosis: five-year clinical trial follow-up. *Arch Neurol.* 2011;68:1421–1427.

32. Iaffaldano P, Viterbo RG, Paolicelli D, *et al.* Impact of natalizumab on cognitive performances and fatigue in relapsing multiple sclerosis: a prospective, open-label, two years observational study. *PLoS One.* 2012;7(4):e35843.

33. Krupp LB, Christodoulou C, Melville P, *et al.* Donepezil improved memory in multiple sclerosis in a randomized clinical trial. *Neurology.* 2004;63:1579–85.

34. Cader S, Palace J, and Matthews PM. Cholinergic agonism alters cognitive processing and enhances brain functional connectivity in patients with multiple sclerosis. *J Psychopharmacol.* 2009;23:686–96.

35. Morrow SA, Smerbeck A, Patrick K, *et al.* Lisdexamfetamine dimesylate improves processing speed and memory in cognitively impaired MS patients: a phase II study. *J Neurol.* 2012 Sep 23.

36. O'Brien AR, Chiaravalloti N, Goverover Y, *et al.* Evidenced-based cognitive rehabilitation for persons with multiple sclerosis: a review of the literature. *Arch Phys Med Rehabil.* 2008;89:761–9.

37. Chiaravalloti ND, Wylie G, Leavitt V, *et al* Increased cerebral activation after behavioral treatment for memory deficits in MS. *J Neurol.* 2012; 259:1337–46.

CHAPTER 28

Autoimmune encephalitis

Sarosh R. Irani, Thomas D. Miller, and Angela Vincent

Introduction

The field of autoimmune encephalitis has grown rapidly over the last decade, an expansion principally driven by the description of a variety of new antibody targets (Fig. 28.1). The detection of novel antibodies has, in turn, led to the recognition of a broader spectrum of phenotypes, and all appear responsive to immunotherapies. These phenotypes show some clear overlaps and also some marked differences which are often related to the antibody specificity. The clinical lessons emerging from patients has drawn attention to the prevalence and importance of autoimmune disease affecting cognition and behaviour, including in those patients who are currently 'negative' for known antibodies, in serum and/or CSF.

Various terms have been used to describe the main neurocognitive syndrome associated with these autoantibodies, including autoimmune encephalitis, autoimmune encephalopathy, limbic encephalopathy (LE), limbic encephalitis, autoimmune dementia, and rapidly progressive dementia (RPD).[4–6] These terms probably reflect the varied rapidity of disease onset, the disease localization, the paraclinical evidence for inflammation, and the background of the author. Although the term autoimmune encephalopathy is probably the most inclusive, 'autoimmune encephalitis' (AE) has been most widely accepted and is the term we will use throughout this chapter.

Although the first description of AE is often attributed to Corsellis and Brierley in the 1960s,[7,8] von Economo's description of encephalitis lethargica (EL) in 1910 fits within this entity and he himself disputed the direct relationship between EL and influenza and suggested the probable immune basis of the disorder.[9,10] AE can be considered as a syndrome encompassing a number of more specific diagnoses. Many patients present with a rapid onset, typically over days or weeks, of amnesia, behavioural change, psychosis, disorientation, and seizures. Therefore, a number of differential diagnoses are initially considered including infective encephalitis (especially herpes virus family-related), drug or toxin overdoses, Creutzfeldt–Jakob disease (CJD), Wernicke–Korsakoff syndrome, non-convulsive status epilepticus, and also the controversial entity of Hashimoto's encephalopathy.[11–13] Because the details of the clinical and paraclinical features vary significantly with antibody specificity, each syndrome is discussed based on its antigenic target (Table 28.1).

We begin by discussing the clinical and paraclinical features associated with the voltage-gated potassium channel (VGKC) complex antibody-related disorders, most importantly the conditions associated with antibodies to leucine-rich glioma inactivated 1 (LGI1) or contactin-associated protein 2 (CASPR2). We then describe the encephalitis associated with N-methyl D-aspartate

(NMDA)-receptor antibodies. Subsequently, we briefly review the rarer entities associated with antibodies to the glycine, gamma-aminobutyric acid (GABA) and α-amino-3-hydroxy-5-methyl-4-isoxazolepropionic acid (AMPA) receptors. We illustrate treatment principles, available evidence for immunotherapies, and address pathophysiological hypotheses for both antibody access to the brain and the mechanisms by which CNS-bound antibodies act. Finally, we address these diseases as models to study the neuroscience of memory and psychosis.

Location, location, location

The subcellular distribution of the target antigen appears key to determining the likely antibody pathogenicity (Fig. 28.1). The main distinction made in the literature is between cell-surface and intracellular antigens. Traditionally, intracellular antigenic targets (including Hu, Yo, Ri, CV2/CRMP5) were associated

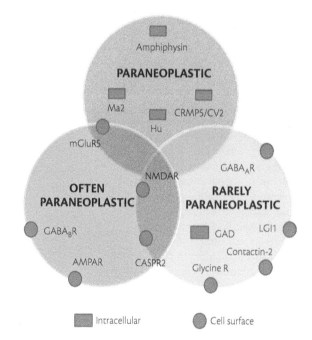

Fig. 28.1 Subcellular locations and paraneoplastic associations of neural antibodies.[162] Antigens with intracellular (blue rectangles) and extracellular (blue circles) localizations. Antibody targets which are 'classically' paraneoplastic (blue circle), often paraneoplastic (peach circle), and rarely paraneoplastic (green circle). Adapted with *Arq Neuropsiquiatr.* 70(10), Machado S, Pinto AN, and Irani SR, What should you know about limbic encephalitis? pp. 817–22, Copyright (2012), with permission from the Brazilian Academy of Neurology, reproduced under the Creative Commons CC BY-NC 4.0 License.

Table 28.1 Additional features of limbic encephalitis associated with the commonest CNS cell-surface directed antibodies

	NMDAR	LGI1	CASPR2	AMPAR	Glycine	GABA_B
Frequent clinical associations	Diffuse encephalitis with psychiatric features with cognitive impairment, seizures, movement disorder, dysautonomia, and reduction in consciousness	LE with faciobrachial dystonic seizures, and serum hyponataremia	Morvan's syndrome with psychiatric features, insomnia, dysautonomia, and neuromyotonia (often with LGI1-antibodies). Less frequently, LE	LE	LE, PERM but also some SPS-spectrum syndromes	LE
Tumour/Infectious associations	Ovarian teratoma in about 30%; Relapses post-HSV encephalitis with NMDAR antibodies	<10% (various tumours described)	Thymoma (~30%)	Lung, breast, thymoma (~50%)	Thymoma rarely (<10%)	Lung (~50%)
Expanding phenotypic spectrum	Few cases with purely psychotic features; predominant movement disorder; few with predominant cryptogenic epilepsy syndrome	Cryptogenic epilepsies	Cryptogenic epilepsies; Guillain-Barre-like syndrome	Atypical psychosis	LE, brainstem encephalitis; Cryptogenic epilepsies	
Approximate number of reported cases since first description	>700 in 6 years	~250 in 3 years	~30 in 3 years	~25 in 4 years	~35 in 5 years	~30 in 3 years
Prevalence in clinically-defined tested cohorts; controls variable but generally <1%	9/48 (19%) with unknown encephalitis	6/62 (10%) with unknown encephalitis	21/27 (78%) with Morvan's syndrome	15/410 (4%) with suspected autoimmune encephalitis	Mainly seen in PERM; 10/81 (12%) with SPS; 1/48 (2%) of pediatric encephalopathies	10/70 (14%) of LE cases.
Primary cell type/ Antigenic target	Neuron/NR1 subunit	Neuron	Neuron	Neuron/ GluR1/2	Neuron/α1 receptor	Neuron/ B1 subunit

Limbic encephalitis (LE) produces amnesia, confusion and seizures (additional features noted above within each antibody specificity). Opsoclonus-myoclonus syndrome (OMS); stiff-person syndrome (SPS); status epilepticus (SE); first episode psychosis (FEP); basal ganglia (BG); progressive encephalomyelitis with rigidity and myoclonus (PERM).

Adapted from *Ann Neurol.* 76(1), Dahm L, Ott C, Steiner J, et al. Seroprevalence of autoantibodies against brain antigens in health and disease, pp. 82–94, Copyright (2014), with permission from John Wiley and Sons; *Ann Neurol.* 76(2), Irani SR, Gelfand JM, Al-Diwani A, et al. Cell-surface central nervous system autoantibodies: Clinical relevance and emerging paradigms, pp. 168–84, Copyright (2014), with permission from John Wiley and Sons, reproduced under the Creative Commons CC BY-NC-ND License.

with paraneoplastic diseases, often with a very poor prognosis, and where the antibody titre was unrelated to the severity of the illness.[14–16]

By contrast, more contemporary literature discusses antibodies against neuronal surface-directed antibody (NSAbs) which are accessible to the circulating antibodies *in vivo*. These diseases are associated with a far better prognosis, even up to near-complete recovery, a lower rate of tumours, and a stricter correlation between antibody levels and clinical state. The cell-surface antibody classification appears to be more important in prognostication than the presence of a tumour.[1–3] Interestingly, the defined targets of many of these antibodies are ion channels (NMDA, GABA, AMPAR, glycine receptors) or proteins which co-associate with channels (LGI1, CASPR2, contactin-2, and DPPX) but may also have other roles in neuronal biology.[17]

One antibody target, glutamic acid decarboxylase (GAD), lies in a hinterland. GAD is an intracellular enzyme and its levels do not correlate well with disease activity. However, there are few tumours observed in patients with GAD antibodies and the associated diseases may respond to immunotherapies. A partial resolution to this intracellular cell-surface antigen discrepancy may be that many patients with GAD-antibodies also harbour other NSAbs, as has been shown in a few studies.[18–20]

Antibody-detection methods

The assays used to detect the autoantibodies are critical to disease definitions and are increasingly scrutinized (Fig. 28.2). While some of the arguments below have been summarized elsewhere,[2,17,21] the assay differences are so integral to the syndrome definition that the related controversies are briefly reviewed here. The main controversies surround whether antibody detection in cerebrospinal fluid (CSF) or serum is more important, the relevance of intrathecal synthesis, and the methodological and technical details of the assay itself which include the sample concentrations, possible exposure to intracellular epitopes, and the use of more than one assay to diagnose a single antibody.

There are conflicting reports as to the relative importance of CSF and serum antibodies.[21,22] In our experience, the levels of NSAbs are almost always higher in the serum than the CSF. In patients with NMDAR (NMDA receptor) and LGI1 antibodies for instance, absolute antibody levels are between 5 and 100 times higher in absolute terms in serum. This difference suggests the antibody is

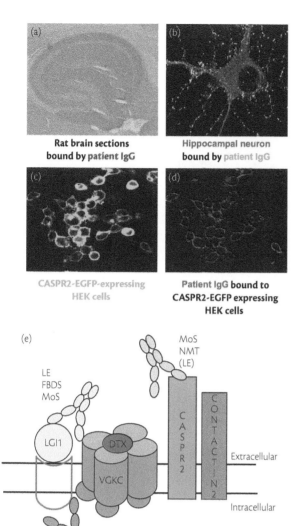

Rat brain sections bound by patient IgG

Hippocampal neuron bound by patient IgG

CASPR2-EGFP-expressing HEK cells

Patient IgG bound to CASPR2-EGFP expressing HEK cells

(e)

MoS
NMT
(LE)

LE
FBDS
MoS

LGI1

DTX

VGKC

C A S P R 2

C O N T A C T I N 2

Extracellular

Intracellular

Fig. 28.2 (a) Sagittal rat brain section showing binding of patient serum NMDAR antibody (IgG). (b) Hippocampal neuronal cultures labelled with LGI1-IgG antibody (green) and intracellularly stained with MAP2, a neuronal marker (red). (c) Enhanced green fluorescent protein (EGFP)-tagged antigen (in this case CASPR2, green) is bound by patient IgG (d red). (e) Depiction of the voltage-gated potassium channel (VGKC)-complex labelled with dendrotoxin (DTX) to show antibodies known to bind the extracellular domains of LGI1 (in patients with limbic encephalitis (LE), faciobrachial dystonic seizures (FBDS), and Morvan syndrome (MoS)), and CASPR2 in patients with MoS more frequently than in neuromyotonia (NMT) or LE. Contactin-2 antibodies are rare. Some antibodies may bind the intracellular domains of some molecules within the VGKC-complex (blue antibody).

peripherally generated. However, if normalized to total immunoglobulin G (IgG) concentrations, which are around 400 times higher in the serum, the concentration of antigen-specific antibody in the CSF relative to that in serum, is often >1, indicating intrathecal synthesis of the antibodies. This is particularly common in patients with NMDAR antibodies. These findings indicate secondary generation of the NSAb within the intrathecal space, not due to simple

diffusion across the blood–brain barrier, and it is unclear whether this intrathecally derived IgG is similarly or more pathogenic than serum IgG. This question may be confounded by the likely differences between intraventricular and lumbar CSF constituents.

Methodological assay differences are also of potential importance (Fig. 28.2). Traditionally, rodent brain sections have been stained with patient serum and/or CSF (Fig. 28.2a). This technique allows antibodies access to both intracellular and extracellular epitopes but can show highly distinctive patterns of binding with different antibodies. In order to detect only NSAbs, and therefore antibodies with pathogenic potential, live neuronal cultures have been used as they express native neuronal proteins and deny antibodies access to intracellular epitopes (Fig. 28.2b). In cell-based assays, cells transfected with the defined antigen are probed with the patient sera to determine antigenic specificity (Fig. 28.2c-d), but different studies use permeabilized or live cells to perform this diagnostic test. Also, some groups use brain sections and/or live hippocampal neuronal binding *plus* a cell-based assay approach to diagnoses NSAbs,[21,23] whereas others rely on the cell-based assay, with absence of binding to a related cell-expressed antigen as a marker of specificity.[18,19,24–26]

In summary, currently due to unresolved differences in methodological approaches, it is prudent to send both serum and CSF for diagnosis. Nevertheless, critically, the presence of the antibody should be understood in the context of the clinical presentation.

LGI1 and CASPR2: VGKC-complex antigens

The two commonest antibodies found in patients with cognitive and behavioural deficits are directed against LGI1 and the NMDA receptor (Fig. 28.3 and 28.4). The syndrome associated with

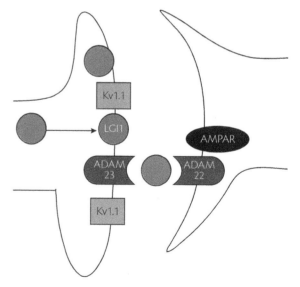

Fig. 28.3 Illustration of the VGKC-complexes: the association of Kv1s and LGI1 (leucine-rich glioma-inactivated 1) and other components of the synaptic complex including Kv1s (blue, such as Kv1.1), LGI1 (red) and α-amino-3-hydroxy-5-methyl-4-isoxazolepropionic acid receptors (AMPAR) and ADAM22/23 (a disintegrin and metalloproteinase 22/23) (brown) anchored at postsynaptic membranes.

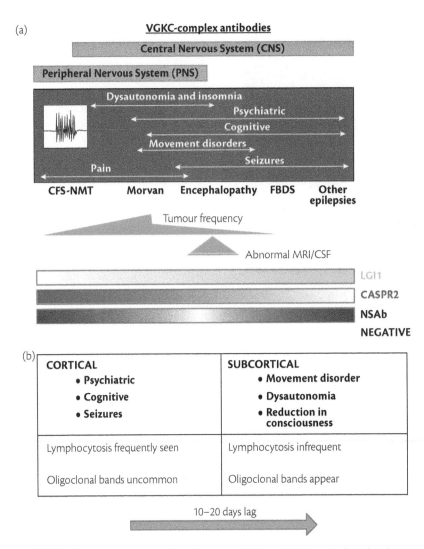

Fig. 28.4 (a) The phenotype spread of VGKC (voltage-gated potassium channel)-complex, LGI1 and CASPR2 antibodies. The relative proportions of patients with LGI1- and CASPR2-antibodies and those who remain without a known antigenic target ('seronegative') are depicted in the gradient bars. Movement disorders include ataxia, chorea, and parkinsonism.[55,163,164] A number of patients, especially those with cramp-fasciculation syndrome-neuromyotonia (CFS–NMT; high-frequency discharges shown) and epilepsy (excluding faciobrachial dystonic seizures, FBDS) currently have no defined antigenic target ('NSAb negative') although their sera precipitate VGKC-complexes in the radioimmunoassay. Reproduced with permissions from Irani et al. 2014.[2] (b) The temporal progression of patients with NMDAR-antibody encephalitis. The disease usually begins with psychiatric and cognitive features plus seizures and, after a lag of 10–20 days, a movement disorder, dysautonomia, and reduction in consciousness are seen. CSF pleocytosis occurs earlier than CSF oligoclonal bands. In addition, EEG spikes occur prior to diffuse slowing. Adapted from *Curr Neurol Neurosci Rep.* 11(3), Irani SR and Vincent A, NMDA receptor antibody encephalitis, pp. 298–304, Copyright (2011), with permission from Springer.

VGKC-complex antibodies has been serologically and clinically reclassified in recent years (Fig. 28.2e and Fig. 28.3). It has become clear that these autoantibodies only rarely target the VGKCs themselves, but that many are directed against proteins which are tightly complexed with the VGKCs, most frequently LGI1 and CASPR2.[24] Around 80 per cent of cases with a purely CNS-localized syndrome have LGI1 antibodies,[24,27] with a minority having CASPR2-antibodies.[24] Antibodies against contactin-2 are rare and tend to coexist with either LGI1 or CASPR2 antibodies in patients with AE.[24] The original radioimmunoassay detects over 95 per cent of patients with CASPR2 or LGI1 antibodies, but also detects antibodies against uncharacterized antigenic targets of the VGKC-complex.[4,24,26,28,29] Some of these are unlikely to be pathogenic antibodies (for detailed discussion see references 2 and 30) but collectively, the term VGKC-complex antibodies is used to describe the detection of these multiple specificities within a single

diagnostic assay (Fig. 28.2e),[24,26,31] although this radioactive test is not widely available except at specialist centres.

The VGKC-complex antibody-associated encephalopathy is now well known to neurologists and consists of the acute to subacute presentation of amnesia, disorientation, and seizures.[4,29,32,33] This is usually seen in adults over 50 years of age, with a slight male predominance. The pattern of cognitive impairment is detailed later, but retrograde and anterograde deficits are present in the acute phase, often with a dense gap around the illness and for several years prior to illness onset.[34–36] Disorientation and frontal dysexecutive features are often seen acutely. The observation of a more insidious onset amnestic syndrome in association with VGKC-complex/LGI1 antibodies,[5,37] without MRI or CSF markers of inflammation, has led to the adoption of the term autoimmune dementia by some authors.[38] In addition to an absence of inflammation, these antibody-associated dementias have been reported to show a more chronic presentation and a good immunotherapy response. These should be considered in the differential diagnosis of more typically neurodegenerative presentations such as CJD and rapid forms of Lewy body dementia and Alzheimer's disease.[5,6,13]

Seizures

Seizures are found in 80–90 per cent of patients with VGKC-complex antibodies. While sometimes seen in isolation, they are often associated with cognitive impairment,[37,39–44] and generalized convulsions rarely pose a clinical problem. The seizures are often frequent and with focal onset. Abdominal, olfactory and visual auras, limb automatisms and jerking have all been reported. More recently, three distinctive semiologies have been described, the most characteristic of which are faciobrachial dystonic seizures (FBDS).

FBDS are of particular importance as they illustrate paradigms for both prevention and treatment of antibody-mediated CNS disease.[31,37,41,45,46] FBDS are short (often < 3 seconds) dystonic events which usually affect the arm and ipsilateral face, and occur at a high frequency (median 50 times, but up to 350 times per day). Many patients with FBDS who were refractory to standard antiepileptic drugs (AEDs) showed an excellent, and often rapid, response to immunotherapy, especially corticosteroids. Retrospective and prospective studies suggest that the onset of FBDS is predictive of the occurrence of a more typical LGI1-antibody associated encephalopathy, with a median lag of around five weeks. These observations led to the hypothesis that successful treatment of the FBDS may prevent an incipient encephalopathy. While this has been substantiated in one small prospective study and several case reports, this is yet to be proven in a blinded or randomized manner.[37,47,48]

Some patients with VGKC-complex antibodies develop ictal bradycardia and pilomotor seizures. The former are present in around 0.5 per cent of seizures on a telemetry unit[49] and, when seen in the context of LGI1 antibodies, may precede the onset of cognitive impairment.[50] Pilomotor seizures show a high specificity for the diagnosis of a LE, mostly associated with LGI1 antibodies.[51,52]

Patients with LGI1 antibodies often have a serum hyponatraemia,[4,29] which can be a diagnostic clue and, along with seizures, provide two reasons to dissuade from the diagnosis of CJD.[53] Hyponatraemia may arise from the modulation of LGI1 expressed in the ADH-secreting neurons of the hypothalamus.[54] Other features found in association with this encephalopathy include dysautonomia (hyperhidrosis, lacrimation, and cardiovascular instability), sleep rhythm disturbances (including REM sleep-behaviour disorder and insomnia), neuropathic pain (often associated with CASPR2 antibodies), cerebellar ataxia (also often CASPR2 antibody related), hallucinations, and depression.[4,55–57] Many of these features are more prominent and common in Morvan's syndrome (MoS).[54,58–60]

Morvan's syndrome and peripheral nerve hyperexcitability

MoS is a rare syndrome, even with the greater recognition over the last few years. The majority have VGKC-complex antibodies, most commonly associated with CASPR2 antibodies but often with coexistent LGI1 antibodies. Patients with MoS have peripheral nerve hyperexcitability (PNH)[61] but also a number of central nervous system manifestations, most commonly profound insomnia, agitation, delusions, and hallucinations. These patients also have a multisystem dysautonomia, pronounced neuropathic pain, significant weight loss, and often normal MR imaging and cerebrospinal fluid examinations. MoS shows an approximately 30 per cent rate of associated thymomas, which are rare in patients with the LE associated with LGI1 or CASPR2 antibodies.[54,58] Patients with MoS have a roughly 30 per cent mortality rate, but this is usually related to metastatic thymoma, and those without a malignancy often respond well to immunotherapy.

It is of interest that patients with 'isolated' PNH have traditionally been reported to have a high rate of anxiety and depression,[62] suggesting a spectrum of cognitive involvement from very mild changes in traditionally pure peripheral nerve disorders, through to the florid cognitive impairment seen in patients with LE (Fig. 28.4a).

Cognitive sequelae of VGKC-complex antibody LE

Early clinical studies of VGKC-complex antibody LE performed cognitive testing in the acute phase of disease and showed global impairment across several domains including memory, executive function and language as measured either by formal neuropsychometry[4,32,33] or by the Addenbrooke's Cognitive Examination–Revised (ACE–R).[37,63] Studies that assessed the cognitive profile following resolution of the illness usually indicated that the executive function and language dysfunction had resolved[4,32] but that patients showed residual anterograde or retrograde memory deficits.[4,32,33,64,65]

Memory has several anatomically and functionally distinct components. Considering retrograde memory, VGKC-complex antibody LE patients were found to have deficits in the recent episodic memories but not personal semantic memories.[65] Another study found that three patients with VGKC-complex antibody LE were impaired on measures of famous faces and famous news events, and measures of anterograde paired-associate learning, with some improvement being observed after immunotherapy.[64] Recognition memory and list-learning, however, were almost universally preserved following resolution of the illness.[4,64,65] Each of these distinct functions are believed to have separate anatomical localizations. Paired-associate learning,[66–68] stimulus requiring association (i.e. the components constituting the narrative of a story)[69,70] and recent episodic memories[71] are particularly reliant on the hippocampus, whereas list-learning/single-item memory, recognition memory, and semantic memory[72–74] depend on extra-hippocampal structures.

However, these studies are either cross-sectional studies or a case series limited to the period of time after treatment. Frisch and colleagues[75] used standardized measures of anterograde memory (the verbal learning and memory test: free recall and recognition of a learnt word list) and executive function (the Epitrack battery: trail-making tasks, response inhibition, digit span backwards, word fluency, and a maze test) and showed significant deficits in executive functioning and verbal and visual memory at presentation in 15 patients. At follow-up, after immunotherapies, there was a resolution in the dysexecutive features but a significant deficit in visual and verbal memory persisted.[75]

Using a larger battery of standardized neuropsychological tests in 20 patients, Butler and colleagues demonstrated that acute VGKC-complex antibody LE likewise impaired anterograde verbal and visual memory, but was also associated with impaired processing speed and executive function.[35] At follow-up, there was normalization in processing speed and executive function but enduring deficits in anterograde memory. A final study[34] described 12 patients with VGKC-complex antibody LE (eight with LGI1 antibody specificity, four not further classified) with tests of anterograde verbal (California verbal learning test, CVLT) and visual (Benson figure) memory, letter fluency (D-words), category fluency (animals), and visual fluency (design fluency), working memory (digits backwards), task switching (modified trails), inhibition (Stroop inhibition), visual localization and construction (visual object space perception) and naming (Boston naming test), single-word comprehension (Peabody picture vocabulary test, PPVT) and sentence repetition. The authors undertook a cross-sectional and a longitudinal cognitive performance study. The cross-sectional work revealed that patients had mild to moderate impairment on anterograde memory as defined by a group average Z score of -1.9, but this was probably driven by verbal memory performance. A mild impairment in executive functions and language were found with normal visuospatial function. 83 per cent were impaired on the CVLT, 64 per cent on category fluency, 55 per cent on letter fluency, whereas very few performed poorly on Stroop inhibition (11 per cent), figure copy (8 per cent), or repetition (18 per cent). This study suggested that the long-term sequelae might include dysexecutive problems. Category fluency requires a search through conceptual knowledge store for semantic extensions derived from a target word.[76] Some argue that this also requires normal frontal lobe functioning[77] to organize retrieval strategies, initiate verbal response, to monitor responses, and to inhibit some responses.[78] Moreover, functional MRI studies have demonstrated that both measures access temporal lobe semantic memory stores[79,80] and a study in amnesic mild cognitive impairment (aMCI) has shown that patients with otherwise normal cognitive profile suffer from deficits on both letter and fluency tasks,[81] whereas there was a relative preservation of switching tasks. These results may represent a deficit in the semantic network for problems with fluency tasks but suggests switching tasks require a higher executive burden which is ostensibly normal in aMCI patients.[81] Therefore, the findings of Bettcher and colleagues[34] may be interpreted as MTL dysfunction within the cortical network supporting category fluency.

These longitudinal studies are often limited by the relatively small number of neuropsychological tests administered and by their lack of integration with localized brain atrophy. Nonetheless, these studies consistently demonstrate that in the acute phase of VGKC-complex antibody LE there is evidence of deficits in executive function, language, processing speed, and both verbal and visual memories. In the more chronic phase there is a resolution in those functions without MTL-dependence, and the most conspicuous residual deficits are MTL-dependent associative anterograde and retrograde memories.

Clinical neuroimaging studies in VGKC-complex antibody LE

The majority of clinical MRI studies undertaken in acute VGKC-complex antibody LE demonstrate an active inflammatory process (as shown by high signal on T2 sequences and/or swelling) predominantly confined to the MTL structures.[4,29,82,83] However, as a number of clinically distinctive features are being better characterized, there is increasing reported normality of MR imaging.[5,37] Longitudinal scanning often demonstrates focal atrophy of the MTL structures in at least 48 per cent of patients.[84] This medial temporal lobe sclerosis may act as a potential focus for subsequent adult-onset epileptogenesis.[82–84] In addition, atrophy has been reported outside of the MTL.[46,85] Table 28.2 provides a summary of reported longitudinal imaging findings.

Volumetric MRI analysis in VGKC-complex antibody encephalitis

Volumetric analyses have also been used to provide a quantitative assessment of cortical and hippocampal volume change during and after VGKC-complex antibody-related syndromes. Irani and colleagues imaged eight patients at convalescence who had normal medial temporal lobe imaging on clinical scans (except for one patient with putaminal high signal). Patients were found to have significantly smaller combined hippocampal/total intracranial volumes and brain/total intracranial volume ratios than controls. Regression analysis found a significant negative association between brain/total intracranial volume and increasing age for both patients and controls, but no association between either hippocampal/total intracranial volume or brain/total intracranial volume with either cognitive impairment or the dosage of corticosteroids received.[37] One potential confound in this study is that more than 50 per cent of the patients were older than the oldest control. However, these results are in keeping with an early volumetric study.[33] Examples of these imaging abnormalities are shown in Fig. 28.5.

A second study[86] quantified the longitudinal structural changes in volumes of both the hippocampus and amygdalae following autoimmune encephalitis using a fully automated software package. They imaged 15 patients with VGKC-complex antibody encephalitis and all had larger amygdalae and hippocampal volumes on their first MRI. At the second MRI, the patients (n = 13) experienced a 14.0 per cent reduction in amygdala volume and a 6.0 per cent reduction in hippocampal volume. Between first and third MRIs (n = 8) there was an 18.3 per cent reduction in amygdala and a 10.7 per cent reduction in hippocampal volumes. There were no differences in any other cortical or subcortical volumes. The MTL atrophy was in excess of the resolution of swelling and high signal change seen during acute imaging, and this has been corroborated by histopathological studies.[4,87,88]

NMDAR-antibody encephalitis

The encephalitis associated with IgG directed against the NR1 subunit of the NMDAR has a very different phenotype and affected demographic to VGKC-complex antibody CNS illnesses (Fig. 28.4b). The disease is associated with benign ovarian teratomas and is especially seen in females between the ages of 12 and 40 years.[89,90] However, young and old men are now reported and the frequency of teratomas is, partly consequentially, decreasing.[25,91]

Patients usually present with a classical sequence of multifocal neurological deficits.[25,89] The typical onset is over a few days with psychiatric symptoms; patients develop delusions, psychosis, and hallucinations, usually without a background history of psychiatric disease. This may be accompanied by other cognitive features

Table 28.2 Clinical magnetic resonance features in acute and chronic VGKC-complex antibody encephalitis

Reference	No. of patients	Acute features	Chronic features
Buckley et al.[32]	2	1 × N MTL	–
		1 × L HPC abnormality	–
Vincent et al.[4]	10	1 × ↑ signal BL HPC	–
		1 × ↑ signal BL HPC	MTL atrophy, ↑ L HPC swelling, ↑ signal R insula
		1 × N	↑ signal esp. L HPC
		1 × atrophy with ↑ signal R insula	↑ signal normalized
		1 × N	N
		1 × N	BL HPC atrophy
		1 × ↑ signal HPC L > R	N
		1 × ↑ HPC and anterior TL signal	Minimal signal change in HPC
		1 × ↑ L MTL sclerosis and R TL abnormalities	HPC change
		1 × ↑ volume and signal in L HPC and AMYG	Atrophy and signal change L > R
Bien et al.[83]	4	1 × HPC swelling	N then atrophy with ↑ signal
Urbach et al.[151]	3	–	1 × BL MTL atrophy
		–	1 × L > R MTL atrophy
		–	1 × L HPC atrophy
Chan et al.[36]	3	1 × ↑ signal BL HPC	Mild BL MTL atrophy
		1 × ↑ in HPC and AMYG	R HPC atrophy
Thieben et al.[29]	7	6 × ↑ signal BL MTL	–
		1 × ↑ signal L MTL	–
Jacobs et al.[85]	2	–	1 × BL HPC atrophy and ↑ signal R MTL
		1 × ↑ signal hypothalamus and MTL	–
Sekiguchi et al.[152]	1	↑ signal HPC	Hypothalamic ↑ signal
Khan et al.[88]	1	L HPC atrophy	–
Chatzikonstantinou et al.[153]	1	↑ signal and diffuse swelling of R HPC	R HPC atrophy
Kaymakamzade et al.[154]	1	↑ signal BL HPC and AMYG	–
Kapina et al.[155]	1	L HPC lesion	–
Kartsounis et al.[65]	1	↑ BL HPC signal	–
Wong et al.[63]	7	7 × ↑ signal and oedema BL HPC	–
Ballater et al.[156]	2	2 × ↑ signal BL MTL	–
Schott et al.[33]	1	↑ signal BL HPC	22.6% L HPC atrophy, 39.6% R HPC atrophy; 11.4% whole-brain volume loss
Harrower et al.[157]	2	1 × N	–
Irani et al.[46]	3	1 × ↑signal R caudate and putamen	1 × mild R caudate atrophy
		1 × N	1 × N
		1 × ↑ signal in BL HPC	1 × N
Irani et al.[37]	8	8 × N MTL	–
		1 × ↑ putaminal signal	

AMYG: amygdala; BL: bilateral; HPC: hippocampus; L: left; MTL: medial temporal lobe; N: normal; R: right; ↑: increased.

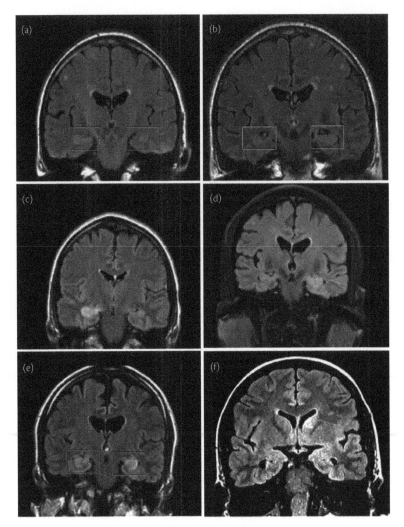

Fig. 28.5 Acute neuroimaging features in VGKC-complex encephalitis. (a & b) Longitudinal imaging from a single patient demonstrating A. Bilateral hippocampal swelling and mild signal change (red boxes). (b) Marked hippocampal atrophy following resolution of the illness (red boxes). (c) Unilateral signal change in the left hippocampus (red arrowhead). (d) Unilateral signal change in the right hippocampus (right arrowhead). E: Bilateral signal change and swelling (red boxes). (f) Caudate head signal change (red arrowhead).

such as amnesia, disorientation, behavioural disturbances, and dysphasia. In a number of patients, particularly males, the presenting symptom can be seizures.[91] However, only occasionally are seizures a severe or recurrent problem.

Subsequently, and typically with the lag of 10 to 20 days, patients develop a movement disorder, dysautonomia, and, sometimes, central hypoventilation.[25,89,90] These are distinctive features, in particular the movement disorder. When hyperkinetic, this movement disorder often shows prominent orofacial dyskinesias, particularly centred around the lips, and stereotyped, antigravity movements of arms and legs.[92] These movements can persist for several hours per day over a period of many weeks and have been likened to status dissociatus.[93] However, the movement disorder can also be hypokinetic, and highly reminiscent of Von Economo's description of one form of EL, with a predominant parkinsonian disorder, bradyphrenia, and bradykinesia.[94] The dysautonomia can often cause tachycardia and labile blood pressure and may be the cause of the fluctuating fever. Some patients have required pacemaker insertion. The central hypoventilation is a less common feature but may necessitate intensive care unit admission which is itself a poor prognostic factor.[90]

The CSF is usually lymphocytic, especially early on in the illness, and oligoclonal bands develop at later time points. In addition, the EEG appearances usually follow a temporal trend from spikes to diffuse slowing (Fig. 28.3b). Alongside this, the dichotomy of the timings of lymphocytosis and oligoclonal band appearances lend support to two major stages to the disease process. The first is characterized by cortical features (neuropsychiatric impairment, seizures, CSF lymphocytosis, and EEG spikes) and the second by a more subcortical process with a movement disorder, dysautonomia, and loss of awareness with diffuse EEG slowing.[25] Some patients do not fit this model but it does offer a framework to consider the biology of the, frequently distinctive, temporal progression of the disease.

More recently, patients have been described with relatively limited presentations. This includes patients with status epilepticus, a predominant movement disorder, or isolated psychiatric features.[95–97] Indeed one controversial question is how often patients with early psychosis have NMDAR antibodies.[98–100] The literature is divided on this subject, probably partly due to the differences in assays used to define the presence of the antibody described above.[2]

The NMDAR antibodies are IgG, but a few recent reports have described phenotypes associated with IgA and IgM NMDAR-directed antibodies.[101,102] These appear to be diseases with an indolent form of cognitive impairment. While the antibodies may have effector functions *in vitro*, clear evidence supporting an immunotherapy response is lacking. Perhaps these antibodies are generated secondary to an alternative primary CNS pathology and, indeed, NMDAR–IgG or VGKC-complex antibodies have been described in occasional patients with neurodegenerative dementias[103] and in a small number (<5%) of patients with proven CJD.[104–106]

Neuroimaging and cognitive studies in NMDA-receptor antibody encephalitis

Patients with NMDAR-antibody encephalitis often have normal MR imaging in the acute phase but 10–20 per cent of patients have hyperintensities on MRI which may localize to the hippocampi (the typical picture of limbic encephalitis), neocortical structures, and/or subcortical regions.[25,89] The latter are often in white matter tracts and appear demyelinating, generating interest in the recently redefined overlap between demyelination and NMDAR-antibody encephalitis.[107,108] Studies reporting imaging from two or more patients are summarized in Table 28.3.

Only two formal studies have been performed to examine the neuropsychological consequences of NMDA-receptor antibody encephalitis. In the first,[109] nine patients were tested at a median time of 43 months (range: 23–69), with five receiving immunomodulatory treatment within three months of symptom onset, three receiving immunomodulation late in the disease, and one patient receiving no treatment. The authors tested attention (dual-task paradigm), working memory (digit span forwards and backwards), verbal memory (Rey auditory verbal learning test, RAVLT), non-verbal memory (Rey–Osterreith complex figure), executive function (category fluency, letter fluency, Stroop inhibition test, behavioural assessment of the dysexecutive syndrome, Tower of London task) and a delayed-matching-to-sample (DMTS) task in which patients had to remember the colour, location, or the association between the colour and location of visual stimuli across either a 900 ms or a 5000 ms delay. This study found that attention was impaired in four patients, working memory was impaired in four patients, verbal memory in two patients, non-verbal memory in one patient, and executive function in five patients. Five patients were impaired in up to four tests, mainly affecting attention or working memory processes, but two patients had extensive neuropsychological impairments across a number of neuropsychological domains (attention, working memory, memory and executive function). Five patients were impaired on the DMTS task, four on the localization aspect of the task, one on the colour aspect, and all patients on the associative component of the task; these were deficits previously shown to be sensitive to hippocampal lesions.[110,111] The authors found a significant positive effect of early treatment on cognitive performance at follow-up and there was also a correlation between the delay in treatment and cognitive outcome.

A second study[112] found evidence of executive dysfunction (as measured by the digit span backwards, Stroop inhibition, and word fluency) but also anterograde memory impairment (as measured by

Table 28.3 Clinical magnetic resonance imaging findings in NMDA-receptor antibody encephalitis. Inclusion of studies reporting imaging from two or more patients

Reference	No. of patients	Acute features
Dalmau et al.[158]	91	46 × N
		22 × ↑ MTL signal change
		22 × cortical change
		6 × CBM change
		6 × BS change
		5 × BG change
		14 × contrast enhancement (cortex, meninges, BG)
		4 × corpus callosum change
		2 × hypothalamic change
		1 × pericallosal change
		1 × multifocal WM change
Iizuka et al.[159]	4	3 × N
		1 × ↑ signal MTL
Irani et al. 2010[24]	44	34 × N throughout
		6 × WM ↑ signal
		4 × ↑ MTL signal change
		1 × hippocampal sclerosis
Baumgartner et al.[160]	2	1 × ↑ signal BL MTL
		1 × ↑ signal Occipt.
Finke et al.[109]	8	8 × N
		1 × ↑ signal L insula, L frontal lobe, and L periventricular regions
Finke et al.[112] (at 3-T)	24	10 × N
		5 × frontal WM lesions
		2 × L frontal WM lesions
		1 × L frontoparietal WM lesion
		1 × L insular WM lesions
		1 × WM lesions in R palladium, L insula, R frontotemporal regions
		1 × R temporal, L trigonal, L frontal horn, L central WM lesions
		1 × L frontal and R frontotemporal WM lesions
		1 × BL frontobasal WM lesions
		1 × L frontal and L temporoparietal WM lesions
Sarkis et al.[161]	5	3 × N
		2 × ↑ signal subcortex
Viaccoz et al.[91]	10	6 × N
		2 × ↑ signal L HPC
		1 × ↑ signal BL HPC, and Occipt.
		1 × ↑ signal BL HPC, putamen, and CBM

BG: basal ganglia; BL: bilateral; BS: brainstem; CBM: cerebellum; L: left; MTL: medial temporal lobe; N: normal; Occipt.: occipital cortex; WM: white matter; ↑: increased.

the RAVLT sum score, immediate-recall and delayed-recall measures) against age-matched controls. They also found evidence of bilaterally reduced hippocampal connectivity in the anterior default mode network but no changes in the sensorimotor, primary visual, or auditory resting state networks. This suggests that the cognitive sequelae in

NMDA-receptor antibody encephalitis are due to a functional dissociation of the hippocampi from this memory network and, surprisingly, not due to regional atrophy.[113–115] Diffusion tensor imaging (DTI) also found evidence of white matter atrophy in the cingulum bilaterally, a finding that correlated with disease severity (as measured by the modified Rankin score).[112]

Rarer antibodies

Recently, a number of less common autoantibodies have been described in the context of a number of central nervous system diseases, typically a limbic encephalitis. These include antibodies to CASPR2 (part of the VGKC complex),[24,116] the glycine receptor,[18,117] GABA$_A$ and GABA$_B$ receptors,[23,118] the AMPA receptor,[119] GAD,[120] and, more rarely, AQP4.[121] Each antibody-associated syndrome has a few particularly prominent clinical features and associations (Table 28.1).

Some important features include the presence of small cell lung cancer (SCLC), thymomas, and breast cancers in patients with AMPA receptor antibodies. Patients with GABA$_B$R antibodies often have frequent refractory seizures and SCLC. The encephalopathy associated with glycine receptor antibodies has traditionally been termed PERM (progressive encephalomyelitis with rigidity and myoclonus). This describes the variable presence of cognitive disturbance with few seizures, but more specifically oculomotor difficulties, ataxia, and a stiff-person-like phenotype (often startle, spasms, and ridgity). An AQP4-antibody associated encephalopathy can occur in children, sometimes with a longitudinally extensive transverse myelitis and/or optic neuritis.

Treatments

Symptomatic

A number of symptomatic therapies are useful in patients with AE. This is especially relevant to those with NMDAR-antibody encephalitis who often have a protracted clinical course, with agitation or seizures, and require intensive care unit admission.

Atypical antipsychotics, especially olanzapine, quetiapine, and benzodiazepines are used to sedate agitated, psychotic patients. Haloperidol should be avoided if possible as it can worsen parkinsonism and may precipitate oculogyric crises. Electroconvulsive therapy should be reserved for the most refractory cases.[122] Benzodiazepines may also be used for seizure control, as should other antiepileptic agents, but often immunotherapies are more effective at achieving seizure control (see following for more details). For those patients admitted to ITU, especially those with NMDAR-antibody encephalitis, long-term ventilation is often required. A thiopental coma may be induced and empirical therapies for control of blood pressure, bradycardia/asystole, and dyskinesias are often administered.

Immunotherapies

The mainstay of disease modification in patients with AE is immunotherapies with evidence principally based on expert clinician experience and respective observational data.

The largest dataset exists for patients with NMDAR-antibody encephalitis. This disease is thought to have a natural history showing a chronic course, often over several years with relapses. A retrospective series of 501 patients with NMDAR-antibody encephalitis has offered a number of recommendations.[90] This series showed

that 53 per cent of patients respond to steroids, IVIG and/or plasma exchange. 57 per cent of the non-responsive patients were subsequently either treated with additional immunotherapy (cyclophosphamide and/or rituximab) or no incremental immunotherapies. The group who were offered further immunosuppressive agents had a better outcome (p = 0.012). Overall, at two years, 394/501 (79 per cent) patients had a good outcome (modified Rankin score, mRS < 3). Patients who were not offered any treatment had a 13 per cent mortality rate compared to 8 per cent in those treated with any immunotherapy. Furthermore, relapse rates were reduced in patients offered additional immunotherapies. The message is consistent with other studies: treat early and upscale immunotherapy if there is a limited response.[25,123] A similar message emerges from the literature around patients with LGI1-antibody encephalitis. Data show that time to reach baseline or improved function (measured by mRS) is expedited with early treatment, in particular corticosteroids.[4,31,37] However, as for NMDAR-antibody encephalitis, it is not clear whether treatments for VGKC-complex antibody LE alter long-term outcomes. Indeed, a recent retrospective analysis suggested identical outcomes at four years in 64 patients with LGI1-antibodies treated with corticosteroids alone, corticosteroids plus IVIG, or corticosteroids plus IVIG and PLEX.[2] As many patients do well with first-line immunotherapies, data regarding second-line immunotherapies in VGKC-complex antibody LE are limited to two recent retrospective reports which suggest a response to rituximab in a minority of corticosteroid-refractory patients.[124,125]

Pathophysiological hypotheses

Our understanding of the pathophysiology of these diseases is based upon clinical and serological observations, in addition to recent *in vitro* and *in vivo* studies. As discussed earlier, antibodies are likely to be peripherally generated. The cells, and limited amounts of antibodies, then migrate across the blood–brain barrier.

Postmortem studies have suggested that sometimes, especially in cases with VGKC-complex antibodies, there is complement fixation by bound antibodies.[87] In NMDAR-antibody encephalitis, complement appears to play less of a role. In this disease, the receptors are internalized by the divalent antibodies and this appears to be the major pathogenic mechanism.[126] These differences may explain the atrophy seen in many patients with VGKC-complex antibody disease, and offers a potential reason for why the patients with NMDAR antibodies may make an almost complete recovery with less brain atrophy.[112] Antibodies may also directly affect channel function although this appears to be a minor mechanism (Fig. 28.6).

However, many questions related to pathophysiology remain unanswered, including why the antibodies modulate hippocampal regions specifically given the widespread antigen distribution,[127] why these diseases differ from those associated with genetic or pharmacological manipulations of the antigenic target,[17] how neuronal plasticity may account for patient recovery from the disease, and the relevance of IgM and IgA subclasses of autoantibodies.

The autoimmune encephalitides as models for the neurobiology of disease

VGKC-complex antibody-associated LE as a model of hippocampal function

Extensive pathological series have not been undertaken in VGKC-complex antibody LE but case reports describe lesions confined to either the amygdala and/or adjacent hippocampi with only mild

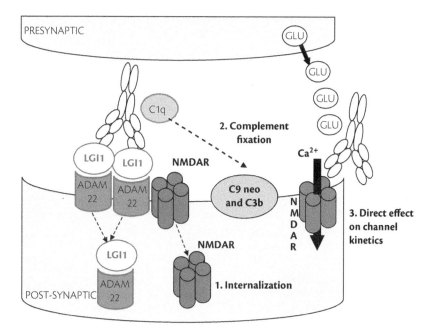

Fig. 28.6 Potential pathogenic mechanisms of neuronal surface directed antibodies (NSAbs). (1) Internalization of receptors has been demonstrated *in vitro* using NMDAR (*N*-methyl-D-aspartate receptor), AMPAR (α-amino-3-hydroxy-5-methylisoxazole-4-propionic acid receptor), and GABA$_A$R (γ-aminobutyric acid A receptor) antibodies. Here the LGI1–DAM22 interaction is shown as a possible unit for cointernalization, as is the NMDAR. (2) Antibody-mediated complement fixation and complement-mediated membrane receptor disruption is another possible mechanism as is direct alteration of ion channel molecular function (3).

Reproduced from *J Neurol.* 262(4), Varley J, Vincent A, and Irani SR, Clinical and experimental studies of potentially pathogenic brain-directed autoantibodies: current knowledge and future directions, pp. 1081–95, Copyright (2014), with permission from Springer, reproduced under the Creative Commons Attribution License.

infiltration, if any, of the surrounding MTL structures.[88,128,129] One pathological report even describes damage restricted to just the CA4 region of the hippocampus with relative sparing of regions CA1–3.[88] Combined with the imaging and behavioural features discussed earlier there is strong evidence to suggest that VGKC-complex antibody encephalopathy is a disease limited to the MTL structures.

One potential implication regarding the apparent restricted MTL pathology following VGKC-complex antibody LE is that these patients could serve as a human model of focal MTL damage. Given the retained phylogeny of the mammalian hippocampus across species[130] there are several mnemonic[71,130–132] and computational accounts[133] of the hippocampus that have yet to be studied in humans.

As cited earlier, three VGKC-complex antibody LE patients were studied for evidence of retrograde amnesia for episodic events and faces (i.e. those that occurred as a single event like the fall of the Berlin Wall).[36] These patients were found to have a temporally ungraded amnesia (i.e. extensive for more than 20 years), greater than might otherwise be expected according to current models of memory consolidation.[71] However, no measures of episodic memories for personal events were reported, and as such these results can only relate to our understanding of the neural basis of semantic memory. The questions asked were highly episodic in nature and so demonstrate the requirement of episodic neural apparatus for semantic recall, especially if relations between object and time are needed.[134,135] Hippocampal pathology associated with VGKC-complex antibody LE has also been reported to impair future imagining, a constructional process believed to be reliant upon the hippocampus.[136,137]

The hippocampus is often conceptualized as a structure that binds items and their locations or contexts into a single mnemonic entity.[132,138] Within this model, focal lesions to the MTL would generate behavioural deficits on tasks requiring associations between several different stimuli. A series of VGKC-complex antibody LE patients were found to have deficits on a visual working memory task that required the binding of multiple items in space but not single items.[139] One intriguing possibility will be to investigate whether VGKC-complex antibody LE results in hippocampal subfield pathology, especially given that the theoretical models of hippocampal function rely on the functional heterogeneity of these regions.[132,133]

The glutamate hypofunction theory of psychosis

Published studies have reported conflicting results about the rates of NMDAR-antibodies in schizophrenic patients or those with first episode psychosis, versus controls. This is probably in part due to discrepancies in assay methodologies, as mentioned earlier. Nevertheless, the close association of psychotic features at the onset of NMDAR-antibody encephalitis lends weight to the importance of glutamate, and the NMDAR, in the pathogenesis of schizophrenia. Research spanning 50 years supports the similarities between models of human NMDAR dysfunction and schizophrenia. Indeed, the NMDAR hypofunction hypothesis of schizophrenia is a model built around observations that low doses of NMDAR antagonists, like ketamine and phencyclidine, produced psychotic and negative symptoms alongside concomitant cognitive impairments.[140,141] Whilst the neurochemical alterations responsible for schizophrenia are complex and involve several neurotransmitter systems including dopamine, glutamate, and 5-hydroxytryptamine, the role of glutamate appears to be key in this process.[142]

In vivo, NMDAR antagonism causes an increase in the firing rate of pyramidal neurons and increased mRNA expression of the immediate-early gene c-fos. In turn, this causes an increased release of other cortical neurotransmitters like glutamate, dopamine, and 5-HT[143,144] but also of GABA.[145] It appears paradoxical that NMDAR blockage would lead to the emergence of the facilitatory actions of these other neurotransmitter systems and produce the positive symptoms observed in schizophrenia. However, disinhibition of the GABA-ergic system induces cognitive, behavioural, and dopaminergic alterations commonly seen in schizophrenia,[146] and it has been proposed that the NMDAR antibodies are predominantly acting on GABA-ergic neurons. Similarly, the seizures likely to be caused by NMDAR-antibody-induced NMDAR downregulation suggest that the NMDAR antibodies may be mediating an effect via disinhibition of GABAergic systems.

Single photon emission computed tomography (SPECT) studies with NMDAR ligands have shown a reduction in NMDARs in the hippocampi of medication-free schizophrenic patients,[147] a finding replicated with ketamine and one that was strongly correlated with negative symptoms.[148] This reduction in NMDARs is also seen in the few available postmortems of patients with NMDAR antibodies.[126] These converging pieces of evidence suggest there are two phases to NMDA dysfunction in the emergence of symptoms suggestive of schizophrenia: an acute phase charaterized by cortical disinhibition resembling first-episode psychosis and a sustained phase of NMDA receptor hypofunction believed to simulate the chronic, negative symptoms of schizophrenia.[149] Maybe the latter can also be responsible for the movement disorder and brainstem dysfunction commonly associated with NMDAR-antibody encephalitis. Diffusion tensor imaging (DTI) has demonstrated that chronic administration of ketamine causes abnormalities in frontal callosal fibres in patterns not unlike schizophrenia,[150] or indeed in NMDAR-antibody encephalitis.[112] These changes could underlie the emergence of the chronic symptoms of schizophrenia[142] and could underlie the cognitive changes seen secondary to NMDAR-antibody encephalitis.[112]

While NMDA hypofunction is not the sole cause of schizophrenia, several related strands of research suggest that glutamate dysfunction is an important contributor to the emergence of positive and negative symptoms associated with schizophrenia. The overlaps with NMDAR-antibody encephalitis patients support a shared pathophysiological mechanism with schizophrenia.

Conclusion

The autoimmune encephalopathies associated with antibodies directed against cell surface neuronal proteins are an expanding group of immunotherapy-responsive conditions with distinctive clinical features and major potential implications for neurobiology studies. Future studies will offer insights as to how specific prolonged receptor dysfunction is reversible, the mechanisms of plasticity, and the neuronal networks engaged in the disease process and recovery. Furthermore, the differing focality of these diseases may offer novel insights into functional localizations. Novel antibody targets are likely to emerge in diseases with cognitive and psychiatric overlaps. Knowledge of their biology will feed into the diseases with known antibody targets and further inform a number of brain neurotransmitter systems and neuronal populations.

References

1. Vincent A, Bien CG, Irani SR, *et al*. Autoantibodies associated with diseases of the CNS: new developments and future challenges. *Lancet Neurol*. 2011;10:759–72.
2. Irani SR, Gelfand JM, Al-Diwani A, *et al*. Cell-surface central nervous system autoantibodies: clinical relevance and emerging paradigms. *Ann Neurol*. 2014 Aug;76(2):168–84.
3. Lancaster E and Dalmau J. Neuronal autoantigens—pathogenesis, associated disorders and antibody testing. *Nat Rev Neurol*. 2012;8:380–90.
4. Vincent A, Buckley C, Schott JM, *et al*. Potassium channel antibody-associated encephalopathy: a potentially immunotherapy-responsive form of limbic encephalitis. *Brain*. 2004;127:701–12.
5. Flanagan EP, McKeon A, Lennon VA, *et al*. Autoimmune dementia: clinical course and predictors of immunotherapy response. *Mayo Clin Proc*. 2010;85:881–97.
6. Geschwind MD, Shu H, Haman A, *et al*. Rapidly progressive dementia. *Ann Neurol*. 2008;64:97–108.
7. Brierley J, Corsellis JAN, Hierons R, *et al*. Subacute encephalitis of later adult life. Mainly affecting the limbic areas. *Brain*. 1960;83:357–70.
8. Corsellis JA, Goldberg GJ, and Norton AR. 'Limbic encephalitis' and its association with carcinoma. *Brain*. 1968;91:481–96.
9. Pearce JM. Baron Constantin von Economo and encephalitis lethargica. *J Neurol Neurosur Ps*. 1996;60:167.
10. Berger JR and Vilensky JA. Encephalitis lethargica (von Economo's encephalitis). *Handb Clin Neurol*. 2014;123:745–61.
11. Castillo P, Woodruff B, Caselli R, *et al*. Steroid-responsive encephalopathy associated with autoimmune thyroiditis. *Arch Neurol*. 2006;63:197–202.
12. Geschwind MD. Rapidly progressive dementia: prion diseases and other rapid dementias. *Continuum (Minneap Minn)*. 2010;16:31–56.
13. Chitravas N, Jung RS, Kofskey DM, *et al*. Treatable neurological disorders misdiagnosed as Creutzfeldt–Jakob disease. *Ann Neurol*. 2011;70:437–44.
14. Graus F, Keime-Guibert F, Rene R, *et al*. Anti-Hu-associated paraneoplastic encephalomyelitis: analysis of 200 patients. *Brain*. 2001;124:1138–48.
15. Gultekin SH, Rosenfeld MR, Voltz R, *et al*. Paraneoplastic limbic encephalitis: neurological symptoms, immunological findings and tumour association in 50 patients. *Brain*. 2000;123 (Pt 7):1481–94.
16. McKeon A and Pittock SJ. Paraneoplastic encephalomyelopathies: pathology and mechanisms. *Acta Neuropathol*. 2011;122:381–400.
17. Varley J, Vincent A, and Irani SR. Clinical and experimental studies of potentially pathogenic brain-directed autoantibodies: current knowledge and future directions. *J Neurol*. 2015;262(4):1081–95.
18. Carvajal-Gonzalez A LM, Waters P, *et al*. Glycine receptor antibodies in PERM and related syndromes: characteristics, clinical features and outcomes. *Brain*. 2014;137:2178–90.
19. McKeon A, Martinez-Hernandez E, Lancaster E, *et al*. Glycine receptor autoimmune spectrum with stiff-man syndrome phenotype. *JAMA Neurol*. 2013;70:44–50.
20. Saiz A, Blanco Y, Sabater L, *et al*. Spectrum of neurological syndromes associated with glutamic acid decarboxylase antibodies: diagnostic clues for this association. *Brain*. 2008;131:2553–63.
21. Gresa-Arribas N, Titulaer MJ, Torrents A, *et al*. Antibody titres at diagnosis and during follow-up of anti-NMDA receptor encephalitis: a retrospective study. *Lancet Neurol*. 2014;13:167–77.
22. Zandi MS, Paterson RW, Ellul MA, *et al*. Clinical relevance of serum antibodies to extracellular *N*-methyl-D-aspartate receptor epitopes. *J Neurol Neurosur Ps*. 2015 Jul;86(7):708–13.
23. Lancaster E, Lai M, Peng X, *et al*. Antibodies to the GABA(B) receptor in limbic encephalitis with seizures: case series and characterisation of the antigen. *Lancet Neurol*. 2010;9:67–76.
24. Irani SR, Alexander S, Waters P, *et al*. Antibodies to Kv1 potassium channel-complex proteins leucine-rich, glioma inactivated 1 protein

and contactin-associated protein-2 in limbic encephalitis, Morvan's syndrome and acquired neuromyotonia. *Brain.* 2010;133:2734–48.

25. Irani SR, Bera K, Waters P, *et al.* N-methyl-D-aspartate antibody encephalitis: temporal progression of clinical and paraclinical observations in a predominantly non-paraneoplastic disorder of both sexes. *Brain.* 2010;133:1655–67.

26. Klein CJ, Lennon VA, Aston PA, *et al.* Insights from LGI1 and CASPR2 potassium channel complex autoantibody subtyping. *JAMA Neurol.* 2013;70:229–34.

27. Lai M, Huijbers MG, Lancaster E, *et al.* Investigation of LGI1 as the antigen in limbic encephalitis previously attributed to potassium channels: a case series. *Lancet Neurol.* 2010;9:776–85.

28. Hart IK, Waters P, Vincent A, *et al.* Autoantibodies detected to expressed K+ channels are implicated in neuromyotonia. *Ann Neurol.* 1997;41:238–46.

29. Thieben MJ, Lennon VA, Boeve BF, *et al.* Potentially reversible autoimmune limbic encephalitis with neuronal potassium channel antibody. *Neurology.* 2004;62:1177–82.

30. Paterson RW, Zandi MS, Armstrong R, *et al.* Clinical relevance of positive voltage-gated potassium channel (VGKC)-complex antibodies: experience from a tertiary referral centre. *J Neurol Neurosur Ps.* 2014;85:625–30.

31. Shin YW, Lee ST, Shin JW, *et al.* VGKC-complex/LGI1-antibody encephalitis: clinical manifestations and response to immunotherapy. *J Neuroimmunol.* 2013;265:75–81.

32. Buckley C, Oger J, Clover L, *et al.* Potassium channel antibodies in two patients with reversible limbic encephalitis. *Ann Neurol.* 2001;50:73–78.

33. Schott JM, Harkness K, Barnes J, *et al.* Amnesia, cerebral atrophy, and autoimmunity. *Lancet.* 2003;361:1266.

34. Bettcher BM, Gelfand JM, Irani SR, *et al.* More than memory impairment in voltage-gated potassium channel complex encephalopathy. *Eur J Neurol.* 2014.

35. Butler CR, Miller TD, Kaur MS, *et al.* Persistent anterograde amnesia following limbic encephalitis associated with antibodies to the voltage-gated potassium channel complex. *J Neurol Neurosur Ps.* 2014;85:387–91.

36. Chan D, Henley SM, Rossor MN, *et al.* Extensive and temporally ungraded retrograde amnesia in encephalitis associated with antibodies to voltage-gated potassium channels. *Arch Neurol.* 2007;64:404–10.

37. Irani SR, Stagg CJ, Schott JM, *et al.* Faciobrachial dystonic seizures: the influence of immunotherapy on seizure control and prevention of cognitive impairment in a broadening phenotype. *Brain.* 2013;136:3151–62.

38. McKeon A, Lennon VA, and Pittock SJ. Immunotherapy-responsive dementias and encephalopathies. *Continuum (Minneap Minn).* 2010;16:80–101.

39. Brenner T, Sills GJ, Hart Y, *et al.* Prevalence of neurologic autoantibodies in cohorts of patients with new and established epilepsy. *Epilepsia.* 2013;54:1028–35.

40. Irani SR, Bien CG, and Lang B. Autoimmune epilepsies. *Curr Opin Neurol.* 2011;24:146–53.

41. Irani SR, Michell AW, Lang B, *et al.* Faciobrachial dystonic seizures precede Lgi1 antibody limbic encephalitis. *Ann Neurol.* 2011;69:892–900.

42. Lilleker JB, Jones MS, and Mohanraj R. VGKC complex antibodies in epilepsy: diagnostic yield and therapeutic implications. *Seizure.* 2013;22:776–9.

43. Quek AM, Britton JW, McKeon A, *et al.* Autoimmune epilepsy: clinical characteristics and response to immunotherapy. *Arch Neurol.* 2012;69:582–93.

44. Vincent A, Irani SR, Lang B. The growing recognition of immunotherapy-responsive seizure disorders with autoantibodies to specific neuronal proteins. *Curr Opin Neurol.* 2010;23:144–50.

45. Barajas RF, Collins DE, Cha S, *et al.* Adult-onset drug-refractory seizure disorder associated with anti-voltage-gated potassium-channel antibody. *Epilepsia.* 2010;51:473–7.

46. Irani SR, Buckley C, Vincent A, *et al.* Immunotherapy-responsive seizure-like episodes with potassium channel antibodies. *Neurology.* 2008;71:1647–48.

47. Boesebeck F, Schwarz O, Dohmen B, *et al.* Faciobrachial dystonic seizures arise from cortico-subcortical abnormal brain areas. *J Neurol.* 2013;260:1684–86.

48. Yoo JY and Hirsch LJ. Limbic encephalitis associated with anti-voltage-gated potassium channel complex antibodies mimicking creutzfeldt-jakob disease. *JAMA Neurol.* 2014;71:79–82.

49. Marynissen T, Govers N, and Vydt T. Ictal asystole: case report with review of literature. *Acta Cardiol.* 2012;67:461–64.

50. Naasan G, Irani SR, Bettcher BM, *et al.* Episodic bradycardia as neurocardiac prodrome to voltage-gated potassium channel complex/leucine-rich, glioma inactivated 1 antibody encephalitis. *JAMA Neurol.* 2014.

51. Rocamora R, Becerra JL, Fossas P, *et al.* Pilomotor seizures: an autonomic semiology of limbic encephalitis? *Seizure.* 2014;23:670–73.

52. Wieser S, Kelemen A, Barsi P, *et al.* Pilomotor seizures and status in non-paraneoplastic limbic encephalitis. *Epileptic Disord.* 2005;7:205–11.

53. Geschwind MD, Tan KM, Lennon VA, *et al.* Voltage-gated potassium channel autoimmunity mimicking Creutzfeldt–Jakob disease. *Arch Neurol.* 2008;65:1341–46.

54. Irani SR, Pettingill P, Kleopa KA, *et al.* Morvan syndrome: clinical and serological observations in 29 cases. *Ann Neurol.* 2012;72:241–55.

55. Becker EB, Zuliani L, Pettingill R, *et al.* Contactin-associated protein-2 antibodies in non-paraneoplastic cerebellar ataxia. *J Neurol Neurosur Ps.* 2012;83:437–40.

56. Iranzo A, Graus F, Clover L, *et al.* Rapid eye movement sleep behavior disorder and potassium channel antibody-associated limbic encephalitis. *Ann Neurol.* 2006;59:178–81.

57. Klein CJ, Lennon VA, Aston PA, *et al.* Chronic pain as a manifestation of potassium channel-complex autoimmunity. *Neurology.* 2012;79:1136–44.

58. Abou-Zeid E, Boursoulian LJ, Metzer WS, *et al.* Morvan syndrome: a case report and review of the literature. *J Clin Neuromuscul Dis.* 2012;13:214–27.

59. Liguori R, Vincent A, Clover L, *et al.* Morvan's syndrome: peripheral and central nervous system and cardiac involvement with antibodies to voltage-gated potassium channels. *Brain.* 2001;124:2417–26.

60. Madrid A, Gil-Peralta A, Gil-Neciga E, *et al.* Morvan's fibrillary chorea: remission after plasmapheresis. *J Neurol.* 1996;243:350–53.

61. Loscher WN, Wanschitz J, Reiners K, *et al.* Morvan's syndrome: clinical, laboratory, and *in vitro* electrophysiological studies. *Muscle Nerve.* 2004;30:157–63.

62. Hart IK, Maddison P, Newsom-Davis J, *et al.* Phenotypic variants of autoimmune peripheral nerve hyperexcitability. *Brain.* 2002;125:1887–95.

63. Wong SH, Saunders MD, Larner AJ, *et al.* An effective immunotherapy regimen for VGKC antibody-positive limbic encephalitis. *J Neurol Neurosur Ps.* 2010;81:1167–69.

64. Addis DR, Moscovitch M, and McAndrews MP. Consequences of hippocampal damage across the autobiographical memory network in left temporal lobe epilepsy. *Brain.* 2007;130:2327–42.

65. Kartsounis LD and de Silva R. Unusual amnesia in a patient with VGKC-Ab limbic encephalitis: a case study. *Cortex.* 2011;47:451–59.

66. Achim AM and Lepage M. Neural correlates of memory for items and for associations: an event-related functional magnetic resonance imaging study. *J Cogn Neurosci.* 2005;17:652–67.

67. Kirwan CB and Stark CE. Medial temporal lobe activation during encoding and retrieval of novel face–name pairs. *Hippocampus.* 2004;14:919–30.

68. Law JR, Flanery MA, Wirth S, *et al.* Functional magnetic resonance imaging activity during the gradual acquisition and expression of paired-associate memory. *J Neurosci.* 2005;25:5720–29.

69. Frisk V and Milner B. The role of the left hippocampal region in the acquisition and retention of story content. *Neuropsychologia.* 1990;28:349–59.

70. Zola-Morgan S, Squire LR, and Amaral DG. Human amnesia and the medial temporal region: enduring memory impairment following a

bilateral lesion limited to field CA1 of the hippocampus. *J Neurosci.* 1986;6:2950–67.

71. Squire LR, Stark CE, and Clark RE. The medial temporal lobe. *Annu Rev Neurosci.* 2004;27:279–306.

72. Brown MW and Aggleton JP. Recognition memory: what are the roles of the perirhinal cortex and hippocampus? *Nat Rev Neurosci.* 2001;2:51–61.

73. Tulving E and Markowitsch HJ. Episodic and declarative memory: role of the hippocampus. *Hippocampus.* 1998;8:198–204.

74. Yonelinas AP. The nature of recollection and familiarity: a review of 30 years of research. *J Mem Lang.* 2002;46:441–517.

75. Frisch C, Malter MP, Elger CE, *et al.* Neuropsychological course of voltage-gated potassium channel and glutamic acid decarboxylase antibody related limbic encephalitis. *Eur J Neurol.* 2013;20:1297–304.

76. Taler V and Phillips NA. Language performance in Alzheimer's disease and mild cognitive impairment: a comparative review. *J Clin Exp Neuropsychol.* 2008;30:501–56.

77. Lezak MD, Howieson DB, Loring DW, *et al. Neuropsychological Assessment.* New York, NY: Oxford University Press, 2004.

78. Henry JD, Crawford JR, and Phillips LH. Verbal fluency performance in dementia of the Alzheimer's type: a meta-analysis. *Neuropsychologia.* 2004;42:1212–22.

79. Birn RM, Kenworthy L, Case L, *et al.* Neural systems supporting lexical search guided by letter and semantic category cues: a self-paced overt response fMRI study of verbal fluency. *Neuroimage.* 2010;49:1099–107.

80. Mummery CJ, Patterson K, Hodges JR, *et al.* Nonliner regression in parametric activation studies. *Neuroimage.* 1996;4:60–66.

81. Nutter-Upham KE, Saykin AJ, Rabin LA, *et al.* Verbal fluency performance in amnestic MCI and older adults with cognitive complaints. *Arch Clin Neuropsychol.* 2008;23:229–41.

82. Bien CG, Schulze-Bonhage A, Deckert M, *et al.* Limbic encephalitis not associated with neoplasm as a cause of temporal lobe epilepsy. *Neurology.* 2000;55:1823–28.

83. Bien CG, Urbach H, Schramm J, *et al.* Limbic encephalitis as a precipitating event in adult-onset temporal lobe epilepsy. *Neurology.* 2007;69:1236–44.

84. Kotsenas AL, Watson RE, Pittock SJ, *et al.* MRI findings in autoimmune voltage-gated potassium channel complex encephalitis with seizures: one potential etiology for mesial temporal sclerosis. *Am J Neuroradiol.* 2014;35: 84–9.

85. Jacob S, Irani SR, Rajabally YA, *et al.* Hypothermia in VGKC antibody-associated limbic encephalitis. *J Neurol Neurosur Ps.* 2008;79:202–204.

86. Wagner J, Witt JA, Helmstaedter C, *et al.* Automated volumetry of the mesiotemporal structures in antibody-associated limbic encephalitis. *J Neurol Neurosur Ps.* 2014.

87. Bien CG, Vincent A, Barnett MH, *et al.* Immunopathology of autoantibody-associated encephalitides: clues for pathogenesis. *Brain.* 2012;135:1622–38.

88. Khan NL, Jeffree MA, Good C, *et al.* Histopathology of VGKC antibody-associated limbic encephalitis. *Neurology.* 2009;72:1703–705.

89. Dalmau J, Tuzun E, Wu HY, *et al.* Paraneoplastic anti-*N*-methyl-D-aspartate receptor encephalitis associated with ovarian teratoma. *Ann Neurol.* 2007;61:25–36.

90. Titulaer MJ, McCracken L, Gabilondo I, *et al.* Treatment and prognostic factors for long-term outcome in patients with anti-NMDA receptor encephalitis: an observational cohort study. *Lancet Neurol.* 2013;12:157–65.

91. Viaccoz A, Desestret V, Ducray F, *et al.* Clinical specificities of adult male patients with NMDA receptor antibodies encephalitis. *Neurology.* 2014;82:556–63.

92. Kleinig TJ, Thompson PD, Matar W, *et al.* The distinctive movement disorder of ovarian teratoma-associated encephalitis. *Mov Disord.* 2008;23:1256–61.

93. Stamelou M, Plazzi G, Lugaresi E, *et al.* The distinct movement disorder in anti-NMDA receptor encephalitis may be related to Status Dissociatus: a hypothesis. *Mov Disord.* 2012;27:1360–63.

94. Baizabal-Carvallo JF, Stocco A, Muscal E, *et al.* The spectrum of movement disorders in children with anti-NMDA receptor encephalitis. *Mov Disord.* 2013;28:543–47.

95. Johnson N, Henry C, Fessler AJ, *et al.* Anti-NMDA receptor encephalitis causing prolonged nonconvulsive status epilepticus. *Neurology.* 2010;75:1480–82.

96. Kayser MS, Titulaer MJ, Gresa-Arribas N, *et al.* Frequency and characteristics of isolated psychiatric episodes in anti-*N*-methyl-D-aspartate receptor encephalitis. *JAMA Neurol.* 2013 Sep 1;70(9):1133–9.

97. Rubio-Agusti I, Dalmau J, Sevilla T, *et al.* Isolated hemidystonia associated with NMDA receptor antibodies. *Mov Disord.* 2011;26:351–52.

98. Zandi MS, Deakin JB, Morris K, *et al.* Immunotherapy for patients with acute psychosis and serum *N*-methyl-D-aspartate receptor (NMDAR) antibodies: a description of a treated case series. *Schizophr Res.* 2014;160:193–95.

99. Dahm L, Ott C, Steiner J, *et al.* Seroprevalence of autoantibodies against brain antigens in health and disease. *Ann Neurol.* 2014.

100. Masdeu JC, Gonzalez-Pinto A, Matute C, *et al.* Serum IgG antibodies against the NR1 subunit of the NMDA receptor not detected in schizophrenia. *Am J Psychiatry.* 2012;169:1120–21.

101. Pruss H, Holtje M, Maier N, *et al.* IgA NMDA receptor antibodies are markers of synaptic immunity in slow cognitive impairment. *Neurology.* 2012;78:1743–53.

102. Steiner J, Walter M, Glanz W, *et al.* Increased prevalence of diverse *N*-methyl-D-aspartate glutamate receptor antibodies in patients with an initial diagnosis of schizophrenia: specific relevance of IgG NR1a antibodies for distinction from *N*-methyl-D-aspartate glutamate receptor encephalitis. *JAMA Psychiatry.* 2013;70:271–78.

103. Doss S, Wandinger KP, Hyman BT, *et al.* High prevalence of NMDA receptor IgA/IgM antibodies in different dementia types. *Ann Clin Transl Neurol.* 2014;1:822–32.

104. Mackay G, Ahmad K, Stone J, *et al.* NMDA receptor autoantibodies in sporadic Creutzfeldt–Jakob disease. *J Neurol.* 2012;259:1979–81.

105. Angus-Leppan H, Rudge P, Mead S, *et al.* Autoantibodies in sporadic Creutzfeldt–Jakob disease. *JAMA Neurol.* 2013;70:919–22.

106. Rossi M, Mead S, Collinge J, *et al.* Neuronal antibodies in patients with suspected or confirmed sporadic Creutzfeldt–Jakob disease. *J Neurol Neurosur Ps.* 2015 Jun;86(6):692–4.

107. Titulaer MJ, Hoftberger R, Iizuka T, *et al.* Overlapping demyelinating syndromes and anti-*N*-methyl-D-aspartate receptor encephalitis. *Ann Neurol.* 2014;75:411–28.

108. Hacohen Y, Absoud M, Hemingway C, *et al.* NMDA receptor antibodies associated with distinct white matter syndromes. *Neurol Neuroimmunol Neuroinflamm.* 2014;1:e2.

109. Finke C, Kopp UA, Pruss H, *et al.* Cognitive deficits following anti-NMDA receptor encephalitis. *J Neurol Neurosur Ps.* 2012;83:195–98.

110. Braun M, Finke C, Ostendorf F, *et al.* Reorganization of associative memory in humans with long-standing hippocampal damage. *Brain.* 2008;131:2742–50.

111. Finke C, Braun M, Ostendorf F, *et al.* The human hippocampal formation mediates short-term memory of colour-location associations. *Neuropsychologia.* 2008;46:614–23.

112. Finke C, Kopp UA, Scheel M, *et al.* Functional and structural brain changes in anti-*N*-methyl-D-aspartate receptor encephalitis. *Ann Neurol.* 2013;74:284–96.

113. Hayes SM, Salat DH, and Verfaellie M. Default network connectivity in medial temporal lobe amnesia. *J Neurosci.* 2012;32:14622–629.

114. Kahn I, Andrews-Hanna JR, Vincent JL, *et al.* Distinct cortical anatomy linked to subregions of the medial temporal lobe revealed by intrinsic functional connectivity. *J Neurophysiol.* 2008;100:129–39.

115. Maguire EA. Neuroimaging studies of autobiographical event memory. *Philos Trans R Soc Lond B Biol Sci.* 2001;356:1441–51.

116. Malter MP, Frisch C, Schoene-Bake JC, *et al*. Outcome of limbic encephalitis with VGKC-complex antibodies: relation to antigenic specificity. *J Neurol*. 2014;261:1695–705.

117. Hutchinson M, Waters P, McHugh J, *et al*. Progressive encephalomyelitis, rigidity, and myoclonus: a novel glycine receptor antibody. *Neurology*. 2008;71:1291–92.

118. Petit-Pedrol M, Armangue T, Peng X, *et al*. Encephalitis with refractory seizures, status epilepticus, and antibodies to the GABA receptor: a case series, characterisation of the antigen, and analysis of the effects of antibodies. *Lancet Neurol*. 2015 Jun;86(6):692–4.

119. Lai M, Hughes EG, Peng X, *et al*. AMPA receptor antibodies in limbic encephalitis alter synaptic receptor location. *Ann Neurol*. 2009;65:424–34.

120. Malter MP, Helmstaedter C, Urbach H, *et al*. Antibodies to glutamic acid decarboxylase define a form of limbic encephalitis. *Ann Neurol*. 2010;67:470–78.

121. Stubgen JP. Subacute encephalopathy associated with aquaporin-4 autoantibodies: a report of 2 adult cases. *Clin Neurol Neurosurg*. 2012;114:1110–13.

122. Braakman HM, Moers-Hornikx VM, Arts BM, *et al*. Pearls & Oysters: electroconvulsive therapy in anti-NMDA receptor encephalitis. *Neurology*. 2010;75:e44–46.

123. Dalmau J, Lancaster E, Martinez-Hernandez E, *et al*. Clinical experience and laboratory investigations in patients with anti-NMDAR encephalitis. *Lancet Neurol*. 2011;10:63–74.

124. Irani SR, Gelfand JM, Bettcher BM, *et al*. Effect of rituximab in patients with leucine-rich, glioma-inactivated 1 antibody-associated encephalopathy. *JAMA Neurol*. 2014;71:896–900.

125. Brown JW, Martin PJ, Thorpe JW, *et al*. Long-term remission with rituximab in refractory leucine-rich glioma inactivated 1 antibody encephalitis. *J Neuroimmunol*. 2014;271:66–68.

126. Hughes EG, Peng X, Gleichman AJ, *et al*. Cellular and synaptic mechanisms of anti-NMDA receptor encephalitis. *J Neurosci*. 2010;30:5866–75.

127. Chang T, Alexopoulos H, Pettingill P, *et al*. Immunization against GAD induces antibody binding to GAD-independent antigens and brainstem GABAergic neuronal loss. *PLoS One*. 2013;8:e72921.

128. Dunstan EJ and Winer JB. Autoimmune limbic encephalitis causing fits, rapidly progressive confusion and hyponatraemia. *Age Ageing*. 2006;35:536–37.

129. Park DC, Murman DL, Perry KD, *et al*. An autopsy case of limbic encephalitis with voltage-gated potassium channel antibodies. *Eur J Neurol*. 2007;14:e5–6.

130. Manns JR and Eichenbaum H. Evolution of declarative memory. *Hippocampus*. 2006;16:795–808.

131. Nadel L and Moscovitch M. Memory consolidation, retrograde amnesia and the hippocampal complex. *Curr Opin Neurobiol*. 1997;7:217–27.

132. Ranganath C. A unified framework for the functional organization of the medial temporal lobes and the phenomenology of episodic memory. *Hippocampus*. 2010;20:1263–90.

133. Rolls ET. The mechanisms for pattern completion and pattern separation in the hippocampus. *Front Syst Neurosci*. 2013;7:74.

134. McKenzie S and Eichenbaum H. Consolidation and reconsolidation: two lives of memories? *Neuron*. 2011;71:224–33.

135. Waidergoren S, Segalowicz J, and Gilboa A. Semantic memory recognition is supported by intrinsic recollection-like processes: 'The butcher on the bus' revisited. *Neuropsychologia*. 2012;50:3573–87.

136. Schacter DL, Addis DR, Hassabis D, *et al*. The future of memory: remembering, imagining, and the brain. *Neuron*. 2012;76:677–94.

137. Hassabis D, Kumaran D, Vann SD, *et al*. Patients with hippocampal amnesia cannot imagine new experiences. *Proc Natl Acad Sci USA*. 2007;104:1726–31.

138. Leutgeb S, Leutgeb JK, Treves A, *et al*. Distinct ensemble codes in hippocampal areas CA3 and CA1. *Science*. 2004;305:1295–98.

139. Pertzov Y, Miller TD, Gorgoraptis N, *et al*. Binding deficits in memory following medial temporal lobe damage in patients with voltage-gated potassium channel complex antibody-associated limbic encephalitis. *Brain*. 2013;136:2474–85.

140. Luby ED, Cohen BD, Rosenbaum G, *et al*. Study of a new schizophrenomimetic drug; sernyl. *AMA Arch Neurol Psychiatry*. 1959;81:363–69.

141. Javitt DC and Zukin SR. Recent advances in the phencyclidine model of schizophrenia. *Am J Psychiatry*. 1991;148:1301–08.

142. Adell A, Jimenez-Sanchez L, Lopez-Gil X, *et al*. Is the acute NMDA receptor hypofunction a valid model of schizophrenia? *Schizophr Bull*. 2012;38:9–14.

143. Moghaddam B and Adams BW. Reversal of phencyclidine effects by a group II metabotropic glutamate receptor agonist in rats. *Science*. 1998;281:1349–52.

144. Lopez-Gil X, Babot Z, Amargos-Bosch M, *et al*. Clozapine and haloperidol differently suppress the MK-801-increased glutamatergic and serotonergic transmission in the medial prefrontal cortex of the rat. *Neuropsychopharmacology*. 2007;32:2087–97.

145. Olney JW and Farber NB. Glutamate receptor dysfunction and schizophrenia. *Arch Gen Psychiatry*. 1995;52:998–1007.

146. Enomoto T, Tse MT, and Floresco SB. Reducing prefrontal gamma-aminobutyric acid activity induces cognitive, behavioral, and dopaminergic abnormalities that resemble schizophrenia. *Biol Psychiatry*. 2011;69:432–41.

147. Pilowsky LS, Bressan RA, Stone JM, *et al*. First *in vivo* evidence of an NMDA receptor deficit in medication-free schizophrenic patients. *Mol Psychiatry*. 2006;11:118–19.

148. Stone JM, Erlandsson K, Arstad E, *et al*. Relationship between ketamine-induced psychotic symptoms and NMDA receptor occupancy: a [(123)I]CNS-1261 SPET study. *Psychopharmacology (Berl)*. 2008;197:401–408.

149. Jentsch JD and Roth RH. The neuropsychopharmacology of phencyclidine: from NMDA receptor hypofunction to the dopamine hypothesis of schizophrenia. *Neuropsychopharmacology*. 1999;20:201–25.

150. Liao Y, Tang J, Ma M, *et al*. Frontal white matter abnormalities following chronic ketamine use: a diffusion tensor imaging study. *Brain*. 2010;133:2115–22.

151. Urbach H, Soeder BM, Jeub M, *et al*. Serial MRI of limbic encephalitis. *Neuroradiology*. 2006;48:380–86.

152. Sekiguchi Y, Takahashi H, Mori M, *et al*. Potassium channel antibody-associated encephalitis with hypothalamic lesions and intestinal pseudo-obstruction. *J Neurol Sci*. 2008;269:176–79.

153. Chatzikonstantinou A, Szabo K, Ottomeyer C, *et al*. Successive affection of bilateral temporomesial structures in a case of non-paraneoplastic limbic encephalitis demonstrated by serial MRI and FDG-PET. *J Neurol*. 2009;256:1753–55.

154. Kaymakamzade B, Kansu T, Tan E, *et al*. LGI1 related limbic encephalitis and response to immunosuppressive therapy. *J Neurol*. 2011;258:2075–77.

155. Kapina V, Vargas M, Vulliemoz S, *et al*. VGKC antibody-associated encephalitis, microbleeds and progressive brain atrophy. *J Neurol*. 2010;257:466–68.

156. Bataller L, Kleopa KA, Wu GF, *et al*. Autoimmune limbic encephalitis in 39 patients: immunophenotypes and outcomes. *J Neurol Neurosur Ps*. 2007;78:381–85.

157. Harrower T, Foltynie T, Kartsounis L, *et al*. A case of voltage-gated potassium channel antibody-related limbic encephalitis. *Nat Clin Pract Neurol*. 2006;2:339–43; quiz following 343.

158. Dalmau J, Gleichman AJ, Hughes EG, *et al*. Anti-NMDA-receptor encephalitis: case series and analysis of the effects of antibodies. *Lancet Neurol*. 2008;7:1091–98.

159. Iizuka T, Sakai F, Ide T, *et al*. Anti-NMDA receptor encephalitis in Japan: long-term outcome without tumor removal. *Neurology*. 2008;70:504–11.

160. Baumgartner A, Rauer S, Mader I, *et al*. Cerebral FDG-PET and MRI findings in autoimmune limbic encephalitis: correlation with autoantibody types. *J Neurol*. 2013;260:2744–53.

161. Sarkis RA, Nehme R, and Chemali ZN. Neuropsychiatric and seizure outcomes in nonparaneoplastic autoimmune limbic encephalitis. *Epilepsy Behav*. 2014;39C:21–25.

162. Machado S, Pinto AN, and Irani SR. What should you know about limbic encephalitis? *Arq Neuropsiquiatr*. 2012;70:817–22.

163. Tan KM, Lennon VA, Klein CJ, *et al*. Clinical spectrum of voltage-gated potassium channel autoimmunity. *Neurology*. 2008;70:1883–90.

164. Tofaris GK, Irani SR, Cheeran BJ, *et al*. Immunotherapy-responsive chorea as the presenting feature of LGI1-antibody encephalitis. *Neurology*. 2012;79:195–96.

CHAPTER 29

Pathology of degenerative dementias

Tamas Revesz, Tammaryn Lashley, and Janice L. Holton

Introduction

The term neurodegenerative disease is used to describe a large group of neurological conditions characterized by relentless clinical deterioration due to gradual loss of neuronal function.

The pathological processes underlying neurodegenerative disorders often selectively affect anatomically interconnected, functionally related systems and networks giving rise to characteristic, often overlapping clinical presentations such as different forms of dementia, akinetic or hyperkinetic movement disorders, or cerebellar degenerations. As the distribution of the pathological changes determines the clinical presentation, several diseases may result in a similar clinical presentation. The examples include frontotemporal dementia (FTD) and corticobasal syndrome, which may be caused by one of a number of diverse pathologies.[1,2]

In order to be able to execute their functions, newly produced proteins need to acquire a specific three-dimensional structure, which is the result of a process that takes place under stringent quality control. Central to the pathomechanism of the neurodegenerative dementias to be discussed in this chapter is that they are characterized by age-dependent misfolding, abnormal aggregation and deposition of disease-specific proteins, hence the often used terms protein folding or conformational disorders, proteinopathies, or proteopathies.[3] The initial phase of the protein aggregation process is the conversion of random-coil secondary structures of soluble native proteins into β-sheet-rich conformations, which initially self-associate into oligomers, consisting of only a few protein molecules, followed by formation of protofibrillar intermediate ensembles and, finally, fibrils.[4] There are several mechanisms, which are known to be able to destabilize the secondary structure of soluble native proteins, and these include increased protein concentration and genetic as well as post-translational modifications of proteins.

Duplication or triplication of genes are associated with increased protein concentration while missense mutations in the coding region of a gene results in an amino acid substitution, which can alter the aggregation potential of a disease protein. Another genetic mechanism is represented by the suprathreshold expansion of an unstable cytosine–adenine–guanine (CAG) repeat region, which takes place in the huntingtin (HTT) gene resulting in the formation of an expanded polyglutamine stretch predisposing the huntingtin protein to aggregation in Huntington's disease.[5]

Mutations may also cause disease via haploinsufficiency such as in familial FTD with parkinsonism due to mutations of the GRN gene (FTDP-17GRN), leading to reduced levels of progranulin protein,[6] although the link to the formation of the TAR DNA-binding protein-43 (TDP-43) inclusions is still not clear. Mutations in noncoding intronic sequences may change the process of alternative splicing of a disease-related protein such as that of the microtubule-associated protein tau, which is the main component of neurofibrillary tangles in Alzheimer's disease and a number of primary tauopathies (see also following).[7]

Repeat expansion of a GGGGCC hexanucleotide repeat, present in a noncoding region of the C9orf72 gene, has been identified as a major cause of familial motor neuron disease/amyotrophic lateral sclerosis (MND/ALS) and also FTD. Data indicate that there is at least 50 per cent loss of at least one of three C9orf72 transcripts. The mechanisms that may be responsible for disease in the C9orf72 cases include haploinsufficiency, RNA gain of function with the formation of nuclear RNA foci, or the expanded non-coding GGGGCC repeats are translated via repeat-associated non-ATG translation process.[8]

The most common risk factor for sporadic protein-folding disorders is age, which is thought to result in altered protein homeostasis (proteostasis), possibly due to changes in cellular protein levels and/or failure of cellular machinery responsible for eliminating damaged, misfolded proteins.[3] Genome-wide association studies have also demonstrated genetic variants which carry an increased risk for developing sporadic neurodegenerative diseases such as Alzheimer's disease, frontotemporal lobar degeneration with TDP-43 inclusions (FTLD-TDP), Parkinson's disease, and progressive supranuclear palsy.[9]

As pathologically altered proteins, characteristic for each disease or group of diseases, form extracellular deposits and/or intracellular inclusions in neurons and in some instances also in glia, these protein aggregates provide a valuable tool in the everyday neuropathological diagnosis. Although the aetiology of the majority of neurodegenerative diseases remains elusive, the significant increase in knowledge about genetic background, cellular events, and biochemical changes has allowed the introduction of molecular classifications of neurodegenerative diseases, including dementias, which will be followed in this chapter (Table 29.1).

Diseases with extracellular protein aggregates and neurofibrillary degeneration

This group of diseases are all characterized by formation of extracellular amyloid plaques composed of different disease-specific amyloid peptides, accompanied by neurofibrillary degeneration. In this

Table 29.1 Molecular classification of neurodegenerative dementias

Disease	Type of protein deposit	Toxic protein	Precursor protein	Genes+	Risk factors
Diseases with amyloid plaques and NFT					
Alzheimer's disease	Senile plaques CAA	Aβ	APP	APP, PS1, PS2	Yes*
	NFT	tau	tau		
Familial British dementia	Amyloid plaques CAA	ABri	ABriPP	BRI2	No
	NFT	tau	tau		
Familial Danish dementia	Amyloid plaques CAA	ADan	ADanPP	BRI2	No
	NFT	tau	tau		
Prion diseases	Amyloid plaques CAA**	PrP	PrP	PRNP	Yes
	NFT	tau	tau		
Synucleinopathies					
Dementia with Lewy bodies	Lewy body	αSyn	αSyn	SNCA	Yes*
	Amyloid plaques	Aβ	APP		
Parkinson's disease with dementia	Lewy body	αSyn	αSyn	SNCA	
	Amyloid plaques	Aβ	APP		
Frontotemporal lobar degenerations					
FTLD-TDP					
Type A	NCI, NII, DN, GI	TDP-43	TDP-43	GRN, C9orf72	Yes*
Type B	NCI	TDP-43	TDP-43	C9orf72	
Type C	DN	TDP-43	TDP-43	-	
Type D	NII, DN	TDP-43	TDP-43	VCP	
FTLD-FUS					
aFTLD-U	NCI, NII, GI	FUS	FUS	-	No
NIFID	NCI, NII, GI	FUS	FUS	-	
BIBD	NCI, NII, GI	FUS	FUS	-	
FTLD-tau					
Pick's disease	Pick body, GI	tau	tau	-	
CBD	NFT, NT, GI-AP	tau	tau	-	MAPT, H1
PSP	NFT, NT, GI-TA	tau	tau	-	MAPT, H1
GGT	NFT, NT, GGI	tau	tau	-	
AGD	NFT, NT, GI	tau	tau	-	
FTDP-17MAPT	NFT, NT, GI	tau	tau	MAPT	
Polyglutamine diseases					
Huntington disease	NII, CP	Huntingtin	Huntingtin	HTT	No

αSyn: α-synuclein; Aβ: amyloid-β; APP: amyloid precursor protein; ABri: amyloid-Bri; ABriPP: amyloid-Bri precursor protein; ADan: amyloid-Dan; ADanPP: amyloid-Dan precursor protein; aFTLD-U: atypical FTLD with ubiquitin-positive, tau and TDP-43-negative inclusions; AGD: argyrophilic grain disease; AP: astrocytic plaque, BIBD: basophilic inclusion body disease; CAA: cerebral amyloid angiopathy; CBD: corticobasal degeneration; CP: cytoplasmic positivity; DN: dystrophic neurites; FTDP-17MAPT: frontotemporal dementia with parkinsonism linked to chromose 17 due to mutation of the MAPT gene. FTLD: frontotemporal lobar degeneration; FUS: fused in sarcoma; GGI: globular glial inclusion; GI: glial inclusion; GGT: globular glial tauopathy; NCI: neuronal cytoplasmic inclusion; NIFID: neuronal intermediate filament inclusion disease; NII: neuronal intranuclear inclusion; NFT: neurofibrillary tangle; NT: neuropil thread; PrP: prion protein; PSP: progressive supranuclear palsy; TA: tufted astrocyte; TDP-43: TAR DNA-binding protein-43. For gene abbreviations see: <http://www.ncbi.nlm.nih.gov/omim/>; *For review see reference 9; ** CAA is a rare manifestation in prion diseases; for review see reference 4.

group, Alzheimer's disease and the *BRI2* gene-related dementias will be discussed and, although some of the familial prion diseases would also fall into this category, they will be discussed elsewhere.

Alzheimer's disease

Alzheimer's disease, by far the most common neurodegenerative disease, is characterized microscopically by two cardinal features: (1) deposition of the amyloid-β peptide (Aβ) in cerebral parenchyma as senile plaques and in blood vessels as cerebral amyloid angiopathy, and (2) formation of neurofibrillary tangles, which are composed of abnormally hyperphosphorylated tau, which is a microtubule-associated protein.

Aβ is produced by multistep processing of the amyloid precursor protein (APP) with the initial step being a β-secretase cleavage, which releases a 99-amino-acid-long C-terminal fragment (C99). This is followed by a second, intramembranous cleavage by the γ-secretase complex, which produces 40- or 42-amino-acid-long peptides (Aβ40 and Aβ42).[10] Soluble Aβ is considered the precursor of disease-associated Aβ deposited in the brain.

Neurofibrillary tangles are due to intraneuronal accumulation of abnormally hyperphosphorylated tau filaments in the cell soma of neurons. Tau filaments also deposit in dendrites as neuropil threads and in axons surrounding amyloid plaques as plaque-associated neurites.

Macroscopic changes

Based on the investigation of large cohorts of cases at postmortem, an overall reduction in brain weight is a typical feature of Alzheimer's disease, although in individual cases the severity of substance loss is variable and may overlap with age-matched controls. Brain atrophy is usually most severe in medial temporal lobe structures, including the hippocampus (Fig. 29.1). It is also prominent in the inferior temporal, middle, and superior frontal gyri while the inferior frontal and orbitofrontal gyri and the occipital lobe are preserved.[11] In early-onset and familial (autosomal-dominant) cases, brain atrophy may be more severe. Inspection of coronal slices of the cerebral hemispheres also demonstrates thinning of the cerebral cortex, reduction in bulk of subcortical white matter, enlargement of the ventricles (Fig. 29.1) and pallor of the locus coeruleus. Data provided by *in vivo* studies using serial MRI have provided insight into the time course of brain atrophy in Alzheimer's disease.[12]

Microscopic changes

The diagnosis of Alzheimer's disease at postmortem depends on the recognition of senile/neuritic plaques and neurofibrillary degeneration in brains of individuals with dementia. Both the Aβ (Fig. 29.1E and 29.1F) and neurofibrillary tangle pathologies (Fig. 29.1C and 29.1D) follow a stereotypic progression from early stages of subclinical Alzheimer's disease to full-blown disease. The Braak and Braak scheme proposes six different stages of hierarchical progression, reflected in the distribution and severity of neurofibrillary degeneration. According to this, the transentorhinal and entorhinal cortices are affected in stages I and II, the hippocampus and other limbic structures in stages III and IV, while isocortical areas are involved in stages V and VI.[13,14]

Aβ plaque accumulation in different brain areas has also been shown to advance in a hierarchical manner and according to

the scheme recommended by Thal and colleagues this can be separated into five distinct phases.[15] In phase 1 Aβ deposits are restricted to the neocortex; in phase 2 additional involvement of allocortical regions including the hippocampus and entorhinal region is seen; in phase 3 the Aβ pathology extends into diencephalic nuclei, the striatum, and cholinergic nuclei of the basal forebrain; in phase 4 brainstem nuclei are affected, and finally in phase 5 Aβ deposition also takes place in the cerebellum.

The most up-to-date neuropathological diagnostic criteria of Alzheimer's disease include the establishment of a CERAD (Consortium to Establish a Registry for Alzheimer's Disease) neuritic plaque-score (none, sparse, moderate, or frequent), the Braak and Braak neurofibrillary pathology stage (0–VI), and Thal Aβ deposition phase (0–5). Consideration of all three components allows the neuropathologist to establish an ABC score, and finally the level of Alzheimer's disease neuropathological change (none, low, intermediate, and high levels) is provided.[16]

Cerebral amyloid angiopathy (CAA)

Amyloid deposition takes place in leptomeningeal and parenchymal small blood vessels, including arteries, arterioles, and capillaries in over 80 per cent of all Alzheimer's patients (Fig. 29.1G).[17] The ApoE ε4 allele is more prevalent when capillary amyloid is also present (type 1) than in cases without capillary Aβ deposition (type 2).[18] Hypoperfusion and occlusion of capillaries due to cerebral amyloid angiopathy are possible additional mechanisms, which adversely affect the brain in Alzheimer's disease.[19]

Other diseases coexisting with Alzheimer's disease

Lewy body disease, TDP-43 inclusions, argyrophilic grain disease, vascular brain injury, and hippocampal sclerosis are the most common comorbidities in Alzheimer's disease.[20]

Alzheimer's disease neuropathology after Aβ42 immunotherapy

Postmortem examination of brains of Alzheimer patients treated with *active Aβ42* immunotherapy showed lower Aβ load with evidence that plaques had been removed, a reduced tau burden in neuronal processes, but no evidence of a beneficial effect on synapses. The pathological side-effects included an increased microglial activation and increased CAA.[21]

Familial British dementia and familial Danish dementia

Mutations of the *BRI2* gene cause the two, closely related rare hereditary, autosomal dominant neurodegenerative diseases, familial British dementia and familial Danish dementia (*BRI2* gene-related dementias).[22,23] Clinically, patients present with a 'dementia and spasticity' syndrome, but cerebellar ataxia is also characteristic.[24]

Neuropathologically, both familial British dementia (Fig. 29.1H-J) and familial Danish dementia (Fig. 29.1K-M) show a striking resemblance to Alzheimer's disease as in both there are widespread cerebral parenchymal amyloid plaques, severe CAA and neurofibrillary tangles, although the ABri and ADan amyloid peptides, have no homology with the Aβ peptide.[25,26]

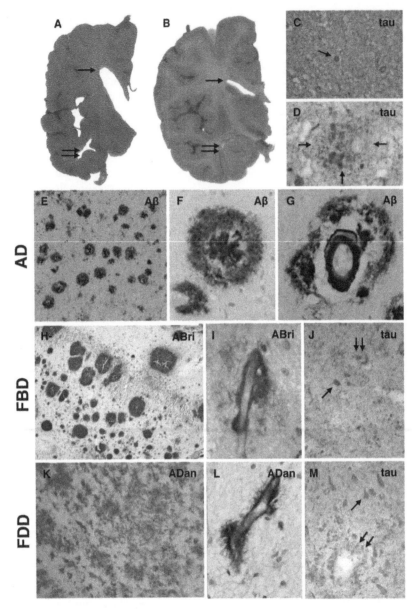

Fig. 29.1 Pathological features of neurodegenerative diseases with extracellular protein deposition. A: A macroscopic coronal slice from a case with Alzheimer's disease and B: Brain slice from a matched control case. The Alzheimer case shows enlargement of the lateral ventricle (arrow) and a reduced sized hippocampus (double arrows). Please also note the narrowing of the cortical ribbon and the reduced bulk of the hemispheric deep white matter in Alzheimer's disease. C: Tau immunohistochemistry shows neurofibrillary tangles (arrow) and numerous neuropil threads, and D: Plaque-associated abnormal neurites (arrows) while Aβ immunohistochemistry (E–G) demonstrates diffuse and mature plaques (E and F), and a blood vessel with cerebral amyloid angiopathy (G) in the cerebral cortex in Alzheimer's disease (AD). H–J: Familial British dementia (FBD) is characterized by deposition of the ABri peptide in amyloid and preamyloid plaques (H) and blood vessel walls resulting in severe cerebral amyloid angiopathy (I). J: Neurofibrillary tangles (arrow), neuropil threads and ABri plaque-associated neurites (double arrow) are also present. K–M: In familial Danish dementia (FDD), the parenchymal ADan deposits are of the diffuse, preamyloid type (K) and, as in familial British dementia, the cerebral amyloid angiopathy is widespread and severe (L). M: Tau immunohistochemistry demonstrates neurofibrillary tangles (arrow), neuropil threads, and abnormal, tau-positive neurites, which are seen around amyloid-laden blood vessels (double arrow) in this disease.

Frontotemporal dementias

After Alzheimer's disease, FTD is the second most common form of dementia in the presenium (disease onset <65 years). The term frontotemporal lobar degeneration (FTLD) is used by neuropathologists for this clinically, genetically, and pathologically diverse group of diseases. A common feature is degeneration of the frontal and temporal lobes with the canonical clinical presentations being behavioural variant FTD (bvFTD), progressive non-fluent aphasia (PNFA), and semantic dementia (SD). An important aspect of FTLDs is that degeneration of motor neurons may also occur, which highlights the aetiological link between FTLDs and MND)/ALS (FTLD–ALS spectrum). The major genes currently known to be involved in familial FTDs include the *MAPT, GRN, C9orf72, TARDBP, VCP,* and *CHMP2B* genes (see chapter 35).[6]

Classification of frontotemporal lobar degenerations

The discovery of tau, TDP-43, and the fused in sarcoma protein (FUS) as the disease proteins composing pathological inclusions and the identification of several genes associated with familial

Table 29.2 FTLD-tau

Predominant tau isoforms in inclusions		
3R-tau	**4R-tau**	**3R-tau and 4R-tau**
Pick's disease	PSP	PART
FTDP-17*MAPT*	CBD	FTDP-17*MAPT*
	AGD	
	GGT	
	FTDP-17*MAPT*	

3R-tau: 3-repeat tau; 4R-tau: 4-repeat tau; AGD: argyrophilic grain disease; CBD: corticobasal degeneration; FTLD: frontotemporal lobar degeneration; FTDP-17*MAPT*: frontotemporal dementia with parkinsonism linked to chromosome 17 due to mutations in the *MAPT* gene; FTLD-tau: frontotemporal lobar degeneration with tau-positive inclusions; GGT: globular glial tauopathy; PART: primary age-related tauopathy.

forms of FTLD have provided the foundation of a molecular classification of FTLDs.[27,28] Three of the four major disease groups are characterized by specific proteinaceous inclusions (FTLD-tau, FTLD-TDP, and FTLD-FUS) while in the fourth group the protein component of the ubiquitin-positive inclusions remains unidentified, hence the term FTLD-UPS. Within each of the three groups in which the proteinaceous nature of the inclusions is known there are several subtypes or separate diseases (Table 29.1).

Tau

Tau is a microtubule-associated protein and its main function is to promote assembly and stabilization of microtubules. In the adult human brain, six tau isoforms are expressed by alternative splicing from the *MAPT* gene.[29] The isoforms are different from one another on the basis of the presence or absence of 29- or 58-amino-acid-long N-terminal inserts and whether they possess a fourth 31-amino-acid-long repeat in the microtubule-binding domain of tau. On the basis of presence or absence of this fourth repeat sequence, there are two major classes of tau isoforms. Three isoforms contain three repeats (3R-tau) with the remaining three having four repeats (4R-tau) in the microtubule-binding domain of tau. In some diseases such as progressive supranuclear palsy, corticobasal degeneration, and certain forms of FTDP-17 due to mutations of the *MAPT* gene (FTDP-17*MAPT*), the inclusions are predominantly composed of 4R-tau, while in Pick's disease and some forms of FTDP-17*MAPT* they are composed of 3R-tau. Both 3R-tau and 4R-tau are present in a third group, which includes Alzheimer's disease, familial British dementia, familial Danish dementia, and certain forms of FTDP-17*MAPT* (Table 29.2).[30]

Frontotemporal lobar degenerations with tau-positive inclusions (FTLD-tau)

Pick's disease

Pick's disease is a rare cause of FTD of all dementia cases (~5 per cent) in large autopsy series.[31] It is characterized by severe circumscribed lobar atrophy with marked neuronal loss with accompanying gliosis, presence of swollen achromatic neurons (Pick cells), and compact, rounded, argyrophilic and tau-positive neuronal cytoplasmic inclusions, known as Pick bodies. The distribution of the localized cortical atrophy correlates with the clinical phenotype

of Pick's disease; it is frontotemporal in bvFTD cases, frontoparietal in cases when apraxia is also a feature, and peri-Sylvian in cases with PNFA.[32]

Pick bodies are particularly common in the granule cells of the dentate fascia and pyramidal neurons of the hippocampus, but they are widespread. Pick bodies are composed mainly of 3R-tau isoforms, which can be confirmed with both biochemical methods[33] and immunohistochemistry (Fig. 29.2A).[34] Tau-positive glial pathology of variable severity is a feature of PiD and these include oligodendroglial cytoplasmic inclusions (Fig. 29.2C) and astrocytic inclusions (ramified astrocytes) (Fig. 29.2B). There is diffuse tau immunoreactivity in the neuropil of affected grey matter.

Corticobasal degeneration (CBD)

Corticobasal degeneration (CBD), which is a cause of corticobasal syndrome, is a 4R-tauopathy with neuronal and glial tau inclusions in cerebral cortex, basal ganglia, brainstem, and cerebellar nuclei.[35] Macroscopically, there is cortical atrophy affecting the posterior frontal lobe and the parietal region, with involvement of the precentral and postcentral gyri in cases presenting with corticobasal syndrome. The atrophy may be asymmetrical with the more severe changes being found contralateral to the most severely affected limbs.[32]

The cortical atrophy is more generalized in cases with frontal dementia or primary progressive aphasia.[36–38] Affected cerebral cortices show neuronal and glial inclusions, neuronal loss with astrocytosis and superficial spongiosis. Pick cells are a feature of CBD.[37] There is significant loss of neurons in the substantia nigra. Neuronal loss, astrocytosis, and occasional swollen neurons are variable in subcortical grey nuclei. The corticospinal tracts may show evidence of degeneration.[39,40]

4R-tau-positive neuronal inclusions are usually prominent in areas of superficial microvacuolation in moderately affected cortex and are seen in subcortical grey nuclei, substantia nigra, other brainstem nuclei, and cerebellar dentate nucleus.[37,41,42] Tau-positive coiled bodies (oligodendroglial inclusions) are widespread in cortices and white matter (Fig. 29.2D).[42–44] The characteristic lesion is the 'astrocytic plaque', comprising a distinct annular array of short, tau-positive stubby processes (Fig. 29.2E)[43,45,46] most easily identified in the premotor, prefrontal, and orbital cortical regions and also in the striatum.[47] Tau-positive neuropil threads are also frequent.[2,35]

Progressive supranuclear palsy (PSP)

PSP is the most common primary tauopathy with the common clinical presentation being atypical parkinsonism (Richardson's syndrome, PSP–RS).[48] However, some patients may have a clinical presentation, which deviates from that seen in PSP–RS and these include parkinsonism resembling initially Parkinson's disease (PSP–P), corticobasal syndrome (PSP–CBS),[49–51] bvFTD,[52,53] or speech and language impairment (PSP–FTD).[48,54–57]

Atrophy of the subthalamic nucleus, midbrain and pontine tegmentum and marked pallor of the substantia nigra are characteristic in the majority of the PSP cases. Atrophy of the superior cerebellar peduncle is also common. The globus pallidus and cerebellar dentate nucleus are atrophied in a significant proportion of the cases and dilatation of the third and fourth ventricles and the cerebral aqueduct is common. Mild generalized or predominantly

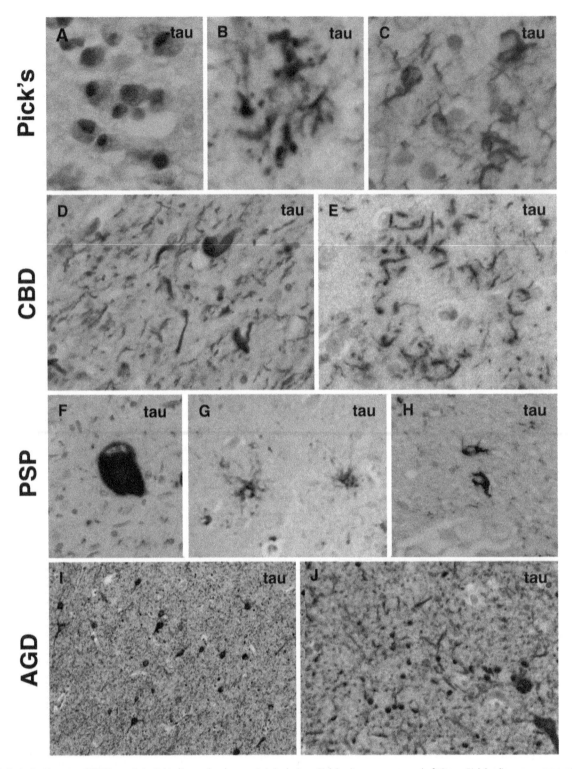

Fig. 29.2 Pathological features of FTLD-tau. A: In Pick's disease the characteristic inclusions, Pick bodies, are composed of 3R-tau. Pick bodies are numerous in the granule cells of the dentate fascia. B and C: Tau-positive glial pathology in the form of ramified astrocytes (B) and oligodendroglial cytoplasmic inclusions (C) is also characteristic. D: In corticobasal degeneration (CBD), subcortical white matter areas are particularly rich in tau-positive neuritic processes. E: The hallmark lesion is the astrocytic plaque in CBD. F–H: Progressive supranuclear palsy (PSP) is characterized by accumulation of hyperphosphorylated 4R-tau in neurons (F) and glia (G and H). G: The stellate shaped tufted astrocytes are the hallmark lesions in PSP and oligodendroglial, coiled bodies are also common (H). I: Widespread deposition of 4R-tau in affected grey matter in argyrophilic grain disease. J: In this condition argyrophilic, tau-positive grains are characteristic, which represent tau deposition in neuronal apical dendrites.

frontal atrophy with involvement of the precentral and postcentral gyri may be seen. The microscopic pathology of progressive supranuclear palsy is characterized by accumulation of hyperphosphorylated 4R-tau in neurons and glia, neuronal loss in basal ganglia, brainstem, and cerebellar nuclei with astrocytosis.[41,58] The neuronal tau pathology includes both neurofibrillary tangles and pretangles (Fig. 29.2F). The tufted astrocytes (Fig. 29.2G) or glial fibrillary tangles, which are tau-positive stellate-shaped astrocytes possessing fine radiating processes, are highly characteristic for this disease.[41,58] Deposition of fibrillar tau in oligodendroglia gives rise to coiled bodies (Fig. 29.2H).[41] Neuropil threads are also present in both grey and white matter. In PSP–RS, the tau burden is usually greater in the basal ganglia and brainstem structures than in neocortex. In contrast, PSP–CBS and PSP–FTD variants are associated with an increased neocortical tau load.[49–51,54]

Argyrophilic grain disease (AGD)

Argyrophilic grain disease (AGD) is a sporadic 4R-tauopathy occurring in the elderly with or without clinical dementia. Young-onset disease has been documented to present clinically as FTD,[59] but AGD does not have a consistent phenotype and is therefore not diagnosable during life.

The pathological hallmark lesions are the argyrophilic and tau-positive grains, which are comma- or spindle-shaped small 4–8 micron structures, occurring in apical dendrites (Fig. 29.2I, J). Other tau-positive lesions such as coiled bodies, pretangles, and bushy astrocytes are also features.[60] Balloon neurons are also a characteristic, albeit non-specific feature of the pathology.

The neuropathological changes are mostly restricted to the medial temporal lobe, but structures such as orbitofrontal cortex, insular cortex, hypothalamic lateral tuberal nucleus, and nucleus accumbens may also be affected. A diffuse form, associated with frontal lobe dementia, has been documented.[60] Staging of AGD, reflecting progression of the disease, has been proposed.[61] AGD is seen to occur in association with other neurodegenerative disease such as Alzheimer's disease, CBD, PSP, Pick's disease, and FTDP-17*MAPT*.

Tangle-predominant dementia

Tangle-predominant dementia or primary age-related tauopathy (PART) also occurs in elderly individuals and neuropathology is characterized by neurofibrillary tangles composed of 3R- and 4R-tau with no or mostly diffuse Aβ plaques. The tangle pathology may be relatively restricted to the medial temporal lobe with ghost, extracellular tangles often being a feature.

Globular glial tauopathy

A form of sporadic tauopathy has been identified in which, in addition to neuronal tau inclusions, there are widespread characteristic 'globular' oligodendroglial and astrocytic inclusions composed of 4R-tau. The cases have been described under a number of different names and have been reported to be associated with a range of clinical presentations including FTD,[62] MND/ALS,[63] or a combination of both FTD and MND/ALS.[64] Recently the overarching term of globular glial tauopathy has been recommended.[65]

Frontotemporal dementia with parkinsonism linked to chromosome 17 due to mutations of the *MAPT* gene (FTDP-17*MAPT*)

There are over 40 different mutations which have been identified as a cause of FTDP-17*MAPT*. A group of mutations affect alternative splicing of tau pre-mRNA while the primary effect of others is at protein level, resulting in reduced ability of tau to interact with microtubules.[66]

Although the severity of the macroscopic changes is dependent on the length of the disease duration, cases with intermediate and late disease stages show frontotemporal atrophy of variable severity,

enlargement of the lateral and third ventricles, reduction in bulk of the white matter of the centrum semiovale and temporal lobes, atrophy of the basal ganglia with pallor of the substantia nigra and locus coeruleus.[67]

Microscopically there is superficial spongiosis and a variable degree of nerve cell loss in the affected cortical regions accompanied by astrogliosis. Swollen, achromatic neurons may be present. Nerve cell loss is usually seen in affected basal ganglia and brainstem nuclei. Tau-positive inclusions are widely distributed in cerebral cortex, subcortical grey matter structures, brainstem nuclei, and cerebellum, and may be seen in the spinal cord. The pattern of tau pathology is variable and depends on the type of the *MAPT* mutation, which also determines whether tau deposition takes place in neurons or in both neurons and glia.

Neuronal inclusions include pretangles, neurofibrillary tangles, and Pick body-like inclusions. The spectrum of glial inclusions includes oligodendroglial coiled bodies, tufted astrocytes, and astrocytic plaques. In some of the mutations such as V337M and R406W, neurofibrillary tangles predominate. In these variants the biochemical characteristics of insoluble tau and the ultrastructural features of the tau filaments are similar to Alzheimer tau.[68,69] A number of mutations such as K257T, G272V, Q336R, and G389R result in a pathological phenotype in which Pick bodies are characteristic. As in cases of sporadic Pick's disease, in these mutants Pick bodies are primarily composed of 3R-tau isoforms, although in some cases inclusions also contain 4R-tau.

The impact of mutations in intron 10 (+3, +11, +12, +13, +14) or exon 10 (N279K, N296N, N296H, and G303V) on alternative splicing of tau is such that 4R-tau is more abundant and forms the inclusions.[67] In another group of cases such as those with P301L or P301S mutations, the tau filaments are also formed by 4R-tau, but the mutations' primary effect is at protein rather than pre-mRNA level. The pathological phenotype in these variants is neuronal and glial, and importantly glial pathology reminiscent of progressive supranuclear palsy and corticobasal degeneration has been documented.[70]

Frontotemporal lobar degenerations with TDP-43-positive inclusions (FTLD-TDP)

Pathologically, FTLD-TDP is defined by the presence of inclusions, composed of the disease-associated form of TDP-43.[71–73] TDP-43 is a highly conserved RNA/DNA binding protein, which is widely expressed and predominantly found in the nucleus. It shuttles between the cytoplasm and nucleus and its major functions include transcription and splicing regulation, microRNA processing, apoptosis, cell division, and stabilization of messenger RNA.[74]

FTLD-TDP includes both sporadic and familial forms and, being responsible for ~50 per cent of all FTLD, is the largest FTLD type.[75] The altered TDP-43 protein is N-terminally truncated, hyperphosphorylated, and ubiquitinated. A further important feature of the pathology is that inclusion-harbouring nerve cells lose the diffuse nuclear TDP-43 staining, which is seen in normal neuronal nuclei (Fig. 29.3A).[71,76] In FTLD-TDP the typical postmortem macroscopic finding is frontotemporal cerebral atrophy. This is asymmetrical in some cases such as in those with *GRN* gene mutations, in which involvement of the parietal lobe is also found. The asymmetry observed by *in vivo* imaging in cases with SD may not be seen in

Table 29.3 FTLD-TDP

	Type A	Type B	Type C	Type D
Neuronal cytoplasmic inclusions	+ + +	+ +	+	+
Neuronal intranuclear inclusions	0/+ +	0	0	+ + +
Dystrophic neurites	+ + +	+	+ + +	+ + +
Major clinical manifestations	bvFTD, CBS, PNFA	FTD with MND/ALS, bvFTD	SD	IBMPFD
Mutations in genes*	GRN, C9orf72	C9orf72	–	VCP

0 = absent; + = sparse; + + = moderate; + + + = frequent; bvFTD: behavioural variant frontotemporal dementia; CBS: corticobasal syndrome; FTD: frontotemporal dementia; FTLD-TDP: frontotemporal lobar degeneration with TDP-43-positive inclusions; IBMPFD: inclusion body myopathy with Paget disease of the bone and frontotemporal dementia; MND/ALS: motor neuron disease/amyotrophic lateral sclerosis; PNFA: progressive non-fluent aphasia; SD: semantic dementia * for gene mutations see <http://www.ncbi.nlm.nih.gov/omim/>

Adapted from *Lancet Neurol.* 9(10), Mackenzie IR, Rademakers R, and Neumann M, TDP-43 and FUS in amyotrophic lateral sclerosis and frontotemporal dementia, pp. 995–1007, Copyright (2010), with permission from Elsevier.

end-stage disease at postmortem. Involvement of the basal ganglia may be noted in some cases and the deep white matter of the frontotemporal area is often significantly reduced in bulk. A marked dilatation of the lateral and third ventricles is seen. The major microscopic TDP-43 lesion types are neuronal cytoplasmic inclusions (NCIs) (Fig. 29.3A), neuronal intranuclear inclusions (NIIs) (Fig. 29.3C and 29.3D), and dystrophic neurites (DNs) (Fig. 29.3B), although delicate neurites in the CA1 hippocampal subregion and 'pre-inclusions with a granular staining pattern' have also been described.[77–79]

The currently known genes, associated with familial forms of FTLD with TDP-43 pathology, are the progranulin (*GRN*), valosin-containing protein (*VCP*), and *C9orf72* genes (for a review see reference 6).

On the basis of morphological features and distribution of the TDP-43 inclusions four subtypes of FTLD-TDP are distinguished with some overlap between subtypes. According to a current harmonized classification[27] 'type A' pathology is present in about 40 per cent of all FTLD-TDP cases and consists of a combination of NCIs, rather short and often comma-shaped DNs and NIIs. 'Type B' pathology is responsible for about one-third of all FTLD-TDP with NCIs being characteristic. If present at all, DNs are sparse. In 'type C', which occurs in about 25 per cent of FTLD-TDP, there are rather long and thicker DNs characteristic with NCIs being either absent or rare. In the very rare 'type D', associated with mutations in the *VCP* gene, NIIs and DNs predominate and NCIs are rare or entirely absent.[27,80] There is correlation between pathological subtype, clinical presentation, and genetics in FTLD-TDP (Table 29.3).

An additional pathology is present in FTLD-TDP cases carrying the *C9orf72* expansion repeat. P62 positive 'star-like' inclusions are found in neurons predominanlty in the hippocampus and cerebellum (Fig. 29.3E and 29.3F).[81]

Concomitant TDP-43 pathology, often limited to the medial temporal lobe, may be seen in a number of neurodegenerative disorders such as Alzheimer's disease, Lewy body disorders, Guamanian ALS parkinsonism/dementia complex, and also in cases with hippocampal sclerosis.[75]

Frontotemporal lobar degenerations with FUS-positive inclusions (FTLD-FUS)

FUS shuttles between the nucleus and cytoplasm and shows both nuclear and cytoplasmic expression. Its functions are poorly characterized but they include cell proliferation, DNA repair, transcription regulation, and RNA and microRNA processing.[74]

The FTLD-FUS group includes three sporadic entities, atypical FTLD with ubiquitin-positive, tau- and TDP-43-negative inclusions (aFTLD-U), neuronal intermediate filament inclusion disease (NIFID), and basophilic inclusion body disease (BIBD).[82–84]

In aFTLD-U, the major disease protein of the ubiquitin-positive NCIs and NII is FUS (Fig. 29.3G and 29.3H). Inclusions are seen in frontotemporal cortices, hippocampus, striatum, thalamus, and brainstem nuclei, and spinal cord motor neurons.[82,85] A characteristic feature of aFTLD-U is the presence of NIIs, which can be of different morphological subtypes and may appear as twisted vermiform, ring-like, straight, or curved structures (Fig. 29.3G).

NIFID, also described as neurofilament inclusion body disease,[86] is characterized by the presence of NCIs (Fig. 29.3I and 29.3J), which are often eosinophilic and display variable immunoreactivity for ubiquitin, but are often strongly positive for p62. NIIs also occur in NIFID[86] (Fig. 29.3J) and a proportion of the FUS-positive inclusions are also positive for α-internexin and neurofilament proteins.[86,87]

The term BIBD derives from the pathological observation that inclusions appear basophilic on the haematoxylin and eosin preparation and, as in NIFID, they are variably positive for ubiquitin, but, unlike in NIFID, they are negative for α-internexin or neurofilament.

FUS belongs to the family of FET proteins, which also includes Ewing's sarcoma protein (EWS) and TATA-binding protein-associated factor 15 (TAF15). The FUS-positive inclusions in all FTLD-FUS subtypes, but not those in ALS due to mutations in *FUS*, also contain EWS, TAF15, and transportin, which is responsible for the nuclear transport of the FET proteins.[88,89]

Frontotemporal lobar degeneration due to mutation in the *CHMP2B* (FTLD-UPS)

Mutations in charged multivesicular body protein 2B (*CHMP2B*) are associated with familial FTLD (90) with bvFTD and extrapyramidal symptoms.[91] In the Danish pedigree, the neuronal intracytoplasmic inclusions are ubiquitin-positive, but negative for TDP-43 and FUS.[92] CHMP2B is a component of the endosomal-sorting complex required for transport-III (ESCRT-III), which is involved in the degradation of proteins in the endocytic and autophagic pathways.

Clinicopathological correlations in frontotemporal dementia

Large clinicopathological series have allowed the identification of certain relatively specific associations.[57,80] SD is predominantly associated with the FTLD-TDP type C while FTD and MND/ALS with TDP-43 type B pathology. PNFA is most commonly due to a tauopathy, although can be caused by Alzheimer's disease. The

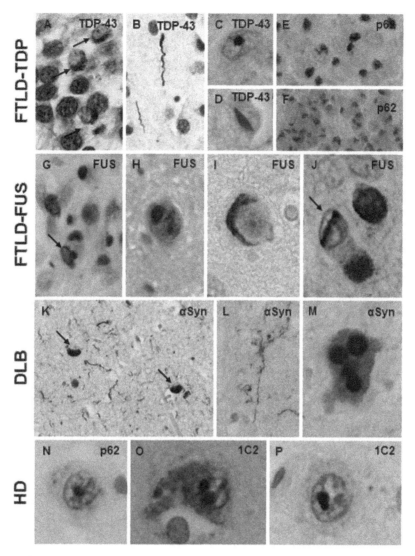

Fig. 29.3 Pathological characteristics of FTLD-TDP, FTLD-FUS, dementia with Lewy bodies, and Huntington's disease. A: The major microscopic TDP-43 immunoreactive lesion types are neuronal cytoplasmic inclusions (arrows), B: dystrophic neurites and C and D: neuronal intranuclear inclusions occurring in characteristic combinations in the different FTLD-TDP subtypes. E and F: In addition to TDP-43 positive inclusions, characteristic p62-positive 'star-like' neuronal cytoplasmic inclusions are also present in neurons of the granule cell layer of the dentate fascia (E) and the cerebellar granule cells (F) in cases carrying the *C9orf72* expansion repeat mutation. G–J: FTLD-FUS is characterized by the presence of FUS-positive neuronal cytoplasmic inclusions and neuronal intranuclear inclusions of different morphological subtypes (G–J). Please note that some neurons with cytoplasmic inclusions show preserved nuclear expression of the FUS protein (H) while this is lost in others (I). NIIs also show different morphological phenotypes (G and J, arrows) including ring-like and vermiform structures (G). K and L: The major microscopic feature of dementia with Lewy bodies and Parkinson's disease with dementia is the presence of extensive cortical Lewy pathology including Lewy bodies (K, arrows) and Lewy neurites (L). Multiple Lewy bodies are shown in a neuron of the substantia nigra in a case of Parkinson's disease with dementia (M). N: In Huntington's disease (HD) the intranuclear inclusions are readily demonstrated with p62 immunohistochemistry (N). The 1C2 antibody, recognizing expanded polyglutamine repeats, labels intranuclear inclusions, the neuronal cytoplasm of affected neurons (O and P), and dystrophic neurites (not shown) in HD.

bvFTD syndrome is almost equally associated with FTLD-tau and FTLD-TDP;[80] very young-onset (apparently sporadic) bvFTD is closely associated with FTLD-FUS.[57,80]

Of the familial FTLDs (see chapters 34 and 35), patients with a *MAPT* mutation most frequently present with bvFTD with or without associated parkinsonian signs. bvFTD may also be associated with SD in some cases.[80] The neuropathological finding in cases with a *GRN* mutation is FTLD-TPD type A and the clinical presentation may be bvFTD, PNFA, or corticobasal syndrome. Cases with *VCP* mutations present with bvFTD[93] as do those with *CHMP2B* mutations[91] or *TARDBP* mutations.[94] There is substantial clinical heterogeneity in cases with *C9orf72* mutation, although bvFTD has been documented in ~50 per cent and MND/ALS in 60 per cent of the cases.[95]

Dementia with Lewy bodies and Parkinson's disease with dementia

These common and closely related diseases are both α-synucleinopathies with widespread Lewy body pathology. Dementia with Lewy bodies (DLB) is the second most common neurodegenerative dementia in the elderly, and dementia is a common non-motor manifestation of late Parkinson's disease, for which the term Parkinson's disease with dementia (PDD) is used (see chapter 36).[96] Longitudinal studies indicate that about 50 per cent of Parkinson's disease patients at 15 years and more than 80 per cent at 20 years follow-up have dementia.[97] In PDD and DLB the clinical presentation may be similar; separation of the two disorders is arbitrarily based on the one-year rule. The guidelines of the DLB Consensus Consortium for clinical diagnosis have been prospectively validated, which included postmortem confirmation of diagnosis.[98]

DLB is a sporadic disorder, although the E46K point mutation and triplication of *SNCA* gene have been described to be associated with a DLB-like picture.[99] *SNCA* gene point mutations such as G51D[100] and duplication[101] are associated with a PDD clinical phenotype.

Neuropathological diagnosis

Diffuse cerebral atrophy may be seen and pallor of the substantia nigra and locus coeruleus is a feature. Atrophy of medial temporal lobe structures may indicate the presence of associated Alzheimer-type pathology.

The cardinal microscopic feature of both DLB and PDD is the presence of often widespread, including cortical, Lewy bodies (Fig. 29.3K and 29.3M) and Lewy neurites (Fig. 29.3L). The severity of the Lewy pathology has been found to correlate with the severity of dementia.[102,103] There are Consensus pathological guidelines for the diagnosis of DLB and the revised criteria require that the severity and distribution of Lewy type α-synuclein pathology are assessed in 10 different anatomical regions.

A case is finally categorized as belonging to one of three available categories, 'brainstem-predominant', limbic (transitional), and neocortical (diffuse). Aβ parenchymal plaques and neurofibrillary tangle tau pathology are consistently found in DLB[102] and comorbid Alzheimer-type pathology is also common in PDD.[104–106] This is also recognized by the DLB Consensus guidelines, and the probability that the clinical dementia is caused by Lewy pathology is dependent on the severity of the Alzheimer's disease-type pathology.[103] In PDD, a combination of cortical Lewy bodies, cortical Aβ plaques, and neurofibrillary pathology stages has been found to be the most robust neuropathological substrate of clinical dementia.[104] Data indicate that coexistent Lewy body and Alzheimer pathology may promote each other.[106,107]

A slightly modified diagnostic approach has been suggested for neuropathological assessment and clinicopathological correlations by the National Institute on Aging–Alzheimer's Association recent guidelines for the neuropathological assessment of Alzheimer's disease.[20] These also recommend that the overarching term 'Lewy body disease' is used for DLB and PDD and distinguish the brainstem, limbic, neocortical, and amygdala predominant categories. This latter is most commonly seen in association with Alzheimer's disease.

Huntington's disease

Huntington's disease is an autosomal dominantly inherited condition caused by an expanded CAG repeat in the N-terminus of the *HTT* gene resulting in an extended polyglutamine stretch in the huntingtin protein.[108]

Macroscopically, very early cases may be normal while advanced cases show atrophy of the entire brain and, in particular, of the neostriatum.[109] The scheme proposed by Vonsattel and colleagues is based on the macroscopic and microscopic pathology of the neostriatum and recognizes five different stages of disease progression.[110]

The most severe microscopic changes are seen in the neostriatum where the medium spiny neurons expressing encephalin and

dopamine D2 receptor in the striosomal compartment are the most vulnerable. Other basal ganglia structures and the cerebral cortex are also affected. Antibodies recognizing expanded polyglutamine stretches highlight widespread neuronal lesions, including intranuclear inclusions, cytoplasmic and neuritic aggregates (Fig. 29.3N-P).[109,111] The density of neocortical intranuclear inclusions correlates with the CAG repeat length.[112]

Conclusion

Identification of disease-associated proteins forming intracellular and, in some instances, extracellular aggregates has significantly contributed to understanding the pathological changes associated with each disease. Although no disease-modifying therapies are as yet available for neurodegenerative dementias, major aspects of their pathomechanisms have been clarified. Understanding mechanisms in one disease type may reveal pathways relevant to several disorders such as the novel concept of prion-like spread of α-synuclein pathology in Parkinson's disease or tau pathology in tauopathies. Clinicopathological studies have identified subgroups in some of the conditions such as Parkinson's disease, progressive supranuclear palsy, and FTLDs, which will be important when effects of potential disease modifying therapies are to be assessed.

References

1. Sieben A, Van Langenhove T, Engelborghs S, et al. The genetics and neuropathology of frontotemporal lobar degeneration. *Acta Neuropathol.* 2012;124(3):353–72. Epub 2012/08/15.
2. Ling H, O'Sullivan SS, Holton JL, et al. Does corticobasal degeneration exist? A clinicopathological re-evaluation. *Brain.* 2010;133(Pt 7):2045–57. Epub 2010/06/30.
3. Walker LC and LeVine H III. Corruption and spread of pathogenic proteins in neurodegenerative diseases. *J Biol Chem.* 2012;287(40):33109–15. Epub 2012/08/11.
4. Revesz T, Holton JL, Lashley T, et al. Genetics and molecular pathogenesis of sporadic and hereditary cerebral amyloid angiopathies. *Acta Neuropathol.* 2009;118(1):115–30.
5. Ross CA. Polyglutamine pathogenesis: emergence of unifying mechanisms for Huntington's disease and related disorders. *Neuron.* 2002;35(5):819–22. Epub 2002/10/10.
6. Rademakers R, Neumann M, and Mackenzie IR. Advances in understanding the molecular basis of frontotemporal dementia. *Nat Rev Neurol.* 2012;8(8):423–34. Epub 2012/06/27.
7. Goedert M and Jakes R. Mutations causing neurodegenerative tauopathies. *Biochim Biophys Acta.* 2005;1739(2–3):240–50. Epub 2004/12/24.
8. Ash PE, Bieniek KF, Gendron TF, et al. Unconventional translation of C9ORF72 GGGGCC expansion generates insoluble polypeptides specific to c9FTD/ALS. *Neuron.* 2013;77(4):639–46. Epub 2013/02/19.
9. Bras J, Guerreiro R, and Hardy J. Use of next-generation sequencing and other whole-genome strategies to dissect neurological disease. *Nat Rev Neurosci.* 2012;13(7):453–64. Epub 2012/06/21.
10. Selkoe DJ. Alzheimer's disease. *Cold Spring Harb Perspect Biol.* 2011;3(7). Epub 2011/05/18.
11. Halliday GM, Double KL, Macdonald V, et al. Identifying severely atrophic cortical subregions in Alzheimer's disease. *Neurobiol Aging.* 2003;24(6):797–806. Epub 2003/08/21.
12. Fox NC and Schott JM. Imaging cerebral atrophy: normal ageing to Alzheimer's disease. *Lancet.* 2004;363(9406):392–4. Epub 2004/04/13.
13. Braak H and Braak E. Neuropathological staging of Alzheimer-related changes. (Review). *Acta Neuropathol.* 1991;82(4):239–59.
14. Braak H, Alafuzoff I, Arzberger T, et al. Staging of Alzheimer disease-associated neurofibrillary pathology using paraffin sections and immunocytochemistry. *Acta Neuropathol.* 2006;112(4):389–404.

15. Thal DR, Rub U, Orantes M, *et al.* Phases of A beta-deposition in the human brain and its relevance for the development of AD. *Neurology.* 2002;58(12):1791–800. Epub 2002/06/27.

16. Montine TJ, Phelps CH, Beach TG, *et al.* National Institute on Aging–Alzheimer's Association guidelines for the neuropathologic assessment of Alzheimer's disease: a practical approach. *Acta Neuropathol.* 2012;123(1):1–11. Epub 2011/11/22.

17. Ellis RJ, Olichney JM, Thal LJ, *et al.* Cerebral amyloid angiopathy in the brains of patients with Alzheimer's disease: the CERAD experience, Part XV. *Neurology.* 1996;46(6):1592–6.

18. Thal DR, Ghebremedhin E, Rub U, *et al.* Two types of sporadic cerebral amyloid angiopathy. *J Neuropathol Exp Neurol.* 2002;61(3):282–93.

19. Thal DR, Griffin WS, de Vos RA, *et al.* Cerebral amyloid angiopathy and its relationship to Alzheimer's disease. *Acta Neuropathol.* 2008;115(6):599–609.

20. Hyman BT, Phelps CH, Beach TG, *et al.* National Institute on Aging–Alzheimer's Association guidelines for the neuropathologic assessment of Alzheimer's disease. *Alzheimers Dement.* 2012;8(1):1–13. Epub 2012/01/24.

21. Boche D, Denham N, Holmes C, *et al.* Neuropathology after active Abeta42 immunotherapy: implications for Alzheimer's disease pathogenesis. *Acta Neuropathol.* 2010;120(3):369–84. Epub 2010/07/16.

22. Vidal R, Frangione B, Rostagno A, *et al.* A stop-codon mutation in the BRI gene associated with familial British dementia. *Nature.* 1999;399(6738):776–81.

23. Vidal R, Revesz T, Rostagno A, *et al.* A decamer duplication in the 3' region of the BRI gene originates an amyloid peptide that is associated with dementia in a Danish kindred. *Proc Natl Acad Sci USA.* 2000;97(9):4920–5.

24. Plant GT, Revesz T, Barnard RO, *et al.* Familial cerebral amyloid angiopathy with nonneuritic amyloid plaque formation. *Brain.* 1990;113(3):721–47.

25. Holton JL, Ghiso J, Lashley T, *et al.* Regional Distribution of Amyloid-Bri Deposition and Its Association with Neurofibrillary Degeneration in Familial British Dementia. *Am J Pathol.* 2001;158(2):515–26.

26. Holton JL, Lashley T, Ghiso J, *et al.* Familial Danish dementia: a novel form of cerebral amyloidosis associated with deposition of both amyloid-Dan and amyloid-beta. *J Neuropathol Exp Neurol.* 2002;61(3):254–67.

27. Mackenzie IR, Neumann M, Baborie A, *et al.* A harmonized classification system for FTLD-TDP pathology. *Acta Neuropathol.* 2011;122(1):111–3. Epub 2011/06/07.

28. Halliday G, Bigio EH, Cairns NJ, *et al.* Mechanisms of disease in frontotemporal lobar degeneration: gain of function versus loss of function effects. *Acta Neuropathol.* 2012;124(3):373–82. Epub 2012/08/11.

29. Goedert M, Spillantini MG, Jakes R, *et al.* Multiple isoforms of human microtubule-associated protein-tau—sequences and localization in neurofibrillary tangles of Alzheimer's disease. *Neuron.* 1989;3:519–26.

30. Goedert M. Tau protein and neurodegeneration. *Semin Cell Dev Biol.* 2004;15(1):45–9.

31. Barker WW, Luis CA, Kashuba A, *et al.* Relative frequencies of Alzheimer disease, Lewy body, vascular and frontotemporal dementia, and hippocampal sclerosis in the State of Florida Brain Bank. *Alzheimer Dis Assoc Disord.* 2002;16(4):203–12. Epub 2002/12/07.

32. Dickson DW, Kouri N, Murray ME, *et al.* Neuropathology of frontotemporal lobar degeneration-tau (FTLD-tau). *J Mol Neurosci.* 2011;45(3):384–9. Epub 2011/07/02.

33. Buee L and Delacourte A. Comparative biochemistry of tau in progressive supranuclear palsy, corticobasal degeneration, FTDP-17 and Pick's disease. *Brain Pathol.* 1999;9(4):681–93. Epub 1999/10/12.

34. de Silva R, Lashley T, Gibb G, *et al.* Pathological inclusion bodies in tauopathies contain distinct complements of tau with three or four microtubule-binding repeat domains as demonstrated by new specific monoclonal antibodies. *Neuropathol Appl Neurobiol.* 2003;29(3):288–302. Epub 2003/06/06.

35. Kouri N, Whitwell JL, Josephs KA, *et al.* Corticobasal degeneration: a pathologically distinct 4R tauopathy. *Nat Rev Neurol.* 2011;7(5):263–72. Epub 2011/04/14.

36. Bergeron C, Pollanen MS, Weyer L, *et al.* Cortical degeneration in progressive supranuclear palsy. A comparison with cortical-basal ganglionic degeneration. *J Neuropathol Exp Neurol.* 1997;56:726–34.

37. Dickson DW, Bergeron C, Chin SS, *et al.* Office of Rare Diseases neuropathologic criteria for corticobasal degeneration. *J Neuropathol Exp Neurol.* 2002;61(11):935–46. Epub 2002/11/15.

38. Ikeda K, Akiyama H, Iritani S, *et al.* Corticobasal degeneration with primary progressive aphasia and accentuated cortical lesion in superior temporal gyrus: case report and review. *Acta Neuropathol.* 1996;92:534–9.

39. Tokumaru AM, Saito Y, Murayama S, *et al.* Imaging-pathologic correlation in corticobasal degeneration. *Am J Neuroradiol.* 2009;30(10):1884–92. Epub 2009/10/17.

40. Tsuchiya K, Murayama S, Mitani K, *et al.* Constant and severe involvement of Betz cells in corticobasal degeneration is not consistent with pyramidal signs: a clinicopathological study of ten autopsy cases. *Acta Neuropathol.* 2005;109(4):353–66. Epub 2005/03/01.

41. Dickson DW, Hauw JJ, Agid Y, *et al.* Progressive Supranuclear Palsy and Corticobasal Degeneration. In: DW Dickson and RO Weller (eds). *Neurodegeneration: The Molecular Pathology of Dementia and Movement Disorders.* 2nd edn. Oxford: Wiley-Blackwell, 2011, pp. 135–55.

42. Wakabayashi K, Oyanagi K, Makifuchi T, *et al.* Corticobasal degeneration: etiopathological significance of the cytoskeletal alterations. *Acta Neuropathol.* 1994;87:545–53.

43. Feany MB and Dickson DW. Widespread cytoskeletal pathology characterizes corticobasal degeneration. *Am J Pathol.* 1995;146(6):1388–96. Epub 1995/06/01.

44. Ksiezak-Reding H, Morgan K, Mattiace LA, *et al.* Ultrastructure and biochemical composition of paired helical filaments in corticobasal degeneration. *Am J Pathol.* 1994;145:1496–508.

45. Ikeda K, Akiyama H, Arai T, *et al.* Glial tau pathology in neurodegenerative diseases: Their nature and comparison with neuronal tangles. *Neurobiol Aging.* 1998;19:S85–S91.

46. Komori T. Tau-positive glial inclusions in progressive supranuclear palsy, corticobasal degeneration and Pick's disease. *Brain Pathol.* 1999;9:663–79.

47. Hattori M, Hashizume Y, Yoshida M, *et al.* Distribution of astrocytic plaques in the corticobasal degeneration brain and comparison with tuft-shaped astrocytes in the progressive supranuclear palsy brain. *Acta Neuropathol.* 2003;106(2):143–9.

48. Williams DR, de Silva R, Paviour DC, *et al.* Characteristics of two distinct clinical phenotypes in pathologically proven progressive supranuclear palsy: Richardson's syndrome and PSP-parkinsonism. *Brain.* 2005;128(Pt 6):1247–58.

49. Dickson DW, Ahmed Z, Algom AA, *et al.* Neuropathology of variants of progressive supranuclear palsy. *Curr Opin Neurol.* 2010;23(4):394–400. Epub 2010/07/09.

50. Ling H, de Silva R, Massey LA, *et al.* Characteristics of progressive supranuclear palsy presenting with corticobasal syndrome: a cortical variant. *Neuropathol Appl Neurobiol.* 2013. Epub 2013/02/26.

51. Tsuboi Y, Josephs KA, Boeve BF, *et al.* Increased tau burden in the cortices of progressive supranuclear palsy presenting with corticobasal syndrome. *Mov Disord.* 2005;20(8):982–8.

52. Donker Kaat L, Boon AJ, Kamphorst W, *et al.* Frontal presentation in progressive supranuclear palsy. *Neurology.* 2007;69(8):723–9. Epub 2007/08/22.

53. Hassan A, Parisi JE, and Josephs KA. Autopsy-proven progressive supranuclear palsy presenting as behavioral variant frontotemporal dementia. *Neurocase.* 2011. Epub 2011/12/21.

54. Josephs KA, Boeve BF, Duffy JR, *et al.* Atypical progressive supranuclear palsy underlying progressive apraxia of speech and nonfluent aphasia. *Neurocase.* 2005;11(4):283–96.

55. Josephs KA, Petersen RC, Knopman DS, *et al.* Clinicopathologic analysis of frontotemporal and corticobasal degenerations and PSP. *Neurology.* 2006;66(1):41–8.

56. Josephs KA and Duffy JR. Apraxia of speech and nonfluent aphasia: a new clinical marker for corticobasal degeneration and progressive supranuclear palsy. *Curr Opin Neurol.* 2008;21(6):688–92. Epub 2008/11/08.

57. Rohrer JD, Lashley T, Schott JM, *et al.* Clinical and neuroanatomical signatures of tissue pathology in frontotemporal lobar degeneration. *Brain.* 2011;134(Pt 9):2565–81. Epub 2011/09/13.

58. Dickson DW, Rademakers R, and Hutton ML. Progressive supranuclear palsy: pathology and genetics. *Brain Pathol.* 2007;17(1):74–82. Epub 2007/05/12.

59. Ishihara K, Araki S, Ihori N, *et al.* Argyrophilic grain disease presenting with frontotemporal dementia: a neuropsychological and pathological study of an autopsied case with presenile onset. *Neuropathology.* 2005;25(2):165–70. Epub 2005/05/07.

60. Ferrer I, Santpere G, and van Leeuwen FW. Argyrophilic grain disease. *Brain.* 2008;131(Pt 6):1416–32. Epub 2008/02/01.

61. Saito Y, Ruberu NN, Sawabe M, *et al.* Staging of argyrophilic grains: an age-associated tauopathy. *J Neuropathol Exp Neurol.* 2004;63(9):911–8.

62. Kovacs GG, Majtenyi K, Spina S, *et al.* White matter tauopathy with globular glial inclusions: a distinct sporadic frontotemporal lobar degeneration. *J Neuropathol Exp Neurol.* 2008;67(10):963–75. Epub 2008/09/19.

63. Josephs KA, Katsuse O, Beccano-Kelly DA, *et al.* Atypical progressive supranuclear palsy with corticospinal tract degeneration. *J Neuropathol Exp Neurol.* 2006;65(4):396–405. Epub 2006/05/13.

64. Fu YJ, Nishihira Y, Kuroda S, *et al.* Sporadic four-repeat tauopathy with frontotemporal lobar degeneration, Parkinsonism, and motor neuron disease: a distinct clinicopathological and biochemical disease entity. *Acta Neuropathol.* 2010;120(1):21–32. Epub 2010/02/09.

65. Ahmed Z, Doherty KM, Silveira-Moriyama L, *et al.* Globular glial tauopathies (GGT) presenting with motor neuron disease or frontotemporal dementia: an emerging group of 4-repeat tauopathies. *Acta Neuropathol.* 2011;122(4):415–28. Epub 2011/07/21.

66. Spillantini MG and Goedert M. Tau pathology and neurodegeneration. *Lancet Neurol.* 2013;12(6):609–22. Epub 2013/05/21.

67. Ghetti B, Wszolek EK, Boeve BF, *et al.* Frontotemporal Dementia and Parkinsonism Linked to Chromosome 17. In: DW Dickson and RO Weller (eds). *Neurodegeneration: The Molecular Pathology of Dementia and Movement Disorders.* 2nd edn. Oxford: Wiley-Blackwell, 2011, pp. 110–34.

68. van Swieten JC, Stevens M, Rosso SM, *et al.* Phenotypic variation in hereditary frontotemporal dementia with tau mutations (in process citation). *Ann Neurol.* 1999;46(4):617–26.

69. Spillantini MG, Crowther RA, and Goedert M. Comparison of the neurofibrillary pathology in Alzheimer's disease and familial presenile dementia with tangles. *Acta Neuropathol.* 1996;92:42–8.

70. Goedert M. Tau gene mutations and their effects. *Mov Disord.* 2005;20 Suppl 12:S45-S52.

71. Neumann M, Sampathu DM, Kwong LK, *et al.* Ubiquitinated TDP-43 in frontotemporal lobar degeneration and amyotrophic lateral sclerosis. *Science.* 2006;314(5796):130–3.

72. Mackenzie IR, Neumann M, Bigio EH, *et al.* Nomenclature for neuropathologic subtypes of frontotemporal lobar degeneration: consensus recommendations. *Acta Neuropathol.* 2009;117(1):15–8. Epub 2008/11/19.

73. Mackenzie IR, Neumann M, Bigio EH, *et al.* Nomenclature and nosology for neuropathologic subtypes of frontotemporal lobar degeneration: an update. *Acta Neuropathol.* 2010;119(1):1–4. Epub 2009/11/20.

74. Lagier-Tourenne C, Polymenidou M, *et al.* TDP-43 and FUS/TLS: emerging roles in RNA processing and neurodegeneration. *Hum Mol Genet.* 2010;19(R1):R46-R64.

75. Mackenzie IR, Rademakers R, and Neumann M. TDP-43 and FUS in amyotrophic lateral sclerosis and frontotemporal dementia. *Lancet Neurol.* 2010;9(10):995–1007.

76. Arai T, Hasegawa M, Akiyama H, *et al.* TDP-43 is a component of ubiquitin-positive tau-negative inclusions in frontotemporal lobar degeneration and amyotrophic lateral sclerosis. *Biochem Biophys Res Commun.* 2006;351(3):602–11.

77. Neumann M, Kwong LK, Truax AC, *et al.* TDP-43-positive white matter pathology in frontotemporal lobar degeneration with ubiquitin-positive inclusions. *J Neuropathol Exp Neurol.* 2007;66(3):177–83.

78. Brandmeir NJ, Geser F, Kwong LK, *et al.* Severe subcortical TDP-43 pathology in sporadic frontotemporal lobar degeneration with motor neuron disease. *Acta Neuropathol.* 2008;115(1):123–31. Epub 2007/11/16.

79. Hatanpaa KJ, Bigio EH, Cairns NJ, *et al.* TAR DNA-binding protein 43 immunohistochemistry reveals extensive neuritic pathology in FTLD-U: a Midwest-Southwest consortium for FTLD study. *J Neuropathol Exp Neurol.* 2008;67(4):271–9. Epub 2008/04/02.

80. Josephs KA, Hodges JR, Snowden JS, *et al.* Neuropathological background of phenotypical variability in frontotemporal dementia. *Acta Neuropathol.* 2011;122(2):137–53. Epub 2011/05/27.

81. Al-Sarraj S, King A, Troakes C, *et al.* p62 positive, TDP-43 negative, neuronal cytoplasmic and intranuclear inclusions in the cerebellum and hippocampus define the pathology of C9orf72-linked FTLD and MND/ALS. *Acta Neuropathol.* 2011;122(6):691–702. Epub 2011/11/22.

82. Neumann M, Rademakers R, Roeber S, *et al.* A new subtype of frontotemporal lobar degeneration with FUS pathology. *Brain.* 2009;132:2922–31.

83. Neumann M, Roeber S, Kretzschmar HA, *et al.* Abundant FUS-immunoreactive pathology in neuronal intermediate filament inclusion disease. *Acta Neuropathol.* 2009;118:605–16.

84. Munoz DG, Neumann M, Kusaka H, *et al.* FUS pathology in basophilic inclusion body disease. *Acta Neuropathol.* 2009 Nov;118(5):617–27.

85. Lashley T, Rohrer JD, Bandopadhyay R, *et al.* A comparative clinical, pathological, biochemical and genetic study of fused in sarcoma proteinopathies. *Brain.* 2011;134:2548–64. Epub 2011/07/15.

86. Josephs KA, Holton JL, Rossor MN, *et al.* Neurofilament inclusion body disease: a new proteinopathy? *Brain.* 2003;126(Pt 10):2291–303. Epub 2003/07/24.

87. Cairns NJ, Uryu K, Bigio EH, *et al.* alpha-Internexin aggregates are abundant in neuronal intermediate filament inclusion disease (NIFID) but rare in other neurodegenerative diseases. *Acta Neuropathol.* 2004;108(3):213–23.

88. Brelstaff J, Lashley T, Holton JL, *et al.* Transportin1: a marker of FTLD-FUS. *Acta Neuropathol.* 2011;122(5):591–600. Epub 2011/08/19.

89. Neumann M, Bentmann E, Dormann D, *et al.* FET proteins TAF15 and EWS are selective markers that distinguish FTLD with FUS pathology from amyotrophic lateral sclerosis with FUS mutations. *Brain.* 2011;134(Pt 9):2595–609. Epub 2011/08/23.

90. Skibinski G, Parkinson NJ, Brown JM, *et al.* Mutations in the endosomal ESCRTIII-complex subunit CHMP2B in frontotemporal dementia. *Nat Genet.* 2005;37(8):806–8. Epub 2005/07/26.

91. Gydesen S, Brown JM, Brun A, *et al.* Chromosome 3 linked frontotemporal dementia (FTD-3). *Neurology.* 2002;59(10):1585–94. Epub 2002/11/27.

92. Holm IE, Isaacs AM, and Mackenzie IR. Absence of FUS-immunoreactive pathology in frontotemporal dementia linked to chromosome 3 (FTD-3) caused by mutation in the CHMP2B gene. *Acta Neuropathol.* 2009;118(5):719–20. Epub 2009/10/22.

93. Watts GD, Wymer J, Kovach MJ, *et al.* Inclusion body myopathy associated with Paget disease of bone and frontotemporal dementia is caused by mutant valosin-containing protein. *Nat Genet.* 2004;36(4):377–81. Epub 2004/03/23.

94. Benajiba L, Le Ber I, Camuzat A, *et al.* TARDBP mutations in motoneuron disease with frontotemporal lobar degeneration. *Ann Neurol.* 2009;65(4):470–3. Epub 2009/04/08.

95. Mahoney CJ, Beck J, Rohrer JD, *et al.* Frontotemporal dementia with the C9ORF72 hexanucleotide repeat expansion: clinical, neuroanatomical and neuropathological features. *Brain.* 2012;135(Pt 3):736–50. Epub 2012/03/01.

96. Ince PG. Dementia with Lewy Bodies and Parkinson's Disease Dementia. In: DW Dickson and RO Weller (eds). *Neurodegeneration: The Molecular Pathology of Dementia and Movement Disorders,* 2nd edn. Oxford: Wiley-Blackwell, 2011, pp. 224–37.

97. Hely MA, Reid WG, Adena MA, *et al.* The Sydney multicenter study of Parkinson's disease: the inevitability of dementia at 20 years. *Mov Disord.* 2008;23(6):837–44. Epub 2008/03/01.

98. McKeith IG, Ballard CG, Perry RH, *et al.* Prospective validation of consensus criteria for the diagnosis of dementia with Lewy bodies. *Neurology.* 2000;54(5):1050–8.

99. Zarranz JJ, Alegre J, Gomez-Esteban JC, *et al.* The new mutation, E46K, of alpha-synuclein causes Parkinson and Lewy body dementia. *Ann Neurol.* 2004;55(2):164–73.

100. Kiely AP, Asi YT, Kara E, *et al.* alpha-Synucleinopathy associated with G51D SNCA mutation: a link between Parkinson's disease and multiple system atrophy? *Acta Neuropathol.* 2013;125(5):753–69. Epub 2013/02/14.

101. Ikeuchi T, Kakita A, Shiga A, *et al.* Patients homozygous and heterozygous for SNCA duplication in a family with parkinsonism and dementia. *Arch Neurol.* 2008;65(4):514–9. Epub 2008/04/17.

102. Lippa CF, Duda JE, Grossman M, *et al.* DLB and PDD boundary issues: diagnosis, treatment, molecular pathology, and biomarkers. *Neurology.* 2007;68(11):812–9.

103. McKeith IG, Dickson DW, Lowe J, *et al.* Diagnosis and management of dementia with Lewy bodies: third report of the DLB Consortium. *Neurology.* 2005;65(12):1863–72. Epub 2005/10/21.

104. Compta Y, Parkkinen L, O'Sullivan SS, *et al.* Lewy- and Alzheimer-type pathologies in Parkinson's disease dementia: which is more important? *Brain.* 2011;134(Pt 5):1493–505. Epub 2011/05/21.

105. Irwin DJ, White MT, Toledo JB, *et al.* Neuropathologic substrates of Parkinson disease dementia. *Ann Neurol.* 2012;72(4):587–98. Epub 2012/10/06.

106. Lashley T, Holton JL, Gray E, *et al.* Cortical alpha-synuclein load is associated with amyloid-beta plaque burden in a subset of Parkinson's disease patients. *Acta Neuropathol.* 2008;115(4):417–25. Epub 2008/01/11.

107. Brown DF, Dababo MA, Bigio EH, *et al.* Neuropathologic evidence that the Lewy body variant of Alzheimer disease represents coexistence of Alzheimer disease and idiopathic Parkinson disease. *J Neuropathol Exp Neurol.* 1998;57:39–46.

108. Bates GP. History of genetic disease: the molecular genetics of Huntington disease—a history. *Nat Rev Genet.* 2005;6(10):766–73. Epub 2005/09/02.

109. Hedreen JC and Roos RAC. Huntington's Disease. In: DW Dickson and RO Weller (eds). *Neurodegeneration: The Molecular Pathology of Dementia and Movement Disorders*, 2nd edn. Oxford: Wiley-Blackwell, 2011, pp. 258–72.

110. Vonsattel JP, Myers RH, Stevens TJ, *et al.* Neuropathological classification of Huntington's disease. *J Neuropathol Exp Neurol.* 1985(44):559–77.

111. Ince PG, Clark B, Holton JL, *et al.* Disorders of Movement and System Degenerations. In: S Love, DN Louis, and DW Ellison (eds). *Greenfield's Neuropathology*, Vol 1. London: Arnold, 2008, pp. 889–1030.

112. Becher MW, Kotzuk JA, Sharp AH, *et al.* Intranuclear neuronal inclusions in Huntington's disease and dentatorubral and pallidoluysian atrophy: correlation between the density of inclusions and IT15 CAG triplet repeat length. *Neurobiol Dis.* 1998;4(6):387–97.

CHAPTER 30

Genetics of degenerative dementias

Rita Guerreiro and Jose Bras

Introduction

The adult-onset forms of degenerative dementias are said to be sporadic. In reality these diseases, from which Alzheimer's disease (AD) is the most common, are complex disorders, most probably resulting from a combination of genetic and environmental factors. A small proportion of dementia cases have a familial basis and early onset. Most of these cases have a well-defined molecular genetic lesion and pattern of inheritance. However, some atypical situations are known to occur and we are still learning how to interpret genetic variability and how to use genetic risk factors to predict disease (see Box 30.1, Fig. 30.1).

The identification of genes associated with different forms of dementia, and particularly the identification of genes causative for mendelian forms, was an essential first step for the understanding of the molecular pathological processes underlying these diseases.

Over the past three decades different genetic techniques have been used to identify genes associated with dementias. Recently the development and implementation of new genotyping and sequencing technologies have allowed the interrogation of the whole genome with an unprecedented resolution. We are now able to detect more subtle genetic effects by replacing or complementing the more traditional molecular techniques with these recently developed technologies Box 30.2.

The identification of dementia-associated genes has also led to an increased interest in the inclusion of genetic information in diagnosis, clinical evaluation, and management of dementias, which has emphasized the need for a deeper understanding of the multidimensional issues associated with genetic testing for dementias.

In this chapter we will briefly review the molecular techniques used in the field and the genes and genetic risk factors currently known to be associated with degenerative dementias. We will also discuss the gaps and uncertainties preventing the effective translation of genetic findings into the clinical practice.

Overview of recent genetic technologies

In the past decade, many of the advances in our understanding of the molecular aetiology of different dementias were tightly linked with the introduction of novel technologies.[1] In particular, the last five years has seen an almost exponential increase in our knowledge of genes involved in these diseases.

The most common type of genetic study prior to the introduction of these advances, were candidate gene case-control association studies. In these, researchers would select a gene of interest and test a few markers in that gene in a group of cases and a group of controls to determine if there was a difference in the frequency of those markers. If a marker was more frequently seen in cases than in controls,

---

Box 30.1 Causative mutations versus risk factors

Mendelian diseases are defined by the occurrence in families with a pattern (autosomal dominant or recessive and X-linked, see Fig. 30.1) that reflects the inheritance of mutations at an individual locus.

To understand mendelian inheritance one needs to collect detailed information on the family under study by correctly identifying which family members are affected and which ones are not. It is easier to identify a mendelian pattern of inheritance in multigenerational pedigrees than in families with a small number of cases, particularly if the information collected for the extended family is accurate and detailed.

Mendelian diseases are usually caused by mutations occurring in the coding part of the genome, more specifically in a gene. These 'disease genes' will normally have an important biological function that is abrogated or altered in some way by the mutation leading to the disease status.

Mutations are generally defined as variants that occur in the population with a frequency of less than 1 per cent, and polymorphisms as those variants occurring at a frequency greater than 1 per cent. Not all variants with a frequency below 1 per cent are pathogenic and not all polymorphisms are benign. The distinction between pathogenic and benign variants is not always clear. Currently the interpretation and prediction of the effects of genetic variants is one of the most studied topics in human genetics.

In addition to mendelian diseases, many common disorders have a genetic component. These disorders are referred to as complex, polygenic, or multifactorial conditions, and result from the combined action of multiple genes and environmental factors. In these cases, genetic variants are not causative of, but rather modulate (either increasing or decreasing) the risk for the development of the diseases.

It is not always easy to determine the type of transmission of a determined phenotype, with several factors such as genetic heterogeneity, variable expressivity, incomplete penetrance, and occurrence of *de novo* mutations contributing to a more complex evaluation.

(continued)

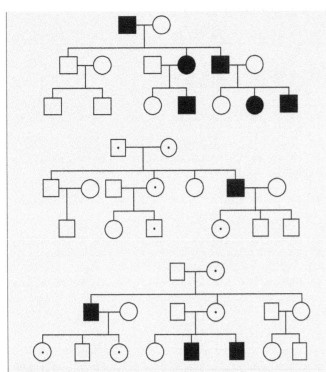

Fig. 30.1 Examples of inheritance patterns of mendelian diseases. From top to bottom: Autosomal dominant; autosomal recessive; X-linked recessive. Black symbols represent affected individuals; white symbols represent healthy family members, and a central dot in a symbol represents carriers.

Top panel: The autosomal dominant pattern of inheritance is the most common pattern for mendelian disorders. The disease occurs in both males and females and often affects many individuals throughout the pedigree. Inheritance of one copy of the affected gene is sufficient to cause disease and the risk of disease transmission from an affected individual is 50 per cent.

Middle panel: The autosomal recessive pattern of inheritance is also common and it occurs when two healthy individuals are carriers for the same recessive mutation. Typically, autosomal recessive mutations are rare, and affected individuals will often not present a family history of the disease, but when they do, all other affected individuals are in the same generation. The risk of disease transmission is 25 per cent, and half of the unaffected offspring will be carriers for the mutation. Given these characteristics, some times families can present with only one affected member that can be easily mistaken as sporadic.

Lower panel: X-linked recessive conditions usually occur only in males, while females are carriers (the second X chromosome in females provides a normal allele). Occasionally females can also show a degree of affectedness. Female carriers will transmit the mutation to all their sons (they inherit only their mother's X chromosome and will become affected) and to half their daughters. Affected males will transmit the mutation to all their daughters (all of whom will be carriers). Sons of affected males receive only their father's Y chromosome, thus they will not inherit the disease.

Very rare examples also exist of inheritance in X-linked dominant and Y-linked patterns. Also of note, some inherited conditions (non-mendelian) are caused by mutations in the mitochondrial DNA. These often show maternal inheritance (reflecting the inheritance pattern of mitochondria).

derived from small cohorts, gene selection bias, and imperfect control selection, based on population genetic background differences (commonly referred to as population stratification) (for a thorough review see reference 2). With the exception of *APOE*, no other gene was replicated by a case-control study to be a bona-fide risk factor for AD. The same is true for Parkinson's disease, where the exception is *GBA*.[3]

The introduction of genome-wide genotyping (and the subsequent reduction in cost) completely changed the playing field for association studies. With this technology, researchers were able to test the complete genome in an (almost) unbiased manner. A large number of markers (currently > 1 million) was selected from the genome and samples were assayed for all markers in a single experiment. In the first iterations of these assays, the markers were selected largely based on how much information of the surrounding genetic landscape they could provide (e.g. because markers that are physically close together are generally more likely to be inherited together, a single marker can work as a proxy for others, allowing a researcher to test a single marker and still obtain information on a larger number of nearby genetic positions). The design of these assays was only possible thanks to the efforts of large-scale projects like the HapMap project and, later, the 1000Genomes project, which have created maps of genetic variability in the human population. More recently, and because of the continued development of these projects, it has become possible to design assays that include specific variants of interest and not only those that are proxies for surrounding markers. One of the most common array that makes use of this type of content is the Illumina ExomeChip that targets markers present almost exclusively in the coding portion of the genome.[4]. It was through genome-wide genotyping that researchers were able to conduct genome-wide association studies (GWAS). Here, all markers in those assays were tested in large numbers of cases and controls (usually > 2000 each), and the frequency of each one of those markers was compared between the two cohorts. When a marker's frequency was found to be statistically different between groups, the marker was considered to be associated with the development of disease. This approach has been widely used for a variety of diseases and results have allowed for a better understanding of the molecular pathways involved in those diseases; Alzheimer's disease is a prime example of the application of GWAS to improve our understanding of the molecular events involved in this pathology.[5–7]

The other remarkable advance in genomic technology was massively parallel sequencing (also called next-generation sequencing or sequencing by synthesis). It allowed researchers to move from sequencing ~500–1000 base pairs of the genome in one experiment to being able to sequence an entire human genome. An enormous amount of effort has been dedicated to applying this technology to the understanding of disease, with great success. However, there are two aspects that still prevent a more widely application of sequencing: the first is cost—it is currently very expensive to sequence large numbers of genomes; the second is interpretability—although our understanding of the human genome has grown greatly in the last years, we are still not able to interpret the vast majority of genetic variability in the context of human biology. Nevertheless, massively parallel sequencing has been at the basis of the identification of many rare causes of disease and this trend is expected to continue over the next few years.

These two technological advances have allowed us to start creating maps of the genetic architecture of disease: GWAS enabled us to identify common genetic variability that exerts small to moderate effects on phenotype, while sequencing allowed us to identify rare

it was said to be a risk factor. The main problem with this approach was the fact that a gene was pre-selected; this is particularly relevant in diseases for which the complete molecular pathobiological events are not fully understood. For the most part, these studies did not yield replicable results and most reports were, in fact, false positive findings variants with large effect sizes. It is likely that the era of GWAS is now coming to an end for many diseases; recently the largest studies for Parkinson's and Alzheimer's diseases were published and each contained over 70 000 individuals.[5,8] Any subsequent studies will face the law of diminishing returns where any large increase in sample size will only identify risk factors with very minute effects. On the other hand, sequencing of large numbers of individuals is only getting started. Over the next 10 years we will witness the identification of novel causative mutations and genetic risk factors for a variety of diseases. The issue then will be to understand how these genetic factors impart their effect on biological pathways and ultimately on disease.

Alzheimer's disease

Alzheimer's disease can have an early (when occurring before 65 years of age) or late (after 65 years) onset. It can also be hereditary (when the disease is present in several members of the same family) or sporadic. The most common form of the disease has a late-onset and is sporadic. The genetic study of the rarer familial, early-onset forms of disease has led to the identification of the genes currently known to cause mendelian forms of AD. These findings have also allowed the development of a hypothesis for the molecular pathogenesis of AD that is thought to apply to all forms of the disease (see following).

APP, PSEN1, and PSEN2

The use of traditional genetic linkage approaches to study multigenerational families with AD has led to the identification, in the early 1990s, of three genes associated with AD. Mutations in the amyloid precursor gene (*APP*),[9] the presenilin 1 (*PSEN1*),[10] and the presenilin 2 (*PSEN2*)[11,12] genes are mainly associated with early-onset and familial forms of the disease. The most commonly mutated gene in AD is *PSEN1* with over 200 mutations identified so far.[13] Mutations

in this gene are fully penetrant and present an age at onset ranging from 24–78 years. The second more commonly mutated gene is *APP*, associated with ages at onset ranging from 30–75 years. Mutations in *PSEN2* are rarer when compared with the other two genes. Ages at onset associated with *PSEN2* mutations range from 44–80 years of age. Figure 30.2 represents a practical approach for genetic testing of patients with a familial form of AD, noting that next-generation sequencing is emerging as a means of assessing multiple genes concurrently and at far lower costs than conventional sequencing. From a clinical point of view, early-onset AD and late-onset AD are similar entities and alterations in any of these genes may, theoretically, have implications for both forms of the disease.

Mutations in these three genes usually have a typical autosomal dominant pattern of inheritance, however one recessive mutation (p.A673V) in *APP* has been identified with dominant-negative effect on amyloidogenesis.[21] Recently, a rare variant in the same amino acid position (p.A673T) was shown to result in an approximately 40 per cent reduction in the formation of amyloidogenic peptides *in vitro* and consequently reported as protective for the risk of development of AD.[22] The p.A673T protective variant seems to be primarily found in Northern Europe, particularly in the Icelandic and Scandinavian populations, being extremely rare in other populations.[23] If independently replicated, the finding of such a protective effect has major implications for AD: (1) it links for the first time both early- and late-onset forms of AD; (2) it provides important evidence to support the amyloid cascade hypothesis of AD; and (3) it has substantial implications for the development of new drug therapies aimed at reducing APP β-cleavage (beta secretase (BACE) activity), thereby reducing production of toxic amyloidogenic Aβ peptides.

All pathogenic point mutations identified in *APP* are located in exons 16 or 17, which correspond to the amyloid beta portion of the full amyloid precursor protein. In addition to early-onset AD, these mutations are known to cause other related phenotypes: cerebral amyloid angiopathy and hereditary cerebral haemorrhage with amyloidosis.[20] In addition to missense mutations, AD has been found to be caused by chromosomal duplications that include the *APP* locus. These quantitative changes were also linked to cerebral amyloid angiopathy and hereditary cerebral haemorrhage with amyloidosis.[14]

It is important to recognize that not all genetic variants present in these genes will invariably lead to dementia. Several mutations (classified as such because they have a frequency of less than 1 per cent in the general population) may be benign, with no deleterious effects in the function of the respective protein. Other changes may be frequent enough to be considered polymorphisms. Polymorphisms are usually not pathogenic but may contribute to the risk of developing the disease (either protective or pathologic).[17]

One of the main factors preventing the inclusion of genetic testing in the diagnosis and clinical management of early-onset AD patients is the true pathogenicity of mutations found on these genes. The evaluation of the pathogenicity of these variants is of extreme importance but in some cases very difficult or even impossible to accomplish. Several attempts to predict the effect of these variants have been devised, but still the most precise assessment of pathogenicity comes from the combination of segregation analyses (where several members of the family are tested and the variant is said to be pathogenic if present in affected and absent in unaffected family members) and functional analyses (where the amyloidogenic effect of the specific mutation is tested in cell lines, for example). Pathogenicity has wrongly been attributed to some variants

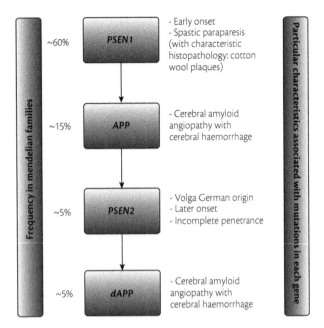

Fig. 30.2 Strategy for the screening of mutations in the known AD mendelian genes. If a patient/family presents any of the characteristics shown in the right part of the figure, the sequence of genes to be analysed should be adjusted accordingly. When a mutation is found in one of these genes, it should be determined if it is a novel mutation or if it has been previously described. This can be done by checking the Alzforum mutations database (<http://www.alzforum.org/mutations>). If the mutation found is deemed to be novel, one needs to evaluate its pathogenicity, as it may be a variant with no clinical significance. A systematic decision tree can be used to evaluate the probable pathogenicity of such variants.[13–20] dAPP:duplication of the *APP* locus.

identified in these genes. Although these variants cannot be considered as the cause of disease in the cases where they are found, they can increase the risk for the development of AD.[17]

Genetic risk factors in AD

The linkage analyses of multigenerational families used to identify AD causative genes have also identified a strong risk factor for the development of the disease. The E4 allele of the apolipoprotein E (*APOE*) gene is the strongest risk factor for all forms of AD.[24,25] This effect has been consistently replicated by different groups in many populations (Table 30.1).

The development of whole-genome genotyping platforms has allowed the identification of common genetic variants with low effects in the risk for the development of the late-onset form of AD (Table 30.2). Although exerting small effects in the risk for disease, these variants have been essential to uncovering the molecular pathways underlying the aetio-pathogenic processes of the disease. The three main pathways identified so far have been the 1) immunological/inflammatory response, 2) endocytosis (clathrin mediated and synaptic), and 3) cholesterol and lipid metabolism.[27]

More recently the integration of whole-genome sequencing and genotyping techniques allowed the identification of a rare variant (p.R47H) in *TREM2* that was shown to increase the risk for AD with odds ratio of ~3. In addition to being the strongest risk factor for AD after APOE, this finding also confirmed the involvement of immunological and inflammatory pathways in the beginning of the pathological processes.[28,29]

The analyses of AD cases and controls at the whole-genome level has led to the identification of other rare variants associated with the disease (in genes: *AKAP9, PLD3, UNC5C*).[30,31] None of these has yet been independently replicated and it is expected that at least some will be deemed as false positives by future analyses.

Molecular pathways identified by genetic findings

The amyloid cascade hypothesis was proposed in 1991 and suggested that the alterations caused by mutations in *APP* to the amyloid beta metabolism were the initiating events of a series of steps leading to the full development of dementia.[32] These steps include the aggregation of Aβ, formation of neuritic plaques and NFTs, disruption of synaptic connections, neuronal death and dementia. Since its proposal, the amyloid cascade hypothesis has been improved, changed, and extended with the inclusion of other factors now known to be part of the molecular signature of AD, and many different versions of the amyloid cascade are used today (see Fig. 30.3).[33] This is still the main hypothesis forming a framework for AD research, allowing for several new research questions to be formulated. The identification of mutations in *APP*, and later *PSEN1* and *PSEN2*, were the first and essential observations for the formulation of the first possible molecular pathway in AD. As discussed, findings from genome-wide association studies and exome sequencing have identified a large number low risk genetic loci which nonetheless provide important clues to pathogenesis, implicating cholesterol and lipid metabolism, immune system and inflammatory responses, and vesicle transport and endocytosis. How these various pathways interact with one another and with environmental factors to cause clinical AD is the subject of intense current research.

Frontotemporal dementia

Frontotemporal dementia (FTD) is an umbrella term used to cover a range of specific diseases. These disorders are characterized by progressive degeneration of the frontal and/or temporal lobes. Clinically, FTD is characterized by a progressive degradation in behaviour, speech, or language. Usually, memory and visuospatial functions are relatively spared. It can be subdivided into three clinical subtypes: 1) behavioural-variant frontotemporal dementia;

Table 30.1 Different genotypes at the rs429358 and rs7412 single nucleotide polymorphisms (SNPs), respective *APOE* alleles, and odds ratios (OR) for developing AD

APOE genotype	rs429358	rs7412	OR
E2/E2	TT	TT	0.23
E2/E3	TT	TC	0.32
E2/E4	TC	TC	1.23
E3/E3	TT	CC	0.50
E3/E4	TC	CC	1.79
E4/E4	CC	CC	6.90

Reproduced from *Hum Mol Genet*. 19(16), Corneveaux JJ, Myers AJ, Allen AN, *et al*. Association of CR1, CLU, and PICALM with Alzheimer's disease in a cohort of clinically characterized and neuropathologically verified individuals, pp. 3295–301, Copyright (2010), with permission from Oxford University Press.

Table 30.2 Genetic risk factors for Alzheimer's disease

Gene official symbol	Gene name	Location
Risk genes		
APOE	Apolipoprotein E	19q13.2
TREM2	Triggering receptor expressed on myeloid cells 2	6p21.1
Risk loci		
CLU	Clusterin	8p21–p12
PICALM	Phosphatidylinositol binding clathrin assembly protein	11q14
CR1	Complement component (3b/4b) receptor 1 (Knops blood group)	1q32
BIN1	Bridging integrator 1	2q14
MS4A6A	Membrane-spanning 4-domains, subfamily A, member 6A	11q12.1
MS4A4E	Membrane-spanning 4-domains, subfamily A, member 4E	11q12.2
CD33	CD33 molecule	19q13.3
ABCA7	ATP-binding cassette, subfamily A (ABC1), member 7	19p13.3
CD2AP	CD2-associated protein	6p12
EPHA1	EPH receptor A1	7q34
HLA-DRB5 and DRB1	Major histocompatibility complex, class II, DR beta 5 and DR beta 1	6p21.3
SORL1	Sortilin-related receptor, L(DLR class) A repeats containing	11q23.2–q24.2
PTK2B	Protein tyrosine kinase 2 beta	8p21.1
SLC24A4	Solute carrier family 24 (sodium/potassium/calcium exchanger), member 4	14q32.12
ZCWPW1	Zinc finger, CW type with PWWP domain 1	7q22.1
CELF1	CUGBP, Elav-like family member 1	11p11
FERMT2	Fermitin family member 2	14q22.1
CASS4	Cas scaffolding protein family member 4	20q13.31
INPP5D	Inositol polyphosphate-5-phosphatase, 145kDa	2q37.1
MEF2C	Myocyte enhancer factor 2C	5q14.3
NME8	NME/NM23 family member 8	7p14.1

2) progressive non-fluent aphasia; and 3) semantic dementia. Frontotemporal dementia is not only a heterogeneous syndrome from a clinical perspective, it also presents heterogeneous imaging features, neuropathology, and genetics. Additionally, it can overlap with other neurodegenerative diseases, mainly parkinsonism syndromes and motor neuron disease.[34,35] Family history of dementia and related disorders can be found in ~40–50 per cent of people with FTD, but only ~10–40 per cent will have an autosomal dominant pattern of inheritance.[36] The relation between mutations and the clinical subtype of FTD is not as strong as the relation with the neuropathology features of the different FTD subtypes, with mutations in one gene usually leading to one hystopathological subtype but possibly causing a range of different clinical phenotypes.[37,38]

Mutations in several genes are known to cause FTD, with mutations in the microtubule-associated tau (*MAPT*), Progranulin (*GRN*) and *C9orf72* being the most frequent and explaining ~80 per cent of familial FTD cases.[39] There are also several genes known to cause rarer forms of FTD and genes associated with FTD-plus syndromes.

MAPT, GRN, and C9ORF72

MAPT was the first gene to be discovered in association with FTD by means of positional cloning in families linked to chromosome 17 who presented with frontotemporal dementia and parkinsonism.[40] Currently, over 40 mutations in *MAPT* are represented in the AD/FTD mutation database.[15] Tau is a microtubule-binding protein able to modulate the stability of axonal microtubules and consequently the transport of organelles and other cellular components. Different tau proteins originate from the alternative splicing of the *MAPT* gene. Six of these isoforms are expressed in human brain and they differ in the number of microtubule-binding domains, which are encoded by the alternative splicing of exons 2, 3, and 10.[41] Mutations in *MAPT* can either cause a disruption in the structure of the tau protein, or they can alter the proportion of the different tau isoforms available. These changes lead to impaired microtubule assembly and impaired axonal transport, promoting pathological tau filament aggregation.[42,43]

Soon after the identification of *MAPT* it was recognized that many chromosome-17-linked FTD families did not have mutations in this gene and had a rather different neuropathology, presenting ubiquitin abnormalities and not tau-associated changes. These families were later found to carry mutations in *GRN*. Currently there are close to 70 mutations described in this gene, the vast majority being loss of function mutations associated with nonsense mediated decay of the mutant *GRN* mRNA and consequent reduced expression of the protein.[15,44,45] This allows for mutation carriers to be detected by measuring their serum concentration of GRN.[46] Although the exact role of progranulin in the neurodegenerative processes occurring in FTD is not clear, granulins are known to be a family of secreted, glycosylated peptides involved in the regulation of cell growth. Recently, homozygous mutations in *GRN* were found to cause neuronal ceroid lipofuscinosis (NCL11).[47] Given the well-established link between NCL and proteins affecting the lysosomal processing, these results associating *GRN* mutations with a form of NCL suggest that progranulin has a lysosomal function.[48]

The last gene harbouring common mutations in FTD to be identified was *C9ORF72*, in several families presenting linkage to chromosome 9 and a phenotype of FTD, ALS, or FTD/ALS.[49,50] Even though many chromosome 9-linked families were studied for a long period of time, the gene underlying the disease in these cases remained elusive for several years. This happened because the mutation found to be the cause of disease in these cases was not a typical coding variant but was instead an intronic GGGGCC hexanucleotide repeat expansion. The typical pathogenic *C9ORF72* expansions have hundreds of repeats (usually ranging from 400 to more than 4 400 repeats on one allele), with healthy controls usually having less than 30 repeats. Exceptions occur with individuals harbouring more than 30 repeats not presenting any cognitive changes: pathogenicity of the intermediate range (from around 20–100 repeats)

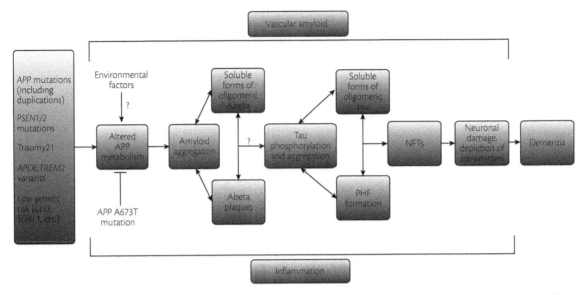

Fig. 30.3 Amyloid cascade hypothesis. This hypothesis supports the idea that amyloid-β (Aβ) peptide plays a central and probably causative role in Alzheimer's disease. It was originally developed for familial forms of AD, but it is possibly transversal to all forms of the disease (as depicted here). All three AD mendelian genes are involved in amyloid-β production. Other genetic, environmental, vascular, and inflammatory factors probably also play a part in the pathogenesis of Alzheimer's disease in general. The amyloid peptide is cleaved from its precursor protein and deposited as senile plaques. Brains with AD typically harbour senile plaques consisting of insoluble aggregates of Aβ. Different assemblies of Aβ, including fibrils, soluble dimers, trimers, and dodecamers, may differentially contribute to AD pathogenesis. Senile plaques trigger oxidative injury and synaptic loss; these, in turn, bring about hyperphosphorylation of tau protein, which leads to formation of tangles, triggering widespread neuronal dysfunction and dementia.
APP: amyloid precursor protein; NFT: neurofibrillary tangles; PHF: paired helical filaments.

continues unproven and although penetrance is probably high by age 80, partial penetrance has been proposed.[51,52] Somatic instability can cause variability in the expansions sizes in the same tissue between patients and between tissues in one patient.[53] Although the function of the C9orf72 protein is still unclear, the results of sensitive homology suggested that it may be related to differentially expressed in normal and neoplastic (DENN)-like proteins, which act as GDP/GTP exchange factors that activate Rab-GTPases. In this way, C9orf72 is predicted to regulate vesicular trafficking in conjunction with Rab-GTPases.[54]

Rare genetic causes of FTD

Mutations in *MAPT*, *GRN*, and *C9ORF72* cause disease associated with an autosomal dominant pattern of inheritance. Similarly, a mutation in *CHMP2B* has been found in a large autosomal dominant Danish frontotemporal dementia family. Mutation of this gene is very rare and associate with unusual ubiquitin-positive but TDP-negative and FUS-negative pathological abnormalities.[55]

Recently, mutations in *TREM2* have been found to be the cause of FTD in families presenting an autosomal recessive form of disease.[56] Mutations in *TREM2* were originally found to cause Nasu–Hakola disease, a rare form of dementia characterized by the presence of bone cysts and fractures.[57] Several families have now been identified with *TREM2* mutations but without any bone-related phenotypes, presenting only what resembles behavioural FTD.[58,59] Additionally, *PRKAR1B* was identified as the cause of an FTD-like neurodegenerative disorder with a unique neuropathological phenotype, displaying abundant neuronal inclusions by haematoxylin and eosin staining throughout the brain with immunoreactivity for intermediate filaments.[60]

The presence of linkage in some families with FTD associated with other disorders (mainly motor neuron disease) has also led to the identification of mutations in other genes (*VCP*, *CHCHD10*, *SQSTM1*, *UBQLN2*, and *OPTN*) in which mutations are rare. Some ALS genes (*FUS*, *TARDBP*) have also been found mutated in FTD cases, but the genetic evidence for the segregation of mutations in these genes with FTD is not strong.[34]

Genetic risk factors in FTD

Genome-wide association studies have recently identified two loci associated with FTD (Table 30.3). The first GWAS was performed on FTD patients with TDP-43 pathology and identified a genome-wide associated locus at 7p21 with the strongest associated SNPs lying in or close to *TMEM106B*.[61] The second finding resulted from a two-stage GWAS on clinical FTD where separate association analyses were performed for each FTD subtype (behavioural variant FTD, semantic dementia, progressive non-fluent aphasia, and FTD overlapping with motor neuron disease) as well as a meta-analysis of the entire dataset. The authors identified a genome-wide associated locus at 6p21.3 (HLA locus) in the subtype meta-analysis and a suggestive association at 11q14 (including *RAB38* and *CTSC*) for the behavioural FTD subtype.[62] The use of subphenotypes in this GWAS also allowed the identification of a strong association between the *C9ORF72* locus and the FTD-MND subgroup.[62,63] Ataxin-2 polyglutamine expansions with intermediate repeat sizes (≥ 29 CAG) have also been recently associated with FTD-MND.[64] Diekstra and colleagues used GWAS data on ALS and FTD-TDP cases, performed a joint meta-analysis and replicated the most associated hits of one disease in the other to identify the *C9ORF72* locus and one SNP in *UNC13A* (rs12608932, 19p13.11) as shared susceptibility loci between ALS and FTD-TDP.[65] Subsequently, rs12608932 in *UNC13A* was found to be a significant

Table 30.3 Genetic risk genes and loci for frontotemporal dementia

Gene official symbol	Gene name	Location
TMEM106B	Transmembrane protein 106B	7p21.3
HLA	Human leukocyte antigen locus	6p21.3
C9orf72*	Chromosome 9 open reading frame 72	9p21.2
UNC13A/ KCNN1*	Unc-13 homolog A (C. elegans)/potassium channel, calcium-activated intermediate/ small conductance subfamily N alpha, member 1	19p13.11/ 19p13.1
ATXN2*	Ataxin 2	12q24.1

*Loci mainly associated with FTD-MND.

exon-level cis-eQTL for *KCNN1* in frontal cortex, with region-specific eQTL data indicating *KCNN1* instead of *UNC13A* as the most probable relevant gene at this locus.[66]

A GWAS of plasma GRN levels in a cohort of healthy controls has led to the identification of two SNPs in chromosome 1p13.3 (near *SORT1*) with genome-wide significant association with plasma GRN levels. This can be considered a possible risk locus for FTD under the hypothesis that factors associated with reduced levels of plasma GRN can increase the risk of developing FTD.[67]

A rare variant (p.A152T) in *MAPT* has also been shown to be a risk factor for frontotemporal dementia spectrum disorders,[68] with different studies describing carriers with phenotypes comprising progressive supranuclear palsy, bvFTD, nonfluent variant primary progressive aphasia, corticobasal syndrome, Parkinson's disease, and clinical Alzheimer's disease.[69,70]

Dementia with Lewy bodies

Lewy bodies (LB) are commonly known as the neuropathological hallmark of Parkinson's disease (PD). They are protein inclusions, formed of insoluble polymers of alpha-synuclein that are present in the neuronal body, forming round lamellated eosinophilic cytoplasmic inclusions.[71]

DLB shares significant phenotypical characteristics with PD and AD; additionally, the disease can also present in a very similar fashion to PD with dementia (PDD), differing only in the earliest symptoms. There is no molecular data that allows for a distinction between DLB and PDD.[72]

There is limited information on the genetic aspects of DLB, mainly because there have been only a few sufficiently powered genetic studies performed to date.

DLB is mainly considered to be a sporadic disease. However, as with other neurodegenerative diseases, the fact that disease onset generally occurs late in life means that in many cases, there are no longer living relatives from previous generations which can lead to cases being potentially mislabelled as sporadic.

Rare cases of aggregation of the disease in families have been identified. To date, there has been a single genome-wide linkage study for DLB. Looking at an autosomal dominant family with autopsy-confirmed DLB, the authors identified a region on chromosome 2 that segregated with the disease.[73] However, follow-up studies searching for pathogenic mutations in the linked locus did not identify a single candidate mutation that could be responsible for the phenotype in that family.[74] It is not clear if the linkage pointed to the wrong locus or if the causal mutation is

complex and thus more difficult to identify than the typical pathogenic mutation (e.g. a mutation similar to those seen in *C9ORF72* FTD/ALS would be difficult to identify using standard methodologies).

The gene encoding the protein alpha-synuclein is currently the only replicated genetic cause of DLB. *SNCA* triplications and the missense mutations p.E46K and p.A53T are associated with clinical and pathological phenotypes ranging from PD to PD with dementia to DLB.

Other studies have attempted to identify pathogenic mutations in kindreds presenting with DLB, particularly looking at genes known to be involved in PD or AD, but so far no segregating mutations have been identified.[75]

The search for genetic risk factors of DLB has been slightly more productive. *APOE*, the strongest risk factor for AD, has also been shown by several groups to be a risk factor for DLB. This has been shown in clinical as well as in pathological confirmed cases.[76] It appears as though the association is virtually indistinguishable from that seen in AD, with the ε-4 allele increasing risk and the ε-2 alleles associated with a decreased risk for disease.[77]

More recently, the gene *GBA*, encoding the protein glucocerebrosidase, was also shown to modulate risk for DLB.[78] *GBA* encodes a lysosomal enzyme that is known to be the cause of a recessive lysosomal storage condition named Gaucher disease, however, when the same mutations are present in a single allele, they increase risk for DLB. This effect was initially identified in PD cases and later replicated in a large multi-centre cohort of DLB cases.

More recently, and through the application of recent genomic technologies, namely genome-wide genotyping, the first large-scale association in DLB was published.[79] In addition to being the largest study in DLB performed to date (700 cases), it also comprised a large number of neuropathologically diagnosed cases, strengthening the diagnostic accuracy and reducing the potential effects of mis-diagnosed samples. Here, the authors confirmed the association of *APOE* with DLB and further identified common genetic variability in *SNCA* to also be involved in disease. A third locus, encompassing the gene *SCARB2*, was identified, showing suggestive levels of association. *SCARB2*, which encodes yet another lysosomal protein, was known as a susceptibility gene for PD but had not been shown to be involved in DLB.

Both associations at *SNCA* and *SCARB2* loci were also seen in PD, however the association profiles in DLB seem to suggest that the associations are, in fact, different than the ones previously seen in PD. These results imply that although the same genes may be involved in both diseases, the manner in which they exert their pathobiological effect may be different. Despite these results, this report is based on a relatively small cohort and further studies are required to replicate these findings.

The results so far show that *APOE* is the strongest genetic risk factor for DLB, acting in a way that seems to be independent from amyloid processing. The involvement of *GBA* and *SCARB2* strongly argue for a role of the lysosome in the pathobiology of this disease, and since the protein α-synuclein has been shown to be degraded by the lysosome,[80] it is possible that this cellular organelle plays a pivotal role in this disease.

Conclusion

The last decade has seen remarkable advances in the identification of novel disease-causing genes and genetic risk factors for neurodegenerative diseases. These have largely been due to novel technological approaches and the accompanying reduction in cost for data generation.

These advances have allowed for unbiased studies that have linked, on a molecular level, diseases that are very dissimilar from a clinical perspective, suggesting that the current disease classification might be improved if these molecular data were to be taken into account. These results have also brought to light novel biological pathways involved in disease, which may, in the future, pave the way for new therapeutic approaches.

Over the next few years we will see these technologies mature and be more widely used in a diagnostic setting. This will be tremendously beneficial to the diagnostic process, where a single test—quick and comparatively inexpensive—will provide information for all genes, instead of clinicians having to perform an educated guess about which gene is more likely to be involved in that specific case. As more data are generated in research and diagnostic settings, we will be able to understand the pathobiology of each syndrome more fully since we will no longer be restricted to analysing only the known genes.

Great strides have also been made in the field of genetic risk prediction. We are now able to estimate the risk a given individual has to develop a neurodegenerative disease over the course of their life based on the genetic make-up of that person. This risk prediction is, however, incomplete, as more information needs to be taken into account to achieve a complete risk profile. We will need multi-scale biological approaches, integrating DNA, RNA, epigenetics, and environment to create adequate risk profiles. In this sense, large-scale, longitudinal studies will be key in allowing us to achieve this goal.

References

1. Bras J, Guerreiro R, and Hardy J. Use of next-generation sequencing and other whole-genome strategies to dissect neurological disease. *Nat Rev Neurosci.* 2012;13(7):453–64.

2. Zondervan KT and Cardon LR. Designing candidate gene and genome-wide case-control association studies. *Nature Protocols.* 2007;2(10):2492–501.

3. Sidransky E, Nalls MA, Aasly JO, *et al.* Multicenter analysis of glucocerebrosidase mutations in Parkinson's disease. *N Engl J Med.* 2009;361(17):1651–61.

4. Guo Y, He J, Zhao S, Wu H, *et al.* Illumina human exome genotyping array clustering and quality control. *Nature Protocols.* 2014;9(11):2643–62.

5. Lambert JC, Ibrahim-Verbaas CA, Harold D, *et al.* Meta-analysis of 74,046 individuals identifies 11 new susceptibility loci for Alzheimer's disease. *Nat Genet.* 2013;45(12):1452–8.

6. Hollingworth P, Harold D, Sims R, *et al.* Common variants at ABCA7, MS4A6A/MS4A4E, EPHA1, CD33 and CD2AP are associated with Alzheimer's disease. *Nat Genet.* 2011;43(5):429–35.

7. Lambert JC, Heath S, Even G, *et al.* Genome-wide association study identifies variants at CLU and CR1 associated with Alzheimer's disease. *Nat Genet.* 2009;41(10):1094–9.

8. Nalls MA, Pankratz N, Lill CM, *et al.* Large-scale meta-analysis of genome-wide association data identifies six new risk loci for Parkinson's disease. *Nat Genet.* 2014;46(9):989–93.

9. Goate A, Chartier-Harlin MC, Mullan M, *et al.* Segregation of a missense mutation in the amyloid precursor protein gene with familial Alzheimer's disease. *Nature.* 1991;349(6311):704–6.

10. Sherrington R, Rogaev EI, Liang Y, *et al.* Cloning of a gene bearing missense mutations in early-onset familial Alzheimer's disease. *Nature.* 1995;375(6534):754–60.

11. Rogaev EI, Sherrington R, Rogaeva EA, *et al.* Familial Alzheimer's disease in kindreds with missense mutations in a gene on chromosome 1 related to the Alzheimer's disease type 3 gene. *Nature.* 1995;376(6543):775–8.

12. Levy-Lahad E, Wasco W, Poorkaj P, *et al.* Candidate gene for the chromosome 1 familial Alzheimer's disease locus. *Science.* 1995;269(5226):973–7.

13. Raux G, Guyant-Marechal L, Martin C, *et al.* Molecular diagnosis of autosomal dominant early onset Alzheimer's disease: an update. *J Med Genet.* 2005;42(10):793–5.

14. Rovelet-Lecrux A, Hannequin D, Raux G, *et al.* APP locus duplication causes autosomal dominant early-onset Alzheimer disease with cerebral amyloid angiopathy. *Nat Genet.* 2006;38(1):24–6.

15. Cruts M, Theuns J, and Van Broeckhoven C. Locus-specific mutation databases for neurodegenerative brain diseases. *Hum Mutat.* 2012;33(9):1340–4.

16. Janssen JC, Beck JA, Campbell TA, *et al.* Early onset familial Alzheimer's disease: Mutation frequency in 31 families. *Neurology.* 2003;60(2):235–9.

17. Guerreiro RJ, Baquero M, Blesa R, *et al.* Genetic screening of Alzheimer's disease genes in Iberian and African samples yields novel mutations in presenilins and APP. *Neurobiol Aging.* 2010;31(5):725–31.

18. Jayadev S, Leverenz JB, Steinbart E, *et al.* Alzheimer's disease phenotypes and genotypes associated with mutations in presenilin 2. *Brain.* 2010;133(Pt 4):1143–54.

19. Karlstrom H, Brooks WS, Kwok JB, *et al.* Variable phenotype of Alzheimer's disease with spastic paraparesis. *J Neurochem.* 2008;104(3):573–83.

20. Roks G, Van Harskamp F, De Koning I, *et al.* Presentation of amyloidosis in carriers of the codon 692 mutation in the amyloid precursor protein gene (APP692). *Brain.* 2000;123 (Pt 10):2130–40.

21. Di Fede G, Catania M, Morbin M, *et al.* A recessive mutation in the APP gene with dominant-negative effect on amyloidogenesis. *Science.* 2009;323(5920):1473–7.

22. Jonsson T, Atwal JK, Steinberg S, *et al.* A mutation in APP protects against Alzheimer's disease and age-related cognitive decline. *Nature.* 2012;488(7409):96–9.

23. Wang LS, Naj AC, Graham RR, *et al.* Rarity of the Alzheimer Disease-Protective APP A673T Variant in the United States. *JAMA Neurol.* 2014.

24. Saunders AM, Strittmatter WJ, Schmechel D, *et al.* Association of apolipoprotein E allele epsilon 4 with late-onset familial and sporadic Alzheimer's disease. *Neurology.* 1993;43(8):1467–72.

25. Corder EH, Saunders AM, Strittmatter WJ, *et al.* Gene dose of apolipoprotein E type 4 allele and the risk of Alzheimer's disease in late onset families. *Science.* 1993;261(5123):921–3.

26. Corneveaux JJ, Myers AJ, Allen AN, *et al.* Association of CR1, CLU and PICALM with Alzheimer's disease in a cohort of clinically characterized and neuropathologically verified individuals. *Hum Mol Genet.* 2010;19(16):3295–301.

27. Jones L, Holmans PA, Hamshere ML, *et al.* Genetic evidence implicates the immune system and cholesterol metabolism in the aetiology of Alzheimer's disease. *PLoS One.* 2010;5(11):e13950.

28. Guerreiro R, Wojtas A, Bras J, *et al.* TREM2 variants in Alzheimer's disease. *N Engl J Med.* 2013;368(2):117–27.

29. Jonsson T, Stefansson H, Steinberg S, *et al.* Variant of TREM2 associated with the risk of Alzheimer's disease. *N Engl J Med* 2013;368(2):107–16.

30. Cruchaga C, Karch CM, Jin SC, *et al.* Rare coding variants in the phospholipase D3 gene confer risk for Alzheimer's disease. *Nature.* 2014;505(7484):550–4.

31. Logue MW, Schu M, Vardarajan BN, *et al.* Two rare AKAP9 variants are associated with Alzheimer's disease in African Americans. *Alzheimer's & Dementia.* 2014;10(6):609–18 e11.

32. Hardy J and Allsop D. Amyloid deposition as the central event in the aetiology of Alzheimer's disease. *Trends Pharmacol Sci.* 1991;12(10):383–8.

33. Haass C. Initiation and propagation of neurodegeneration. *Nat Med.* 2010;16(11):1201–4.

34. Hardy J and Rogaeva E. Motor neuron disease and frontotemporal dementia: sometimes related, sometimes not. *Exp Neurol.* 2014;262 Pt B:75–83.

35. Seelaar H, Rohrer JD, Pijnenburg YA, *et al.* Clinical, genetic and pathological heterogeneity of frontotemporal dementia: a review. *J Neurol Neurosur Ps.* 2011;82(5):476–86.

36. Rohrer JD, Guerreiro R, Vandrovcova J, *et al.* The heritability and genetics of frontotemporal lobar degeneration. *Neurology.* 2009;73(18):1451–6.

37. Rohrer JD and Warren JD. Phenotypic signatures of genetic frontotemporal dementia. *Curr Opin Neurol.* 2011;24(6):542–9.

38. See TM, LaMarre AK, Lee SE, *et al.* Genetic causes of frontotemporal degeneration. *J Geriatr Psych Neur.* 2010;23(4):260–8.

39. Mahoney CJ, Beck J, Rohrer JD, *et al.* Frontotemporal dementia with the C9ORF72 hexanucleotide repeat expansion: clinical, neuroanatomical and neuropathological features. *Brain.* 2012;135(Pt 3):736–50.

40. Hutton M, Lendon CL, Rizzu P, *et al.* Association of missense and 5'-splice-site mutations in tau with the inherited dementia FTDP-17. *Nature.* 1998;393(6686):702–5.

41. Kar A, Kuo D, He R, Zhou J, *et al.* Tau alternative splicing and frontotemporal dementia. *Alzheimer Dis Assoc Disord.* 2005;19 Suppl 1:S29–36.

42. Brandt R, Hundelt M, and Shahani N. Tau alteration and neuronal degeneration in tauopathies: mechanisms and models. *Biochimica et Biophysica Acta.* 2005;1739(2–3):331–54.

43. Spillantini MG, Van Swieten JC, and Goedert M. Tau gene mutations in frontotemporal dementia and parkinsonism linked to chromosome 17 (FTDP-17). *Neurogenetics.* 2000;2(4):193–205.

44. Baker M, Mackenzie IR, Pickering-Brown SM, *et al.* Mutations in progranulin cause tau-negative frontotemporal dementia linked to chromosome 17. *Nature.* 2006;442(7105):916–9.

45. Cruts M, Gijselinck I, van der Zee J, *et al.* Null mutations in progranulin cause ubiquitin-positive frontotemporal dementia linked to chromosome 17q21. *Nature.* 2006;442(7105):920–4.

46. Finch N, Baker M, Crook R, *et al.* Plasma progranulin levels predict progranulin mutation status in frontotemporal dementia patients and asymptomatic family members. *Brain.* 2009;132(Pt 3):583–91.

47. Smith KR, Damiano J, Franceschetti S, *et al.* Strikingly different clinico-pathological phenotypes determined by progranulin-mutation dosage. *Am J Hum Genet.* 2012;90(6):1102–7.

48. Gotzl JK, Mori K, Damme M, *et al.* Common pathobiochemical hallmarks of progranulin-associated frontotemporal lobar degeneration and neuronal ceroid lipofuscinosis. *Acta Neuropathologica.* 2014;127(6):845–60.

49. Dejesus-Hernandez M, Mackenzie IR, Boeve BF, *et al.* Expanded GGGGCC hexanucleotide repeat in noncoding region of C9ORF72 causes chromosome 9p-Linked FTD and ALS. *Neuron.* 2011;72(2):245–56.

50. Renton AE, Majounie E, Waite A, *et al.* A hexanucleotide repeat expansion in C9ORF72 is the cause of chromosome 9p21-Linked ALS-FTD. *Neuron.* 2011;72(2):257–68.

51. Beck J, Poulter M, Hensman D, *et al.* Large C9orf72 hexanucleotide repeat expansions are seen in multiple neurodegenerative syndromes and are more frequent than expected in the UK population. *Am J Hum Genet.* 2013;92(3):345–53.

52. Galimberti D, Arosio B, Fenoglio C, *et al.* Incomplete penetrance of the C9ORF72 hexanucleotide repeat expansions: frequency in a cohort of geriatric non-demented subjects. *J Alzheimers Dis.* 2014;39(1):19–22.

53. Woollacott IO and Mead S. The C9ORF72 expansion mutation: gene structure, phenotypic and diagnostic issues. *Acta Neuropathologica.* 2014;127(3):319–32.

54. Levine TP, Daniels RD, Gatta AT, *et al.* The product of C9orf72, a gene strongly implicated in neurodegeneration, is structurally related to DENN Rab-GEFs. *Bioinformatics.* 2013;29(4):499–503.

55. Skibinski G, Parkinson NJ, Brown JM, *et al.* Mutations in the endosomal ESCRTIII-complex subunit CHMP2B in frontotemporal dementia. *Nat Genet.* 2005;37(8):806–8.

56. Guerreiro RJ, Lohmann E, Bras JM, *et al.* Using exome sequencing to reveal mutations in TREM2 presenting as a frontotemporal dementia-like syndrome without bone involvement. *JAMA Neurol.* 2013;70(1):78–84.

57. Paloneva J, Manninen T, Christman G, *et al.* Mutations in two genes encoding different subunits of a receptor signaling complex result in an identical disease phenotype. *Am J Hum Genet.* 2002;71(3):656–62.

58. Guerreiro R, Bilgic B, Guven G, *et al.* Novel compound heterozygous mutation in TREM2 found in a Turkish frontotemporal dementia-like family. *Neurobiol Aging.* 2013;34(12):2890 e1–5.

59. Giraldo M, Lopera F, Siniard AL, *et al.* Variants in triggering receptor expressed on myeloid cells 2 are associated with both behavioral variant frontotemporal lobar degeneration and Alzheimer's disease. *Neurobiol Aging.* 2013;34(8):2077 e11–8.

60. Wong TH, Chiu WZ, Breedveld GJ, *et al.* PRKAR1B mutation associated with a new neurodegenerative disorder with unique pathology. *Brain.* 2014;137(Pt 5):1361–73.

61. Van Deerlin VM, Sleiman PM, Martinez-Lage M, *et al.* Common variants at 7p21 are associated with frontotemporal lobar degeneration with TDP-43 inclusions. *Nat Genet.* 2010;42(3):234–9.

62. Ferrari R, Hernandez DG, Nalls MA, *et al.* Frontotemporal dementia and its subtypes: a genome-wide association study. *Lancet Neurol.* 2014;13(7):686–99.

63. Girard SL and Rouleau GA. Genome-wide association study in FTD: divide to conquer. *Lancet Neurol.* 2014;13(7):643–4.

64. Lattante S, Millecamps S, Stevanin G, *et al.* Contribution of ATXN2 intermediary polyQ expansions in a spectrum of neurodegenerative disorders. *Neurology.* 2014;83(11):990–5.

65. Diekstra FP, Van Deerlin VM, van Swieten JC, *et al.* C9orf72 and UNC13A are shared risk loci for amyotrophic lateral sclerosis and frontotemporal dementia: a genome-wide meta-analysis. *Ann Neurol.* 2014;76(1):120–33.

66. Ramasamy A, Trabzuni D, Guelfi S, *et al.* Genetic variability in the regulation of gene expression in ten regions of the human brain. *Nature Neurosci.* 2014;17(10):1418–28.

67. Carrasquillo MM, Nicholson AM, Finch N, *et al.* Genome-wide screen identifies rs646776 near sortilin as a regulator of progranulin levels in human plasma. *Am J Hum Genet.* 2010;87(6):890–7.

68. Coppola G, Chinnathambi S, Lee JJ, *et al.* Evidence for a role of the rare p.A152T variant in MAPT in increasing the risk for FTD-spectrum and Alzheimer's diseases. *Hum Mol Genet.* 2012;21(15):3500–12.

69. Lee SE, Tartaglia MC, Yener G, *et al.* Neurodegenerative disease phenotypes in carriers of MAPT p.A152T, a risk factor for frontotemporal dementia spectrum disorders and Alzheimer disease. *Alzheimer Dis Assoc Disord.* 2013;27(4):302–9.

70. Kara E, Ling H, Pittman AM, *et al.* The MAPT p.A152T variant is a risk factor associated with tauopathies with atypical clinical and neuropathological features. *Neurobiol Aging.* 2012;33(9):2231 e7–e14.

71. George S, Rey NL, Reichenbach N, Steiner JA, *et al.* alpha-Synuclein: the long distance runner. *Brain Pathology.* 2013;23(3):350–7.

72. Lippa CF, Duda JE, Grossman M, *et al.* DLB and PDD boundary issues: diagnosis, treatment, molecular pathology, and biomarkers. *Neurology.* 2007;68(11):812–9.

73. Bogaerts V, Engelborghs S, Kumar-Singh S, *et al.* A novel locus for dementia with Lewy bodies: a clinically and genetically heterogeneous disorder. *Brain.* 2007;130(Pt 9):2277–91.

74. Meeus B, Nuytemans K, Crosiers D, *et al.* Comprehensive genetic and mutation analysis of familial dementia with Lewy bodies linked to 2q35–q36. *J Alzheimers Dis.* 2010;20(1):197–205.

75. Meeus B, Verstraeten A, Crosiers D, *et al.* DLB and PDD: a role for mutations in dementia and Parkinson disease genes? *Neurobiol Aging.* 2012;33(3):629 e5- e18.

76. Tsuang D, Leverenz JB, Lopez OL, *et al.* APOE epsilon4 increases risk for dementia in pure synucleinopathies. *JAMA Neurol.* 2013;70(2):223–8.

77. Berge G, Sando SB, Rongve A, *et al.* Apolipoprotein E epsilon2 geno-type delays onset of dementia with Lewy bodies in a Norwegian cohort. *J Neurol Neurosur Ps.* 2014;85(11):1227–31.

78. Nalls MA, Duran R, Lopez G, *et al.* A multicenter study of glucocer-ebrosidase mutations in dementia with Lewy bodies. *JAMA Neurol.* 2013;70(6):727–35.

79. Bras J, Guerreiro R, Darwent L, *et al.* Genetic analysis implicates APOE, SNCA and suggests lysosomal dysfunction in the etiology of dementia with Lewy bodies. *Hum Mol Genet.* 2014;23(23):6139–46.

80. Mak SK, McCormack AL, Manning-Bog AB, *et al.* Lysosomal degrada-tion of alpha-synuclein in vivo. *J Biol Chem.* 2010;285(18):13621–9.

CHAPTER 31

Other genetic causes of cognitive impairment

Davina J. Hensman Moss, Nicholas W. Wood, and Sarah J. Tabrizi

Huntington's disease

Introduction

Huntington's disease is a devastating progressive neurodegenerative condition characterized by movement, behavioural, and cognition problems. The condition is autosomal dominantly inherited, and while relatively rare, is the most common identified genetic cause of cognitive impairment. George Huntington originally described the disease in 1872[1] in what remains one of the best descriptions of the condition. He noted three 'marked peculiarities in this disease; (I) its hereditary nature; (II) a tendency to insanity and suicide; and (III) its manifesting itself as a grave disease only in adult life'. Years before Mendel's work was recognized, Huntington astutely observed the genetic nature of the disorder: 'If the thread is broken then the grandchildren of the original shakers may be assured that they are free from the disease.'

Prevalence

The prevalence of HD is generally given as 4–10 per 100 000 in populations of Western European descent;[2] prevalence is thought to be lower in Asian, Japanese, Finnish, and South African populations.[3,4] However, due to the stigma and complex psychosocial issues surrounding the disease this is likely an underestimate: a prevalence of at least 12.4 per 100 000 in the UK population is thought to be more reflective of the true rate.[5] The highest prevalence in the world is in Venezuela near Lake Maracaibo: 700 per 100 000, and it is the collaboration of people in this region and an international group of researchers that was crucial in the identification of the HD gene.

Genetics of HD

HD is inherited in an autosomal dominant manner, and is caused by a trinucleotide repeat expansion in the huntingtin (*HTT*) gene on the short arm of chromosome 4 at 4p16.3. The disease is found in individuals with greater than 36 and up to 121 CAG repeats (Table 31.1); the mean repeat number is 40, but there is a marked skew to the right in this distribution. 50–70 per cent of the variability of age of onset is accounted for by CAG repeat length and age, with higher CAG being associated with more aggressive disease (Table 31.1). The size of CAG repeat can therefore be used to give a prediction of the age of motor onset in premanifest individuals.[6,7] and this index is what has been widely used in the research setting.

However, the relationship is not sufficiently uniform to predict onset age for a given individual in a clinical context. The onset variability not accounted for by CAG is thought to be partly genetically determined,[8] supporting the concept of disease modifiers in HD.[9]

CAG repeat lengths vary from generation to generation, with both expansion and contraction of the number of repeats occurring, but with an overall tendency towards expansion. Large expansions are associated with transmission down the male line,[10] and there is a familial tendency towards large expansions: 90 per cent of juvenile HD cases inherit the *HTT* gene through the paternal line. The tendency of the CAG expansion to expand during transmission underlies the phenomenon of *anticipation* observed in Huntington's and other neurodegenerative conditions such as SCAs 1, 2, 3, 6, 7, and dentatorubral-pallidoluysian atrophy (DRPLA), in which there is an increased severity of disease in successive generations.

Clinical presentation of adult-onset HD

Typically symptoms develop between 35 and 45 years of age, but onset has been described between 2 and 87 years of age. HD can produce a wide range of phenotypic presentations, and as the disease progresses the signs and symptoms change.

By consensus, disease onset is defined as the point when a person who carries a CAG-expanded *HTT* allele develops 'the unequivocal presence of an otherwise unexplained extrapyramidal movement disorder' (eg chorea, dystonia, bradykinesia, rigidity).[11,12] However, the transition from premanifest to manifest HD is not as abrupt as previously assumed. There may be more subtle features evident to the careful observer prior to this in the perisymptomatic or prodromal phases of HD. These include delayed initiation of saccades, slower saccades particularly on vertical eye movements, irregular finger tapping, and a generalized restlessness. Psychiatric symptoms and cognitive changes often occur before motor onset.[13–15]

It is thought that neuronal dysfunction starts many years prior to disease onset, but that neural plasticity and compensatory mechanisms may be responsible for the lag between neural damage and symptom onset (see Fig. 31.1).

Motor features

The cardinal motor symptoms of HD are chorea and dystonia which are present in 90 per cent[2] and 95 per cent[16] of symptomatic patients respectively. The ad hoc Committee on Classification of the

Table 31.1 Relationship between size of CAG repeat expansion and clinical outcome

CAG repeat length	<27	27–35	36–39	≥40	≥55–60
Clinical manifestation	Normal Not unstable	Intermediate repeat allele Not pathogenic May expand into disease range in future generations in paternal line	Reduced penetrance but pathogenic	Fully penetrant	Usually have juvenile onset

World Federation of Neurology[17] defined chorea as 'a state of excessive, spontaneous movements, irregularly timed, non-repetitive, randomly distributed and abrupt in character. These movements may vary in severity from restlessness with mild, intermittent exaggeration of gesture and expression, fidgeting movements of the hands, unstable dance-like gait to a continuous flow of disabling violent movements.' Chorea may affect face, trunk, or limbs, and although the pattern of the movements may differ between patients, they occur in individuals in a stereotyped manner. Choreic movements are continuously present during waking hours, and are often exacerbated by stress.[18] Dystonia is characterized by involuntary, sustained or spasmodic and patterned contractions of muscles, frequently causing twisting and posturing[19] and may affect face, trunk, or limbs.

Gait is impaired, not only due to the chorea and dystonia but also due to impairment in motor control and postural reflexes, making patients prone to falling. Hypophonia, dysarthria, and dysphagia all cause significant morbidity in HD and are important to enquire about and address clinically. Dysphagia with choking episodes is reported even in early disease. At this stage dysphagia is usually related to impulsive, disordered eating, whilst later disease mechanical disintegration of swallowing plays a greater role in disability. Eye movement abnormalities occur early. As the disease progresses, head thrusting is used to initiate gaze shifts, pursuit is impaired with saccadic instructions, and there is gaze impersistence (difficulty in maintaining fixation on an item in the visual scene).

Psychiatric features

Psychiatric problems, particularly anxiety and depression, are a major cause of morbidity in HD and may occur many years before symptom onset. A survey of 2835 patients with HD found that 40 per cent had symptoms of depression, and 50 per cent reported having sought treatment for depression at some stage in the past.[20] The frequency of psychiatric problems and their potential amenability to treatment means that psychiatric symptoms are particularly important to address clinically.

Suicide in HD is much higher than the general population both in the manifest and premanifest stages: in a survey of 4171 gene carriers, 17.5 per cent had suicidal thought at or around the time of assessment, and 10 per cent had made at least one suicide attempt in the past.[21] Suicidal ideation is highest in gene carriers around the time of diagnosis, with manifest disease, and those beginning to lose independence: risk factors include depression, loneliness, and impulsivity.[21,22] Psychosis, despite being relatively well recognized in HD, is in fact quite rare. Additional familial factors may predispose to schizophrenia-like symptoms in HD.[23] Hypomania and, more rarely, mania are seen.[24]

Irritability, a mood state characterized by a reduction in control over temper, is common (65.4 per cent)[25] and some patients become aggressive. Apathy, which is defined as a disorder of motivation, with diminished goal-directed behaviour, cognition, and emotion[26,27] is prevalent in symptomatic HD (55.8 per cent),[25,28] and prior to motor onset.[29] It should be noted that while apathy may be related to depression, it may also be a feature of HD independent of mood disturbance. Obsessions and compulsions, for example about bowel habit, food, or infidelity of spouse, can be features of HD, and can be challenging for loved ones to cope with.

The combination of low mood, apathy, obsessiveness, and irritability can precipitate social isolation, and a negative spiral in the patient's condition. In addition to addressing these issues and considering pharmacological management, it is also important to provide multidisciplinary support to not only the patient themselves but also to families and carers.

Cognitive features

The severity of cognitive involvement in HD is variable and becomes more prevalent and marked as the disease progresses. Individuals who are many years from predicted motor diagnosis[6] show few, if any, overt signs of cognitive decline. There often are subtle cognitive differences detectable more than a decade prior to predicted

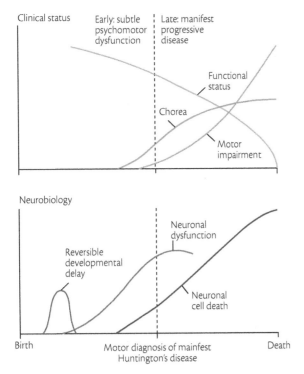

Fig. 31.1 Outline of the clinicopathological progression of HD.
Reproduced from *Lancet Neurol.* 10(1), Ross CA and Tabrizi SJ. Huntington's disease: from molecular pathogenesis to clinical treatment, pp. 83–98, Copyright (2011), with permission from Elsevier.

motor onset which gradually decline as motor onsets approaches (Fig. 31.3).[30,31] These presymptomatic changes are likely to relate to abnormalities on MRI such as caudate atrophy which can be seen in cross-sectional studies up to 15 years prior to predicted motor onset, and the increased rates of whole-brain, caudate, and putaminal atrophy observed up to 15 years before predicted onset and controls (Fig. 31.2).[13,15] An important research question is what, if any, compensatory mechanisms exist to minimize cognitive dysfunction at this stage. Thanks to the availability of presymptomatic genetic diagnosis enabling the study of individuals many years from symptom onset, these very early signs of HD are amenable to investigation, and large-scale studies such as TrackOn-HD aim for a better understanding of these mechanisms.

Many of the cognitive changes in HD represent disruption to frontostriatal circuits, evident in the key cognitive abnormalities observed in these patients (see chapters 2, 3, 7, and 8).[24] Cognitive deficits are particularly apparent in executive functioning, including the ability to plan, organize, and monitor behaviour, and to show mental flexibility and set-shifting.[32] There are also impairments in attention, verbal fluency, psychomotor speed, memory and visuospatial functioning (see reference 24 for a comprehensive review).

There is no accepted cognitive battery for the cognitive assessment of HD although most HD centres rely on the Unified Huntington's Disease Rating Scale (UHDRS) for routine clinical practice, which incorporates the symbol digit modality test, the

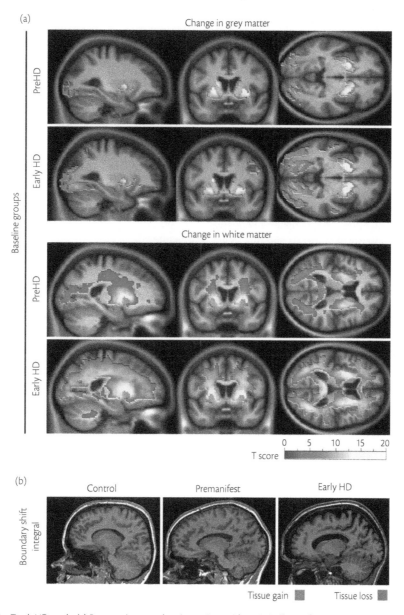

Fig. 31.2 Imaging changes from the Track-HD study. (a) Parametric maps showing regions with statistically significant atrophy in grey matter (top) and white matter (bottom) over 24 months, relative to controls. (b) The brain boundary shift integral, a quantification of whole-brain volume change estimated through measurement of shift at the brain–CSF boundary over 12 months within each subject group.

(a) Adapted from *Lancet Neurol.* 10(1), Tabrizi SJ, Scahill RI, Durr A, *et al.* Biological and clinical changes in premanifest and early stage Huntington's disease in the TRACK-HD study: the 12-month longitudinal analysis, pp. 31–42, Copyright (2011), with permission from Elsevier. (b) Adapted from *Lancet Neurol,* 11(1), Tabrizi SJ, Reilmann R, Roos RA, *et al.* Potential endpoints for clinical trials in premanifest and early Huntington's disease in the TRACK-HD study: analysis of 24 month observational data, pp. 42–53, Copyright (2012), with permission from Elsevier.

Stroop colour word test, and a verbal fluency test as part of a comprehensive examination.[33]

One of the challenges in interpreting cognitive examination findings in HD is evaluating premorbid intellect.[34] Commonly used single-word reading tests such as the Wide Range Achievement Test (WRAT) Reading subset and the National Adult Reading Test (NART)[35] test reading ability, which may itself be affected early in the course of disease, resulting in an underestimation of premorbid IQ. In comparing test-based versus demographic-based estimates of premorbid intellect in mild and moderate HD subjects, O'Rouke and colleagues[36] found that demographic-based estimates were less confounded by disease progression and may reflect a more valid indicator of prior cognitive capacity.

The earliest detected cognitive deficit described in premanifest HD is impairment of emotion recognition, which is significantly different from controls in expansion-positive cases more than 15 years from predicted motor onset,[34] shows longitudinal change,[15] and can cause considerable distress to patients and their families. Timing[15,37,38] and speeded tapping[15,30] are also affected early in disease and deteriorate longitudinally making them potential biomarkers for clinical trials. The Track-HD study found cognitive decline in 10 out of 12 outcome measures in 116 early-HD subjects relative to controls over 24 months, with greatest sensitivity in symbol digit, circle tracing (direct and indirect), and Stroop word reading tasks,[39] see Fig. 31.3.

The concept of mild cognitive impairment (MCI),[40] a transitional stage between normal cognition and dementia, is being increasingly used to describe early cognitive changes in HD.[34] MCI is operationally defined by subjective cognitive complaints and objective cognitive deficits, but with the absence of dementia and functional impairment.[41,42] Duff and colleagues[43] tested episodic memory, processing speed, executive functioning, and visuospatial perception in 575 prodromic gene carriers and found the prevalence of MCI was 38 per cent, and this increased as participants approached the estimated age of diagnosis (far = 27.3 per cent, mid = 42.3 per cent, near = 54.1 per cent; p < 0.0001 for trend).

While some argue against the use of the term dementia in HD on the basis that the cognitive changes are more circumscribed than dementia implies, the term is still widely used. Criteria for HD dementia have been based largely on features of the dementia associated with Alzheimer's disease (AD), however the pattern of spared and impaired cognitive abilities observed in HD is distinct from that in AD.[44,45]

Typically, HD patients have a 'subcortical' as opposed to cortical cognitive pattern of deficits.[46] HD memory performance is affected by slowed retrieval largely independent of the ability to store information and motor slowing.[47] Peavy and colleagues[44] showed that speed of processing, initiation and attention measures defined the onset of HD dementia better than traditional definitions created for AD which required memory deficits. In early HD, language is relatively spared with preservation of lexical abilities, however studies show that the application of syntactic movement rules is impaired.[48,49] As the disease progresses communication is also compromised by both dysphasia and dysarthria.

Other features of HD

Mutant huntingtin protein is ubiquitously expressed in the body. Thus Huntington's disease has peripheral effects not all of which are secondary to brain dysfunction (reviewed in reference 50). It causes metabolic symptoms, which include catabolic weight loss, skeletal muscle atrophy, endocrine dysfunction, and sleep disturbance. Weight loss, which is thought to be related to the chorea, procatabolic nature of the condition, xerostomia, and feeding difficulties, is associated with poor outcome and is important to recognize and address proactively.[18] Sleep is often disturbed due to disturbed circadian rhythms (reviewed in reference 51) and negatively impacts on quality of life (see Box 31.1).

Juvenile HD

This is also known as the Westphal variant of HD, and is characterized by *onset* before 20 years of age, although cases with young-adult onset and a primarily rigid phenotype are also described as having the Westphal variant. The extrapyramidal features of rigidity, bradykinesia, and akinesia develop early in these patients, and many have a history of learning impairments at school. Unlike in adult-onset HD, seizures can be a feature and are more common in those with very young onset.

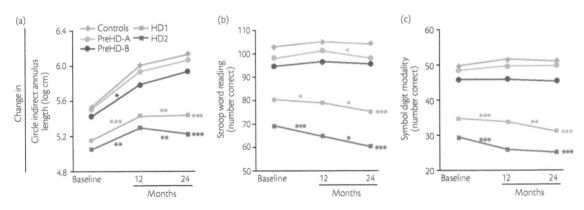

Fig. 31.3 Longitudinal changes in cognitive measures from the Track-HD study over 24 months. Significant change differences relative to controls over 0–12, 12–24, and 0–24 months are represented by *p < 0.05, **p < 0.01, and ***P < 0.001. Groups determined at start of study; PreHD-A: more than 10.8 years from predicted onset; PreHD-B: less than 10.8 years from predicted onset; HD1: early HD and less symptomatic on total functional capacity scale (TFC); HD2: early HD and more symptomatic on TFC.

Adapted from *Lancet Neurol.* 11(1), Tabrizi SJ, Reilmann R, Roos RA, *et al.* Potential endpoints for clinical trials in premanifest and early Huntington's disease in the TRACK-HD study: analysis of 24 month observational data, pp. 42–53, Copyright (2012), with permission from Elsevier.

A 55-year-old man was brought to see the general practitioner by his wife. She explained that her husband had been healthy and active when younger but that his ability to function independently had declined over the previous few years to the point where she was now helping him with all activities of daily living. If she did not help or prompt her husband, he would not wash or dress himself and would sit on the sofa all day doing nothing. Her husband had no history of physical illness but had suffered from recurrent bouts of depression for many years and had developed obsessive–compulsive behaviours over the last 15 years. These included picking litter up from the street and arranging his belongings in lines. On questioning about illness in the family, the patient explained that he thought that his mother had been diagnosed with Alzheimer's disease in her 40s.

On examination, the patient had occasional involuntary movements in his arms. Examination of the limbs was otherwise normal. He was fully orientated and scored 26/30 on the mini mental state examination.

After counselling of the patient and his family at a specialist genetics centre, the patient underwent genetic testing and the diagnosis of Huntington's disease was confirmed.

After a full assessment of his care needs, this patient began regularly attending his local day centre; this led to a dramatic improvement in his behaviour and mood. He enjoyed the mental stimulation and social contact of the day centre, and benefited from the structure and routine of going there every day (having a specific goal such as leaving the house and going to a day centre is a good way to combat apathy). He also started taking fluoxetine; this led to his obsessive–compulsive behaviours improving to a more manageable level. The patient's wife greatly appreciated the support and time by herself that resulted from her husband's attendance at the day centre, and she also made contact with, and received support from, the Huntington's Disease Association (<www.hda.org.uk>), an organization which provides invaluable support for those affected by Huntington's disease. The relatives of the patient (those now known to be at risk of carrying the abnormal Huntington's disease gene themselves) were offered information and support, including genetic counselling and information about predictive testing for Huntington's disease for those who wanted it.

Adapted from *BMJ*. 343, Novak MJ and Tabrizi SJ, A man with deteriorating ability to live independently, Copyright (2011), with permission from the BMJ Publishing Group Ltd.

Molecular pathogenesis of HD

HD is caused by an expanded CAG triplet repeat encoding a polyglutamine (polyQ) expansion in exon 1 of the huntingtin (*HTT*) gene. The protein HTT is large (~350 kDa) and highly conserved, and is necessary for embryonic development.[52–54] It is expressed widely in the central nervous system and peripheral tissues and in most intracellular compartments. It has been shown to interact with numerous other intracellular proteins. Huntingtin's exact intracellular functions are incompletely understood but it is known to be involved in vesicular transport, cytoskeletal anchoring, neuronal transport, postsynaptic signalling, cytoprotection, and transcriptional regulation.[55]

Key features of Huntington's disease pathogenesis have been consistently described (Fig. 31.4) (reviewed in reference 55):

- Mutant *HTT* has the propensity to form abnormal conformations, including β-sheet structures (although *HTT* in large inclusions is not the primary pathogenic species in HD).

- Systems for handling abnormal proteins are impaired in cells and tissues from Huntington's disease patients and in experimental models.

- *HTT* is truncated and gives rise to toxic N-terminal fragments.

- Post-translational modifications of *HTT* influence toxicity, via conformational changes, aggregation propensity, cellular localization, and clearance.

- Nuclear translocation of mutant *HTT* enhances toxic effects of the protein, in part via transcription-related effects.

- Cellular metabolic pathways are impaired in samples from Huntington's disease patients and models.

Histologically, there is massive striatal neuronal cell death, with up to 95 per cent loss of GABAergic medium spiny projection neurons which project to the globus pallidus and the substantia nigra. There is relative sparing of large cholinergic interneurons and specific loss in layers V and VI of the cerebral cortex.[56,57] Microglial activation is seen from early in disease.[58] From a macroscopic perspective, there is generalized brain atrophy, particularly involving the caudate nucleus and to a lesser extent the putamen, with atrophy of the internal segment of the globus pallidus and substantia nigra pars reticulata.[13,57] White matter tracts are affected in HD from premanifest stages,[13–15,59,60] see Fig. 31.2 (also referred to in the cognitive section earlier in this chapter).

Genetic testing in HD

Genetic testing is performed by measuring the CAG repeat length in the *HTT* gene; a positive test refers to a CAG length in the fully penetrant range (see Table 31.1 reference 61 for an overview). Testing may be diagnostic in an individual with symptoms to confirm or refute a diagnosis of HD, or predictive in an individual known to be at risk of disease because of their family history. Most people at risk of HD choose *not* to undergo predictive testing. Predictive testing for HD requires expert counselling; it is performed in specialist genetic centres and follows internationally agreed guidelines.[62] Similar principles are adopted in the genetic testing for the other neurodegenerative diseases covered in this chapter.

Management of HD

The cornerstone of the clinical management of HD is a multidisciplinary approach since the needs of patients are diverse and change over time (for a detailed overview on management see reference 61). Most HD clinics are run by a combination of clinical geneticists, neurologists, neuro-psychiatrists, nurse specialists with support from physiotherapists, speech and language therapists, and dieticians. The role of the general practitioner and sometimes social worker is also important, liaising with the specialist team, and providing regular and local input. HD organizations, such as the Huntington's disease association in the United Kingdom (HDA; <http://www.hda.org.uk>) provide valuable support via regional care advisors, and also provide a wealth of information on their website and via booklets.

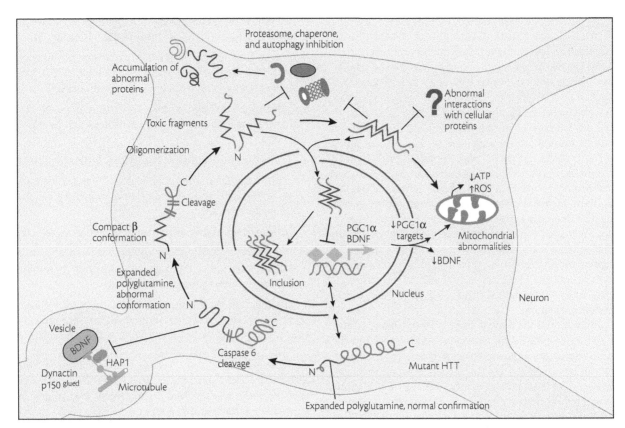

Fig. 31.4 Postulated intracellular pathogenesis of Huntington's disease. Mutant HTT (shown as a helical structure) with an expanded polyglutamine repeat (shown in green) undergoes a conformational change and interferes with cellular trafficking, especially of BDNF. Mutant HTT is cleaved at several points to generate toxic fragments with abnormal compact β conformation. Pathogenic species can be monomeric or, more likely (and as shown), form small oligomers. Toxic effects in the cytoplasm include inhibition of chaperones, proteasomes, and autophagy, which can cause accumulation of abnormally folded proteins and other cellular constituents. There may be direct interactions between mutant HTT and mitochondria. Other interactions between mutant HTT and cellular proteins in the cytoplasm are still poorly understood. Pathognomonic inclusion bodies are found in the nucleus (and small inclusions are also found in cytoplasmic regions). However, inclusions are not the primary pathogenic species. A major action of mutant HTT is interference with gene transcription, in part via PGC1α, leading to decreased transcription of BDNF and nuclear-encoded mitochondrial proteins. ROS: reactive oxygen species.
Adapted from *Lancet Neurol.* 10(1), Tabrizi SJ, Scahill RI, Durr A, *et al.* Biological and clinical changes in premanifest and early stage Huntington's disease in the TRACK-HD study: the 12-month longitudinal analysis, pp. 31–42, Copyright (2011), with permission from Elsevier.

Management of motor symptoms

Though common, chorea is rarely functionally disabling for patients with HD, however in some cases it causes embarrassment and thereby increases risk of social isolation. The side-effects of the antichorea medications, and the fact that they are rarely very efficacious, means that antichoreic medications should be used sparingly. Tetrabenazine can be an effective option[63–65] but should be avoided in patients with psychosis, active depression, aggressive behaviours, and non-compliance. Side-effects include depression, anxiety, sedation, parkinsonism, and cognitive impairment.[63] For patients with coexisting psychosis, depression, and aggression, antipsychotic agents such as olanzapine, sulpiride, or rispiridone should be considered as the first-line option. In some cases amantadine or riluzole may be effective.[64] In all cases these medications require careful evaluation prior to initiation of treatment and ongoing monitoring of response.

Impairment of voluntary motor function and gait disturbances are challenging to treat but can benefit from physiotherapy assessment and exercises. The European Huntington's Disease Network has some helpful physiotherapy guidelines.[66] Walking aids and wheelchairs often become necessary as symptoms progress, and involving an occupational therapist to review a patient's home environment can prove useful. In the later stages, rigidity and dystonia become more dominant; in some cases antispasticity drugs can assist but often afford no functional benefit.

Speech and swallowing can be early and debilitating problems in HD and are important to enquire about; affected patients should be referred for speech and language therapy input.[2] Dysarthria contributes to communication difficulties, and as the disease progressive patients can become mute. Ultimately, feeding via gastrostomy with the option of small amounts of oral feeding for pleasure is sometimes the best option.

Management of psychiatric problems

Much of our current practice is based on anecdotal evidence. The most useful drugs for depression are the serotonin-selective reuptake inhibitors (SSRIs). Anecdotal reports and our own practice suggest that citalopram and mirtazapine are effective, particularly when anxiety is a co-factor. SSRIs are also the first-line option for obsessive–compulsive behaviours in HD.[67] Irritability, aggression, and impulsivity may be ameliorated by antipsychotic agents such as olanzapine, rispiridone, and quetiapine.[68] These newer

Table 31.2 Principal causes of Huntington's disease phenocopy syndromes

Condition	Gene	Protein	Inheritance	Notes
Familial prion disease	PRNP	Prion	AD	Includes HDL1
HDL2	JPH3	Junctophilin 3	AD	African ancestry
HDL3	Unknown	Unknown	AR	Two pedigrees only
SCA17	TBP	TATA-binding protein	AD	Cerebellar atrophy and ataxia, see below
SCA1	ATXN1	Ataxin 1	AD	
SCA2	ATXN2	Ataxin 2	AD	
SCA3	ATXN3	Ataxin 3	AD	
DRPLA	ATN1	Atrophin 1	AD	Myoclonic epilepsy, see below
PKAN (NBIA1)	PANK2	Pantothenate kinase	AR	MRI 'eye-of-the tiger sign'; pigmentary retinopathy
Neuroferritinopathy	FTL	Ferritin light chain	AD	Early dysarthria and persistent asymmetry
Chorea-acanthocytosis	CHAC	Chorein	AR	Mutilating orofacial dystonia
Macleod syndrome	XK	Krell antigen	XR	Systemic features
Wilson's disease	ATP7B	Copper-transporting ATPase	AR	Kayser–Fleischer rings, etc.
Friedreich's ataxia	FRDA	Frataxin	AR	Rarely resembles HD, see below
Mitochondrial disease	mtDNA or nuclear mitochondrial genes, see below			
Benign hereditary chorea	TITF1	Thyroid transcription factor 1	AD	Non-choreic features rare
Acquired causes	e.g. Sydenham's chorea, anti-basal ganglia antibodies, neuro-SLE, thyrotoxicosis, vascular disease, and medications			

AD: autosomal dominant; AR: autosomal recessive; XR: X-linked recessive.

antipsychotics have an improved side-effect profile in terms of extrapyramidal symptoms and are also useful for severe anxiety and motor symptoms. Mood-stabilizing drugs such as valproate and carbamazepine are useful for symptoms of mania. Benzodiazepines can be useful in the short-term treatment of anxiety and long-term agitation in advanced disease. Sleep disturbance is routinely managed with sleep hygiene measures and hypnotics; melatonin may also help.

Management of cognitive symptoms
Formal neuropsychometric testing can be useful to quantify impairments and inform optimal management and care of patients with cognitive impairment, particularly when insight is also impaired. There are no therapeutic agents with proven efficacy for the cognitive impairment in HD. Environmental enrichment, which enhances mental and physical activity levels, has been found to induce beneficial effects in rodent models of HD,[69] and there is some evidence that MCI due to Alzheimer's disease can respond to cognitive stimulation.[70] In our clinical experience there is anecdotal support for cognitive stimulation and a strong social network benefiting our patients, and it will be interesting to see whether this is supported experimentally in the future. In the meantime, providing a safe and supportive environment are cornerstones in managing cognitive HD symptoms.

Huntington's disease phenocopy syndromes

In around 1–3 per cent of cases where Huntington's disease is suspected clinically, patients lack the CAG repeat expansion that causes HD.[11,71–73] Such individuals are said to have Huntington's disease

phenocopy syndromes,[74] reviewed in reference 73. The known causes of HD phenocopies are summarized in Table 31.2. In a case series of 285 patients with HD phenocopy syndromes, 8 patients (2.8 per cent) were identified as having other inherited neurological diseases including SCA17, HDL2, PRNP (familial prion disease), and FA (Friedreich's ataxia).[75] Several of these syndromes are described below; Huntington's disease-like syndrome 1 (HDL1) and Huntington's disease-like 2 (HDL2) will be discussed here.

Huntington's disease-like syndrome 1 (HDL1) is a rare autosomal dominant condition causing personality change, dementia, and chorea. It is caused by eight extra octapeptide repeats inserted within the prion protein (PrP).[74] This and other familial prion diseases are described in chapter 38. Huntington's disease-like syndrome 2 (HDL2) is caused by GTC/CAG triplet repeat expansions in the JPH3 gene encoding junctophilin-3. The condition is phenotypically similar to HD with similar cognitive and psychiatric profile, although dystonia is more marked than chorea. It is more prevalent among populations of African ancestry.[76,77]

Hereditary cerebellar causes of cognitive impairment

The role of the cerebellum in motor control is long established, but its role in cognition has been more controversial (see chapter 26). Schmahmann and colleagues[78] coined the term 'cerebellar cognitive affective syndrome' (CCAS) which is characterized by: disturbances of executive functioning, impaired spatial cognition, inappropriate affect, and linguistic difficulties. There are numerous identified genetic causes of cerebellar impairment, which we outline in the following. Known cognitive symptoms will be highlighted, though it should be noted that for some of the rarer ataxias detailed neuropsychologial studies are limited.

Autosomal recessive ataxias

Friedreich's ataxia (FRDA)

Friedreich's ataxia (FRDA) is the most common of the cerebellar ataxias among Indo-Caucasian populations with a prevalence of 2 in 100 000,[79] and it is inherited in an autosomal recessive manner. The FRDA gene, on chromosome 9q13, codes for a 210 amino acid protein called frataxin. In more than 97 per cent of cases the condition is caused by a homozygous triplet GAA expansion (> 40 repeats) in the first intron of the frataxin gene; however, about 3 per cent of such cases are compound heterozygous for the expansion with the second allele carrying a point mutation.[80,81] Frataxin is a mitochondrial membrane protein involved in iron distribution. The neuropathological changes of FRDA involve the spinal cord, with degeneration of posterior columns and spinocerebellar tracts, the dentate nucleus of the cerebellum, and the heart.[79,82]

FRDA causes progressive neurological disability and classically presents by 25 years of age. Unsteadiness of gait is the most common presenting symptom;[82] there is progressive ataxia (cerebellar and sensory),[83] limb weakness, spasticity, absent lower limb reflexes, extensor plantars, posterior sensory changes, and dysarthria.[82] Systemically, FRDA causes a hypertrophic cardiomyopathy, increased risk of diabetes mellitus, and skeletal abnormalities are common; a multidisciplinary approach is therefore key to management.

Although primarily a movement disorder with systemic features, cognitive impairments may be observed in FRDA. There are reports of slow information-processing speed,[84–86] and some suggest verbal span and letter fluency are impaired.[87] Emotional lability and depression have also been recorded.[82] The cognitive impairments observed may be due to cerebellar impairment disrupting cerebro-ponto-cerebello-thalamo-cerebral loops, direct cortical pathology, or a combination of the two.[88]

Autosomal recessive spastic ataxia of Charlevoix–Saguenay (ARSACS)

Autosomal recessive spastic ataxia of Charlevoix–Saguenay (ARSACS) is a rare neurodegenerative disorder characterized by early-onset cerebellar ataxia, lower limb spasticity, sensorimotor axonal neuropathy, and atrophy of the superior cerebellar vermis. It has been associated with normal IQ but impaired visuospatial functioning.[89] There are reports of impaired goal directed action, apathy, and impulsivity associated with the condition.[90]

Autosomal dominant cerebellar ataxias (spinocerebellar ataxias)

The progressive autosomal dominant cerebellar ataxias are usually labelled spinocerebellar ataxia (SCA), followed by a number to denote the gene locus. They have an overall prevalence of 1–4 in 100 000.[91] Dentatorubral-pallidoluysian atrophy (DRPLA) does not have a SCA designation but bears similarities to the SCAs and so will be included here. The SCAs exhibit many phenotypic similarities so it can be almost impossible to diagnose the genotype from the phenotype alone,[92] although there are features making one or another SCA more likely (see Table 31.3).

Penetrance of the SCAs is generally complete. Patients typically display limb and truncal ataxia, dysarthria, dysphagia, pyramidal signs, extrapyramidal signs (dystonia, rigidity, bradykinesia), and autonomic disorders. Patients may develop other neurological signs that can evolve over the course of years. There may be non-cerebellar oculomotor features such as slow saccades, oculomotor palsy, blepharospasm, an ocular stare, and ptosis. There may be signs of brainstem disease such as facial atrophy and fasciculations, temporal muscle atrophy, tongue atrophy and fasciculations, poor cough, and dysphagia.

There are a variety of mutations responsible for the SCAs; unstable CAG repeat expansions cause SCA1, SCA2, SCA3 (Machado–Joseph Disease), SCA6, SCA7, SCA17, and DRPLA. Analogously to HD, there is an overall tendency for the expansions to expand intergenerationally, age at onset usually has an inverse relation with number of repeats, and earlier onset is generally associated with a more florid phenotype.

Harding[93] observed significant cognitive impairment in 25 per cent patients with autosomal dominant cerebellar ataxias. As mutations have become better characterized, their cognitive attributes have been examined,[94] although it is not yet clear to what extent these features are specific to each disorder, or are more general features relating to the brain areas damaged. Severity of cognitive deficit generally correspond with severity of pathological and clinical features.[95] Table 31.3 summarizes the autosomal dominant ataxias, with known genetic mutations and well-documented cognitive features as part of the disease.

There are currently no effective curative treatments for the inherited ataxias. As with Huntington's disease, the management is supportive and specialist clinics have a multidisciplinary approach involving physical, occupational, and speech therapy. Unfortunately there are currently no medications which help the balance disturbance of cerebellar ataxia. It is, however, important to consider appropriate and targeted symptomatic treatments for the additional features that may arise. These medications are well reviewed in Ataxia UK's guidelines, available at: (<http://www.ataxia.org.uk/data/files/ataxia_guidelines_web.pdf>).

Hereditary vasculopathies

Vascular causes of cognitive impairment are varied, and are the focus of chapter 25. In this section we provide an overview of the hereditary vasculopathies which cause arteriopathy and microvascular disintegration leading to vascular cognitive impairment. For more detail, the reader is referred to reference 113.

Cerebral autosomal dominant arteriopathy with subcortical infarcts and leukoencephalopathy (CADASIL)

Cerebral autosomal dominant arteriopathy with subcortical infarcts and leukoencephalopathy (CADASIL) typically presents in youth and adulthood with migraine, subcortical transient ischaemic attacks or strokes, psychiatric disorders, and subcortical and frontal cognitive impairment.[113,114] Systemic involvement with ocular, cardiac, and peripheral nerve features have been reported. The disease is caused by dominant mutations within the *NOTCH3* gene[115] which is expressed in vascular smooth muscle cells. There is microangiopathy with granular osmophilic deposits in the basement membrane, and abnormal responsiveness to vasoactive agents.[116] On MRI there is generalized brain atrophy[117] and focal

Table 31.3 Autosomal dominant ataxias with known gene loci showing phenotype and cognitive impairment where cognitive features are well documented

Disease	Gene/locus	Mutation (pathogenic range)	General features in addition to those of cerebellar ataxia	Cognitive features
SCA 1	6p/ataxin 1	CAG expansion (45–83)	Bulbar dysfunction, somatosensory and oculomotor dysfunctions, pyramidal signs, visual impairments, electrophysiological abnormalities[92]	Executive dysfunction, verbal memory impairment[96,97]
SCA 2	12q/ataxin 2	CAG expansion[33–64] (33–500)	Slowed ocular movements, peripheral neuropathy, postural and action tremor, myoclonus and hyporeflexia	Dementia in 19–42%[97] (higher than SCA1, 3, 6, 7), in those with dementia-impaired attention, memory, frontal executive functions[95,98,99]
SCA 3	14q/ataxin 3	CAG expansion (52–87)	Pyramidal involvement, opthalmoplegia, peripheral neuropathy, parkinsonism in some	Cognitive dysfunction including attention difficulties[96,100]
SCA 6	19p/CACNA1	CAG expansion (20–33)	Ataxia, occasional extrapyramidal and sensory effects	Impaired executive function and visual memory[95,101,102]
SCA 7	3p/ataxin 7	CAG expansion (37–460)	Ataxia, retinal degeneration, opthalmoplegia, seizures	Impaired executive function,[95] dementia
SCA 8	13q	CTG expansion (107–127)	Dysarthria with a characteristic drawn-out slowness of speech and gait instability Neuropsychiatric problems	Frequent impairments of attention, information processing and executive functions[103,104]
SCA 10	22q	ATTCT expansion (1000–4000)	Ataxia, epilepsy Predominant Latin American origin	Cognitive dysfunction and behavioural disturbances noted[105]
SCA 12	5q/PPP2R2B	CAG expansion (66–78)	Tremors; common in India	Dementia[106]
SCA 13	10q/KCNC3	Point mutations	Childhood onset ataxia of slow progression	Mental retardation
SCA 14	19q/PKCγ	Conventional mutations including missense and deletions		Cognitive impairment
SCA 17	6q/TBP	CAG expansion (49–66)	Psychiatric features, extrapyramidal signs, seizures, dementia	Apraxia, dementia[107,108]
SCA 19	1p/KCND3	Missense mutations	Adult onset ataxia, postural tremor, myoclonus, sensory impairment	Frontal executive dysfunction, global impairment as disease progresses[109]
SCA 21	7p	Not known	Ataxia, extrapyramidal features	Mild to severe cognitive deficit[110]
SCA 27	FGF 14	Point mutations	Tremor, dyskinesia	Some cognitive impairment recorded
DRPLA	12p/atrophin	CAG expansion (48–93)	Ataxia, myoclonus, epilepsy, chorea, psychiatric symptoms	Dementia[111,112]

white matter abnormalities, which can be apparent prior to symptom onset.[118] Changes are particularly apparent in frontal, parietal, and anterior temporal lobes and the external capsule.[113]

Cerebral autosomal recessive arterioapthy with subcortical infarcts and leukoencephalopathy (CARASIL)

CARASIL, also known as Maeda syndrome, is clinically similar to CADASIL but with earlier onset and more systemic features such as arthropathy, lower back pain, spondylosis deformans, disc herniation, and alopecia, and an autosomal recessive rather than dominant family history.[113] It is more common in Asian regions, and has a male to female predominance of 3:1. The disease has been linked to a mutation in *HTRA1*. There is damage to vascular smooth muscle fibres and arterioscleotic changes.

Small vessel disease associated with COL4A1 mutation

COL4A1 mutations results in a defect of type IV collagen with resulting vascular pathology. Mutations in the COL4A1 gene are associated with proencephaly and infantile hemiparesis but have more recently been linked to small vessel disease which can present later in life.[119] Features include ischaemic stroke, haemorrhage, lacunar infarction, leukariosis, and microbleeds, and systemic involvement of the eye, kidneys, and muscle. Depending on the age of onset, affected individuals present with infantile hemiparesis, seizures, visual loss, dystonia, strokes, migraine, mental retardation, cognitive impairment, and dementia.[113]

Other familial amyloid angiopathies

Familial British dementia with amyloid angiopathy (FBD) is an autosomal dominant condition characterized by a dementia, progressive spastic tetraparesis and cerebellar ataxia with onset in the sixth decade. A point mutation in the *BRI* gene has been shown to be the causative genetic abnormality.[120] Familial Danish dementia is an early-onset autosomal dominant disorder due to *CHMP2B* truncation mutations.[121] It is clinically characterized by ataxia and a frontotemporal dementia with early personality change, apathy, hyperorality, early dyscalculia, and stereotyped behaviours; as the disease manifests, individuals develop a florid motor syndrome with pyramidal and extrapyramidal features.[122]

Fabry disease

Fabry disease is a progressive, X-linked inherited disorder of glycosphingolipid metabolism due to a deficient or absent lysosomal α-galactosidase A activity. The classic form of the disease, presenting in males with no detectable α-Gal A activity, is characterized by angiokeratomas, acroparesthesia, hypohidrosis, corneal opacity, and progressive vascular disease of the central nervous system, heart, and kidneys. In contrast, mild forms may manifest only in adulthood with cardiac and renal disease.[113] Neurologically it is associated with both peripheral and central nervous system involvement, with large and small vessel ischaemic strokes, and there are reports of mild cognitive deficits.[123]

Primary mitochondrial disorders and cognitive impairment

Mitochondria are intracellular organelles whose major function is the generation of the energy carrier ATP. From a clinical genetics perspective, mitochondria are passed only down the female line,[124–126] though in very rare cases there may be paternal transmission.[127] Mitochondrial mutations may be present in some (heteroplasmy) or all (homoplasmy) mitochondria within a cell, with corresponding variations in severity.

Mitochondrial disorders present as multi-system diseases. Central nervous system manifestations of mitochondrial disorders include stroke-like episodes, epilepsy, migraine, ataxia, spasticity, movement and psychiatric disorders, cognitive decline, and dementia. Other features include myopathy, deafness, progressive external opthalmoplegia, diabetes, bone marrow involvement. The manifestations of mitochondrial disease are highly variable, and it should be noted that patients may suffer from some but not other characteristic features.[128] There have been relatively few neuropsychological studies on cognitive impairment in mitochondrial diseases but cognitive impairment and dementia are well recognized in these conditions.[129,130]

Mitochondrial encephalopathy lactic acidosis and stroke-like episodes (MELAS)

MELAS is characterized by parieto-occipital stroke-like episodes, often associated with concurrent encephalopathy and elevated plasma and CSF lactate. The stroke-like episodes are not due to thromboembolic disease but respiratory chain dysfunction within cerebral tissues,[128,131] consequently the focal deficit often develops over hours or even days, and they may be associated with headache, nausea, and encephalopathic features. Radiological lesions may extend over multiple vascular territories. Seizures commonly accompany the focal episodes. Other symptoms such as deafness, diabetes, myopathy, or a pigmentary retinopathy may be present. In a study of 31 symptomatic MELAS with the m.3243A>G mutation, Kaufmann and colleagues[132] found that the global neuropsychological score decreased over annual visits but there was no decline in asymptomatic carrier relatives. Cognitive decline may relate to neurodegeneration rather than just being secondary to stroke-like episodes.[133]

Myoclonic epilepsy with ragged red fibres (MERRF)

There is progressive myoclonus, focal and generalized epilepsy, cerebellar ataxia, cognitive impairment, and myopathy. Proximal weakness, sensory ataxia, proprioceptive and pyramidal signs abnormalities also occur. In the later stages of the disease, severe cognitive impairment is common and often exhibits prominent frontal features.[128]

Conclusion

In this chapter we have provided an overview of a wide range of genetically determined causes of cognitive impairment, and highlighted their key cognitive features. While curative treatments are not yet available for these conditions, their genetic nature make them amenable to study, and it is hoped that through detailed understanding of the mechanisms by which mutations are linked with disease that therapeutic targets may be identified and rational treatments developed.

References

1. Huntington G. On Chorea. *The Medical and Surgical Reporter, Philadelphia.* 1872;26(15):317–21.
2. Wild EJ and Tabrizi SJ. Huntington's disease. In: NW Wood (ed.). *Neurogenetics: A Guide for Clinicians.* Cambridge: Cambridge University Press, 2012.
3. Pringsheim T, Wiltshire K, Day L, *et al.* The incidence and prevalence of Huntington's disease: a systematic review and meta-analysis. *Mov Disord.* 2012;27(9):1083–91. Epub 2012/06/14.
4. Harper P. The epidemiology of Huntington's disease. In: GP Bates, P Harper, and L Jones (eds). *Huntington's Disease.* Oxford: Oxford University Press, 2002.
5. Rawlins M. Huntington's disease out of the closet? *Lancet.* 2010;376(9750):1372–3.
6. Langbehn DR, Brinkman RR, Falush D, *et al.* A new model for prediction of the age of onset and penetrance for Huntington's disease based on CAG length. *Clin Genet.* 2004;65(4):267–77. Epub 2004/03/18.
7. Langbehn DR, Hayden MR, and Paulsen JS. CAG-repeat length and the age of onset in Huntington disease (HD): A review and validation study of statistical approaches. *Am J Med Gen B.* 2009;9999B:n/a-n/a.
8. Wexler NS, Lorimer J, Porter J, *et al.* Venezuelan kindreds reveal that genetic and environmental factors modulate Huntington's disease age of onset. *Proc Natl Acad Sci USA.* 2004;101(10):3498–503. Epub 2004/03/03.
9. Gusella J and MacDonald, ME. Huntington's disease: the case for genetic modifiers. *Genome Medicine.* 2009;1(80).
10. Telenius HKH, Theilmann J, Andrew SE, *et al.* Molecular analysis of juvenile Huntington disease: the major influence on (CAG)n repeat length is the sex of the affected parent. *Hum Mol Genet.* 1993;2:1535–40.
11. Group THsDCR. A novel gene containing a trinucleotide repeat that is expanded and unstable on Huntington's disease chromosomes. The Huntington's Disease Collaborative Research Group. *Cell.* 1993;72(6):971–83. Epub 1993/03/26.
12. Hogarth P, Kayson E, Kieburtz K, *et al.* Interrater agreement in the assessment of motor manifestations of Huntington's disease. *Mov Disord.* 2005;20(3):293–7. Epub 2004/12/08.
13. Tabrizi SJ, Langbehn DR, Leavitt BR, *et al.* Biological and clinical manifestations of Huntington's disease in the longitudinal TRACK-HD study: cross-sectional analysis of baseline data. *Lancet Neurol.* 2009;8(9):791–801. Epub 2009/08/04.
14. Tabrizi SJ, Scahill RI, Durr A, *et al.* Biological and clinical changes in premanifest and early stage Huntington's disease in the

TRACK-HD study: the 12-month longitudinal analysis. *Lancet Neurol.* 2011;10(1):31–42. Epub 2010/12/07.

15. Tabrizi SJ, Reilmann R, Roos RA, *et al.* Potential endpoints for clinical trials in premanifest and early Huntington's disease in the TRACK-HD study: analysis of 24 month observational data. *Lancet Neurol.* 2012;11(1):42–53. Epub 2011/12/06.

16. Louis ED, Lee P, Quinn L, *et al.* Dystonia in Huntington's disease: prevalence and clinical characteristics. *Mov Disord.* 1999;14(1):95–101. Epub 1999/01/26.

17. Barbeau A, Duvoisin RC, Gerstenbrand F, *et al.* Classification of extrapyramidal disorders. Proposal for an international classification and glossary of terms. *J Neurol Sci.* 1981;51(2):311–27. Epub 1981/08/01.

18. Kremer B. Clinical neurology of Huntington's disease. In: GP Bates, P Harper, and L Jones (eds). *Huntington's Disease.* Oxford: Oxford University Press, 2002.

19. Tarsy D and Simon DK. Dystonia. *N Engl J Med..* 2006;355(8):818–29. Epub 2006/08/25.

20. Paulsen JS, Nehl C, Hoth KF, *et al.* Depression and stages of Huntington's disease. *J Neuropsychiatry Clin Neurosci.* 2005;17(4):496–502. Epub 2006/01/03.

21. Paulsen JS, Hoth KF, Nehl C, *et al.* Critical periods of suicide risk in Huntington's disease. *Am J Psychiat.* 2005;162(4):725–31. Epub 2005/04/01.

22. Lipe H, Schultz A, and Bird TD. Risk factors for suicide in Huntington's disease: a retrospective case controlled study. *Am J Med Genet.* 1993;48(4):231–3. Epub 1993/12/15.

23. Lovestone S, Hodgson S, Sham P, *et al.* Familial psychiatric presentation of Huntington's disease. *J Med Genet.* 1996;33(2):128–31. Epub 1996/02/01.

24. Craufurd D and Snowden J. Neuropsychological and neuropsychiatric aspects of Huntington's disease. In: GP Bates, P Harper, and L Jones (eds). *Huntington's Disease.* Oxford: Oxford University Press, 2002.

25. Paulsen JS, Ready RE, Hamilton JM, *et al.* Neuropsychiatric aspects of Huntington's disease. *J Neurol Neurosur Ps.* 2001;71(3):310–4. Epub 2001/08/21.

26. Marin RS. Apathy: a neuropsychiatric syndrome. *J Neuropsychiatry Clin Neurosci.* 1991;3(3):243–54. Epub 1991/01/01.

27. Starkstein SE and Leentjens AF. The nosological position of apathy in clinical practice. *J Neurol Neurosur Ps.* 2008;79(10):1088–92. Epub 2008/01/12.

28. Reedeker N BJ, van Duijn E, Giltay EJ, *et al.* Incidence, Course, and Predictors of Apathy in Huntington's Disease: A Two-Year Prospective Study. *J Neuropsychiatry Clin Neurosci.* 2011;23(4):434–41.

29. Duff K, Paulsen JS, Beglinger LJ, *et al.* 'Frontal' behaviors before the diagnosis of Huntington's disease and their relationship to markers of disease progression: evidence of early lack of awareness. *J Neuropsychiatry Clin Neurosci.* 2010;22(2):196–207. Epub 2010/05/14.

30. Paulsen JS, Langbehn DR, Stout JC, *et al.* Detection of Huntington's disease decades before diagnosis: the Predict-HD study. *J Neurol Neurosur Ps.* 2008;79(8):874–80. Epub 2007/12/22.

31. Paulsen JS, Zhao H, Stout JC, *et al.* Clinical markers of early disease in persons near onset of Huntington's disease. *Neurology.* 2001;57(4):658–62.

32. Brandt J and Butters N. The neuropsychological characteristics of Huntington's disease. *Tremds Neurosci.* 1986;9(118–120).

33. Group HS. Unified Huntington's disease rating scale: reliability and consistency. *Mov Disord.* 1996;11:136–42.

34. Paulsen JS. Cognitive impairment in Huntington disease: diagnosis and treatment. *Current Neurology and Neuroscience Reports.* 2011;11(5):474–83. Epub 2011/08/24.

35. Nelson HE and Willison JR. The Revised National Adult Reading Test (NART): Test Manual. indsor: NRER-Nelson, 1991.

36. O'Rourke JJ, Adams WH, Duff K, *et al.* Estimating premorbid functioning in huntington's disease: the relationship between disease progression and the wide range achievement test reading subtest. *Arch Clin Neuropsych.* 2011;26(1):59–66. Epub 2010/12/15.

37. Hinton SC, Paulsen JS, Hoffmann RG, *et al.* Motor timing variability increases in preclinical Huntington's disease patients as estimated onset of motor symptoms approaches. *JINS.* 2007;13(3):539–43. Epub 2007/04/21.

38. Rowe KC, Paulsen JS, Langbehn DR, *et al.* Self-paced timing detects and tracks change in prodromal Huntington disease. *Neuropsychology.* 2010;24(4):435–42. Epub 2010/07/08.

39. Stout JC, Jones R, Labuschagne I, *et al.* Evaluation of longitudinal 12 and 24 month cognitive outcomes in premanifest and early Huntington's disease. *J Neurol Neurosur Ps.* 2012;83(7):687–94. Epub 2012/05/09.

40. Boeve BF, Boylan KB, Graff-Radford NR, *et al.* Characterization of frontotemporal dementia and/or amyotrophic lateral sclerosis associated with the GGGGCC repeat expansion in C9ORF72. *Brain.* 2012;135(Pt 3):765–83. Epub 2012/03/01.

41. Petersen RC, Stevens JC, Ganguli M, *et al.* Practice parameter: early detection of dementia: mild cognitive impairment (an evidence-based review). Report of the Quality Standards Subcommittee of the American Academy of Neurology. *Neurology.* 2001;56(9):1133–42. Epub 2001/05/09.

42. Winblad B, Palmer K, Kivipelto M, *et al.* Mild cognitive impairment—beyond controversies, towards a consensus: report of the International Working Group on Mild Cognitive Impairment. *J Int Med.* 2004;256(3):240–6. Epub 2004/08/25.

43. Duff K, Paulsen J, Mills J, *et al.* Mild cognitive impairment in prediagnosed Huntington disease. *Neurology.* 2010;75(6):500–7. Epub 2010/07/09.

44. Peavy GM, Jacobson MW, Goldstein JL, *et al.* Cognitive and functional decline in Huntington's disease: dementia criteria revisited. *Mov Disord.* 2010;25(9):1163–9. Epub 2010/07/16.

45. Salmon DP, Kwo-on-Yuen PF, Heindel WC, *et al.* Differentiation of Alzheimer's disease and Huntington's disease with the Dementia Rating Scale. *Arch Neurol.* 1989;46(11):1204–8. Epub 1989/11/01.

46. Salmon DP, Hamilton JM, and Peavy GM. Neuropsychological deficits in Huntington's disease: Implications for striatal function in cognition. *Handbook of Neuropsychology,* 2nd edn. Amsterdam: Elsevier, 2001.

47. Rohrer D, Salmon DP, Wixted JT, *et al.* The disparate effects of Alzheimer's disease and Huntington's disease on semantic memory. *Neuropsychology.* 1999;13(3):381–8. Epub 1999/08/14.

48. Teichmann M, Gaura V, Demonet JF, *et al.* Language processing within the striatum: evidence from a PET correlation study in Huntington's disease. *Brain.* 2008;131(Pt 4):1046–56. Epub 2008/03/13.

49. Teichmann M, Dupoux E, Cesaro P, *et al.* The role of the striatum in sentence processing: evidence from a priming study in early stages of Huntington's disease. *Neuropsychologia.* 2008;46(1):174–85. Epub 2007/09/15.

50. van der Burg JM, Bjorkqvist M, and Brundin P. Beyond the brain: widespread pathology in Huntington's disease. *Lancet Neurol.* 2009;8(8):765–74. Epub 2009/07/18.

51. Morton AJ. Circadian and sleep disorder in Huntington's disease. *Exp Neurol.* 2012;243:34–44. Epub 2012/10/27.

52. Duyao MP, Auerbach AB, Ryan A, *et al.* Inactivation of the mouse Huntington's disease gene homolog Hdh. *Science.* 1995;269(5222):407–10. Epub 1995/07/21.

53. Nasir J, Floresco SB, O'Kusky JR, *et al.* Targeted disruption of the Huntington's disease gene results in embryonic lethality and behavioral and morphological changes in heterozygotes. *Cell.* 1995;81(5):811–23. Epub 1995/06/02.

54. Zeitlin S, Liu JP, Chapman DL, *et al.* Increased apoptosis and early embryonic lethality in mice nullizygous for the Huntington's disease gene homologue. *Nature Gen.* 1995;11(2):155–63. Epub 1995/10/01.

55. Ross CA and Tabrizi SJ. Huntington's disease: from molecular pathogenesis to clinical treatment. *Lancet Neurol.* 2011;10(1):83–98.

56. Ferrante RJ, Kowall NW, Beal MF, *et al.* Selective sparing of a class of striatal neurons in Huntington's disease. *Science.* 1985;230(4725):561–3. Epub 1985/11/01.

57. Gutekunst C-A, Norflus F, and Hersch SM. The neuropathology of Huntington's disease. In: GP Bates, P Harper, and L Jones (eds). *Huntington's Disease*. Oxford: Oxford University Press, 2002.

58. Sapp E, Kegel KB, Aronin N, *et al.* Early and progressive accumulation of reactive microglia in the Huntington disease brain. *J Neuropath Exp Neur* 2001;60(2):161–72. Epub 2001/03/29.

59. Dumas EM, van den Bogaard SJ, Ruber ME, *et al.* Early changes in white matter pathways of the sensorimotor cortex in premanifest Huntington's disease. *Hum Brain Map.* 2012;33(1):203–12. Epub 2011/01/26.

60. Rosas HD, Lee SY, Bender AC, *et al.* Altered white matter microstructure in the corpus callosum in Huntington's disease: implications for cortical 'disconnection'. *NeuroImage.* 2010;49(4):2995–3004. Epub 2009/10/24.

61. Novak MJU and Tabrizi SJ. Huntington's disease. *BMJ.* 2010;340(Jun 30):c3109–c.

62. Guidelines for the molecular genetics predictive test in Huntington's disease. International Huntington Association (IHA) and the World Federation of Neurology (WFN) Research Group on Huntington's Chorea. *Neurology.* 1994;44(8):1533–6. Epub 1994/08/01.

63. Group HS. Tetrabenazine as antichorea therapy in Huntington disease: a randomized controlled trial. *Neurology.* 2006;66(3):366–72. Epub 2006/02/16.

64. Armstrong MJ and Miyasaki JM. Evidence-based guideline: pharmacologic treatment of chorea in Huntington disease: report of the guideline development subcommittee of the American Academy of Neurology. *Neurology.* 2012;79(6):597–603. Epub 2012/07/21.

65. Burgunder JM, Guttman M, Perlman S, *et al.* An International Survey-based Algorithm for the Pharmacologic Treatment of Chorea in Huntington's Disease. *PLoS Currents.* 2011;3:RRN1260. Epub 2011/10/07.

66. European Huntington's Disease Network Physiotherapy Guidance Document.Group EPW. Physiotherapy Guidance Document 2009. Available at: <http://www.euro-hd.net/html/disease/huntington/pub-docs/physiotherapy-guidance-doc-2009.pdf?eurohdsid=16190857de79 31911227b257dc3f4b7a>.

67. Anderson K, Craufurd D, Edmondson MC, *et al.* An international survey-based algorithm for the pharmacologic treatment of obsessive-compulsive behaviors in Huntington's disease. *PLoS Currents.* 2011;3:RRN1261. Epub 2011/09/29.

68. Groves M, van Duijn E, Anderson K, *et al.* An international survey-based algorithm for the pharmacologic treatment of irritability in Huntington's disease. *PLoS Currents.* 2011;3:RRN1259. Epub 2011/10/07.

69. Nithianantharajah J and Hannan AJ. Enriched environments, experience-dependent plasticity and disorders of the nervous system. *Nature RNeurosci.* 2006;7(9):697–709. Epub 2006/08/23.

70. Zanetti O, Binetti G, Magni E, *et al.* Procedural memory stimulation in Alzheimer's disease: impact of a training programme. *Acta Neurol Scand.* 1997;95(3):152–7.

71. Andrew SEGYP, Kremer B, Squitieri F, *et al.* Huntington Disease without CAG Expansion: Phenocopies or Errors in Assignment? *Am J Hum Genet.* 1994;54:852–63.

72. Persichetti F, Kanaley L, Ge P, *et al.* Huntingtton's disease CAG trinucleotide repeats in pathologically confirmed post-mortem brains. *Neurobiology of Disease.* 1994;1:159–66.

73. Wild EJ and Tabrizi ST. Huntington's disease phenocopy syndromes. *Curr Opin Neurol.* 2007;20:681–7.

74. Moore RCXF, Monaghan J, Han D, *et al.* Huntington's Disease Phenocopy Is a Familiar Prion Disease. *Am J Hum Genet.* 2001;69:1385–8.

75. Wild EJ, Mudanohwo EE, Sweeney MG, *et al.* Huntington's disease phenocopies are clinically and genetically heterogeneous. *Mov Disord.* 2008;23(5):716–20. Epub 2008/01/09.

76. Margolis RL, Holmes SE, Rosenblatt A, *et al.* Huntington's Disease-like 2 (HDL2) in North America and Japan. *Ann Neurol.* 2004;56(5):670–4. Epub 2004/10/07.

77. Magazi DS, Krause A, Bonev V, *et al.* Huntington's disease: genetic heterogeneity in black African patients. *South Afr Med J.*2008;98(3):200–3. Epub 2008/03/20.

78. Schmahmann JD. Disorders of the cerebellum: ataxia, dysmetria of thought, and the cerebellar cognitive affective syndrome. *J Neuropsychiatry Clin Neurosci.* 2004;16(3):367–78. Epub 2004/09/21.

79. Pandolfo M. Friedreich ataxia. *Seminars in Pediatric Neurology.* 2003;10(3):163–72.

80. Durr AC, Agid Y, Campuzano V, *et al.* Clinical and Genetic Abnormalities in Patients with Friedreich's Ataxia. *New Engl J Med.* 1996;335(16).

81. Campuzano V, Montermini L, Molto MD, *et al.* Friedreich's ataxia: autosomal recessive disease caused by an intronic GAA triplet repeat expansion. *Science.* 1996;271(5254):1423–7. Epub 1996/03/08.

82. Harding AE. *Freidreich's Ataxia. The Hereditary Ataxias and Related Disorders*. London: Churchill Livingstone, 1984.

83. Pandolfo M. Friedreich ataxia: the clinical picture. *J Neurol* 2009;256 Suppl 1:3–8. Epub 2009/04/11.

84. White M and Botez-Marquard T. Neuropsychologic and neuropsychiatric characteristics of patients with Friedreich's ataxia. *Acta Neurol Scand.* 2000;102:222–6.

85. Corben LA, Georgiou-Karistianis N, Fahey MC, *et al.* Towards an understanding of cognitive function in Friedreich ataxia. *Brain Res Bull.* 2006;70(3):197–202. Epub 2006/07/25.

86. Nieto A, Correia R, de Nobrega E, *et al.* Cognition in Friedreich Ataxia. *Cerebellum.* 2012;11(4):834–44. Epub 2012/02/22.

87. Wollmann T, Barroso J, Monton F, *et al.* Neuropsychological test performance of patients with Friedreich's ataxia. *J Clin Exp Neuropsyc.* 2002;24(5):677–86. Epub 2002/08/21.

88. Corben LA, Akhlaghi H, Georgiou-Karistianis N, *et al.* Impaired inhibition of prepotent motor tendencies in Friedreich ataxia demonstrated by the Simon interference task. *Brain Cognition.* 2011;76(1):140–5. Epub 2011/03/01.

89. Bouchard JP, Barbeau A, Bouchard R, *et al.* Autosomal Recessive Spastic Ataxia of Charlevoix–Saguenay. *Can J Neurol Sci.* 1978;5(1):61–9.

90. Verhoeven WM, Egger JI, Ahmed AI, *et al.* Cerebellar cognitive affective syndrome and autosomal recessive spastic ataxia of charlevoix-saguenay: a report of two male sibs. *Psychopathology.* 2012;45(3):193–9. Epub 2012/03/24.

91. Manto MU. The wide spectrum of spinocerebellar ataxias (SCAs). *Cerebellum.* 2005;4(1):2–6. Epub 2005/05/18.

92. Subramony S. The Ataxias. In: NW Wood (ed.). *Neurogenetics A Guide for Clinicians*. Cambridge: Cambridge University Press, 2012, pp. 52–63.

93. Harding AE. *Autosomal Dominant Cerebellar Ataxias. The Hereditary Ataxias and Related Disorders*. London: Churchill Livingstone, 1984.

94. Geschwind DH. Focusing attention on cognitive impairment in spinocerebellar ataxia. *Arch Neurol.* 1999;56(1):20–2. Epub 1999/01/29.

95. Sokolovsky N, Cook A, Hunt H, *et al.* A preliminary characterisation of cognition and social cognition in spinocerebellar ataxia types 2, 1, and 7. *Behavioural Neurology.* 2010;23(1–2):17–29. Epub 2010/08/18.

96. Burk K, Globas C, Bosch S, *et al.* Cognitive deficits in spinocerebellar ataxia type 1, 2, and 3. *J Neurol.* 2003;250(2):207–11. Epub 2003/02/08.

97. Kawai Y, Suenaga M, Watanabe H, *et al.* Cognitive impairment in spinocerebellar degeneration. *Eur Neurol.* 2009;61(5):257–68. Epub 2009/03/20.

98. Burk K, Globas C, Bosch S, *et al.* Cognitive deficits in spinocerebellar ataxia 2. *Brain.* 1999;122:769–77.

99. Storey E, Forrest SM, Shaw JH, *et al.* Spinocerebellar ataxia type 2: clinical features of a pedigree displaying prominent frontal-executive dysfunction. *Arch Neurol.* 1999;56(1):43–50. Epub 1999/01/29.

100. Maruff P, Tyler P, Burt T, *et al.* Cognitive deficits in Machado–Joseph disease. *Ann Neurol.* 1996;40(3):421–7. Epub 1996/09/01.

101. Kawai Y, Suenaga M, Watanabe H, *et al.* Prefrontal hypoperfusion and cognitive dysfunction correlates in spinocerebellar ataxia type 6. *J Neurol Sci.* 2008;271(1–2):68–74. Epub 2008/05/10.

102. Globas C, Bosch S, Zuhlke C, *et al.* The cerebellum and cognition. Intellectual function in spinocerebellar ataxia type 6 (SCA6). *J Neurol.* 2003;250(12):1482–7. Epub 2003/12/16.

103. Torrens L, Burns E, Stone J, *et al.* Spinocerebellar ataxia type 8 in Scotland: frequency, neurological, neuropsychological and neuropsychiatric findings. *Acta Neurol Scand.* 2008;117(1):41–8. Epub 2007/12/22.

104. Lilja A, Hamalainen P, Kaitaranta E, *et al.* Cognitive impairment in spinocerebellar ataxia type 8. *J Neurol Sci.* 2005;237(1–2):31–8. Epub 2005/06/17.

105. Matsuura T and Ashizawa T. Spinocerebellar Ataxia Type 10. In: RA Pagon, TD Bird, CR Dolan, K Stephens, *et al.* (eds). *GeneReviews.* Seattle, WA: University of Washington, Seattle, 1993. Available at: <http://www.ncbi.nlm.nih.gov/books/NBK1175/>.

106. O'Hearn E, Holmes SE, Calvert PC, *et al.* SCA-12: Tremor with cerebellar and cortical atrophy is associated with a CAG repeat expansion. *Neurology.* 2001;56(3):299–303. Epub 2001/02/15.

107. Schneider SA, van de Warrenburg BP, Hughes TD, *et al.* Phenotypic homogeneity of the Huntington disease-like presentation in a SCA17 family. *Neurology.* 2006;67(9):1701–3. Epub 2006/11/15.

108. Rolfs A, Koeppen AH, Bauer I, *et al.* Clinical features and neuropathology of autosomal dominant spinocerebellar ataxia (SCA17). *Ann Neurol.* 2003;54(3):367–75. Epub 2003/09/04.

109. Schelhaas HJ, van de Warrenburg BP, Hageman G, *et al.* Cognitive impairment in SCA-19. *Acta Neurologica Belgica.* 2003;103(4):199–205. Epub 2004/03/11.

110. Zoghbi HY and Orr HT. Glutamine repeats and neurodegeneration. *Annu Rev Neurosci.* 2000;23:217–47. Epub 2000/06/09.

111. Wardle M, Majounie E, Williams NM, *et al.* Dentatorubral pallidoluysian atrophy in South Wales. *J Neurol Neurosur Ps.* 2008;79(7):804–7. Epub 2007/10/30.

112. Tsuji S. Dentatorubral-pallidoluysian atrophy (DRPLA): clinical features and molecular genetics. *Adv Neurosci.* 1999;79:399–409. Epub 1999/10/09.

113. Federico A, Di Donato I, Bianchi S, *et al.* Hereditary cerebral small vessel diseases: a review. *J Neurol Sci.* 2012;322(1–2):25–30. Epub 2012/08/08.

114. Dominguez-Sanchez FJ, Lasa-Aristu A, and Goni-Imizcoz M. Intelligence impairment, personality features and psychopathology disturbances in a family affected with CADASIL. *Spanish Journal of Psychology.* 2011;14(2):936–43. Epub 2011/11/09.

115. Joutel A, Corpechot C, Ducros A, *et al.* Notch3 mutations in CADASIL, a hereditary adult-onset condition causing stroke and dementia. *Nature.* 1996;383(6602):707–10. Epub 1996/10/24.

116. Ruchoux MM and Maurage CA. Endothelial changes in muscle and skin biopsies in patients with CADASIL. *Neuropath Appl Neuro.* 1998;24(1):60–5. Epub 1998/04/29.

117. Peters N, Holtmannspotter M, Opherk C, *et al.* Brain volume changes in CADASIL: a serial MRI study in pure subcortical ischemic vascular disease. *Neurology.* 2006;66(10):1517–22. Epub 2006/05/24.

118. Stromillo ML, Dotti MT, Battaglini M, *et al.* Structural and metabolic brain abnormalities in preclinical cerebral autosomal dominant arteriopathy with subcortical infarcts and leucoencephalopathy. *J Neurol Neurosur Ps.* 2009;80(1):41–7. Epub 2008/10/03.

119. Lanfranconi S and Markus HS. COL4A1 mutations as a monogenic cause of cerebral small vessel disease: a systematic review. *Stroke.* 2010;41(8):e513–8. Epub 2010/06/19.

120. Mead S, James-Galton M, Revesz T, *et al.* Familial British dementia with amyloid angiopathy: early clinical, neuropsychological and imaging findings. *Brain.* 2000;123 (Pt 5):975–91. Epub 2000/04/25.

121. Isaacs AM, Johannsen P, Holm I, *et al.* Frontotemporal dementia caused by CHMP2B mutations. *Current Alzheimer Research.* 2011;8(3):246–51. Epub 2011/01/13.

122. Gydesen S, Brown JM, Brun A, *et al.* Chromosome 3 linked frontotemporal dementia (FTD-3). *Neurology.* 2002;59(10):1585–94. Epub 2002/11/27.

123. Schiffmann R, Moore DF. Neurological manifestations of Fabry disease. In: A Mehta, M Beck, G Sunder-Plassmann (eds). *Fabry Disease: Perspectives from 5 Years of FOS.* Oxford: Oxford PharmaGenesis, 2006. Available at: <http://www.ncbi.nlm.nih.gov/books/NBK11586/>.

124. Taylor RW, McDonnell MT, Blakely EL, *et al.* Genotypes from patients indicate no paternal mitochondrial DNA contribution. *Ann Neurol.* 2003;54(4):521–4. Epub 2003/10/02.

125. Filosto M, Mancuso M, Vives-Bauza C, *et al.* Lack of paternal inheritance of muscle mitochondrial DNA in sporadic mitochondrial myopathies. *Ann Neurol.* 2003;54(4):524–6. Epub 2003/10/02.

126. Schwartz M and Vissing J. No evidence for paternal inheritance of mtDNA in patients with sporadic mtDNA mutations. *J Neuro Sci.* 2004;218(1–2):99–101. Epub 2004/02/05.

127. Schwartz M and Vissing J. Paternal inheritance of mitochondrial DNA. *New Engl J Med.* 2002;347(8):576–80. Epub 2002/08/23.

128. McFarland R, Taylor R, Schaefer A, Turnbull D. Mitochondrial disorders. In: NW Wood (ed.). *Neurogenetics: A Guide for Clinicians.* Cambridge: Cambridge University Press, 2012, pp. 188–211.

129. Kaufmann P, Shungu DC, Sano MC, *et al.* Cerebral lactic acidosis correlates with neurological impairment in MELAS. *Neurology.* 2004;62(8):1297–302. Epub 2004/04/28.

130. Finsterer J. Mitochondrial disorders, cognitive impairment and dementia. *J Neuro Sci.* 2009;283(1–2):143–8. Epub 2009/03/10.

131. Yeh HL, Chen YK, Chen WH, *et al.* Perfusion status of the stroke-like lesion at the hyperacute stage in MELAS. *Brain Dev.* 2013 Feb;35(2)158–64.

132. Kaufmann P, Engelstad K, Wei Y, *et al.* Natural history of MELAS associated with mitochondrial DNA m.3243A>G genotype. *Neurology.* 2011;77(22):1965–71. Epub 2011/11/19.

133. Salsano E, Giovagnoli AR, Morandi L, *et al.* Mitochondrial dementia: a sporadic case of progressive cognitive and behavioral decline with hearing loss due to the rare m.3291T>C MELAS mutation. *J Neuro Sci.* 2011;300(1–2):165–8. Epub 2010/10/15.

CHAPTER 32

Changing concepts and new definitions for Alzheimer's disease

Bruno Dubois and Olga Uspenskaya-Cadoz

Alzheimer's disease (AD) is a progressive neurodegenerative disorder with cognitive, behavioural and functional abnormalities. AD is the most prevalent form of dementia: it accounts for approximately 70 per cent of cases of progressive cognitive impairment in aged individuals,[4] age being the single most important risk factor. The prevalence of AD doubles every 5 years after the age of 60 and reaches 40 per cent after 90.[5] The disease is linked with ageing but it is not due to ageing, as exemplified by early-onset cases, usually defined as symptoms starting before 65.[6]

The dementia syndrome associated with advanced AD has characteristic clinical features usually including various combinations of memory impairment, language abnormalities, impaired gestural skills (apraxia), disturbances of visuospatial functions, and executive deficits. These cognitive and behavioural abnormalities interfere with functional activities of daily living (ADL), with ADL impairment being a marker and core criterion for the diagnosis of a dementia syndrome.[7]

A number of bedside tests, for example the Mini Mental Status Examination, can be used to provide a global quantification of the deficits and is useful for characterizing the stage of cognitive decline.[8] However, more detailed neuropsychological testing with standardized assessment of attention, memory, language, executive functions, and visuospatial abilities is required for quantifying the deficits of AD and may aid distinguishing AD from other degenerative dementias.

In addition, various neuropsychiatric disturbances can be observed in patients with AD: apathy, dysphoria, and agitation are common during the course of the disease.[9] Apathy, characterized by a lack of interest in unusual or interpersonal activities, can occur very early in the course of the disease, in the absence of depression. In contrast, psychosis (delusions or hallucinations), where present, is observed in the more advanced phases of the disease.

The clinical diagnosis of AD has traditionally required exclusion of alternative explanations for cognitive decline using blood testing, brain neuroimaging including computerized tomography (CT) or magnetic resonance imaging (MRI), and, on some occasions, cerebrospinal fluid (CSF) examination, but has not employed biomarkers to help certify a positive diagnosis.

There are no established disease-modifying treatments for AD. Cholinesterase inhibitors (ChE-Is) and memantine have proven benefits in placebo-controlled trials and may be useful for individual patients, but overall their effects are limited;[10] and trials using potential disease-modifying treatments have not yet demonstrated significant effect, at least on clinical outcomes. Psychotropic agents, including mood-stabilizing anticonvulsants and neuroleptics, should be used with parsimony for behavioural disturbances and neuropsychiatric symptoms, although depression should always be considered and treated as appropriate. Education of and support for caregivers is important for optimal care of the patients.

The historical concept of AD

We have learned—and many still teach—that AD is a clinicopathological entity: the diagnosis of AD cannot be confirmed on clinical grounds alone and definite diagnosis needs histological confirmation based on cerebral biopsy or postmortem examination, the exception being in rare cases where autosomal dominantly inherited genetic mutation in the *APP*, *presenilin 1*, or *presenilin 2* genes identified. In the absence of such histological, or genetic, evidence, the clinical diagnosis of AD can only be *probable* and should only be made when the disease is advanced and reaches the threshold of dementia.

AD as a dementia

Based on the original NINCDS–ADRDA criteria,[11] the diagnosis of probable AD requires a two-step procedure. First, a *dementia syndrome* must be invoked by clinical examination, documented by mental status questionnaire, and confirmed by neuropsychological testing: there must be deficit in two or more areas of cognition, including memory with a progressive worsening over time responsible for a significant impact on activities of daily living. There must be no disturbance of consciousness at the time of the assessment and no evidence of systemic or other brain diseases that could account for a dementia syndrome. Second, a *process of exclusion* should rule out other possible aetiologies of a dementia syndrome with blood investigations (for excluding infectious, inflammatory, or metabolic diseases), brain neuroimaging—CT scan or MRI (for excluding small vessel disease, strategic lacunar infarcts, large vessel infarcts, and/or cerebral haemorrhages, brains tumour, hydrocephalus, etc.), and where appropriate additional investigations such as CSF examination.

The concept of MCI

Considering AD only as a 'dementia' has obvious limitations, the most obvious being that it precludes diagnosis of patients with early memory problems that have not yet become disabling. This in turn has led to concept of mild cognitive impairment (MCI), a label that refers to objective memory and/or cognitive impairment not severe enough to impact on daily living activity. The concept of MCI was introduced by Flicker and colleagues[12] and the Mayo Clinic group[13] to fill the gap between the cognitive changes of normal ageing and those associated with dementia (be it due to vascular disease, neurodegeneration, or other causes). The mild symptomatic phase of AD, which precedes the fully developed clinical syndrome of dementia, was also included within the MCI spectrum.

Whilst the concept of MCI offers advantages, it also has several limitations. As used today, MCI is a clinical syndrome syndrome with a number of different pathological aetiologies. To decrease the clinical and pathological heterogeneity, subtyping MCI has been proposed (see chapter 21). However, the aetiologic heterogeneity of MCI remains problematic,[14] with only ~70 per cent of amnestic MCI cases who progress to dementia actually meet neuropathological criteria for AD.[15]

From a clinical point of view, in a given patient the most important thing for the clinician is not just to recognize the syndrome but to identify as far as possible the underlying *disease* as this may have significant impact in terms of prognosis or treatment. An obvious example is the need to distinguish MCI associated with depression and that due to AD, where management (including treatment) and prognosis are very different. From a research point of view, the heterogeneity of MCI may dilute the potential for a significant treatment effect and may have contributed to the negative outcomes in several MCI trials aiming to delay time to dementia.[16] This is particularly the case as novel approaches or drug compounds currently under development (including immunotherapy, γ- or β-secretase inhibitors, α-secretase activators) are AD-specific, and would not be expected to alter the disease process in other forms of cognitive impairment.

Revisiting the current concept of AD

Considering AD as a dementia is too late

AD pathology is already well advanced by the time patients present with their first cognitive symptoms, even if these are not sufficient to meet current criteria for dementia. There are a number of reasons for attempting to diagnose AD before dementia, including that:

- There is no reason to link the diagnosis of a disease with a certain threshold of severity and to exclude a large number of patients who are not yet expressing a full-blown dementia from diagnosis and treatment.

- There is no justification to anchor the diagnosis of AD to a dementia syndrome. By analogy with Parkinson's disease, the diagnosis should not hinge on a level of severity (e.g. when the patient is bedridden), but on the presence of the earliest motor symptoms (e.g. a limited resting tremor of one hand). The same should apply for AD.

- Earlier diagnosis may allow for earlier therapeutic interventions. Selecting patients with functional disability may be too late because at this stage amyloid burden is already extremely

widespread as shown by *in vivo* amyloid PET studies,[17] and there is also considerable irreversible neuronal loss. This may explain why clinical trials of disease-modifying treatments in patients with AD dementia have not proven effective, at least on meaningful clinical outcomes. There is therefore considerable interest in using a biomarker-based strategy to identify individuals with prodromal AD in whom therapies might be more effective, and where there is the potential to prevent the onset of symptoms.

The low specificity of the NINCDS–ADRDA criteria for AD

Performance of NINCDS–ADRDA criteria is low because at the time (1984) these criteria were established the clinical phenotype of AD was not specified and no reference to biomarkers was proposed. This explains why AD was frequently misdiagnosed with other neurodegenerative diseases that can fulfil the NINCDS–ADRDA criteria.[18]

Progress since the original NINCDS–ADRDA criteria

The clinical phenotype of AD

In more than 85 per cent of cases, AD presents as a progressive amnestic disorder. Episodic memory deficit is a highly prevalent and reliable neuropsychological marker of AD.[14] Early episodic memory impairment in underpinned by postmortem studies of AD patients which typically show that the early disease process appear to affect medial temporal lobe structures (entorhinal cortex, hippocampal formations, parahippocampal gyrus),[19] areas known to be critical for long-term episodic memory.

This pattern explains the typically rather homogeneous clinical presentation of AD, which can be divided into two main stages. The first consists of a progressive and predominantly amnestic syndrome related to the early involvement of medial temporal structures. The second is characterized by the spread of cognitive symptoms to other domains, including executive (conceptualization, judgment, problem-solving) and instrumental (language, praxis, face or object recognition) functions and of psycho-behavioural changes, due to the progressive spread of neuronal pathology to involve neocortical areas.[20] All these symptoms progressively impact on the patient's ability to continue their ADLs, as required to make a diagnosis of dementia.

A better characterization of other dementias

Diagnostic accuracy of Alzheimer's disease (AD) has also improved in recent years because of identification and definition of new dementia conditions through specific criteria, including the frontotemporal dementias, corticobasal degeneration, and dementia with Lewy bodies (DLB). Individualization of these diseases, which were often previously confused with AD, has consequently decreased its apparent heterogeneity.

The development of reliable biomarkers

Biomarkers for AD are now available at least in expert centres. These biomarkers can be divided into those that can demonstrate facets of the underlying pathophysiology, and those that are topographical/downstream markers.[2,21,22]

Pathophysiological markers. These target the underlying aetiological process that characterizes Alzheimer pathology. They include increased amyloid-PET imaging and CSF studies.

Amyloid-PET imaging is a very sensitive means of demonstrating Aβ plaque burden *in vivo*. Several different compounds are in various stages of clinical development and use, with one compound (Florbetapir) now licensed for the detection of fibrillar amyloid, and thus as a potential rule in/out of AD in cognitively impaired individuals. Amyloid-PET has shown very high post-mortem validation for the presence of fibrillar amyloid pathology,[23,24] good predictability for progression to AD dementia,[21,25] but low sensitivity to change in the clinical stages.[26] An important and as yet unresolved issue is that a significant minority of cognitively normal elderly individuals are amyloid-PET positive.[27]

Typical CSF findings in AD include decreased Aβ1-42 and increased total- and phopho-tau levels, although tau elevation may also be seen in other neurodegenerative diseases.[3] These CSF changes have a good specificity for AD: they significantly increase diagnostic accuracy in cases with clinically doubtful diagnoses[28] and are highly correlated with postmortem AD changes.[29,30] It should be noted that there is a large variability in CSF biomarker levels between techniques[31] and centres.[32]

Topographical/downstream markers. These evaluate less specific and downstream brain changes that result from AD pathology. They include medial temporal lobe atrophy[33] and reduced glucose metabolism in temporal parietal regions on FDG-PET.[34]

♦ Medial temporal atrophy, and hippocampal atrophy in particular,[35] are the most useful prodromal MRI biomarkers of a further progression to AD dementia. Hippocampal atrophy can be determined either by visual assessment[36] or quantification (e.g. by manual segmentation or automated software). The specificity of hippocampal volume for AD is influenced by several conditions, such as ageing, and in particular other neurological conditions or dementias which are associated with hippocampal volume loss (e.g. hippocampal sclerosis, Lewy body pathology, argyrophilic grain disease, and frontotemporal dementia). The reliability of volumetric measures obtained from repeated MRI scans is

high,[37] allowing the rate of atrophy over time to be assessed. This measure is a good diagnostic marker for early AD as the progression of hippocampal loss is approximately two to four times faster in AD patients than in age-matched normal controls.[38]

♦ FDG-PET has also proven to have a good sensitivity to detect brain dysfunction and early changes in AD[34] and to follow its evolution over time.[39] FDG uptake is reduced, predominantly in temporoparietal association areas including the precuneus and posterior cingulate cortex, and these changes are closely related to cognitive impairment as demonstrated in crosssectional and longitudinal studies.

AD biomarkers therefore demonstrate different facets of the disease, and have different clinical functions. Some are specific markers of AD pathology (CSF Aβ1-42 and amyloid-PET) but do not provide useful information about severity. Topographical/downstream markers (e.g. atrophy) by contrast can be used to show the effect of neurodegeneration or, when acquired serially, to quantify change over time (i.e. as markers of progression). They have been shown consistently to predict AD dementia in MCI cohorts and to correlate with disease severity. Recent advances in knowledge, natural history, and time course of these biomarkers have significantly changed our view of the disease. Amyloid markers become dynamic first before the occurrence of the clinical phase whereas tau markers and structural changes (hippocampal volume) are more linked to the prodromal/dementia phases of the disease. The temporal trajectory of each marker has been illustrated in a hypothetical model by Jack and colleagues (see Fig. 32.1).

To conclude this historical perspective, the classical definition of AD, based on the NINCDS–ADRDA diagnostic criteria,[11] had two major limitations: 1) they do not take into account specific features of the disease (i.e. the specific clinical phenotype and positive biomarkers), and 2) they can only be invoked when the dementia threshold is reached. The new conceptual framework for the diagnosis of AD recently proposed by the International Working

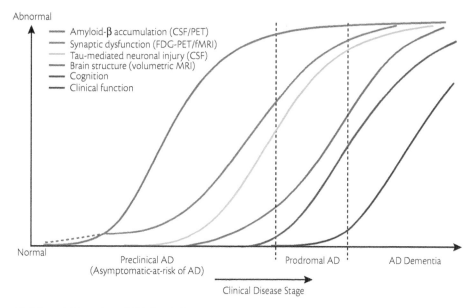

Fig. 32.1 Hypothetical model of dynamic biomarkers of Alzheimer's disease.

Table 32.1 The new concept of Alzheimer's disease

The NINCDS–ADRA concept of AD diagnosis (1984)	The IWG concept of AD diagnosis (2007)
◆ The diagnosis of AD **cannot be certified** clinically and needs a postmortem confirmation to be ascertained:	◆ Pathological biomarkers can be considered as **surrogate** markers of the underlying AD pathology:
◆ Therefore, the clinical diagnosis of AD can only be '**probable**'	◆ Therefore, the clinical diagnosis can be established *in vivo*
◆ and can only be made when the disease is advanced and reaches the threshold of **dementia**	◆ And **no more reference** to dementia is needed

Group (IWG)[1] [and latterly by the NIA/Alzheimer's Association (NIA/AA)][3] is based on two requirements: (1) to be earlier, and (2) to be more specific, even at an early stage of the disease. The differences between the old and new criteria are summarized in Table 32.1.

New concepts of AD

The reliable identification of biomarkers of AD is responsible for a major change in the conceptualization and diagnosis of the disease. Importantly, the new diagnostic criteria proposed by the IWG or by the NIA/AA both now use paraclinical investigations (MRI, CSF) not only for excluding other aetiologies of a dementia syndrome but also as part of the diagnostic procedure. However, the NIA/AA criteria have the advantage of being applicable when no supportive biomarkers are available, albeit at the expense of diagnostic specificity.

Considering biomarkers not to be linked to a stage of severity but rather to the disease process, these criteria potentially allow identification of Alzheimer's disease at a prodromal/MCI stage and even at a preclinical stage of the disease. Both sets of criteria recognize preclinical states of AD necessarily based on pathophysiological biomarkers since cognition remains normal (see Table 32.1 for a summary).

The IWG/Dubois criteria identify these individuals as 'asymptomatic at risk for AD'. This neutral nomenclature was chosen to acknowledge that not all these individuals progress to symptomatic AD. The NIA/AA criteria describe this state as 'preclinical AD'. This nomenclature may have more of an implication for progression, suggesting that 'preclinical' is the predecessor state for 'clinical' AD. The symptomatic phase of AD described in both sets of criteria embraces the same clinical entities, though with different terminologies and emphases. Differences in the classification of the stages of AD between the two sets of criteria can be found in Table 32.3.

IWG criteria emphasize a single clinical-biological approach that includes all symptomatic phases of AD and they use the same diagnostic algorithm across the spectrum of symptomatic disease consisting of:

◆ *A specific clinical phenotype.* As stated earlier, episodic memory disorders are the keystone of the clinical syndrome of typical AD. However, it should be reminded that a free recall deficit is common to many brain diseases. One way to disentangle the different diseases is to keep in mind the three stages of episodic memory

(see Box 32.1). Adequate memory tests that control for encoding and facilitate retrieval processing by the use of semantic cues can qualify the nature of the memory deficit. They can distinguish genuine memory storage impairment (e.g. failure of information storage and new memory formation as in AD) from attention or retrieval disorders. Memory tests, such the Free and Cued Selective Reminding Test (FCSRT) which controls encoding and retrieval processes,[40] can identify the 'amnesic syndrome of the hippocampal type' observed in AD,[14] which is defined by a very poor free recall (as in any memory disorder) and, crucially, decreased total recall even when given cues (i.e. insufficient effect of cueing).

Of course, an amnestic presentation may not always be present and other clinical phenotypes can be associated with postmortem evidence of AD pathology.[41] Therefore, the IWG has highlighted the concept of *atypical forms of AD* with specific clinical phenotypes that include non-amnestic focal cortical syndromes, such as logopenic aphasia, bi-parietal atrophy, posterior cortical atrophy, and frontal variant AD (Table 32.3).

◆ *Presence of AD biomarkers.* Biomarkers are *supportive* features of a diagnostic framework that is anchored around a core clinical phenotype. The AD diagnosis, evoked in case of a specific clinical phenotype (either typical or atypical), needs confirmation from the presence of one or several AD biomarkers. Among these, *in vivo* evidence of AD pathology (CSF changes of Aβ and tau levels or positive amyloid-PET) is the most specific and should be required for research purposes or atypical cases.

For the IWG, the diagnosis of AD is made on the basis of both clinical and biological evidence, with a high level of specificity and predictive validity. The diagnostic algorithm begins with a characteristic clinical phenotype (typical or atypical) and then requires supporting biomarkers that reflect the underlying AD process or pathology. The availability of specific *in vivo* biomarkers of AD pathology has moved the definition of AD from a *clinicopathological* entity to a *clinicobiological* entity. As biomarkers can be considered as surrogate markers of the histopathological changes, the clinical diagnosis can now be established *in vivo* and reference to dementia may no longer be needed.

The NIA/AA criteria

also divide the clinical phase of AD into MCI and AD dementia but employ different approaches to the diagnosis in each stage of the illness.

◆ *MCI due to AD.* The clinical criteria for MCI are the same as those previously published.[42] The NIA/AA criteria stratify the diagnosis of MCI with biomarkers to determine the likelihood that the syndrome is due to AD. A single positive biomarker of either amyloid abnormalities or neurodegeneration supports intermediate likelihood of MCI being due to AD, while two biomarkers—one of amyloid type and one of neurodegeneration type—support high likelihood of MCI being due to AD.

◆ *AD dementia.* The NIA/AA criteria apply an approach to diagnosis of dementia and AD dementia that differs from the approach to MCI due to AD.[43] Diagnostic standards for all causes of dementia are provided and 10 categories of dementia of the AD type are established including probable AD dementia, possible AD dementia, probable or possible AD dementia with evidence of the AD pathophysiological process.

Table 32.2 Different stages and classification of AD subtypes across NIA–AA and IWG criteria

NIA–AA criteria	IWG criteria	Comments
Preclinical AD Asymptomatic cerebral amyloidosis (ACA) ACA + evidence of neuronal injury (NI) ACA + NI + subtle cognitive decline	**Asymptomatic at risk with AD pathology**[1] **Presymptomatic AD**[2]	[1] Normal cognition with a pathophysiological marker [2] Normal cognition with an autosomal dominant AD-causing mutation
MCI due to AD MCI due to AD high likelihood[1] MCI due to AD intermediate likelihood[2] MCI possibly due to AD[3] MCI unlikely due to AD[4]	**Prodromal AD**[5]	[1] Biomarkers of amyloidosis and neuronal injury are positive [2] Biomarker of amyloidosis positive or biomarker of neuronal injury untested [3] Biomarker of amyloidosis positive and biomarker of neuronal injury are untested or give conflicting results [4] Biomarker of amyloidosis positive and biomarker of neuronal injury are negative [5] Episodic memory impairment or atypical AD-compatible syndrome with one pathophysiological marker (CSF or abnormal amyloid imaging)
Dementia caused by AD Probable AD dementia with increased level of certainty • AD dementia with documented clinical decline • AD dementia with an autosomal dominant AD-causing mutation Possible AD dementia • AD dementia with an atypical course • AD dementia with evidence of mixed aetiology Probable AD dementia with evidence of AD pathophysiological process • High likelihood of AD aetiology (biomarkers of amyloid abnormalities and neurodegeneration both present) • Intermediate likelihood of AD aetiology (biomarker of amyloid abnormalities or neurodegeneration is present) Possible AD dementia with evidence of the AD pathophysiological process • High likelihood of AD aetiology (biomarkers of amyloid abnormalities and neurodegeneration both present) • Intermediate likelihood of AD aetiology (biomarker of amyloid abnormalities or neurodegeneration is present) Pathophysiologically proved AD dementia (clinical phenotype of probable AD with neuropathology findings indicative of AD)	**AD dementia**[1]	[1] Episodic memory impairment or atypical AD phenotype with impaired activities of daily living AND at least one of the following biomarkers: • CSF changes (low Aβ and high tau p-tau) • abnormal amyloid imaging • medial temporal atrophy on MRI • bilateral parietal hypometabolism on FDG–PET • PS1, PS2, APP mutation carrier

Proposal for a new lexicon for AD

The new conceptual framework of AD suggests redefining a common lexicon[2] concerning AD and related entities (see Box 32.2).

Alzheimer's disease

AD should now be a label defining the clinical disorder which starts with the onset of the first specific clinical symptoms of the disease and which crucially encompasses both the predementia and dementia phases. AD now refers to the whole spectrum of the clinical phase of the disease and is not restricted to the dementia syndrome. The clinical diagnosis can be established *in vivo* and relies on a dual clinical-biological entity that requires the evidence of an amnestic syndrome of the hippocampal type (defined by a free recall deficit that is not normalized by cueing) and the presence of pathophysiological markers of AD. Distinguishing prodromal AD and dementia stages within the whole spectrum of AD might be still useful for individual patients, and in the wider socio-economic context.

AD dementia

It is likely to still be meaningful to identify the *dementia* threshold as a severity milestone in the course of disease. The presence of a dementia adds a set of management issues for the clinician to address including those related to patient autonomy such as driving and financial capacity as well as those related to care and daily living. The transition between the two states may be arbitrary when the underlying disease is a continuous process. Individual clinician's experience in dementia diagnosis and quality of information they receive or obtain on the cognitive and functional status of the patient will impact significantly on the threshold of detection of the transition to AD.

Prodromal AD

Prodromal AD refers to the early symptomatic predementia phase of the disease, characterized by a specific clinical phenotype of the amnestic syndrome of the hippocampal type with positive pathophysiological biomarkers. The memory disorders can be isolated or associated with other cognitive or behavioural changes that may

Box 32.1 Three stages of long-term memory

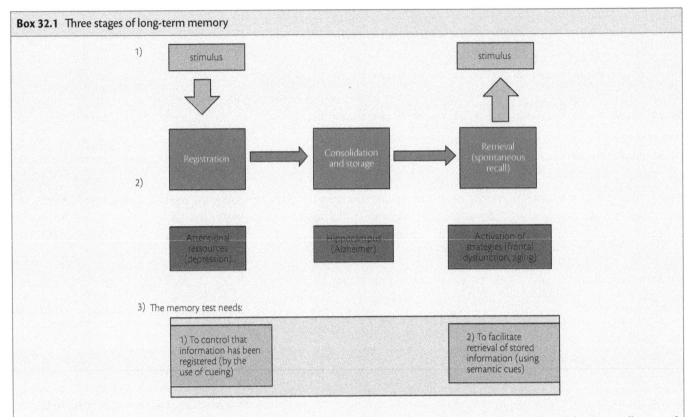

1) Episodic memory is currently evaluated by the recall of a list of items (words, sentences, drawings) after a delay (generally around 5–15 minutes).

2) To be recalled, the items should go through three successive stages:

   a. **Registration**, which mainly relies on attention resources. This stage is impaired in conditions that interfere with attention processes: e.g. depression, anxiety, sleep disorders, drugs (anticholinergics, benzodiazepines), ageing.

   b. The second stage is **storage**, i.e. transformation of perceived events into memory traces. This stage mainly relies on the hippocampus and related structures. This stage is impaired in Alzheimer's disease.

   c. The last stage is **retrieval**: this mainly relies on the ability to activate strategic processes to retrieved stored information, considered to be highly dependent on the functioning of the frontal lobes. This stage is impaired in case of frontal lesions/dysfunctions (frontotemporal dementias, subcorticofrontal dementias, or even normal ageing where activation of retrieval strategies is decreased and effortful).

3) There is a need to use memory tests that can dissociate different conditions by controlling for registration and by facilitating retrieval. This can be made with semantic cues as in the Free and Cued Selective Reminding Test.[40]

not be severe enough to interfere significantly with activities of daily living.

Atypical AD

This refers to less common clinical phenotypes that occur with AD pathology. There are well-defined clinical phenotype variant presentations of AD that do not follow the typical pattern of an amnestic syndrome of the hippocampal type. These include cortical syndromes of logopenic aphasia, posterior cortical atrophy, and frontal variants of AD. The diagnosis of atypical AD is established when the well-characterized clinical presentations (Table 32.3) are supported by a positive pathophysiological biomarkers of AD.

Mixed AD

This is defined by the co-occurrence of Alzheimer's pathology with other biological causes of cognitive decline, mainly cerebrovascular

disease or Lewy body pathology. Mixed pathologies are highly prevalent in the elderly and account for most dementia cases in the very old.[44] The label of 'mixed AD' is reserved to cases where both clinical features and diagnostic markers point to a mixed aetiology. Patients should fulfil the diagnostic criteria for typical AD and additionally present with clinical *and* brain imaging/biological evidence of other comorbid disorders such as cerebrovascular disease or Lewy body diseases.

Preclinical states of AD

There is a growing interest in the long preclinical phase of AD.[22] This preclinical phase refers to cognitively normal individuals with biomarker evidence of Alzheimer pathology. Positive retention of amyloid-PET or low Aβ level in the CSF is being reported in up to 30 per cent of older normal controls.[45] These healthy individuals may or may not later convert to prodromal AD. Such evolution to

Table 32.3 The specific phenotypes of Alzheimer's disease

Specific clinical phenotype of typical AD	◆ early, predominant amnestic syndrome of hippocampal type—isolated or associated with other cognitive changes
biparietal variant of AD	◆ impaired limb praxis skills—and features of the Gerstmann syndrome
logopenic variant of AD	◆ impaired single word retrieval—and repetition of sentences
posterior variant of AD	◆ impaired visuospatial functions—and/or of visual identification of objects, symbols, or visages
frontal variant of AD	◆ impaired executive functions—with the presence of a primary progressive apathy

a clinical disease may depend on several factors including genetic (such as ApoE genotype), other risk factors (e.g. vascular) or protective factors (diet, cognitive reserve), and comorbidities (e.g. diabetes). In the absence of knowledge about what factors combine to influence conversion, these normal individuals who are

---

Box 32.2   Terminology

1) **Alzheimer's Disease (AD)**: the whole clinical phase, no longer restricted to the dementia syndrome.

2) **Prodromal AD**: the early symptomatic, predementia phase of AD.

3) **AD dementia**: when cognitive symptoms interfere with activity of daily living.

4) **Typical AD**: the most common clinical phenotype of AD, characterized by an amnestic syndrome of the hippocampal type.

5) **Atypical AD**: less common but well-characterized clinical phenotypes that occur with Alzheimer's pathology. The diagnosis of AD needs in vivo evidence of pathophysiological markers.

6) **Mixed AD**: patients who fulfil the criteria for AD and additionally present with clinical and biomarkers evidence of other comorbid disorders.

7) **Asymptomatic at risk:** cognitively normal individuals with positive pathophysiological biomarkers.

8) **Presymptomatic AD**: cognitively normal individuals with a proven AD autosomal dominant mutation.

9) **Alzheimer's pathology**: underlying neurobiological changes responsible for AD.

10) **Pathophysiological markers**: biological changes that reflect the underlying AD pathology (CSF changes; PET-amyloid). They are markers of diagnosis.

11) **Topographical biomarkers**: downstream markers of neurodegeneration that can be structural (MRI) or metabolic (FDG-PET). They are markers of progression.

10) **Mild cognitive impairment (MCI)**: patients for whom there is no disease clearly identified.

---

biomarker-positive have been defined as 'asymptomatic, at risk for AD' or 'asymptomatic amyloidosis' rather than preclinical or presymptomatic because a large percentage of them will not progress to a symptomatic clinical condition.

This is not the case for cognitively normal individuals sharing an autosomal dominant monogenic AD mutation[46] Because of the full penetrance of the mutations, these individuals will inevitably develop a clinical AD if they live long enough. They are at a 'presymptomatic state for AD'.

Research versus clinical criteria

Whilst these newer criteria aim both to allow for diagnosis of AD earlier and more accurately, they depend on availability of suitable biomarkers. According to a report of AD International,[47] 58 per cent of people with dementia live in low- and middle-income countries. Even in developed countries, there is still a lack of availability of high-tech investigations for biomarkers outside tertiary or research centres. Therefore, the diagnostic approach proposed here can be applied only in expert centres with facilities to assess a large spectrum of biomarkers, viable assessment procedures, and with access to normative data. In this context, they may be useful for complex diagnosis such as in case of young-onset AD, posterior cortical atrophy, or logopenic aphasias where biomarkers may increase diagnostic accuracy.

When these biomarkers are not affordable, the older NINCDS–ADRDA criteria can be used in a clinical setting. However, in any case, it is still possible to refer to the new conceptual framework of AD according to which AD refers to the whole spectrum of the clinical phase of the disease, starting with the onset of the first specific clinical symptoms and encompassing both the prodromal/predementia and dementia phases.

References

1. Dubois B, Feldman HH, Jacova C, *et al.* Research criteria for the diagnosis of Alzheimer's disease: revising the NINCDS–ADRDA criteria. *Lancet Neurol.* 2007;6, 734–746.

2. Dubois B, Feldman HH, Jacova C, *et al.* Revising the definition of Alzheimer's disease: a new lexicon. *Lancet Neurol.* 2010 Nov;9(11):1118–27.

3. Jack CR, Albert MS, Knopman DS, *et al.* Introduction to the recommendations from the National Institute on Aging and the Alzheimer's Association workgroup on diagnostic guidelines for Alzheimer's disease. *Alzheimers Dement.* 2011 May;7(3):257–62.

4. Ferri CP, Prince M, Brayne C, *et al.* Global prevalence of dementia: a Delphi consensus study. Alzheimer's Disease International. *Lancet.* 2005 Dec 17;366(9503):2112–7.

5. Brookmeyer R, Evans DA, Hebert L *et al.* National estimates of the prevalence of Alzheimer's disease in the United States, *Alzheimers Dement.* 2011;7(1):61–73.

6. Rossor MN, Fox NC, Mummery CJ *et al.* The diagnosis of young-onset dementia. *Lancet Neurol.* 2010 Aug;9(8):793–806.

7. American Psychiatric Association. *Diagnostic and Statistical Manual of Mental Disorders, Fourth Edition—Text Revision (DSM–IV–TR).* Washington, DC: American Psychiatric Publishing, Inc., 2000.

8. Folstein MF, Folstein SE, and McHugh PR. 'Mini-mental state'. A practical method for grading the cognitive state of patients for the clinician. *J Psychiatr Res.* 1975;12(3):189–98.

9. Mega MS, Cummings JL, Fiorello T, *et al.* The spectrum of behavioral changes in Alzheimer's disease. *Neurology.* 1996;46 (1):130–135.

10. Birks J. Cholinesterase inhibitors for Alzheimer's disease. *Cochrane Database Syst Rev.* 2006;25;(1):CD005593.

11. McKhann G, Drachman DA, Folstein M. *et al.* Clinical diagnosis of Alzheimer's disease—Report of the the NINCDS–ADRDA Work Group under the auspices of Department of Health and Human Services Task Force on Alzheimer's disease. *Neurology.* 1984;34:939–944.

12. Flicker C, Ferris SH, and Reisberg B. Mild cognitive impairment in the elderly: predictors of dementia. *Neurology.* 1991 July;41:1006–9.

13. Petersen RC, Smith GE, Waring SC, *et al.* Mild cognitive impairment: Clinical characterization and outcome. *Arch Neurol.* 1999 March;56:303–8.

14. Dubois B and Albert ML. Amnestic MCI or prodromal Alzheimer's disease? *Lancet Neurol.* 2004 April;3(4):246–8.

15. Jicha GA, Parisi JE, Dickson DW, *et al.* Neuropathologic outcome of mild cognitive impairment following progression to clinical dementia. *Arch Neurol.* 2006 May;63(5):674–81.

16. Jelic V, Kivipelto M, and Winblad B. Clinical trials in mild cognitive impairment: lessons for the future. *J Neurol Neurosur Ps.* 2006 April;77(4):429–38.

17. Jack CR, Lowe VJ, Weigand SD, *et al.* Serial PIB and MRI in normal, mild cognitive impairment and Alzheimer's disease: implications for sequence of pathological events in Alzheimer's disease. *Brain.* 2009 May;132(Pt 5):1355–65.

18. Varma AR, Snowden JS, Lloyd JJ, *et al.* Evaluation of the NINCDS–ADRDA criteria in the differentiation of Alzheimer's disease and frontotemporal dementia. *J Neurol Neurosur Ps.* 1999 February;66(2):184–8.

19. Delacourte A. The natural and molecular history of Alzheimer's disease. *J Alzheimers Dis.* 2006;9(3 Suppl):187–94.

20. Braak H and Braak E. Neuropathological stageing of Alzheimer-related changes. *Acta Neuropathologica.* 1991; 82 (4): 239–59.

21. Jack CR, Knopman DS, Jagust WJ, *et al.* Hypothetical model of dynamic biomarkers of the Alzheimer's pathological cascade. *Lancet Neurol.* 2010; 9(1): 119–28.

22. Sperling RA, Aisen PS, Beckett LA, *et al.*Toward defining the preclinical stages of Alzheimer's disease: recommendations from the National Institute on Aging–Alzheimer's Association workgroups on diagnostic guidelines for Alzheimer's disease. *Alzheimers Dement.* 2011 May;7(3):280–92.

23. Clark CM, Schneider JA, Bedell BJ, *et al.* Use of florbetapir-PET for imaging beta-amyloid pathology. *JAMA.* 2011; Jan 19;305(3):275–83.

24. Ikonomovic MD, Klunk WE, Abrahamson EE, *et al.* Post-mortem correlates of in vivo PiB–PET amyloid imaging in a typical case of Alzheimer's disease. *Brain.* 2008;131(Pt 6):1630–45.

25. Koivunen J, Scheinin N, Virta JR, *et al.* Amyloid PET imaging in patients with mild cognitive impairment: a 2-year follow-up study. *Neurology.* 2011;76:1085–90.

26. Ossenkoppele R, Tolboom N, Foster-Dingley JC, *et al.* Longitudinal imaging of Alzheimer pathology using [11C]PIB, [18F] FDDNP and [18F]FDG PET. *Eur J Nucl Med Mol Imaging.* 2012 Jun;39(6):990–1000.

27. Aizenstein HJ, Nebes RD, Saxton JA, *et al.* Frequent amyloid deposition without significant cognitive impairment among the elderly. *Arch Neurol.* 2008 Nov;65(11):1509–17.

28. Le Bastard N, Martin JJ, Vanmechelen E, *et al.* Added diagnostic value of CSF biomarkers in differential dementia diagnosis. *Neurobiol Aging.* 2010 Nov;31(11):1867–76.

29. Buerger K, Ewers M, Pirttilä T, *et al.* CSF phosphorylated tau protein correlates with neocortical neurofibrillary pathology in Alzheimer's disease. *Brain.* 2006 Nov;129(Pt 11):3035–41.

30. Tapiola T, Alafuzoff I, Herukka SK, *et al.* Cerebrospinal fluid (beta)-amyloid 42 and tau proteins as biomarkers of Alzheimer-type pathologic changes in the brain. *Arch Neurol.* 2009 Mar;66(3):382–9.

31. Fagan AM, Shaw LM, Xiong C, *et al.* Comparison of analytical platforms for cerebrospinal fluid measures of β-amyloid 1-42, total tau, and p-tau181 for identifying Alzheimer disease amyloid plaque pathology. *Arch Neurol.* 2011 Sep;68(9):1137–44.

32. Verwey NA, van der Flier WM, Blennow K, *et al.* A worldwide multicentre comparison of assays for cerebrospinal fluid biomarkers in Alzheimer's disease. *Ann Clin Biochem.* 2009 May;46 (Pt 3):235–40.

33. Sabuncu MR, Desikan RS, Sepulcre J, *et al.* The dynamics of cortical and hippocampalatrophy in Alzheimer disease. *Arch Neurol.* 2011 Aug;68(8):1040–8.

34. Mosconi L. Brain glucose metabolism in the early and specific diagnosis of Alzheimer's disease.FDG–PET studies in MCI and AD. *Eur J Nucl Med Mol Imaging.* 2005;32:486–510.

35. Risacher SL, Saykin AJ, West JD, *et al.* Baseline MRI predictors of conversion from MCI to probable AD in the ADNI cohort. *Curr Alzheimer Res.* 2009 Aug;6(4):347–61.

36. Scheltens P, Leys D, Barkhof F, *et al.* Atrophy of medial temporal lobes on MRI in 'probable' Alzheimer's disease and normal ageing: diagnostic value and neuropsychological correlates. *J Neurol Neurosur Ps.* 1992 Oct;55(10):967–72.

37. Giedd JN, Kozuch P, Kaysen D, *et al.* Reliability of cerebral measures in repeated examinations with magnetic resonance imaging. *Psychiatry Res.* 1995;61:113–19.

38. Lo RY, Hubbard AE, Shaw LM, *et al*; for the Alzheimer's Disease Neuroimaging Initiative. Longitudinal change of biomarkers in cognitive decline. *Arch Neurol.* 2011 Oct;68(10):1257–66.

39. de Leon MJ, Convit A, Wolf OT, *et al.* Prediction of cognitive decline in normal elderly subjects with 2-[(18)F]fluoro-2-deoxy-D-glucose/poitron-emission tomography (FDG/PET). *Proc Natl Acad Sci USA.* 2001 Sep 11;98(19):10966–71.

40. Grober E, Buschke H, Crystal H, *et al.* Screening for dementia by memory testing. *Neurology.* 1988 Jun;38(6):900–3.

41. Murray ME, Graff-Radford NR, Ross OA, *et al.* Neuropathologically definedsubtypes of Alzheimer's disease with distinct characteristics: a restropective study. *Lancet Neurol.* 2011 Sep; 10(9):785–96.

42. Albert MS, DeKosky ST, Dickson D, *et al.* The diagnosis of mild cognitive impairment due to Alzheimer's disease: recommendations from the National Institute on Aging–Alzheimer's Association workgroups on diagnostic guidelines for Alzheimer's disease. *Alzheimers Dement.* 2011;7(3):270–9.

43. McKhann GM, Knopman DS, Chertkow H, *et al.* The diagnosis of dementia due to Alzheimer's disease: recommendations from the National Institute on Aging–Alzheimer's Association workgroups on diagnostic guidelines for Alzheimer's disease. *Alzheimers Dement.* 2011;7(3):263–9.

44. Jellinger KA and Attems J. Prevalence of dementia disorders in the oldest-old: an autopsy study. *Acta Neuropathol.* 2010 Apr;119(4):421–33.

45. Rowe C, Ellis K, Brown B, *et al.* Cognition, hippocampal volume and fibrillar Aβ burden as predictors of cognitive decline: three-year follow-up results from AIBL. Abstracts of AAIC 2012. *Alzheimers Dement.* 2012(Suppl):P433.

46. Bateman RJ, Xiong C, Benzinger TL, *et al.* Clinical and biomarker changes in dominantly inherited Alzheimer's disease. *N Engl J Med.* 2012 Aug 30;367(9):795–804.

47. Alzheimer's Disease International. World Alzheimer Report (2009). Available at https://www.alz.co.uk/research/files/WorldAlzheimerReport.pdf.

CHAPTER 33

Presentation and management of Alzheimer's disease

Susan Rountree and Rachelle S. Doody

Clinical features of AD through the disease process (mild/moderate/severe)

Introduction

Alzheimer disease (AD) is a syndrome of cognitive and functional decline associated with variable noncognitive or behavioural manifestations. These changes are correlated with biochemical and neuropathological changes in the brain that relentlessly worsen over time in conjunction with symptom progression.

AD is a feared risk of the ageing process and is the most common cause of dementia in adults 65 years of age or older.[1] The majority of cases are sporadic and causality is attributed to both genetic predisposition and environmental risk factors. Ageing in the context of increasing longevity is the primary risk factor for the development of AD, not confined to industrialized nations, and is the basis of global concern about an impending epidemic of this disease. Susceptibility genes have been identified, including the apolipoprotein E isoform epsilon 4 (APOE ε4) on chromosome 19; this inherited allele was found to increase the risk of developing AD from 20 per cent to 90 per cent in families with one or more APOE ε4 alleles,[2] suggesting a functional role of the isoform in the pathogenesis of late-onset AD.[3] Although the ε4 allele is neither necessary nor sufficient to cause the illness, it decreases the age of onset.[4] Several other genes have been identified through large genome-wide association studies (including *PICALM CR1 CLU, BIN1*) that are associated with the development of common or sporadic AD but they account for only a fraction of the increased risk.[5,6] These genes may however, serve as biomarkers or suggest pathogenic mechanisms or therapeutic targets.

Environmental risk factors are thought to be equally important in triggering AD. It is unknown whether vascular ageing has a causal role in AD pathogenesis but there are data consistent with causation.[7] Longitudinal studies suggest that some vascular risk factors during midlife (age 40–60) are associated with the propensity to develop AD dementia[8,9] and include diabetes mellitus[10] or elevated serum glucose levels,[11] high cholesterol,[12] high plasma homocysteine,[13] and obesity[14,15] or the metabolic syndrome.[16] Although the observation of cerebrovascular disease is a common finding in elderly individuals with dementia, a neuropathological study controlling for age and gender found concomitant cerebrovascular disease was observed more frequently in AD subjects compared with other neurodegenerative disorders, suggesting that[17] cerebrovascular disease may lower the threshold for AD and treatment of

vascular risk factors may be an effective preventative or delaying strategy. Low vitamin D levels are associated with a higher risk of AD.[18] The mechanisms underlying these associations are not completely understood. It is hypothesized that changes in the cerebrovascular endothelium affect the permeability of the blood–brain barrier, increasing free radical production and oxidative stress.[9,19] Dysregulation of insulin signalling in the brain is thought to be an early and common feature of AD,[20] and insulin is thought to reduce β-amyloid accumulation by multiple mechanisms[21] as well as be neuroprotective. Although type II diabetes and peripheral elevation of insulin have been associated with the development of cognitive impairment later in life, elevation of peripheral insulin was reported to be cognitively protective following the diagnosis of AD.[22] Other investigations have reported synergy of putative risk factors in multiplying the risk of AD, particularly the presence of both diabetes and the APOE-ε4 genotype,[23] or traumatic brain injury and APOE-ε4 allele.[24] On the other hand, some life-style factors may protect against cognitive decline in the elderly including exercise[25] and engaging in stimulating leisure activity.[26,27]

The pathogenesis of AD is incompletely understood but prevailing theories point to failure of β-amyloid clearance mechanisms as central to the process.[28,29] With ageing and metabolic disorders, amylin amyloid accumulates in cerebral blood vessels and grey matter and may induce failure of β-amyloid clearance.[30] APOE mediates the clearance of β-amyloid and the ε4 allele is less effective than other alleles.[31,32] Age-related changes in cerebral blood vessels may also impair the clearance of amyloid from the brain.[33] In the oldest old, aged 90 years or more, AD dementia frequently coexists with other conditions that affect cognition.[34] An autopsy series of clinically diagnosed AD cases found that elderly individuals frequently had mixed neuropathological conditions. In cases where the clinical diagnosis of AD was not accurate, the most frequent findings included tangle-only dementia, frontotemporal degeneration, cerebrovascular disease, Lewy body disease, and hippocampal sclerosis. Another autopsy series of incident dementia cases found AD neuropathology in 77 per cent of cases yet only 42 per cent had pure AD. AD neuropathology was mixed with changes of vascular dementia in 11 per cent of the cases overall yet the occurrence of pure vascular dementia was rare, occurring in only 3 per cent of the cases.[35] Individuals who develop symptoms of dementia before age 65 may have early-onset AD but other commonly diagnosed conditions that mimic AD occurring in younger individuals include human immunodeficiency virus (HIV), traumatic brain injury, or alcohol abuse.[36]

β-amyloid is an abnormally conformed protein aggregation found in 100 per cent of people with AD and in up to 30 per cent of elderly people without cognitive symptoms.[37] Cognitive impairment in AD is thought to be related to the burden of neocortical neurofibrillary tangles composed of hyperphosphorylated tau protein per se rather than accumulation of neuritic plaques of aggregated β-amyloid peptides. It is now recognized that the time course of the illness extends over many decades (see chapter 32) and includes a long preclinical or asymptomatic phase of illness postulated to occur due to a temporal lag between the deposition and accumulation of β-amyloid and hyperphosphorylated tau in the brain and the development of clinical dementia.[28]

In a 2013 publication, the Alzheimer Association estimated that 25 per cent of prevalent AD dementia cases involve younger people (< 65 year old).[38] Rarely (1 per cent) is the disease actually caused by an autosomal dominant inherited mutation in the amyloid precursor protein (APP), presenilin 1, or presenilin 2 genes causing alterations in amyloid processing that lead to AD with complete penetrance.[39] Individuals with Down syndrome or trisomy 21 who have an extra copy of the *APP* gene develop neuropathological changes of AD and cerebral amyloid angiopathy typically in their mid-30s,[40] although the clinical evidence of dementia and the development of neurofibrillary tangles and senile plaques is not always concordant.[41] In autosomal dominant AD, changes are recognized to occur in the brain at least two decades before the onset of clinical symptoms.[39] All of these mutations increase the production of β-amyloid throughout life. These rare monogenic forms of the illness have helped elucidate the pathogenesis of AD and suggest therapeutic targets. While AD occurring in younger individuals is highly polygenic, it is thought that 90 per cent of these cases maybe triggered by autosomal recessive mechanisms.[42]

Sporadic and genetic cases share the same neuropathological findings.[43] By the time symptoms of dementia become evident, pathological changes in the brain are extensive and well established. Individuals experience variable rates of disease progression, and some elderly people with pathological changes found on autopsy may have functioned normally during life or seem resistant to the development of dementia.[44] Although the reasons for this are poorly understood, the clinical expression of the disease may be influenced or mitigated by cognitive reserve[45] or, more specifically, brain reserve. Factors that could potentially augment neuronal reserve by either increasing the density or the connectivity of neurons include premorbid brain size,[46,47] premorbid verbal IQ,[48] head circumference,[49] and educational or occupational attainment.[50] Although not universally accepted, the cognitive reserve hypothesis is bolstered by longitudinal studies that report low linguistic ability early in life, assessed by idea density in autobiographies, is related to the development of dementia late in life[51] and the severity of AD neuropathology found at autopsy in the neocortex.[52]

An accurate diagnosis is vitally important to ensure proper treatment of patients and to assist with prognosis. The diagnosis of dementia due to AD remains a clinical challenge since biomarkers of AD and neuropathological changes found at autopsy are imperfectly related to cognition or function.

Staging of AD: Mild/moderate/severe

The symptomatic phase of AD is arbitrarily divided into mild, moderate, and severe stages. In many cases, functional and cognitive abilities are disparate, and behavioural problems are not universally predictable, although neuropsychiatric symptoms will occur at some stage during the illness in most people with AD.[53] Cognition and function progressively decline during the symptomatic or dementia phase of the illness.

Clinicians caring for individuals with AD should ideally make a baseline evaluation of cognition, function, and behaviour with input from a person who knows the patient well or the caregiver. Patients should also be followed longitudinally to monitor progression and, where applicable, treatment response.

The designation of mild, moderate, and severe stage has been useful in the design and implementation of clinical research trials. Most research cites the 30-point Mini-Mental Status Examination (MMSE)[54] score as the basis for staging the illness; a score of 0–10 points indicating severe-, 11–20 points moderate-, and 21–30 points mild-stage disease. The MMSE tests several cognitive domains but the test is not very sensitive to changes that occur in the early[55,56] or advanced phase of the illness.[57] We consider examples of each stage in the following.

Mild-stage AD

Current clinical criteria for a diagnosis of dementia due to Alzheimer's disease rely upon the recognition of functional decline leading to loss of independence in daily living and cognitive dysfunction as ascertained from history, interview of an informant, and objective cognitive testing.[58] Outside of established research centres, the use of biomarkers of AD to identify prodromal or preclinical AD is not currently feasible owing to lack of validation studies.[59,60] Cognitive profiles typically found in the mild stage usually include impairments of episodic memory or delayed recall, attentional deficits in speed of processing information, problems with abstract reasoning and executive function, impaired visuospatial performance, and language problems involving word- or name-finding difficulty. Anomia and word-finding problems are common in early AD. Later in the course of the illness auditory comprehension becomes defective.

Behavioural problems may or may not be apparent but usually personality change is noted in affected individuals that may include irritability, anxiety, or depression when episodic memory problems and mild functional impairments first arise.[61] Delusions of theft occur in up to half of those with mild-stage disease.[62] A typical case of sporadic AD is presented in Box 33.1. An atypical case in a younger individual with a subtle memory deficit, at least initially, is also presented. However, note that the initial clinical presentation of a younger individual with AD may differ from an older individual with sporadic AD in many respects, as we discuss in the following.

In case 2, executive dysfunction and socially inappropriate behaviour raise the possibility of a diagnosis of frontotemporal dementia (FTD) rather than AD, especially in a younger individual. Individuals with mild-stage AD may seem normal in causal social situations. Magnetic resonance imaging (MRI) scanning may be normal in very early AD, but usually shows early, symmetrical medial temporal lobe atrophy with excess global volume loss progressing as the disease advances. Positron emission tomography (PET) studies of cerebral metabolism with fluorodeoxyglucose (FDG) may help to distinguish between AD and FTD.[63] FDG-PET in AD usually shows hypometabolism in the association and limbic cortex including the posteriomedial parietal (precuneus) and posterior cingulate gyrus, inferior parietal lobe, posterolateral portions of the temporal lobe and the hippocampus and medial temporal cortex.[64] Hypometabolism in the posterior cingulate is often

Box 33.1 Mild-stage AD

Case 1

A 76-year-old right-handed male presented with a two-year history of memory loss characterized by misplacing personal belongings, forgetting appointments, and repeating himself during conversations. He retired from teaching at the university where he was a professor of accounting, due to cognitive difficulty; he became prone to confusion while lecturing. He acknowledged forgetting recent conversations or at least their details but his wife reported forgetting entirely about plans that had been discussed multiple times (e.g. that she was leaving for a trip). He distorted aspects of past events and believed these distorted versions with great conviction. Over the last year there had been difficulty recalling driving routes and recently the police escorted him home after they found him walking around a parking lot searching for his automobile.

Family history: Maternal grandmother developed memory loss at age 95

Medical history: Hypertension

Social history: Shares a bottle of wine with wife at dinner every evening

Neuroradiological tests

- MRI generalized volume loss without lobar predominance, diffuse white matter changes
- PET distribution of FDG was abnormal with hypometabolism present in the posterior cingulate gyri and parietotemporal lobes bilaterally, uptake was well preserved in the basal ganglia, thalami, occipital, and frontal lobes (see Fig. 33.1)

Neuropsychological testing

- MMSE score 24/30 points with 'world' and 22/30 points serial seven subtractions
- Learning rate was mildly reduced and delayed recall was impaired to severely deficient with no benefit from reduced retrieval demand or cueing
- Orientation was impaired for place and time
- Semantic fluency was low-average to impaired
- Visuoperceptual skills impaired on clock test, did not differentiate between hour- and minute-hand length, unable to reproduce a cube but average performance on complex figure copy

Neurobehavioural assessment

- Personality changes: anxiety, dependency upon wife

Clinical diagnosis: Mild AD

Case 2

64-year-old right-handed self-employed businessman attended with a four-year history of cognitive difficulty. Three years previously he had consulted a neurologist and underwent neuropsychological testing that found executive dysfunction and impaired visuoperceptual skills; however, visual and verbal memory tests were reportedly intact. The diagnostic impression an unspecified cognitive impairment associated with anxiety and depression. Cognitive/behavioural psychotherapy was recommended and a selective serotonin reuptake inhibitor (SSRI) was prescribed for six months.

One year after the initial evaluation, the family noticed he had increased difficulty remembering conversations or the names of people, misplacing personal objects, and had word-finding difficulty so he returned for re-evaluation. He had difficulty estimating the cost of services, executing contracts with customers, and ruminated excessively over deadlines or conflicts in the workplace. His wife became concerned about his judgment. For example, he tried to locate a gas leak in their utility room by using a lighter and said: 'only the excess gas would flare up if there was a leak'. She was concerned about escalating behavioural problems including agitation and irritability. Occasionally he thought that his wife and daughter were plotting against him and that his daughter misspent funds from the family business. He lost interest in golf and in spending time with friends and grandchildren. His wife reported that over the preceding few years, there were many instances of inappropriate sexual comments made to friends or family members. Recently he inappropriately kissed one of his wife's friends on the lips.

Family history: Father died with a clinical diagnosis of Alzheimer's disease aged 77

Medical history: Diabetes mellitus type II, hyperlipidemia

Social history: No alcohol or illicit drug use

Neuroradiological testing

- MRI demonstrated nonspecific white matter intensities and no other intracranial abnormalities (e.g. focal atrophy)
- FDG-PET normal

(continued)

Neuropsychological testing

- MMSE score 27/30 points, recall 1/3 words following a brief delay
- Immediate and delayed recall of verbal information impaired (previously average)
- Delayed recall of visual information impaired (previously low-average)
- Semantic fluency low-average to impaired
- Orientation was impaired for place
- Executive dysfunction (graphomotor speed)
- Visuoperceptual skills impaired (complex figure copy)
- Normal activities of daily living

Neurobehavioural assessment

- Delusional: believes others are stealing from him
- Personality changes: anxious, prefers staying home, stubborn, and resists changes in routine
- Aggression: lashes out when others offer help, insults others, easily loses temper, threatens others, is bossy, expresses dissatisfaction with most things
- Disinhibition: lack of social manners, makes insensitive statements to others, inappropriate sexual comments, flirts, sarcasm, talks loudly

Clinical diagnosis: Mild AD, frontal subtype.

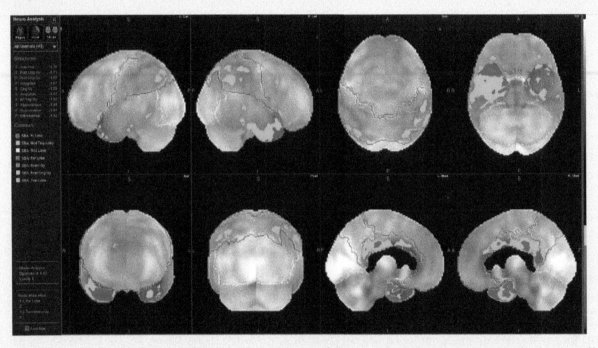

Fig. 33.1 FDG-PET in mild-stage AD. The distribution of FDG is abnormal, with hypometabolism present in the posterior cingulate gyri and parietotemporal lobes bilaterally. The findings are typical of Alzheimer's disease. Uptake was well preserved in the basal ganglia, thalami, occipital and frontal lobes.
Courtesy of James L Fleckenstein MD.

present in early AD,[65] while frontal cortex is relatively spared until later stages of the disease.[66] FDG-PET, however, may be negative or not be helpful in evaluating patients with the earliest symptoms of AD. PET ligands are now available to detect underlying brain amyloid pathology with high sensitivity and a positive scan would suggest that AD is the most likely diagnosis in a person with dementia. Amyloid imaging does not exclude the presence of other pathology in the brain. This individual did not have functional impairment in basic self-maintenance or complex instrumental activities of daily living. It is estimated that if functional impairment is required to diagnose AD, a clinical diagnosis could be delayed for over a year in more than 56 per cent of patients undergoing an initial evaluation at an academic medical centre.[67]

Finally, younger individuals with AD are more likely to have a non-amnestic presentation than older individuals with sporadic AD (64 per cent versus 7 per cent).[68] Memory may appear intact or only marginally impaired on formal neuropsychological testing. The phenotype of early onset AD frequently presents with isolated impairment in language, visuospatial, or executive function, and they seldom carry the APOE ε4 allele.[69]

Moderate-stage AD

As AD progresses individuals continue to decline cognitively and functionally which leads to loss of independence or the ability to live safely alone. The recognition of a cognitive impairment should be apparent even during a casual interview. The presence of agitation, dysphoria, anxiety, apathy, and aberrant motor behaviour increases over time with disease progression.[70] Agitated behaviour may include both motor restlessness and aggressive behaviours.

Box 33.2 describes a case of moderate-stage AD. This patient had multiple vascular risk factors associated with AD and presented classically with an amnestic disorder seven years previously. Several years after the onset of the amnestic disorder she developed loss of sense of direction and problems handling complex activities of daily living (finances, operating an automobile), suggesting a moderately advanced AD dementia. There was no medical evaluation or treatment until two years prior to diagnosis. Many individuals resist seeking help when they initially experience the onset of memory problems due to fear or concern of negative social stigma associated with the diagnosis of AD. Alzheimer's Disease International (see <http://www.alz.co.uk>) released a global survey of dementia patients and their care provider and reported that they experience distress leading to feelings of isolation and marginalization. About 25 per cent of respondents with AD had concealed their diagnosis and 40 per cent withdrew from social activities due to stigma surrounding the disease.

Box 33.2 Moderate-stage AD, a case history

A 70-year-old right-handed registered nurse presented with a seven-year history of cognitive decline. In 2005, she retired from working full time as a school nurse because she worried about making mistakes. She had to double-check students' medications in order to dispense the correct dose and forgot to renew her nursing license. The family noted over the next several years progressive worsening of verbal and visual memory function that included forgetting conversations, repeating herself during conversations, and misplacing personal items. She would call her niece thinking it was her husband's phone number and leave messages for him to contact her. Later she became confused and got lost while shopping at the mall.

In 2009, there were problems handling financial matters including writing cheques on a closed bank account and forgetting to pay bills. In 2010 she seemed detached emotionally, and did not seem particularly affected by the death of her daughter-in-law. She got lost driving and was unable to return home without assistance. Afterwards, a geriatric specialist prescribed a cholinesterase inhibitor (ChE-I) and a month later added memantine.

She was referred to an academic centre in 2012 to be evaluated for participation in a clinical research trial. At that visit she expressed fear that her family was planning to put her in a nursing home and was reluctant to undergo neuropsychological testing. The spouse commented that she had been sleeping excessively. The patient denied memory problems but said her family frequently pointed out instances of memory failure and acknowledged getting lost driving an automobile.

Family history: Negative for dementia

Medical history: Morbid obesity, hypertension, hyperlipidemia, atrial fibrillation

Social history: No illicit drug or alcohol use

Laboratory testing: Elevated plasma homocysteine 25.6 UMOL/L (5.0–12.0)

Neuroradiological testing

- Computerized axial tomography (CT) brain normal
- FDG-PET showing hypometabolism symmetrically in posterior cingulate gyrus, right parietal and right temporal lobes and right frontal lobe, metabolism relatively preserved in the left cerebral hemisphere and in the basal ganglia and thalami and in the occipital lobes (see Fig. 33.2)

Neuropsychological testing

- MMSE score 19/30 points, recall 1/3 words following a brief delay, disoriented for date, place, unable to draw intersecting pentagons
- Attention and concentration defective
- Delayed verbal recall nil, delayed recall of visual information impaired
- Semantic fluency impaired
- Visuoconstruction and conceptual abilities impaired
- Basic self-care activities of daily living intact
- Complex or instrumental activites of daily living impaired

Neurobehavioural assessment

- Delusional: believes others are out to get her/watch her, accusing others of abandonment
- Personality changes: apathy
- Mood: overwhelmed by change in routine, makes negative self comments, cries excessively, worries about insignificant things
- Motor: restlessness, can't sit still

(continued)

- ◆ Perseveration: repeats statements and questions, hides things, searches through closets
- ◆ Disturbance of biological rhythms: excessive sleep, poor nutritional habits, reduced appetite
- ◆ Agnosagnosia: limited insight into deficits

Clinical diagnoses: 1) Moderate AD, asymmetrical variant of AD on FDG-PET, 2) hyperhomocysteinemia, 3) behavioural and psychological symptoms of dementia (BPSD)

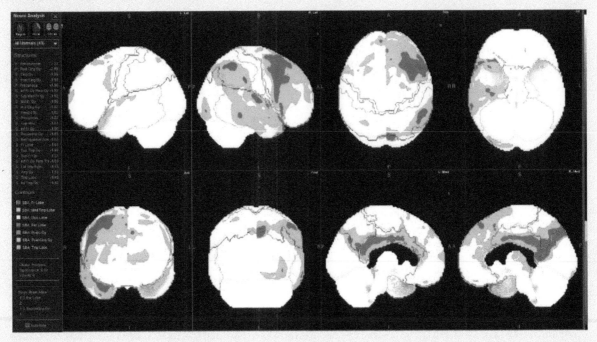

Fig. 33.2 FDG-PET in moderate-stage AD. The distribution of FDG is abnormal with hypometabolism symmetrically apparent in the posterior cingulate gyri, right parietal and right temporal lobes, and right frontal lobe, metabolism relatively preserved in the left cerebral hemisphere and in the basal ganglia and thalami and in the occipital lobes.

Courtesy of James L Fleckenstein MD.

Behavioural and psychological symptoms of dementia (BPSD) is an umbrella term coined by the International Psychogeriatric Association in 1996 to describe fluctuating noncognitive symptoms. Emotional instability is not unique to AD and occurs in 60–93 per cent of individuals with any type of dementia during some portion of their illness.[71]

In AD, distinct changes in personality and affective symptoms are frequent and they often remit spontaneously. Apathy is the most common behavioural symptom. Dysphoria, apathy, and aberrant motor behaviour seem to be associated with the severity of cognitive impairment.[70] Most delusions in AD dementia are paranoid or persecutory in nature and commonly include delusions of theft or abandonment. Delusions of spousal infidelity are particularly distressing to the caregiver.[72] Capgras syndrome is a delusional misidentification where the patient believes that an identical appearing imposter has replaced a person familiar to them. Phantom boarder is another common delusional misidentification where the patient believes that someone else is in their home. In the advanced stages of the illness patients may fail to recognize their reflection in the mirror or have the delusion that the house is not their home. This may trigger agitation or elopement.

As the disease advances, visual or auditory hallucinations may occur but tactile hallucinations are rare in AD. If visual hallucinations arise during the mild stage of dementia, consideration should be given to another diagnosis such as dementia with Lewy bodies (DLB) in which delusions such as those described above are also very common. More commonly, patients may have mixed pathology with

features of *both* conditions. In a retrospective study of 100 autopsy-proven AD cases, the majority (74 per cent) had experienced BPSD by the time of the initial medical evaluation. BPSD was associated with significantly decreased median survival time and greater functional rather than cognitive impairment compared with AD cases without BPSD.[73] The treatment of BPSD is empiric or based on the observed symptoms. Symptoms may not necessarily require treatment unless there is significant distress or the problem threatens well-being of the patient or the care provider. Long-term treatment with antipsychotic drugs, both conventional and newer drugs, should be minimized because these medications have potentially severe toxicities associated with their use,[74–77] and are reported to be associated with an increased risk of death in elderly patients with dementia.[78,79] It is recommended that patients with BPSD receive optimal treatment with available anti-dementia drugs (see later this chapter) and if feasible, undergo environmental modification or non-drug therapy. Low doses of antipsychotic drugs should not be ruled out however.[80]

Severe-stage AD: Case history

Next we consider a case of severe AD (Box 33.3). The history demonstrates progression of cognitive, functional, and neurobehavioural symptoms with the onset of parkinsonism occurring during the advanced stage of the illness. The neurological examination should be completely normal or non-focal in early stages of AD. Abnormalities of motor examination at the onset of cognitive decline including prominent asymmetric limb apraxia, gait and balance

---

Box 33.3 Severe-stage AD, a case history

A 79-year-old right-handed homemaker presented with problems dating back eight years. Her first symptoms included difficulties remembering appointments and decline in organizational skills. The husband noted changes in personality including mood swings and irritability. She became very argumentative. Over a holiday she was confused and unable to prepare a meal and afterwards arranged to be evaluated by a physician; AD was suspected and a cholinesterase inhibitor (ChE-I) was started on two occasions, but at both times she was intolerant (nausea, insomnia, and muscle cramps) and discontinued the drug. Memantine was prescribed and according to her husband reduced mood swings.

Neuropsycholgical testing performed two years into her illness was consistent with mild stage AD. MMSE score was 21/30 points. She was disoriented for time and place and recalled 0/3 words. There were deficits in executive functioning. Delayed recall of verbal and visual material was defective. Language was intact for auditory comprehension but there was impaired semantic fluency and naming to confrontation. Visuoconstruction was impaired and she could only copy basic figures. Attention span and working memory were both average. Motor inhibition and praxis were intact but she was unable to perform a bimanual alternating movement and finger-tapping speed was slowed bilaterally. Complex or instrumental activities of daily living were mildly impaired for managing finances and medication. On the NPI-Q (neuropsychiatric inventory questionnaire) and there were moderate levels of agitation and mild levels of dysphoria that were minimally distressing.

Neuroradiological testing included a brain MRI demonstrating global cerebral atrophy and nonspecific white matter changes.

ChE-I medication was prescribed the third time and tolerated. Three years into her illness, cognition and function were stable but behavioural problems or panic attacks were reported. An SSRI was begun to control anxiety and mood swings. Four years there was moderate AD with declines in cognition (nonverbal IQ, word recognition memory, graphomotor sequencing) and instrumental activities of daily living (food preparation, transportation). MMSE score was 14/30 points. Donepezil was increased to high dose (10 mg twice daily) and tolerated by the patient. Five years later, the MMSE was 12/30. Self-maintenance or basic ADLs were normal but complex or instrumental ADLs declined further. BPSD was controlled by the SSRI. At six years there was stability overall in cognition, function, and behaviour. Seven years into her illness there were declines in overall severity, confrontation naming, visuospatial, simple motor speed, praxis, and functional ability declined overall including new impairments in self-care ADLs (toilet, feeding, dressing, grooming, and bathing). The MMSE was 10/30. Recently she fell getting out of bed. Her husband noted 'weakness' or, more specifically, that the gait was abnormal: she drags the right foot and does not swing her arms. Motor examination disclosed mild hypomimia and bradykinesia with cogwheel rigidity of the right upper extremity. Strength was normal. She was unable to arise from chair without use of hands but no postural instability was present.

Brain MRI indicated there progression of cerebral atrophy, now moderate to severe, and ventriculomegaly, and the development of left greater than right hippocampal atrophy.

Clinical diagnosis: 1) Severe AD with secondary parkinsonism, 2) mood disorder with depression, anxiety, and emotional lability.

---

difficulties, supranuclear gaze palsy, or parkinsonism signify the likelihood of another neurodegenerative condition including corticobasal degeneration, progressive supranuclear palsy, Parkinson's disease dementia, Lewy body disease, or multiple system atrophy.

Sporadic AD patients may develop extrapyramidal findings as the disease progresses; this is referred to as secondary parkinsonism and is not generally responsive to dopaminergic medication. Judicious administration or a trial of low-dose (100 mg/25 mg) levo-dopa/carbidopa can be helpful in differentiating mixed dementia (AD plus PD) from secondary parkinsonism associated with advanced AD. These patients may have cardinal symptoms of PD including bradykinesia, cogwheel rigidity, and abnormal balance but typically do not have a resting tremor. The condition is due to the spread of neuropathological changes of AD to the substantia nigra.[81]

Myoclonic jerks and frontal release reflexes along with gait disturbance may occur in advanced disease. Eventually patients may lose the ability to stand erect or walk without assistance (camptocormia), and terminally they may become bedridden and develop flexion contractures. Dysphagia leading to aspiration pneumonia is the most common cause of death in AD patients[82] and is associated with advancing dementia, silent brain infarction in the basal ganglia, the use of psychotropic drugs, and male rather than female gender.[83]

Atypical phenotyptes and disease presentation

It is increasingly recognized that there are atypical presentations of AD which do not present in a classical way with predominantly episodic memory impairment. These phenotypes are far more common in early-onset AD.

Posterior cortical atrophy (PCA) variant AD

Box 33.4 describes two cases of the posterior cortical atrophy (PCA) variant of AD which is associated with early visual perceptual (both spatial and object recognition) deficits that develop before more widespread cognitive deficits become apparent.

Hypometabolism patterns on FDG-PET are reported to vary across the variants or phenotypes of AD, with greater parieto-occipital involvement in posterior cortical atrophy thought to reflect specific impairments of functional networks. In contrast, amyloid binding patterns are found to be diffuse and similar across most AD syndromes.[84] In the first case, although the PET scan showed hypometabolism in the posterior parietal regions with lesser involvement of the occipital regions there were no other features to support the diagnosis of dementia with Lewy bodies (DLB) including parkinsonism, fluctuations, or vivid visual hallucinations. In the same case, several cognitive domains were affected at the time that neuropsychological testing was initially performed but disorders of visuospatial processing may be the initial and only manifestation of AD for several years.

Language or logopenic variant of AD

Primary progressive aphasia (PPA) may be due to underlying pathological changes of FTD or AD. There are three recognized syndromes

Box 33.4 Posterior cortical atrophy (PCA) variant of AD

Case 1

A 49-year-old right-handed school secretary presented with a three-year history. The family noted inattentiveness which they attributed to stress and anxiety because her son got divorced shortly after his wedding ceremony. She was demoted at work for poor performance. The school principal noted errors in her work, including poor sentence structure and misspelled words in e-mails. She wrote a cheque upside down and on another occasion she wrote a cheque incorrectly for $660.00 rather than $60.00. Initially, alexia or inabililty to read and other problems with visual processing were attributed to eye problems. At home she began having difficulty setting the table, mixing together two different types of flatware, and would often get in on the wrong side of the car. She was initially treated for depression and anxiety by the primary care physician with an SSRI and hormone replacement, suspecting the symptoms were post-menopausal.

Family history: Hypercholesterolemia, hysterectomy, and oophorectomy 2006

Medical history: Paternal aunt (one of 13 siblings) diagnosed with AD age 75

Social history: No illicit drug or alcohol use

Neuroradiological testing

- MRI brain mild nonspecific scattered white matter changes on FLAIR images, mild diffuse volume loss greater than expected for patient's age
- FDG-PET indicated mild nonspecific hypometabolism in the inferior temporal regions with significant and severe hypometabolism in the posterior parietal regions, cuneus, and to a lesser extent hypometabolism of the occipital lobes; the cingulate and posterior cingulate appeared normal (see Figs 33.3 and 33.4)

Neuropsychological testing

- MMSE score 18/30 points, recall 1/3 words following a brief delay, disoriented for the date, unable to draw intersecting pentagons, reverse spell 'world', serially subtract seven from 100, write a sentence, or name a watch
- Verbal and visual memory was deficient for immediate recall with nil delayed recall
- Inability to complete any items with a visuospatial component including written information to assess processing speed and reproduction of simple designs
- Language, naming to confrontation, and semantic or category fluency were deficient
- Motor, mild transitive and intransitive apraxia was noted for performance and imitation of gestures
- Able to care for physical self-maintenance activities but requires help with use of telephone, shopping, food preparation, and handling finances or complex activites

Neurobehavioural assessment

- Depressive symptoms of mild degree were self-reported

Treatment was initiated with a cholinesterase inhibitor. At the first annual follow-up there were increasing visual perceptual difficulties. The husband reported when dressing she would hold things upside down and could not hang up clothes properly. Simultanagnosia and optic ataxia were noted on examination; she was unable to count the number of apothecary jars on a desk in the examination room and groped for things in front of her. She was no longer able to read or recognize faces. The MMSE declined to 15/30 with 'world' and 14/30 with serial sevens. Interim decline on neuropsychological testing were found in orientation, visuospatial construction ability but there was improvement on a verbal list learning task. A repeat MRI was performed which did not show any focal atrophy or structural lesions and memantine was prescribed. At a follow-up visit although the visual symptoms continued to progress cognition improved with MMSE 19/20 'world' and 17/30 with serial sevens. At the second comprehensive there was moderate AD with MMSE 14/30 with both methods of scoring. Impairments were worsening in basic self-maintenance and complex activities of daily living. High-dose donepezil was prescribed.

Clinical diagnosis: Posterior cortical atrophy due to AD.

Case 2

A 53-year-old female reported having trouble with her vision. Three years ago her husband noted an episode where she picked up a piece of paper to read it and was holding it upside down. From that time forward she noticed increased effort necessary for reading. An optometrist evaluated the patient and found a refractive error. Several years later she had difficulty reading a clock face and began relying on digital clocks to tell time. Recently she has been forgetful and confused and is unable to perform complex visual tasks. There are problems with calculations, and declines in judgment and problem solving. She misplaces things and has word-finding difficulty.

Family history: Negative for dementing disorders

Medical history: Benign ovarian tumour surgically removed

Social history: No drug or alcohol use

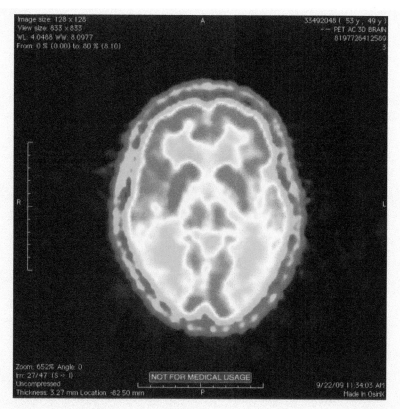

Fig. 33.3 FDG-PET in posterior cortical atrophy (PCA) variant AD. The distribution of FDG is abnormal with mild non-specific hypometabolism in the inferior temporal regions with significant and severe hypometabolism in the posterior parietal regions, cuneus, and to a lesser extent hypometabolism of the occipital lobes; the cingulate and posterior cingulate appeared normal.

Courtesy of Javier R Villanueva-Meyer MD.

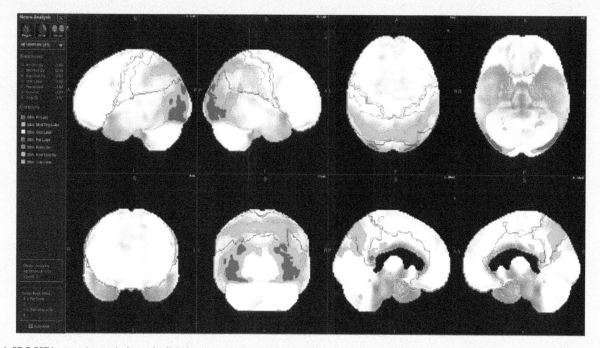

Fig. 33.4 FDG-PET in posterior cortical atrophy (PCA) variant AD. The distribution of FDG is abnormal with hypometabolism being particularly prominent in the occipital lobes with mesial sparing.

Courtesy of James L Fleckenstein MD.

(continued)

Neuroradiological testing

- MRI brain with disproportionate volume loss in the parietal area (precuneus) bilaterally but otherwise unremarkable
- FDG-PET abnormal hypometabolism in the occipital lobes with mesial sparing

  Neuropsychological testing confounded by foreign birth, English as second language

- MMSE score 21/30, disoriented for place, recalled 1/3 words following a brief delay, unable to draw intersecting pentagons, spell 'world' backwards, or perform serial seven subtractions
- Memory impaired for rote verbal learning and delayed recall, recall of stories was low-average immediately and following a 30-minute delay
- Visuospatial impaired clock drawing, drawing intermediate figures, and block construction
- Language fluency impaired for confrontation naming/category fluency
- Executive function, unable to complete a graphomotor task requiring mental tracking and visual scanning

Neurobehavioural assessment

- Depression, apathy, and anxiety

of PPA including progressive nonfluent aphasia (PFNA), semantic dementia (SD), and logopenic progressive aphasia (LPA), although PNFA and LPA may overlap in many respects.[85] AD can present with isolated language difficulty, but other cognitive domains eventually become affected.[86] Box 33.5 describes such a case. The initial diagnosis was PPA due to FTD. In this patient, the age, pattern of speech impairment, and other affected cognitive domains made the logopenic variant of AD a more likely diagnosis than FTD. Most cases of logopenic aphasia are due to Alzheimer rather than frontotemporal pathology,[87] so treatment with a cholinesterase inhibitor may be indicated in such cases. There are no approved medications indicated for treatment of FTD although memantine is frequently prescribed.[88] In FTD, use of cholinesterase-inhibitor (ChE-I) drugs may increase behavioural problems and are not thought to improve cognition since there is no recognized cholinergic deficit in FTD.[89,90] When distinguishing FTD from AD some factors to take into consideration are age at onset, since FTD generally presents before the 60, and the first symptoms are often related to personality changes, language, or executive functioning.[91] In comparison with AD, patients with FTD have less severe memory deficits and visuoconstructional abilities are usually spared into the most advanced stages of the illness.

Logopenic variant primary progressive aphasia the FDG-PET pattern indicates asymmetric involvement of left temporoparietal region. In AD, neuropsychological tests may show problems with confrontation naming including paraphasic errors and word-finding difficulty with pauses in speech. Later speech may become progressively impaired and patients may utter brief phrases lacking propositional value. Expressive language function is usually impaired before receptive function or comprehension declines but eventually both are defective. In the profound stages of AD an individual may be capable of making only repetitive vocalizations or nonsensical utterances.

Amyloid imaging may help distinguish between FTD and AD.[11C]Pittsburgh Compound B (PiB) is a ligand that is a non-specific marker of Aβ-peptide-related cerebral amyloidosis and it also labels neurofibrillary tangles although the overall intensity of the binding is markedly lower than that associated with β-amyloid. It is not commercially available. The deposition of β-amyloid is a common neuropathological finding in a number of conditions other than AD including vascular dementia and DLB. Positive amyloid tracer binding in healthy elderly adults is frequently reported. In one control group of healthy older adults, 22 per cent were PiB-positive; they performed worse on a test of episodic

---

Box 33.5 Language or logopenic variant of AD, a case history

A 70-year-old retired teacher presented with a five-year history of progressive problems involving speech and language difficulty. Initially she experienced difficulty with word finding, reading numbers, and fluency or expressive language production. She stopped driving and managing her finances due to loss of confidence. A year later she developed forgetfulness and had problems understanding verbal commands and making decisions. She could no longer write but could read aloud. Behavioural changes included irritability. An evaluation at an academic centre reported that fluency was severely limited and language output was agrammatic. Verbal output was confined to single words or short phrases with phonemic ('rhinoterous' for 'rhinoceros') and semantic ('sphinx' for 'pyramid') paraphasic errors. There were many long pauses in speech to find words. Semantic knowledge was preserved as demonstrated by circumlocutory descriptions of pictured objects. Comprehension for complex information was impaired but she understood simple yes or no questions. Anomia for common items was present but she could point to the correct item when named by the examiner. Left–right orientation and calculations were also impaired. Verbal and visual learning was severely impaired for learning but recall reflected retention of learned words and geometric figures. She was able to copy figures accurately. Attention and executive functioning indicated severe impairment with slow performance. It was thought she had a language-dominant variant of FTD, so no therapy was prescribed.

Three years later aphasia worsened and psychiatric problems including agitation, anxiety, and paranoia began. An SSRI was prescribed by the primary care physician. There were visual hallucinations and care providers reported she began arguing with her reflection in the mirror. She became distrustful and uncooperative, and refused to go places. She would hide objects for fear they would be stolen, engaged in repetitive activity of packing a suitcase. Low-dose olanzapine was prescribed and slowly titrated to 5 mg twice daily which resolved her symptoms.

Afterwards the patient had two generalized seizures and was admitted to the hospital. Medications were discontinued but she remained resistant, agitated, and angry so quetiapine was started and titrated to 150 mg daily. Combativeness was reduced. The caregiver stopped all antipsychotic medications after reading literature on the potential adverse effects of these drugs.

Medical history: Post thyroidectomy for carcinoma

Family history: Negative for dementia

Neuroradiological tests:

♦ FDG-PET abnormal distribution with hypometabolism symmetrically apparent in the posterior cingulate gyrus, bilateral parietal lobes, and both frontal lobes; temporal hypometabolism was apparent on the left with extension of parietal hypometabolism into the left occipital lobe. The pattern suggested severe AD.

The patient was uncooperative and could not undergo formal neuropsychological testing.

Treatment with cholinesterase inhibitor was started and memantine was added a month latter. At a follow-up visit there was less aggression but occasional episodes of agitation and a quick temper continued to be problematic for the care provider.

Clinical diagnosis: Language-variant AD with active BPSD symptoms.

memory compared with PiB-negative controls, raising the possibility that amyloid tracers may be able to detect preclinical AD.[92] The significance of the 10–20 per cent of individuals diagnosed with AD dementia who are PiB-negative is as yet unknown.[93]

Florbetapir or [18F]AV45 is a different tracer that was approved by the FDA in the United States in 2011 and in Europe in 2013 to rule out the presence of pathologically significant levels of β-amyloid in the brain. A positive study does not establish an AD diagnosis, only the presence of neuritic plaques. This radioligand has been quantitatively correlated with the density of β-amyloid plaques found on human autopsy brain tissue,[94] but evidence of AD pathophysiological process does not exclude another cause of dementia. Florbetapir positivity has substantial overlap in cases of probable AD, mild cognitive impairment (MCI), and elderly individuals with normal cognition.[95] If available, amyloid imaging may assist in making a clinical diagnosis of AD in cases where there is uncertainly about the cause of dementia. If the amyloid imaging test is negative, it decreases but does not completely rule out the possibility that cognitive impairment is due to AD. Where amyloid imaging is not available, cerebrospinal fluid (CSF) examination and measurement of AB1-42 (low in AD) and tau/phosphorylated tau (high in AD) can provide *in vivo* evidence for AD pathology and correlates inversely with amyloid-PET load.

Management: Current pharmacologic and non-pharmacologic treatments

Pharmacological therapy

Treatment options for AD include two different types of medications, both of which modulate levels of neurotransmitters. Cholinesterase inhibitors (ChE-Is) including donepezil, rivastigmine, and galantamine work by increasing the levels of acetylcholine in the neuronal synaptic cleft and decreasing hydrolysis of acetylcholine by blocking the enzyme acetylcholinesterase. The uncompetitive N-methyl-D-aspartate (NMDA) receptor antagonist memantine modulates glutamate activity at the postsynaptic membrane and reduces calcium influx into cells.

Most of the commercially available anti-dementia drugs (ChE-Is and memantine) require titration to achieve the therapeutic dose and can be associated with adverse reactions (see Table 33.1). Side-effects of the anti-dementia drugs are more frequent during titration than during the maintenance phase of therapy. Adverse reactions are less frequent when the drugs are titrated slowly. ChE-Is are reported to be equivalent as regards efficacy,[96] so the use of any ChE-I over another based upon tolerability and ability to escalate the drug to the optimal or therapeutic dose.

Donepezil is a synthetic drug that reversibly binds selectively and inhibits acetylcholinesterase. In randomized controlled trials (RCTs) lasting six months[97,98] to one year, donepezil[99,100] was found to improve cognition, stabilize patient function, and reduce the risk of functional decline in patients with mild to moderate AD. Donepezil is reported to be effective in both early[101] and severe AD.[102,103] Although both 5 mg and 10 mg are therapeutic doses, higher doses of donepezil are reported to improve cognitive functioning in moderate to severe AD patients (23 mg daily compared with 10 mg daily).[104] Donepezil treatment compared with placebo reduced behavioural problems including depression and apathy in both mild to moderate and moderate to severe AD,[105,106] and anxiety in moderate to severe AD.[107]

Galantamine is proposed to potentiate the effect of acetylcholine on nicotinic receptors by allosteric modulation as well as inhibiting acetylcholinesterase. In RCTs lasting six months, galantamine compared with placebo slowed decline of functional ability and cognition in mild to moderate AD.[108,109] In a five-month trial, galantamine also benefitted behaviour; the placebo-treated patients had significantly worsening on the neuropsychiatric inventory.[110] The optimal or therapeutic dose of galantamine is one 24 mg extended-release capsule daily or a 12 mg capsule twice daily.

Rivastigmine binds pseudoirreversibly to both acetylcholinesterase and butytylcholinesterase with a similar degree of affinity. Rivastigmine compared with placebo improved cognition, activities of daily living, and global functioning in mild to moderate AD,[111] and has also proven beneficial in the treatment of Parkinson's disease dementia.[112] In open-label studies of nursing home residents, rivastigmine reduced the emergence of activity disturbances[113] and the concomitant use of antipsychotic medications.[114] It is the only anti-dementia drug available in a transdermal patch (4.6, 9.5, or 13.3 mg/24 hours). The 9.5 mg/24-hour patch is reported to have better tolerability than the highest or optimal dose of oral rivastigmine (12 mg twice daily), but it also represents a lower average dose.[115]

Table 33.1 Current pharmacologic therapies in Alzheimer disease (AD)

Generic and brand name®	Formulation	Effective dose	Mode of action	Approved indication	Most common adverse effects leading to discontinuation in clinical studies
Generic donepezil or Aricept®	5 mg, 10 mg (tablet) or 5 mg, 10 mg (orally disintegrating tablet) or 1 mg/ml (solution) 23 mg (tablet)	5–10 mg QD *Titrate from 5 mg QD to 10 mg QD after 4–6 weeks* 23 mg QD *Titrate from 10 mg QD to 23 mg QD after 3 months; maximum oral dose 23 mg daily*	AChE inhibitor	Mild to moderate AD and severe AD Moderate to severe AD	Nausea Vomiting Diarrhoea With 23 mg QD increased frequency of nausea, vomiting, stomach ulcers, gastrointestinal bleeding, and weight loss *Precautions: increased frequency of AEs individuals whose body weight ≤ 55 kg or 121 lbs* *See precautions for all ChE-Is*
Generic rivastigmine or Exelon®	1.5 mg, 3 mg, 4.5 mg, 6 mg (capsule) or 2 mg/ml (solution) 4.6 mg/24 hrs (5 cm²), 9.4 mg/24 hrs (10 cm²), 13.3 mg/24 hrs (15 cm²) (transdermal patch)	3–6 mg BID *Titrate dose (1.5→3→4.5→6mg BID) at 2–4 week intervals as tolerated; maximum oral dose 6 mg twice daily* 9.4–13.3 mg/24 hrs *Titrate patch from 4.6→9.4 mg/ 24 hr after 4 weeks if tolerated; replace old patch with new patch every 24 hrs* Maximum dose is 13.3 mg/24 hrs daily	AChE inhibitor and BChE inhibitor	Mild to moderate AD and Parkinson's disease Dementia	Nausea Vomiting Anorexia Dizziness Extrapyramidal symptoms increased in Parkinson's disease Pruritis with transdermal patch Increase frequency of all AEs with 13.3 mg/24 hr versus 9.5 mg/24-hr patch *Precaution: Increase frequency of AEs if body weight ≤ 50 kg or 110 lbs* *See precautions for all ChEIs*
Generic galantamine or Razadyne®	4 mg, 8 mg, 12 mg (tablet) 4 mg/ml (solution) 8 mg, 16 mg, 24 mg ER (extended-release tablet)	8–12 mg BID *Titrate dose (4 → 8 → 12 mg BID) at 4 week intervals as tolerated; maximum oral dose 12 mg BID* 16–24 mg ER *Titrate dose (8 →16→ 24 mg ER QD) at 4 week intervals as tolerated; maximum dose 24 mg ER daily*	AChE inhibitor and allosteric modulator nicotinic receptor	Mild- to moderate-stage AD	Nausea Vomiting Anorexia Dizziness Syncope *See precautions for all ChE-Is*
Generic memantine Namenda®	5 or 10 mg (capsule) or 2 mg /ml (solution) 7,14, 21, and 28 mg ER (extended release capsules)	10 mg BID *Titrate dose by 5 mg per week until taking 10 mg BID* *Titrate dose (7→14→21→28 mg ER QD) at 1 week intervals as tolerated; maximum dose 28 mg ER daily*	NMDA receptor antagonist	Moderate- to severe-stage AD	None reported** Dizziness

*Precautions for all ChE-Is: generalized cholinomimetic effect may exacerbate or cause extrapyramidal symptoms; lead to bladder outlet obstruction, syncope due to bradycardia or heart block, worsen COPD or asthma, increase gastric acid secretion leading to ulcers or gastrointestinal bleeding, induce convulsions, potentiate cholinergic agonists (succinylcholine or similar neuromuscular blockers during anesthaesia), interfere with anticholinergic drugs; renal or hepatic impairment reduce clearance of drugs.

**Adverse reaction for memantine in clinical trials at a higher frequency than placebo group include fatigue, pain, hypertension, dizziness, headache, constipation, vomiting, back pain, confusion, somnolence, hallucination, coughing, dyspnea.

AChE: acetylcholinesterase; BChE: butyrylcholinesterase; NMDA:N-methyl-D-aspartate.

Adapted from Susan D Rountree and Jeffrey L Cummings 'Current Management of Alzheimer's Disease', In: RS Doody (ed.). *Alzheimer's Dementia*. pp. 45–95, Copyright (2008), with permission from Carma Publishing.

The only ChE-I RCT lasting more than one year that has been published was conducted in the UK.[116] Donepezil was compared with placebo and no differences were found in rates of institutionalization at one or three years or in behavioural or psychological symptoms of dementia at any time point. Donepezil treatment was associated with improved patient function after 12 weeks at all time points and cognitive benefits that persisted 2 years. This study was controversial due to its design and execution (which disadvantaged finding a drug benefit), and was excluded from a Cochrane Library review of ChE-Is in AD.[96]

Memantine is the only commercially available glutamate moderator and has been approved in the US and Europe to treat moderate to severe AD. Memantine requires titration and the daily dose should be adjusted in patients with renal insufficiency. The usual maintenance dose is a 10 mg tablet taken twice daily and the maximum dosage is 30 mg every day. An extended-release or once-daily formulation is available (7 mg, 14 mg, 21mg, or 28 mg). Abnormal signalling of glutamate occurs in AD along with tonic activation of the NMDA receptor. This is thought to disrupt NMDA-mediated learning and memory caused by a decrease in the signal to noise ratio. Two six-month RCTs that evaluated the efficacy of memantine monotherapy compared with placebo in mild to moderate AD found conflicting results. One study reported benefits in cognition, global status, and behaviour,[117] but another reported no treatment benefit.[118]

Combination therapy or the use of donepezil and memantine in moderate to severe AD was reported to significantly benefit cognition, activities of daily living, global function, and behaviour compared with donepezil alone.[119] In this study the use of both memantine and donepezil compared with donepezil seemed to mitigate caregiver burden. Combination therapy, however, or the addition of memantine to a ChE-I was not clearly beneficial in a study involving mild to moderate AD patients.[120] The DOMINO-AD[121] is a long-term RCT conducted by the UK Medical Research Council and Alzheimer's Society to evaluate the use of both donepezil and memantine in moderate or severe AD (MMSE range 5–13 points) over the course of 12 months. Patients taking a ChE-I were assigned to donepezil, memantine, memantine and donepezil, or placebo. Those taking donepezil compared with no treatment had significantly slowed cognitive decline (32 per cent) and functional loss (23 per cent), while memantine treatment compared with no treatment slowed cognitive decline (20 per cent) and functional decline (11 per cent). Memantine compared to no treatment was significantly associated with fewer neuropsychiatric symptoms (83 per cent). Subgroup analyses did not show treatment benefits of adding memantine to donepezil by pre-stated criteria, but combination treatment was numerically better.

The results of these RCTs suggest that the benefit of memantine may not be consistent in mild to moderate AD, yet long-term observational controlled studies (LTOCs) suggest that combination therapy (ChE-I and memantine) is more effective than ChE-I monotherapy, and both regimens are more effective than no anti-dementia drug treatment in slowing functional and cognitive decline in AD,[122] and reduce the risk of nursing home placement.[123] In an observational study, higher mean doses of any ChE-I (monotherapy) were associated with slower functional decline.[124] Combination therapy probabilistically provides the best chance to diminish the rate of cognitive and functional decline compared with ChE-I monotherapy or no drug treatment.[122] In another LTOC, persistent therapy or earlier treatment from the onset of clinical symptoms in AD dementia using any regimen of anti-dementia drugs was associated with better cognitive and functional outcomes even in the most advanced or profound stages of illness.[125]

Short-term studies show modest treatment effects for the use of ChE-Is in all stages of AD. Initiation of therapy may be associated with a period of stabilization[126] followed by modest reductions in the rate of cognitive and functional decline compared with no treatment. In short-term studies, memantine does not seem to have a consistent or large treatment effect in mild to moderate AD but is beneficial in moderate to severe stages of the illness. LTOCs address the long-term benefit of the anti-dementia drug therapy in clinical practice and suggest that combination therapy has advantages over ChE-I monotherapy regardless of the stage when drug therapy is initiated.[127] Although there are no guidelines that address duration of therapy, anti-dementia drugs are thought to continue to benefit patients as long as they are taken. No studies indicate that treatment influences or prolongs survival.

Recommendations for use of anti-dementia drugs

Our current recommendation is to start ChE-I when AD dementia is diagnosed and slowly titrate the drug to the optimal or therapeutic dose. Individual patients may have differences in tolerability so if one drug cannot be escalated another ChE-I should be prescribed. The use of more than one ChE-I at a time is contraindicated. Donepezil may have an advantage because the higher dose can enhance cholinergic function when patients decline to a more advanced stage of the illness, and it is has simple titration and once-daily dosing. Short-term studies suggest the addition of memantine should be considered when the patient progresses or declines functionally or cognitively to moderate or severe AD, but LTOCs suggest that combination therapy should not be tied to the clinical stage of the illness.[128] Generally anti-dementia drugs are thought to be helpful in management of behavioural disturbances as they seem to decrease the emergence of problem behaviours.

Non-pharmacological treatment

Many non-pharmacologic treatments are reported to be at least temporarily beneficial and associated with reduction in psychological distress. Potential interventions include cognitive exercises and rehabilitation of function, including language or speech therapy. Cognitive exercises and social programs may temporarily benefit the patient and provide the caregiver with much needed respite from their duties. Environmental or sensory stimulation in dementia patients may be temporarily effective in reducing anxiety or activity disturbances.

Holistic therapies or alternative therapies like therapeutic touch[129] seem to reduce behavioural problems in AD patients and aromatherapy is reported to lessen agitated behaviours.[130]

Sleep disorders are common and worsen as the disorder progresses; they are hypothesized to arise from a breakdown of the circadian sleep–wake cycle. Sleep architecture changes and AD patients may have fragmented sleep–wake patterns. Waking at night and episodes of confusion in the afternoon or evening known as 'sundowning' are thought to arise from circadian rhythm disturbances. The use of sedative drugs to treat sleep disruption may increase behavioural problems or confusion and generally should be avoided. Bright-light therapy may help improve sleep derangements along with diurnal activity programmes and restricting time spent in bed.[131]

Music therapy is reported to benefit all stages of dementia and even improve autobiographical memory in those with mild AD.[132,133] Multifactorial interventions including both motor and cognitive stimulation exercises and practising activities of daily living were found to stabilize cognitive and functional abilities in dementia patients residing in a nursing home over a 12-month period.[134] Non-pharmacologic treatment should be considered psychological support and an adjunct to anti-dementia drug treatment.

In advanced AD, urinary incontinence is a common problem. If there is no underlying urological problem, incontinence may be improved by a behavioural strategy involving scheduled toileting or prompted voiding,[135] and medications can be used at night. Note that early onset of urinary difficulty may suggest another diagnosis such as normal pressure hydrocephalus rather than or in addition to AD dementia.

Techniques for communication with dementia patients are another important facet of non-pharmacologic therapy, especially in the later stages of the illness. Early on, AD patients frequently mispronounce words or make semantic or phonemic paraphasic errors and speech may be interrupted by word-finding difficulties. The caregiver can improve communication by using simple sentences but talking slowly is not reported to improve communication.[136] Some caregivers may inadvertently increase agitation by trying to correct faulty recollection of events or encouraging the person with AD to remember something from the past. It is fruitless to argue about misperceptions or delusions. The 3Rs, 'repeat, reassure, and redirect', can in some cases limit behavioural problems and the need for psychoactive medication.[137]

Practical issues: Driving, legal, behaviour, effects on carers

Most patients with AD live at home and are cared for by family members. Caregiving creates a significant burden on the care provider as the person with AD requires increased supervision. Although care providers generally have positive feeling about their role, they may become isolated and depressed. If they are young, the role can impact employment and financial security. Research indicates that a caregiver's emotional state can trigger or worsen behavioural problems in a patient with dementia and certain characteristics of the care provider can be linked to the development of specific behavioural problems in dementia patients.[138]

Strategies that enable caregivers to cope with dementia patients were found to improve the life of community-dwelling dementia patients, and in a controlled trial, recreational or occupational activity in mild to moderate AD were found to improve the mood of both patients and their caregivers.[139] Following the diagnosis of AD dementia, the patient and family should establish who will have the legal authority to manage financial and healthcare matters. Many patients will still have the ability to make decisions or the capacity to participate actively in this process. National patient's associations such as the Alzheimer's Association (<http://www.alz.org>) and the US Alzheimer's Disease Education & Referral Center (ADEAR) funded by the National Institute on Aging (<http://www.alzheimers.org>) are excellent resources, and provide information and support services to individuals with AD and their families.

Long-term placement

With the loss of functional ability, it becomes increasingly difficult for those with dementia to remain independent or for their caregiver to meet their needs. During the moderate stage of the illness it is no longer safe for the patient to live alone. There are new concerns about managing finances and using appliances in the home. The individual may have increased confusion. Those with severe AD require assistance with basic or self-care activities. In the severe stage of illness, problems with language or the ability to

communicate, judgment, and significant changes in personality necessitate continuous care be available around the clock.

If adequate help in the home is not available residential care becomes a necessity. The burden on the caregiver is thought to be a major factor in the decision to make long-term care placement. The availability of long-term care services for AD patients with dementia varies worldwide and is also influenced by a host of factors including prevailing geopolitical concerns and socio-economic resources. Long-term care facilities vary widely in their ability to provide specialized services for people with dementia. Ideally the components of long-term care would be tailored to an individual patient and include structured cognitive and recreational activities along with self-care assistance. Generally it is unwise to select a facility that is unlicensed since there is no oversight of services provided.

Delirium

Change or stress in the environment can precipitate a behavioural disturbance because the demands of change may exceed the individual ability to cope so behavioural symptoms may arise. If new behavioural disturbances arise, consider the possibility of physical illnesses like an infection or metabolic problem, discomfort, or injury, and drug side-effects. The development of an acute or subacute behavioural disturbance with inattention signifies delirium. Those with dementia are at a higher risk for developing delirium.[140] One observational study reported that 25 per cent of AD patients developed delirium during hospitalization and delirium was associated with higher risk of adverse outcomes overall including death, institutionalization, and cognitive decline.[141] Appropriate treatment requires identifying and treating the cause of the delirium. Any ongoing anti-dementia therapies should be maintained.

Driving and medication management

Following the diagnosis of dementia due to AD, safety concerns should be considered and discussed. The actual recommendations should take into account the individual's functional and/or cognitive status. Most patients will resist any change that threatens their independence and some may lack insight about the necessity to make life-style changes. The care provider must be included in all conversations since AD patients have poor or incomplete recall of discussions. It is advantageous to provide a written summary of what is covered during the meeting to the patient and their family.

Driving and medication management should be reviewed with all newly diagnosed patients. Discussing loss of driving privileges may generate conflict and when individuals with dementia should stop driving is a very controversial issue. In the US, there are no consistent state laws regulating driving that address this issue and most states do not have mandatory reporting, and different countries have different regulations. An evidence-based review concerning the risk of driving in AD found that there was increased risk of being in a collision, impaired driving performance, and problems with visual processing relevant to driving.[142] A more recent systemic review found that a Clinical Dementia Rating scale greater that 1 or MMSE score less than 24 identified patients at increased risk for unsafe driving. Other characteristics associated with unsafe driving include a caregiver's rating of a patient's driving ability as marginal or unsafe, a history of crashes or traffic citations, and self-imposed avoidance of driving, and aggressive or impulsive personality characteristics.[143] The recommendations from the 2010 practice parameter is that clinicians should inform AD patients and their caregivers that those with mild dementia (CDR of 1) are at a substantially higher risk for unsafe driving and should consider discontinuing driving or at least prepare for the eventuality of driving cessation. Driving performance evaluations may not adequately address navigational skills, direction sense, or intact processing of visuospatial information. Many care providers erroneously believe that they could prevent an accident from occurring if they ride in the car with the patient.

Medication management should be discussed at the time of the initial diagnosis. Amnestic deficits lead to a dangerous situation where too much of a medication or too little may be ingested. Frequently patients are 'non-compliant' because they forget to take scheduled doses. Solutions to this problem may be as simple as a having the spouse oversee that medication is dispensed properly or a medication manager should be designated. Those without a live-in caregiver may use an automatic monitored medication dispenser or have a friend or relative drop by to dispense the medication. Social circumstances including financial resources and the presence of a capable care provider also affect the ability to make necessary changes in life-style to ensure safety.

End-of-life care

Life expectancy in people diagnosed with AD before age 75 is shorter overall than expected in the general population and is influenced by factors that predict survival in the general population that include age, sex, and general debility.[144–146] The rate of cognitive decline following the onset of symptoms is also significantly associated with increased risk of death.[147] The majority of patients succumb to coexisting medical illnesses before reaching a profound or terminal stage of the disease. In the US, palliative care is provided by hospice programs when life expectancy is estimated to be less than six months. Hospice care focuses on relief of symptoms and patient support. Information concerning the availability of this resource may be obtained from the National Hospice and Palliative Care Organization (<http://www.nhpco.org/>). Anti-dementia drug therapy can be withdrawn when there are no residual functional or cognitive abilities.

Emerging and future treatments

AD is a multimodal condition for which there are likely to be several treatment strategies. The task of drug discovery and development is daunting. It is estimated that three to six years elapse between drug discovery and clinical trials, and another six to seven years between the clinical trials and drug approval. Out of 1000 potential drugs only 1 may reach the clinical testing phase. The approval rate for AD drugs has been dismally low and the last drug approved in the US to treat AD was memantine in 2003. Some current research involves additional neurotransmitter-based therapies. Muscarininc M1 agonists or nicotinic agonists specific for either the α7 or α2 β4 receptors may potentially have greater tolerability, so they can be given in higher doses than the currently available ChE-Is. Serotonin 5HT6 antagonists may improve cognition, learning, and memory, and are being developed as novel treatments for AD and other forms of dementia.

Risk-factor modification

No-one knows how to prevent AD. It is estimated that a strategy to delay the onset of the disease for just one or two years would reduce the worldwide prevalence of AD by 12–23 per cent overall.[148] There have been multiple research attempts to modify risk factors in AD dementia with no apparent benefit. Factors that reduce risk or prevent AD may not affect people with established disease. Modulation of risk factors must be timed appropriately, including dietary and pharmacologic interventions. Although one study found hormone replacement therapy (HRT) in women over 65 significantly increased risk of cognitive decline and dementia, early HRT prior to age 65 was associated with a substantial reduction in AD during the study follow-up.[149] HRT may be beneficial if taken during a critical window near menopause.[150] Studies involving strategies to lower homocysteine with vitamins,[151] lower high cholesterol with HMG-CoA redutase inhibitors,[152] reduce insulin resistance[153] or inflammation,[154] and supplement with docosahexanoic acid (DHA) have been uniformly negative in those with established AD dementia.

Anti-β-amyloid therapy

Strategies to inhibit the production or enhance clearance of β-amyloid have to date not been successful in those with established AD dementia. γ-secretase inhibitors[155,156] semagacestat and tarenflurbil, and the antifibrillilzation or anti-aggregation agent tramiprosate[157] failed in phase 3 trials to benefit established AD dementia. β-secretase inhibitors may have greater tolerability in humans compared with γ-secretase inhibitors that affect notch processing with potentially adverse systemic effects.

Other trials have involved either active immunotherapy (vaccination with β-amyloid antigens) or passive immunotherapy (administration of anti-β-amyloid antibodies). AN1972 was a polyclonal vaccine consisting of human β-amyloid and an adjuvant to enhance immune response or an active immunization strategy failed in phase 3 trial: 6 per cent of the vaccine recipients developed meningoencephalitis[158] due to T-cell reactivity that may have caused brain inflammation. Human monoclonal antibodies have been developed to avoid the autoimmune encephalitis. Two phase 3 trials of intravenous bapineuzumab, an antibody directed against the N-terminus of the β-amyloid peptide, were completed on apolipoprotein ε4 carriers and non-carriers with mild to moderate AD. Topline results announced by the sponsors indicate the treatment failed to prevent cognitive and functional decline. The human monoclonal antibody solanezumab binds to the central region of β-amyloid and binds soluble amyloid peptide.[156] In two phase 3 trials involving mild to moderate AD, the drug failed its primary clinical endpoints but subgroup analysis reported possible slowing of cognitive decline, especially in participants with mild AD. Phase 3 trials in mild AD are now underway, as are phase 2 trials with other anti-amyloid antibody therapies.

Gammaglobulin or pooled human immunoglobulin (IVIG) contains natural anti-amyloid human antibodies, and patients given IVIG maintained, and in some cases may have slowed, cognitive loss over a period of six months,[159] although the number of subjects studied was small and they were also receiving antidementia drug therapy. Epidemiological evidence suggests that individuals who have ever received IVIG for any medical condition have a significantly reduced risk of dementia diagnosis compared with age matched controls,[160] but recent topline results of a phase 3 multicentre study were negative.

Studies are now underway to evaluate experimental therapy in individuals with presymptomatic disease, including individuals with autosomal dominant forms of AD. For example, an extended family from Colombia that carries a PSEN1 (presenilin-1) mutation is undergoing treatment with crenezumab, a monoclonal human antibody directed against β-amyloid. The DIAN (Dominantly Inherited Alzheimer Network) study, which involves families with APP (amyloid precursor protein), PSEN1 and PSEN2 mutations, is planning to test solenezumab, gantanerumab, and a β-site APP cleaving enzyme (BACE) inhibitor for the prevention of clinical disease. When reliable biomarkers of the disease are validated, individuals with presymptomatic disease could one day be offered primary prevention or treatment.

Neurofibrillary tangle formation

It is speculated that agents will be required to block the development of neurofibrillary tangles in addition to interfering with β-amyloid effectively to prevent the development of AD dementia. Agents that inhibit tau kinase similar to valproate and minocycline are under development. Methylthioninium chloride, commonly known as methylene blue, blocks the hyperphosphorylation of microtubule-associated protein tau *in vitro*. This agent was reported to reduce cognitive decline in a phase 2 study over a period of 50 weeks and is currently in phase 3 trial in the UK.[161] Passive immunization studies with anti-tau antibodies have been successfully conducted in two transgenic mouse models[162] which may lead to therapeutic treatment of AD and other dementias involving toxic aggregation of tau protein.

Insulin therapy and metabolic approaches

AD has been referred to as 'type 3' diabetes. Brain insulin deficiency and insulin resistance are present in AD, although it is unclear if this is a cause or a result of the disease state. Early on deficits in brain energy metabolism occur and are detectable by a pattern of reduced uptake of fludeoxyglucose F-18 on brain PET scan and these metabolic problems invariably worsens as the disease progresses. Intranasal administration of insulin may be a safe and effective way of delivering insulin to the brain and avoiding hypoglycaemia. In a pilot study of mild to moderate AD, treatment was associated with improvements in delayed memory function and seemed to preserve functional ability and cognition in younger patients over a period of four months. Cognitive improvement was correlated with correction of AD biomarkers in the CSF including more favourable β-amyloid 1-42 levels and tau:β-amyloid 1-42 ratio. Glucose brain metabolism was stabilized in participants who received insulin compared with placebo treatment.[163]

Neuroprotective therapies

A phase 3 trial is ongoing evaluating another neutraceutical, resveratrol, which is a polyphenol or phytoestrogen found in red wine or grape skins and other fruits. The effects of the drug in humans are unknown but it is reported to lower blood sugar. In animal models the drug is reported to improve exercise tolerance and have antidiabetic, anticancer, antiviral, and anti-inflammatory properties. It is hypothesized to activate the sirtuin 1 gene, associated with improving insulin resistance and modulating cellular reaction to stress and influencing longevity. Neuroprotective effects include reducing β-amyloid plaque formation in a transgenic mice model of AD although the exact mechanisms underlying plaque reduction are unknown.[164] Resveratrol is an inhibitor of monoamine oxidase A so the hypothesized neuroprotective effects could be mediated in part by antioxidant activity. Glial modulators may also help mitigate the consequences of chronic brain inflammation induced by the neuropathology of AD.

Other therapeutics

Nerve growth factor (NGF) has been demonstrated to increase survival and function of cholinergic neurons. Regeneration with NGF-producing cells implanted into the basal nucleus of Meynert using autologous fibroblasts[165] resulted in significant morbidity, so a safer method is under development utilizing a viral vector to carry a gene for NGF. This might increase production regionally in the brain. Stem cells are unlikely to provide direct benefit for AD since the cells could not be placed in all brain regions where replacement cells are needed. The development of system-specific regeneration may one day lead to a therapy that could stimulate new cells to develop. Small molecules that stimulate neurogenesis are also in preclinical stages of testing.

Researchers now hypothesize that experimental interventions should be given earlier during the course of the illness, or before the brain is too damaged to benefit from therapy. The currently available anti-dementia drugs (ChE-Is and NMDA receptor antagonist) are considered to be symptomatic rather than disease-modifying, although some question this distinction.[166] Drugs with the potential to delay greatly or modify the cause of AD are under development. It is unclear what impact disease-modifying drugs will have on the course of the illness or the regenerative capacity of the brain. These drugs may or may not improve cognition so may be utilized along with symptomatic drugs to treat AD. In the future it will be possible to identify early or even preclinical stage illness (see chapter 32) and use therapy earlier to prevent cognitive decline, but treatments are not likely to prevent all cases of AD, and symptomatic therapies are likely to continue to play a role in treatment or symptomatic patients.

References

1. Alzheimer's Association. 2011 Alzheimer's disease facts and figures. *Alzheimers Dement.* 2011;7(2):208–44.
2. Corder EH, Saunders AM, Strittmatter WJ, *et al.* Gene dose of apolipoprotein E type 4 allele and the risk of Alzheimer's disease in late onset families. *Science.* 1993;261(5123):921–3.
3. Strittmatter WJ, Saunders AM, Schmechel D, *et al.* Apolipoprotein E: high-avidity binding to beta-amyloid and increased frequency of type 4 allele in late-onset familial Alzheimer disease. *Proc Natl Acad Sci USA.* 1993;90(5):1977–81.
4. Slooter AJ, Cruts M, Kalmijn S, *et al.* Risk estimates of dementia by apolipoprotein E genotypes from a population-based incidence study: the Rotterdam Study. *Arch Neurol.* 1998;55(7):964–8.
5. Hollingworth P, Harold D, Jones L, *et al.* Alzheimer's disease genetics: current knowledge and future challenges. *Int J Geriatr Psychiatry.* 2011;26(8):793–802.
6. Chapuis J, Hansmannel F, Gistelinck M, *et al.* Increased expression of BIN1 mediates Alzheimer genetic risk by modulating tau pathology. *Mol Psychiatry.* 2013;18(11):1225–34.
7. Roher AE, Tyas SL, Maarouf CL, *et al.* Intracranial atherosclerosis as a contributing factor to Alzheimer's disease dementia. *Alzheimers Dement.* 2011;7(4):436–44.
8. Kivipelto M, Helkala EL, Laakso MP, *et al.* Midlife vascular risk factors and Alzheimer's disease in later life: longitudinal, population based study. *BMJ.* 2001;322(7300):1447–51.
9. Middleton LE and Yaffe K. Promising strategies for the prevention of dementia. *Arch Neurol.* 2009;66(10):1210–5.
10. Arvanitakis Z, Wilson RS, Bienias JL, *et al.* Diabetes mellitus and risk of Alzheimer disease and decline in cognitive function. *Arch Neurol.* 2004;61(5):661–6.

11. Ohara T, Doi Y, Ninomiya T, *et al*. Glucose tolerance status and risk of dementia in the community: the Hisayama study. *Neurology*. 2011;77(12):1126–34.

12. Reiman EM, Chen K, Langbaum JB, *et al*. Higher serum total cholesterol levels in late middle age are associated with glucose hypometabolism in brain regions affected by Alzheimer's disease and normal aging. *Neuroimage*. 2010;49(1):169–76. .

13. Seshadri S, Beiser A, Selhub J, *et al*. Plasma homocysteine as a risk factor for dementia and Alzheimer's disease. *N Engl J Med*. 2002;346(7):476–83.

14. Whitmer RA, Gustafson DR, Barrett-Connor E, *et al*. Central obesity and increased risk of dementia more than three decades later. *Neurology*. 2008;71(14):1057–64.

15. Kivipelto M, Ngandu T, Fratiglioni L, *et al*. Obesity and vascular risk factors at midlife and the risk of dementia and Alzheimer disease. *Arch Neurol*. 2005;62(10):1556–60.

16. Yaffe K, Kanaya A, Lindquist K, *et al*. The metabolic syndrome, inflammation, and risk of cognitive decline. *JAMA*. 2004;292(18):2237–42.

17. Toledo JB, Arnold SE, Raible K, *et al*. Contribution of cerebrovascular disease in autopsy confirmed neurodegenerative disease cases in the National Alzheimer's Coordinating Centre. *Brain*. 2013;136(9):2697–706.

18. Balion C, Griffith LE, Strifler L, *et al*. Vitamin D, cognition, and dementia: a systematic review and meta-analysis. *Neurology*. 2012;79(13):1397–405.

19. Akinyemi RO, Mukaetova-Ladinska EB, Attems J, *et al*. Vascular risk factors and neurodegeneration in ageing related dementias: Alzheimer's disease and vascular dementia. *Curr Alzheimer Res*. 2013;10(6):642–53.

20. Talbot K, Wang HY, Kazi H, *et al*. Demonstrated brain insulin resistance in Alzheimer's disease patients is associated with IGF-1 resistance, IRS-1 dysregulation, and cognitive decline. *J Clin Invest*. 2012;122(4):1316–38.

21. Pandini G, Pace V, Copani A, *et al*. Insulin has multiple antiamyloidogenic effects on human neuronal cells. *Endocrinology*. 2013;154(1):375–87.

22. Pavlik V, Massman P, Barber R, *et al*. Differences in the association of peripheral insulin and cognitive function in non-diabetic Alzheimer's disease cases and normal controls. *J Alzheimers Dis*. 2013;34(2):449–56.

23. Irie F, Fitzpatrick AL, Lopez OL, *et al*. Enhanced risk for Alzheimer disease in persons with type 2 diabetes and APOE epsilon4: the Cardiovascular Health Study Cognition Study. *Arch Neurol*. 2008;65(1):89–93.

24. Mayeux R, Ottman R, Maestre G, *et al*. Synergistic effects of traumatic head injury and apolipoprotein-epsilon 4 in patients with Alzheimer's disease. *Neurology*. 1995;45(3 Pt 1):555–7.

25. Angevaren M, Aufdemkampe G, Verhaar HJ, *et al*. Physical activity and enhanced fitness to improve cognitive function in older people without known cognitive impairment. *Cochrane Database Syst Rev*. 2008(3):CD005381.

26. Akbaraly TN, Portet F, Fustinoni S, *et al*. Leisure activities and the risk of dementia in the elderly: results from the Three-City Study. *Neurology*. 2009;73(11):854–61.

27. Landau SM, Marks SM, Mormino EC, *et al*. Association of lifetime cognitive engagement and low beta-amyloid deposition. *Arch Neurol*. 2012;69(5):623–29.

28. Sperling RA, Aisen PS, Beckett LA, *et al*. Toward defining the preclinical stages of Alzheimer's disease: recommendations from the National Institute on Aging–Alzheimer's Association workgroups on diagnostic guidelines for Alzheimer's disease. *Alzheimers Dement*. 2011;7(3):280–92.

29. Mormino EC, Kluth JT, Madison CM, *et al*. Episodic memory loss is related to hippocampal-mediated beta-amyloid deposition in elderly subjects. *Brain*. 2009;132(Pt 5):1310–23.

30. Jackson K, Barisone GA, Diaz E, *et al*. Amylin deposition in the brain: A second amyloid in Alzheimer's disease? *Ann Neurol*. 2013; 74(4):517–26.

31. Schmechel DE, Saunders AM, Strittmatter WJ, *et al*. Increased amyloid beta-peptide deposition in cerebral cortex as a consequence of apolipoprotein E genotype in late-onset Alzheimer disease. *Proc Natl Acad Sci USA*. 1993;90(20):9649–53.

32. Kim J, Basak JM, and Holtzman DM. The role of apolipoprotein E in Alzheimer's disease. *Neuron*. 2009;63(3):287–303.

33. Weller RO, Preston SD, Subash M, *et al*. Cerebral amyloid angiopathy in the aetiology and immunotherapy of Alzheimer disease. *Alzheimers Res Ther*. 2009;1(2):6.

34. James BD, Bennett DA, Boyle PA, *et al*. Dementia from Alzheimer disease and mixed pathologies in the oldest old. *JAMA*. 2012;307(17):1798–800.

35. Barker WW, Luis CA, Kashuba A, *et al*. Relative frequencies of Alzheimer disease, Lewy body, vascular and frontotemporal dementia, and hippocampal sclerosis in the State of Florida Brain Bank. *Alzheimer Dis Assoc Disord*. 2002;16(4):203–12.

36. McMurtray A, Clark DG, Christine D, *et al*. Early-onset dementia: frequency and causes compared to late-onset dementia. *Dement Geriatr Cogn Disord*. 2006;21(2):59–64.

37. Mortimer JA. The Nun Study: risk factors for pathology and clinical-pathologic correlations. *Curr Alzheimer Res*. 2012;9(6):621–7.

38. Alzheimer's Association. 2013 Alzheimer's disease facts and figures. *Alzheimers Dement*. 2013;9(2):208–45.

39. Bateman RJ, Xiong C, Benzinger TL, *et al*. Clinical and biomarker changes in dominantly inherited Alzheimer's disease. *N Engl J Med*. 2012;367(9):795–804.

40. Schweber MS. Alzheimer's disease and Down syndrome. *Prog Clin Biol Res*. 1989;317:247–67.

41. Cork LC. Neuropathology of Down syndrome and Alzheimer disease. *Am J Med Genet Suppl*. 1990;7:282–6.

42. Wingo TS, Lah JJ, Levey AI, *et al*. Autosomal recessive causes likely in early-onset Alzheimer disease. *Arch Neurol*. 2012;69(1):59–64.

43. Castellani RJ, Lee HG, Zhu X, *et al*. Neuropathology of Alzheimer disease: pathognomonic but not pathogenic. *Acta Neuropathol*. 2006;111(6):503–9.

44. Katzman R, Terry R, DeTeresa R, *et al*. Clinical, pathological, and neurochemical changes in dementia: a subgroup with preserved mental status and numerous neocortical plaques. *Ann Neurol*. 1988;23(2):138–44.

45. Stern Y. Cognitive reserve and Alzheimer disease. *Alzheimer Dis Assoc Disord*. 2006;20(3 Suppl 2):S69–74.

46. Mori E, Hirono N, Yamashita H, *et al*. Premorbid brain size as a determinant of reserve capacity against intellectual decline in Alzheimer's disease. *Am J Psychiatry*. 1997;154(1):18–24.

47. Erten-Lyons D, Woltjer RL, Dodge H, *et al*. Factors associated with resistance to dementia despite high Alzheimer disease pathology. *Neurology*. 2009;72(4):354–60.

48. Pavlik VN, Doody RS, Massman PJ, *et al*. Influence of premorbid IQ and education on progression of Alzheimer's disease. *Dement Geriatr Cogn Disord*. 2006;22(4):367–77.

49. Perneczky R, Wagenpfeil S, Lunetta KL, *et al*. Head circumference, atrophy, and cognition: implications for brain reserve in Alzheimer disease. *Neurology*. 2010;75(2):137–42.

50. Stern Y, Albert S, Tang MX, *et al*. Rate of memory decline in AD is related to education and occupation: cognitive reserve? *Neurology*. 1999;53(9):1942–7.

51. Riley KP, Snowdon DA, Desrosiers MF, *et al*. Early life linguistic ability, late life cognitive function, and neuropathology: findings from the Nun Study. *Neurobiol Aging*. 2005;26(3):341–7.

52. Snowdon DA, Greiner LH, and Markesbery WR. Linguistic ability in early life and the neuropathology of Alzheimer's disease and cerebrovascular disease. Findings from the Nun Study. *Ann NY Acad Sci*. 2000;903:34–8.

53. Lyketsos CG, Carrillo MC, Ryan JM, *et al*. Neuropsychiatric symptoms in Alzheimer's disease. *Alzheimers Dement*. 2011;7(5):532–9.

54. Folstein MF, Folstein SE, and McHugh PR. 'Mini-mental state'. A practical method for grading the cognitive state of patients for the clinician. *J Psychiatr Res*. 1975;12(3):189–98.

55. Tang-Wai DF, Knopman DS, Geda YE, *et al*. Comparison of the short test of mental status and the mini-mental state examination in mild cognitive impairment. *Arch Neurol*. 2003;60(12):1777–81.

56. Spering CC, Hobson V, Lucas JA, *et al.* Diagnostic accuracy of the MMSE in detecting probable and possible Alzheimer's disease in ethnically diverse highly educated individuals: an analysis of the NACC database. *J Gerontol A Biol Sci Med Sci.* 2012;67(8):890–6.

57. Doody RS, Strehlow SL, Massman PJ, *et al.* Baylor profound mental status examination: a brief staging measure for profoundly demented Alzheimer disease patients. *Alzheimer Dis Assoc Disord.* 1999;13(1):53–9.

58. McKhann GM, Knopman DS, Chertkow H, *et al.* The diagnosis of dementia due to Alzheimer's disease: recommendations from the National Institute on Aging-Alzheimer's Association workgroups on diagnostic guidelines for Alzheimer's disease. *Alzheimers Dement.* 2011;7(3):263–9.

59. Dubois B, Feldman HH, Jacova C, *et al.* Research criteria for the diagnosis of Alzheimer's disease: revising the NINCDS-ADRDA criteria. *Lancet Neurol.* 2007;6(8):734–46.

60. Visser PJ, Vos S, van Rossum I, *et al.* Comparison of International Working Group criteria and National Institute on Aging–Alzheimer's Association criteria for Alzheimer's disease. *Alzheimers Dement.* 2012;8(6):560–3.

61. Cummings JL. Alzheimer's disease. *N Engl J Med.* 2004;351(1):56–67.

62. Hwang JP, Yang CH, Tsai SJ, *et al.* Delusions of theft in dementia of the Alzheimer type: a preliminary report. *Alzheimer Dis Assoc Disord.* 1997;11(2):110–2.

63. Foster NL, Heidebrink JL, Clark CM, *et al.* FDG-PET improves accuracy in distinguishing frontotemporal dementia and Alzheimer's disease. *Brain.* 2007;130(Pt 10):2616–35.

64. Johnson KA, Fox NC, Sperling RA, *et al.* Brain imaging in Alzheimer disease. *Cold Spring Harbor Perspectives in Medicine.* 2012;2(4):a006213.

65. Minoshima S, Giordani B, Berent S, *et al.* Metabolic reduction in the posterior cingulate cortex in very early Alzheimer's disease. *Ann Neurol.* 1997;42(1):85–94.

66. Foster NL, Chase TN, Mansi L, *et al.* Cortical abnormalities in Alzheimer's disease. *Ann Neurol.* 1984;16(6):649–54.

67. Park KW, Pavlik VN, Rountree SD, *et al.* Is functional decline necessary for a diagnosis of Alzheimer's disease? *Dement Geriatr Cogn Disord.* 2007;24(5):375–9.

68. Mendez MF, Lee AS, Joshi A, *et al.* Nonamnestic presentations of early-onset Alzheimer's disease. *Am J Alzheimers Dis Other Demen.* 2012;27(6):413–20.

69. van der Flier WM, Pijnenburg YA, *et al.* Early-onset versus late-onset Alzheimer's disease: the case of the missing APOE ε4 allele. *Lancet Neurol.* 2011;10(3):280–8.

70. Mega MS, Cummings JL, Fiorello T, *et al.* The spectrum of behavioral changes in Alzheimer's disease. *Neurology.* 1996;46(1):130–5.

71. Sink KM, Holden KF, and Yaffe K. Pharmacological treatment of neuropsychiatric symptoms of dementia: a review of the evidence. *JAMA.* 2005;293(5):596–608.

72. Tsai SJ, Hwang JP, Yang CH, *et al.* Delusional jealousy in dementia. *J Clin Psychiatry.* 1997;58(11):492–4.

73. Weiner MF, Hynan LS, Bret ME, *et al.* Early behavioral symptoms and course of Alzheimer's disease. *Acta Psychiatr Scand.* 2005;111(5):367–71.

74. Arana GW. An overview of side effects caused by typical antipsychotics. *J Clin Psychiatry.* 2000;61 Suppl 8:5–11; discussion 12–3.

75. Masand PS. Side effects of antipsychotics in the elderly. *J Clin Psychiatry.* 2000;61 Suppl 8:43–9; discussion 50–1.

76. Dolder CR and Jeste DV. Incidence of tardive dyskinesia with typical versus atypical antipsychotics in very high risk patients. *Biol Psychiatry.* 2003;53(12):1142–5.

77. Cowan C and Oakley C. Leukopenia and neutropenia induced by quetiapine. *Prog Neuropsychopharmacol Biol Psychiatry.* 2007;31(1):292–4.

78. Schneider LS, Dagerman KS, and Insel P. Risk of death with atypical antipsychotic drug treatment for dementia: meta-analysis of randomized placebo-controlled trials. *JAMA.* 2005;294(15):1934–43.

79. Wang PS, Schneeweiss S, Avorn J, *et al.* Risk of death in elderly users of conventional vs. atypical antipsychotic medications. *N Engl J Med.* 2005;353(22):2335–41.

80. Devanand DP, Mintzer J, Schultz SK, *et al.* Relapse risk after discontinuation of risperidone in Alzheimer's disease. *N Engl J Med.* 2012;367(16):1497–507.

81. Liu Y, Stern Y, Chun MR, *et al.* Pathological correlates of extrapyramidal signs in Alzheimer's disease. *Ann Neurol.* 1997;41(3):368–74.

82. Kalia M. Dysphagia and aspiration pneumonia in patients with Alzheimer's disease. *Metabolism.* 2003;52(10 Suppl 2):36–8.

83. Wada H, Nakajoh K, Satoh-Nakagawa T, *et al.* Risk factors of aspiration pneumonia in Alzheimer's disease patients. *Gerontology.* 2001;47(5):271–6.

84. Lehmann M, Ghosh PM, Madison C, *et al.* Diverging patterns of amyloid deposition and hypometabolism in clinical variants of probable Alzheimer's disease. *Brain.* 2013;136(Pt 3):844–58.

85. Amici S, Gorno-Tempini ML, Ogar JM, *et al.* An overview on Primary Progressive Aphasia and its variants. *Behav Neurol.* 2006;17(2):77–87.

86. Leyton CE, Hsieh S, Mioshi E, *et al.* Cognitive decline in logopenic aphasia: more than losing words. *Neurology.* 2013;80(10):897–903.

87. Gefen T, Gasho K, Rademaker A, *et al.* Clinically concordant variations of Alzheimer pathology in aphasic versus amnestic dementia. *Brain.* 2012;135(Pt 5):1554–65.

88. Bei H, Ross L, Neuhaus J, *et al.* Off-label medication use in frontotemporal dementia. *Am J Alzheimers Dis Other Demen.* 2010;25(2):128–33.

89. Boxer AL and Miller BL. Clinical features of frontotemporal dementia. *Alzheimer Dis Assoc Disord.* 2005;19 Suppl 1:S3–6.

90. Mendez MF, Shapira JS, McMurtray A, *et al.* Preliminary findings: behavioral worsening on donepezil in patients with frontotemporal dementia. *Am J Geriatr Psychiatry.* 2007;15(1):84–7.

91. Neary D, Snowden JS, Gustafson L, *et al.* Frontotemporal lobar degeneration: a consensus on clinical diagnostic criteria. *Neurology.* 1998;51(6):1546–54.

92. Pike KE, Savage G, Villemagne VL, *et al.* Beta-amyloid imaging and memory in non-demented individuals: evidence for preclinical Alzheimer's disease. *Brain.* 2007;130(Pt 11):2837–44.

93. Jagust WJ, Bandy D, Chen K, *et al.* The Alzheimer's Disease Neuroimaging Initiative positron emission tomography core. *Alzheimers Dement.* 2010;6(3):221–9.

94. Clark CM, Pontecorvo MJ, Beach TG, *et al.* Cerebral PET with florbetapir compared with neuropathology at autopsy for detection of neuritic amyloid-beta plaques: a prospective cohort study. *Lancet Neurol.* 2012;11(8):669–78.

95. Fleisher AS, Chen K, Liu X, *et al.* Using positron emission tomography and florbetapir F18 to image cortical amyloid in patients with mild cognitive impairment or dementia due to Alzheimer disease. *Arch Neurol.* 2011;68(11):1404–11.

96. Birks J. Cholinesterase inhibitors for Alzheimer's disease. *Cochrane Database Syst Rev.* 2006;(1):CD005593.

97. Rogers SL, Farlow MR, Doody RS, *et al.* A 24-week, double-blind, placebo-controlled trial of donepezil in patients with Alzheimer's disease. Donepezil Study Group. *Neurology.* 1998;50(1):136–45.

98. Rogers SL, Doody RS, Mohs RC, *et al.* Donepezil improves cognition and global function in Alzheimer disease: a 15-week, double-blind, placebo-controlled study. Donepezil Study Group. *Arch Intern Med.* 1998;158(9):1021–31.

99. Winblad B, Engedal K, Soininen H, *et al.* A 1-year, randomized, placebo-controlled study of donepezil in patients with mild to moderate AD. *Neurology.* 2001;57(3):489–95.

100. Mohs RC, Doody RS, Morris JC, *et al.* A 1-year, placebo-controlled preservation of function survival study of donepezil in AD patients. *Neurology.* 2001;57(3):481–8.

101. Seltzer B, Zolnouni P, Nunez M, *et al.* Efficacy of donepezil in early-stage Alzheimer disease: a randomized placebo-controlled trial. *Arch Neurol.* 2004;61(12):1852–6. Erratum in: *Arch Neurol.* 2005;62(5):825.

102. Winblad B, Kilander L, Eriksson S, *et al.* Donepezil in patients with severe Alzheimer's disease: double-blind, parallel-group, placebo-controlled study. *Lancet.* 2006;367(9516):1057–65. Erratum in: *Lancet.* 2006;367(9527):1980; *Lancet.* 2006;368(9548):1650.

103. Black SE, Doody R, Li H, *et al.* Donepezil preserves cognition and global function in patients with severe Alzheimer disease. *Neurology.* 2007;69(5):459–69.

104. Farlow MR, Salloway S, Tariot PN, *et al.* Effectiveness and tolerability of high-dose (23 mg/d) versus standard-dose (10 mg/d) donepezil in moderate to severe Alzheimer's disease: A 24-week, randomized, double-blind study. *Clin Ther.* 2010;32(7):1234–51.

105. Holmes C, Wilkinson D, Dean C, *et al.* The efficacy of donepezil in the treatment of neuropsychiatric symptoms in Alzheimer disease. *Neurology.* 2004;63(2):214–9.

106. Feldman H, Gauthier S, Hecker J, *et al.* A 24-week, randomized, double-blind study of donepezil in moderate to severe Alzheimer's disease. Neurology. 2001;57(4):613–20.

107. Gauthier S, Feldman H, Hecker J, *et al.* Efficacy of donepezil on behavioral symptoms in patients with moderate to severe Alzheimer's disease. *Int Psychogeriatr.* 2002;14(4):389–404.

108. Wilcock GK, Lilienfeld S, and Gaens E. Efficacy and safety of galantamine in patients with mild to moderate Alzheimer's disease: multicentre randomised controlled trial. Galantamine International-1 Study Group. *BMJ.* 2000;321(7274):1445–9.

109. Raskind MA, Peskind ER, Wessel T, *et al.* Galantamine in AD: A 6-month randomized, placebo-controlled trial with a 6-month extension. The Galantamine USA-1 Study Group. *Neurology.* 2000;54(12):2261–8.

110. Tariot PN, Solomon PR, Morris JC, *et al.* A 5-month, randomized, placebo-controlled trial of galantamine in AD. The Galantamine USA-10 Study Group. *Neurology.* 2000;54(12):2269–76.

111. Rosler M, Anand R, Cicin-Sain A, *et al.* Efficacy and safety of rivastigmine in patients with Alzheimer's disease: international randomised controlled trial. *BMJ.* 1999;318(7184):633–8.

112. Maidment I, Fox C, and Boustani M. Cholinesterase inhibitors for Parkinson's disease dementia. *Cochrane Database Syst Rev.* 2006(1):CD004747.

113. Cummings JL, Koumaras B, Chen M, *et al.* Effects of rivastigmine treatment on the neuropsychiatric and behavioral disturbances of nursing home residents with moderate to severe probable Alzheimer's disease: a 26-week, multicenter, open-label study. *Am J Geriatr Pharmacother.* 2005;3(3):137–48.

114. Edwards K, Koumaras B, Chen M, *et al.* Long-term effects of rivastigmine treatment on the need for psychotropic medications in nursing home patients with Alzheimer's disease: results of a 52-week open-label study. *Clin Drug Investig.* 2005;25(8):507–15.

115. Winblad B, Cummings J, Andreasen N, *et al.* A six-month double-blind, randomized, placebo-controlled study of a transdermal patch in Alzheimer's disease—rivastigmine patch versus capsule. *Int J Geriatr Psychiatry.* 2007;22(5):456–67.

116. Courtney C, Farrell D, Gray R, *et al.* Long-term donepezil treatment in 565 patients with Alzheimer's disease (AD2000): randomised double-blind trial. *Lancet.* 2004;363(9427):2105–15.

117. Peskind ER, Potkin SG, Pomara N, *et al.* Memantine treatment in mild to moderate Alzheimer disease: a 24-week randomized, controlled trial. *Am J Geriatr Psychiatry.* 2006;14(8):704–15.

118. Bakchine S and Loft H. Memantine treatment in patients with mild to moderate Alzheimer's disease: results of a randomised, double-blind, placebo-controlled 6-month study. *J Alzheimers Dis.* 2008;13(1):97–107.

119. Tariot PN, Farlow MR, Grossberg GT, *et al.* Memantine treatment in patients with moderate to severe Alzheimer disease already receiving donepezil: a randomized controlled trial. *JAMA.* 2004;291(3):317–24.

120. Porsteinsson AP, Grossberg GT, Mintzer J, *et al.* Memantine treatment in patients with mild to moderate Alzheimer's disease already receiving a cholinesterase inhibitor: a randomized, double-blind, placebo-controlled trial. *Curr Alzheimer Res.* 2008;5(1):83–9.

121. Howard R, McShane R, Lindesay J, *et al.* Donepezil and memantine for moderate-to-severe Alzheimer's disease. *N Engl J Med.* 2012;366(10):893–903.

122. Atri A, Shaughnessy LW, Locascio JJ, *et al.* Long-term course and effectiveness of combination therapy in Alzheimer disease. *Alzheimer Dis Assoc Disord.* 2008;22(3):209–21.

123. Lopez OL, Becker JT, Wahed AS, *et al.* Long-term effects of the concomitant use of memantine with cholinesterase inhibition in Alzheimer disease. *J Neurol Neurosurg Psy.* 2009;80(6):600–7.

124. Wattmo C, Wallin AK, Londos E, *et al.* Long-term outcome and prediction models of activities of daily living in Alzheimer disease with cholinesterase inhibitor treatment. *Alzheimer Dis Assoc Disord.* 2011;25(1):63–72.

125. Rountree SD, Chan W, Pavlik VN, *et al.* Persistent treatment with cholinesterase inhibitors and/or memantine slows clinical progression of Alzheimer disease. *Alzheimers Res Ther.* 2009;1(2):7.

126. Mayeux R. Clinical practice. Early Alzheimer's disease. *N Engl J Med.* 2010;362(23):2194–201. Erratum in: N Engl J Med. 2010.363(12):1190.

127. Rountree SD, Atri A, Lopez OL, *et al.* Effectiveness of antidementia drugs in delaying Alzheimer disease progression. *Alzheimers Dement.* 2013;9(3):338–45.

128. Fillit HM, Doody RS, Binaso K, *et al.* Recommendations for best practices in the treatment of Alzheimer's disease in managed care. *Am J Geriatr Pharmacother.* 2006;4 Suppl A:S9-S24; quiz S25-S28.

129. Woods DL, Craven RF, and Whitney J. The effect of therapeutic touch on behavioral symptoms of persons with dementia. *Altern Ther Health Med.* 2005;11(1):66–74.

130. Lin PW, Chan WC, Ng BF, *et al.* Efficacy of aromatherapy (Lavandula angustifolia) as an intervention for agitated behaviours in Chinese older persons with dementia: a cross-over randomized trial. *Int J Geriatr Psychiatry.* 2007;22(5):405–10.

131. Burns A, Byrne J, Ballard C, *et al.* Sensory stimulation in dementia. *BMJ.* 2002;325(7376):1312–3.

132. Holmes C, Knights A, Dean C, *et al.* Keep music live: music and the alleviation of apathy in dementia subjects. *Int Psychogeriatr.* 2006;18(4):623–30.

133. Irish M, Cunningham CJ, Walsh JB, *et al.* Investigating the enhancing effect of music on autobiographical memory in mild Alzheimer's disease. *Dement Geriatr Cogn Disord.* 2006;22(1):108–20.

134. Graessel E, Stemmer R, Eichenseer B, *et al.* Non-pharmacological, multicomponent group therapy in patients with degenerative dementia: a 12-month randomizied, controlled trial. *BMC Med.* 2011;9:129.

135. Doody RS, Stevens JC, Beck C, *et al.* Practice parameter: management of dementia (an evidence-based review). Report of the Quality Standards Subcommittee of the American Academy of Neurology. *Neurology.* 2001;56(9):1154–66.

136. Small JA, Gutman G, Makela S, *et al.* Effectiveness of communication strategies used by caregivers of persons with Alzheimer's disease during activities of daily living. *J Speech Lang Hear Res.* 2003;46(2):353–67.

137. Cummings JL. Treatment of Alzheimer's disease. *Clinical Cornerstone.* 2001;3(4):27–39.

138. Sink KM, Covinsky KE, Barnes DE, *et al.* Caregiver characteristics are associated with neuropsychiatric symptoms of dementia. *J Am Geriatr Soc.* 2006;54(5):796–803.

139. Farina E, Mantovani F, Fioravanti R, *et al.* Efficacy of recreational and occupational activities associated to psychologic support in mild to moderate Alzheimer disease: a multicenter controlled study. *Alzheimer Dis Assoc Disord.* 2006;20(4):275–82.

140. Khan BA, Zawahiri M, Campbell NL, *et al.* Delirium in hospitalized patients: implications of current evidence on clinical practice and future avenues for research—a systematic evidence review. *J Hosp Med.* 2012;7(7):580–9.

141. Fong TG, Jones RN, Marcantonio ER, *et al.* Adverse outcomes after hospitalization and delirium in persons with Alzheimer disease. *Ann Intern Med.* 2012;156(12):848–56, W296.

142. Dubinsky RM, Stein AC, and Lyons K. Practice parameter: risk of driving and Alzheimer's disease (an evidence-based review): report of the quality standards subcommittee of the American Academy of Neurology. *Neurology.* 2000;54(12):2205–11.

143. Iverson DJ, Gronseth GS, Reger MA, *et al*. Practice parameter update: evaluation and management of driving risk in dementia: report of the Quality Standards Subcommittee of the American Academy of Neurology. *Neurology*. 2010;74(16):1316–24.

144. Brookmeyer R, Corrada MM, Curriero FC, *et al*. Survival following a diagnosis of Alzheimer disease. *Arch Neurol*. 2002;59(11):1764–7.

145. Heyman A, Peterson B, Fillenbaum G, *et al*. The consortium to establish a registry for Alzheimer's disease (CERAD). Part XIV: Demographic and clinical predictors of survival in patients with Alzheimer's disease. *Neurology*. 1996;46(3):656–60.

146. Larson EB, Shadlen MF, Wang L, *et al*. Survival after initial diagnosis of Alzheimer disease. *Ann Intern Med*. 2004;140(7):501–9.

147. Rountree SD, Chan W, Pavlik VN, *et al*. Factors that influence survival in a probable Alzheimer disease cohort. *Alzheimers Res Ther*. 2012;4(3):16.

148. Brookmeyer R, Johnson E, Ziegler-Graham K, *et al*. Forecasting the global burden of Alzheimer's disease. *Alzheimers Dement*. 2007;3(3):186–91.

149. Shumaker SA, Legault C, Kuller L, *et al*. Conjugated equine estrogens and incidence of probable dementia and mild cognitive impairment in postmenopausal women: Women's Health Initiative Memory Study. *JAMA*. 2004;291(24):2947–58.

150. Shao H, Breitner JC, Whitmer RA, *et al*. Hormone therapy and Alzheimer disease dementia: new findings from the Cache County Study. *Neurology*. 2012;79(18):1846–52.

151. Ford AH and Almeida OP. Effect of homocysteine lowering treatment on cognitive function: a systematic review and meta-analysis of randomized controlled trials. *J Alzheimers Dis*. 2012;29(1):133–49.

152. McGuinness B, O'Hare J, Craig D, *et al*. Statins for the treatment of dementia. *Cochrane Database Syst Rev*. 2010(8):CD007514.

153. Harrington C, Sawchak S, Chiang C, *et al*. Rosiglitazone does not improve cognition or global function when used as adjunctive therapy to AChE inhibitors in mild-to-moderate Alzheimer's disease: two phase 3 studies. *Curr Alzheimer Res*. 2011;8(5):592–606.

154. Jaturapatporn D, Isaac MG, McCleery J, *et al*. Aspirin, steroidal and non-steroidal anti-inflammatory drugs for the treatment of Alzheimer's disease. *Cochrane Database Syst Rev*. 2012;2:CD006378.

155. Green RC, Schneider LS, Amato DA, *et al*. Effect of tarenflurbil on cognitive decline and activities of daily living in patients with mild Alzheimer disease: a randomized controlled trial. *JAMA*. 2009;302(23):2557–64.

156. Doody RS, Raman R, Farlow M, *et al*. A phase 3 trial of semagacestat for treatment of Alzheimer's disease. *N Engl J Med*. 2013;369(4):341–50.

157. Aisen PS, Gauthier S, Ferris SH, *et al*. Tramiprosate in mild-to-moderate Alzheimer's disease—a randomized, double-blind, placebo-controlled, multi-centre study (the Alphase Study). *Arch Med Sci*. 2011;7(1):102–11.

158. Orgogozo JM, Gilman S, Dartigues JF, *et al*. Subacute meningoencephalitis in a subset of patients with AD after A beta 42 immunization. *Neurology*. 2003;61(1):46–54.

159. Dodel RC, Du Y, Depboylu C, *et al*. Intravenous immunoglobulins containing antibodies against beta-amyloid for the treatment of Alzheimer's disease. *J Neurol Neurosurg Psych*. 2004;75(10):1472–4.

160. Fillit H, Hess G, Hill J, Bonnet P, *et al*. IV immunoglobulin is associated with a reduced risk of Alzheimer disease and related disorders. *Neurology*. 2009;73(3):180–5.

161. Rafii MS and Aisen PS. Recent developments in Alzheimer's disease therapeutics. *BMC Med*. 2009;7:7.

162. Chai X, Wu S, Murray TK, *et al*. Passive immunization with anti-Tau antibodies in two transgenic models: reduction of Tau pathology and delay of disease progression. *J Biol Chem*. 2011;286(39):34457–67.

163. Craft S, Baker LD, Montine TJ, *et al*. Intranasal insulin therapy for Alzheimer disease and amnestic mild cognitive impairment: a pilot clinical trial. *Arch Neurol*. 2012;69(1):29–38.

164. Karuppagounder SS, Pinto JT, Xu H, *et al*. Dietary supplementation with resveratrol reduces plaque pathology in a transgenic model of Alzheimer's disease. *Neurochem Int*. 2009;54(2):111–8.

165. Tuszynski MH, Thal L, Pay M, *et al*. A phase 1 clinical trial of nerve growth factor gene therapy for Alzheimer disease. *Nat Med*. 2005;11(5):551–5.

166. Doody RS. We should not distinguish between symptomatic and disease-modifying treatments in Alzheimer's disease drug development. *Alzheimers Dement*. 2008;4(1 Suppl 1):S21–5.

CHAPTER 34

Primary progressive aphasia

Jonathan D. Rohrer and Jason D. Warren

The term primary progressive aphasia (PPA) has been used to encompass all patients with progressive language impairment as the initial feature of a degenerative disorder.[1-3] A number of subtypes have been described, the current criteria defining three: a nonfluent variant, or progressive nonfluent aphasia (PNFA), a semantic variant, or semantic dementia (SD), and a logopenic variant, or logopenic aphasia (LPA).[4] While early PNFA can resemble Broca's aphasia and early LPA may resemble conduction aphasia (reviewed in reference 5), the PPA subtypes do not correspond closely with the acute aphasia syndromes of stroke, due to differing functional and structural neuroanatomical patterns of involvement and the progressive nature of the disease. There is clinical, genetic, and pathological overlap with the frontotemporal dementia spectrum:[6,7] some patients develop behavioural symptoms similar to behavioural variant FTD,[8,9] or motor features consistent with corticobasal syndrome (CBS),[10,11] progressive supranuclear palsy (PSP),[12,13] or less commonly, motor neuron disease (MND).[14-16]

History of the concept

Pick, Serieux and others first described patients with progressive language impairment in the late nineteenth century.[17] While progressive language problems were largely neglected in the West during the middle part of the twentieth century, in Japan the disorder Gogi (literally 'word meaning') aphasia (now equated with SD) was described in the 1940s.[18] Warrington[19] and Mesulam[20] provided the first modern accounts of the progressive language disorders in Western literature. Warrington described progressive selective impairment of semantic memory in a group of patients with conjoint deficits of transcortical aphasia and visual agnosia, though the term 'semantic dementia' was coined a number of years later.[21,22] Mesulam independently described a group of patients who presented with progressive language problems including patients with both impaired speech production and comprehension and progressive word deafness. He later went on to coin the term 'primary progressive aphasia',[1] distinguishing this group of language-led dementias with relative preservation of other cognitive capacities from neurodegenerative diseases such as Alzheimer's disease (AD) that are accompanied by aphasia. The Lund–Manchester criteria (1994) (updated in 1998 and often known as the Neary criteria) later defined two variants of progressive aphasia: PNFA and SD.[6,23] Separate criteria for PPA were described by Mesulam in 2001.[2] The first detailed description of the third LPA subtype was provided in 2004,[24] followed by revised clinical criteria describing the three subtypes, currently designated the nonfluent, semantic, and logopenic variants of PPA.[4] These new criteria have not settled but rather stimulated nosological debate: many patients have overlap forms of PPA or otherwise do not fall clearly into a single canonical subtype, while additional candidate subtypes have been described, for example, an aphasic syndrome associated with mutations in the progranulin (GRN) gene.[25]

Epidemiology

The incidence and prevalence of PPA and its variants are unclear as there are no large epidemiological studies. Onset is usually in the sixth or seventh decades although the incidence in older people has almost certainly been underestimated. There are few studies of age at onset although for SD, in a series of 100 cases the mean age of onset was 60.3 years with a range of 40–79 years.[26] PPA most often occurs sporadically but in around a quarter of patients there is a family history of PPA or one of the other disorders in the FTD spectrum.[27,28] However, genetic predisposition varies among PPA subtypes, PNFA being much more commonly familial than SD or LPA.[28] The most common genetic cause of PPA is a mutation in the GRN gene.[29-31] More rarely, hexanucleotide expansions in the C9ORF72 gene have been described as causing PPA.[32-35] No clear genetic or other risk factors for sporadic PPA have been identified: findings from studies of apolipoprotein E (ApoE) and prion protein (PRNP) codon 129 genotypes, and microtubule-associated protein tau (MAPT) haplotype[24,36-41] have been inconsistent, while one study showed an increased frequency of early-life learning disability in PPA patients and their first-degree relatives.[42,43]

Classification

Traditionally, PPA has been classified by the clinical syndrome rather than by the neuroanatomical phenotype or underlying molecular pathology. Initially, akin to stroke aphasic syndromes, PPA syndromes were characterized as fluent versus nonfluent based on output speech features. Patients with SD tend to present with a 'fluent' aphasia whilst other PPA patients are 'nonfluent', however, in practice this categorization is too simplistic and fluency is difficult to operationalise, variously encompassing reduced speech output, word-finding difficulty, anomia, agrammatism and the effortful speech seen in patients with apraxia of speech.[5] The nonfluent variant of PPA identified in current consensus criteria encompasses a relatively heterogeneous group of subjects.[4,44]

Classification by clinical syndrome

Table 34.1 summarizes and contrasts the clinical features of the main three PPA syndromes, whilst Figure 34.1 gives a schema for diagnosis of the underlying PPA syndrome at the bedside. Figure 34.2 shows typical brain imaging features of the different clinical syndromes.

Table 34.1 Clinical, neuropsychological, and neuroanatomical features of the major progressive aphasia clinical subtypes

	Semantic variant	Nonfluent variant	Logopenic variant
Spontaneous speech	Normal rate but fluent, empty, and circumlocutory Semantic errors	Slow with hesitancy and effortfulness due to motor speech disorder and/or agrammatism Phonetic/apraxic errors Phonemic errors	Slow spontaneous speech with word-finding pauses Occasional phonemic errors
Semantic knowledge/ single word comprehension	Impaired secondary to verbal semantic impairment	Initially intact but later becomes affected	Relatively intact
Word retrieval/naming	Severe anomia	May be normal initially, later anomia	Anomia
Grammar/sentence comprehension	Normal initially but becomes impaired as single word comprehension deteriorates	Impaired for complex sentences	Impaired for simple and complex sentences
Single word repetition	Normal	Impaired with phonetic/apraxic errors	Relatively intact
Sentence repetition	Often normal initially but can make transposition errors	Often impaired	Impaired
Motor speech mpairment/Apraxia of speech	None	Present	None
Reading	Surface dyslexia	Phonological dyslexia	Phonological dyslexia
Other cognitive domains involved	Non-verbal semantic impairment, e.g. visual agnosia or prosopagnosia	Dominant parietal impairment (dyscalculia, limb apraxia) particularly if associated with corticobasal syndrome	Phonological memory deficit with reduced digit span. Early dominant parietal impairment and verbal memory deficit
Behavioural symptoms	Disinhibition, appetite change	Apathy, irritability	Apathy, depression, anxiety
Neurological examination	Usually normal	May be associated with CBS, PSP, or MND/ALS Orofacial apraxia	Usually normal
Neuroimaging	Asymmetrical antero-inferior temporal lobe involvement Spread to contralateral temporal lobe, frontal and anterior cingulate cortices	Asymmetrical left inferior frontal and insula atrophy Spread to middle and superior frontal lobes, temporal lobe, particularly superiorly, and anterior parietal lobe	Asymmetrical left greater than right temporoparietal junction atrophy Spread anteriorly in the temporal lobe, hippocampal atrophy and posterior cingulate

CBS: corticobasal syndrome; MND/ALS: motor neurone disease/amyotrophic lateral sclerosis; PSP: progressive supranuclear palsy.

Source data from *Curr Alzheimer Res.* 8(3), Rohrer JD and Schott JM, Primary progressive aphasia: defining genetic and pathological subtypes, pp. 266–72, Copyright (2011), with permission from Bentham Science Publishers.

The semantic variant or semantic dementia (SD)

SD is characterized by loss of semantic or conceptual knowledge and commonly presents as a nominal aphasia.[21,22,26,45,46] Typically, the patient complains of word-finding difficulty and will ask the meaning of familiar words, or may appear selectively 'deaf'. On examination, there is profound anomia, reduced comprehension of single words, impaired generation of words and categories, and regularization errors on reading words aloud (e.g. sounding the English word 'yacht' as 'yatsht'), resulting from the inappropriate use of 'surface' rules of sound–print correspondence ('surface dyslexia'). Speech articulation, phonology, syntax, and prosody are intact and repetition of words and phrases and comprehension of grammatical relations (within the limits of single word comprehension) are normal. Initially, speech is generally copious, garrulous, and circumlocutory but the relentless erosion of vocabulary leads ultimately to mutism.

During the course of SD, the meaning of objects in other sensory domains is generally also lost with supervening agnosia for visual,[47] auditory,[48] tactile,[49] and chemosensory[50] stimuli: the deficit in these cases particularly affects object recognition or the association of the sensory percept with meaning ('associative agnosia'), while perceptual encoding and discrimination (i.e. the ability to distinguish objects even without understanding of what they are) are relatively (or entirely) spared. In some patients, nonverbal deficits dominate the clinical presentation: of these nonverbal presentations, the best defined is selective impairment of face recognition (progressive prosopagnosia), and such cases usually develop significant aphasia later in the course. From one perspective, the development of deficits extending across modalities in SD implies an underlying essentially 'pan-modal' defect of semantic memory. Integral to the SD syndrome is initially intact (or relatively preserved) performance in a range of other cognitive domains, including episodic (autobiographical) memory and perceptual, spatial, praxis, and nonverbal executive functions.[45]

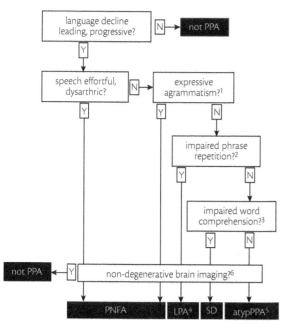

Fig. 34.1 Bedside assessment of the progressive aphasias. The figure presents a simple algorithm (informed by current consensus criteria for progressive aphasia) for syndromic diagnosis of patients presenting with progressive language decline at the bedside. The clinical syndromic diagnosis should be supplemented by neuropsychological assessment, brain MRI, and ancillary investigations including CSF examination (see text). atyp: atypical; LPA: logopenic progressive aphasia; PNFA: progressive nonfluent aphasia; PPA: primary progressive aphasia; SD: semantic dementia. 1: Terse, telegraphic phrasing with errors of tense or function words. 2: Disproportionate to repetition of single (polysyllabic) words. 3: This can be probed by having the patient select a nominated item from an array or supply a definition. Associated semantic defects should also be sought: in other language channels (surface dyslexia and dysgraphia—a tendency when reading aloud or writing to 'regularize' words according to superficial rules of phonemic correspondence rather than learned vocabulary, e.g. sounding 'sew' as 'soo') and other semantic domains (e.g. by asking the patient to list visual attributes of an object or to indicate the purpose of a familiar household item from sight). 4: Third major subtype of progressive aphasia,[10] in most cases due to Alzheimer's pathology. Patients present with hesitant (but grammatical) speech marred by word-finding pauses, anomia, and impaired phonological working memory manifesting as disproportionate difficulty repeating phrases over single words; more widespread deficits similar to those accompanying other Alzheimer phenotypes emerge later in the course, and brain MRI often shows predominantly left-sided temporoparietal atrophy.[18] 5: Atypical PPA variants represent a substantial minority of cases, including patients presenting with 'pure anomia', deficits affecting language channels other than speech, or relatively pure dysprosody. 6: Non-degenerative pathologies (e.g. brain tumours) should always be excluded on brain imaging.

Behavioural disturbances are not usually prominent at presentation in SD but often become significant as the disease evolves and include obsessionality and mental rigidity, clock-watching, preoccupation with games and puzzles, irritability and disinhibition, alterations of eating behaviour with odd food preferences, and loss of emotional understanding and responsiveness.[8,9,51,52] These behaviours overlap closely with those seen in behavioural variant frontotemporal dementia and are likely to arise both from impaired understanding of social signals and spread of disease to extratemporal areas, in particular orbitofrontal cortex.

In contrast to PNFA, features of parkinsonism or MND rarely develop in association with SD but a parkinsonian syndrome may emerge later in the course of the disease.[53–55]

Patients with SD tend to have longer survival from symptom onset than those with other PPA syndromes, one study showing a median survival of 12.8 years.[26]

Neuroimaging

The majority of patients with SD have selective, asymmetrical left greater than right anterior temporal lobe atrophy at presentation (see Fig. 34.2). The reverse anatomical pattern with right greater than left temporal lobe atrophy is well recognized.[56–58] This right temporal lobe variant of SD appears to be less common than the left temporal variant, although this may represent an ascertainment bias. Patients with the right temporal variant often have initial behavioural symptoms rather than a progressive aphasia,[57] with the development of verbal semantic impairment only later in the illness, leading some authors to argue that this right temporal variant should be distinguished from the primary progressive aphasias.[59] These patients tend to show a regional atrophy profile that mirrors that of the left temporal lobe variant.[60]

The pattern of regional grey matter atrophy in SD has been established in detail from numerous studies over the last 20 years. Initial voxel-based morphometry (VBM) studies corroborated the asymmetrical (predominantly left-sided) pattern of atrophy affecting mainly the anterior, inferior, and lateral temporal lobes.[61,62] The findings of these studies were extended by region of interest studies of temporal lobe structures which showed that the temporal pole, fusiform gyrus, entorhinal cortex, inferior temporal gyrus, amygdala, and hippocampus were the most affected areas with relative preservation of the superior temporal gyrus and an anteroposterior gradient relatively sparing posterior cortical areas.[63,64] Further VBM studies showed that there may be involvement of areas outside the temporal lobes in SD, particularly orbitofrontal, insular, and anterior cingulate cortices.[65,66]

Over time, there is increasing involvement of the less affected contralateral temporal lobe as well as spread within the same hemisphere to affect more posterior temporal areas and the orbitofrontal, anterior insula, inferior frontal, and anterior cingulate lobes.[60,67–69]

Studies investigating white matter integrity in SD using diffusion tensor imaging (DTI) have tended to show concordant findings, with asymmetrical (left more than right) changes affecting the inferior longitudinal fasciculus and uncinate fasciculus in particular, with relatively sparing of the superior longitudinal fasciculus (although with some studies showing that the arcuate fasciculus subcomponent may be affected).[70–76] White matter tract changes in SD appear more extensive than the relatively circumscribed distribution of grey matter atrophy, underlining the concept that SD results from disintegration of a large-scale brain network centred on the anterior temporal lobes.[46] The network basis of SD has been addressed using both resting-state[77] and activation[78,79] functional MRI. Functional alterations include abnormally enhanced activation of cortices beyond the zone of structural damage,[79] underlining the fact that this is a syndrome of abnormal semantic reorganization and disintegration.

Pathology and genetics

The majority of patients with clinically and radiologically typical SD have a particular subtype (type C) of TDP-43 pathology at

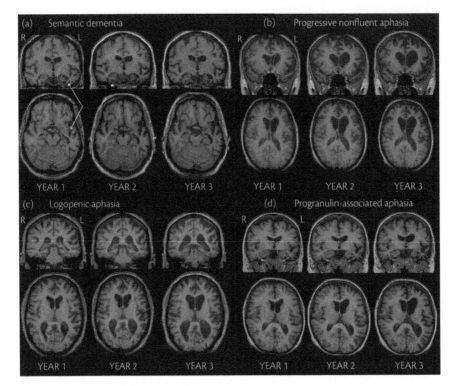

Fig. 34.2 Longitudinal imaging of PPA syndromes. Longitudinal series of representative coronal (top) and axial (bottom) T1-weighted MR images from patients with pathologically confirmed (a) SD (TDP-43-positive pathology type C), (b) PNFA (tau-positive Pick's disease), (c) LPA (Alzheimer's disease pathology), and (d) PPA secondary to a progranulin mutation. Three scans, registered into the same space and separated by approximately one year, are shown in order to highlight the progression of atrophy, (earlier scans shown on the left in each panel). Brain images are shown in radiological convention, that is, left (L) hemisphere on the right (R) of the picture.
(a) In SD, there is focal left anterior temporal lobe atrophy (circled) in the initial scan with the inferior aspects (arrows) affected more than superior. Over time the left temporal lobe becomes increasingly affected with the subsequent involvement of the right temporal lobe.
(b) In PNFA, there is focal atrophy of the left inferior frontal lobe (circled) initially which spreads with progression to involve the middle and superior frontal lobes on the left and, to a lesser extent, the right hemisphere.
(c) In LPA, there is focal atrophy of the posterior temporal lobe and inferior parietal lobe (circled) in the first scan. With progression the atrophy spreads more anteriorly and also to involve the temporoparietal junction on the right.
(d) In PPA due to a progranulin mutation there is left hemisphere atrophy initially involving the temporal lobe (circled) in this example, with spread to involve the left frontal, temporal, and parietal lobes over time.
Adapted from *Eur Neurol J*. 1(1), Rohrer JD and Fox NC, Neuroimaging in primary progressive aphasia, pp. 1–9, Copyright (2009), San Lucas Medical Ltd.

postmortem (originally characterized as ubiquitin-positive inclusions prior to the discovery of the TDP-43 protein's involvement in FTD, and its subtyping).[26,80–82] Cases of SD leading with right temporal lobe atrophy also tend to have TDP-43 type C pathology.[83] A minority of cases of SD have tau-positive Pick's disease or Alzheimer's disease.[26,81,84] There are rare reports of SD associated with mutations in the *C9ORF72*[34] or *VCP* genes.[85] It is unclear whether these different underlying pathologies produce a common pattern of macroscopic brain damage. One small VBM study of pathologically confirmed cases found that patterns of atrophy were similar in SD cases associated with both ubiquitin-positive and tau-positive pathology while in the rare cases with Alzheimer's pathology, there was mainly left hippocampal atrophy;[86] however, another study showed more parietal lobe involvement in patients with Pick's disease compared to TDP type C pathology.[81]

The nonfluent variant or progressive nonfluent aphasia (PNFA)

PNFA is a substantially more heterogeneous clinical syndrome than SD. It is usually defined by the presence of agrammatism and/or

hesitant, effortful speech secondary to a motor speech impairment characterized as an apraxia of speech (AOS).[4,87] However, there are cases described presenting with pure agrammatism and pure AOS as well as both deficits.[44,80,88,89] Whether to include cases of primary progressive AOS within the PNFA spectrum remains controversial, although longitudinal studies tend to show that patients presenting with AOS tend to develop aphasia over time. This is perhaps unsurprising as both AOS and agrammatism are related to left inferior frontal/insular atrophy.[90]

AOS is a deficit of planning articulation with the key features of difficulty initiating speech and trial and error groping towards the correct word, leading to dysprosodic, hesitant, and effortful speech output.[91] Errors in patients with AOS are speech sound distortions (often duplications or misarticulations) termed 'apraxic' or 'phonetic' errors. In practice, these can be difficult to distinguish from phonemic errors due to the incorrectly selected syllable, although it is likely that phonetic and phonemic errors co-occur in PNFA. Most patients eventually become mute, although non-speech vocalizations, such as laughter, may be present even when there is no speech.[92]

Expressive agrammatism is usually manifest as the loss of function words such as 'the', 'and', and 'or' in conversational speech, imparting a terse, 'telegraphic' quality. Tenses may be used incorrectly or words incorrectly pluralized. In addition, patients commonly have receptive agrammatism with a sentence comprehension deficit particularly for syntactically more complex sentences.[93–95]

Other aphasic features including anomia are usually initially relatively mild, but may be profound. In general (and in contrast to SD), naming of verbs tends to be affected more than nouns.[96] Single word comprehension is usually essentially normal at presentation but becomes affected later in the course.[97] There is commonly early difficulty with repetition of polysyllabic words and sentences, extending over time also to monosyllables. As the syndrome evolves, reading and writing also become impaired with deficits analogous to those affecting speech, including phonological errors (e.g. particular difficulty reading non-words, 'phonological dyslexia') and agrammatism. Non-linguistic domains also involved relatively early in the course include calculation and limb praxis,[98] whilst episodic memory and visuospatial skills are generally relatively intact initially. Behavioural features similar to frontotemporal dementia frequently emerge but are not usually prominent at presentation.[8]

Features of an atypical parkinsonian syndrome may develop in association with PNFA, more commonly CBS,[10,11] although patients with PSP have also been described.[12,13] Less commonly, PNFA may be associated with MND.[14–16]

Neuroimaging

Brain MRI in individual patients with PNFA often shows asymmetric (predominantly left-sided) atrophy of cortices surrounding the Sylvian fissure, however this varies in extent and severity. In group studies of grey matter atrophy in PNFA, the most significantly affected areas are in the left inferior frontal lobe (particularly the frontal opercular region) and anterior insula.[68,87,99,100] AOS is associated with atrophy of premotor and supplementary motor areas[88] as well as the insula and basal ganglia.[87] Progression of the PNFA syndrome is associated with spread of atrophy from the left inferior frontal and insular cortices to involve the superior temporal, middle and superior frontal, and anterior parietal lobes as well as the caudate.[68,69,99] More posterior atrophy, particularly of the left anterior parietal lobe, may be associated clinically with CBS.[99]

DTI studies have chiefly shown involvement of more dorsal language pathways, that is the subcomponents of the left superior longitudinal fasciculus, and particularly the arcuate fasciculus.[71–76,101] In patients with predominantly apraxia of speech rather than agrammatism, the premotor components of the SLF appear to be affected more than other regions.[89] As for SD, recent work has implicated a large-scale dominant language hemisphere network in the pathogenesis of the PNFA syndrome, with abnormal functional reorganization.[102]

Pathology and genetics

Around a third of patients with PNFA have a family history of a disorder in the frontotemporal lobar degeneration spectrum.[28] Mutations in *GRN* are the most common genetic cause, with a smaller number having expansions in the *C9ORF72* gene (although mutations in both these genes present more commonly with behavioural variant FTD).[29–34] There are some suggestions that the PNFA phenotype of patients with *GRN* mutations is distinct, with earlier and more prominent anomia and expressive agrammatism without AOS.[25,103]

Pathologically, PNFA has been associated with both tau and TDP-43 pathologies, and somewhat less frequently with AD pathology.[80,81,104] Tau subtypes include corticobasal degeneration, progressive supranuclear palsy and Pick's disease. Some studies have suggested that these tau subtypes are particularly associated with an AOS phenotype.[12] TDP-43 subtypes include type A (which includes patients with *GRN* mutations and some *C9ORF72* expansions) and type B (which includes most patients with *C9ORF72* expansions). Patients with TDP-43 pathology may be more likely to have agrammatism (and/or anomia) without a motor speech disorder.[44,80]

The logopenic variant or logopenic aphasia (LPA)

LPA is associated with spontaneous speech containing long word-finding pauses, but without expressive agrammatism or motor speech impairment.[4,24,105] Sentence-level processing is affected early, leading to deficits in repetition and comprehension of both simple and complex sentences.[4,44,105] This is likely to be attributable to impaired verbal or phonological short-term memory (reflected in reduced auditory digit span).[105] Single word processing is relatively intact but does become affected with disease progression.[106] At presentation, naming tends to be affected to a greater extent than in PNFA but less prominently than in SD. Reading is often affected, manifesting as phonological dyslexia.[107]

As the disease progresses there is episodic memory impairment[106] and more widespread cognitive impairment. As with PNFA, behavioural features are generally not salient early in LPA but may emerge later.[8,9]

There are usually no additional neurological features in LPA, and in particular (in contrast to PNFA) associated parkinsonism or MND appear rare.[108]

Neuroimaging

Individual patients with LPA may show posterior predominantly left-sided peri-Sylvian atrophy, but (as in PNFA) there is considerable variation in atrophy profiles between individuals. Group studies of LPA have shown grey matter involvement in the left posterior superior temporal and inferior parietal lobes and, to a lesser extent, precuneus, posterior cingulate and middle/inferior temporal lobes.[24,106] Over time, atrophy spreads forwards in the left hemisphere particularly to affect the medial temporal lobes, as well as corresponding areas in the right hemisphere (i.e. the temporoparietal junction and precuneus/posterior cingulate.[106]

Using T2*-weighted MRI around a third of patients with LPA have cerebral microhaemorrhages[109] which may signify amyloid angiopathy.

DTI studies of white matter integrity in LPA have yielded variable findings, tending to find less white matter tract involvement than in other PPA subtypes. Involvement of the posterior parts of the inferior longitudinal fasciculus, and posterior parts of the superior longitudinal fasciculus has been demonstrated.[71–73] With reference to the emerging network paradigm of PPA, an important issue concerns the extent to which LPA has a distinct profile of large-scale network disintegration or instead reflects a particular anatomical emphasis within a network that also participates in the pathogenesis of other AD variant syndromes.[110]

Pathology and genetics

LPA is usually sporadic and most commonly associated with AD pathology.[104,111] It is often considered an atypical variant of AD and has been referred to as the 'language variant' of AD. Such terms are however not ideal, given that PNFA accounts for an important minority of language-led cases of AD, while a substantial minority of cases of LPA in published series lack markers of AD pathology. These observations provide a rationale for using neuroimaging and CSF biomarkers (where available) in order to assess the likelihood of underlying AD pathology in LPA or PNFA, with potential implications for treatment (see following).

Other clinical phenotypes and the problem of classification

Recent consensus criteria for PPA have allowed studies to survey the PPA spectrum to determine the proportion of cases meeting consensus definitions if strictly applied. One study found that around 40 per cent of cases did not fit neatly into one of the three subtypes[112] and had features of 'mixed' PPA. This chimes with the experience of many clinicians who care for these patients.

Classification of PPA by clinical syndrome remains challenging even for experienced clinicians. Future disease-modifying therapies for PPA are likely to target particular molecular pathologies: accurate classification of PPA and reliable prediction of underlying tissue pathology in particular PPA syndromes are therefore problems of potential practical as well as neurobiological importance. Ultimately, this pathologically motivated classification would entail the distinction of PPA associated with TDP, tau, and AD (see Table 34.2), and further, stratification of TDP-associated PPA into type A (with or without a *GRN* mutation or *C9ORF72* expansion), type B (with or without a *C9ORF72* expansion), and type C subtypes, and stratification of tau-associated PPA into CBD, PSP, and Pick's subtypes. Currently, however, *in vivo* biomarkers that would support such a classification are lacking.

Clinically, the presence of a PSP syndrome usually indicates underlying tau pathology but the emergence of a PSP syndrome often occurs a number of years after initial presentation with PPA, making this less helpful for selecting patients for clinical trials. The presence of MND features usually indicates TDP-43 pathology but MND is an uncommon association of PPA. SD is strongly associated with TDP-43 type C pathology, particularly where typical neuroimaging features are present: one study of pathologically confirmed SD showed that the classical pattern of knife-edge anterior temporal lobe atrophy is associated with TDP-43 or less commonly tau pathology, but not AD pathology.[86] For the majority of LPA cases and a minority of SD and PNFA cases the underlying pathology is AD. Increasingly biomarkers are available with high sensitivity and specificity for AD pathology. Brain imaging with amyloid PET tracers such as Pittsburgh Compound B (PiB) and florbetapir commonly reveals amyloid deposition in LPA whereas only a minority of PNFA or SD cases have a positive scan.[113–115] Ligands binding to tau are now in development and are likely to be helpful in defining patients with tau pathology.[116] CSF biomarkers of neurodegeneration are increasingly entering specialist clinical practice: the combination of elevated total or phosphorylated tau levels with decreased amyloid beta1-42 fraction (Aβ42) shows high sensitivity and specificity for differentiating AD from other

Table 34.2 Biomarkers and diagnostic features of tissue pathologies in the primary progressive aphasia spectrum

Diagnosis	Current biomarker	Future biomarker	Other highly suggestive features
PPA-TDP	GRN mutation analysis Plasma GRN	TDP-43 in CSF or plasma	MND/ALS clinical syndrome Semantic dementia syndrome with characteristic imaging pattern
PPA-tau	MAPT mutation analysis*	Tau forms in CSF Tau ligand PET brain scan	Progressive AOS clinical syndrome PSP clinical syndrome
PPA-AD	Amyloid PET brain scan CSF: raised tau, low Aβ42	None currently identified	None currently identified

*uncommon association but may be indicated if compatible family history or neuroimagng features; Aβ42: amyloid beta1-42 fraction; AOS: apraxia of speech; CSF: cerebrospinal fluid; GRN: progranulin gene; MAPT: microtubule-associated protein tau gene; MND–ALS: motor neurone disease–amyotrophic lateral sclerosis; PET: positron emission tomography; PPA-AD: primary progressive aphasia associated with Alzheimer's disease pathology; PPA = TDP: primary progressive aphasia associated with TDP-43 pathology; PPA-tau: primary progressive aphasia associated with tau pathology; PSP: progressive supranuclear palsy.

Source data from *Curr Alzheimer Res.* 8(3), Rohrer JD and Schott JM, Primary progressive aphasia: defining genetic and pathological subtypes, pp. 266–72, Copyright (2011), with permission from Bentham Science Publishers.

pathologies.[117] Currently available tau and Aβ42 assays do not, however, allow subclassification of pathologies in the frontotemporal lobar degeneration spectrum. This may be refined by application of novel CSF markers, such as neurofilament levels. There are fewer studies looking at blood-based biomarkers. However, screening for *GRN* mutations (TDP-43 pathology) may in future be based on assays of plasma progranulin which can reliably predict *GRN* mutations.[118,119]

Aside from the identification of new biomarkers, we would also emphasize the ongoing importance of clinical phenotyping in PPA. Historically, the major PPA syndromes were each originally identified and defined by astute clinical observers. There remains a relative dearth of information about important aspects of PPA: for example, the natural history of the canonical subtypes, and the core cognitive deficit underpinning LPA. Recent work has identified important deficits beyond the domain of language that extend across the PPA spectrum: for example, impairments of nonverbal sound processing.[48,120] Such impairments may cut across traditional syndromic boundaries. Cognitive information processing accounts of PPA have yet to be worked out in detail but may inform future pathophysiological classification schemes that may resolve some of the issues around the current diagnostic criteria.

Management

There are currently no proven symptomatic or curative pharmacological therapies for any of the PPA syndromes. Small trials have yielded inconclusive results, for example using bromocriptine[121] and galantamine,[122] and there are unsubstantiated single case reports of the use of a variety of drugs. Many patients find speech and language therapy helpful for communication strategies, although there is little evidence for its efficacy. Cognitive rehabilitation strategies have been used reportedly with some success in individual patients, but are likely to come into their own as an adjunct to disease-modifying therapies: it is important to appreciate that neurorehabilitation models relevant to stroke may not apply in these relentlessly progressive disorders, and patients should be helped to maximize useful function within their limited capacities. Assessment of swallowing safety and (where indicated) dietary modification are important considerations in more advanced disease. It is important to monitor patients clinically for emergence of other neurological (especially extrapyramidal and motor neuron) features as these may warrant symptomatic management in their own right. Genetic counselling is important in those with a family history and/or a known *GRN* mutation or *C9ORF72* expansion.

Acknowledgements

Jonathan Rohrer is an MRC Clinician Scientist. Jason Warren is supported by a Wellcome Trust Senior Clinical Research Fellowship.

References

1. Mesulam M-M. Primary progressive aphasia—differentiation from Alzheimer's disease. *Ann Neurol.* 1987;22(4):533–34.
2. Mesulam M-M. Primary progressive aphasia. *Ann Neurol.* 2001;49(4):425–32.
3. Mesulam M-M. Primary progressive aphasia—a language-based dementia. *N Engl J Med.* 2003;349(16):1535–42.
4. Gorno-Tempini ML, Hillis AE, Weintraub S, et al. Classification of primary progressive aphasia and its variants. *Neurology.* 2011;76(11):1006–14.
5. Rohrer J, Knight WD, Warren JE, et al. Word-finding difficulty: a clinical analysis of the progressive aphasias. *Brain.* 2008;131(Pt 1): 8–38.
6. Neary D, Snowden JS, Gustafson L, et al. Frontotemporal lobar degeneration: a consensus on clinical diagnostic criteria. *Neurology.* 1998;51(6):1546–54.
7. Seelaar H, Rohrer J, Pijnenburg YAL, et al. Clinical, genetic and pathological heterogeneity of frontotemporal dementia: a review. *J Neurol Neurosur Ps.* 2011;82(5):476–86.
8. Rohrer J and Warren JD. Phenomenology and anatomy of abnormal behaviours in primary progressive aphasia. *J Neurol Sci.* 2010;293(1–2):35–38.
9. Rosen HJ, Allison SC, Ogar JM, et al. Behavioral features in semantic dementia vs other forms of progressive aphasias. *Neurology.* 2006;67(10):1752–56.
10. Graham NL, Bak TH, Patterson K, et al. Language function and dysfunction in corticobasal degeneration. *Neurology.* 2003;61(4):493–99.
11. McMonagle P, Blair M, and Kertesz A. Corticobasal degeneration and progressive aphasia. *Neurology.* 2006;67(8):1444–51.
12. Josephs KA and Duffy JR. Apraxia of speech and nonfluent aphasia: a new clinical marker for corticobasal degeneration and progressive supranuclear palsy. *Curr Opin Neurol.* 2008;21(6):688–92.
13. Rohrer J, Paviour D, Bronstein AM, et al. Progressive supranuclear palsy syndrome presenting as progressive nonfluent aphasia: a neuropsychological and neuroimaging analysis. *Mov Disord.* 2010;25(2):179–88.
14. Caselli RJ, Windebank AJ, Petersen RC, et al. Rapidly progressive aphasic dementia and motor neuron disease. *Ann Neurol.* 1993;33(2):200–207.
15. Bak TH and Hodges JR. The effects of motor neurone disease on language: Further evidence. *Brain Lang.* 2004;89(2):354–61.
16. da Rocha AJ, Valério BCO, Buainain RP et al. Motor neuron disease associated with non-fluent rapidly progressive aphasia: case report and review of the literature. *Eur J Neurol.* 2007;14(9):971–75.
17. Mesulam M-M. Primary progressive aphasia: a 25-year retrospective. *Alz Dis Assoc Dis.* 2007;21(4):S8–S11.
18. Tanabe H. The uniqueness of Gogi aphasia owing to temporal lobar atrophy. *Alz Dis Assoc Dis.* 2007;21(4):S12–3.
19. Warrington EK. The selective impairment of semantic memory. *Q J Exp Psychol.* 1975;27(4):635–57.
20. Mesulam M-M. Slowly progressive aphasia without generalized dementia. *Ann Neurol.* 1982;11(6):592–98.
21. Snowden JS, Goulding PJ, and Neary D. Semantic dementia: A form of circumscribed cerebral atrophy. *Behavioural Neurology.* 1989;2(3):167–82.
22. Hodges JR, Patterson K, Oxbury S, et al. Semantic dementia. Progressive fluent aphasia with temporal lobe atrophy. *Brain.* 1992;115 (Pt 6):1783–806.
23. Brun A, Englund B, Gustafson L, et al. Clinical and neuropathological criteria for frontotemporal dementia. The Lund and Manchester Groups. *J Neurol Neurosur Ps.* 1994;57(4):416–18.
24. Gorno-Tempini ML, Dronkers NF, Rankin KP, et al. Cognition and anatomy in three variants of primary progressive aphasia. *Ann Neurol.* 2004;55(3):335–46.
25. Rohrer J, Crutch SJ, Warrington EK, et al. Progranulin-associated primary progressive aphasia: a distinct phenotype? *Neuropsychologia.* 2010;48(1):288–97.
26. Hodges JR, Mitchell J, Dawson K, et al. Semantic dementia: demography, familial factors and survival in a consecutive series of 100 cases. *Brain.* 2009;133(Pt 1):300–6.
27. Goldman JS, Farmer JM, Wood EM, et al. Comparison of family histories in FTLD subtypes and related tauopathies. *Neurology.* 2005;65(11):1817–19.
28. Rohrer J, Guerreiro R, Vandrovcova J, et al. The heritability and genetics of frontotemporal lobar degeneration. *Neurology.* 2009;73(18):1451–56.
29. Snowden JS, Pickering-Brown SM, Mackenzie IR, et al. Progranulin gene mutations associated with frontotemporal dementia and progressive non-fluent aphasia. *Brain.* 2006;129(Pt 11):3091–102.
30. Mesulam M-M, Johnson N, Krefft TA, et al. Progranulin mutations in primary progressive aphasia: the PPA1 and PPA3 families. *Arch Neurol.* 2007;64(1):43–47.
31. Beck J, Rohrer J, Campbell T, et al. A distinct clinical, neuropsychological and radiological phenotype is associated with progranulin gene mutations in a large UK series. *Brain.* 2008;131(Pt 3):706–20.
32. Hsiung GYR, DeJesus-Hernandez M, Feldman HH, et al. Clinical and pathological features of familial frontotemporal dementia caused by C9ORF72 mutation on chromosome 9p. *Brain.* 2012;135(Pt 3):709–22.
33. Mahoney CJ, Beck J, Rohrer J, et al. Frontotemporal dementia with the C9ORF72 hexanucleotide repeat expansion: clinical, neuroanatomical and neuropathological features. *Brain.* 2012;135(3):736–50.
34. Simón-Sánchez J, Dopper EGP, Cohn-Hokke PE, et al. The clinical and pathological phenotype of C9orf72 hexanucleotide repeat expansions. *Brain.* 2012;135(Pt 3):723–35.
35. Snowden JS, Rollinson S, Thompson JC, et al. Distinct clinical and pathological characteristics of frontotemporal dementia associated with C9ORF72 mutations. *Brain.* 2012;135(Pt 3):693–708.
36. Acciarri A, Masullo C, Bizzarro A, et al. APOE epsilon2-epsilon4 genotype is a possible risk factor for primary progressive aphasia. *Ann Neurol.* 2006;59(2):436–37.
37. Daniele A, Matera MG, Seripa D, et al. APOE epsilon 2/epsilon 4 genotype a risk factor for primary progressive aphasia in women. *Arch Neurol.* 2009;66(7):910–12.
38. Li X, Rowland LP, Mitsumoto H, et al. Prion protein codon 129 genotype prevalence is altered in primary progressive aphasia. *Ann Neurol.* 2005;58(6):858–64.
39. Rohrer J, Mead S, Omar R, et al. Prion protein (PRNP) genotypes in frontotemporal lobar degeneration syndromes. *Ann Neurol.* 2006;60(5):616;author reply 617.
40. Seripa D, Bizzarro A, Panza F, et al. The APOE gene locus in frontotemporal dementia and primary progressive aphasia. *Arch Neurol.* 2011;68(5):622–28.

41. Sobrido M-J, Abu-Khalil A, Weintraub S, *et al.* Possible association of the tau H1/H1 genotype with primary progressive aphasia. *Neurology.* 2003;60(5):862–64.

42. Rogalski EJ, Johnson N, Weintraub S, *et al.* Increased frequency of learning disability in patients with primary progressive aphasia and their first-degree relatives. *Arch Neurol.* 2008;65(2):244–48.

43. Rogalski E, Weintraub S, and Mesulam M-M. Are there susceptibility factors for primary progressive aphasia? *Brain Lang.* 2013;127(2):135–8.

44. Rohrer J, Rossor MN, and Warren JD. Syndromes of nonfluent primary progressive aphasia: a clinical and neurolinguistic analysis. *Neurology.* 2010;75(7):603–10.

45. Hodges JR, and Patterson K. Semantic dementia: a unique clinicopathological syndrome. *Lancet Neurol.* 2007;6(11):1004–14.

46. Fletcher PD and Warren JD. Semantic Dementia: a specific networkopathy. *J Mol Neurosci.* 2011;45(3):629–36.

47. Bozeat S, Lambon Ralph MA, Patterson K, *et al.* Non-verbal semantic impairment in semantic dementia. *Neuropsychologia.* 2000;38(9):1207–15.

48. Goll JC, Crutch SJ, Loo JHY, *et al.* Non-verbal sound processing in the primary progressive aphasias. *Brain.* 2010;133(Pt 1):272–85.

49. Coccia M, Bartolini M, Luzzi S, *et al.* Semantic memory is an amodal, dynamic system: Evidence from the interaction of naming and object use in semantic dementia. *Cognitive Neuropsychology.* 2004;21(5):513–27.

50. Piwnica-Worms KE, Omar R, Hailstone JC, *et al.* Flavour processing in semantic dementia. *Cortex.* 2009;46(6):761–8.

51. Edwards-Lee T, Miller BL, Benson DF, *et al.* The temporal variant of frontotemporal dementia. *Brain.* 1997;120 (Pt 6):1027–40.

52. Snowden JS, Bathgate D, Varma A, *et al.* Distinct behavioural profiles in frontotemporal dementia and semantic dementia. *J Neurol Neurosur Ps.* 2001;70(3):323–32.

53. Kim S, Seo S, Go S, *et al.* Semantic dementia combined with motor neuron disease. *J Clin Neurosci.* 2009;16(12):1683–5.

54. Josephs KA, Whitwell JL, Murray ME, *et al.* Corticospinal tract degeneration associated with TDP-43 type C pathology and semantic dementia. *Brain.* 2013;136(Pt 2):455–70.

55. Kremen SA, Mendez MF, Tsai P-H, *et al.* Extrapyramidal signs in the primary progressive aphasias. *American Journal of Alzheimer's Disease and Other Dementias.* 2011;26(1):72–7.

56. Chan D, Anderson VM, Pijnenburg Y, *et al.* The clinical profile of right temporal lobe atrophy. *Brain.* 2009;132(Pt 5):1287–98.

57. Seeley WW, Bauer AM, Miller BL, *et al.* The natural history of temporal variant frontotemporal dementia. *Neurology.* 2005;64(8):1384–90.

58. Thompson SA, Patterson K, and Hodges JR. Left/right asymmetry of atrophy in semantic dementia: behavioral-cognitive implications. *Neurology.* 2003;61(9):1196–203.

59. Mesulam M-M, Rogalski EJ, Wieneke C, *et al.* Neurology of anomia in the semantic variant of primary progressive aphasia. *Brain.* 2009;132(Pt 9):2553–65.

60. Brambati SM, Rankin KP, Narvid J, *et al.* Atrophy progression in semantic dementia with asymmetric temporal involvement: a tensorbased morphometry study. *NeurobiolAging.* 2009;30(1):103–11.

61. Mummery CJ, Patterson K, Wise RJ, *et al.* Disrupted temporal lobe connections in semantic dementia. *Brain.* 1999;122 (Pt 1):61–73.

62. Mummery C, Patterson K, Price CJ, *et al.* A voxel-based morphometry study of semantic dementia: relationship between temporal lobe atrophy and semantic memory. *Ann Neurol.* 2000;47(1):36–45.

63. Chan D, Fox NC, Scahill RI, *et al.* Patterns of temporal lobe atrophy in semantic dementia and Alzheimer's disease. *Ann Neurol.* 2001;49(4):433–42.

64. Galton CJ, Patterson K, Graham K, *et al.* Differing patterns of temporal atrophy in Alzheimer's disease and semantic dementia. *Neurology.* 2001;57(2):216–25.

65. Rosen HJ, Gorno-Tempini ML, Goldman WP, *et al.* Patterns of brain atrophy in frontotemporal dementia and semantic dementia. *Neurology.* 2002;58(2):198–208.

66. Boxer AL, Rankin KP, Miller BL, *et al.* Cinguloparietal atrophy distinguishes Alzheimer disease from semantic dementia. *Arch Neurol.* 2003;60(7):949–56.

67. Bright P, Moss HE, Stamatakis EA, *et al.* Longitudinal studies of semantic dementia: The relationship between structural and functional changes over time. *Neuropsychologia.* 2008;46(8):2177–88.

68. Rogalski EJ, Cobia D, Harrison TM, *et al.* Progression of language decline and cortical atrophy in subtypes of primary progressive aphasia. *Neurology.* 2011;76(21):1804–10.

69. Rohrer J, Warren JD, Modat M, *et al.* Patterns of cortical thinning in the language variants of frontotemporal lobar degeneration. *Neurology.* 2009;72(18):1562–69.

70. Acosta-Cabronero J, Patterson K, Fryer TD, *et al.* Atrophy, hypometabolism and white matter abnormalities in semantic dementia tell a coherent story. *Brain.* 2011;134(Pt 7):2025–35.

71. Agosta F, Scola E, Canu E, *et al.* White matter damage in frontotemporal lobar degeneration spectrum. *Cerebral Cortex.* 2012;22(12):2705–14.

72. Galantucci S, Tartaglia MC, Wilson SM, *et al.* White matter damage in primary progressive aphasias: a diffusion tensor tractography study. *Brain.* 2011;134(Pt 10):3011–29.

73. Mahoney CJ, Malone IB, Ridgway GR, *et al.* White matter tract signatures of the progressive aphasias.*Neurobiol Aging.* 2013;34(6):1687–99.

74. Schwindt GC, Graham NL, Rochon E, *et al.* Whole-brain white matter disruption in semantic and nonfluent variants of primary progressive aphasia. *Hum Brain Map.* 2011;34(4):973–84.

75. Whitwell JL, Avula R, Senjem ML, *et al.* Gray and white matter water diffusion in the syndromic variants of frontotemporal dementia. *Neurology.* 2010;74(16):1279–87.

76. Zhang Y, Tartaglia MC, Schuff N, *et al.* MRI signatures of brain macrostructural atrophy and microstructural degradation in frontotemporal lobar degeneration subtypes. *Journal of Alzheimer's Disease.* 2013;33(2):431–44.

77. Seeley WW, Crawford RK, Zhou J, *et al.* Neurodegenerative diseases target large-scale human brain networks. *Neuron.* 2009;62(1):42–52.

78. Agosta F, Henry RG, Migliaccio R, *et al.* Language networks in semantic dementia. *Brain.* 2010;133(Pt 1):286–99.

79. Goll JC, Ridgway GR, Crutch SJ, *et al.* Nonverbal sound processing in semantic dementia: a functional MRI study. *Neuroimage.* 2012;61(1):170–80.

80. Deramecourt V, Lebert F, Debachy B, *et al.* Prediction of pathology in primary progressive language and speech disorders. *Neurology.* 2010;74(1):42–49.

81. Rohrer J, Lashley T, Schott JM, *et al.* Clinical and neuroanatomical signatures of tissue pathology in frontotemporal lobar degeneration. *Brain.* 2011;134(Pt 9):2565–81.

82. Snowden JS, Neary D, and Mann DMA. Frontotemporal lobar degeneration: clinical and pathological relationships. *Acta Neuropathologica.* 2007;114(1):31–38.

83. Rohrer J, Geser F, Zhou J, *et al.* TDP-43 subtypes are associated with distinct atrophy patterns in frontotemporal dementia. *Neurology.* 2010;75(24):2204–11.

84. Chow TW, Varpetian A, Moss T, *et al.* Alzheimer's disease neuropathologic changes in semantic dementia. *Neurocase.* 2010 Feb;16(1):15–22.

85. Kim E-J, Park Y-E, Kim D-S, *et al.* Inclusion body myopathy with Paget disease of bone and frontotemporal dementia linked to VCP p.Arg155Cys in a Korean family. *Arch Neurol.* 2011;68(6):787–96.

86. Pereira JMS, Williams GB, Acosta-Cabronero J, al. Atrophy patterns in histologic vs clinical groupings of frontotemporal lobar degeneration. *Neurology.* 2009;72(19):1653–60.

87. Ogar JM, Dronkers NF, Brambati SM, *et al.* Progressive nonfluent aphasia and its characteristic motor speech deficits. *Alz Dis Assoc Dis.*2007;21(4):S23–30.

88. Josephs KA, Duffy JR, Strand EA, *et al.* Clinicopathological and imaging correlates of progressive aphasia and apraxia of speech. *Brain.* 2006;129(Pt 6):1385–98.

89. Josephs KA, Duffy JR, Strand EA, *et al.* Characterizing a neurodegenerative syndrome: primary progressive apraxia of speech. *Brain.* 2012;135(Pt 5):1522–36.

90. Wilson SM, Henry ML, Besbris M, *et al.* Connected speech production in three variants of primary progressive aphasia. *Brain.* 2010;133(Pt 7):2069–88.

91. Ogar JM, Slama H, Dronkers NF, *et al.* Apraxia of speech: an overview. *Neurocase.* 2005;11(6):427–32.

92. Rohrer J, Warren JD, and Rossor MN. Abnormal laughter-like vocalisations replacing speech in primary progressive aphasia. *J Neurol Sci.* 20W09;284(1–2):120–3.

93. Cooke A, DeVita C, Gee J, *et al.* Neural basis for sentence comprehension deficits in frontotemporal dementia. *Brain Lang.* 2003;85(2):211–21.

94. Grossman M andMoore P. A longitudinal study of sentence comprehension difficulty in primary progressive aphasia. *J Neurol Neurosur Ps.* 2005;76(5):644–49.

95. Peelle JE, Cooke A, Moore P, *et al.* Syntactic and thematic components of sentence processing in progressive nonfluent aphasia and nonaphasic frontotemporal dementia. *Journal of Neurolinguistics.* 2007;20(6):482–94.

96. Hillis AE, Oh S, and Ken L. Deterioration of naming nouns versus verbs in primary progressive aphasia. *Ann Neurol.* 2004;55(2):268–75.

97. Blair M, Marczinski CA, Davis-Faroque N, *et al.* A longitudinal study of language decline in Alzheimer's disease and frontotemporal dementia. *JINS.* 2007;13(2):237–45.

98. Joshi A, Roy EA, Black SE, *et al.* Patterns of limb apraxia in primary progressive aphasia. *Brain Cogn.* 2003;53(2):403–7.

99. Gorno-Tempini M-L, Murray RC, *et al.* Clinical, cognitive and anatomical evolution from nonfluent progressive aphasia to corticobasal syndrome: a case report. *Neurocase.* 2004;10(6):426–36.

100. Nestor PJ, Graham NL, Fryer TD, *et al.* Progressive non-fluent aphasia is associated with hypometabolism centred on the left anterior insula. *Brain.* 2003;126(Pt 11):2406–18.

101. Grossman M, Powers J, Ash S, *et al.* Disruption of large-scale neural networks in non-fluent/agrammatic variant primary progressive aphasia associated with frontotemporal degeneration pathology. *Brain Lang.* 2012;127(2):106–20.

102. Sonty SP, Mesulam M-M, Thompson CK, *et al.* R. Primary progressive aphasia: PPA and the language network. *Ann Neurol.* 2003;53(1):35–49.

103. Snowden JS, Pickering-Brown SM, Du Plessis D, *et al.* Progressive anomia revisited: focal degeneration associated with progranulin gene mutation. *Neurocase.* 2007;13(5):366–77.

104. Mesulam M-M, Wicklund AH, Johnson N, *et al.* Alzheimer and frontotemporal pathology in subsets of primary progressive aphasia. *Ann Neurol.* 2008;63(6):709–19.

105. Gorno-Tempini ML, Brambati SM, Ginex V, *et al.* The logopenic/phonological variant of primary progressive aphasia. *Neurology.* 2008;71(16):1227–34.

106. Rohrer J, Caso F, Mahoney C, *et al.* Patterns of longitudinal brain atrophy in the logopenic variant of primary progressive aphasia. *Brain Lang.* 2013;127(2):121–6.

107. Brambati SM, Ogar J, Neuhaus J, *et al.* Reading disorders in primary progressive aphasia: a behavioral and neuroimaging study. *Neuropsychologia.* 2009;47(8–9):1893–900.

108. Graff-Radford J, Duffy JR, Strand EA, *et al.* Parkinsonian motor features distinguish the agrammatic from logopenic variant of primary progressive aphasia. *Parkinsonism Relat D.* 2012;18(7):890–2.

109. Whitwell JL, Jack CR, Duffy JR, *et al.* Microbleeds in the logopenic variant of primary progressive aphasia. *Alzheimer's and Dementia.* 2013;10(1):62–6.

110. Warren JD, Fletcher PD, and Golden HL. The paradox of syndromic diversity in Alzheimer disease. *Nature Neurol.* 2012;8(8):451–64.

111. Rohrer J, Rossor MN, and Warren JD. Alzheimer's pathology in primary progressive aphasia. *Neurobiol Aging* 2012;33(4):744–52.

112. Sajjadi SA, Patterson K, Arnold RJ, *et al.* Primary progressive aphasia: A tale of two syndromes and the rest. *Neurology.* 2012;78(21):1670–7.

113. Rabinovici GD, Jagust WJ, Furst AJ, *et al.* Abeta amyloid and glucose metabolism in three variants of primary progressive aphasia. *Ann Neurol.* 2008;64(4):388–401.

114. Leyton CE, Villemagne VL, Savage S, *et al.* Subtypes of progressive aphasia: application of the International Consensus Criteria and validation using β-amyloid imaging. *Brain.* 2011;134(Pt 10):3030–43.

115. Leyton CE, Hsieh S, Mioshi E, *et al.* Cognitive decline in logopenic aphasia: more than losing words. *Neurology.* 2013;80(10):897–903.

116. Chien DT, Bahri S, Szardenings AK, *et al.* Early clinical PET imaging results with the novel PHF-tau radioligand [F-18]-T807. *JAD.* 2013;34(2):457–68.

117. Bian H, Van Swieten JC, Leight S, *et al.* CSF biomarkers in frontotemporal lobar degeneration with known pathology. *Neurology.* 2008;70(19 Pt 2):1827–35.

118. Coppola, G, Karydas, A, Rademakers, R, *et al.* Gene expression study on peripheral blood identifies progranulin mutations. *Ann Neurol.* 2008;64(1):92–6.

119. Finch, N, Baker, M, Crook, R, *et al.* Plasma progranulin levels predict progranulin mutation status in frontotemporal dementia patients and asymptomatic family members. *Brain.* 2009;132(Pt 3):583–91.

120. Rohrer, J, Sauter, D, Scott, S, *et al.* Receptive prosody in nonfluent primary progressive aphasias. *Cortex.* 2010;48(3):308–16.

121. Reed, DA, Johnson NA, Thompson C, *et al.* A clinical trial of bromocriptine for treatment of primary progressive aphasia. *Ann Neurol.* 2004;56(5):750.

122. Kertesz A, Morlog D, Light M, *et al.* Galantamine in frontotemporal dementia and primary progressive aphasia. *Demtnia Geriat Cogn.* 2008;25(2):178–85.

CHAPTER 35

Frontotemporal dementia

Bruce Miller and Soo Jin Yoon

Introduction

Neurodegenerative diseases selectively attack specific neural circuits. Hippocampal volume loss has been implicated in episodic memory loss in Alzheimer's disease (AD), while frontal lobe deficits such as social disinhibition, loss of empathy, and apathy are the dominant clinical manifestations of FTD. With all forms of FTD, symptoms start insidiously and progress gradually; however, the pathological process begins even before the very early clinical changes of the disease. In recent years, many remarkable advances in this field have been made in the areas of neuroimaging, pathology, and genetics that have facilitated diagnosis and stimulated a better understanding of FTD.

The three clinical subtypes of FTD are diagnosed according to newly derived consensus criteria: behavioural variant FTD (bvFTD), nonfluent/agrammatic variant primary progressive aphasia (nfvPPA), and semantic variant primary progressive aphasia (svPPA).[1,2] Asymmetric but bilateral involvement of the right fronto-insular brain regions is the most likely degenerative pattern to produce bvFTD. bvFTD results in a deterioration of social conduct, emotion, and personality. By contrast, left-side brain degeneration produces clinical presentations associated with progressive language disturbance, so-called primary progressive aphasia (PPA), which is covered in detail in chapter 34.

Epidemiology

To date, there are few epidemiological studies of FTD; however, FTD is a common type of dementia in individuals younger than the age of 65 and may be more prevalent than AD in individuals under 60. Additionally, in persons over the age of 65, FTD, which was thought to be a rare cause of dementia, appears to be more common than previously assumed.[3–8] The average age at onset is about 50–60 years although approximately 10 per cent of FTD patients exhibit an age of onset of over 70 years. A diagnosis of FTD is usually made three to four years after symptom onset. There is a wide range in duration of illness (less than 1 year up to 20 years), partly reflecting different underlying pathologies and problems with misdiagnosis. This condition affects both sexes equally. bvFTD is the most common diagnostic subgroup of FTD and accounts for more than half of all FTD cases. Of bvFTD cases, 9 per cent are also diagnosed as having possible or probable MND. Individuals with an FTD-MND phenotype have a fulminant course with a mean survival of less than three years.[5,7,9]

Clinical pathogenesis

bvFTD is characterized by insidious changes in personality, social conduct, and emotional modulation. The anterior insula (AI) and anterior cingulate cortex (ACC), especially in the right hemisphere,

are the most likely targets of pathogenesis in bvFTD.[10–15] The insula is sometimes classified as a limbic sensory cortex because of its association with the sense of the physiological condition of the body (interoception), whereas the ACC can be regarded as a limbic motor cortex because its output is particularly important for autonomic and emotional control.[16] The insula and ACC both connect with the amygdala, hypothalamus, orbitofrontal cortex, and brainstem homeostatic regions to provide substrates for the feelings and behaviour associated with social interactions.[17]

In addition, the right AI is integral for the subjective evaluation of one's condition, including emotional states, and it plays an important role in interoceptive representation of internal visceral states, a process thought to be foundational for self-awareness.[16,18,19] In particular, the ventral AI (fronto-insula) seems to play an especially important role in social-emotional functions such as emotional processing and empathy.[19,20]

The target neural network is different depending on the specific neurodegenerative disease. Figure 35.1 shows that neurodegenerative diseases (including bvFTD, SD (svPPA), and PNFA (nfvPPA)) target large-scale brain networks.[21] There is also a direct link between intrinsic connectivity, the degree to which distributed brain regions co-activate regardless of task, and grey matter volume—that is, normal connectivity profiles resemble disease-specific brain atrophy patterns.[21] The toxic proteins associated with neurodegenerative diseases spread transneuronally through neuronal networks.[10] Early bvFTD disrupts complex social-emotional functions that rely on the ACC and ventral AI as well as the amygdala and striatum. These regions constitute a large-scale intrinsic connectivity network in healthy subjects, referred to as the 'salience network' because of its consistent activation in response to emotionally significant internal and external stimuli.[21,22]

Additionally, there is a reciprocal and inverse relationship between the salience network and the default mode network (DMN).[23,24] The DMN is important for memory and includes a network anchored by the precuneus, hippocampus, and medial prefrontal cortex. The salience network is disrupted in bvFTD but enhanced in AD; whereas DMN is disrupted in AD, but shows bvFTD-related enhancements within parietal DMN regions.

Seeley and colleagues explored the relationship between a layer 5b neuron, called Von Economo neurons (VENs), which are found only in the ACC and AI and are 30 per cent more abundant in the right hemisphere.[13,25] These VENs are crucial in the development and maintenance of social cognition, and at the time of autopsy are depleted in bvFTD patients but not so in AD.

Pathology

FTD refers to clinical syndromes, while frontotemporal lobar degeneration (FTLD) refers to pathological changes. FTLD

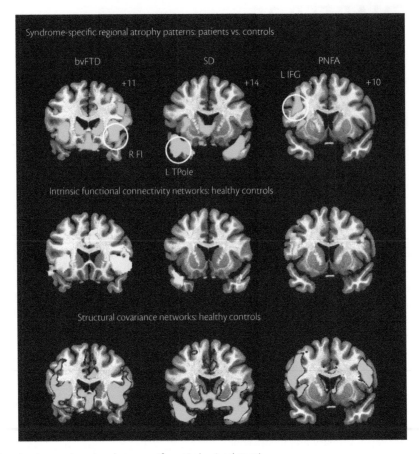

Fig. 35.1 Large-scale intrinsic functional networks and syndrome-specific cortical regional atrophy.
Reproduced from Neuron, 62(1), Seeley WW, Crawford RK, Zhou J, Miller BL, Greicius MD, Neurodegenerative diseases target large-scale human brain networks, pp. 42–52, Copyright (2009), with permission from Elsevier.

presents with gross bilateral frontotemporal atrophy, synapse loss, microvacuolation, reactive astroglial proliferation, and ultimately neuron loss, especially in the superficial laminar layers of frontal and temporal regions (Fig. 35.2).[14,26]

The subtypes of underlying pathological changes in patients with FTD are classified on the basis of the pattern of abnormal protein accumulation (Fig. 35.2). According to the different pathological intracellular inclusion proteins, the involved brain regions, clinical symptoms, and prognoses may be different (Fig. 35.3).

Inclusions of microtubule-associated protein tau are present in approximately 40 per cent of FTLD cases (FTLD-tau). Tau protein is normally localized to the axon, and its main functions include stabilizing neuronal microtubules and facilitating axonal transport. Further subclassification is based on morphological criteria and the predominance of either tau with three microtubule-binding repeats (3R-tau) or four microtubule-binding repeats (4R-tau). The clinical spectrum of FTLD-tau includes Pick's disease, corticobasal degeneration (CBD), progressive supranuclear palsy (PSP), FTDP-17, and other nonspecific tauopathies.[7,27] Pick's disease is a 3R-tau protein disease; and CBD, PSP, and FTDL-17 are 4R-tau protein disorders.

Most of the remaining cases are tau negative, ubiquitin positive, and have inclusions comprising the 43 kDa TAR DNA-binding protein (TDP-43; FTLD-TDP). A minority (~5–10 per cent) are negative for both tau and TDP-43 proteins and in many of those cases inclusions of RNA-binding protein fused in sarcoma (FUS) have

been found (FTLD-FUS). A small proportion of cases have either no inclusions or show ubiquitin-positive inclusions that are TDP-43 and FUS negative, suggesting that additional protein abnormalities remain to be found in FTLD.[3]

Whereas physiological TDP-43, a nuclear protein that appears to be involved in transcription regulation, is localized to the nucleus of neuronal and glial cells, under pathological conditions, immunodetection of nuclear TDP-43 is reduced in inclusion-bearing neuronal and glial cells and TDP-43 is redistributed to accumulate in neuronal and glial cell bodies and processes, a consequence of which may be loss of TDP-43 nuclear function.[28,29]

FTLD-TDP is the most frequent pathological FTLD subtype (~50 per cent of cases) and can present with any of the major clinical phenotypes of FTD syndromes (Table 35.1),[30] including bvFTD with/without MND, svPPA, nfvPPA, and familial inclusion body myopathy with Paget disease of the bone and frontotemporal dementia (IBMPFD). FTLD-TDP type B is the main pathological substrate of most FTD cases with MND, and in rare cases, FTLD-FUS is present.

Behavioural variant frontotemporal dementia

Diagnostic criteria and clinical manifestations

Diagnosing FTD begins with a detailed clinical assessment, including a history from family members and caregivers, determination

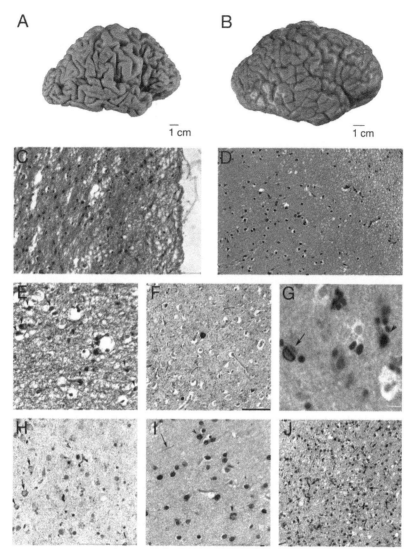

Fig. 35.2 Gross and microscopic pathological changes in FTLD. A: FTLD brain with frontotemporal atrophy: anterior portion—image right side. B: Normal brain: anterior portion—image right side. C: Pick's disease: haematoxylin and eosin (H & E) staining revealed microvacuolation, gliosis, and neuron loss. D: H & E staining in a normal cortex. E: Immunohistochemical stain for tau proteins revealed Pick bodies (arrowhead); cytoplasmic hyperphosphorylated tau inclusions in Pick's disease, shown in insula neurons. F: FTDP-17 case—tau-positive inclusions detected in immunohistochemical stains for tau protein. G: FUS neuropathology, FUS immunohistochemical stains revealed a normal cell with a nuclear signal (arrowhead) and an affected cell with a signal in the cytoplasm (arrow). H: *GRN* mutations—TDP-43 immunohistochemical insula stains disclosed many neuronal cytoplasmic inclusions (NCIs, arrow) and short dystrophic neuritis (DN, arrowhead), consistent with FTLD-TDP type A pathology. Intranuclear inclusion—red arrow. I: C9 mutations—inferior temporal gyrus (ITG) TDP-43 stains revealed moderate NCIs (arrow) throughout the cortex thickness, and scarce DN (arrowhead), indicating FTLD-TDP type B pathology. C9 mutations can either present as TDP type A or B pathology. J: svPPA—ITG TDP-43 stains disclosed many long DNs (arrowhead) and few NCIs (arrow), which are compatible with FTLD-TDP type C pathology. Scale bar: 100 μm except (G) which is 10 μm.

Courtesy of Dr Lea T Grinberg, University of California, San Francisco.

of genetic background, a behavioural and functional assessment, a neurological examination, neuropsychological tests, laboratory tests, and brain imaging. Reports from the Lund and Manchester Groups in 1994, Neary and colleagues in 1998, McKhann and colleagues in 2001, Knopman and colleagues in 2008, along with recent international consensus criteria for bvFTD demonstrate that diagnostic criteria for FTD continues to evolve (Table 35.2).[1,26,31–33]

According to recently proposed bvFTD diagnostic criteria, patients should show progressive behavioural and/or cognition deterioration. At the early stages of the disease, executive dysfunction may be subtle in contrast to prominent behavioural symptoms.[34] There are three levels of diagnostic certainty: possible,

probable, and definite. Patients qualify for possible bvFTD on the basis of three or more persistent or recurrent core behavioural or cognitive features out of six symptoms. A diagnosis of probable bvFTD requires meeting possible criteria for bvFTD and significant functional decline as well as frontotemporal neuroimaging abnormalities. The term 'definite' is reserved for those with neuropathology-proven FTLD or a pathogenic gene mutation.[1]

There are some patients who display a bvFTD-like syndrome but show little or no progression over a decade. Such patients are considered to have a bvFTD 'phenocopy syndrome', manifesting characteristic behavioural features without actively progressing to outright dementia. These 'phenocopy syndrome' cases are

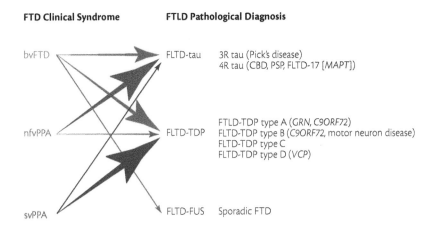

FTD Clinical Syndrome   **FTLD Pathological Diagnosis**

FLTD-tau   3R tau (Pick's disease)
4R tau (CBD, PSP, FLTD-17 [MAPT])

FLTD-TDP   FTLD-TDP type A (GRN, C9ORF72)
FTLD-TDP type B (C9ORF72, motor neuron disease)
FLTD-TDP type C
FLTD-TDP type D (VCP)

FLTD-FUS   Sporadic FTD

Fig. 35.3 Correlations between the pathological types of frontotemporal lobar degeneration and the clinical syndromes of frontotemporal dementia.

predominantly male and usually show normal structural and functional brain imaging, no or very subtle executive dysfunction, intact activities of daily living, and preserved social cognition.[35] While some of these patients suffer from primary psychiatric disorders, others suffer from slow (sometimes genetic forms) of bvFTD.[36]

bvFTD patients commonly display disinhibition, engage in overspending, hoarding behaviour, and a range of socially embarrassing behaviours (e.g. stealing, public urination, or sexually inappropriate comments and gestures), often despite retained knowledge of those rules.[37] Disinhibition is related to the dysfunction of orbitobasal frontal cortex. Patients often also exhibit apathy, which is manifest by a lack of motivation, reduced interest in previous hobbies, diminished activity as well as progressive social isolation. It is associated with the ACC and medial frontal function.[38]

In AD, core social-emotional processes often persist, and patients may even demonstrate enhancement of emotional warmth and sensitivity. While the families of patients with AD describe their loved ones as 'still the same person as they were before', those of patients with bvFTD note profound deficits in empathy and interpersonal warmth. Empathy depends upon intact integrity of the medial frontal lobe and anterior temporal lobe.[39] In FTD, patients may exhibit stereotyped or ritualized behaviours including repetition of a story or phrase and repetitive organization of objects. Repetitive

simple motor movements such as finger or foot tapping, hand or leg rubbing, and clapping, indicate basal ganglia involvement while more complex compulsive routines may also involve right dorsal ACC and left premotor cortex.[40,41]

Disruption to this orbitofrontal-insular-striatal circuit may also contribute to the hyperorality and weight gain commonly observed in FTD.[34,42] Some patients with bvFTD pick up garbage, drink beverages found on the street, eat out of trash cans, and sample food from strangers' plates in restaurants, behaviours that suggest deficits in disgust reactivity.[34,43] Lastly, the neuropsychological profile of bvFTD is executive/generation deficits, which is associated with atrophy of the dorsolateral and prefrontal cortex.[34,40,44]

Cognitively, patients with AD show severe impairment in delayed recall and orientation, however, in contrast, usually bvFTD shows mild memory impairment and high recognition memory scores due to decreased attention in the early stage of the disease. AD patients have more impaired orientation, while bvFTD patients have preserved orientation for time and place.[45] Copying is usually

Table 35.1 FTLD-TDP subtypes

	Cortical pathology	Phenotype	Genetic defects
Type A	Many NCI, Many short DN, predominantly layer 2, lentiform NII	bvFTD, nfvPPA	GRN, C9ORF72
Type B	Moderate NCI, few DN, All layers	bvFTD, FTD-MND	C9ORF72
Type C	Many long DN, few NCI, predominantly layer 2	svPPA, bvFTD	
Type D	Many short DN, many lentiform NII, few NCI, all layers	Familial IBMPFD	VCP

NCI: neuronal cytoplasmic inclusions, DN: dystrophic neuritis, NII: neuronal intra-nuclear inclusions.

Table 35.2 International consensus diagnostic criteria for bvFTD

Possible bvFTD	Early behavioural disinhibition
	Early apathy
	Early loss of sympathy or empathy
	Early perseverative, stereotyped, or compulsive/ritualistic behaviour
	Hyperorality and dietary changes
	Neuropsychological profile: executive/generation deficits with relative sparing of memory and visuospatial functions
Probable bvFTD	Meets criteria for possible bvFTD
	Exhibits significant functional decline
	Frontal and/or anterior temporal atrophy on MRI or CT or frontal and/or anterior temporal hypoperfusion or hypometabolism on PET or SPECT
Definite bvFTD	Meets criteria for possible or probable bvFTD
	Histopathological evidence of FTLD on biopsy or at postmortem
	Presence of a known pathogenic mutation

The term 'early' indicates symptom presentation within the first three years.

spared in bvFTD but when it is abnormal it is not caused by spatial perception dysfunction and attention, as seen in AD cases, but a failure of spatial planning and working memory.[46]

Consensus guidelines for FTD emphasize early behavioural abnormalities and personality changes as a feature of the disease, and patients are noted to have little insight or self-awareness regarding these changes.[47] In addition, bvFTD patients may even develop shifts in long-held core aspects of their personal identity. Changes in hobbies, ideology, religious beliefs, and aesthetic preferences may occur in this disease.[4,48-50]

Although blunted affect and reduced emotional expression are common in FTD, some patients show an elevation of mood (euphoria), inappropriate jocularity, and exaggerated self-esteem. Delusions are not uncommon in bvFTD, and tend to be jealous, somatic, religious, or bizarre, but are less likely to be persecutory. In patients with combined FTD-MND and in young-onset FTLD-FUS, psychotic symptoms are especially common and present in up to 50 per cent of cases.[3,51-53]

Patients with bvFTD typically retain visuospatial function, and some patients may even develop new visual creativity. Diminished language function seen in neurodegenerative diseases that target the left frontal or left anterior temporal lobes can lead to the emergence of previously unrecognized visual and musical creativity, possibly through facilitation of posterior brain regions.[54-56] The enhancement of right posterior brain function may account for the heightened interest in visuospatially-based activities in FTD patients, such as the tendency to solve jigsaw puzzles, design beautiful gardens, fix sprinklers, or even create visual art.

Neuroimaging

In bvFTD, brain CT and MRI may show atrophy in the frontal and/or temporal regions (especially, anterior cingulate, frontoinsular, striatal, and frontopolar areas), which is more involved in the right hemisphere than the left.[3,12,40,57] Single photon emission computed tomography (SPECT) and positron emission tomography (PET) reveal decreased perfusion or glucose metabolism in those same areas, often before structural changes can be appreciated.[3,57]

The clinical and the pathological heterogeneity of FTLD pose a significant diagnostic challenge, and *in vivo* phenotypic characterization of these patients can be improved by the use of imaging biomarkers (Table 35.3).[58-61] A specific pattern of focal grey matter atrophy might be predictive of the underlying pathological process of bvFTD; severe bilateral prefrontal atrophy may be suggestive of Pick's disease; marked atrophy of the caudate nucleus may predict FTLD-FUS; and the asymmetric involvement of a hemisphere may suggest progranulin-associated FTLD. However, patterns of atrophy seem to relate more closely to clinical features than to specific pathological changes.

The recent development of amyloid binding PET tracers that enable *in vivo* measurement of the cerebral amyloid load can help to separate patients in whom AD accounts for the underlying neuropathology. Several studies have already shown that clinically diagnosed FTD patients are much less likely to show amyloid deposition relative to AD patients.[62,63]

Genetic and pathological profiles

Approximately 30–50 per cent of FTD patients have a family history of the disorder with approximately 10 per cent exhibiting an autosomal dominant pattern of inheritance. For the purposes of genetic screening, it is imperative to collect a detailed and thorough family history as well as determine the clinical subtype of the patient. Familial FTD is associated with mutations in genes encoding tau (*MAPT*), progranulin (*GRN*), c9orf72 protein (*C9ORF72*), and the less common valosin-containing protein (*VCP*), chromatin-modifying protein 2B (*CHMP2B*), transactive DNA-binding protein (*TARDBP*), and fused-in-sarcoma (*FUS*). Sometimes a mutation *de novo* without family history of dementia is found.

In 1998, mutations in *MAPT* were shown to cause familial FTD with parkinsonism linked to chromosome 17q21 (FTDP-17).

Table 35.3 The pathology, MRI findings, and clinical manifestations according to genetic mutation

Gene symbol (chromosomal locus)	Pathology (FTLD)	Brain MRI findings	Clinical manifestations
C9ORF72 (chromosome 9)	TDP type A and B	Symmetric widespread cortical atrophy including cerebellum (sensorimotor cortices—when combined with MND)	Onset age: 33–72 years old Mean illness duration: 3–10 years Survival is shorter when combined MND is present. Phenotype: bvFTD, FTD-MND, nonfluent aphasia, rarely mixed svPPA with frontal features, psychosis, memory impairment, parietal dysfunction, mild parkinsonism
GRN (chromosome 17)	TDP type A	Asymmetric frontal, temporal, and parietal atrophy	Onset age: 35–89 years old Mean illness duration: 3–12 years Phenotype: bvFTD, nfvPPA, or a mixed aphasia, CBS, early parietal lobe impairment, frequent hallucinations and delusions, episodic memory deficits
MAPT (chromosome 17)	Tau	Symmetric anteromedial temporal lobe and orbitofrontal atrophy	Onset age: 45–65 years old Mean illness duration: 9 years Phenotype: bvFTD, CBD, PSP, Klüver–Bucy symptom Prominent episodic memory impairment presented initially with behavioural symptoms, semantic impairment, nfvPPA

The neuropathology of such cases is characterized by cytoplasmic neurofibrillary inclusions composed of hyperphosphorylated tau. Inherited FTLD-tau accounts for less than 5 per cent of all cases of FTD and less than 25 per cent of familial FTD cases. Patients with *MAPT* mutations commonly present with bvFTD with or without parkinsonism. Although patients may become anomic or develop a paucity of speech output, typical svPPA or nfvPPA are not common in association with *MAPT* mutations.

The progranulin gene encodes for the growth factor associated with cell proliferation, repair, and anti-inflammatory effects. *GRN* mutations, discovered in 2006 as a cause for FTD, occur at a rate similar to *MAPT* mutations. In *GRN*-related FTD, the penetrance is about 90 per cent by age 75 and there is no evidence of genetic anticipation. *GRN* mutations exert their pathogenic effect through reduced progranulin protein levels. These mutations are pathogenic for ubiquitin immunoreactive and TDP-43 positive neuronal intra-nuclear inclusions.[28,64,65]

The clinical manifestations of *GRN* mutations vary, even within one family: bvFTD is the most common *GRN* mutation presentation, and others include progressive aphasia, episodic memory loss (10–30 per cent), parietal deficits presenting with dyscalculia, visuospatial dysfunction; and CBS (corticobasal syndrome) and MND.[64,66–69] Using a progranulin ELISA in plasma, pathogenic *GRN* mutations can be detected in symptomatic and asymptomatic carriers.[70]

The most recently discovered pathogenic mutation associated with the autosomal dominant FTD-MND phenotype is the *C9ORF72* mutation and it is the most common cause of familial bvFTD in individuals with European ancestry.[5,60,68,71] Psychosis, appetite/eating changes, and parkinsonism are common. PPA and CBS appear can be associated with this mutation.[60] All *C9ORF72* mutation cases have TDP-43 positive pathology, with some having features most consistent with harmonized FTLD-TDP type A pathology, and others having features most consistent with type B pathology.

FTLD-FUS is rare, but has been characterized by a very early onset age (<40 years old), bvFTD with a negative family history and severe caudate atrophy on brain MRI.[41,72–74] Visual hallucinations and delusions can also occur. The FUS protein is a nuclear protein related to DNA repair and regulation of RNA splicing. *FUS* gene mutations on chromosome 16 are associated with the clinicopathological spectrum of FTD and MND. Pathologically, ubiquitin-positive and TDP-43-negative inclusions are found. In bvFTD, any of the histological variants can be found in FTLD-TDP and FTLD-tau, and in a small proportion of FTLD-FUS cases.[3]

Rare *VCP* mutations and charged multivesicular body protein 2B (*CHMP2B*) mutations also contribute to the development of FTD.[75] Mutations in *VCP* on chromosome 9 are associated with IBMPFD, adult-onset proximal and distal muscle weakness, early-onset Paget's disease of the bone, and FTD. Mutations in *CHMP2B* on chromosome 3 have been identified in individuals with autosomal dominant FTD, parkinsonism, dystonia, pyramidal signs, myoclonus, and are mostly confined to a large Danish cohort with FTD.

When considering the genetic aspects of bvFTD, it is important to determine which cases should undergo genetic screening, and whilst there is no consensus, the following are important factors to take into account. First, a strong family history of dementia and psychiatric symptoms that may be compatible with genetic bvFTD should be sought. Second, if a patient has symptoms and signs of MND,

the possibility of a *C9ORF72* mutation associated with FTLD-TDP type B should be considered. Third, salient parietal symptoms with asymmetrical brain atrophy may suggest a *GRN* mutation. Fourth, bvFTD patients who have parkinsonism (PSP, CBS), hyperorality (Klüver–Bucy syndrome), or prominent disinhibition should be considered for *MAPT* mutations related to tau pathology. Fifth, psychotic features raise the possibility of FTLD-TDP pathology related to *C9ORF72* or *GRN* mutations. Lastly, in young age-onset FTD, *MAPT* mutations may be more common, whereas *GRN* mutations are more commonly seen in older age cases; however, the onset age of patients with *GRN* mutations widely vary.[58]

A study of patients' presymptomatic family members with a FTD syndrome suggests that subtle frontal-executive dysfunction and/or behavioural abnormalities may begin in childhood or adolescence and later develop into FTD. This dysfunction might reflect the native cognitive capacities of affected subjects.[76]

Management

Currently, there are no curative or disease-modifying drug treatments for FTD, nor is there any evidence for the potential neuroprotective effects of neurotransmitter augmentation strategies. Consequently, treatment largely remains supportive and involves a combination of nonpharmacological and pharmacological measures aimed at reducing the effect of distressing symptoms.

To treat the behavioural symptoms of FTD successfully, it is imperative to first discover the cause of the abnormal behaviour. Every abnormal behaviour need not be controlled by medication. Some behavioural symptoms may respond to drugs, even though large, randomized, placebo-controlled trials are limited. Antidepressants can be used as a first-line treatment to reduce the behavioural symptoms associated with FTD. Behavioural symptoms such as apathy, impulsivity, and compulsiveness may respond to selective serotonin reuptake inhibitors, while irritability, agitation, depression, and eating disorders may respond better to trazodone. Roaming, prominent agitation, aggressive behaviour, or psychosis may respond best to antipsychotic medications; however, usage of antipsychotics may increase the chances of mortality in FTD patients because of the dysfunction of the basal ganglia and motor neurons in these individuals. Therefore, extreme caution must be considered when using atypical antipsychotics.[3] Genetic discoveries have invigorated the search for effective FTD treatments, but none yet exist.

Caregiver burden in FTD is greater than in AD, and behavioural changes rather than the level of disability, seem to be correlated with caregiver distress and burden in bvFTD.[77] Although treatments for FTD are not well developed, an early and accurate diagnosis remains essential to help patients and families plan for the future and avoid inappropriate and counterproductive interventions.

References

1. Rascovsky K, Hodges JR, Knopman D, *et al.* Sensitivity of revised diagnostic criteria for the behavioural variant of frontotemporal dementia. *Brain.* 2011;134(Pt 9):2456–77.
2. Gorno-Tempini ML, Hillis AE, Weintraub S, *et al.* Classification of primary progressive aphasia and its variants. *Neurology.* 2011;76(11):1006–14.
3. Piguet O, Hornberger M, Mioshi E, *et al.* Behavioural-variant frontotemporal dementia: diagnosis, clinical staging, and management. *Lancet Neurol.* 2011;10(2):162–72.

4. Boxer AL and Miller BL, Clinical features of frontotemporal dementia. *Alzheimer Dis Assoc Disord.* 2005;19 Suppl 1:S3–6.

5. Seelaar H, Rohrer JD, Pijnenburg YA, *et al.* Clinical, genetic and pathological heterogeneity of frontotemporal dementia: a review. *J Neurol Neurosur Ps.* 2011;82(5):476–86.

6. Premi E, Padovani A, and Borroni B. Frontotemporal Lobar Degeneration. *Adv Exp Med Biol.* 2012;724:114–27.

7. Johnson JK, Diehl J, Mendez MF, *et al.* Frontotemporal lobar degeneration: demographic characteristics of 353 patients. *Arch Neurol.* 2005;62(6):925–30.

8. Galimberti D and Scarpini E. Clinical phenotypes and genetic biomarkers of FTLD. *J Neural Transm.* 2012;119(7):851–60.

9. Olney RK, Murphy J, Forshew D, *et al.* The effects of executive and behavioral dysfunction on the course of ALS. *Neurology.* 2005;65(11):1774–7.

10. Zhou JG, ennatas ED, Kramer JH, *et al.* Predicting regional neurodegeneration from the healthy brain functional connectome. *Neuron.* 2012;73(6):1216–27.

11. Seeley WW. Anterior insula degeneration in frontotemporal dementia. *Brain Struct Funct.* 2010;214(5–6):465–75.

12. Seeley WW, Crawford R, Rascovsky K, *et al.* Frontal paralimbic network atrophy in very mild behavioral variant frontotemporal dementia. *Arch Neurol.* 2008;65(2):249–55.

13. Seeley WW. Selective functional, regional, and neuronal vulnerability in frontotemporal dementia. *Curr Opin Neurol.* 2008;21(6):701–7.

14. Broe M, Hodges JR, Schofield E, *et al.* Staging disease severity in pathologically confirmed cases of frontotemporal dementia. *Neurology.* 2003;60(6):1005–11.

15. Rosen HJ, Gorno-Tempini ML, Goldman WP, *et al.* Patterns of brain atrophy in frontotemporal dementia and semantic dementia. *Neurology.* 2002;58(2):198–208.

16. Craig AD. How do you feel—now? The anterior insula and human awareness. *Nat Rev Neurosci.* 2009;10(1):59–70.

17. Mega MS, Cummings JL, Salloway S, *et al.* The limbic system: an anatomic, phylogenetic, and clinical perspective. *J Neuropsychiatry Clin Neurosci.* 1997;9(3):315–30.

18. Craig AD. Emotional moments across time: a possible neural basis for time perception in the anterior insula. *Philos Trans R Soc Lond B Biol Sci.* 2009;364(1525):1933–42.

19. Kurth F, Zilles K, Fox PT, *et al.* A link between the systems: functional differentiation and integration within the human insula revealed by meta-analysis. *Brain Struct Funct.* 2010;214(5–6):519–34.

20. Abu-Akel A and Shamay-Tsoory S. Neuroanatomical and neurochemical bases of theory of mind. *Neuropsychologia.* 2011;49(11):2971–84.

21. Seeley WW, Crawford RK, Zhou J, *et al.* Neurodegenerative diseases target large-scale human brain networks. *Neuron.* 2009;62(1):42–52.

22. Seeley WW, Menon V, Schatzberg AF, *et al.* Dissociable intrinsic connectivity networks for salience processing and executive control. *J Neurosci.* 2007;27(9):2349–56.

23. Zhou J, Greicius MD, Gennatas ED, *et al.* Divergent network connectivity changes in behavioural variant frontotemporal dementia and Alzheimer's disease. *Brain.* 2010;133(Pt 5):1352–67.

24. Seeley WW, Allman JM, Carlin DA, *et al.* Divergent social functioning in behavioral variant frontotemporal dementia and Alzheimer disease: reciprocal networks and neuronal evolution. *Alzheimer Dis Assoc Disord.* 2007;21(4):S50–7.

25. Seeley WW, Zhou J, and Kim EJ. Frontotemporal Dementia: What Can the Behavioral Variant Teach Us about Human Brain Organization? *Neuroscientist.* 2012;18(4):373–85.

26. Clinical and neuropathological criteria for frontotemporal dementia. The Lund and Manchester Groups. *J Neurol Neurosur Ps.* 1994;57(4):416–8.

27. Cairns NJ, Bigio EH, Mackenzie IR, *et al.* Neuropathologic diagnostic and nosologic criteria for frontotemporal lobar degeneration: consensus of the Consortium for Frontotemporal Lobar Degeneration. *Acta Neuropathol.* 2007;114(1):5–22.

28. Neumann M, Kwong LK, Truax AC, *et al.* TDP-43-positive white matter pathology in frontotemporal lobar degeneration with ubiquitin-positive inclusions. *J Neuropathol Exp Neurol.* 2007;66(3):177–83.

29. Mackenzie IR, Rademakers R, and Neumann M. TDP-43 and FUS in amyotrophic lateral sclerosis and frontotemporal dementia. *Lancet Neurol.* 2010;9(10):995–1007.

30. Mackenzie IR, Neumann M, Baborie A, *et al.* A harmonized classification system for FTLD-TDP pathology. *Acta Neuropathol.* 2011;122(1):111–13.

31. Neary D, Snowden JS, Gustafson L, *et al.* Frontotemporal lobar degeneration: a consensus on clinical diagnostic criteria. *Neurology.* 1998;51(6):1546–54.

32. McKhann GM, Albert MS, Grossman M, *et al.* Clinical and pathological diagnosis of frontotemporal dementia: report of the Work Group on Frontotemporal Dementia and Pick's Disease. *Arch Neurol.* 2001;58(11):1803–9.

33. Knopman DS, Kramer JH, Boeve BF, *et al.* Development of methodology for conducting clinical trials in frontotemporal lobar degeneration. *Brain.* 2008;131(Pt 11):2957–68.

34. Wittenberg D, Possin KL, Rascovsky K, *et al.* The early neuropsychological and behavioral characteristics of frontotemporal dementia. *Neuropsychol Rev.* 2008;18(1):91–102.

35. Kipps CM, Hodges JR, and Hornberger M. Nonprogressive behavioural frontotemporal dementia: recent developments and clinical implications of the 'bvFTD phenocopy syndrome'. *Curr Opin Neurol.* 2010;23(6):628–32.

36. Khan BK, Yokoyama JS, Takada LT, *et al.* Atypical, slowly progressive behavioural variant frontotemporal dementia associated with C9ORF72 hexanucleotide expansion. *J Neurol Neurosur Ps.* 2012;83(4):358–64.

37. Miller BL, Cummings JL, Villanueva-Meyer J, *et al.* Frontal lobe degeneration: clinical, neuropsychological, and SPECT characteristics. *Neurology.* 1991;41(9):1374–82.

38. Rankin KP, Santos-Modesitt W, Kramer JH, *et al.* Spontaneous social behaviors discriminate behavioral dementias from psychiatric disorders and other dementias. *J Clin Psychiatry.* 2008;69(1):60–73.

39. Rankin KP, Kramer JH, and Miller BL. Patterns of cognitive and emotional empathy in frontotemporal lobar degeneration. *Cogn Behav Neurol.* 2005;18(1):28–36.

40. Rosen HJ, Allison SC, Schauer GF, *et al.* Neuroanatomical correlates of behavioural disorders in dementia. *Brain.* 2005;128(Pt 11):2612–25.

41. Lee SE, Seeley WW, Poorzand P, *et al.* Clinical characterization of bvFTD due to FUS neuropathology. *Neurocase.* 2012;18(4):305–17.

42. Woolley JD, Gorno-Tempini ML, Seeley WW, *et al.* Binge eating is associated with right orbitofrontal-insular-striatal atrophy in frontotemporal dementia. *Neurology.* 2007;69(14):1424–33.

43. Eckart JA, Sturm VE, Miller BL, *et al.* Diminished disgust reactivity in behavioral variant frontotemporal dementia. *Neuropsychologia.* 2012;50(5):786–90.

44. Kramer JH, Jurik J, Sha SJ, *et al.* Distinctive neuropsychological patterns in frontotemporal dementia, semantic dementia, and Alzheimer disease. *Cogn Behav Neurol.* 2003;16(4):211–8.

45. Hornberger M, Piguet O, Graham AJ, *et al.* How preserved is episodic memory in behavioral variant frontotemporal dementia? *Neurology.* 2010;74(6):472–9.

46. Possin KL, Laluz VR, Alcantar OZ, *et al.* Distinct neuroanatomical substrates and cognitive mechanisms of figure copy performance in Alzheimer's disease and behavioral variant frontotemporal dementia. *Neuropsychologia.* 2011;49(1):43–8.

47. Rankin KP, Baldwin E, Pace-Savitsky C, *et al.* Self awareness and personality change in dementia. *J Neurol Neurosur Ps.* 2005;76(5):632–9.

48. Miller BL, Seeley WW, Mychack P, *et al.* Neuroanatomy of the self: evidence from patients with frontotemporal dementia. *Neurology.* 2001;57(5):817–21.

49. Sturm VE, Rosen HJ, Allison S, *et al.* Self-conscious emotion deficits in frontotemporal lobar degeneration. *Brain.* 2006;129(Pt 9):2508–16.

50. Sturm VE, Ascher EA, Miller BL, *et al*. Diminished self-conscious emotional responding in frontotemporal lobar degeneration patients. *Emotion*. 2008;8(6):861–9.

51. Snowden JS, Rollinson S, Thompson JC, *et al*. Distinct clinical and pathological characteristics of frontotemporal dementia associated with C9ORF72 mutations. *Brain*. 2012;135(Pt 3):693–708.

52. Mendez MF, Shapira JS, Woods RJ, *et al*. Psychotic symptoms in frontotemporal dementia: prevalence and review. *Dement Geriatr Cogn Disord*. 2008;25(3):206–11.

53. Lillo P, Garcin B, Hornberger M, *et al*. Neurobehavioral features in frontotemporal dementia with amyotrophic lateral sclerosis. *Arch Neurol*. 2010;67(7):826–30.

54. Viskontas IV, Boxer AL, Fesenko J, *et al*. Visual search patterns in semantic dementia show paradoxical facilitation of binding processes. *Neuropsychologia*. 2011;49(3):468–78.

55. Flaherty AW, Frontotemporal and dopaminergic control of idea generation and creative drive. *J Comp Neurol*. 2005;493(1):147–53.

56. Mell JC, Howard SM, and Miller BL. Art and the brain: the influence of frontotemporal dementia on an accomplished artist. *Neurology*. 2003;60(10):1707–10.

57. Boccardi M, Sabattoli F, Laakso MP, *et al*. Frontotemporal dementia as a neural system disease. *Neurobiol Aging*. 2005;26(1):37–44.

58. Whitwell JL, Weigand SD, Boeve BF, *et al*. Neuroimaging signatures of frontotemporal dementia genetics: C9ORF72, tau, progranulin and sporadics. *Brain*. 2012;135(Pt 3):794–806.

59. Whitwell JL, Przybelski SA, Weigand SD, *et al*. Distinct anatomical subtypes of the behavioural variant of frontotemporal dementia: a cluster analysis study. *Brain*. 2009;132(Pt 11):2932–46.

60. Boeve BF, Boylan KB, Graff-Radford NR, *et al*. Characterization of frontotemporal dementia and/or amyotrophic lateral sclerosis associated with the GGGGCC repeat expansion in C9ORF72. *Brain*. 2012;135(Pt 3):765–83.

61. Rohrer JD, Warren JD, Barnes J, *et al*. Mapping the progression of progranulin-associated frontotemporal lobar degeneration. *Nat Clin Pract Neurol*. 2008;4(8):455–60.

62. Rabinovici GD, Furst AJ, O'Neil JP, *et al*. 11C-PIB PET imaging in Alzheimer disease and frontotemporal lobar degeneration. *Neurology*. 2007;68(15):1205–12.

63. Engler H, Santillo AF, Wang SX, *et al*. In vivo amyloid imaging with PET in frontotemporal dementia. *Eur J Nucl Med Mol Imaging*. 2008;35(1):100–6.

64. Josephs KA, Ahmed Z, Katsuse O, *et al*. Neuropathologic features of frontotemporal lobar degeneration with ubiquitin-positive inclusions with progranulin gene (PGRN) mutations. *J Neuropathol Exp Neurol*. 2007;66(2):142–51.

65. Mackenzie IR, Baker M, Pickering-Brown S, *et al*. The neuropathology of frontotemporal lobar degeneration caused by mutations in the progranulin gene. *Brain*. 2006;129(Pt 11):3081–90.

66. Kelley BJ, Haidar W, Boeve BF, *et al*. Prominent phenotypic variability associated with mutations in Progranulin. *Neurobiol Aging*. 2009;30(5):739–51.

67. Boeve BF, Baker M, Dickson DW, *et al*. Frontotemporal dementia and parkinsonism associated with the IVS1+1G→A mutation in progranulin: a clinicopathologic study. *Brain*. 2006;129(Pt 11):3103–14.

68. DeJesus-Hernandez M, Mackenzie IR, Boeve BF, *et al*. Expanded GGGGCC hexanucleotide repeat in noncoding region of C9ORF72 causes chromosome 9p-linked FTD and ALS. *Neuron*. 2011;72(2):245–56.

69. Rohrer JD, Crutch SJ, Warrington EK, *et al*. Progranulin-associated primary progressive aphasia: a distinct phenotype? *Neuropsychologia*. 2010;48(1):288–97.

70. Finch N, Baker M, Crook R, *et al*. Plasma progranulin levels predict progranulin mutation status in frontotemporal dementia patients and asymptomatic family members. *Brain*. 2009;132(Pt 3):583–91.

71. Renton AE, Majounie E, Waite A, *et al*. A hexanucleotide repeat expansion in C9ORF72 is the cause of chromosome 9p21-linked ALS-FTD. *Neuron*. 2011;72(2):257–68.

72. Josephs KA, Whitwell JL, Parisi JE, *et al*. Caudate atrophy on MRI is a characteristic feature of FTLD-FUS. *Eur J Neurol*. 2010;17(7):969–75.

73. Rohrer JD, Lashley T, Holton J, *et al*. The clinical and neuroanatomical phenotype of FUS associated frontotemporal lobar degeneration. *J Neurol Neurosur Ps*. 2011;82(12):1405–7.

74. Seelaar H, Klijnsma KY, de Koning I, *et al*. Frequency of ubiquitin and FUS-positive, TDP-43-negative frontotemporal lobar degeneration. *J Neurol*. 2010;257(5):747–53.

75. Nalbandian A, Donkervoort S, Dec E, *et al*. The multiple faces of valosin-containing protein-associated diseases: inclusion body myopathy with Paget's disease of bone, frontotemporal dementia, and amyotrophic lateral sclerosis. *J Mol Neurosci*. 2011;45(3):522–31.

76. Geschwind DH, Robidoux J, Alarcon M, *et al*. Dementia and neurodevelopmental predisposition: cognitive dysfunction in presymptomatic subjects precedes dementia by decades in frontotemporal dementia. *Ann Neurol*. 2001;50(6):741–6.

77. Boutoleau-Bretonniere C, Vercelletto M, Volteau C, *et al*. Zarit burden inventory and activities of daily living in the behavioral variant of frontotemporal dementia. *Dement Geriatr Cogn Disord*. 2008;25(3):272–7.

CHAPTER 36

Dementia with Lewy bodies and Parkinson's disease dementia

Haşmet A. Hanağası, Başar Bilgiç, and Murat Emre

Introduction

Dementia with Lewy bodies (DLB) and Parkinson's disease dementia (PDD) are Lewy body-(LB) related neurodegenerative dementias affecting cognition, behaviour, movement and autonomic function. In terms of molecular pathology, they are both synucleinopathies, characterized by accumulation of misfolded α-synuclein protein in the form of Lewy bodies and Lewy neurites.

DLB and PDD have overlapping clinical, neurochemical, and pathological findings; when the clinical picture is fully developed they are practically indistinguishable.[1,2] The main difference is the temporal sequence of symptoms; motor symptoms precede dementia in PDD whereas it coincides with or follows dementia in DLB. They are believed to represent two entities on the same disease spectrum, with pathological and imaging evidence suggesting that there is more concomitant amyloid pathology in DLB.[2-5] Consensus guidelines proposed an arbitrary cut-off with regard to chronology of symptoms to distinguish these two disorders. Patients who develop dementia after one year following the onset of parkinsonian symptoms should be diagnosed as PDD, whereas those who develop dementia and parkinsonism concomitantly or within one year of each other should be diagnosed as DLB.[4] This one year rule is perhaps more appropriately used for research purposes: in practice, patients who are diagnosed with PD first and subsequently develop dementia should be given the diagnosis of PDD, whereas those who develop dementia first followed by parkinsonism should be designated as DLB.

Dementia with Lewy bodies

Whilst historically other terms including diffuse Lewy body disease, Lewy body dementia, the Lewy body variant of Alzheimer's disease, senile dementia of Lewy body type, and dementia associated with cortical Lewy bodies have been used, the term DLB was proposed at a consensus meeting in 1996[6] and is now widely used. This consortium also described the consensus guidelines for DLB followed by two revisions.[7,8]

Epidemiology

DLB is the second most common cause of neurodegenerative dementias after Alzheimer's disease (AD), accounting for 15–30 per cent of all dementia cases in autopsy series.[9-12] In a systematic review, prevalence rates were found to vary widely between <1–5 per cent of the general population, and <1–30.5 per cent of dementia patients.[13] A study in the United States of America revealed an incidence rate of 3.2 per cent among all incident dementia cases and 0.1 per cent in the general population;[14] in a Finnish community study, in patients with dementia over 75 years the prevalence rates was 21.9 per cent.[15] Lower prevalence rates have been reported in Asian countries[16]

The mean age of onset is between 60 and 80 years,[8] with onset before the age of 60 being rare. Mean survival time (range 2–20 years) and rate of cognitive decline are similar to that seen in AD, although some patients may show rapid progression to death within 1–2 years.[17] DLB has been associated with neuroleptic sensitivity which can be fatal, leading to a two to threefold increase in mortality,[18] and it can be classified as mild (reversible side-effects such as drowsiness) or severe (worsening parkinsonism, irreversible cognitive decline, delirium, and features of neuroleptic malignant syndrome). Compared to AD, patients with DLB were found to have a greater risk of hospital admissions commonly due to fall-related injuries and bronchopneumonia.[19]

Genetics

DLB is more frequent among those with a positive family history of dementia compared to those without.[20,21] The syndrome and its core features tend to aggregate in families.[22] The first chromosomal locus for DLB was mapped at 2q35–q36 in an autopsy-confirmed Belgian family across three generations with different phenotypes including dementia and/or parkinsonism.[23] Molecular genetic analysis did not reveal a simple pathogenic or gene dosage mutation that cosegregated with DLB in this pedigree.[24] The findings on apolipoprotein ε (APOE) polymorphisms in DLB are inconclusive. In some studies, an increased APOE4 allele frequency was reported, whereas others found no such difference.[25-27] Duplications or triplications of α-synuclein gene are known to cause familial forms of PD, PDD, or DLB. Gene multiplications may lead to a gene dose-dependent increase in the expression of α-synuclein, severity of the disease, and a decrease in the age of onset.[28,29] Glucoserebrosidase (GBA) mutations have also been associated with pathologically 'pure' Lewy body disorders, characterized by more extensive, cortical Lewy body pathology.[30] Presence of GBA mutations has been reported in 6.8 per cent of cases with a pathological diagnosis of diffuse Lewy body disease.[31]

Clinical features of DLB

Cognitive features

The central clinical feature is progressive cognitive decline that interferes with normal social and occupational function.[8] The cognitive profile is characterized by particularly severe deficits in executive, visuospatial functions and attention.[32,33] Prominent memory impairments may be absent in the early stages but usually appear as the disease progresses. Patients with concurrent Alzheimer-type pathology may show prominent memory deficits already in the early stages.

A core feature of DLB is fluctuation in cognitive performance, occurring in 50 per cent to 75 per cent of patients.[8] Fluctuation is defined as pronounced variations in attention and alertness, varying from hour-to-hour to day-to-day, and seemingly occurs regardless of the severity of cognitive impairment.[34] There is often no consistent fluctuation pattern even within the same patient. Fluctuations in cognition are reported to be associated with cholinergic deficits[34] and can be assessed with neuropsychological evaluations, for example using computerized tests such as choice reaction time (which reveals momentary fluctuations in the performance during the testing period) or with fluctuation rating scales to capture fluctuations within a day or across days.[35,36]

Behavioural features

Visual hallucinations are the most common psychiatric symptom, and are seen in at least two-thirds of patients.[8] They are usually present early in the disease courses, are often recurrent, and consist of well-formed, detailed, mute images.[37] Patients may have preserved insight into their hallucinations both during and after they occur. Auditory, olfactory, and tactile hallucinations are less common and they usually occur together with concomitant visual hallucinations. Visual illusions may also occur. Delusions are less prevalent,[38] but the phantom boarder phenomenon (the conviction that there are strangers living in the patient's home) and a broader feeling of 'presence' are common; delusions of persecution, theft, and infidelity may also occur. Psychotic symptoms have been associated with differential perfusion changes on single photon emission computed tomography (SPECT) imaging, with visual hallucinations observed with dysfunction of the parietal and ventral occipital cortices, misidentifications with dysfunction of the limbic-paralimbic structures, and delusions with dysfunction of the frontal cortices.[39] Depression and anxiety may appear years before the onset of dementia, with up to 34 per cent of DLB patients experiencing a major depressive episode as a presenting symptom of DLB.[20]

Motor, autonomic, and other associated features

Presence of spontaneous parkinsonism is another core feature of DLB, occurring in 70–100 per cent of cases,[8] but it is not universally present: in a clinicopathological study, absence of parkinsonism was the most common reason for failure to diagnose DLB.[41] Parkinsonism varies in severity, with symptoms including rigidity and bradykinesia, shuffling gait, stooped posture, and masked faces. Conversely, resting tremor is uncommon. Postural instability can already be prominent in the early stages. More than 50 per cent of patients have severe sensitivity to neuroleptics,[18] which is not dose-related and may present with as rapid and irreversible worsening of parkinsonism, cognitive decline, drowsiness, or occasionally with a neuroleptic malignant syndrome-like presentation with profound autonomic instability (see Box 36.1).

Other associated features include a range of sleep disturbances. Rapid eye movement (REM) sleep behaviour disorder is characterized by loss of normal skeletal muscle atonia during REM sleep and vivid dreams with simple or complex motor behaviour.[42] It is

---

Box 36.1 Case presentation

A 70-year-old man was assessed for difficulties in walking and cognitive complaints. Over the previous three years he had become forgetful, with difficulties remembering names, appointments, and finding words, and his gait had become increasingly slow and shuffling. His complaints had become more prominent during the past year with increased slowing, forgetfulness, and occasional hallucinations. He had urge incontinence for the last few years, his wife reported shouting and movements during sleep. Neurological examination revealed a symmetrical akinetic-rigid parkinsonism, while cognitive assessment demonstrated prominent impairments in attention, executive, and visual-spatial functions with mild impairment of memory which improved on cueing. His MRI showed prominent parieto-occipital and slight hippocampal atrophy. He was diagnosed with DLB, treatment with a cholinesterase inhibitor and levodopa was initiated with moderate improvement of gait and cognition.

---

present in nearly 70 per cent of DLB patients and may occur many years before the onset of dementia or parkinsonism.[42] As the disease progresses, it may become less frequent or less symptomatic.[43] It has been suggested that inclusion of REM sleep behaviour disorder (RBD) as a core clinical feature improves the diagnostic accuracy of autopsy-confirmed DLB patients.[44] Disturbed sleep–wake cycle and excessive daytime sleepiness are also common features.

LB pathology and neuronal loss in the autonomic nervous system,[8] giving rise to a range of autonomic abnormalities such as orthostatic hypotension, impotence, urinary incontinence, and constipation are may be seen in DLB.[45] Urinary incontinence is the most frequent autonomic symptom, followed by constipation.[8]

Repeated falls, syncope, and transient loss of consciousness may occur and constitute supporting features for diagnosis. Unprovoked falls may be related to postural instability or autonomic dysfunction. Transient and otherwise unexplained lapses of consciousness, with or without falls, may represent orthostatic syncope.

Pathological and biochemical correlates

The core pathological hallmarks include Lewy bodies (LBs) in neuronal cytoplasm and Lewy neurites. They can be seen in the brainstem nuclei, amygdala, limbic-paralimbic cortices, basal ganglia and cerebral cortex, medulla and peripheral autonomic nervous system may also be involved.[46] Gliosis and neuronal loss are also present in these regions. LBs are usually found in the deeper layers of the neocortex: α-synuclein is the major protein component;[47] neurofilaments, ubiquitin, torsin A, and parkin minor constituents.[48] Morphologically, LBs are divided into brainstem and cortical types.[46] 'Brainstem-' type LBs, easily detected by standard histological methods such as haematoxylin–eosin staining, are spherical intraneuronal cytoplasmic inclusions characterized by hyaline eosinophilic core, concentric lamellar band, and a narrow pale halo. Cortical LBs occur in limbic and neocortical regions, mainly in the layer II, III, V, VI of the cortex. They are not readily identifiable with classical histological stainings, and immunohistochemistry with anti-α-synuclein antibodies is required to detect them. DLB Consortium criteria for a pathological diagnosis of DLB proposes a classification system using α-synuclein immunohistochemistry with semiquantitative grading of Lewy-related pathology (mild, moderate, severe, very severe) in brainstem, limbic, and diffuse neocortical areas rather than counting LBs in various brain regions.[8]

In addition to LB pathology, 75–90 per cent of patients have concomitant amyloid plaques and many meet pathological criteria for Alzheimer's disease (AD) according to the Consortium to Establish a Registry of Alzheimer's Disease (CERAD) criteria.[49–51] Although concomitant amyloid plaques are common, neurofibrillary tangles are rare. Vascular pathology can be found in up to 30 per cent of DLB patients.[52] Concomitant AD-type or vascular pathology may have an impact on the clinical presentation,[53] with the presence of significant AD pathology being associated with more severe memory impairment compared to cases with purer LB pathology which are associated with more severe executive and visuospatial dysfunction.

Biochemically DLB is associated with severe dopaminergic and cholinergic deficiency,[54] the latter typically being more prominent in DLB than in AD.[55] In DLB there is loss of cholinergic neurons in the nucleus basalis of Meynert[56] and reductions in markers of cholinergic activity (choline acetyltransferase levels) in temporal and parietal cortex. Reduction of choline acetyltransferase activity in the temporal lobe is correlated with the degree of the cognitive impairment.[57] Cholinergic deficits are greater in the temporal cortices of patients with visual hallucinations as compared to those without.[58] Muscarinic M1 postsynaptic receptor binding in the temporal lobe may be increased in patients with delusional thinking.[59]

Dopaminergic deficit is the other prominent neurochemical feature. Reduction in postsynaptic D2 receptor density in striatum is greater in DLB than in PD or healthy controls, which may contribute to the weak response to dopaminergic drugs or neuroleptic sensitivity.[60] LB pathology also occurs in the dorsal raphe nucleus, leading to marked reduction of serotonin levels in the basal ganglia and cerebral cortices. Deficits in serotoninergic and noradrenergic systems may contribute to cognitive and behavioural symptoms.[61]

Auxiliary investigations

In structural magnetic resonance imaging (MRI), hippocampus and medial temporal lobes are relatively well-preserved compared with AD patients,[62] although mild hippocampal atrophy (10–20 per cent) can be seen compared to controls.[63] The utility of MRI in differential diagnosis is, however, limited. Atrophy in other cortical and subcortical structures has also been reported, including striatum, substantia innominata, hypothalamus, and dorsal midbrain.[64] In longitudinal MRI studies, the rate of cerebral atrophy was found to be 1.4 per cent per year, three times more than that seen in controls, but less than that seen in AD.[65]

In one MR spectroscopy (MRS) study, no changes were found in the grey matter N-acetyl aspartate/Creatinine (NAA/Cr) ratio—considered to be a marker of neuronal integrity—in DLB patients compared to healthy controls.[66] In another study of proton MRS focusing on posterior cingulate gyri and inferior precunei, NAA/Cr levels were reduced in all dementia groups (AD, vascular dementia, frontotemporal dementia (FTD)) except for DLB, suggesting relative preservation of posterior cingulate cortex neuronal integrity in DLB.[67] In a diffusion tensor imaging (DTI) study, changes (increased diffusion (D) and decreased fractional anisotropy (FA) values) in corpus callosum and pericallosal areas were found in DLB patients compared to normal controls.[68] White matter was also affected in the frontal, parietal, and occipital areas with less involvement of the temporal lobe. Areas of reduced FA in DLB versus controls were also observed primarily in parietooccipital white matter tracts where the changes were more diffuse in AD; compared to AD, DLB was also associated with reduced FA in pons and left thalamus.[69] Resting state functional MRI (fMRI) studies suggest increased functional connectivity between the right posterior cingulate and other brain areas.[70,71] These imaging studies would suggest relatively preserved neuronal integrity, diffuse white matter tract breakdown and disrupted connectivity in DLB patients.

SPECT and positron emission tomography (PET) studies have demonstrated decreased glucose metabolism and perfusion deficits in parietal and occipital cortices.[72,73] Occipital hypometabolism is, however, not always present and FDG-PET changes may be similar to that seen in AD (Fig. 36.1). Reduced uptake of ^{18}F-fluorodopa in the striatum may distinguish DLB from AD with high sensitivity and specificity.[74] ^{123}I-β-CIT SPECT demonstrates reduced dopamine transporter binding in the caudate and posterior putamen in DLB compared to AD patients.[75,76] SPECT using ^{123}I-metaiodobenzylguanidine (MIBG), a marker of postganglionic cardiac sympathetic innervation, shows reduced cardiac MIBG uptake in DLB and PD patients as opposed to normal findings in AD.[77] Using Pittsburgh compound B (PiB), an in vivo marker of β-amyloid burden, as predicted by pathological studies, 80 per cent of DLB cases were found to have increased amyloid load.[78–80]

Electro-encephalography (EEG) may show slowing of background activity in DLB patients in early stages, and epoch-by-epoch analysis may demonstrate fluctuations. Frontal intermittent delta activity and transient temporal slow waves are other changes which can occur more commonly in DLB than in AD.[81,82]

Biomarkers

Currently, there are no blood or cerebrospinal fluid (CSF) markers that can be reliably used for diagnosis, to follow disease progression, or as an outcome measure for therapeutic interventions. CSF α-synuclein has been studied as a potential biomarker for DLB but results have been controversial.[83,84] Several studies reported lower amyloid β40–42 levels in DLB compared to controls and PDD cases.[85,86] CSF amyloid β38 was suggested as a diagnostic biomarker for DLB;[87] Aβ42:Aβ38 ratio discriminated AD from with a sensitivity of 78 per cent and a specificity of 67 per cent.

Diagnosis of DLB

The central feature required for the diagnosis of DLB is progressive cognitive decline that interferes with the social and occupational functionality of the patient (Table 36.1).[8] Core features

(a)   (b)

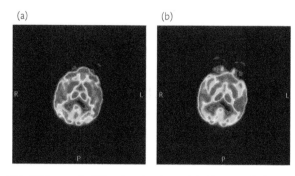

Fig. 36.1 PET image of a DLB patient showing occipital hypometabolism.

Table 36.1 Revised criteria for the clinical diagnosis of dementia with Lewy bodies

---

1. Central feature (essential for a diagnosis of possible or probable DLB)

- Dementia defined as progressive cognitive decline that interferes with social and occupational function
- Prominent or persistent memory impairment may not necessarily occur in the early stages but is usually evident with progression.
- Deficits on tests of attention, executive function, and visuospatial ability may be especially prominent.

2. Core features (two core features are sufficient for a diagnosis of probable DLB, one for possible DLB)

- Fluctuating cognition with pronounced variation in attention and alertness.
- Recurrent visual hallucinations
- Spontaneous features of parkinsonism

3. Suggestive features (1 or more + a core feature = Probable DLB, any 1 alone = Possible DLB)

- REM sleep behaviour disorder
- Severe neuroleptic sensitivity
- Low dopamine transporter uptake in basal ganglia demonstrated by SPECT or PET imaging

4. Supportive features (commonly present but lacking diagnostic value)

- Repeated falls and syncope
- Transient, unexplained loss of consciousness
- Severe autonomic dysfunction, e.g. orthostatic hypotension, urinary incontinence
- Hallucinations in other modalities
- Systematized delusions
- Depression
- Relative preservation of medial temporal lobe on CT or MRI scan
- Decreased tracer uptake on SPECT or PET imaging in occipital regions
- Abnormal (low uptake) MIBG myocardial scintigraphy
- Prominent slow waves on EEG with temporal lobe transient sharp waves

5. A diagnosis of DLB is less likely

- In the presence of cerebrovascular disease evident as focal neurologic signs or on brain imaging
- In the presence of any other physical illness or brain disorder sufficient to account in part or in total for the clinical picture
- If parkinsonism only appears for the first time at a stage of severe dementia

6. Temporal sequence of symptoms

- DLB should be diagnosed when dementia occurs before or concurrently with parkinsonism (if it is present). The term Parkinson's disease dementia (PDD) should be used to describe dementia that occurs in the context of well-established Parkinson's disease. In a practice setting, the term that is most appropriate to the clinical situation should be used and generic terms such as LB disease are often helpful. In research studies in which distinction needs to be made between DLB and PDD, the existing one-year rule between the onset of dementia and parkinsonism DLB continues to be recommended. Adoption of other time periods will simply confound data pooling or comparison between studies. In other research settings that may include clinicopathologic studies and clinical trials, both clinical phenotypes may be considered collectively under categories such as LB disease or α-synucleinopathy.

Reproduced from *Neurology*. 65(12), McKeith IG, Dickson DW, Lowe J, *et al*. Diagnosis and management of dementia with Lewy bodies: third report of the DLB Consortium, pp. 1863–72, Copyright (2005), with permission from Wolters Kluwer Health, Inc.

include fluctuation in cognition with pronounced variation in attention and alertness, recurrent and persistent visual hallucinations, and spontaneous (i.e. not drug-induced) parkinsonism. Consensus guidelines recommend that two of the core clinical features have to be present for a diagnosis of probable and one for a diagnosis of possible DLB.[4] Suggestive and supportive features may increase diagnostic accuracy; they are more frequent than in other dementing diseases but their specifity is low. Suggestive features include REM sleep behaviour disorder, severe neuroleptic sensitivity, and decreased dopamine transporter binding in striatum. Possible DLB can be diagnosed if one or more suggestive features are present in a patient with dementia even in the absence of any core features. Supportive features include repeated falls and syncope, transient or unexplained loss of consciousness, severe autonomic dysfunction, systematized delusions, hallucinations in other modalities (i.e. auditory and tactile), depression, relative preservation of medial temporal lobe on computed tomography (CT) or MRI scan, decreased tracer uptake on SPECT or PET imaging in occipital regions, abnormal ^{123}I-MIBG scintigraphy, prominent slow waves on EEG with transient sharp waves in temporal lobe.

The diagnosis of DLB is principally based on clinical features and exclusion of other diagnoses. A history of stroke, focal neurological signs, and the presence of significant comorbid physical illness and other brain disorders reduce the certainty of diagnosis.

Management

Both nonpharmacological and pharmacological interventions can be used in management. Recognition and amelioration of sensory impairments such as impaired vision or hearing, environmental optimization such as improving lighting, may reduce hallucinations, delusions, and falls. Education of caregivers is important: behavioural symptoms may be relieved or reduced by an appropriate approach to patients, and can reduce use of antipsychotics.

Consideration should be given to discontinuation of drugs with anticholinergic effects such as tricyclic antidepressants, anticholinergics or antispasmodics as they may impair cognition, exacerbate psychotic symptoms, and cause orthostatic hypotension.[38] Levodopa is the drug of choice to treat motor symptoms and should be started at low doses and increased slowly to the minimum required dose. Response to levodopa can be limited, partly due to primary unresponsiveness and partly due to the predominance of symptoms (such as postural instability) known to be unresponsive to levodopa.[88,89] Potential side-effects of levodopa include visual hallucinations, delusions, orthostatic hypotension, and nausea.

Orthostatic hypotension can be treated with hydration, increased salt intake, avoiding prolonged bed rest, thigh-high compression stockings, efforts to stand up slowly, and minimizing or discontinuing medication that contributes to orthostasis. In refractory cases fludrocortisone and midodrine can be considered. Constipation may benefit from exercise, increased dietary fibre, increased water intake, and laxatives. REM sleep behaviour disorder can be treated with low dose clonazepam (0.25–1.0 mg) at bedtime; however, this can worsen the symptoms of obstructive sleep apnoea or may cause daytime sleepiness and unsteadiness.[42] Melatonin may also be used at a dose of 3–12 mg, either as monotherapy or in conjunction with clonazepam.[90] Modafinil and methylphenidate can be considered to treat excessive daytime sleepiness although there is no direct evidence for its use in DLB. Serotonin reuptake inhibitors (SSRIs) and serotonin-norepinephrine reuptake inhibitors (SNRIs) can be used to treat depressive symptoms.

Although being often the most troubling neuropsychiatric feature, visual hallucinations may not require drug treatment if they are not frightening. Neuroleptics should be used with great caution to treat psychotic features as some patients may show severe neuroleptic sensitivity which is not predictable.[18] In addition, antipsychotics may increase the risk of cerebrovascular events and death in elderly patients with dementia.[91] As reductions in cholinergic activity correlate with hallucinations, cholinesterase inhibitors may be considered for management of mild hallucinations and delusions before using neuroleptics,[92,93] and are often very effective (see following). Classical neuroleptics such as haloperidol are contraindicated, risperidone and olanzapine can also worsen parkinsonism, and so when required quetiapine and clozapine are the neuroleptics which can be considered. Initial doses should be low and the dose should be titrated slowly while monitoring for adverse effects. Neuroleptics can cause orthostatic hypotension and blood pressure should be monitored.

As patients with DLB have severe cholinergic deficits, cholinesterase inhibitors rivastigmine and donepezil were tested in randomized, placebo-controlled trials. In the study with rivastigmine (6–12 mg/day) there were no statistically significant differences from placebo on mean mini-mental state examination (MMSE) score, clinician-assessed global change from baseline and mean neuropsychiatric inventory (NPI, 10 items) score. More than twice as many patients on rivastigmine (63.4 per cent) than on placebo (30.0 per cent) showed at least a 30 per cent improvement from baseline in their NPI-4 scores ($P \leq 0.001$), with psychotic features resolving almost completely in over half of the treated patients. Apathy, anxiety, delusions, and hallucinations showed most response. There was also a significant improvement in a computerized test of attention. Nausea, vomiting, anorexia and somnolence were the most common side-effects. Worsening of parkinsonism was not reported, except for emergent tremor in four rivastigmine-treated patients.[92] In the study with donepezil,[93] patients given 5 mg or 10 mg donepezil showed greater improvement in the majority of the cognitive and behavioural scales, including the MMSE and NPI; 10 mg was also associated with improved global function and reduced caregiver burden. Patients taking donepezil were less apathetic, less anxious, had less cognitive fluctuation, and fewer delusions and hallucinations compared to placebo patients. Adverse effects (AEs) were usually mild to moderate.

Some changes in glutamatergic activity have been reported in patients with DLB[94] and the uncompetitive N-methyl-D-aspartate antagonist memantine was tested in two randomized controlled studies with inconsistent results.[95,96] In the larger study with 121 PDD and 78 DLB patients,[96] those treated with memantine had greater improvements in clinicans global impression of change score compared to placebo; improvements were predominantly in the DLB group. Likewise, behavioural symptoms as assessed with NPI total score significantly improved in the DLB group only. Cognitive tests, activities of daily living, or caregiver burden scores did not show significant improvements in either patient group. Adverse events in the two treatment groups were similar except for slightly more sedation in the memantine group. In another, smaller randomized trial of memantine including both patients with DLB or PDD, significantly improved mean global impression of change

score was observed in the total population; the difference was, however, driven by a larger efficacy in the PDD group.[95] NPI scores showed a statistically significant improvement under memantine in the DLB group, but not in the PDD population. No statistically significant differences were observed for individual cognitive tests, activities of daily living, or caregiver burden scores.

Based on the available evidence, cholinesterase inhibitors such as rivastigmine and donepezil should be considered in patients with a diagnosis with DLB, taking into account potential benefits and risks. The data on benefits of memantine are less clear, perhaps being considered in patients with prominent behavioural symptoms.

Parkinson's disease dementia

Although considered primarily a motor disorder, non-motor symptoms may accompany Parkinson's disease (PD) from early stages and be present even before the manifestation of motor symptoms. Due to advances in treatment and increased life expectancy, cognitive impairment and dementia in PD have become increasingly more recognized.

Epidemiology

Subtle cognitive deficits may be detected even in the early stages of PD if appropriate neuropsychological tests are administered. In the majority of patients, however, overt cognitive impairment becomes manifest in the late stages of the disease, especially in old age. In a community-based study, 36 per cent of newly diagnosed patients were found to have cognitive impairment at the time of diagnosis, while 57 per cent of this cohort developed cognitive deficits within 3.5 (+/-0.7) years; the incidence of dementia was estimated to be 38.7 per 1000 person-years of observation.[97] In another study, 24 per cent of 115 newly diagnosed PD patients displayed impaired performance on at least three neuropsychological tests and were classified as cognitively impaired.[98] A pooled analysis comprising 1346 non-demented PD patients from 8 centres showed that 25.8 per cent of patients had fulfilled criteria for mild cognitive impairment (MCI).[99]

Both the prevalence and incidence of dementia are increased in PD. In a systematic review, the point prevalence of dementia was 24–31 per cent. The prevalence of PDD in the general population aged 65 years and over was calculated to be 0.3–0.5 per cent, and 3–4 per cent of all dementias were estimated to be due to PDD.[100]

The incidence of dementia in PD was reported to be 1.7–5.9 times higher compared to controls.[101,102] In the Sydney cohort, 48 per cent of surviving patients with PD had developed dementia 15 years after the diagnosis[103] and the cumulative incidence had risen to 83 per cent 20 years after the diagnosis.[104] In a study in Norway, the 8-year cumulative prevalence of dementia was 78.2 per cent (26 per cent of cases being demented at baseline).[105] In a door-to-door survey, 15 per cent of PD patients developed dementia compared to 4.9 per cent of the control group.[101]

The most established risk factors for PDD include age and disease severity. Old age at disease onset or at the time of evaluation are significant risk factors. In one study, older patients (mean age 79 years) with more severe disease had a 12-fold increased dementia risk compared to younger patients with mild disease;[106] severe motor disability, long disease duration, atypical neurological features such as early autonomic impairment, symmetrical disease presentation, and unsatisfactory response to dopaminergic treatment were additional risk factors.

Low cognitive scores at baseline, early development of confusion or hallucinations on dopaminergic medication, axial involvement including speech impairment and postural imbalance and excessive daytime sleepiness may also be associated with increased risk of dementia in PD. REM sleep behaviour disorder (RBD) is frequently seen in PD: in one study, PD patients with RBD had a sixfold higher occurrence of dementia than those without.[107] Dementia is associated with postural instability and gait disorder phenotype, and tremor-dominant patients have lower risk of developing dementia. Poor verbal fluency, poor performance on verbal memory tests, and subtle impairment in executive functions at baseline were significantly associated with incident dementia.[108] In one cohort, impairment in cognitive tests relying on frontal executive functions were associated with a lower risk of dementia whereas impairment in those tests assessing more posterior cortical functions was associated with a higher risk.[97] White matter hyperintensities were associated with cognitive decline in PD patients.[109] Smoking has been associated with a two- to fourfold higher risk for dementia in PD,[110] but no significant association with head injury or diabetes mellitus has been reported with incident dementia.[111]

Genetic aspects

Siblings of PDD patients have been reported to have a threefold increased risk of history of AD.[112] The data concerning the association of apolipoprotein ε4 (APOE4), a genetic risk factor for AD, with PDD have been inconsistent; along with APOE4, APOE2 has also been suggested to be associated with PDD.[113]

There is some evidence that variations in the tau (*MAPT*) gene seem to be a genetic risk factor, the H1/H1 haplotype being associated with a greater rate of cognitive decline and dementia in PD,[114,115] but not for other neurodegenerative diseases such as DLB and AD.[116]

A significantly higher frequency of heterozygote mutations in the glucocerebrosidase gene (*GBA*) has been reported in PD and DLB. Up to half of PD patients heterozygous for *GBA* mutations developed cognitive impairment later in their disease in one series,[117] and compared to PD patients without mutations PD patients with GBA mutations were found to be at higher risk of dementia with an odds ratio of 5.8.[118]

Altered expression of, or missense mutations in the α-synuclein gene have been linked to familial PD, sometimes associated with dementia. There is, however, a more robust relationship with cognitive decline and α-synuclein duplication, and even more so with the triplication of the α-synuclein gene.[29,119]

Mutations in parkin, *PINK1*, and *DJ-1* genes cause autosomal recessive PD. Dementia rates seem to be lower in patients with *PINK1* and *DJ-1* mutations, with the rate in parkin mutation carriers may be more similar to sporadic PD. G2019S *LRRK2* mutations, a cause of autosomal-dominant PD, may be associated with cognitive impairment,[120] but overall the frequency of dementia in monogenic forms of PD may be lower than in sporadic PD. This observation may in part relate to the relatively younger age of these patients, especially in the case of recessive mutations.[121]

Clinical features of PDD

Cognitive features

In typical cases, the profile of dementia can be best described as a dysexecutive syndrome with prominent impairment of attention,

executive, and visuospatial functions, moderately impaired episodic memory, and associated neuropsychiatric symptoms including apathy and psychosis (Table 36.2).

Cognitive impairments seen in non-demented PD patients (which is designated as PD-MCI) have in general similar profile to those found in patients with dementia, with quantitative rather than qualitative differences. The most common deficits are in executive functions, visuospatial functions, memory, and attention. The profile of cognitive deficits in PD-MCI is variable, the most frequent subtype being single-domain non-amnestic MCI, the most frequent single deficit being episodic memory impairment.[99]

Impairment of attentional functions and working memory is an early and prominent feature in PDD. Attentional fluctuations occur in a similar way to patients with DLB. PDD patients tend to be more apathetic compared to AD patients, and impaired attention is an important determinant of ability to undertake activities of daily living in PDD.[122]

Impairment in executive functions is one of the early and prominent cognitive features of PDD. Using the Mattis Dementia Rating Scale which is sensitive to executive function, PDD patients were found to have lower initiation, perseverance, and construction, but higher memory subscores compared to patients with AD.[123] Insight is usually relatively preserved in PDD, in contrast to many patients with AD.

Working memory, explicit visual and verbal memory, and implicit memory such as procedural learning can all be impaired in PDD. The relative severity of memory impairment as compared to general level of cognitive dysfunction, and the profile of impairment usually differ from that seen in AD. In typical cases, the memory impairment is characterized by a deficit in free recall with relatively preserved recognition. Memory scores in patients with PDD were found to correlate with performance in executive function tests, suggesting that impairment of memory in PDD may partly be due to difficulties in developing search strategies, although this view has been recently challenged.[124] Memory impairment resembling that seen in typical AD can also be seen in a subpopulation of PDD patients.[125]

Another early cognitive deficit in PDD is impairment in visuospatial functions. Impairment, especially in visuoperceptual abilities, is typically more severe than patients with typical, amnestic AD.[126] Visuospatial abilities such as object assembly are often more impaired in PDD, whereas visuospatial memory tasks are worse in AD. Deficits in visuospatial functions may be more evident in more complex tasks, which require planning, sequencing of response, or generation of strategies, suggesting that these deficits may be, at least partly, due to problems in sequential organization of behaviour (i.e. executive dysfunction).

Core language functions are largely preserved in PDD. Where present, deficits usually consist of word finding difficulties, pauses in spontaneous speech, or relate to difficulties understanding complex sentences.

Several structured scales, some specifically developed for PD, can be used for screening cognitive impairment. The Montreal Cognitive Assessment (MoCA), with a high test–re-test and inter-rater reliability, can be used as a screening instrument, with a cut off score of 21/30 yielded a sensitivity of 90 per cent in PDD patients compared to non-demented PD patients.[127] Both the MoCA and cognitive screening instruments specifically developed

Table 36.2 Clinical features of dementia associated with PD

I Core features

1) Diagnosis of Parkinson's disease according to Queen Square Brain Bank criteria

2) A dementia syndrome with insidious onset and slow progression, developing within the context of established Parkinson's disease and diagnosed by history, clinical, and mental examination, defined as:
   - Impairment in more than one cognitive domain
   - Representing a decline from premorbid level
   - Deficits severe enough to impair daily life (social, occupational, or personal care), independent of the impairment ascribable to motor or autonomic symptoms

II Associated clinical features

1) Cognitive features:
   - Attention: Impaired. Impairment in spontaneous and focused attention, poor performance in attentional tasks; performance may fluctuate during the day and from day to day
   - Executive functions: Impaired. Impairment in tasks requiring initiation, planning, concept formation, rule finding, set-shifting or set maintenance; impaired mental speed (bradyphrenia)
   - Visuospatial functions: Impaired. Impairment in tasks requiring visual-spatial orientation, perception, or construction
   - Memory: Impaired. Impairment in free recall of recent events or in tasks requiring learning new material, memory usually improves with cueing, recognition is usually better than free recall
   - Language: Core functions largely preserved. Word finding difficulties and impaired comprehension of complex sentences may be present

2) Behavioural features:
   - Apathy: Decreased spontaneity; loss of motivation, interest, and effortful behaviour
   - Changes in personality and mood including depressive features and anxiety
   - Hallucinations: Mostly visual, usually complex, formed visions of people, animals or objects
   - Delusions: Usually paranoid, such as infidelity, or phantom boarder (unwelcome guests living in the home) delusions
   - Excessive daytime sleepiness

III Features which do not exclude PDD but make the diagnosis uncertain

- Coexistence of any other abnormality which may by itself cause cognitive impairment, but judged not to be the cause of dementia, e.g. presence of relevant vascular disease in imaging
- Time interval between the development of motor and cognitive symptoms not known

IV Features suggesting other conditions or diseases as cause of mental impairment which, when present, make it impossible to reliably diagnose PDD

- Cognitive and behavioural symptoms appearing solely in the context of other conditions such as:
  Acute confusion due to
  a) Systemic diseases or abnormalities
  b) Drug intoxication
  Major Depression according to DSM IV
- Features compatible with "Probable Vascular dementia" criteria according to NINDS-AIREN (dementia in the context of cerebrovascular disease as indicated by focal signs in neurological exam such as hemiparesis, sensory deficits, and evidence of relevant cerebrovascular disease by brain imaging AND a relationship between the two as indicated by the presence of one or more of the following: onset of dementia within three months after a recognized stroke, abrupt deterioration in cognitive functions, and fluctuating, stepwise progression of cognitive deficits)

for PD including Mini Mental Parkinson and the Parkinson neuropsychometric dementia assessment (PANDA) may be more sensitive than the MMSE to detect cognitive impairment in PD.[128,129] More elaborate cognitive scales for in depth assessment include the general cognitive scales such as Mattis Dementia Rating Scale and the Cambridge Cognition–Revised (CAMCOG–R), as well as PD-specific scales such as SCales for Outcomes of PArkinson's disease-cognition (SCOPA-Cog) and PD Cognitive Rating Scale (PD-CRS).[130]

Behavioural features

A wide range of neuropsychiatric symptoms are seen in PDD, the most common are hallucinations, apathy, depression, anxiety, and insomnia. At least one neuropsychiatric symptom is present in more than 90 per cent of the patients.[131] Hallucinations and delusions may result *de novo* following treatment with dopaminergic agents, but do so more frequently in patients with pre-existing dementia. When minor forms such as feeling of presence are included, hallucinations occur in 70 per cent of patients with PDD, as compared to 25 per cent of those with AD.[132] Visual hallucinations are similar to those seen in in DLB, with well-formed figures of humans or animals, often with preserved insight. Delusional misidentification syndromes (the house not being their real home, individuals being replaced by a double, i.e. the impostor or Capgras syndrome) are found in 17 per cent of PDD patients.[133] Apathy is common in the earlier stages while delusions increase with more severe motor and cognitive dysfunction. Depression is more common in PDD than in AD.

Motor, autonomic, and other associated features

In PDD motor symptoms are typically symmetrical with predominance of bradykinesia, rigidity, and postural instability. In a cross-sectional study, postural-instability gait difficulty (PIGD) subtype was over-represented with 88 per cent in patients with PDD in contrast to 38 per cent in non-demented patients.[134] A transition from tremor dominant to PIGD-type is associated with higher risk of dementia.[135] PD patients with falls are more likely to have lower MMSE scores and also are more likely to have dementia. L-dopa-responsiveness may diminish as cognitive impairment emerges; potential underlying mechanisms may include the development of α-synuclein pathology in striatum and loss of striatal dopamine D2 and D3 receptors, or predominance of non-dopaminergic axial features, such as postural instability.

Autonomic disturbances include constipation, urinary incontinence, orthostatic and postprandial hypotension, and can result in syncope and falls, excessive sweating, reduced heart rate variability predisposing to ventricular arrhythmias, and sexual dysfunction. In a comparative study, cardiovascular autonomic dysfunction was more frequent in patients with PDD as compared to those with DLB, vascular dementia, and AD, PDD, due to both impairment of parasympathetic and sympathetic function.[136]

REM sleep behaviour disorder (RBD) is common in PDD. Presence of RBD in non-demented patients with PD is also associated with cognitive deficits, specifically on measures of episodic verbal memory, executive function, and visuospatial and visuoperceptual processing.[137] RBD can be an early indicator of incipient dementia and may predate the onset of dementia by many decades. Excessive daytime sleepiness (EDS) and poor sleep quality are also common in patients with PDD (see Box 36.2).

Box 36.2 Case presentation

A 63-year-old man was admitted to the movement disorders clinic because of parkinsonism and cognitive impairment. At age 52 he noticed resting tremor on his right hand; within one year, he developed rigidity and bradykinesia, more on the right side and was diagnosed to have Parkinson's disease (PD), his symptoms improved under dopaminergic treatment. His extrapyramidal symptoms slowly worsened over the next few years and he started experiencing wearing-off phenomenon. Eight years after dopaminergic treatment was initiated, he started developing cognitive dysfunction, apathy, and vivid hallucinations. He became inattentive and forgetful, his thinking became slower, he subsequently developed problems navigating in his own home. His past medical history revealed REM sleep behaviour disorder, starting almost 10 years before the onset of motor symptoms. Neuropsychological testing showed marked impairment in attention/concentration, verbal fluency, visuospatial/visuoconstructional tests (Fig. 36.2), cognitive flexibility, and other tasks of executive functions. He was diagnosed with dementia associated with Parkinson's disease (PDD) and treatment with a cholinesterase inhibitor was started.

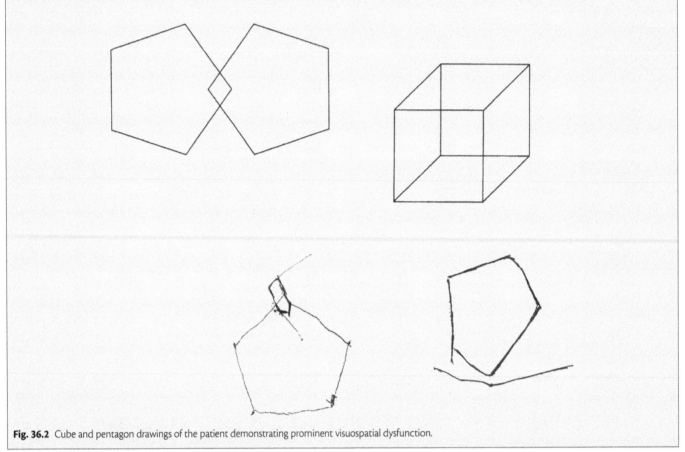

Fig. 36.2 Cube and pentagon drawings of the patient demonstrating prominent visuospatial dysfunction.

Pathological and biochemical correlates

PDD is characterized by variable combination of degeneration in subcortical nuclei, cortical AD-type pathology and Lewy body (LB)-type degeneration.[2] Combination of LB-type and AD-type pathology was found to be a better predictive of dementia than the severity of the single pathology.[138] It is probably the topographical and temporal sequence of neuronal loss rather than the type of protein aggregation which ultimately determine the clinical phenotype. AD-type and LB-pathology do not need to be mutually exclusive as there are interactions between different protein aggregations: α-synuclein can induce phosphorylation and fibrillization of tau; and β-amyloid may promote the aggregation of α-synuclein-exacerbating α-synuclein-induced neuronal dysfunction.[139]

In contrast to earlier studies with ubiquitin staining, recent studies using the more sensitive α-synuclein immunohistochemistry revealed that dementia best correlates with LB pathology, although some degree of AD-type pathology (more plaques than tangles) usually coexists. The fact that families with α-synuclein gene duplications and triplications develop dementia more often also supports a primary and possibly a 'dose-dependent' role of synuclein-based pathology in development of PDD.

Dementia usually develops later in the disease course and may be related to an ascending order of pathological changes.[140,141] Some support for this 'bottom-up' hypothesis is also provided by other studies:[142] PD patients with relatively long disease duration prior to dementia onset had lower levels of cortical cholinergic activity than those with a short disease duration before developing dementia, implying greater loss of ascending cholinergic projections in the former group. A more 'top-down' pathological process, with greater burden of cortical pathology in PD patients with a more rapid disease course and short time before dementia onset, has also been described.[141,142] Younger patients who developed dementia late in the disease process seem to have a predominance of α-synuclein pathology with little amyloid pathology whereas those with a late age of onset and rapid progression to dementia seem to have mixed α-synuclein and amyloid pathology, typically with both severe neocortical Lewy body disease, and high amyloid burden.[141] Approximately 55 per cent of subjects with widespread α-synuclein pathology (Braak PD stages 5–6) lacked clinical signs of dementia or extrapyramidal signs before death:[143] it is unclear why these subjects could 'tolerate' high levels of synuclein deposition without having symptoms.

Biochemically, degeneration of the subcortical nuclei results in various neurochemical changes including cholinergic, dopaminergic, serotoninergic, and noradrenergic deficits, of which cholinergic loss is most prominent. Loss of cholinergic cells in the nucleus basalis of Meynert (nbM) greater than that observed in AD occurs in patients with PDD. LBs are frequently found in nbM cells. Cholinacetyltransferase activity is markedly decreased in the frontal cortex of PDD and DLB when compared to normal controls and patients with AD. In contrast to AD, PDD is also associated with neuronal loss in the pedunculopontine cholinergic nuclei which project to structures such as thalamus. Using vesicular acetylcholine transporter ([123I]-iodobenzovesamicol, IBVM) as a marker of cholinergic integrity, SPECT studies demonstrate reductions in parietal and occipital cortices in non-demented PD patients, while demented PD cases have a more extensive decrease in cortical binding.[144] Functional imaging studies with PET have shown that that, compared to controls, mean cortical AChE activity was lowest in patients with PDD, followed by patients with PD without dementia and AD patients.[145] The degree of cortical cholinergic deficits correlated particularly well with typical cognitive deficits found in PDD, (e.g. impaired performance on tests of attention and executive functions).[146]

The noradrenergic locus coeruleus shows neuronal loss especially in demented and depressed PD patients.[147] Degeneration in serotonergic dorsal raphe nucleus has been reported and may contribute to affective symptoms.[148] Neuronal loss was also observed in ventral tegmental areal, which provides dopaminergic input to meso-limbic and prefrontal cortex and medial substantia nigra.[149]

Correlates in neuroimaging

MRI studies reveal frontal, occipital, and parietal grey matter loss and an increased rate of whole brain atrophy in PDD patients compared with control subjects. Atrophy of grey and white matter is typically less prominent than in DLB patients. A volumetric study revealed a relationship between decrease in caudate volume (but not in hippocampus) and cognitive decline.[150] Although there are studies showing atrophy of medial temporal lobe structures such as the hippocampus in PDD, these are not as prominent as in AD. Supratentorial white matter hyperintensities were also found to be independently associated with cognitive decline in PDD patients.[109]

Reduced fractional anisotropy (FA) was found in the substantia nigra of non-demented PD patients with DTI. PDD patients showed significant FA reduction in the bilateral posterior cingulate bundles compared with non-demented PD patients;[151] both FA and mean diffusivity values in cingulate and corpus callosum showed significant correlations with cognitive parameters.[151,152] In a resting state functional MRI study, corticostriatal connectivity was found to be selectively disrupted in PDD patients.[153]

PET usually shows hypometabolism in parietal and temporal cortex similar to that seen in AD, with hypometabolism in visual areas and frontal lobe also described.[154] In PET with N-[11C]-methyl-4-piperidyl acetate (MP4A) and 18F-fluorodopa (FDOPA), which assesses cholinergic innervation of cortex, PDD patients exhibited a severe cholinergic deficit in various cortical regions including frontal and temporoparietal cortices.[155] In PET studies with PiB, in PDD mean cortical amyloid load was comparable to controls and non-demented PD patients.[156] In another study, 83 per cent of PDD patients had 'normal' PiB uptake whereas 85 per cent of DLB patients had *significantly* increased amyloid load in one or more cortical regions.[78]

Regional cerebral blood flow (rCBF) SPECT studies have shown frontal hypoperfusion or bilateral temporoparietal deficits in PDD.[157] Perfusion deficits in precuneus and inferior lateral parietal regions have also been described. [123I]-MIBG is a marker of postganglionic sympathetic cardiac innervation: SPECT studies with this compound demonstrate innervation deficits both in PDD and DLB but not in AD. The integrity of nigro-striatal dopaminergic terminals can be assessed using markers of dopamine transporter, such as [123I]-FP-CIT SPECT. Significant reductions were found in [123I]-FP-CIT binding in the caudate, anterior, and posterior putamen in subjects with DLB and PDD compared to those with AD and controls.

Diagnosis of PDD

Clinical diagnostic criteria for PDD and and practical recommendations for diagnosis have been described by a Movement Disorder Society task force.[158,159] Clinical features of PDD are shown in Table 36.2 and diagnostic criteria for probable and possible PDD are given in Table 36.3. Diagnostic criteria for mild cognitive impairment in PD (PD-MCI) have also been recently published by a task force of the Movement Disorder Society.[160]

Diagnosis of dementia in PD can be confounded by several factors, not least the coexistence of motor and speech dysfunction. When severe motor impairment is present it may be difficult to discern the presence and magnitude of cognitive deficits and to what extent they contribute to functional impairment. Depression, other systemic disorders, or adverse effects of drugs may mimic symptoms of dementia. The mode of onset, speed of progression, the type of behavioural symptoms, pattern of cognitive deficits, and the clinical context in which these symptoms occur are helpful in differentiating dementia from its mimickers such as acute confusion or pseudo-dementia. Once a dementia syndrome with parkinsonism is established, differential diagnosis include DLB, AD associated with drug-induced parkinsonism, other degenerative diseases such as progressive supranuclear palsy, corticobasal syndrome or FTDP-17, cerebrovascular disease, hydrocephalus, intoxications, metabolic, endocrine, systemic disorders, or infections. A detailed history specifically inquiring the features known to be associated with PDD, a comprehensive neuropsychological assessment, neurological and systemic examination, a review of current medication, and use of appropriate auxiliary investigations are helpful in differential diagnosis.

Management of patients with PDD

Non-pharmacological measures include education of the family about disease symptoms and appropriate care (which can reduce behavioural symptoms and unnecessary use of

Table 36.3 Diagnostic criteria for PDD

Probable PDD

A. Core features: Both must be present

B. Associated clinical features:

- Typical profile of cognitive deficits including impairment in at least two of the four core cognitive domains (impaired attention which may fluctuate, impaired executive functions, impairment in visuospatial functions, and impaired free recall memory which usually improves with cueing)

- The presence of at least one behavioural symptom (apathy, depressed or anxious mood, hallucinations, delusions, excessive daytime sleepiness) supports the diagnosis of probable PDD; lack of behavioural symptoms, however, does not exclude the diagnosis

C. None of the group III features present

D. None of the group IV features present

Possible PDD

A. Core features: Both must be present

B. Associated clinical features:

- Atypical profile of cognitive impairment in one or more domains, such as prominent or receptive-type (fluent) aphasia, or pure storage-failure-type amnesia (memory does not improve with cueing or in recognition tasks) with preserved attention

- Behavioural symptoms may or may not be present

OR

C. One or more of the group III features present

D. None of the group IV features present

Reproduced from *Mov Disord.* 22(12), Emre M, Aarsland D, Brown R, *et al.* Clinical diagnostic criteria for dementia associated with Parkinson's disease, pp. 1689–707, Copyright (2007), with permission from John Wiley and Sons.

psychopharmacological medication), providing and promoting sufficient mental and physical activities. Before initiating pharmacological treatment conditions including systemic diseases, depression and adverse events of medication should be considered and managed appropriately. In particular, treatments with anticholinergics, tricyclic antidepressants, and benzodiazepines should be minimized and ideally discontinued where possible. The need for pharmacological intervention should be determined based on symptom frequency, severity, and burden.

Based on the prominent cholinergic deficits associated with PDD, cholinesterase inhibitors (ChE-Is) have been investigated in PDD patients. There have been two large randomized placebo-controlled trials, one with rivastigmine and the other with donepezil. In the rivastigmine trial, both cognitive and general status scales showed significant improvements compared to placebo; there were also benefits in the behavioural, attentional, and executive function test scores.[161] Except for slightly more patients having worsening of tremor there were no significant effects on motor symptoms as compared to placebo; the beneficial effects seemed to last for at least six months;[162] a subanalysis revealed consistent benefits on all aspects of attention.[163] In the large placebo-controlled trial, donepezil 10 mg was also associated with beneficial effects in cognitive and overall scales, with no significant differences on ADLs or behavioural scores. In a smaller randomized placebo-controlled trial in non-demented PD patients, galantamine did not show any significant benefits on cognitive function tests.[164] In a Cochrane meta-analysis, cholinesterase inhibitors in PDD were concluded to be associated with a positive impact on global assessment, cognitive

function, behavioural disturbance, and activities of daily living rating scales.[165] Based on the two large randomized controlled trials and the results of meta-analysis, treatment with cholinesterase inhibitors such as rivastigmine or donepezil should be considered in patients with PDD, taking into account expected benefits and risks.

Memantine, a partial NMDA receptor antagonist used in the treatment of AD, was tested in patients with DLB or PDD in two randomized controlled trials. In one, there was a significant difference in favor of memantine only in the global outcome scale, where patients with PDD had more benefits as compared to those with DLB.[95] In the larger study the global outcome scale and behavioural scores were significantly better with memantine in the DLB group, whereas there were no significant differences in the PDD population.[166] These results suggest that memantine may have mild beneficial effects in patients with Lewy body-related dementias, possibly more so in the DLB population, in global status and for behavioural symptoms.

Patients with mild psychotic symptoms such as hallucinations should be first treated with ChE-I before considering neuroleptics as ChE-I may improve these symptoms.[161] Nevertheless, neuroleptic treatment may become necessary in patients with severe psychosis or agitation. Classical neuroleptics are contraindicated as they worsen motor function and may result in life-threatening neuroleptic hypersensitivity. In a systematic review of atypical neuroleptics for the treatment of psychosis in PD, clozapine was concluded to be the only drug with proven efficacy and acceptable tolerability, although in practice this is not straightforward as regular blood monitoring for leucopenia is required.[167] Other atypical neuroleptics such as olanzapine and risperidone can worsen motor function. The efficacy of quetiapine is not well demonstrated although it may be considered under monitoring for side-effects.

Tricyclic antidepressants such as amitriptyline and nortriptiline may be effective in PD depression but should not be used in patients with PDD, due to their anticholinergic effects. Selective serotonin reuptake inhibitors such as paroxetine, or mixed serotonin and noradrenalin reuptake inhibitors such as venlafaxine, have been shown to be effective in PD depression.[168] Sedating antidepressants such as trazodone can be considered to treat sleep disturbances. Melatonin or very low doses of clonazepam may be used to treat RBD; daytime somnolence, however, should be monitored. EDS may be treated with modafinil, although there are no studies in PDD patients.[169]

References

1. Aarsland D, Londos E, and Ballard C. Parkinson's disease dementia and dementia with Lewy bodies: different aspects of one entity. *Int Psychogeriatr.* 2009 Apr;21(2):216–9.
2. Emre M. What causes mental dysfunction in Parkinson's disease? *Mov Disord.* 2003 Sep;18 Suppl 6:S63–71.
3. Lippa CF, Duda JE, Grossman M, *et al.* DLB and PDD boundary issues: diagnosis, treatment, molecular pathology, and biomarkers. *Neurology.* 2007 Mar 13;68(11):812–9.
4. McKeith IG and Mosimann UP. Dementia with Lewy bodies and Parkinson's disease. *Parkinsonism Relat Disord.* 2004 May;10 Suppl 1:S15–18.
5. McKeith I. Dementia with Lewy bodies and Parkinson's disease with dementia: where two worlds collide. *Pract Neurol.* 2007 Nov;7(6):374–82.

6. McKeith IG. Consensus guidelines for the clinical and pathologic diagnosis of dementia with Lewy bodies (DLB): report of the Consortium on DLB International Workshop. *J Alzheimers Dis.* 2006;9(3 Suppl):417–23.

7. McKeith IG, Perry EK, and Perry RH. Report of the second dementia with Lewy body international workshop: diagnosis and treatment. Consortium on Dementia with Lewy Bodies. *Neurology.* 1999 Sep 22;53(5):902–5.

8. McKeith IG, Dickson DW, Lowe J, *et al.* Diagnosis and management of dementia with Lewy bodies: third report of the DLB Consortium. *Neurology.* 2005 Dec 27;65(12):1863–72.

9. Okazaki H, Lipkin LE, and Aronson SM. Diffuse intracytoplasmic ganglionic inclusions (Lewy type) associated with progressive dementia and quadriparesis in flexion. *J Neuropathol Exp Neurol.* 1961 Apr;20:237–44.

10. Barker WW, Luis CA, Kashuba A, *et al.* Relative frequencies of Alzheimer disease, Lewy body, vascular and frontotemporal dementia, and hippocampal sclerosis in the State of Florida Brain Bank. *Alzheimer Dis Assoc Disord.* 2002 Dec;16(4):203–12.

11. Hulette C, Mirra S, Wilkinson W, *et al.* The Consortium to Establish a Registry for Alzheimer's Disease (CERAD). Part IX. A prospective cliniconeuropathologic study of Parkinson's features in Alzheimer's disease. *Neurology.* 1995 Nov;45(11):1991–5.

12. Lim A, Tsuang D, Kukull W, *et al.* Clinico-neuropathological correlation of Alzheimer's disease in a community-based case series. *J Am Geriatr Soc.* 1999 May;47(5):564–9.

13. Zaccai J, McCracken C, and Brayne C. A systematic review of prevalence and incidence studies of dementia with Lewy bodies. *Age Ageing.* 2005 Nov;34(6):561–6.

14. Miech RA, Breitner JCS, Zandi PP, *et al.* Incidence of AD may decline in the early 90s for men, later for women: The Cache County study. *Neurology.* 2002 Jan 22;58(2):209–18.

15. Rahkonen T, Eloniemi-Sulkava U, Rissanen S, *et al.* Dementia with Lewy bodies according to the consensus criteria in a general population aged 75 years or older. *J Neurol Neurosur Ps.* 2003 Jun;74(6):720–4.

16. Chan SSM, Chiu HFK, Lam LCW, *et al.* Prevalence of dementia with Lewy bodies in an inpatient psychogeriatric population in Hong Kong Chinese. *Int J Geriatr Psychiatry.* 2002 Sep;17(9):847–50.

17. Gaig C, Valldeoriola F, Gelpi E, *et al.* Rapidly progressive diffuse Lewy body disease. *Mov Disord.* 2011 Jun;26(7):1316–23.

18. McKeith I, Fairbairn A, Perry R, *et al.* Neuroleptic sensitivity in patients with senile dementia of Lewy body type. *BMJ.* 1992 Sep 19;305(6855):673–8.

19. Hanyu H, Sato T, Hirao K, *et al.* Differences in clinical course between dementia with Lewy bodies and Alzheimer's disease. *Eur J Neurol.* 2009 Feb;16(2):212–7.

20. Papapetropoulos S, Lieberman A, Gonzalez J, *et al.* Family history of dementia: dementia with lewy bodies and dementia in Parkinson's disease. *J Neuropsychiatry Clin Neurosci.* 2006;18(1):113–6.

21. Woodruff BK, Graff-Radford NR, Ferman TJ, *et al.* Family history of dementia is a risk factor for Lewy body disease. *Neurology.* 2006 Jun 27;66(12):1949–50.

22. Nervi A, Reitz C, Tang M-X, *et al.* Familial aggregation of dementia with Lewy bodies. *Arch Neurol.* 2011 Jan;68(1):90–3.

23. Bogaerts V, Engelborghs S, Kumar-Singh S, *et al.* A novel locus for dementia with Lewy bodies: a clinically and genetically heterogeneous disorder. *Brain.* 2007 Sep;130(Pt 9):2277–91.

24. Meeus B, Nuytemans K, Crosiers D, *et al.* Comprehensive genetic and mutation analysis of familial dementia with Lewy bodies linked to 2q35-q36. *J Alzheimers Dis.* 2010;20(1):197–205.

25. Borroni B, Grassi M, Costanzi C, *et al.* APOE genotype and cholesterol levels in lewy body dementia and Alzheimer disease: investigating genotype-phenotype effect on disease risk. *Am J Geriatr Psychiatry.* 2006 Dec;14(12):1022–31.

26. Singleton AB, Wharton A, O'Brien KK, *et al.* Clinical and neuropathological correlates of apolipoprotein E genotype in dementia with Lewy bodies. *Dement Geriatr Cogn Disord.* 2002;14(4):167–75.

27. Engelborghs S, Dermaut B, Goeman J, *et al.* Prospective Belgian study of neurodegenerative and vascular dementia: APOE genotype effects. *J Neurol Neurosur Ps.* 2003 Aug;74(8):1148–51.

28. Chartier-Harlin M-C, Kachergus J, Roumier C, *et al.* Alpha-synuclein locus duplication as a cause of familial Parkinson's disease. *Lancet.* 2004 Oct 25;364(9440):1167–9.

29. Farrer M, Kachergus J, Forno L, *et al.* Comparison of kindreds with parkinsonism and alpha-synuclein genomic multiplications. *Ann Neurol.* 2004 Feb;55(2):174–9.

30. Clark LN, Kartsaklis LA, Wolf Gilbert R, *et al.* Association of glucocerebrosidase mutations with dementia with lewy bodies. *Arch Neurol.* 2009 May;66(5):578–83.

31. Nishioka K, Ross OA, Vilariño-Güell C, *et al.* Glucocerebrosidase mutations in diffuse Lewy body disease. *Parkinsonism Relat Disord.* 2011 Jan;17(1):55–7.

32. Calderon J, Perry RJ, Erzinclioglu SW, *et al.* Perception, attention, and working memory are disproportionately impaired in dementia with Lewy bodies compared with Alzheimer's disease. *J Neurol Neurosur Ps.* 2001 Feb;70(2):157–64.

33. Walker Z, Allen RL, Shergill S, *et al.* Neuropsychological performance in Lewy body dementia and Alzheimer's disease. *Br J Psychiatry.* 1997 Feb;170:156–8.

34. Ferman TJ, Smith GE, Boeve BF, *et al.* DLB fluctuations: specific features that reliably differentiate DLB from AD and normal aging. *Neurology.* 2004 Jan 27;62(2):181–7.

35. Walker MP, Ayre GA, Cummings JL, *et al.* The Clinician Assessment of Fluctuation and the One Day Fluctuation Assessment Scale. Two methods to assess fluctuating confusion in dementia. *Br J Psychiatry.* 2000 Sep;177:252–6.

36. Walker MP, Ayre GA, Cummings JL, *et al.* Quantifying fluctuation in dementia with Lewy bodies, Alzheimer's disease, and vascular dementia. *Neurology.* 2000 Apr 25;54(8):1616–25.

37. Mosimann UP, Rowan EN, Partington CE, *et al.* Characteristics of visual hallucinations in Parkinson disease dementia and dementia with lewy bodies. *Am J Geriatr Psychiatry.* 2006 Feb;14(2):153–60.

38. McKeith I, Mintzer J, Aarsland D, *et al.* Dementia with Lewy bodies. *Lancet Neurol.* 2004 Jan;3(1):19–28.

39. Nagahama Y, Okina T, Suzuki N, *et al.* Neural correlates of psychotic symptoms in dementia with Lewy bodies. *Brain.* 2010 Feb;133(Pt 2):557–67.

40. Auning E, Rongve A, Fladby T, *et al.* Early and presenting symptoms of dementia with lewy bodies. *Dement Geriatr Cogn Disord.* 2011;32(3):202–8.

41. McKeith IG, Ballard CG, Perry RH, *et al.* Prospective validation of consensus criteria for the diagnosis of dementia with Lewy bodies. *Neurology.* 2000 Mar 14;54(5):1050–8.

42. Postuma RB, Gagnon J-F, and Montplaisir JY. REM sleep behavior disorder: from dreams to neurodegeneration. *Neurobiol Dis.* 2012 Jun;46(3):553–8.

43. Postuma RB, Gagnon J-F, Vendette M, *et al.* Idiopathic REM sleep behavior disorder in the transition to degenerative disease. *Mov Disord.* 2009 Nov 15;24(15):2225–32.

44. Ferman TJ, Boeve BF, Smith GE, *et al.* Inclusion of RBD improves the diagnostic classification of dementia with Lewy bodies. *Neurology.* 2011 Aug 30;77(9):875–82.

45. Horimoto Y, Matsumoto M, Akatsu H, *et al.* Autonomic dysfunctions in dementia with Lewy bodies. *J Neurol.* 2003 May;250(5):530–3.

46. Hansen L, Salmon D, Galasko D, *et al.* The Lewy body variant of Alzheimer's disease: a clinical and pathologic entity. *Neurology.* 1990 Jan;40(1):1–8.

47. Spillantini MG, Crowther RA, Jakes R, *et al.* alpha-Synuclein in filamentous inclusions of Lewy bodies from Parkinson's disease and dementia with lewy bodies. *Proc Natl Acad Sci USA.* 1998 May 26;95(11):6469–73.

48. Beyer K, Domingo-Sàbat M, and Ariza A. Molecular pathology of Lewy body diseases. *Int J Mol Sci.* 2009 Mar;10(3):724–45.

49. Mirra SS, Heyman A, McKeel D, *et al*. The Consortium to Establish a Registry for Alzheimer's Disease (CERAD). Part II. Standardization of the neuropathologic assessment of Alzheimer's disease. *Neurology*. 1991 Apr;41(4):479–86.

50. Consensus recommendations for the postmortem diagnosis of Alzheimer's disease. The National Institute on Aging, and Reagan Institute Working Group on Diagnostic Criteria for the Neuropathological Assessment of Alzheimer's Disease. Ball M, Braak H, Coleman P, *et al*. *Neurobiol Aging*. 1997 Aug;18(4 Suppl):S1–2.

51. Lopez OL, Becker JT, Kaufer DI, *et al*. Research evaluation and prospective diagnosis of dementia with Lewy bodies. *Arch Neurol*. 2002 Jan;59(1):43–6.

52. Jellinger KA. Prevalence of vascular lesions in dementia with Lewy bodies. A postmortem study. *J Neural Transm*. 2003 Jul;110(7):771–8.

53. Merdes AR, Hansen LA, Jeste DV, *et al*. Influence of Alzheimer pathology on clinical diagnostic accuracy in dementia with Lewy bodies. *Neurology*. 2003 May 27;60(10):1586–90.

54. Perry RH, Irving D, Blessed G, *et al*. Senile dementia of Lewy body type. A clinically and neuropathologically distinct form of Lewy body dementia in the elderly. *J Neurol Sci*. 1990 Feb;95(2):119–39.

55. Samuel W, Alford M, Hofstetter CR, *et al*. Dementia with Lewy bodies versus pure Alzheimer disease: differences in cognition, neuropathology, cholinergic dysfunction, and synapse density. *J Neuropathol Exp Neurol*. 1997 May;56(5):499–508.

56. Perry EK, Haroutunian V, Davis KL, *et al*. Neocortical cholinergic activities differentiate Lewy body dementia from classical Alzheimer's disease. *Neuroreport*. 1994 Mar 21;5(7):747–9.

57. Lippa CF, Smith TW, and Perry E. Dementia with Lewy bodies: choline acetyltransferase parallels nucleus basalis pathology. *J Neural Transm*. 1999;106(5–6):525–35.

58. Gómez-Isla T, Growdon WB, McNamara M, *et al*. Clinicopathologic correlates in temporal cortex in dementia with Lewy bodies. *Neurology*. 1999 Dec 10;53(9):2003–9.

59. Ballard C, Piggott M, Johnson M, *et al*. Delusions associated with elevated muscarinic binding in dementia with Lewy bodies. *Ann Neurol*. 2000 Dec;48(6):868–76.

60. Piggott MA, Marshall EF, Thomas N, *et al*. Striatal dopaminergic markers in dementia with Lewy bodies, Alzheimer's and Parkinson's diseases: rostrocaudal distribution. *Brain*. 1999 Aug;122 (Pt 8):1449–68.

61. Perry EK, Marshall E, Kerwin J, *et al*. Evidence of a monoaminergic-cholinergic imbalance related to visual hallucinations in Lewy body dementia. *J Neurochem*. 1990 Oct;55(4):1454–6.

62. Burton EJ, Barber R, Mukaetova-Ladinska EB, *et al*. Medial temporal lobe atrophy on MRI differentiates Alzheimer's disease from dementia with Lewy bodies and vascular cognitive impairment: a prospective study with pathological verification of diagnosis. *Brain*. 2009 Jan;132(Pt 1):195–203.

63. Sabattoli F, Boccardi M, Galluzzi S, *et al*. Hippocampal shape differences in dementia with Lewy bodies. *Neuroimage*. 2008 Jul 1;41(3):699–705.

64. Kantarci K, Ferman TJ, Boeve BF, *et al*. Focal atrophy on MRI and neuropathologic classification of dementia with Lewy bodies. *Neurology*. 2012 Aug 7;79(6):553–60.

65. O'Brien JT, Paling S, Barber R, *et al*. Progressive brain atrophy on serial MRI in dementia with Lewy bodies, AD, and vascular dementia. *Neurology*. 2001 May 22;56(10):1386–8.

66. Molina JA, García-Segura JM, Benito-León J, *et al*. Proton magnetic resonance spectroscopy in dementia with Lewy bodies. *Eur Neurol*. 2002;48(3):158–63.

67. Kantarci K, Petersen RC, Boeve BF, *et al*. 1H MR spectroscopy in common dementias. *Neurology*. 2004 Oct 26;63(8):1393–8.

68. Bozzali M, Falini A, Cercignani M, *et al*. Brain tissue damage in dementia with Lewy bodies: an in vivo diffusion tensor MRI study. *Brain*. 2005 Jul;128(Pt 7):1595–604.

69. Watson R, Blamire AM, Colloby SJ, *et al*. Characterizing dementia with Lewy bodies by means of diffusion tensor imaging. *Neurology*. 2012 Aug 28;79(9):906–14.

70. Galvin JE, Price JL, Yan Z, *et al*. Resting bold fMRI differentiates dementia with Lewy bodies vs Alzheimer disease. *Neurology*. 2011 May 24;76(21):1797–803.

71. Kenny ER, Blamire AM, Firbank MJ, *et al*. Functional connectivity in cortical regions in dementia with Lewy bodies and Alzheimer's disease. *Brain*. 2012 Feb;135(Pt 2):569–81.

72. Lobotesis K, Fenwick JD, Phipps A, *et al*. Occipital hypoperfusion on SPECT in dementia with Lewy bodies but not AD. *Neurology*. 2001 Mar 13;56(5):643–9.

73. Albin RL, Minoshima S, D'Amato CJ, *et al*. Fluoro-deoxyglucose positron emission tomography in diffuse Lewy body disease. *Neurology*. 1996 Aug;47(2):462–6.

74. Hu XS, Okamura N, Arai H, *et al*. 18F-fluorodopa PET study of striatal dopamine uptake in the diagnosis of dementia with Lewy bodies. *Neurology*. 2000 Nov 28;55(10):1575–7.

75. O'Brien JT, McKeith IG, Walker Z, *et al*. Diagnostic accuracy of 123I-FP-CIT SPECT in possible dementia with Lewy bodies. *Br J Psychiatry*. 2009 Jan;194(1):34–9.

76. McKeith I, O'Brien J, Walker Z, *et al*. Sensitivity and specificity of dopamine transporter imaging with 123I-FP-CIT SPECT in dementia with Lewy bodies: a phase III, multicentre study. *Lancet Neurol*. 2007 Apr;6(4):305–13.

77. Yoshita M, Taki J, and Yamada M. A clinical role for 123I-MIBG myocardial scintigraphy in the distinction between dementia of the Alzheimer's-type and dementia with Lewy bodies. *J Neurol Neurosur Ps*. 2001 Nov;71(5):583–8.

78. Edison P, Rowe CC, Rinne JO, *et al*. Amyloid load in Parkinson's disease dementia and Lewy body dementia measured with [11C]PIB positron emission tomography. *J Neurol Neurosur Ps*. 2008 Dec;79(12):1331–8.

79. Foster ER, Campbell MC, Burack MA, *et al*. Amyloid imaging of Lewy body-associated disorders. *Mov Disord*. 2010 Nov 15;25(15):2516–23.

80. Gomperts SN, Rentz DM, Moran E, *et al*. Imaging amyloid deposition in Lewy body diseases. *Neurology*. 2008 Sep 16;71(12):903–10.

81. Roks G, Korf ESC, Van der Flier WM, *et al*. The use of EEG in the diagnosis of dementia with Lewy bodies. *J Neurol Neurosur Ps*. 2008 Apr;79(4):377–80.

82. Bonanni L, Thomas A, Tiraboschi P, *et al*. EEG comparisons in early Alzheimer's disease, dementia with Lewy bodies and Parkinson's disease with dementia patients with a 2-year follow-up. *Brain*. 2008 Mar;131(Pt 3):690–705.

83. Mollenhauer B, Cullen V, Kahn I, *et al*. Direct quantification of CSF alpha-synuclein by ELISA and first cross-sectional study in patients with neurodegeneration. *Exp Neurol*. 2008 Oct;213(2):315–25.

84. Ohrfelt A, Grognet P, Andreasen N, *et al*. Cerebrospinal fluid alpha-synuclein in neurodegenerative disorders-a marker of synapse loss? *Neurosci Lett*. 2009 Feb 6;450(3):332–5.

85. Bibl M, Mollenhauer B, Esselmann H, *et al*. CSF amyloid-beta-peptides in Alzheimer's disease, dementia with Lewy bodies and Parkinson's disease dementia. *Brain*. 2006 May;129(Pt 5):1177–87.

86. Parnetti L, Tiraboschi P, Lanari A, *et al*. Cerebrospinal fluid biomarkers in Parkinson's disease and dementia with Lewy bodies. *Biol Psychiatry*. 2008 Nov 15;64(10):850–5.

87. Mulugeta E, Londos E, Ballard C, *et al*. CSF amyloid β38 as a novel diagnostic marker for dementia with Lewy bodies. *J Neurol Neurosur Ps*. 2011 Feb;82(2):160–4.

88. Molloy S, McKeith IG, O'Brien JT, *et al*. The role of levodopa in the management of dementia with Lewy bodies. *J Neurol Neurosur Ps*. 2005 Sep;76(9):1200–3.

89. Lucetti C, Logi C, Del Dotto P, *et al*. Levodopa response in dementia with lewy bodies: a 1-year follow-up study. *Parkinsonism Relat Disord*. 2010 Sep;16(8):522–6.

90. Aurora RN, Zak RS, Maganti RK, *et al*. Best practice guide for the treatment of REM sleep behavior disorder (RBD). *J Clin Sleep Med*. 2010 Feb 15;6(1):85–95.

91. Raedler TJ. Cardiovascular aspects of antipsychotics. *Curr Opin Psychiatry*. 2010 Nov;23(6):574–81.

92. McKeith I, Del Ser T, Spano P, *et al.* Efficacy of rivastigmine in dementia with Lewy bodies: a randomised, double-blind, placebo-controlled international study. *Lancet.* 2000 Dec 16;356(9247):2031–6.

93. Mori E, Ikeda M, and Kosaka K. Donepezil for dementia with Lewy bodies: a randomized, placebo-controlled trial. *Ann Neurol.* 2012 Jul;72(1):41–52.

94. Dalfó E, Albasanz JL, Martin M, *et al.* Abnormal metabotropic glutamate receptor expression and signaling in the cerebral cortex in diffuse Lewy body disease is associated with irregular alpha-synuclein/phospholipase C (PLCbeta1) interactions. *Brain Pathol.* 2004 Oct;14(4):388–98.

95. Aarsland D, Ballard C, Walker Z, *et al.* Memantine in patients with Parkinson's disease dementia or dementia with Lewy bodies: a double-blind, placebo-controlled, multicentre trial. *Lancet Neurol.* 2009 Jul;8(7):613–8.

96. Emre M, Tsolaki M, Bonuccelli U, *et al.* Memantine for patients with Parkinson's disease dementia or dementia with Lewy bodies: a randomised, double-blind, placebo-controlled trial. *Lancet Neurol.* 2010 Oct;9(10):969–77.

97. Williams-Gray CH, Evans JR, Goris A, *et al.* The distinct cognitive syndromes of Parkinson's disease: 5 year follow-up of the CamPaIGN cohort. *Brain.* 2009 Nov;132(Pt 11):2958–69.

98. Muslimovic D, Post B, Speelman JD, *et al.* Cognitive profile of patients with newly diagnosed Parkinson disease. *Neurology.* 2005 Oct 25;65(8):1239–45.

99. Aarsland D, Bronnick K, Williams-Gray C, *et al.* Mild cognitive impairment in Parkinson disease: a multicenter pooled analysis. *Neurology.* 2010 Sep 21;75(12):1062–9.

100. Aarsland D, Zaccai J, and Brayne C. A systematic review of prevalence studies of dementia in Parkinson's disease. *Mov Disord.* 2005 Oct;20(10):1255–63.

101. De Lau LML, Schipper CMA, Hofman A, *et al.* Prognosis of Parkinson disease: risk of dementia and mortality: the Rotterdam Study. *Arch Neurol.* 2005 Aug;62(8):1265–9.

102. Marder K, Tang MX, Cote L, *et al.* The frequency and associated risk factors for dementia in patients with Parkinson's disease. *Arch Neurol.* 1995 Jul;52(7):695–701.

103. Hely MA, Morris JGL, Reid WGJ, *et al.* Sydney Multicenter Study of Parkinson's disease: non-L-dopa-responsive problems dominate at 15 years. *Mov Disord.* 2005 Feb;20(2):190–9.

104. Hely MA, Reid WGJ, Adena MA, *et al.* The Sydney multicenter study of Parkinson's disease: the inevitability of dementia at 20 years. *Mov Disord.* 2008 Apr 30;23(6):837–44.

105. Aarsland D, Andersen K, Larsen JP, *et al.* Prevalence and characteristics of dementia in Parkinson disease: an 8-year prospective study. *Arch Neurol.* 2003 Mar;60(3):387–92.

106. Levy G, Schupf N, Tang M-X, *et al.* Combined effect of age and severity on the risk of dementia in Parkinson's disease. *Ann. Neurol.* 2002 Jun;51(6):722–9.

107. Marion M-H, Qurashi M, Marshall G, *et al.* Is REM sleep behaviour disorder (RBD) a risk factor of dementia in idiopathic Parkinson's disease? *J Neurol.* 2008 Feb;255(2):192–6.

108. Woods SP and Tröster AI. Prodromal frontal/executive dysfunction predicts incident dementia in Parkinson's disease. *JINS.* 2003 Jan;9(1):17–24.

109. Lee S-J, Kim J-S, Yoo J-Y, *et al.* Influence of white matter hyperintensities on the cognition of patients with Parkinson disease. *Alzheimer Dis Assoc Disord.* 2010 Sep;24(3):227–33.

110. Ebmeier KP, Calder SA, Crawford JR, *et al.* Mortality and causes of death in idiopathic Parkinson's disease: results from the Aberdeen whole population study. *Scott Med J.* 1990 Dec;35(6):173–5.

111. Levy G, Tang M-X, Cote LJ, *et al.* Do risk factors for Alzheimer's disease predict dementia in Parkinson's disease? An exploratory study. *Mov Disord.* 2002 Mar;17(2):250–7.

112. Marder K, Tang MX, Alfaro B, *et al.* Risk of Alzheimer's disease in relatives of Parkinson's disease patients with and without dementia. *Neurology.* 1999 Mar 10;52(4):719–24.

113. Huang X, Chen PC, and Poole C. APOE-[epsilon]2 allele associated with higher prevalence of sporadic Parkinson disease. *Neurology.* 2004 Jun 22;62(12):2198–202.

114. Goris A, Williams-Gray CH, Clark GR, *et al.* Tau and alpha-synuclein in susceptibility to, and dementia in, Parkinson's disease. *Ann Neurol.* 2007 Aug;62(2):145–53.

115. Healy DG, Abou-Sleiman PM, Lees AJ, *et al.* Tau gene and Parkinson's disease: a case-control study and meta-analysis. *J Neurol Neurosur Ps.* 2004 Jul;75(7):962–5.

116. Setó-Salvia N, Clarimón J, Pagonabarraga J, *et al.* Dementia risk in Parkinson disease: disentangling the role of MAPT haplotypes. *Arch Neurol.* 2011 Mar;68(3):359–64.

117. Goker-Alpan O, Lopez G, Vithayathil J, *et al.* The spectrum of parkinsonian manifestations associated with glucocerebrosidase mutations. *Arch Neurol.* 2008 Oct;65(10):1353–7.

118. Setó-Salvia N, Pagonabarraga J, Houlden H, *et al.* Glucocerebrosidase mutations confer a greater risk of dementia during Parkinson's disease course. *Mov Disord.* 2012 Mar;27(3):393–9.

119. Sironi F, Trotta L, Antonini A, *et al.* alpha-Synuclein multiplication analysis in Italian familial Parkinson disease. *Parkinsonism Relat Disord.* 2010 Mar;16(3):228–31.

120. Wider C, Dickson DW, and Wszolek ZK. Leucine-rich repeat kinase 2 gene-associated disease: redefining genotype-phenotype correlation. *Neurodegener Dis.* 2010;7(1-3):175–9.

121. Kasten M, Kertelge L, Brüggemann N, *et al.* Nonmotor symptoms in genetic Parkinson disease. *Arch Neurol.* 2010 Jun;67(6):670–6.

122. Bronnick K, Ehrt U, Emre M, *et al.* Attentional deficits affect activities of daily living in dementia-associated with Parkinson's disease. *J Neurol Neurosur Ps.* 2006 Oct;77(10):1136–42.

123. Aarsland D, Litvan I, Salmon D, *et al.* Performance on the dementia rating scale in Parkinson's disease with dementia and dementia with Lewy bodies: comparison with progressive supranuclear palsy and Alzheimer's disease. *J Neurol Neurosur Ps.* 2003 Sep;74(9):1215–20.

124. Brønnick K, Alves G, Aarsland D, *et al.* Verbal memory in drug-naive, newly diagnosed Parkinson's disease. The retrieval deficit hypothesis revisited. *Neuropsychology.* 2011 Jan;25(1):114–24.

125. Weintraub D, Moberg PJ, Culbertson WC, *et al.* Evidence for impaired encoding and retrieval memory profiles in Parkinson disease. *Cogn Behav Neurol.* 2004 Dec;17(4):195–200.

126. Mosimann UP, Mather G, Wesnes KA, *et al.* Visual perception in Parkinson disease dementia and dementia with Lewy bodies. *Neurology.* 2004 Dec 14;63(11):2091–6.

127. Dalrymple-Alford JC, MacAskill MR, Nakas CT, *et al.* The MoCA: well-suited screen for cognitive impairment in Parkinson disease. *Neurology.* 2010 Nov 9;75(19):1717–25.

128. Mahieux F, Boller F, Fermanian J, *et al.* Mini-Mental Parkinson: first validation study of a new bedside test constructed for Parkinson's disease. *Behav Neurology.* 1995;8:15–22.

129. Kalbe E, Calabrese P, Kohn N, *et al.* Screening for cognitive deficits in Parkinson's disease with the Parkinson neuropsychometric dementia assessment (PANDA) instrument. *Parkinsonism Relat Disord.* 2008;14(2):93–101.

130. Kulisevsky J and Pagonabarraga J. Cognitive impairment in Parkinson's disease: tools for diagnosis and assessment. *Mov Disord.* 2009 Jun 15;24(8):1103–10.

131. Aarsland D, Brønnick K, Ehrt U, *et al.* Neuropsychiatric symptoms in patients with Parkinson's disease and dementia: frequency, profile and associated care giver stress. *J Neurol.Neurosur Ps.* 2007 Jan;78(1):36–42.

132. Fénelon G, Mahieux F, Huon R, *et al.* Hallucinations in Parkinson's disease: prevalence, phenomenology and risk factors. *Brain.* 2000 Apr;123 (Pt 4):733–45.

133. Pagonabarraga J, Llebaria G, García-Sánchez C, *et al.* A prospective study of delusional misidentification syndromes in Parkinson's disease with dementia. *Mov Disord.* 2008 Feb 15;23(3):443–8.

134. Burn DJ, Rowan EN, Minett T, *et al.* Extrapyramidal features in Parkinson's disease with and without dementia and dementia with Lewy bodies: A cross-sectional comparative study. *Mov Disord.* 2003 Aug;18(8):884–9.

135. Alves G, Larsen JP, Emre M, *et al.* Changes in motor subtype and risk for incident dementia in Parkinson's disease. *Mov Disord.* 2006 Aug;21(8):1123–30.

136. Allan LM, Ballard CG, Allen J, *et al.* Autonomic dysfunction in dementia. *J Neurol Neurosur Ps.* 2007 Jul;78(7):671–7.

137. Vendette M, Gagnon J-F, Décary A, *et al.* REM sleep behavior disorder predicts cognitive impairment in Parkinson disease without dementia. *Neurology.* 2007 Nov 6;69(19):1843–9.

138. Compta Y, Parkkinen L, O'Sullivan SS, *et al.* Lewy- and Alzheimer-type pathologies in Parkinson's disease dementia: which is more important? *Brain.* 2011 May;134(Pt 5):1493–505.

139. Pletnikova O, West N, Lee MK, *et al.* Abeta deposition is associated with enhanced cortical alpha-synuclein lesions in Lewy body diseases. *Neurobiol Aging.* 2005 Sep;26(8):1183–92.

140. Braak H, Del Tredici K, Rüb U, *et al.* Staging of brain pathology related to sporadic Parkinson's disease. *Neurobiol Aging.* 2003 Apr;24(2):197–211.

141. Halliday G, Hely M, Reid W, *et al.* The progression of pathology in longitudinally followed patients with Parkinson's disease. *Acta Neuropathol.* 2008 Apr;115(4):409–15.

142. Ballard C, Ziabreva I, Perry R, *et al.* Differences in neuropathologic characteristics across the Lewy body dementia spectrum. *Neurology.* 2006 Dec 12;67(11):1931–4.

143. Parkkinen L, Pirttilä T, and Alafuzoff I. Applicability of current staging/categorization of alpha-synuclein pathology and their clinical relevance. *Acta Neuropathol.* 2008 Apr;115(4):399–407.

144. Kuhl DE, Minoshima S, Fessler JA, *et al.* In vivo mapping of cholinergic terminals in normal aging, Alzheimer's disease, and Parkinson's disease. *Ann Neurol.* 1996 Sep;40(3):399–410.

145. Bohnen NI, Kaufer DI, Ivanco LS, *et al.* Cortical cholinergic function is more severely affected in parkinsonian dementia than in Alzheimer disease: an in vivo positron emission tomographic study. *Arch Neurol.* 2003 Dec;60(12):1745–8.

146. Bohnen NI, Kaufer DI, Hendrickson R, *et al.* Cognitive correlates of cortical cholinergic denervation in Parkinson's disease and parkinsonian dementia. *J Neurol.* 2006 Feb;253(2):242–7.

147. Jellinger KA. Morphological substrates of mental dysfunction in Lewy body disease: an update. *J Neural Transm Suppl.* 2000;59:185–212.

148. Jellinger KA. Pathology of Parkinson's disease. Changes other than the nigrostriatal pathway. *Mol Chem Neuropathol.* 1991 Jun;14(3):153–97.

149. Rinne JO, Rummukainen J, Paljärvi L, *et al.* Dementia in Parkinson's disease is related to neuronal loss in the medial substantia nigra. *Ann Neurol.* 1989 Jul;26(1):47–50.

150. Apostolova LG, Beyer M, Green AE, *et al.* Hippocampal, caudate, and ventricular changes in Parkinson's disease with and without dementia. *Mov Disord.* 2010 Apr 30;25(6):687–8.

151. Matsui H, Nishinaka K, Oda M, *et al.* Dementia in Parkinson's disease: diffusion tensor imaging. *Acta Neurol Scand.* 2007 Sep;116(3):177–81.

152. Wiltshire K, Concha L, Gee M, *et al.* Corpus callosum and cingulum tractography in Parkinson's disease. *Can J Neurol Sci.* 2010 Sep;37(5):595–600.

153. Seibert TM, Murphy EA, Kaestner EJ, *et al.* Interregional correlations in Parkinson disease and Parkinson-related dementia with resting functional MR imaging. *Radiology.* 2012 Apr;263(1):226–34.

154. Pavese N. PET studies in Parkinson's disease motor and cognitive dysfunction. *Parkinsonism Relat Disord.* 2012 Jan;18 Suppl 1:S96–99.

155. Hilker R, Thomas AV, Klein JC, *et al.* Dementia in Parkinson disease: functional imaging of cholinergic and dopaminergic pathways. *Neurology.* 2005 Dec 13;65(11):1716–22.

156. Maetzler W, Reimold M, Liepelt I, *et al.* [11C]PIB binding in Parkinson's disease dementia. *Neuroimage.* 2008 Feb 1;39(3):1027–33.

157. Bissessur S, Tissingh G, Wolters EC, *et al.* rCBF SPECT in Parkinson's disease patients with mental dysfunction. *J Neural Transm Suppl.* 1997;50:25–30.

158. Emre M, Aarsland D, Brown R, *et al.* Clinical diagnostic criteria for dementia associated with Parkinson's disease. *Mov Disord.* 2007 Sep 15;22(12):1689–1707; quiz 1837.

159. Dubois B, Burn D, Goetz C, *et al.* Diagnostic procedures for Parkinson's disease dementia: recommendations from the movement disorder society task force. *Mov Disord.* 2007 Dec;22(16):2314–24.

160. Litvan I, Goldman JG, Tröster AI, *et al.* Diagnostic criteria for mild cognitive impairment in Parkinson's disease: Movement Disorder Society Task Force guidelines. *Mov Disord.* 2012 Mar;27(3):349–56.

161. Emre M, Aarsland D, Albanese A, *et al.* Rivastigmine for dementia associated with Parkinson's disease. *N Engl J Med.* 2004 Dec 9;351(24):2509–18.

162. Poewe W, Wolters E, Emre M, *et al.* Long-term benefits of rivastigmine in dementia associated with Parkinson's disease: an active treatment extension study. *Mov Disord.* 2006 Apr;21(4):456–61.

163. Wesnes KA, McKeith I, Edgar C, *et al.* Benefits of rivastigmine on attention in dementia associated with Parkinson disease. *Neurology.* 2005 Nov 22;65(10):1654–6.

164. Grace J, Amick MM, and Friedman JH. A double-blind comparison of galantamine hydrobromide ER and placebo in Parkinson disease. *J Neurol Neurosur Ps.* 2009 Jan;80(1):18–23.

165. Rolinski M, Fox C, Maidment I, *et al.* Cholinesterase inhibitors for dementia with Lewy bodies, Parkinson's disease dementia and cognitive impairment in Parkinson's disease. *Cochrane Database Syst Rev.* 2012;3:CD006504.

166. Emre M, Tsolaki M, Bonuccelli U, *et al.* Memantine for patients with Parkinson's disease dementia or dementia with Lewy bodies: a randomised, double-blind, placebo-controlled trial. *Lancet Neurol.* 2010 Oct;9(10):969–77.

167. Goetz CG, Koller WC, and Poewe W. Drugs to treat dementia and psychosis: management of Parkinson's disease. *Mov Disord.* 2002;17 Suppl 4:S120–127.

168. Richard IH, McDermott MP, Kurlan R, *et al.* A randomized, double-blind, placebo-controlled trial of antidepressants in Parkinson disease. *Neurology.* 2012 Apr 17;78(16):1229–36.

169. Adler CH, Caviness JN, Hentz JG, *et al.* Randomized trial of modafinil for treating subjective daytime sleepiness in patients with Parkinson's disease. *Mov Disord.* 2003 Mar;18(3):287–93.

CHAPTER 37

Corticobasal degeneration, progressive supranuclear palsy, multiple system atrophy, argyrophilic grain disease, and rarer neurodegenerative diseases

Elizabeth A. Coon and Keith A. Josephs

Introduction

Neurodegenerative disorders include a variety of cognitive and motor syndromes with varying clinical presentations and pathologic findings. Tauopathies are a distinct subset due to abnormal deposition of the protein tau and include corticobasal degeneration and progressive supranuclear palsy which will be discussed in this chapter, as well as some forms of frontotemporal lobar degeneration. Abnormal accumulation of the protein alpha synuclein leads to another spectrum of parkinsonian disorders including multiple system atrophy which has prominent autonomic dysfunction.

Corticobasal degeneration

Background

Corticobasal degeneration (CBD) is a rare neurodegenerative disorder with heterogeneous clinical features which can affect motor, sensory, behavioural, and cognitive systems (see Table 37.1). The disorder was originally termed 'corticodentatonigral degeneration with neuronal achromasia' in the initial description by Rebeiz, Kolodny and Richardson.[1] They described a distinctive clinical syndrome of progressive asymmetric, akinetic rigidity, and apraxia accompanied by cortical and subcortical features. Pathology demonstrated degeneration of the cerebral cortex, substantia nigra, and dentate nucleus of the cerebellum with swollen and achromatic neurons.[1]

The terminology has evolved since the initial description. Corticobasal syndrome (CBS) refers to the clinical presentation which most often accounts for CBD pathology. An often elusive clinical presentation can make CBD difficult to diagnose during life and thus the terminology CBD is reserved for neuropathological diagnosis.[2] While the prevalence of CBD is largely unknown, estimates from Eastern European and Asian population studies suggest an annual incidence rate of 0.02 cases per 100 000 individuals.[3]

Clinical features

Corticobasal degeneration has an insidious onset, typically presenting in the 50s to 70s, followed by a slowly progressive course. The average disease duration is less than eight years.[4,5] The core clinical features are progressive asymmetric rigidity and apraxia, accompanied by cortical and extrapyramidal dysfunction.[6] (Table 37.1)

Progressive asymmetric rigidity and apraxia

Focality or asymmetry is a key feature in CBS with most patients presenting with asymmetric limb clumsiness.[4] Examination demonstrates focal ideomotor or ideational apraxia with extrapyramidal features of akinaesia, rigidity, or dystonic posturing. As the disease progresses, the limb becomes useless and other limbs become similarly affected.

Cortical dysfunction

Alien limb phenomenon is manifested in approximately 50 percent of patients at some point in the disease course and is attributed to dysfunction of the supplementary motor area and its connections.[4,5] Patients may describe one limb as 'having a mind of its own' and tend to dissociate themselves from the limb and its actions. There may be involuntary grasping of objects or levitation of a limb. Some patients may manifest mirror movements in association with the alien limb phenomenon.[7] Cortical sensory loss is often evident on examination as agraphaesthesia, astereognosis, impaired joint position sense, and two-point discrimination in the setting of intact primary sensory testing.[6] Myoclonus, when present, tends to be confined to one limb and prominent on voluntary action (action myoclonus) or in response to sensory stimulation (sensory myoclonus).[8]

Extrapyramidal dysfunction

Extrapyramidal dysfunction is most often evident as asymmetric limb rigidity and akinaesia with little significant or sustained improvement from levodopa therapy.[9] Dystonia confined to one

Table 37.1 Proposed corticobasal syndrome diagnostic criteria

Core Features:

♦ Insidious onset and progressive course

♦ No identifiable cause

♦ **Cortical dysfunction** with at least one of the following:

· Focal or asymmetrical ideomotor apraxia

· Alien limb phenomenon

· Cortical sensory loss

· Visual or sensory hemineglect

· Constructional apraxia

· Focal or asymmetric myoclonus

· Apraxia of speech/nonfluent aphasia

♦ **Extrapyramidal dysfunction** with at least one of the following:

· Focal or asymmetrical appendicular rigidity lacking prominent and sustained levodopa response

· Focal or asymmetrical appendicular dystonia

Supportive investigations:

♦ Variable degrees of focal or lateralized cognitive dysfunction with relative preservation of learning and memory

♦ Focal or asymmetric atrophy on structural imaging, typically maximal in parietofrontal cortex

♦ Focal or asymmetric findings on functional imaging, typically maximal in parietofrontal cortex

Adapted from *Ann Neurol*. 54(Suppl 5), Boeve BF, Lang AE, and Litvan I. Corticobasal degeneration and its relationship to progressive supranuclear palsy and frontotemporal dementia, pp. S15–9, Copyright (2003), with permission from John Wiley and Sons.

limb is also common early and progresses to involve other limbs. When tremor is present, it is minimal at rest and often jerky with action. Gait may be initially normal but a disorder characterized by postural instability and bradykinaesia is common later in the disease.[4] Dysarthria is almost always a feature of CBD while dysphagia and corticospinal tract signs can also be seen.[4] The primary eye movement abnormality seen in CBD is increased saccadic latency,[10,11] although one report suggests that a supranuclear gaze palsy, very similar to that in PSP, may also be evident in some cases of pathologically diagnosed CBD.[12]

Cognitive dysfunction

Dementia coexists with motor deficits in approximately half of patients with CBD; it may be an early feature in a small set of patients but is more likely to be present late in disease.[13] Impairment in one or more cognitive domains is often present and insight is typically spared. Comorbid depression is frequent. Frontal lobe type symptoms such as apathy, irritability, disinhibition, or obsessive–compulsive disorder are common and can mistakenly lead to a diagnosis of behavioural variant frontotemporal dementia (bvFTD).[14] Language deficits characterized by agrammatic errors and the motor speech disorder apraxia of speech are associated with CBD and can also occur in PSP.[15]

Clinical heterogeneity

It is important to appreciate that CBS is the presenting clinical syndrome in only approximately half of pathologically confirmed CBD cases. Presentations of bvFTD and a progressive supranuclear palsy (PSP)-like syndrome make up slightly less than a third of the other pathologically confirmed CBD cases.[14,16,17] Affected cortical and subcortical affected areas can vary in CBD, and this most likely accounts for the clinical heterogeneity. When atrophy is predominantly posterior, symptoms of Bálint (or Bálint–Holmes) syndrome (ocular apraxia, optic ataxia, and simultagnosia), Gerstmann syndrome (acalculia, finger agnosia, apraxia, right–left disorientation, and agraphia), visual agnosia, alexia, or transcortical sensory aphasia can be present.[18,19] Aphasia is more often found in patients presenting with motor symptoms involving their dominant limb.[4] Even asymmetry, while characteristic of CBS, is not the rule as patients with symmetric presentations have also been shown to have CBD on neuropathologic examination.[20]

Neuropsychology

Neuropsychometric testing is better characterized in CBS than CBD. The prominent impairment is that of a dysexecutive syndrome with impairments in attention, concentration, and executive function. Testing may also demonstrate an asymmetric praxis disorder as well as language and visuospatial defects.[21,22]

Neuroimaging

Neuroimaging studies have centred on CBS rather than CBD, but it is important to note that there are no absolute diagnostic features. MRI findings are of asymmetric atrophy affecting the posterior frontal cortex, superior parietal cortex, and corpus callosum, with hypointense T1-weighted signal in the putamen and hyperintense T2-weighted signal in the motor cortex or subcortical white matter (Fig. 37.1).[23,24] Imaging in pathologically confirmed CBD demonstrates atrophy which predominantly affects the premotor cortex, posterior superior frontal lobe, and the supplementary motor area.[25,26] Functional neuroimaging demonstrates asymmetric hypoperfusion with single photon emission computed tomography (SPECT) and asymmetric hypometabolism on positron emission tomography (PET) of the parietofrontal cortex with the basal ganglia variably affected (Fig. 37.2).[27,28]

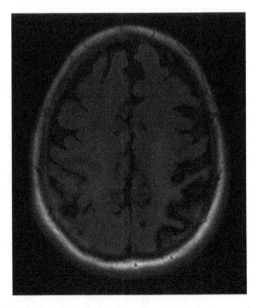

Fig. 37.1 MRI findings in corticobasal syndrome. Magnetic resonance imaging (MRI) T2 fluid-attenuated inversion recovery (FLAIR) image demonstrating asymmetric right frontoparietal cortical atrophy in a patient with CBS.

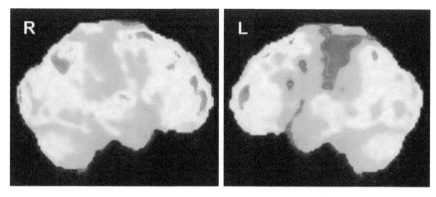

Fig. 37.2 Functional imaging findings in corticobasal syndrome. Positron emission tomography (PET) images from a patient with CBS showing hypometabolism (blue and green) that is more pronounced in the left posterior frontal lobe compared to the right.

Neuropathology

Criteria for the pathologic diagnosis of CBD have been refined. Macroscopically, there is variable frontoparietal and occasionally frontotemporal atrophy which may be asymmetric with pallor of the substantia nigra. Microscopically, the key pathological features are hyperphosphorylated four microtubule-binding repeat (4-R) tau inclusions affecting both neurons and glia in grey and white matter of the cortical, basal ganglia, diencephalon, and rostral brainstem.[29] Astrocytic plaques, tau-positive clusters in distal astrocyte processes, are the hallmarks of CBD (Fig. 37.3). Corticobasal bodies are tau-positive inclusions in the locus ceruleus and substantia nigra while coiled bodies represent bundles of tau-positive fibrils coiled in oligodendroglia nuclei. Neuropil threads are found in grey and white matter. The 'achromatic' or ballooned neurons present in the initial description are typically present but not specific to CBD.[30]

Difficulty arises in neuropathological diagnosis when tau-positive lesions affect the brainstem and cerebellum to a greater extent, overlapping with features of PSP.[30,31] Several mimics present clinically with CBS and have different underlying pathologies including Alzheimer's disease, frontotemporal lobar degeneration with TDP-43 pathology, PSP, and Creutzfeldt-Jakob disease[4,16]

Pathophysiology

Dysfunction of tau is the primary factor in the pathogenesis of CBD yet the mechanism of neurodegeneration is still unclear. Hyperphosphorylation of 4-R tau leads to reduced binding affinity to microtubules and loss of proper microtubule functioning. The dissociated species of tau may possess a toxic gain of function with greater propensity for multimerization.[32] There is also evidence of altered microglia signalling,[33] alterations in kinase pathways,[34] mitochondrial dysfunction, and chronic inflammation,[35] with disruption of synaptic function and excitotoxic signalling in CBD.[36,37]

Management

Symptom management focuses on palliation as therapies directed at tau-mediated degeneration are under development. Pharmacotherapy for parkinsonism should be tried as patients may initially improve. The mainstay of management centres on physical, occupational, and speech therapies. Constraint-induced movement therapy to force the use of the affected side has been successful in a few patients with severely disabled limbs.[38] Tau-directed

therapeutics in development target different mechanisms including

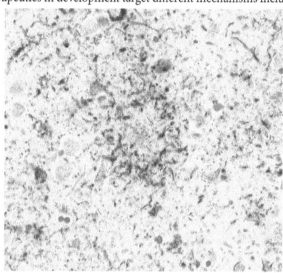

Fig. 37.3 Astrocytic plaque in CBS. Immunostaining with tau reveals astroglial inclusions characteristic of corticobasal syndrome.

inhibiting tau kinases to decrease tau hyperphosphorylation, inhibiting tau aggregation, and utilizing microtubule stabilizing agents.[39]

Progressive supranuclear palsy

Background

Progressive supranuclear palsy (PSP) is a neurodegenerative disorder first described in 1964 by Steele, Richardson, and Olszewski as an 'unusual syndrome' of postural instability, supranuclear gaze palsy, mild dementia, and progressive axial rigidity and bulbar palsy.[40] Pathologically, PSP is characterized by neuronal and glial tau protein accumulation in the basal ganglia, diencephalon, brainstem, and cerebellum with limited cortical involvement.[40–42] Since the initial report, several clinical variants have been described which reflect differences in the distribution in tau pathology.[43]

PSP is the most common cause of parkinsonism after Parkinson's disease (PD), with an estimated prevalence of 6–10 per cent of that of PD.[44,45] Prevalence is age-dependent and estimated at 6.4 per 100 000.[44] Correct diagnosis is often delayed as patients presenting with less distinctive symptoms are often initially considered to have PD or multiple system atrophy.[46]

Clinical features

PSP onset is typically in the 60s and ranges from the mid-40s to 70s with progression to death within 5 to 8 years.[47] Nosologically, PSP is divided into the classic form, PSP syndrome (PSP-S), also known as Richardson's syndrome, and 'atypical PSP' or PSP variants named for their clinical type and associated tau pathology.[47] The National Institute of Neurologic Disease and Stroke (NINDS) criteria for PSP are more specific than sensitive and highlight the most important clinical features for diagnosis,[48] while there are no accepted guidelines for the variants of PSP (Table 37.2).

PSP syndrome (PSP-S)

The classic form of PSP is an akinetic-rigid syndrome of early and prominent postural instability and falls, with visual and ocular disturbances. The most common initial complaint is unsteadiness of gait with unexplained falls as balance is affected early. Axial rigidity is more prominent than appendicular rigidity in contrast to PD and posture is erect rather than stooped. Posture may be extreme with patients developing retrocollis. The gait is described as lurching like that of a 'drunken sailor' or 'dancing bear', while falls are typically backward.[47]

Parkinsonism is manifested as stiffness and bradykinaesia and tremor is typically absent. There is either poor or absent response of parkinsonism to levodopa therapy. Patients inevitably become wheelchair-bound due to motor progression and postural instability.[49,50]

The supranuclear ophthalmoplegia which gives the syndrome its name may initially be subtle or not present until a year or more after disease onset. Slowing of vertical saccadic eye movements and square wave jerks on neurologic exam precede difficulty with down or up gaze.[10,11,49] Classically, down gaze is affected to a greater degree than up gaze. Patients may have difficulty looking down while feeding themselves, leading to messy eating, and the 'dirty-tie' sign. Later, all voluntary eye movements are lost but the supranuclear character can be demonstrated by having the patient fixate on a target and rotating the head to obtain full movements.

Besides oculomotor abnormalities, ocular abnormalities are also common. Spontaneous blink rate is decreased which may lead to complaints of ocular irritation, epiphora, and blurred vision. Retraction of the eye lids and eye lid apraxia leads to a staring gaze (Fig. 37.4).[47,51] The procerus sign refers to a worried expression due to a furrowed brow from contraction of the procerus, frontalis, and corrugator muscles.[52] Faces become masked with mouth held open (Fig. 37.4). Speech becomes slow and slurred with a growling quality and eventually becomes unintelligible.[46] Swallowing is affected early and the most common causes of death is aspiration pneumonia or respiratory failure.[50,53]

Neuropsychiatric manifestations develop in over half of patients within the first two years of disease.[54] Subcortical dementia manifests with cognitive slowing, executive dysfunction, poor recall, and attention. Apathy with irritability and disinhibition may mimic frontal lobe disease. The 'applause sign' or failure to stop clapping after asked to clap only three times has been described in PSP[55] but is not specific. Forced laughing and signs of pseudobulbar palsy eventually become prominent.[50,54]

Table 37.2 NINDS–SPSP clinical criteria for the diagnosis of PSP

Mandatory inclusion criteria

Possible PSP

- Gradually progressive disease onset with onset at age 40 or later
- *Either* vertical supranuclear palsy *or* both slowing of vertical saccades and prominent postural instability with falls in the first year of disease onset
- No evidence of other diseases that could explain the clinical features

Probable PSP

- Gradually progressive disease onset with onset at age 40 or later
- Vertical supranuclear palsy *and* prominent postural instability with falls in the first year of disease onset
- No evidence of other diseases that could explain the clinical features

Definite PSP

- Clinically probable or possible PSP *and* histopathological evidence of typical PSP

Supportive criteria

- Symmetric akinaesia or rigidity, proximal more than distal
- Abnormal neck posture, especially retrocollis
- Poor or absent response of parkinsonism to levodopa therapy
- Early dysphagia and dysarthria
- Early cognitive impairment including at least two of the following: apathy, impairment in abstract thought, decreased verbal fluency, utilization or imitation behaviour, or frontal release signs

Mandatory exclusion criteria

- Recent encephalitis
- Alien limb syndrome, cortical sensory deficits, focal frontal or temporoparietal atrophy
- Hallucinations or delusions
- Cortical dementia of Alzheimer's type
- Prominent early cerebellar symptoms or prominent early unexplained dysautonomia
- Severe asymmetric parkinsonian signs
- Neuroradiologic evidence of relevant structural abnormality
- Whipple's disease confirmed by polymerase chain reaction

Source data from *Neurology*. 47(1), Litvan I, Agid Y, Calne D, *et al.* Clinical research criteria for the diagnosis of progressive supranuclear palsy (Steele–Richardson–Olszewski syndrome): report of the NINDS–SPSP international workshop, pp. 1–9, Copyright (1996), Wolters Kluwer Health, Inc.

PSP–parkinsonism (PSP–P)

PSP with parkinsonism as the predominant finding, PSP–P, is a more indolent form and represents roughly a third of PSP cases.[46] Patients are often initially diagnosed with PD as bradykinaesia, rigidity, and tremor may have an asymmetric onset and initially respond to levodopa. A parkinsonian rest tremor can be present although a jerky postural tremor is also common in these patients. Falls, extraocular abnormalities, and cognitive changes may not be present in the first two years but later overlap with Richardson's syndrome.

PSP–pure akinaesia with gait freezing (PSP–PAGF)

The clinical syndrome of pure akinaesia with gait freezing has a gradual onset and is characterized by difficulty initiating gait or speech and 'freezing' during walking, writing, and speaking. Appendicular rigidity and tremor are often absent, eye movements may be normal, and patients may not have cognitive symptoms.[56]

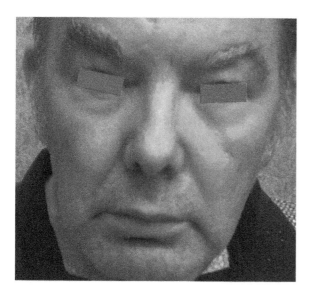

Fig. 37.4 Characteristic facial appearance in PSP. The furrowed brow and eyelid retraction in this patient lead to a characteristic staring, worried expression in PSP (eyes obscured for privacy).

PSP–PAGF can be a differential diagnosis of a normal pressure hydrocephalus phenotype.

PSP–primary progressive apraxia of speech (PSP–PPAOS)

Apraxia of speech characterized by speech production errors such as groping may be the presenting and sole complaint leading to a diagnosis of PSP–PPAOS. PPAOS is associated with supplementary motor area and premotor dysfunction, and typical features of PSP-S may occur later in disease course.[57,58]

PSP–corticobasal syndrome (PSP–CBS)

Some patients may present with progressive asymmetric rigidity and apraxia, dystonia, and cortical sensory loss leading to the clinical diagnosis of CBS with PSP findings at autopsy.[31]

PSP–corticospinal tract dysfunction (PSP–CSTD)

Some patients with PSP may have involvement of the corticospinal tract with predominantly upper motor neuron symptoms in addition to parkinsonism and classic features of PSP.[59]

Clinical heterogeneity

As demonstrated earlier in this chapter, there is great variability in the clinical presentation of PSP. Some patients with pathologic evidence of PSP never manifest eye movement abnormalities.[60,61] Cognitive or behavioural symptoms may be the sole manifestation of disease and cerebellar ataxia may be the initial and main symptoms.[62] Often patients present with a constellation of symptoms which encompass both PSP and CBS. This 'hybrid' presentation correlates to neuroanatomical imaging findings which demonstrate features of both PSP and CBS.[63] Other neurodegenerative disorders may mimic PSP such as primary lateral sclerosis with eye movement abnormalities, gait difficulty, and falls.[64]

Neuropsychology

Early cognitive impairment in PSP can be detected with the dementia rating scale (DRS) with particular impairment on the initiation and perseveration subscale. The frontal assessment battery (FAB) can be helpful in differentiating PSP from other disorders with impairments in lexical fluency and motor series subscores in PSP patients.[65,66]

Neuroimaging

There are no absolute diagnostic features on imaging. Midbrain atrophy may be detected by MRI in advanced cases and leads to the 'hummingbird' or 'penguin' sign on coronal images (Fig. 37.5).[67,68] Atrophy of the dorsal mesencephalon leads to widening of the interpeduncular cistern or 'mouse ears' configuration. Diffusion tensor imaging may demonstrate white matter degeneration of the brainstem, association and commissural fibres.[69] The superior cerebellar peduncles, body of the corpus callosum, and inferior and superior longitudinal fasciculi are predominantly affected with severity of motor function and saccadic impairments correlating to

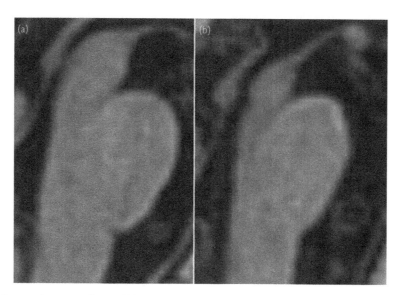

Fig. 37.5 Imaging findings in PSP. Compared to a normal control (a), the midbrain tegmental atrophy with relative preservation of the pons leads to a 'humming-bird' profile (b).

the degeneration of the inferior longitudinal fasciculus and superior longitudinal fasciculus respectively.[69]

Neuropathology

Definite PSP is a pathologic diagnosis.[48] Midbrain atrophy is the most common pathological finding on gross examination of the brain with dilation of the aqueduct of Sylvius and hypopigmentation of the substantia nigra.[31] Histopathologically, tau protein accumulates in neurons as globose, neurofibrillary tangles, and neuropil threads. Tau accumulation in glial cells as tufted astrocytes is almost pathognomonic (Fig. 37.6); coiled bodies may also be present.[41,48,70]

Pathophysiology

Dopaminergic neurons in the nigrostriatal system are affected in PSP along with cholinergic and GABAergic neurons in the basal ganglia, striatum, and brainstem.[71] The pathologic tau in PSP is composed of four repeat-tau protein aggregates with an unclear mechanism leading to accumulation. Hereditary PSP is rare but has been reported in familial frontotemporal dementia with parkinsonism linked to chromosome 17 (FTDP-17).[72] PSP is also associated with the H1 haplotype in the tau gene (*MAPT*).

Management

There is no treatment to slow or halt PSP progression and symptomatic approaches are the mainstay in clinical practice. Levodopa may lead to slight but unsustained benefit, and zolpidem, the GABAergic agonist of benzodiazepine receptors, has been reported to improve akinaesia and rigidity in PSP.[73] Treatment of sleep difficulties and urinary incontinence in combination with occupational, physical, and speech therapy are important for both patient and caregiver. Fall prevention is important with the use of weighted walking aids to reduce the tendency for backwards falls. Ocular care with lubricating drops is recommended and some patients may benefit from bifocals or prisms. Pharmacologic therapies in development

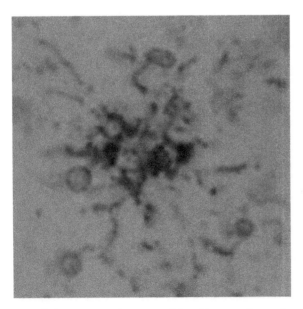

Fig. 37.6 Tufted astrocyte in PSP. Immunostaining with tau reveals extension of tau along distal processes leading to the 'tufted' appearance.

target abnormal aggregation of microtubule-associated protein tau through kinase inhibitors, cytoskeleton stabilizers, and free radical scavengers.[39]

Multiple system atrophy

Background

Multiple system atrophy (MSA) is a progressive neurodegenerative disorder characterized by autonomic failure in combination with pyramidal, extrapyramidal, or cerebellar findings. The term MSA was introduced in 1969 by Graham and Oppenheimer to encompass the disorders of striatonigral degeneration, olivopontocerebellar ataxia, and Shy–Drager syndrome.[74] MSA is an α-synucleinopathy with the different subtypes reflecting selective damage to the basal ganglia (MSA-P) or cerebellum (MSA-C).[75-77] The parkinsonian-type of MSA, MSA-P, is synonymous with striatonigral degeneration and MSA–C refers to olivopontocerebllar ataxia with dominant cerebellar symptoms.[78,79] MSA affects an estimated 0.6 per 100 000 people per year, which increases to 3 per 100 000 people per year in a population over 50 years.[78,80]

Clinical features

MSA typically presents in the 50s and is rapidly progressive with median survival of 7–9 years.[81,82] Autonomic systems are present in the majority of patients at presentation while the predominant motor symptoms of parkinsonism or cerebellar dysfunction lead to the diagnosis of MSA–P or MSA–C respectively.[83] Overlap is common with cerebellar findings found in nearly half of MSA–P patients and parkinsonism in over half of patients with MSA–C.[83,84] Epidemiological studies demonstrate ethnic variation with regard to the incidence of MSA–P and MSA–C. A North American study found a majority of MSA–P (60 per cent) compared to MSA–C (13 per cent), while a Japanese study had a much higher percentage of MSA–C (84 per cent) than MSA–P (16 per cent).[78,85]

Autonomic dysfunction

If not present at onset, autonomic symptoms develop in nearly all patients.[86] Genitourinary dysfunction is the most common initial symptom in women while erectile dysfunction is most common in men.[87] Urinary dysfunction in MSA with constant urge or stress incontinence differs from the frequency and urgency which can also be seen in PD. Severe orthostatic hypotension, defined as a drop in systolic blood pressure of at least 30 mm Hg systolic or 15 mm Hg diastolic within 3 minutes of standing from a recumbent position is common in MSA. Often patients do not have an adequate heart rate increase and may report symptoms of light-headedness, dizziness, weakness, fatigue, darkening of vision, cognitive clouding, or frank syncope. Despite prominent orthostatic hypotension, supine hypertension may be comorbid and complicate treatment. Patients often progress to anhidrosis which can be evaluated with evaluated with thermoregulatory sweat test (Fig. 37.7). Constipation is frequently observed in MSA, similar to other parkinsonian disorders, while faecal incontinence may also be present.[88]

Parkinsonian features

Extrapyramidal features of bradykinaesia, rigidity, and postural instability are the prominent parkinsonian features. However, the relative symmetry of parkinsonism in MSA may help to distinguish it from Parkinson's disease. Additionally, the classic pill-rolling rest tremor of PD is less likely while a postural tremor is present

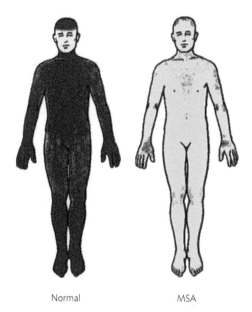

Normal   MSA

Fig. 37.7 Thermoregulatory sweat test in MSA. Sweating is shown in purple while yellow is indicative of anhidrosis. MSA patients typically progress to global anhidrosis.

in roughly half of MSA patients.[78] While parkinsonian symptoms may initially respond to levodopa therapy, the response is rarely maintained. Furthermore, the presence of early parkinsonian features is associated with a more rapid functional decline.[89]

Cerebellar dysfunction

The most common cerebellar feature is ataxia of gait and is often accompanied by an ataxic dysarthria and oculomotor dysfunction including square wave jerks, dysmetric saccades, and jerky pursuit. Limb ataxia is usually less prominent than the disturbances of gait or speech.[79,86]

Non-motor symptoms

In addition to motor and autonomic symptoms, MSA patients may have some form of sleep disruption early in the disease course. Similar to other α-synucleinopathies, rapid eye movement (REM) sleep behaviour disorder is common in MSA patients or patients may have insomnia or restless leg symptoms.[79,88] Of the non-motor features in MSA, respiratory involvement is particularly worrisome. Stridor is important to recognize and serves as a negative prognostic indicator.[88] Stridor occurs in approximately a third of patients and when accompanied by central respiratory failure can lead to severe respiratory insufficiency.[90,91] Nocturnal inspiratory stridor due to laryngeal abductor paralysis and obstructive sleep apnoea can lead to sudden death.

Cognitive symptoms

Significant cognitive impairment excludes a diagnosis of MSA according to current consensus criteria (see Table 37.3), yet dementia can occur.[92,93] When present, cognitive impairment can range from subcortical executive deficits to profound dementia;[66,93] however, the presence of dementia without ataxia is more suggestive of PD with dementia or dementia with Lewy bodies (DLB). Depression is present in less than half of MSA patients yet is more common in those with dementia.[66,78] Anxiety may also be a disabling feature of MSA.[94]

Table 37.3 Diagnostic criteria for MSA

Probable MSA

♦ Sporadic, progressive, adult-onset disease characterized by
  - Autonomic failure involving urinary incontinence with erectile dysfunction in males or an orthostatic decrease of blood pressure within 3 minutes of standing by at least 30 mm Hg systolic or 15 mm Hg diastolic, *and*
  - Poorly levodopa-responsive parkinsonism (bradykinaesia with rigidity, tremor, or postural instability), *or*
  - A cerebellar syndrome (gait ataxia with cerebellar dysarthria, limb ataxia, or cerebellar oculomotor dysfunction)

Possible MSA

♦ Sporadic, progressive, adult-onset disease characterized by
  - Parkinsonism, *or*
  - A cerebellar syndrome, *and*
  - At least one feature suggesting autonomic dysfunction (otherwise unexplained urinary urgency, frequency or incomplete bladder emptying, erectile dysfunction in males, or significant orthostatic blood pressure decline that does not meet the level required in probable MSA), *and*
  - At least one of the additional features

Additional features

Possible MSA–P or MSA–C
  - Babinski sign with hyper-reflexia
  - Stridor

Possible MSA–P
  - Rapidly progressive parkinsonism
  - Poor response to levodopa
  - Postural instability within three years of motor onset
  - Gait ataxia with cerebellar dysarthria, limb ataxia, or cerebellar oculomotor dysfunction
  - Dysphagia within five years of motor onset
  - Atrophy on MRI of putamen, middle cerebellar peduncle, pons, or cerebellum

Possible MSA–C
  - Parkinsonism (bradykinaesia, rigidity)
  - Atrophy on MRI of putamen, middle cerebellar peduncle, or pons
  - Hypometabolism on FTD-PET in putamen
  - Presynaptic nigrostriatal dopaminergic denervation on SPECT or PET

Supporting features
  - Orofacial dystonia
  - Disproportionate antecollis
  - Camptocormia (severe anterior flexion of the spine) and/or Pisa syndrome (severe lateral flexion of the spine)
  - Contractures of hands or feet
  - Inspiratory sighs
  - Severe dysphonia
  - Severe dysarthria
  - New or increased snoring
  - Cold hands and feet
  - Pathologic laughter or crying
  - Jerky, myoclonic postural/action tremor

Non-supporting features
  - Classic pill-rolling rest tremor
  - Clinically significant neuropathy
  - Hallucinations not induced by drugs
  - Onset after age 75 years
  - Family history of ataxia or parkinsonism
  - Dementia
  - White matter lesions suggesting multiple sclerosis

Source data from *Neurology*. 71, Gilman S, Wenning GK, Low PA, *et al*. Second consensus statement on the diagnosis of multiple system atrophy, pp. 670–6, Copyright (2008), Wolters Kluwer Health, Inc.

Neuropsychology

Frontal lobe dysfunction may be found on cognitive testing in MSA.[92] Executive function and verbal memory is impaired with prominent deficits noted in verbal fluency.[66,95]

Neuroimaging

There are no absolute diagnostic features on imaging. MRI may detect putaminal abnormalities and atrophy of the brainstem, middle cerebellar peduncles, and cerebellum.[96] The 'hot cross bun' sign is evident in patients with MSA–C due to loss of transverse pontocerebellar fibers in the basis pontis with preservation of the corticospinal tracts and pontine tegmentum (Fig. 37.8).[97] With functional imaging, MSA patients may show hypometabolism in the striatum, brainstem, and cerebellum.[96]

Neuropathology

Definite diagnosis of MSA requires neuropathologic confirmation. MSA is characterized by neuronal loss with gliosis in the basal ganglia, cerebellum, pons, inferior olivary nuclei, and spinal cord. The hallmark of MSA pathology is the presence of glial cytoplasmic inclusions (GCIs) which are predominantly found in oligodendrocytes (Fig. 37.9).[98] A-synuclein is the major component of GCIs which are also immunoreactive for several other proteins.[98,99] Abnormal accumulation of α- synuclein is seen in cytoplasmic and nuclear inclusions as well as neurites.[100]

Pathophysiology

MSA is presumed to be a primary oligodendrogliopathy with secondary neuronal multisystem degeneration.[82] Deficient release of oligodendroglial glial-derived neurotrophic factor (GDNF) leading to selective neuronal loss has been found in an MSA transgenic mouse model.[101] Molecular mechanisms related to α-synuclein misfolding, aggregation, and fibrillation are hypothesized to play a role in neurodegeneration similar to other α-synucleinopathies.

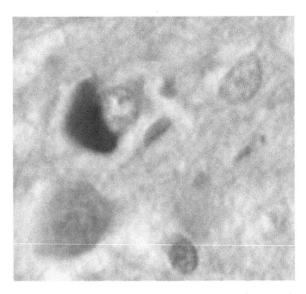

Fig. 37.9 Glial cytoplasmic inclusion in MSA. Immunostaining for α-synuclein showing a cytoplasmic inclusion in an oligodendrocyte.

Management

While current studies focus on neuroprotective agents, there are no established disease modifying therapies in MSA.[39] Symptomatic treatment focuses on improving parkinsonism and dysautonomia. Dopaminergic therapy with levodopa or dopaminergic agonists should be tried. Orthostatic hypotension can be treated with non-pharmacologic interventions such as thigh-high compression stocking and abdominal binders along with high fluid intake and high salt diet with more frequent and smaller meals to reduce postprandial hypotension. Midodrine may improve blood pressure with monitoring for supine hypertension. Urinary dysfunction may benefit from anticholinergic medications, particularly with trospium which is a peripheral acting anticholinergic. Inspiratory stridor should be treated with continuous positive airway pressure (CPAP). Physical, speech, and occupational therapy are also important in the treatment approach to MSA.

Argyrophilic grain disease

Background

Argyrophilic grain disease (AGD) is a sporadic tauopathy characterized by dementia that is diagnosed solely on neuropathologic findings. Argyrophilic grains are small filaments or tubules derived from dendrites and pre-tangle neurons. The presence of argyrophilic grains in a subset of patients with adult-onset dementia was described by Braak and Braak in 1987 as a distinctive degenerative disease.[102] The diagnosis of AGD as a distinct entity is controversial as subsequent studies have shown the association of AGD with multiple other neurodegenerative diseases.[103–105] Furthermore, AGD has been reported in 30 per cent of brains from cognitively normal individuals.[106] One theory hypothesizes that the presence of AGD contributes to the development of dementia by lowering the threshold for cognitive deficits.[107] The proportion of neurodegenerative dementias ascribed to AGD is approximately 5 per cent.[104,105]

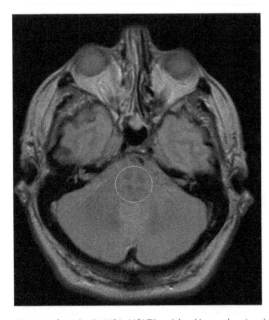

Fig. 37.8 Hot cross bun sign in MSA. MRI T2-weighted image showing the characteristic cross-shaped hyperintensity in the pons in MSA (circled).

Table 37.4 Rarer neurodegenerative diseases

Disorder	Clinical features	Typical clinical presentation	Atypical symptoms	Pathology	Area affected
Neurofilament inclusion disease (NFID)	Rapidly progressive, young onset	FTD or CBS	Parkinsonism, upper motor neuron disease	Neurofilaments +/− FUS positive inclusions	Widespread, predominantly frontotemporal and basal ganglia
Basophilic inclusion body disease (BIBD)	Young onset	FTD and MND	Progressive supranuclear palsy	FUS-positive inclusions, basophilic inclusions on H&E	Frontotemporal cortices, caudate nucleus, substantia nigra
Globular glial tauopathy (GGT)	Mid-late onset	MND and/or FTD	PSP features	Tau, 'globular' oligodendroglial inclusions	Frontotemporal and limbic
Tangle dominant dementia (TDD)	Late onset, female preponderance	Amnestic dementia	Psychiatric symptoms	NFT without neuritic plaques and scarce amyloid plaques	Diffuse cerebral atrophy, severe limbic involvement
Hippocampal sclerosis dementia (HSD)	Late onset	FTD and AD	MND	Severe neuronal loss and gliosis	Hippocampus (CA-1 and subiculum)

AD: Alzheimer's dementia; CBS: corticobasal syndrome; FTD: frontotemporal dementia; FUS: fused in sarcoma; H&E: haematoxylin and eosin stain; MND: motor neuron disease; NF: Neurofilament; NFT: neurofibrillary tangles; PSP: progressive supranuclear palsy.

Clinical features

Cognitive symptoms

A range of clinical symptoms is reported in AGD including cognitive decline, dementia and behavioural abnormalities.[104,108,109] Mild amnestic impairment may be the initial manifestation of AGD[110,111] while episodic memory loss may be present in over half of patients.[109] Amnesia, irritability, and agitation followed by delusions, dysphoria, and apathy may be symptoms of AGD in older patients.[112] The presence of prominent behavioural changes, aggression, or transcortical sensory aphasia has led AGD to be considered as one neuropathological cause of frontotemporal dementia.[113]

Clinical and pathological correlations are important as variability in lesions and accompanying Alzheimer's disease pathology lead to difficulty in ascribing clinical symptoms solely to AGD. AGD has been suggested to act as an additive pathology with the presence of AGD plus mild–moderate AD-type pathology resulting in clinical symptoms.[107,114]

Neuroimaging

Imaging in AGD patients with dementia symptoms has shown focal atrophy of the anterior hippocampus/amygdala complex.[114]

Neuropathology

The neuropathologic hallmarks of AGD are phospho-tau positive argyrophilic grains, pre-neurofibrillary neuronal tangles and coiled bodies in oligodendrocytes.[102] Argyrophilic grains (AG) are named for their affinity for staining using the Gallyas silver iodide method, and are also labelled with antibodies to phospho-tau protein. AGs are mainly present in transentorhinal and entorhinal cortex, CA1 area of the hippocampus and presubiculum.[104] Coiled bodies in oligodendrocytes are associated with AGs yet lack specificity. Pretangle neurons share the same distribution as AGs. Tau-containing astrocytes, ballooned neurons, tangles, and neuropil threads may be present.[115]

Other rarer neurodegenerative diseases

A subset of disorders do not fulfil criteria for any of the commonly described neurodegenerative diseases and are lumped as 'other neurodegenerative disorders' based on atypical clinical or neuropathology features. These rare neurologic disorders are increasingly characterized by their pathologic profiles (Table 37.4).[116–122]

References

1. Rebeiz JJ, Kolodny EH, and Richardson EP, Jr. Corticodentatonigral degeneration with neuronal achromasia: a progressive disorder of late adult life. *Trans Am Neurol Assoc.* 1967;92:23–6.
2. Litvan I, Agid Y, Goetz C, et al. Accuracy of the clinical diagnosis of corticobasal degeneration: a clinicopathologic study. *Neurology.* 1997;48:119–25.
3. Winter Y, Bezdolnyy Y, Katunina E, et al. Incidence of Parkinson's disease and atypical parkinsonism: Russian population-based study. *Mov Disord.* 2010;25:349–56.
4. Wenning GK, Litvan I, Jankovic J, et al. Natural history and survival of 14 patients with corticobasal degeneration confirmed at postmortem examination. *J Neurol Neurosur Ps.* 1998;64:184–9.
5. Rinne JO, Lee MS, Thompson PD, et al. Corticobasal degeneration. A clinical study of 36 cases. *Brain.* 1994;117 (Pt 5):1183–96.
6. Boeve BF, Lang AE, and Litvan I. Corticobasal degeneration and its relationship to progressive supranuclear palsy and frontotemporal dementia. *Ann Neurol.* 2003;54 Suppl 5:S15–9.
7. Gottlieb D, Robb K, and Day B. Mirror movements in the alien hand syndrome. Case report. *Am J Phys Med Rehabil.* 1992;71:297–300.
8. Thompson PD, Day BL, Rothwell JC, et al. The myoclonus in corticobasal degeneration. Evidence for two forms of cortical reflex myoclonus. *Brain.* 1994;117 (Pt 5):1197–207.
9. Kompoliti K, Goetz CG, Boeve BF, et al. Clinical presentation and pharmacological therapy in corticobasal degeneration. *Arch Neurol.* 1998;55:957–61.
10. Rivaud-Pechoux S, Vidailhet M, Gallouedec G, et al. Longitudinal ocular motor study in corticobasal degeneration and progressive supranuclear palsy. *Neurology.* 2000;54:1029–32.
11. Vidailhet M, Rivaud S, Gouider-Khouja N, et al. Eye movements in parkinsonian syndromes. *Ann Neurol.* 1994;35:420–6.
12. Ling H, O'Sullivan SS, Holton JL, et al. Does corticobasal degeneration exist? A clinicopathological re-evaluation. *Brain.* 2010;133:2045–57.
13. Murray R, Neumann M, Forman MS, et al. Cognitive and motor assessment in autopsy-proven corticobasal degeneration. *Neurology.* 2007;68:1274–83.
14. Kertesz A, McMonagle P, Blair M, et al. The evolution and pathology of frontotemporal dementia. *Brain.* 2005;128:1996–2005.

15. Josephs KA and Duffy JR. Apraxia of speech and nonfluent aphasia: a new clinical marker for corticobasal degeneration and progressive supranuclear palsy. *Curr Opin Neurol*. 2008;21:688–92.

16. Boeve BF, Maraganore DM, Parisi JE, *et al*. Pathologic heterogeneity in clinically diagnosed corticobasal degeneration. *Neurology*. 1999;53:795–800.

17. Josephs KA, Petersen RC, Knopman DS, *et al*. Clinicopathologic analysis of frontotemporal and corticobasal degenerations and PSP. *Neurology*. 2006;66:41–8.

18. Kaiser M, Groll M, Siciliano C, *et al*. Binding mode of TMC-95A analogues to eukaryotic 20S proteasome. *Chembiochem*. 2004;5:1256–66.

19. Tang-Wai DF, Josephs KA, Boeve BF, *et al*. Pathologically confirmed corticobasal degeneration presenting with visuospatial dysfunction. *Neurology*. 2003;61:1134–5.

20. Hassan A, Whitwell JL, Boeve BF, *et al*. Symmetric corticobasal degeneration (S-CBD). *Parkinsonism Relat Disord*. 2010;16:208–14.

21. Pillon B, Blin J, Vidailhet M, *et al*. The neuropsychological pattern of corticobasal degeneration: comparison with progressive supranuclear palsy and Alzheimer's disease. *Neurology*. 1995;45:1477–83.

22. Massman PJ, Kreiter KT, Jankovic J, *et al*. Neuropsychological functioning in cortical-basal ganglionic degeneration: differentiation from Alzheimer's disease. *Neurology*. 1996;46:720–6.

23. Soliveri P, Monza D, Paridi D, *et al*. Cognitive and magnetic resonance imaging aspects of corticobasal degeneration and progressive supranuclear palsy. *Neurology*. 1999;53:502–7.

24. Hauser RA, Murtaugh FR, Akhter K, *et al*. Magnetic resonance imaging of corticobasal degeneration. *Journal of Neuroimaging*. 1996;6:222–6.

25. Josephs KA, Whitwell JL, Dickson DW, *et al*. Voxel-based morphometry in autopsy proven PSP and CBD. *Neurobiol Aging*. 2008;29:280–9.

26. Whitwell JL, Jack CR, Jr., Boeve BF, *et al*. Imaging correlates of pathology in corticobasal syndrome. *Neurology*. 2010;75:1879–87.

27. Pirker W, Asenbaum S, Bencsits G, *et al*. [123I]beta-CIT SPECT in multiple system atrophy, progressive supranuclear palsy, and corticobasal degeneration. *Mov Disord*. 2000;15:1158–67.

28. Sawle GV, Brooks DJ, Marsden CD, *et al*. Corticobasal degeneration. A unique pattern of regional cortical oxygen hypometabolism and striatal fluorodopa uptake demonstrated by positron emission tomography. *Brain*. 1991;114 (Pt 1B):541–56.

29. Dickson DW, Bergeron C, Chin SS, *et al*. Office of Rare Diseases neuropathologic criteria for corticobasal degeneration. *J Neuropathol Exp Neurol*. 2002;61:935–46.

30. Dickson D. In: MM Esiri (ed.). *The Neuropathology of Dementia*. Cambridge: Cambridge University Press, 2004, pp. 227–56.

31. Dickson DW. Neuropathologic differentiation of progressive supranuclear palsy and corticobasal degeneration. *J Neurol*. 1999;246 Suppl 2:II6–15.

32. Kouri N, Whitwell JL, Josephs KA, *et al*. Corticobasal degeneration: a pathologically distinct 4R tauopathy. *Nat Rev Neurol*. 2011;7:263–72.

33. Ishizawa K and Dickson DW. Microglial activation parallels system degeneration in progressive supranuclear palsy and corticobasal degeneration. *J Neuropathol Exp Neurol*. 2001;60:647–57.

34. Mandelkow EM, Drewes G, Biernat J, *et al*. Glycogen synthase kinase-3 and the Alzheimer-like state of microtubule-associated protein tau. *FEBS letters*. 1992;314:315–21.

35. Ludolph AC, Kassubek J, Landwehrmeyer BG, *et al*. Tauopathies with parkinsonism: clinical spectrum, neuropathologic basis, biological markers, and treatment options. *Eur J Neurol*. 2009;16:297–309.

36. Ittner LM, Ke YD, Delerue F, *et al*. Dendritic function of tau mediates amyloid-beta toxicity in Alzheimer's disease mouse models. *Cell*. 2010;142:387–97.

37. Hoover BR, Reed MN, Su J, *et al*. Tau mislocalization to dendritic spines mediates synaptic dysfunction independently of neurodegeneration. *Neuron*. 2010;68:1067–81.

38. Boeve BF, Josephs KA, and Drubach DA. Current and future management of the corticobasal syndrome and corticobasal degeneration. *Handb Clin Neurol*. 2008;89:533–48.

39. Wenning GK, Krismer F, and Poewe W. New insights into atypical parkinsonism. *Curr Opin Neurol*. 2011;24:331–8.

40. Steele JC, Richardson JC, and Olszewski J. Progressive Supranuclear Palsy. A Heterogeneous Degeneration Involving the Brain Stem, Basal Ganglia and Cerebellum with Vertical Gaze and Pseudobulbar Palsy, Nuchal Dystonia and Dementia. *Arch Neurol*. 1964;10:333–59.

41. Hauw JJ, Daniel SE, Dickson D, *et al*. Preliminary NINDS neuropathologic criteria for Steele-Richardson-Olszewski syndrome (progressive supranuclear palsy). *Neurology*. 1994;44:2015–9.

42. Litvan I, Agid Y, Calne D, *et al*. Clinical research criteria for the diagnosis of progressive supranuclear palsy (Steele–Richardson–Olszewski syndrome): report of the NINDS–SPSP international workshop. *Neurology*. 1996;47:1–9.

43. Dickson DW, Ahmed Z, Algom AA, *et al*. Neuropathology of variants of progressive supranuclear palsy. *Curr Opin Neurol*. 2010;23:394–400.

44. Schrag A, Ben-Shlomo Y, and Quinn NP. Prevalence of progressive supranuclear palsy and multiple system atrophy: a cross-sectional study. *Lancet*. 1999;354:1771–5.

45. Santacruz P, Uttl B, Litvan I, *et al*. Progressive supranuclear palsy: a survey of the disease course. *Neurology*. 1998;50:1637–47.

46. Williams DR, de Silva R, Paviour DC, *et al*. Characteristics of two distinct clinical phenotypes in pathologically proven progressive supranuclear palsy: Richardson's syndrome and PSP-parkinsonism. *Brain*. 2005;128:1247–58.

47. Williams DR and Lees AJ. Progressive supranuclear palsy: clinicopathological concepts and diagnostic challenges. *Lancet Neurol*. 2009;8:270–9.

48. Litvan I, Hauw JJ, Bartko JJ, *et al*. Validity and reliability of the preliminary NINDS neuropathologic criteria for progressive supranuclear palsy and related disorders. *J Neuropathol Exp Neurol*. 1996;55:97–105.

49. Litvan I, Grimes DA, Lang AE, *et al*. Clinical features differentiating patients with postmortem confirmed progressive supranuclear palsy and corticobasal degeneration. *J Neurol*. 1999;246 Suppl 2:II1–5.

50. Maher ER and Lees AJ. The clinical features and natural history of the Steele-Richardson-Olszewski syndrome (progressive supranuclear palsy). *Neurology*. 1986;36:1005–8.

51. Scaravilli T, Tolosa E, and Ferrer I. Progressive supranuclear palsy and corticobasal degeneration: lumping versus splitting. *Mov Disord*. 2005;20 Suppl 12:S21–8.

52. Romano S and Colosimo C. Procerus sign in progressive supranuclear palsy. *Neurology*. 2001;57:1928.

53. Nath U, Thomson R, Wood R, *et al*. Population based mortality and quality of death certification in progressive supranuclear palsy (Steele-Richardson-Olszewski syndrome). *J Neurol Neurosur Ps*. 2005;76:498–502.

54. Donker Kaat L, Boon AJ, Kamphorst W, *et al*. Frontal presentation in progressive supranuclear palsy. *Neurology*. 2007;69:723–9.

55. Dubois B, Slachevsky A, Pillon B, *et al*. 'Applause sign' helps to discriminate PSP from FTD and PD. *Neurology*. 2005;64:2132–3.

56. Williams DR, Holton JL, Strand K, *et al*. Pure akinesia with gait freezing: a third clinical phenotype of progressive supranuclear palsy. *Mov Disord*. 2007;22:2235–41.

57. Josephs KA, Duffy JR, Strand EA, *et al*. Characterizing a neurodegenerative syndrome: primary progressive apraxia of speech. *Brain*. 2012;135:1522–36.

58. Josephs KA, Boeve BF, Duffy JR, *et al*. Atypical progressive supranuclear palsy underlying progressive apraxia of speech and nonfluent aphasia. *Neurocase*. 2005;11:283–96.

59. Josephs KA, Katsuse O, Beccano-Kelly DA, *et al*. Atypical progressive supranuclear palsy with corticospinal tract degeneration. *J Neuropathol Exp Neurol*. 2006;65:396–405.

60. Davis PH, Bergeron C, and McLachlan DR. Atypical presentation of progressive supranuclear palsy. *Ann Neurol*. 1985;17:337–43.

61. Birdi S, Rajput AH, Fenton M, *et al*. Progressive supranuclear palsy diagnosis and confounding features: report on 16 autopsied cases. *Mov Disord*. 2002;17:1255–64.

62. Kanazawa M, Shimohata T, Toyoshima Y, *et al.* Cerebellar involvement in progressive supranuclear palsy: a clinicopathological study. *Mov Disord.* 2009;24:1312–8.

63. Josephs KA, Eggers SD, Jack CR, Jr, *et al.* Neuroanatomical correlates of the progressive supranuclear palsy corticobasal syndrome hybrid. *Eur J Neurol.* 2012 Nov;19(11):1440–6.

64. Coon EA, Whitwell JL, Jack CR, Jr, *et al.* Primary lateral sclerosis as progressive supranuclear palsy: diagnosis by diffusion tensor imaging. *Mov Disord.* 2012;27:903–6.

65. Paviour DC, Winterburn D, Simmonds S, *et al.* Can the frontal assessment battery (FAB) differentiate bradykinetic rigid syndromes? Relation of the FAB to formal neuropsychological testing. *Neurocase.* 2005;11:274–82.

66. Brown RG, Lacomblez L, Landwehrmeyer BG, *et al.* Cognitive impairment in patients with multiple system atrophy and progressive supranuclear palsy. *Brain.* 2010;133:2382–93.

67. Oba H, Yagishita A, Terada H, *et al.* New and reliable MRI diagnosis for progressive supranuclear palsy. *Neurology.* 2005;64:2050–5.

68. Kato N, Arai K, and Hattori T. Study of the rostral midbrain atrophy in progressive supranuclear palsy. *J Neurol Sci.* 2003;210:57–60.

69. Whitwell JL, Master AV, Avula R, *et al.* Clinical Correlates of White Matter Tract Degeneration in Progressive Supranuclear PalsyWhite Matter Tract Degeneration in PSP. *Arch Neurol.* 2011;68:753–60.

70. Josephs KA, Mandrekar JN, and Dickson DW. The relationship between histopathological features of progressive supranuclear palsy and disease duration. *Parkinsonism Relat Disord.* 2006;12:109–12.

71. Kasashima S and Oda Y. Cholinergic neuronal loss in the basal forebrain and mesopontine tegmentum of progressive supranuclear palsy and corticobasal degeneration. *Acta Neuropathol.* 2003;105:117–24.

72. Rojo A, Pernaute RS, Fontan A, *et al.* Clinical genetics of familial progressive supranuclear palsy. *Brain.* 1999;122 (Pt 7):1233–45.

73. Daniele A, Albanese A, Gainotti G, *et al.* Zolpidem in Parkinson's disease. *Lancet.* 1997;349:1222–3.

74. Graham JG and Oppenheimer DR. Orthostatic hypotension and nicotine sensitivity in a case of multiple system atrophy. *J Neurol Neurosur Ps.* 1969;32:28–34.

75. Burn DJ and Jaros E. Multiple system atrophy: cellular and molecular pathology. *Molecular Pathology.* 2001;54:419–26.

76. Kosaka K. Diffuse Lewy body disease in Japan. *J Neurol.* 1990;237:197–204.

77. Kosaka K, Yoshimura M, Ikeda K, *et al.* Diffuse type of Lewy body disease: progressive dementia with abundant cortical Lewy bodies and senile changes of varying degree—a new disease? *Clin Neuropathol.* 1984;3:185–92.

78. Gilman S, May SJ, Shults CW, *et al.* The North American Multiple System Atrophy Study Group. *J Neural Transm.* 2005;112:1687–94.

79. Gilman S, Low PA, Quinn N, *et al.* Consensus statement on the diagnosis of multiple system atrophy. *J Auton Nerv Syst.* 1998;74:189–92.

80. Geser F, Seppi K, Stampfer-Kountchev M, *et al.* The European Multiple System Atrophy-Study Group (EMSA-SG). *J Neural Transm.* 2005;112:1677–86.

81. Schrag A, Wenning GK, Quinn N, *et al.* Survival in multiple system atrophy. *Mov Disord.* 2008;23:294–6.

82. Wenning GK, Stefanova N, Jellinger KA, *et al.* Multiple system atrophy: a primary oligodendrogliopathy. *Ann Neurol.* 2008;64:239–46.

83. Gilman S, Wenning GK, Low PA, *et al.* Second consensus statement on the diagnosis of multiple system atrophy. *Neurology.* 2008;71:670–6.

84. Kollensperger M, Geser F, Ndayisaba JP, *et al.* Presentation, diagnosis, and management of multiple system atrophy in Europe: final analysis of the European multiple system atrophy registry. *Mov Disord.* 2010;25:2604–12.

85. Yabe I, Soma H, Takei A, *et al.* MSA-C is the predominant clinical phenotype of MSA in Japan: analysis of 142 patients with probable MSA. *J Neurol Sci.* 2006;249:115–21.

86. Wenning GK, Colosimo C, Geser F, *et al.* Multiple system atrophy. *Lancet Neurol.* 2004;3:93–103.

87. Kirchhof K, Apostolidis AN, Mathias CJ, *et al.* Erectile and urinary dysfunction may be the presenting features in patients with multiple system atrophy: a retrospective study. *International Journal of Impotence Research.* 2003;15:293–8.

88. Colosimo C. Nonmotor presentations of multiple system atrophy. *Nat Rev Neurol.* 2011;7:295–8.

89. Watanabe H, Saito Y, Terao S, *et al.* Progression and prognosis in multiple system atrophy: an analysis of 230 Japanese patients. *Brain.* 2002;125:1070–83.

90. Isozaki E, Naito A, Horiguchi S, *et al.* Early diagnosis and stage classification of vocal cord abductor paralysis in patients with multiple system atrophy. *J Neurol Neurosur Ps.* 1996;60:399–402.

91. Glass GA, Josephs KA, and Ahlskog JE. Respiratory insufficiency as the primary presenting symptom of multiple-system atrophy. *Arch Neurol.* 2006;63:978–81.

92. Robbins TW, James M, Lange KW, *et al.* Cognitive performance in multiple system atrophy. *Brain.* 1992;115(Pt 1):271–91.

93. Burk K, Daum I, and Rub U. Cognitive function in multiple system atrophy of the cerebellar type. *Mov Disord.* 2006;21:772–6.

94. Schrag A, Sheikh S, Quinn NP, *et al.* A comparison of depression, anxiety, and health status in patients with progressive supranuclear palsy and multiple system atrophy. *Mov Disord.* 2010;25:1077–81.

95. Bak TH, Crawford LM, Hearn VC, *et al.* Subcortical dementia revisited: similarities and differences in cognitive function between progressive supranuclear palsy (PSP), corticobasal degeneration (CBD) and multiple system atrophy (MSA). *Neurocase.* 2005;11:268–73.

96. Brooks DJ and Seppi K. Proposed neuroimaging criteria for the diagnosis of multiple system atrophy. *Mov Disord.* 2009;24:949–64.

97. Schrag A, Kingsley D, Phatouros C, *et al.* Clinical usefulness of magnetic resonance imaging in multiple system atrophy. *J Neurol Neurosur Ps.* 1998;65:65–71.

98. Ubhi K, Low P, and Masliah E. Multiple system atrophy: a clinical and neuropathological perspective. *Trends Neurosci.* 2011;34:581–90.

99. Wakabayashi K, Yoshimoto M, Tsuji S, *et al.* Alpha-synuclein immunoreactivity in glial cytoplasmic inclusions in multiple system atrophy. *Neurosci Lett.* 1998;249:180–2.

100. Yoshida M. Multiple system atrophy: alpha-synuclein and neuronal degeneration. *Neuropathology.* 2007;27:484–93.

101. Ubhi K, Rockenstein E, Mante M, *et al.* Neurodegeneration in a transgenic mouse model of multiple system atrophy is associated with altered expression of oligodendroglial-derived neurotrophic factors. *J Neurosci.* 2010;30:6236–46.

102. Braak H and Braak E. Argyrophilic grains: characteristic pathology of cerebral cortex in cases of adult onset dementia without Alzheimer changes. *Neurosci Lett.* 1987;76:124–7.

103. Martinez-Lage P and Munoz DG. Prevalence and disease associations of argyrophilic grains of Braak. *J Neuropathol Exp Neurol.* 1997;56:157–64.

104. Braak H and Braak E. Argyrophilic grain disease: frequency of occurrence in different age categories and neuropathological diagnostic criteria. *J Neural Transm.* 1998;105:801–19.

105. Tolnay M, Schwietert M, Monsch AU, *et al.* Argyrophilic grain disease: distribution of grains in patients with and without dementia. *Acta Neuropathol.* 1997;94:353–8.

106. Knopman DS, Parisi JE, Salviati A, *et al.* Neuropathology of cognitively normal elderly. *J Neuropathol Exp Neurol.* 2003;62:1087–95.

107. Thal DR, Schultz C, Botez G, *et al.* The impact of argyrophilic grain disease on the development of dementia and its relationship to concurrent Alzheimer's disease-related pathology. *Neuropathol Appl Neurobiol.* 2005;31:270–9.

108. Tolnay M, Monsch AU, and Probst A. Argyrophilic grain disease. A frequent dementing disorder in aged patients. *Adv Exp Med Biol.* 2001;487:39–58.

109. Ikeda K, Akiyama H, Arai T, *et al.* Clinical aspects of argyrophilic grain disease. *Clin Neuropathol.* 2000;19:278–84.

110. Jicha GA, Petersen RC, Knopman DS, *et al.* Argyrophilic grain disease in demented subjects presenting initially with amnestic mild cognitive impairment. *J Neuropathol Exp Neurol.* 2006;65:602–9.

111. Petersen RC, Parisi JE, Dickson DW, *et al.* Neuropathologic features of amnestic mild cognitive impairment. *Arch Neurol.* 2006;63:665–72.

112. Togo T, Isojima D, Akatsu H, *et al.* Clinical features of argyrophilic grain disease: a retrospective survey of cases with neuropsychiatric symptoms. *Am J Geriatr Psychiatry.* 2005;13:1083–91.

113. Ishihara K, Araki S, Ihori N, *et al.* Argyrophilic grain disease presenting with frontotemporal dementia: a neuropsychological and pathological study of an autopsied case with presenile onset. *Neuropathology.* 2005;25:165–70.

114. Josephs KA, Whitwell JL, Parisi JE, *et al.* Argyrophilic grains: a distinct disease or an additive pathology? *Neurobiol Aging.* 2008;29:566–73.

115. Ferrer I, Santpere G, and van Leeuwen FW. Argyrophilic grain disease. *Brain.* 2008;131:1416–32.

116. Josephs KA, Holton JL, Rossor MN, *et al.* Neurofilament inclusion body disease: a new proteinopathy? *Brain.* 2003;126:2291–303.

117. Page T, Gitcho MA, Mosaheb S, *et al.* FUS immunogold labelling TEM analysis of the neuronal cytoplasmic inclusions of neuronal intermediate filament inclusion disease: a frontotemporal lobar degeneration with FUS proteinopathy. *J Mol Neurosci.* 2011;45:409–21.

118. Yokota O, Tsuchiya K, Terada S, *et al.* Basophilic inclusion body disease and neuronal intermediate filament inclusion disease: a comparative clinicopathological study. *Acta Neuropathol.* 2008;115:561–75.

119. Kovacs GG, Majtenyi K, Spina S, *et al.* White matter tauopathy with globular glial inclusions: a distinct sporadic frontotemporal lobar degeneration. *J Neuropathol Exp Neurol.* 2008;67:963–75.

120. Ahmed Z, Doherty KM, Silveira-Moriyama L, *et al.* Globular glial tauopathies (GGT) presenting with motor neuron disease or frontotemporal dementia: an emerging group of 4-repeat tauopathies. *Acta Neuropathol.* 2011;122:415–28.

121. Jellinger KA. Different tau pathology pattern in two clinical phenotypes of progressive supranuclear palsy. *Neurodegener Dis.* 2008;5:339–46.

122. Blass DM, Hatanpaa KJ, Brandt J, *et al.* Dementia in hippocampal sclerosis resembles frontotemporal dementia more than Alzheimer disease. *Neurology.* 2004;63:492–7.

CHAPTER 38

Prion diseases

Simon Mead, Peter Rudge, and John Collinge

Introduction

Prion diseases are a heterogeneous group of transmissible neurodegenerative disorders including sheep scrapie, mink encephalopathy, chronic wasting disease of cervids, bovine spongiform encephalopathy (BSE) in cattle, felines, and exotic ungulates, and Creutzfeldt–Jakob disease (CJD) in humans.[1] The human conditions are usually classified by the clinical syndrome (CJD, Gerstmann–Sträussler syndrome (GSS), fatal familial insomnia (FFI), and kuru), often accompanied by aetiology: inherited, acquired, or sporadic. Human prion infection is distinctively associated with long, clinically silent, incubation periods which may span over half a century.[2] The transmissibility of the human diseases was demonstrated with the transmission (by intracerebral inoculation with brain homogenates) to chimpanzees, of kuru (1966), CJD (1968), GSS (1981), FFI (1994) and variant CJD (1996).[3–9]

In the last 30 years, attention has increasingly focused on these relatively rare diseases because of the unique biology of prions, the relevance of this mechanism to other neurodegenerative diseases, and the evidence that BSE prions have infected humans causing variant CJD (vCJD). Central to the pathogenesis of these disorders is a normal cell surface glycoprotein (prion protein, PrP^C) which is expressed in most tissues, and at high levels in the nervous system. According to the 'protein-only' hypothesis,[10] the infectious agent of prion disease largely or completely comprises a multimeric and abnormal isoform of the prion protein (termed PrP^{Sc}; 'Sc' for scrapie isoform).[11] Prion replication may be initiated by a pathogenic mutation in the PrP gene (resulting in a PrP^C predisposed to misfold) in inherited prion diseases by exposure to a 'seed' of PrP^{Sc} in acquired cases, or as a result of the spontaneous conversion of PrP^C as a rare stochastic event in sporadic prion disease.

PrP^C has a structured domain comprising the C-terminal half of the protein, whereas the N-terminal domain has no structure in solution (Fig. 38.1). Other features include five repeat motifs between codon 51 and codon 91 (4 octapaptides and one nonapeptide), and high affinity copper binding sites in the N-terminal domain; one disulphide bond, three alpha helices, a short beta strand, and two glycosylation sites in the C-terminal domain. PrP^C is attached to the outer membrane of the cell by a glycosylinositolphosphate anchor. PrP function is unknown although several minor defects in PrP-knockout mice, molecular interactions, and transport functions have been described. PrP^{Sc} is largely of β-sheet structure although the aggregates in disease brain are heterogeneous and the precise structure of the infectious particle or 'prion' remains uncertain. Prions propagate through a process of binding and conversion between PrP^C and PrP^{Sc} termed 'templated misfolding'.

The characteristic microscopic hallmarks of prion disease are spongiform degeneration of the cerebral cortex, neuronal loss, and gliosis associated with PrP deposition, which may be PrP-amyloid in some cases (Fig. 38.2). Typical grey matter vacuoles are 2–20μm but they can expand into much larger structures. Some inherited prion diseases have relatively little or no vacuole formation. There is substantial neuronal loss that increases with time. Understanding the microscopic pathology has been greatly enhanced by the development of PrP immunohistology which shows several abnormalities not apparent on routine stains. In sporadic CJD (sCJD), amyloid plaques occur in about 10 per cent of patients with a dense core and fibrillary halo. Some inherited disorders, such as that associated with the P102L mutation, have numerous plaques in the cerebellum which have a multicentric appearance, while those patients with the octapeptide repeat (OPRI) mutations have a pathognomonic 'tigroid' arrangement in the cerebellum with PrP deposition in a striped pattern perpendicular to the pial surface. Non-plaque PrP deposition occurs in all cases of sCJD. The deposits can be granular, synaptic, perineuronal decorating the

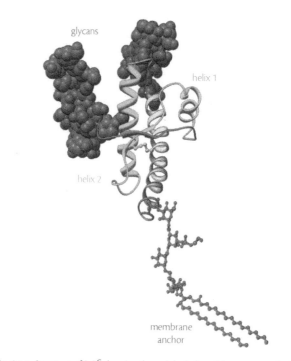

Fig. 38.1 Structure of PrP^C showing three alpha helices (blue, green, and yellow), a single disulphide bond, up to two glycans (red), and attachment to the cell surface via a glycosylinositolphosphate anchor (purple). An N-terminal region is not shown.

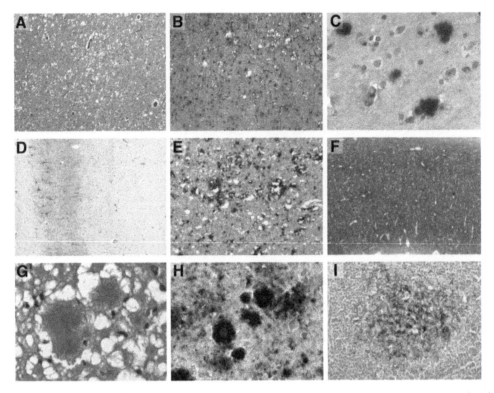

Fig. 38.2 Examples of prion pathology courtesy of Professor Sebastian Brandner, UCL Institute of Neurology. A: spongiform change in sCJD (H&E); B: gliosis and spongiform change in sCJD (GFAP); C: kuru-like plaques in sCJD (ICSM35); D: perineuronal PrP staining in sCJD (ICSM35); E: perivacuolar PrP staining in sCJD (ICSM35); F: synpatic PrP staining in sCJD (ICSM35); G and H: florid plaques in vCJD (H&E, ICSM35); H: PrP deposition in a tonsillar biopsy specimen in vCJD (ICSM35).

neurones, or perivacuolar. Tau inclusions are common in all types of CJD which colocalize with PrP amyloid, but these are distinct from those seen in Alzheimer's disease (in the latter the deposits are thread like whereas in CJD they form minute rods).[12]

In addition to public health concerns, prions have assumed much wider relevance in understanding neurodegenerative and other diseases involving accumulation of misfolded host proteins. These molecular processes, and the emerging and rapidly developing field of protein-misfolding diseases has prion disease as a key paradigm.[13–15] The commonest neurodegenerative diseases can be considered in this category, notably Alzheimer's and Parkinson's diseases. It has long been speculated that other neurodegenerative conditions might be at least experimentally transmissible[16] and experimental transmission of aspects of Alzheimer pathology to primates has been reported.[17] Systemic amyloidosis has been experimentally transmitted by exposure to amyloid fibrils by transfusion or oral exposure in mice.[18,19] Recent work has shown that brain extracts containing β-amyloid deposits taken from either Alzheimer's disease patients or transgenic mice expressing β-amyloid precursor protein (APP) induced β-amyloidosis and related pathology when injected into the brains of presymptomatic APP transgenic mice.[20,21] The morphology of amyloid plaques depended on the source of the injected amyloid in a manner reminiscent of prion strains.

Human prion disease history

Scrapie is a naturally occurring prion disease of sheep and goats, recognized in Europe for over two centuries[22] and present in the sheep flocks of many countries. Scrapie was demonstrated to be transmissible in 1936[23] and the recognition that kuru, and then CJD, resembled scrapie led to the suggestion that these diseases may also be transmissible.[24]

Kuru was an epidemic ataxic syndrome with later dementia in the Fore population in the Eastern Highlands of Papua New Guinea, transmitted by ritual cannibalism. Since the cessation of cannibalism in the late 1950s the disease has steadily declined. Remarkably, however, there have been some presentations in the twenty-first century.[2]

The term Creutzfeldt–Jakob disease was introduced by Spielmeyer in 1922 bringing together the case reports published by Creutzfeldt and Jakob.[25] The incidence of sporadic CJD (sCJD) is around 1–2 million per year and strongly correlated with increasing age, but not gender. It is thought to arise from somatic mutation of *PRNP* or spontaneous conversion of PrP^C to PrP^{Sc} as a rare stochastic event. An alternative hypothesis, that of exposure to an environmental source of either human or animal prions, is not supported by early epidemiological studies,[26] but it is hard to exclude a small proportion of sCJD having an acquired cause. Some more recent studies have suggested a proportion of apparently sporadic CJD may be related to surgery or other iatrogenic routes.[27,28]

Molecular genetics

The human PrP gene (*PRNP*) is located on chromosome 20p is mutated in all familial forms of prion disease. The first mutation to be identified in *PRNP* was in a family with an inherited dementia and consisted of an extra six octapeptide repeats.[29] A second mutation (P102L) was reported in two families with GSS (30). Approximately 15 per cent of prion diseases are inherited and over

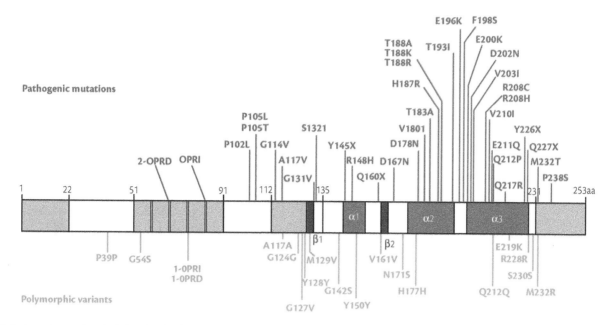

Fig. 38.3 Pathogenic mutations (red, above) and polymorphic changes (green, below) in the prion protein gene are shown on this schematic. The central grey bar also illustrates the secondary structural features of the prion protein.

30 coding mutations in *PRNP* are now recognized,[1] including alteration of the octapeptide repeat motif, point mutations, stop codon mutations, and frameshifts (Fig. 38.3).

A common PrP polymorphism at residue 129, where either methionine or valine can be encoded, is a key determinant of genetic susceptibility in acquired and sporadic forms of prion disease, the large majority of which occur in homozygotes.[31,32] This protective effect of *PRNP* codon 129 heterozygosity is also seen in some of the inherited prion diseases.[33–35] Most prion disease occurs as sCJD where, by definition, there will not be a family history. However, *PRNP* mutations are seen in some apparently sporadic cases, since the family history may not be apparent due to late age of onset, partial penetrance or non-paternity.

Prion biology and strains

The existence of multiple isolates or strains of prions with distinct biological properties has provided a challenge to the 'protein-only' model of prion replication. It is now clear that prion strains can be distinguished by differences in the biochemical properties of PrP^Sc. Prion strain diversity appears to encoded by differences in PrP conformation.[36,37]

Transmission of prion diseases between different mammalian species is restricted by a 'species barrier'.[38] Early studies of the molecular basis of this barrier argued that it resided in differences in PrP primary structure between the species from which the inoculum was derived and the inoculated host. Transgenic mice expressing hamster PrP were, unlike wild type mice, highly susceptible to infection with hamster prions.[39] That most sporadic and acquired CJD occurred in individuals homozygous at *PRNP* polymorphic codon 129 supported the view that prion propagation proceeded most efficiently when the interacting PrP^Sc and PrP^C were of identical primary structure.[31,32] However, prion strain type also affects ease of transmission to another species. Interestingly, with BSE prions this strain component to the barrier seems to predominate, with BSE not only transmitting efficiently to a range of species but also maintaining its transmission characteristics even when passaged through an intermediate species with a distinct PrP gene.[8,40]

According to the *conformational selection model*, the PrP amino acid sequence in a given species is compatible with only a subset of possible mammalian prion strains and the degree of overlap between such preferred conformations between two species will determine the effectiveness of barrier and which strain or strains propagate in the recipient when exposed to a prion from another species.[37,41] Recent advances, including the recognition of subclinical carrier states of prion infection in animal models,[42] suggest that prions themselves are not directly neurotoxic but rather their propagation involves production of toxic species which may be uncoupled from infectivity.[41] A *general model of prion propagation* to encompass these phenomena, centring on the kinetics of prion propagation, has been proposed.[43] A further complexity was introduced by the finding that neuronal tissue grafts not expressing prion protein are resistant to prion toxicity in surrounding diseased tissue.[44] These findings led to the proposal of the *receptor hypothesis* which proposes that cell surface PrP^C is a necessary component of the toxic pathway.

Clinical features

Core features of prion diseases include cognitive dysfunction, ataxia, myoclonus, pyramidal or extrapyramidal signs, and rapid progression. Cognitive decline may remain focal for weeks or even months but ultimately becomes global. Memory, expressive speech, and executive functions are often involved focally early on. Many patients, particularly those with inherited prion diseases associated with insertional mutations, are profoundly apraxic and some have complex articulation and language disturbances. Behavioural change is common which may relate to executive dysfunction, delirium, or more specific psychiatric syndromes. This may require careful management and typically comprises irritability, aggression, or withdrawal from normal social interchange. Sensory loss is not often detected because the patients are frequently not capable of cooperating with the examination. Ultimately most patients enter a state of akinetic mutism. Death generally follows decreasing conscious level and respiratory failure.

Sporadic CJD

sCJD is the most frequent type of prion disease in humans (Box 38.1). The typical phenotype is a rapidly progressive disease characterized by cognitive decline, ataxia, and myoclonus. Typically the age of onset is between 55 and 80 years but many cases occur outside this range; cases in the >75 years range have probably been overlooked in the past but cases under the age of less than 45 years are rare. Only 3 cases of sporadic CJD younger than 30 years old have been identified in the UK since 1970. Median survival is 4 months, with only an atypical 5–10 per cent surviving over two years from onset.

Clinicians have long recognized different phenotypes of sCJD. The Heidenhain variant is not infrequent and is characterized by visual disturbance culminating in cortical blindness. Other phenotypes include an ataxic variant, a thalamic variant, and a panencephalitic type with extensive white matter change, these latter being mainly in the Japanese literature but may merely reflect long

Table 38.1 MRI–CJD Consortium criteria for sporadic Creutzfeldt–Jakob disease

I. Clinical signs (with a symptom duration of less than two years)
Dementia
Cerebellar or visual
Pyramidal or extrapyramidal
Akinetic mutism

II. Tests
Periodic sharp wave complexes on the EEG
14-3-3 protein detection in the CSF
High signal abnormalities in caudate nucleus and putamen or at least two cortical regions (temporal, parietal, or occipital) either in diffusion-weighted imaging (DWI) or fluid-attenuated inversion recovery (FLAIR) MRI

Probable CJD
Two out of I and at least one out of II

Possible CJD
Two out of I and duration less than two years

duration of disease where more grey matter is destroyed. Some case series describe groups with long, pure cognitive and/or psychiatric phases early in the clinical course. Whether or not these different phenotypes represent distinct disease entities or extremes of a range of involvement of different neurological systems is not clear.

The World Health Organisation has drawn up criteria for diagnosing various types of CJD and recently MRI criteria have been recommended to be added (Table 38.1). While these criteria are useful in epidemiological surveys ensuring uniformity of data, they may be restrictive in clinical trials where early diagnosis is essential.

MRI is the most useful modality of imaging in sCJD with sensitivities regularly reported to be over 90 per cent and with high specificity (Fig. 38.4). High signal return from grey matter is characteristic of sCJD and is usually most apparent on diffusion weighted images, less so on FLAIR and least on T2-weighted images. Apparent diffusion coefficient (ADC) maps should be calculated to confirm true restricted diffusion and remove T2-weighted 'shine through'. Enhancement with gadolinium does not occur. In sCJD there is usually high signal return from the basal ganglia, typically the caudate and anterior putamen, which may be asymmetrical. In addition, thalamic signal is often patchily abnormal. The abnormality can include the posterior complex but invariably the thalamic signal should be less intense than that from the caudate nuclei otherwise vCJD is more likely. Cortical 'ribboning' is found in many patients. The distribution can be focal, involving any part of the cortex; care must be taken with areas which are prone to artefact. Little is known about the progression of abnormal signal on serial MRI but it may become more extensive and the signal characteristics may change.

In sCJD, a characteristic abnormality is repetitive (> 5) bi- or triphasic periodic complexes occurring at 0.5–2 second (s) intervals with < 0.5 s variability between complexes and distributed widely over the cortex (Fig. 38.5). Sensitivity is only moderate if a single electro-encephalograph (EEG) is obtained. The prevalence of periodic complexes increases with the age of the patient, codon 129 methionine homozygosity, and short disease duration. This abnormality occurs most frequently if myoclonus is present, and there is phase locking between the complexes and the myoclonic jerks in

---

Box 38.1 Typical case report

An 80-year-old lady worked as a chef until she retired 18 months before presentation. There was no family history of neurodegenerative disease and a past medical history only positive for depression. She was a non-smoker and had minimal alcohol intake.

The patient presented with a six-month history of unsteadiness. She began to have problems walking and had frequent falls. Her symptoms rapidly progressed and she became uncoordinated. Two months after the onset of her balance problems, she began to have difficulties recalling recent events and developed word-finding problems; whilst having a conversation with her husband she would stop mid-sentence and appear blank. She became emotionally labile. She described seeing people who weren't there, namely family members who had died. There was a rapid progression in her symptoms resulting in her becoming bed-bound, secondary to ataxia. She would frequently appear agitated and frightened, her husband also commented on her startling when he came into the room.

Cognitive examination was limited due to marked dysphasia, although she appeared to recognize family members. On neurological examination she was unable to walk due to marked ataxia. There was increased tone present in both the upper and lower limbs. Frontal release signs were also present with bilateral palmomental response and a positive pout reflex. The plantar response was extensor bilaterally. Myoclonus was present spontaneously and with tactile stimulus.

MRI head scan showed high signal in the occipital cortex (ribboning), caudate, and putamen on DWI sequences. Blood tests: Serum blood tests were unremarkable, VGKC Ab were negative, paraneoplastic screen was negative. CSF was positive for 14-3-3 protein. EEG showed periodic sharp wave complexes.

Diagnosis: sporadic Creutzfeldt–Jakob disease.

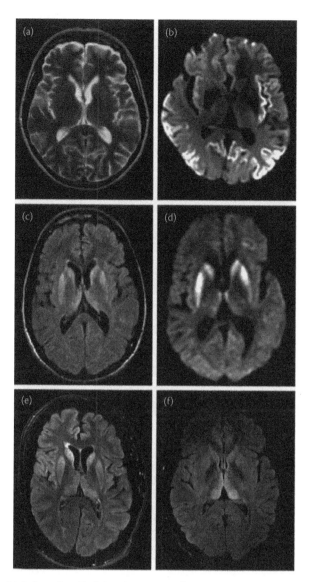

Fig. 38.4 Examples of brain imaging courtesy of Harpreet Hyare, UCLH NHS Trust. (a) T2-weighted axial MRI in sCJD showing subtlety of increased cortical signal. (b) Diffusion-weighted imaging (DWI) showing cortical ribbon in sCJD. (c) FLAIR images, and (d) DWI showing high signal in the caudate, putamen, and less so from the thalamus in sCJD. (e) FLAIR images in iCJD showing cortical, caudate, putamen, and thalamic high signal. (f) FLAIR images showing pulvinar sign in vCJD.

many where the myoclonus is of cortical origin. The specificity of such complexes is fairly high but they do occur with a wide range of pathologies including those that mimic CJD such as metabolic disorders, especially hepatic coma, other neurodegenerative diseases and encephalitides, strokes, and tumours.

In all types of prion disease the cerebrospinal fluid (CSF) typically has a normal cell count of 0–2 cells/mm^3. A pleocytosis suggests an alternative diagnosis, particularly an inflammatory disorder. Total protein level is usually normal or only modestly elevated, and there is no evidence of intrathecal immunoglobulin synthesis. The 14-3-3 proteins comprise a large family of intracellular proteins found in all eukaryotic cells, and constitute about 1 per cent of the total protein content of brain neurons. They are found in the CSF in a variety of conditions where there is rapid and extensive neuronal destruction.[45] They are detected using a qualitative assay, giving a positive,

negative or 'weak positive' result. The 14-3-3 assay is included in the World Health Organization's diagnostic criteria for sCJD. The assay is typically positive in classical, rapidly progressive sCJD, with a sensitivity of over 90 per cent for the MM1 subtype. However, it is less sensitive for longer duration cases, for younger patients, and for the acquired and the more slowly progressive inherited prion diseases. It is positive in only about 40 per cent of cases of vCJD. Interestingly, successive studies over the years have tended to show a reducing sensitivity of the 14-3-3 assay for CJD. This may well be related to the increasing recognition and inclusion of cases with atypical, more slowly progressive clinical features leading to more 'false negative' results in recent studies. The overall specificity of the 14-3-3 assay for prion disease is quite low, at around 70–80 per cent. In patients with clinically suspected CJD, false positive results occur most commonly when the final diagnosis is inflammatory or malignant (including CNS tumours and paraneoplastic syndromes). Other causes of a positive result include recent stroke, infective encephalitis, and subacute sclerosing panencephalitis (SSPE), but these diagnoses can usually be ruled out clinically or on the basis of other tests.

S100b comprise a large family of calcium-binding cytoplasmic proteins found in glia in the CNS, as well as widely outside the CNS. They are detected using a quantitative assay. Their levels are raised in the CSF in a large number of destructive diseases of the nervous system where there is extensive gliosis, including CJD. As with the 14-3-3 proteins, they are more likely to be raised in rapidly progressive disease, where sensitivity is around 90 per cent; however, the specificity is even lower than for 14-3-3, and in practice they rarely add any further useful diagnostic information.

Tau is a microtubule-associated protein, which is found in increased levels in the CSF when there is destruction of neurons. In some disease states the tau protein becomes hyperphosphorylated. The levels of total tau and hyperphosphorylated tau can be measured using quantitative assays. The total tau (T-tau) level in the CSF is elevated in a wide variety of degenerative CNS disorders, including Alzheimer's disease. It is increasingly used, in combination with CSF Aβ_{1-42}, as a diagnostic marker for Alzheimer's disease. In sCJD it can be elevated to a much higher level than in the more common slowly evolving degenerative disorders.[46] If a high threshold is used, the sensitivity is again high for rapidly progressive CJD, and the specificity seems to be similar to that of the 14-3-3 assay.

The only way to obtain a definite diagnosis of CJD, other than the inherited forms, is to obtain tissue. In sCJD, brain biopsy or autopsy are required, biopsy being reserved for atypical cases in whom there are potentially treatable differential diagnoses.

The Real-time Quaking-Induced Conversion Assay (rtQUIC) is becoming available clinically. The concept of this technology is to detect seeding activity of prions in a test CSF sample. The assay employs cycles of shaking and incubation to amplify misfolded PrP *in vitro* which is monitored using fluorescent chemicals which bind to amyloid proteins. In blinded studies, the rtQUIC has achieved high levels of sensitivity and specificity for sCJD.[47]

Inherited prion disease

There are at least 30 different pathological mutations causing inherited prion disease (IPD). There are several types of mutation: alteration of the normal number of octapeptide repeats, point mutations, stop codon mutations, and insertions or deletions causing frameshifts. Phenotypes can be highly variable even in patients with the same mutation and within a family. Some of these cases

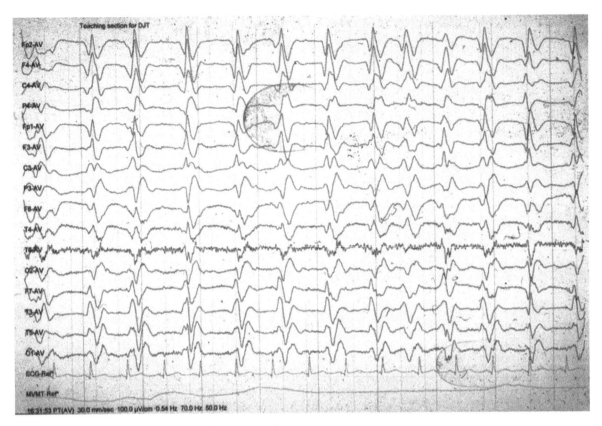

Fig. 38.5 Example EEG recording in sCJD showing periodic sharp wave complexes.

have been transmitted to other species but many have not, particularly those reported from a single family. Failure of transmission in experimental situations does not necessarily mean that transmission will not occur given the appropriate route of inoculation and genetic background of the recipient.

Octapeptide repeat insertion mutation (OPRI)

The largest experience is 6 extra OPR including 100 patients in the UK.[35,48,49] These patients have a mean age of onset of symptoms of 35 (20–53) years and mean age at death of 45 (30–65) years. Interestingly, those with methionine homozygosity at codon 129 have an earlier onset (by about 10 years) than heterozygotes although the duration of the illness is similar between genotypes. Patients present with cortical cognitive deficits encompassing acalculia, language dysfunction, apraxia, and memory impairment together with frontal behavioural disturbance. Physical signs include ataxia, corticospinal, and extrapramidal features. Myoclonus occurs but seizures are rare.

Those involving one, two, or three additional repeats may be coincidental findings, as these have been found in healthy control populations. Four repeat insertions have been reported more frequently associated with a late-onset, short duration course with an absence of family history and so are often mistaken for sCJD.

P102L (typically Gerstmann–Straussler–Scheinkler disease)

In the UK the most frequent point mutation is P102L which usually presents as the GSS syndrome.[30,50] Ataxia is the commonest symptom with cognitive decline, leg weakness, and lower limb pain, especially burning discomfort, occurring later. Additional features

include psychiatric symptoms and pyramidal and extrapyramidal signs in a minority. Myoclonus is uncommon. Occasional CJD-like atypical patients are seen. The age of onset is 27–66 (mean 51) years and death occurs from 33–69 (mean 55) years.

A117V

This mutation was first described in France and subsequently has been reported from a number of countries.[51,52] Parkinsonian features are frequent with dementia and there is a severe loss of ability to speak but with relative preservation of understanding. The age of onset is variable between 20 and 64 years and duration is several years. Amyloid plaques are plentiful and there is often associated tau pathology.

D178N (FFI)

Fatal familial insomnia, due to a mutation most frequently on the 129 methionine allele, was the first described in Italians but occurs extensively. Onset is between 36 and 62 (mean 51) years and the duration is wide, varying between 1 and 6 (mean 2.5) years. Insomnia is said to be the cardinal feature of the disease often preceded by lack of attentiveness. This may soon be accompanied by autonomic symptoms; as the disease progresses dementia, ataxia, pyramidal signs and myoclonus occur, and the syndrome becomes similar to CJD.

D178N mutations can also mimic slowly progressive sCJD and this is said to occur more frequently if the mutation in on the V allele.

E200K

This is the most common mutation worldwide and may be particularly common in localized populations (e.g. in Eastern Europe, North Africa, and Chile), although less common in the UK.[53] E200K patients are on average slightly younger than sCJD subjects but there is great variation. They are indistinguishable from sCJD apart from some having a peripheral neuropathy of mixed axonal and demyelinating type and seizures are more common than in sCJD. There are rare reports of this mutation being on the valine allele where the patients are reported to have a longer course and more ataxia.

Other point mutations

A number of other point mutations have been described often in a single family and therefore clear links with a phenotype have not been made. Typically mutations are associated with a GSS phenotype, CJD, both syndromes, or mixed features. Premature stop codon mutations are associated with vascular deposition of PrP and a range of phenotypes.

Genetic counselling and pre-symptomatic testing

PRNP analysis allows unequivocal diagnosis in patients with inherited prion disease. This has also allowed pre-symptomatic testing of unaffected, but at-risk family members, as well as antenatal testing following appropriate genetic counselling. The effect of codon 129 genotype on the age of onset of disease associated with some mutations also means it is possible to determine within a family whether a carrier of a mutation will have an early or late onset of disease. Most of the well-recognized pathogenic *PRNP* mutations appear fully penetrant; however, experience with some mutations is extremely limited. In families with the E200K mutation there are examples of elderly unaffected gene carriers who appear to have escaped the disease. Families should be counseled to take precautions to avoid iatrogenic transmission of prions by surgery or blood transfusion.

Variant CJD

In 1995–96, there were several extremely young-onset cases with CJD and review of the histology of these cases showed a remarkably consistent and unique pattern.[8,9,36,54,55] These cases were named 'new variant' CJD, subsequently simply 'variant' or 'vCJD'. The striking feature of vCJD is the young age of the patients. The mean age of onset is 29 (range 16–74) years and the mean duration 14 months. Surprisingly, the average age of onset has not progressively increased with time; the reason for this is unknown.

Presentation of vCJD is with behavioural and psychiatric disturbances and, in some cases, sensory disturbance. Initial symptoms are often depression, anxiety, withdrawal, and behavioural change resulting in a psychiatric referral. Suicidal ideation is, however, infrequent and response to antidepressants poor. Delusions, which are complex and unsustained, are common. Other features include emotional lability, aggression, insomnia, and auditory and visual hallucinations. Dysaesthesiae, or pain in the limbs or face, which was persistent rather than intermittent and unrelated to anxiety levels is a frequent early feature, sometimes prompting referral to a rheumatologist. A minority of cases have early memory loss or gait ataxia but in most cases such overt neurological features are not apparent until some months later. Typically, a progressive cerebellar syndrome then develops with gait and limb ataxia followed by dementia and progression to akinetic mutism. Myoclonus is frequent and may be preceded by chorea.

No *PRNP* mutations are present in vCJD and gene analysis is important to exclude pathogenic mutations, as inherited prion

disease can present in this age group and a family history is not always apparent. The codon 129 genotype has uniformly been homozygous for methionine at *PRNP* codon 129 to date in clinical cases with the exception of a recent case thought clinically to be vCJD in an MV heterozygote,[56] although in this case neither tonsil biopsy (see following) nor autopsy was performed.

In vCJD, about 90 per cent of patients in a prospective series have high signal return from the pulvinar and medial areas of the thalamus, particularly adjacent to the ventricle, the so-called hockey stick sign. However, it is unclear when this sign develops and it is not infrequent that the initial scan is reported as normal but becomes clearly abnormal over a few months.

Ante-mortem tissue based diagnosis of vCJD can now be made by tonsil biopsy with detection of characteristic PrP immunostaining and PrPSc type.[57] It has long been recognized that prion replication, in experimentally infected animals, is first detectable in the lymphoreticular system, considerably earlier than the onset of neurological symptoms. Importantly, PrPSc is only detectable in tonsil in vCJD and not other forms of human prion disease studied. To date, tonsil biopsy has proved 100 per cent specific and sensitive for vCJD diagnosis and is well tolerated. Incidence of vCJD has been in decline since 2000; there have been no new presentations since 2010.

In 2011, the MRC Prion Unit developed a blood-based assay for vCJD termed the direct detection assay (DDA).[58] Further development of the DDA has shown high specificity; sensitivity in a blinded study was 71 per cent.[59,60] The test utilizes a capture matrix based on steel powder, followed by highly sensitive immunodetection of PrP. The test is available clinically from the National Prion Clinic in London.

Iatrogenic CJD (iCJD)

While there have been a handful of transmissions in man from neurosurgery (five cases), cortical electroencephalography (two cases), and probably corneal transplants (two cases), the two major causes of iatrogenic CJD are dural grafts and administration of contaminated human growth hormone to children. In addition, transmission of vCJD by blood transfusion has been reported, with a large number of healthy individuals potentially exposed.

Dural graft-associated CJD

There have been 196 cases of CJD following dural grafting mostly from Japan although the incidence is falling. The mean incubation period is 11 years (range 1.4–23 years). The initial symptoms are most frequently a cerebellar syndrome, especially ataxia of gait, rather than cerebral cortical symptoms, although these features ultimately occur in most cases.

Growth hormone-associated CJD

Growth hormone administration to children has resulted in a number of cases of CJD. All the cases have received hormones from pooled cadaver pituitary glands, a manufacturing process that ceased in 1985, when recombinant material became available. In the manufacturing process many hundreds or thousands of pituitaries were pooled thereby greatly increasing the chance of contamination from an infected cadaver.

The total number of cases recorded by 2006 was 194 with the majority occurring in France (107), UK (51), and USA (26). The primary diagnosis requiring hormone replacement was idiopathic growth hormone deficiency or post surgery for hypothalamic or pituitary tumours in most cases. In the UK population, the relative risk of getting iCJD from growth hormone injection was maximal at 9–10 years of age and the lifetime risk to recipients about 3 per cent. The mean incubation period worldwide, assuming a mid-point of administration as the time of infection, is 15 years (range 4–36 years). In 2012, iCJD cases due to cadaver sourced growth hormone administration continued to occur at a frequency of two to five cases per annum in the UK, indicating potentially extremely long incubation period (see kuru, following).

As growth hormone was only administered in children, the mean age of these patients is young. Patients typically present with an ataxia and subsequently develop some cortical features. The disease evolves over a period of months, death typically occurring within 12–18 months. Homozygosity at codon 129 is over-represented in these cases but interestingly, 129VV comprises the majority of the UK cases whilst in the USA and France it is 129MM. The reason for this is unclear but a plausible explanation is that in the UK, a 129VV-infected donor contaminated the product whereas in the other countries it was 129MM, a more frequent phenotype in the general population.

Blood transfusion-associated vCJD

There have been three known transmissions of vCJD infection through the use of red cell transfusion that resulted in iatrogenic vCJD, all from donors who subsequently died of the disease. The clinical syndrome was very similar to vCJD. Two cases resulted from the same blood donor and all occurred with non-leukodepleted blood.

Two additional cases of transmission of prions but not resulting in vCJD are known. One was an elderly patient who received blood from a donor who subsequently developed vCJD. She had PrPSc detectable in the lymphoreticular system and died of an unrelated cause. The other was a patient with haemophilia who had received multiple transfusions of blood products, none of which was known to come from vCJD donor, who was shown to have PrPSc in the lymphoreticular tissue but not the CNS. Interestingly the three vCJD cases were all 129MM as were the donors but the cases of asymptomatic infection the patients were both 129MV.

Kuru

Kuru is a fatal, predominantly ataxic disease confined to a remote region of Papua New Guinea. First recognized at the turn of the twentieth century, it was clearly defined by Alpers in the 1950s and subsequently shown by Gajdusek to be transmissible to other primates by intracerebral inoculation and later to other animals.

Kuru predominantly affected women and children. The disease was transmitted at cannibalistic feasts where tissues with the greatest concentration of prions (e.g. brain) were preferentially eaten by the children and females, the males older than seven years predominantly consuming muscle. The disease is a progressive ataxia and subsequent dementia developing over one to two years, the patient ultimately becoming moribund but cognitive function is preserved.

Banning cannibalistic practices has resulted in a dramatic decline in the prevalence of kuru although a few cases may still occur.

Interestingly, while the early cases were predominantly 129MM and 129VV, in the most recent examples heterozygotes are the majority some with extremely long incubation times (over 50 years). Some elderly women who atteneded cannibalistic feasts but did not get kuru possess a novel genetic resistance factor, G127V, unique to the Fore.

Treatment

There is no therapy that has been shown convincingly to alter the course of any form of prion disease. One trial of flupertine, in which a placebo was also given, claimed a beneficial effect on certain clinical scores but not mortality; this trial was small and of borderline statistical significance. The largest trial to date was PRION-1, a patient preference trial, in which quinacrine had no significant effect on survival or any clinical assessment variables. There have been a number of anecdotal reports concerning tetracycline derivatives claiming benefit but none is convincing. The glycosaminoglycan pentosan administered intraventricularly to animal models of prion disease has been shown to have a beneficial effect. It has been given to a small number of patients with a variety of types of CJD, and long survival has been described in some vCJD patients.

Administration of monoclonal antibodies or small molecules which interfere with conversion of PrPc to PrPSc have been trialled in mouse models of CJD and show some benefit if given prophylactically during the incubation period after intraperitoneal injection of prions.

Some types of symptomatic therapy have been beneficial. This particularly applies to myoclonus (levetiracetam, valproate, and clonazepam), aggression (risperidone), agiatation (diazepines), and hallucinations (centrally acting anticholinesterases). Other symptoms such as insomnia and rigidity are usually resistant to treatment with the standard agents but botulinum injection can be useful in patients with focal rigidity. Supportive therapy, including various forms of parenteral nutrition and vigorous treatment of intercurrent infections, may prolong survival but has little effect on quality-of-life measures.

Good nursing care in conjunction with symptomatic therapy and liaison with carers and relatives is essential in these diseases.

References

1. Collinge J. Prion diseases of humans and animals: their causes and molecular basis. *Annu Rev Neurosci*. 2001;24:519–50.
2. Collinge J, Whitfield J, McKintosh E, *et al*. Kuru in the 21st century—an acquired human prion disease with very long incubation periods. *Lancet*. 2006;367:2068–74.
3. Gajdusek DC, Gibbs CJ Jr, and Alpers MP. Experimental transmission of a kuru-like syndrome to chimpanzees. *Nature*. 1966;209:794–6.
4. Gibbs CJJr, Gajdusek DC, Asher DM,*et al*. Creutzfeldt–Jakob disease (spongiform encephalopathy): transmission to the chimpanzee. *Science*. 1968;161:388–9.
5. Masters CL, Gajdusek DC, and Gibbs CJ Jr. Creutzfeldt–Jakob disease virus isolations from the Gerstmann–Straussler syndrome with an analysis of the various forms of amyloid plaque deposition in the virus-induced spongiform encephalopathies. *Brain*. 1981;104:559–88.
6. Tateishi J, Brown P, Kitamoto T, *et al*. First experimental transmission of fatal familial insomnia. *Nature*. 1995;376:434–5.
7. Collinge J, Palmer MS, Sidle KCL, *et al*. Transmission of fatal familial insomnia to laboratory animals. *Lancet*. 1995;346:569–70.

8. Hill AF, Desbruslais M, Joiner S, *et al*. The same prion strain causes vCJD and BSE. *Nature*. 1997;389:448–50.

9. Bruce ME, Will RG, Ironside JW, *et al*. Transmissions to mice indicate that 'new variant' CJD is caused by the BSE agent. *Nature*. 1997;389:498–501.

10. Griffith JS. Self Replication and scrapie. Nature. 1967;215:1043–4.

11. Prusiner SB. Novel proteinaceous infectious particles cause scrapie. *Science*. 1982;216:136–44.

12. Reiniger L, Lukic A, Linehan J, *et al*. Tau, prions and A beta: the triad of neurodegeneration. *Acta Neuropathol (Berl)*. 2011;121:5–20.

13. Hardy J and Revesz T. The spread of neurodegenerative disease. *N Eng J Med*. 2012;366:2126–8.

14. Li JY, Englund E, Holton JL, *et al*. Lewy bodies in grafted neurons in subjects with Parkinson's disease suggest host-to-graft disease propagation. *Nat Med*. 2008;14:501–3.

15. Frost B, Jacks RL, and Diamond MI. Propagation of tau misfolding from the outside to the inside of a Cell. *J Biol Chem*. 2009;284:12845–52.

16. Gajdusek DC. Transmissible and non-transmissible amyloidoses: autocatalytic post-translational conversion of host precursor proteins to beta- pleated sheet configurations. *J Neuroimmunol*. 1988;20:95–110.

17. Baker HF, Ridley RM, Duchen LW,*et al*. Induction of α(A4)-amyloid in primates by injection of Alzheimer's disease brain homogenate: Comparison with transmission of spongiform encephalopathy. *Mol Neurobiol*. 1994;8:25–39.

18. Solomon A, Richey T, Murphy CL, *et al*. Amyloidogenic potential of foie gras. *Proc Natl Acad Sci USA*. 2007 Jun 26;104(26):10998–1001.

19. Sponarova J, Nystrom SN, and Westermark GT. AA-amyloidosis can be transferred by peripheral blood monocytes. *PLoS One*. 2008;3:e3308.

20. Meyer-Luehmann M, Coomaraswamy J, Bolmont T, *et al*. Exogenous induction of cerebral beta-amyloidogenesis is governed by agent and host. *Science*. 2006;313:1781–4.

21. Walker LC, LeVine H, III, Mattson MP, *et al*. Inducible proteopathies. *Trends Neurosci*. 2006 Aug;29(8):438–43.

22. McGowan JP. Scrapie in sheep. *Scott J Agric*. 1922;5:365–75.

23. Cuillé J and Chelle PL. La maladie dite tremblante du mouton est-elle inoculable? *C R Acad Sci*. 1936;203:1552–4.

24. Hadlow WJ. Scrapie and kuru. *Lancet*. 1959;ii:289–90.

25. Spielmeyer W. Die histopathologische Forschung in der Psychiatrie. *Klin Wochenschrift*. 1922;2:1817–9.

26. Brown P, Cathala F, Raubertas RF, *et al*. The epidemiology of Creutzfeldt–Jakob disease: conclusion of a 15-year investigation in France and review of the world literature. *Neurology*. 1987;37:895–904.

27. Collins S, Law MG, Fletcher A, *et al*. Surgical treatment and risk of sporadic Creutzfeldt–Jakob disease: a case-control study. *Lancet*. 1999;353:693–7.

28. Mahillo-Fernandez I, Pedro-Cuesta J, *et al*. Surgery and risk of sporadic Creutzfeldt–Jakob disease in Denmark and Sweden: registry-based case-control studies. *Neuroepidemiology*. 2008;31:229–40.

29. Owen F, Poulter M, Lofthouse R, *et al*. Insertion in prion protein gene in familial Creutzfeldt–Jakob disease. *Lancet*. 1989;1:51–2.

30. Hsiao K, Baker HF, Crow TJ, *et al*. Linkage of a prion protein missense variant to Gerstmann–Strauss syndrome. *Nature*. 1989;338:342–5.

31. Collinge J, Palmer MS, and Dryden AJ. Genetic predisposition to iatrogenic Creutzfeldt–Jakob disease. *Lancet*. 1991;337:1441–2.

32. Palmer MS, Dryden AJ, Hughes JT,*et al*. Homozygous prion protein genotype predisposes to sporadic Creutzfeldt–Jakob disease. *Nature*. 1991;352:340–2.

33. Baker HE, Poulter M, Crow TJ, *et al*. Amino acid polymorphism in human prion protein and age at death in inherited prion disease (letter). *Lancet*. 1991;337:1286.

34. Hsiao K, Dlouhy SR, Farlow MR, *et al*. Mutant prion proteins in Gerstmann–Sträussler–Sheinker disease with neurofibrillary tangles. *Nature Genet*. 1992;1:68–71.

35. Poulter M, Baker HF, Frith CD,*et al*. Inherited prion disease with 144 base pair gene insertion: I: Genealogical and molecular studies. *Brain*. 1992;115:675–85.

36. Collinge J, Sidle KC, Meads J, *et al*. Molecular analysis of prion strain variation and the aetiology of 'new variant' CJD. Nature. 1996;383:685–90.

37. Collinge J. Variant Creutzfeldt–Jakob disease. *Lancet*. 1999;354:317–23.

38. Pattison IH. Experiments with scrapie with special reference to the nature of the agent and the pathology of the disease. In: CJ Gajdusek, CJ Gibbs, and MP Alpers (eds). *Slow, Latent and Temperate Virus Infections*. NINDB Monograph 2. Washington, DC: US Government Printing, 1965, pp. 249–57.

39. Prusiner SB, Scott M, Foster D, *et al*. Transgenetic studies implicate interactions between homologous PrP isoforms in scrapie prion replication. *Cell*. 1990;63:673–86.

40. Bruce M, Chree A, McConnell I, *et al*. Transmission of bovine spongiform encephalopathy and scrapie to mice: Strain variation and the species barrier. *Philos T Roy Soc B*. 1994;343:405–11.

41. Hill AF and Collinge J. Subclinical prion infection. *Trends Microbiol*. 2003;11:578–84.

42. Hill AF, Joiner S, Linehan J, *et al*. Species barrier independent prion replication in apparently resistant species. *Proc Natl Acad Sci USA*. 2000;97:10248–53.

43. Collinge J, Clarke A. A general model of prion strains and their pathogenicity. *Science*. 2007;318:930–6.

44. Brandner S, Isenmann S, Raeber A, *et al*. Normal host prion protein necessary for scrapie-induced neurotoxicity. *Nature*. 1996;379:339–43.

45. Hsich G, Kenney K, Gibbs CJ, Jr, *et al* The 14-3-3 brain protein in cerebrospinal fluid as a marker for transmissible spongiform encephalopathies. *N Engl J Med*. 1996;335:924–30.

46. Riemenschneider M, Wagenpfeil S, Vanderstichele H, *et al*. Phospho-tau/total tau ratio in cerebrospinal fluid discriminates Creutzfeldt-Jakob disease from other dementias. *Mol Psychiatry*. 2003;8:343–7.

47. McGuire LI, Peden AH, Orru CD, *et al*. Real time quaking-induced conversion analysis of cerebrospinal fluid in sporadic Creutzfeldt-Jakob disease. *Ann Neurol*. 2012;72:278–85.

48. Collinge J, Brown J, Hardy J, *et al*. Inherited prion disease with 144 base pair gene insertion: II: Clinical and pathological features. *Brain*. 1992;115:687–710.

49. Mead S, Poulter M, Beck J, *et al*. Inherited prion disease with six octapeptide repeat insertional mutation—molecular analysis of phenotypic heterogeneity. *Brain*. 2006;129:2297–317.

50. Webb TE, Poulter M, Beck J, *et al*. Phenotypic heterogeneity and genetic modification of P102L inherited prion disease in an international series. *Brain*. 2008;131:2632–46.

51. Tranchant C, Sergeant N, Wattez A, *et al*. Neurofibrillary tangles in Gerstmann–Sträussler–Scheinker syndrome with the A117V prion gene mutation. *J Neurol Neurosur Ps*. 1997;63:240–6.

52. Mallucci G, Campbell TA, Dickinson A, *et al*. Inherited prion disease with an alanine to valine mutation at codon 117 in the prion protein gene. *Brain*. 1999;122:1823–37.

53. Goldfarb LG, Korczyn AD, Brown P, *et al*. Mutation in codon 200 of scrapie amyloid precursor gene linked to Creutzfeldt–Jakob disease in Sephardic Jews of Libyan and non- Libyan origin. *Lancet*. 1990;336:637–8.

54. Tabrizi S, Scaravilli F, Howard RS, *et al*.Creutzfeldt–Jakob disease in a young woman. Report of a Meeting of Physicians and Scientists, St. Thomas' Hospital, London. *Lancet*. 1996;347:945–8.

55. Gore SM. More than happenstance: Creutzfeldt–Jakob disease in farmers and young adults. *BMJ*. 1995;311:1416–8.

56. Kaski D, Mead S, Hyare H, *et al.* Variant CJD in an individual heterozygous for PRNP codon 129. *Lancet.* 2009;374:2128.

57. Hill AF, Zeidler M, Ironside J, *et al.* Diagnosis of new variant Creutzfeldt–Jakob disease by tonsil biopsy. *Lancet.* 1997;349:99–100.

58. Edgeworth JA, Farmer M, Sicilia A, *et al.* Detection of prion infection in variant Creutzfeldt–Jakob disease: a blood-based assay. *Lancet.* 2011;377:487–93.

59. Jackson GS, Burk-Rafel J, Edgeworth JA, *et al.* A highly specific blood test for vCJD. *Blood.* 2014;123:452–3.

60. Jackson GS, Burk-Rafel J, Edgeworth JA, *et al.* Population Screening for Variant Creutzfeldt–Jakob Disease Using a Novel Blood Test: Diagnostic Accuracy and Feasibility Study. *JAMA Neurol.* 2014 Apr;71(4):421–8.

CHAPTER 39

Traumatic brain injury

David J. Sharp, Simon Fleminger, and Jane Powell

Epidemiology

Traumatic brain injury (TBI) is indicated by the combination of head trauma followed by neurological, cognitive, and behavioural or emotional sequelae. It is a common cause of death and disability worldwide.[1,2] There are an estimated 1.7 million TBIs annually in the United States, Of these, about 1.3 million are treated in emergency departments, 300 000 are hospitalized, and around 50 000 die.[2] Patients who survive are often left with long-lasting disability, with enormous social and economic costs.[1] Across Europe, the total direct and indirect costs of moderate/severe TBI in 2010 were estimated to be €33 billion.[1] In the UK, direct costs are around £1 billion/year, with substantial indirect costs increasing the overall economic impact of moderate and severe TBI to around £5 billion per year.[1] TBI rates are highest in men, as well as in young children (0–4 yrs), older adolescents (15–19), and older adults (> 65 yrs).[2] In the civilian population of the US, the commonest causes of TBI are falls (35 per cent), motor vehicle accidents (17 per cent), and assaults (10 per cent),[2] and in recent military conflicts, exposure to explosive devices has become a common cause.[3]

The clinical effects of a TBI can be devastating, and the persistent effects are often under-recognized. Many problems are due to a combination of cognitive, affective, and behavioural disturbances.[4,5] These can often be interrelated and may be produced by a common underlying pathology. The social impact of these impairments can be catastrophic. For example, a recent study of the homeless in one large UK city found that 50 per cent of homeless individuals had previously had a significant TBI, 90 per cent of which had occurred prior to them becoming homeless.[6] Similarly, high levels of TBI are present in prison populations and the resulting behavioural problems appear to be a major factor in determining patterns of re-offending.[7]

Pathophysiology and neuroimaging of TBI

Understanding cognitive impairments after TBI requires a detailed investigation of the patterns of brain injury produced by trauma, and how these relate to cognition. The pathology can be directly caused by the initial injury but can also evolve over time, either due to recovery processes or the evolution of late effects such as neurodegeneration and persistent inflammation (Fig. 39.1). This creates a complex set of factors, which contribute over time to cognitive and psychiatric impairments.

Two main mechanisms of acute injury are thought to be important: direct contact and acceleration/deceleration. Direct injuries result from an object striking the head or the brain striking the inside of the skull. Alternatively, indirect injury can result from rapid acceleration and deceleration, which impart shear, tensile, and compressive strains that mainly damage long-distance white matter connections by producing diffuse axonal injury. Primary injuries include skull fractures, intracranial haematoma, and diffuse axonal injury.[8] Secondary damage is produced by processes that are triggered by the initial injury, including ischaemia, raised intracranial pressure, infection, and inflammation. Primary and secondary injuries interact to produce a complex pattern of damage that evolves over time.

Focal injury

Damage after head injury can be classified as focal or diffuse (Table 39.1). Focal injuries commonly result in intracerebral, extradural, and subdural haematomas, which if large enough produce significant elevations in intracranial pressure. These abnormalities are easily diagnosed with computed tomography (CT) imaging. When neurosurgery is required and performed in a timely fashion, patients often make a very good recovery. Haematomas within the brain substance are also common and these have a complex relationship with persistent cognitive impairment. Focal injuries of this type are most commonly observed in the orbitofrontal, temporal pole and occipital regions.[9] These often are the result of a coup/contra-coup injury; for example, a blow to the occipital region after falling backwards produces the 'coup'. The 'contra-coup' produces contusions in the orbitofrontal cortex and temporal poles and results from the impact of the brain on the internal bony

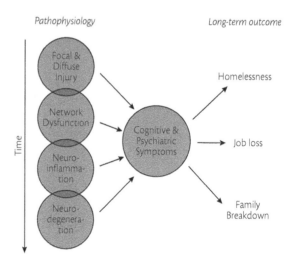

Fig. 39.1 The interaction between pathophysiology, cognitive impairment, and long-term outcome after traumatic brain injury.

Table 39.1 Types of damage after head injury

Focal	Diffuse
Scalp injury	Diffuse traumatic axonal injury
Skull fracture	Hypoxic ischaemic injury
Extradural epidural haematoma	Infection meningitis/encephalitis
Subdural haematoma	Vascular injury arterial/venous
Subarachnoid haemorrhage	Raised intracranial pressure
Intracerebral/intracerebellar haematoma	

surfaces of the skull, including the sphenoid ridge and tentorium cerebelli.[10]

Diffuse injury

There is often a rather poor correlation between the pattern of focal injury and the nature of cognitive impairment observed after TBI.[10] Patients with clear focal injuries sometimes have little if any cognitive impairment, whereas patients with no gross abnormalities may be severely affected. This contrasts with stroke where a clearer mapping between the location of focal brain injury (the infarct) and cognitive dysfunction (the stroke syndrome) is often observed. The presence of diffuse (traumatic) axonal injury (DAI) explains some of this discrepancy. It is commonly seen after TBI but has been difficult to demonstrate specifically with conventional neuroimaging (Fig. 39.2). DAI appears to be a key determinant of persistent cognitive impairment after TBI[11,12] and produces damage to long-distance axonal connections, which are vulnerable to the biomechanical forces produced by TBI.[13,14] In extreme cases, mechanical stress at the time of impact results in axonal shearing. More commonly, axons remain intact but damage to the axolemma around the nodes of ranvier is observed, as well as to neurofilament subunits disrupting axonal transport.

Standard CT and magnetic resonance imaging (MRI) does not demonstrate DAI with sensitivity or specificity, but recent imaging advances have allowed the location and severity of DAI to be identified more clearly.[16] Microbleeds—detectable using susceptibility-weighted MR imaging available on most clinical scanners—are thought to provide a surrogate marker signifying the presence of underlying DAI, but may also signify diffuse vascular injury. Diffusion MRI provides a more sensitive way of assessing the structure of white matter,[17] and of quantifying the location and amount of damage to particular white matter tracts Fig. 39.3.[18] For some types of cognitive impairment there is a relatively straightforward mapping between the location of white matter injury and the type of cognitive impairment. For example, the degree of abnormality of the fornix has been shown to correlate with memory impairment.[11] Diffusion MRI measurements of white matter damage also provide prognostic information that complements standard clinical measures,[19] and can be used to predict cognitive function in individual patients.[12] Currently diffusion MRI is mainly used in the research setting, but it has great potential as a clinical tool, particularly to identify the presence of subtle DAI not visible on conventional imaging.

Neuromodulatory neurotransmitter abnormalities

The cognitive effects of TBI are mediated in part by disruption to neuromodulatory neurotransmitter systems such as dopamine,

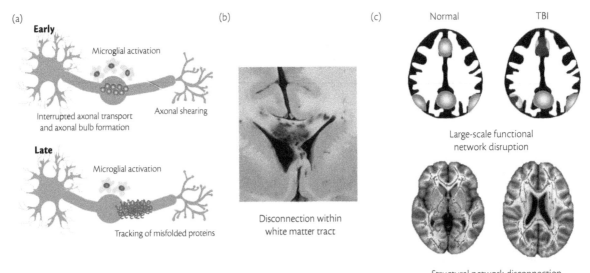

Fig. 39.2 Effects of diffuse axonal injury DAI across spatial scales. (a) Early: at the microscopic scale, diffuse axonal injury can interrupt axonal transport, produce axonal bulbs, and trigger neuroinflammation through microglial activation. Late: these abnormalities can eventually lead to neurodegeneration and persistent neuroinflammation, which might be associated with the abnormal diffusion tracking of misfolded neurodegenerative proteins along axons. (b) At the macroscopic scale, injuries are readily apparent in large white matter tracts on neuropathological examination. Diffuse axonal injury preferentially damages certain white matter tracts, such as the corpus callosum—seen here in a postmortem specimen with black regions of haemorrhage, indicative of underlying damage. (c) At the whole-brain scale, damage to tracts interrupts long-distance communication between brain regions. Damage to white matter tracts is illustrated here as reduced fractional anisotropy red regions within a white matter skeleton. This white matter damage can disrupt interactions between nodes of a brain network, represented here as reduced interactions between nodes in one intrinsic connectivity network, the default mode network red/yellow regions.

Adapted from *Nature Neurol.* 10, Sharp DJ, *et al.* Network dysfunction after traumatic brain injury, pp. 156–166, Copyright 2014, with permission from Nature Publishing Group; Courtesy of DP Agamanolis, http://neuropathology-web.org

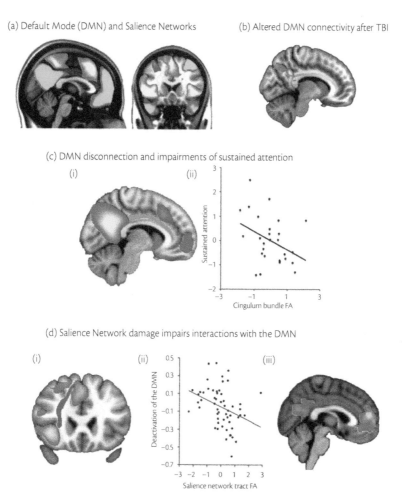

Fig. 39.3 Network abnormalities after TBI. (a) Intrinsic connectivity networks ICNs identified using functional MRI: Default mode network (DMN) in blue and salience network (SN) in red/yellow. These networks often show anti-correlated activity. This is particularly apparent when attention is externally focused, leading to increased SN and decreased DMN activity. (b) Abnormal DMN functional connectivity from the posterior cingulate cortex to the rest of the DMN red/yellow, seen at 'rest' after TBI 30. (c) Damage to the structural connectivity of the DMN predicts sustained attention impairment. (i) The right cingulum bundle green connects anterior and posterior nodes of the DMN, and (ii) damage to this tract measured by reduced fractional anisotropy (FA) correlates with impairments of sustained attention, here measured as reaction time RT change over the course of a choice-reaction time task 27. (d) Damage to the white matter connections of the SN predicts a failure to appropriately deactivate the DMN when cognitive control is required 28. (i) Activation within the SN during successful stopping on the stop signal task is shown in red. The white matter tract connecting these regions is shown in blue. (ii) The correlation between SN tract integrity and DMN deactivation when successfully stopping on the stop signal task. (iii) Brain regions where transient deactivations associated with cognitive control are correlated with SN tract integrity.

acetylcholine, and noradrenaline. Nuclei within the brainstem and basal forebrain appear particularly vulnerable, and DAI may damage their long-distance projections. Catecholamines such as dopamine and noradrenaline influence the cognitive functions typically impaired by TBI, and striatal dopamine dysfunction has been demonstrated using single photon emission computed tomography (SPECT) imaging.[20,21] It has been proposed that the resulting hypo-dopaminergic state produces a specific pattern of cognitive impairments[22] which are distinct from those found in the hypocholinergic state seen after damage to the basal forebrain.[23] Identifying these neurotransmitter abnormalities has practical importance because drugs acting on these systems are available (see treatment section, following).

Network dysfunction

Many of the cognitive impairments seen after TBI cannot be explained merely by considering the functioning of individual brain regions, in part because cognitive functions such as attention and memory require efficient interactions between spatially distinct brain regions.[24] In fact, many aspects of cognitive dysfunction after TBI can be usefully thought of as disorders of brain connectivity, and it is informative to consider the effect of TBI on brain networks.[15] Recent advances in neuroimaging allow both the structure and function of large-scale brain networks to be studied. These networks can be defined by identifying brain regions that show shared functional activity.[15] Large-scale intrinsic connectivity networks (ICNs) have been defined in this way, where coordinated activity is seen across diverse states of behaviour (Fig. 39.3a).[25,26] The interactions of nodes in these ICNs depend on the integrity of highly organized white matter connections. Therefore, DAI may produce cognitive impairment by disrupting connections between nodes in the networks.[27,28] In severe cases this can lead to prolonged impairments of conscious level.[29] More subtle injuries partially disconnect the networks, producing predictable patterns of persistent cognitive impairment.[27,28,30]

Neurodegeneration

TBI is often considered as a static insult but there is compelling evidence that it can trigger neurodegeneration as a late effect.[31] Patients with TBI can unexpectedly deteriorate many years after injury,[32] and show higher than expected rates of Alzheimer's disease AD, Parkinson's Disease, and chronic traumatic encephalopathy (CTE).[33-35] Repetitive mild TBI can lead to CTE, but a single significant injury such as a road traffic accident or exposure to a bomb blast can also predispose individuals to late cognitive decline including AD and CTE.[36-38] Interactions with genetic factors may increase an individual's susceptibility to neurodegeneration. For example, the risk of developing AD[39] and Parkinson's disease[35] is related to apolipoprotein E (APOE) and α-synuclein genotypes respectively. The interaction between the initial injury, protein misfolding, and chronic neuroinflammation appear important in determining how neurodegenerative pathology develops after TBI (Fig. 39.2).[40,41] These observations suggest a prolonged, dynamic element to the pathophysiology of TBI, mediated by an individual's genetic predisposition.

The prevalence of progressive neurodegeneration after TBI is unknown. Recently there has been a resurgence of interest in the link between the repetitive mild TBIs, for example associated with sporting or military activity, and CTE (previously termed dementia puglistica).[34,38] Studies have typically focused on the neuropathological investigation of a relatively small number of such cases (<200). They have shown a characteristic distribution of neurodegenerative changes, in particular hyperphosphorylated tau, in the brains of young people exposed to repeated head injury.[34] This work reinforces the link between head injury and neurodegeneration, but it is currently not clear what the prevalence of CTE is in populations exposed to repeated head injuries, how the 'dose' of head injury relates to the likelihood of developing neurodegeneration, or whether CTE has a distinct cognitive or psychiatric phenotype. It is thus difficult for individuals and their families to make well-informed decisions about the risks of participating in risky leisure or work-based activities. Large-scale longitudinal studies are required to determine the prevalence and characteristics of the various dementia syndromes seen after TBI accurately.

Cognitive impairment

Although the pathophysiology of TBI can be highly variable, there is a characteristic profile of cognitive impairment after TBI, with deficits most commonly seen in the domains of awareness, processing speed, memory, attention, and executive function.[42-46] These cognitive problems not only compromise day-to-day functioning but present challenges to rehabilitation.

Awareness

TBI frequently produces loss of consciousness. In severe cases this can last weeks or months, and may develop into persistent vegetative or minimally conscious states (PVS and MCS).[29] DAI appears to be particularly relevant to the duration of impaired consciousness. It is almost universally present in cases of fatal brain injury[47] and has a characteristic distribution in severe cases where widespread damage is normally seen in the corpus callosum and brainstem.[13] In cases of PVS, the structure of the cortex can appear intact despite marked functional abnormality, whereas damage to the subcortical white matter and/or the thalamic relay nuclei are usually seen.[29] Recent theories of consciousness emphasize the importance of cortico–cortico synchronization coordinated through frontoparietal white matter tracts.[48] This can be disrupted by TBI, resulting in the disconnection of 'hub' regions that support information exchange, such as the posterior cingulate cortex.[49,50] Electro-encephalographic measures of functional connectivity and information exchange can be used to discriminate between patients in different conscious states after TBI,[51] and the willful control of brain activity measured using functional MRI shows promise as a way to clarify conscious level and potentially to communicate with 'locked-in' patients.[52] Impairments of awareness can persist long after injury, with patients often exhibiting impaired self-awareness.[53] This can limit recovery and attempts at rehabilitation and is associated with dysfunction within the salience network—a frontal ICN.[54]

Information-processing speed

TBI patients often complain of slowed thinking, and this is confirmed by slow and variable processing speeds on behavioural indices such as choice reaction times and by simple colour-naming or word-reading scores in the Stroop task.[11,55] Although processing speed influences more complex cognitive functions, it does not completely explain deficits in other domains.[56] Processing speed correlates with the amount of overall white matter injury, but does not usually show a correlation with damage to individual tracts.[11,12]

Attention

Impairments of attention are often present, including deficits in divided, selective, and sustained attention.[57,58] These can manifest as moment-to-moment fluctuations in vigilance *level*, or as a decline in attention paid over time: vigilance *decrement*.[27,59] The latter appears to be particularly sensitive to the effects of brain injury, with lapses in attention producing increased variability in responses as vigilance level declines. These attentional problems can interact to produce highly variable behaviour. Impairments in sustained attention can be sensitively measured by tasks such as the sustained attention to response task (SART).[58] Patients show a failure of attentional control as automatic responding replaces controlled processing. This results in inappropriate responses, which are accompanied by a failure of the α-wave desynchonization that normally accompanies attention control.[60]

Tasks that require an external focus of attention, including most neuropsychological tests, are accompanied by a highly reproducible reduction in activity within the default mode network (DMN) (Fig. 39.3a), with the degree of deactivation increasing with task difficulty.[61] Lapses of attention in healthy individuals are associated with an absence of this task-dependent DMN deactivation.[62] DMN functional connectivity is abnormal after TBI (Fig. 39.3b),[30] and patients with high vigilance decrement show reduced control over DMN activity and damage to structural connections within the DMN (Fig. 39.3c). This is accompanied by a reduction in the functional connectivity of the DMN that predicts the behavioural impairment.[27] Together these results suggest that impairments of sustained attention after TBI are produced by a failure of DMN control, which appears to be a feature of cognitive impairment across a range of disease states, notably Alzheimer's disease.[63]

Executive function

Impairments of executive functions are commonly seen, and include deficits in working memory (holding information 'in mind' for short periods of time), planning, and inhibitory control (the ability to suppress reflexive cognitive and emotional responses). These often combine to cause significant disability, although the impairments themselves can sometimes be difficult to quantify using standard neuropsychological assessments. Patients often have particular problems in completing tasks with multiple competing sub-goals because of the inefficient application of strategies.[64] This is exemplified by difficulties with tasks like the multiple errands test, which involves following competing rules in a real-world setting (Fig. 39.4).

Executive impairments are usually associated with frontal lobe damage as demonstrated by the case Phineas Gage, where a railroad explosion caused bilateral damage to the prefrontal cortices.[65] Phineas made a remarkable physical recovery but was left with dramatic personality and behavioural changes. The degree to which the 'central' executive system responsible for supporting executive

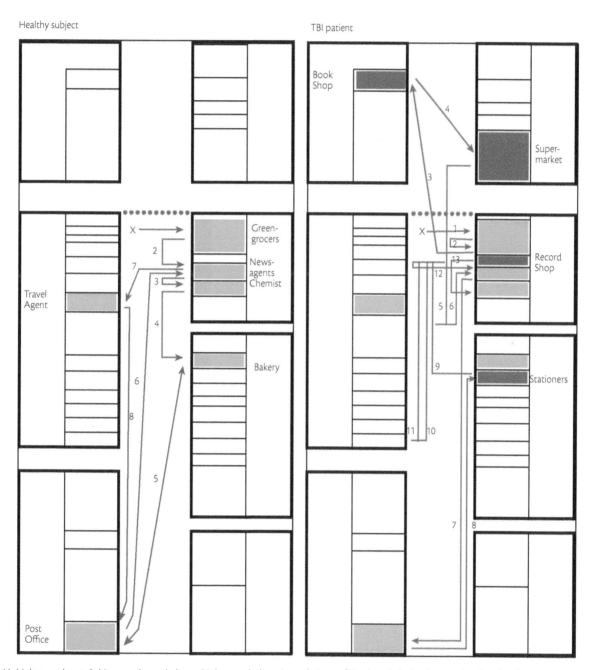

Fig. 39.4 Multiple errands test. Subjects under took the multiple errands shopping task. A set of simple tasks had to be completed, such as buying a newspaper, without breaking any of a set of rules. For example, the dotted line across the street towards the top of the page represents a point beyond which the patients are explicitly told NOT to go. Subjects needed to go into the shops in green, but were not required to go into the shops in red. The performances of a healthy control (left) and a brain-injured patient (right) are illustrated. 'X' indicates the starting point of the test and the numbers indicate the order of subject movements. The patient's dysexecutive problems were not readily measured using formal tests of executive function. As can be seen from the figure, the patient was less efficient doing the task and broke more rules.

Courtesy of Professor Paul Burgess and adapted from David A, Fleminger S, Kopelman M, *et al. Lishman's Organic Psychiatry: A Textbook of Neuropsychiatry*, 4th edn. Copyright 2012, with permission from John Wiley and Sons.

functions can be fractionated into distinct anatomical components is controversial. One theory proposes a single frontoparietal 'multiple demand system' that flexibly supports the assembly of subgoals into complex goal-directed behaviour.[66,67] According to this theory, neural activity within a large frontoparietal system is related to task complexity rather than distinct cognitive processing. In contrast, a detailed analysis of the relationship between lesion location and cognitive function in patients with frontal lobe injury from a variety of causes provides evidence for anatomically and functional independent attentional control processes.[68] It is proposed that superior medial frontal regions support the 'energization' of mental activity, left lateral frontal regions support attentional task setting that generates stimulus response mappings in novel situations, and right lateral frontal regions support monitoring and the signalling of anomalies or unexpected events.

Recent work also demonstrates the importance of network connections between frontal regions for efficient executive function. Impairments of attentional control and motor inhibition have been studied experimentally using tasks such as the stop signal task.[28] TBI patients show impairments of motor control that are related to the degree of damage to the white matter connecting superior medial and right lateral frontal nodes within a frontal ICN, the salience network (SN). The SN and DMN often show coupled and anti-correlated activity (Fig. 39.3a). TBI patients with impairments of response inhibition show abnormal structural connections of the salience network which are strongly associated with a failure of DMN control (Fig. 39.3d).[15,28,69] This illustrates the importance of brain network interactions for efficient cognition, showing how frontal damage can disrupt the network interactions that underlie the moment-to-moment changes in cognitive control which are necessary for efficient behaviour.

Memory

The early period after TBI is often characterized by marked episodic memory dysfunction, with patients usually experiencing a period of post-traumatic amnesia (PTA) during which new memories are not encoded (Box 39.1 and Fig. 39.5). Thus, patients with a significant head injury rarely recall experiencing it or the circumstances in which it occurred. Ongoing PTA is characterized by pronounced impairments of orientation and memory and these are often associated with less obvious deficits in attention, processing speed, and executive function. Other cognitive functions, such as language, often remain intact, so that impairments may not be apparent to the untrained observer. PTA is of variable duration, often ending quite abruptly. It may last for seconds or minutes, but can extend for many days or weeks. Its duration is a significant predictor of long-term functional outcomes, and it is widely used as an indicator of the severity of the brain injury. Formal assessment of PTA should form part of standard TBI care: in addition to its uses for severity classification and prognostication, it is important for determining when a patient is safe to discharge. Validated clinical tools are available for assessing PTA prospectively,[70,71] but when PTA has not been assessed at the time of injury its duration can be reasonably well estimated via a retrospective assessment where the point at which continuous memories start to be formed is estimated by asking patients to recall events in the post-traumatic period.[72] The pathophysiology of PTA is poorly understood, and there does not seem to be a clear relationship with the location of gross structural brain injury.[73] As memory formation depends on hippocampal

---

Box 39.1 Case 1

A 34-year-old was assaulted after trying to intervene in a mugging. He was punched and kicked, sustaining a head injury when he fell to the ground. He has no memory for the attack, and had retrograde amnesia for a few seconds prior to the assault. He was admitted to a major trauma centre. His initial CT imaging performed shortly after arrival in A&E showed bifrontal and bitemporal haemorrhagic contusions, subarachnoid haemorrhage, a shallow subdural haematoma with midline shift, and an occipital fracture (Fig. 39.5). He did not require neurosurgery, but went on to have six weeks of agitation and PTA. He spent two months on an inpatient neurorehabilitation ward, and received cognitive rehabilitation and occupational therapy. He made good progress although his therapy was hampered by self-awareness impairment.

Follow-up MRI four months after his injury showed post-contusional gliotic damage mainly in the left temporal pole and left inferior frontal cortex, including the orbitofrontal cortex. There were also a small number of microhaemorrhages, suggestive of underlying diffuse axonal injury, and extensive superficial siderosis over the left hemisphere, the residual effect of haemorrhage.

His cognitive problems continued after discharge. He had particular problems with memory, finding it difficult to remember new information and recall the names of friends and relatives. He also found it difficult to plan trips when leaving the house and to concentrate for long periods. He had a range of other problems that were prominent in the first months after injury. He was generally anxious, although was not clearly suffering from PTSD. He was anosmic, and had high-tone hearing loss on the left. He had evidence of growth hormone deficiency, which was treated with growth hormone injections, and had had persistent dizziness, with features of benign paroxysmal positional vertigo.

He made a graded return to work after around six months. He had significant problems in the following year at work, with recurrent episodes of sick leave and difficulty communicating with colleagues. These problems were compounded by a return to episodes of binge drinking that had been an issue prior to the injury. He was no longer able to cope as well with this level of alcohol intake, which led to absences from work. Four years later he was still in full-time employment and had made a successful transition to a new job. He has never completely returned to 'normal', but is leading a full and active life.

---

interactions with different brain regions, a functional but reversible disconnection of the hippocampus from these networks is likely to play a role.

PTA is associated with neuropsychiatric problems, including anosognosia (impaired insight or self-awareness of problems), which is often associated with amnesia, disorientation and confabulation (Box 39.2).[74] Delusional misidentifications are common. These often manifest in unfamiliar objects being invested with a sense of familiarity. Patients sometimes show the 'Fregoli delusion', believing that somebody well known to them is dressing up and impersonating other people.[75] Patients may also feel that their hospital has been mislocated to somewhere that has strong emotional memories for them (reduplicative paramnesia).[76] These early confabulatory/delusional states are often associated with abnormalities

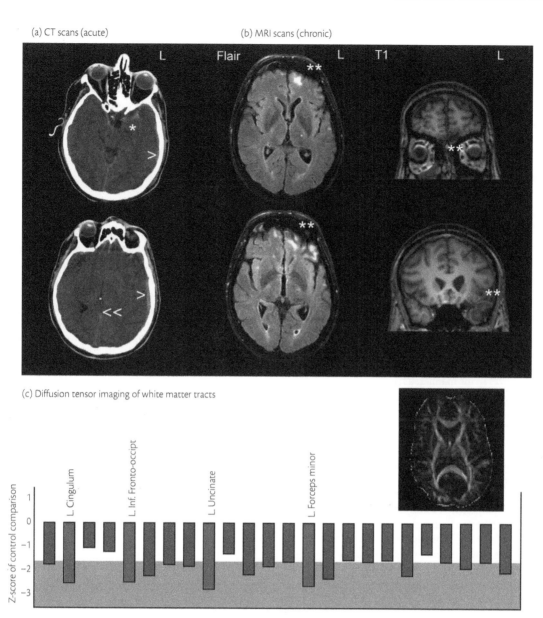

(a) CT scans (acute)

(b) MRI scans (chronic)

(c) Diffusion tensor imaging of white matter tracts

Fig. 39.5 Neuroimaging case 1. (a) CT scan in the acute phase showing haemorrhagic contusion *, shallow subdural haematoma > and midline shift <<. (b) T1 and FLAIR MRI scans in the chronic phase showing predominantly left-sided post-traumatic gliotic change in the inferior frontal lobe and temporal pole **. (c) Diffusion tensor imaging DTI assessment of white matter structure. The graph shows Z-scores for the comparison of fractional anisotropy (FA) in each tract between the patient and controls. The central white area denotes the area of Z < 1.64 p > 0.01 for the control groups FA. Red bars indicate where that tract's FA value was >2.3 standard deviations from the control group mean. This provides evidence for marked left hemisphere tract damage within the left cingulum bundle, left fronto-occipital fasciculus, left uncinate fasciculus, and left forceps minor. The inset shows an illustration of DTI data, where the colour represents the predominant direction of water diffusion.

of mood such that the patient is initially upbeat, being oblivious to their disability. As insight improves, elevated mood often changes to one of depression, a phenomenon seen more generally in the recovery process.[77]

Persistent memory impairments are often observed after TBI, beyond the period at which PTA has resolved.[43] In particular, patients often present with difficulties in remembering specific events (episodic memory), with assimilating and/or retrieving new information to which they have been exposed recently, and with remembering to perform a planned action or intention at the appropriate time ('prospective' memory). Memory difficulties are often associated with, and exacerbated by, attentional and executive dysfunction. This common combination of impairments can have

particularly severe impacts on the patient's daily functioning and it poses a major challenge for rehabilitation.[78]

Injury severity and cognitive outcome

TBI severity is an important determinant of long-term outcome. This is conventionally classified as mild, moderate, or severe, as indicated by durations of loss of consciousness or post-traumatic amnesia (PTA; >24 hours indicates a moderate or severe injury), or by the lowest recorded Glasgow Coma Scale (GCS) score. The GCS is a standardized assessment of consciousness level, based on clinical assessment of motor, verbal, and eye-opening functions.[79] It has considerable clinical utility and is very widely used, but it is not a sensitive tool for detecting specific cognitive impairments[70]

Box 39.2 Case 2

A 28-year-old man was found wandering and confused. CT brain scanning showed severe bilateral frontal contusions, worse on the left and involving the orbitofrontal cortex. He was disorientated and agitated for several days. He then developed a delusional state: for about two weeks he had a persistent belief that he was building a space rocket. He also had a confabulatory memory of having walked into town, when in fact he had not left the ward. Later he absconded from hospital to return home and get tools in order to build his rocket. He was assertive and upbeat in his mood.

This confabulatory delusional state resolved spontaneously, but for several weeks he was agitated, denying he had had problems and demanding to be allowed home. By this time he was by and large orientated, but his memory was unreliable and occupational therapy assessment found that he was disorganized on a shopping task. He was placed on a section of the Mental Health Act. By about two months post injury he was much more settled and discharged home.

He was reviewed in outpatients four months after injury. At this stage he was working as a painter and decorator, although under supervision. On examination, his mood was now subdued and he was rather quiet in his manner; a friend reported that this was much more like his usual self. He admitted that his memory was not as good as it used to be and that he needed a little help at work.

and is limited in its ability to predict long-term outcome.[80] Both GCS scores and PTA duration are predictors of functional recovery by the time of hospital discharge,[81,82] and also of community integration and/or employment several years later.[83,84] PTA duration is better than GCS at predicting the persistence of cognitive impairments a year after TBI,[85] although the correlation with any particular aspect of cognitive functioning is modest.

There are important limitations to the standard approach of classifying TBI severity using clinical measures alone. The information needed is often either unavailable or is of uncertain value;[86] for example, the interpretation of changes in conscious level and cognitive function may be confounded by the presence of medical sedation, paralysis or intoxication. As a result, it is sensible to consider other information, particularly neuroimaging and the presence or absence of ongoing symptoms. One system incorporates this information to classify injury severity as (i) moderate/severe (definite) TBI, (ii) mild (probable) TBI, and (iii) symptomatic (possible) TBI (see Table 39.1).[86] This approach has the advantage of distinguishing subcategories within the large group of patients traditionally classified as 'mild' TBI, and it also acknowledges the fact that moderate and severe injuries can in some ways be viewed as a more homogenous category for the purposes of many clinical management decisions.

Cognitive impairment is generally worst shortly after TBI, and its duration varies depending on the severity of the brain injury. One large meta-analysis demonstrated early cognitive impairment in both mild and moderate/severe TBI.[4] Significant impairment was still present more than two years after injury in the moderate/severe group. By contrast, the mild group as a whole had largely returned to normal by three months. Although the cognitive outcome

of mild TBI is generally benign, a significant minority of these patients develop persistent symptoms, and in some patients long-term outcome can be surprisingly poor. For example, one careful prospective study of a group of patients of all severities injured in Glasgow shows increased mortality and late clinical deterioration, including in patients who were thought initially to have had only 'mild' TBI.[5,87]

Concussion

Concussion is widely used to describe the effects of minor head injury. It is used most commonly in relation to sporting injury.[88] Here it is usually defined as a distinct subset of TBI that results in 'functional disturbance' in the absence of abnormality on conventional CT or MRI. A general assumption is that the neurological dysfunction associated with concussion will be short-lived, usually in the region of minutes, as is commonly observed with most sporting injuries.

Whilst it has been proposed that concussion is distinct from mild TBI,[88] this is controversial and problematic. First, the symptoms and signs of concussion, including headache, cognitive impairment, emotional lability, loss of consciousness, and sleep disturbance, overlap completely with other types of TBI; therefore attempts to separate concussion from other types of TBI on clinical grounds are futile. Second, the term 'concussion' does not have a distinct pathological meaning, and concussive symptoms can arise after various types of focal and diffuse brain injuries. Finally, the underlying assumption that concussions are benign events is increasingly being questioned. There is a wide range of possible outcomes even after apparently trivial head injuries, and catastrophic effects can result from repeated minor injuries (see neurodegeneration section, following). Therefore concussion should be viewed not as a distinct subtype of TBI but rather as a description for the collection of symptoms that can occur after head injuries of all severities.

Personality change

Personality change and challenging behaviours including emotional lability, irritability, self-centredness, and childish behaviour are common after TBI and can be very problematic for family and friends.[89] They are in many cases the behavioural effects of the dysexecutive and attentional impairments described previously.[68,90] For example, (a) disinhibition can produce attention-seeking, socially over-familiar, or inappropriate behaviour; (b) loss of initiative and drive can manifest as apathy; and (c) a failure to monitor and switch between different modes of behaviour in response to social cues can result in behaviour that is perceived as aggressive.[91]

Psychiatric impairment

Psychiatric symptoms are common after TBI. They often coexist with cognitive impairment and can influence clinical outcome, interfere with rehabilitation, and increase mortality.[5,92-94] New psychiatric problems often occur after injury,[95] either through direct neural effects or because of a psychological reaction to the impact of the injury. However, pre-existing disorders are common, and increase the risk of developing a psychiatric disorder after injury, from 45 per cent– ~75 per cent in one study.[95]

Depression

Major depression is common and disabling after TBI.[5,96] Estimates of the prevalence in the first two years vary widely from 12–58 per cent, probably because of differences in diagnostic methodology.[97] Rates can remain elevated many years after injury (~40 per cent),[98] and have been reported as higher following injuries that are clinically more severe,[99] although this is not always the case.[96] There are many possible causes for depressive symptoms after TBI and a clear psychiatric diagnosis is made difficult by the overlap between the non-specific effects of TBI and the psychiatric criteria used to define depression. Clinical tools such as the Beck Depression Inventory can be helpful in screening for depression and have been validated against more detailed psychiatric evaluation.[100] Patients who develop depression after TBI have been shown to have more structural brain injury. Reduced prefrontal[96] and hippocampal volumes[101] have been observed in patients who develop depression after TBI, suggesting that damage in these areas or their connections may be causally linked to depression after TBI.

The presence of depression has an adverse effect on clinical outcome,[5,96] and is associated with greater distress for carers.[102] Patients who are depressed are also likely to have more cognitive impairments across a range of domains.[96,103] However, the direction of causation is often unclear: patients may be depressed because of the impact of their cognitive impairment; their cognitive impairment might be caused by depression; or both depression and cognitive impairment might share a common underlying aetiology, such as neurotransmitter abnormalities or sleep disturbance. A patient's perception of their own cognitive problems is also likely to be influenced by their psychiatric state. This may be a particular issue in mild TBI cases where high levels of distress and premorbid personality traits can substantially influence both the subjective experience of cognitive impairment and a patient's effortful engagement with cognitive assessments.[104]

It might be predicted that treating depression would improve cognitive function following TBI, and there is a small amount of evidence to support this view. Most data are available for intervention in the subacute or chronic phases using selective serotonin reuptake inhibitors (SSRIs).[105,106] For example, a short course of sertraline improved various aspects of cognitive function in a single-blind non-randomized study with mild TBI patients.[106] Psychological treatments for depression may also be helpful, with a recent randomized control trial finding mindfulness-based cognitive therapy to reduce symptoms of post-TBI depression.[107]

Anxiety and post-traumatic stress disorder

Post-traumatic stress disorder (PTSD) can develop after head injuries, and has been a recent focus of work in veterans of the military conflicts in Iran and Iraq.[108] The core features of PTSD involve persistently re-experiencing a traumatic event as intrusive thoughts, dreams or flashbacks, avoiding stimuli that are associated with the event, and developing negative mood and cognitions associated with the event. PTSD in the context of TBI requires a careful diagnostic approach since, as with depression, the two conditions have overlapping symptomatology. Diagnosing PTSD following TBI is particularly problematic when self-report symptom questionnaires are used, and dramatically lower rates of PTSD are reported when diagnosis is based on structured psychiatric interview.[109,110] In general, PTSD is uncommon if patients have no memory of their injury and is less likely with longer periods of loss of consciousness or PTA, although there is controversy about its prevalence in this situation. The presence of PTSD after mild TBI is predictive of cognitive impairment on neuropsychological testing,[108] but is a more powerful predictor of subjective cognitive complaints.[111]

There is less work on general anxiety disorders, although these are also common after TBI. Patients often show features of anxiety about travelling, post-traumatic stress, and agoraphobic symptoms. Estimates of prevalence again vary widely, although one careful longitudinal study provides an estimate of 44 per cent in the first year after TBI.[95] As with depression, anxiety often contributes to complaints of cognitive difficulties, with heightened levels leading patients to focus on perceived cognitive impairments. Psychological treatment with cognitive behaviour therapy (CBT) is likely to be the treatment of choice for anxiety disorders, including PTSD, after TBI.[112] One randomized controlled trial (RCT) found it helpful for preventing PTSD after mild TBI,[113] and another reported that a combination of CBT and neurorehabilitation reduced anxiety symptoms after TBI.[114]

Psychosis

TBI probably produces only a small increase in risk of psychosis, seen particularly in individuals who are genetically susceptible. One recent meta-analysis of case-controlled studies suggested an odds ratio for schizophrenia after TBI of 1.6, with an increased risk in the relatives of schizophrenics but no correlation with the severity of injury.[115] At least some of this increased risk is probably because those who are at increased risk of developing schizophrenia are also at increased risk of suffering a head injury.[116]

Other factors influencing cognitive function after TBI

Psychogenic and financial causes

Some cognitive and psychiatric symptoms are psychogenic in origin. These may relate to psychological reactions, psychosocial stressors, and individual coping strategies. This is particularly relevant to the outcome after mild TBI, where objective evidence of injury may be lacking and many symptoms are non-specific. 'Post-concussion symptoms' frequently follow TBI but are also presented by many patients injured without involvement of the head.[117,118] High levels of post-concussion symptoms have also been reported in those with chronic pain[119] or chronic fatigue,[120] suggesting that post-concussion syndrome has much in common with somatization disorders. It is therefore unsurprising that patients who have negative expectations about the likely consequences of their mild TBI suffer more post-concussion symptoms.[121]

Personality change may be also triggered, exacerbated, or maintained by psychogenic factors including the psychological effects of the trauma of having had a head injury, the stress of changed life circumstances, and premorbid characteristics. Cognitive impairments may limit the individual's functioning in ways that produce frustration and exacerbate behavioural disturbances, and a number of longitudinal studies have demonstrated interrelationships between these presenting symptoms and relationships with psychosocial outcome.[122]

Financial issues can sometimes complicate the assessment of cognition after TBI. Patients with financial incentives such as compensation or disability claims are more symptomatic than matched TBI controls without possible secondary gain.[123] These effects are most prominent in mild TBI. Here, ongoing litigation is sometimes associated with more cognitive symptoms,[124] and can also influence effort expended during cognitive testing.[125] One meta-analysis of mild TBI found persistent cognitive impairment only in patients who were pursuing compensation. Unlike a group of similar patients without financial incentives, the severity of this group's symptoms tended to increase over time.[126] The possible impact of secondary gain should therefore always be considered when assessing cognition following TBI. The issue is of most relevance in cases of mild TBI, where there is a discrepancy between the severity of the initial injury and symptom progression, especially when there are questions over the level of effort that the patient applies during attempts to quantify his/her problems objectively.

Alcohol and drug dependence

Alcohol and drug dependence are a problem for many patients at the time of their head injuries, and frequently play a causative role. However, in the first year after injury, the prevalence of alcohol and drug dependence may reduce, perhaps reflecting hospitalization and reduced social activity. Thus, one study found half the rate of dependence at 12 months post-injury, followed by a gradual return to pre-injury levels of dependence and hazardous substance use.[127] Post-injury substance use may exacerbate some impairments and disabilities, and have greater adverse effects on health than would similar consumption prior to the injury. High levels of alcohol and drug use have been linked to long-term clinical deterioration,[5] and patients should therefore be strongly encouraged to limit alcohol consumption and abstain from using non-prescribed drugs.

Sleep

Sleep disturbance is very common after TBI[128-130] and may be an under-recognized cause of cognitive impairment. A wide range of sleep problems can result from primary damage in regions involved in regulating the sleep cycle such as the hypothalamus, as well as from secondary factors such as pain, depression, and anxiety. One detailed study found that 76 per cent of patients had new onset sleep–wake disturbance 6 months after TBI, with excessive daytime sleepiness, fatigue, and hypersomnolence being particularly common.[129] One mechanism for sleep disturbance following TBI is a reduction in hypothalamic hypocretin (orexin), which plays a role in the regulation of the normal sleep–wake cycle.[131] In addition, TBI patients show a small increased risk of obstructive sleep apnoea,[132] although the mechanism for this is unclear. Sleep disturbance can be assessed easily in clinic using validated scales such as the Epworth sleepiness scale (daytime somnolence) and the Pittsburgh sleep questionnaire (night-time sleep quality).[133,134] However, many patients will require formal assessment with polysomnography for definitive diagnosis.

There is some evidence that sleep disturbance is associated with cognitive impairment after TBI,[135] perhaps mediated in part through increased fatigue in those who are sleep deprived.[136] This is an area where focused intervention could significantly improve patients' quality of life, and several approaches are possible. Endogenous melatonin production can be reduced following TBI.[137] Melatonin supplementation is quite widely used, although there is little clear evidence for its efficacy. A small RCT recently provided evidence that modafinil can reduce excessive daytime sleepiness, although it did not affect fatigue or vigilance.[138] Other treatments for insomnia, such as benzodiazepines and GABA agonists, can exacerbate cognitive impairments, so should be avoided or used with caution.[139] Non-pharmacological approaches include CBT, which has been found effective in reducing insomnia in the general population: a small study with TBI patients has shown improved sleep and reduced fatigue after a brief CBT intervention.[140]

Endocrine dysfunction

Hypothalamo-pituitary dysfunction after TBI can produce endocrine disturbance, which may adversely affect cognition. Hormone abnormalities are very common in the acute phase, but often resolve quickly. However, 10–50 per cent of TBI patients may be persistently affected, with growth hormone deficiency (GHD) the most common abnormality.[141-143]. Estimates vary depending on methods of diagnosis. Our own experience suggests that in civilian TBI the true rate of endocrine problems is closer to 10 per cent, although it is significantly higher following exposure to blast TBI.[144]

Cognitive function may improve with the correction of endocrine abnormalities. For example, in other contexts the cognitive and neuropsychiatric impairments associated with GHD respond to GH replacement.[145-147] Most cases of GHD after TBI are probably undiagnosed and untreated, perhaps because its symptoms are mis-attributed to the brain trauma and GH levels are not routinely measured.[141,148,149] This is unfortunate, since GHD following TBI has been associated with worse cognitive function and quality of life,[150-152] and GH replacement several years after TBI has been shown to have benefits to quality of life that are similar to treatment of adult-onset GHD from other causes.[153] To identify persistent problems, one approach is to screen all patients with baseline pituitary blood tests after TBI around three months after injury, which allows time for acute dysfunction to resolve. Although baseline testing of hormonal levels provide some information about hypothalamo-pituitary function, dynamic endocrine tests are necessary to completely exclude impairment.

Managing cognitive impairment after TBI

Neurosurgical and intensive care management

Prompt neurosurgical and intensive care management can save lives and dramatically reduce cognitive disability after TBI. Patients in the developed world are increasingly seen in the context of major trauma centres, regardless of whether neurosurgical intervention is needed. Organizing services to facilitate high-quality intensive care input and rapid surgery has been shown to save lives after TBI.[154] Much of the early management of TBI is devoted to preventing secondary injury by maintaining tissue perfusion and oxygenation. This can be achieved by limiting the adverse effects of elevated intracranial pressure, as well as treating concurrent problems such as infection and multi-organ injury.[155] Timely neurosurgical intervention is therefore critical for limiting cognitive disability, and rapid treatment of large subdural and extradural haematomas is particularly beneficial. One recent RCT suggests that decompressive craniectomy is not beneficial in the management of diffuse TBI,[156] although at the time of writing another is due to report shortly.[157] Therapeutic hypothermia may improve functional outcomes, and an RCT is ongoing.[158] Despite strong basic science support, trials of acute neuroprotection following TBI have had disappointing results, and currently no neuroprotective agents are routinely used in adult TBI management.

Since optimizing early management is of fundamental importance to long-term outcomes, a solid evidence base is needed to determine how particular treatments relate to later physical, cognitive, and psychosocial function. Large RCTs are warranted in numerous areas to clarify the late effects of early intervention, which may be paradoxical.[156] Such RCTs are challenging to perform and often require substantial investment, but can be highly informative.[156,159] The use of neuroimaging, blood, and CSF biomarkers as surrogate clinical endpoints in early stage phase II studies is likely to enhance the speed and feasibility of assessing novel interventions, and this should improve the likelihood of successfully identifying effective treatments in larger phase III studies.[160]

Managing agitation in the acute period

Agitation is common in the initial period after TBI, and is often seen in the context of PTA. It is surprisingly easy for the causes of agitation and aggression after TBI to be misconstrued if the symptoms of PTA are not appreciated. Agitated patients should be managed in an inpatient setting by experienced staff, ideally in a major trauma centre, applying principles similar to those with delirium of other causes.[161] Stimulation should be limited by using a quiet room that is configured to minimize the risk of injury: for example, placing the mattress on the floor if the patient is at risk of falling. Restraint may be needed, so adequate staff should be available and the legal basis for particular actions should be considered. Other possible causes for post-TBI agitation that should be considered include pain, infection, constipation, side-effects of medication, and the effects of recreational drugs used prior to admission. Alcoholics are at elevated risk of TBI, and acute withdrawal during emergency treatment commonly contributes to their agitation. Therefore, there should be a low threshold for treatment with intravenous thiamine to prevent the Wernicke–Korsakoff syndrome.

Agitation usually lasts less than a week,[162] and validated measures such as the agitated behaviour scale should be used to monitor progress.[163] There is limited evidence for using medication to control agitated behaviour in this early phase,[164,165] and it should probably be avoided if possible. If absolutely necessary, then a rule of thumb is to 'start low and go slow'. Short-acting benzodiazepines may be useful, but occasionally they increase disinhibition or result in paradoxical agitation; it is thus advisable to avoid using them on an 'as-required' basis. Emotionally labile patients may be helped by antidepressants (e.g. SSRIs), and those who are fearful or paranoid can respond to a second-generation antipsychotic such as risperidone, quetiapine, or olanzapine. If epilepsy needs to be treated then mood-stabilizing anticonvulsants such as valproate should be considered. Even where psychotropic medication appears to have been beneficial, the improvement could have reflected spontaneous recovery and so there should always be a plan to reduce and stop the medication as soon as possible.

Rehabilitation

A multidisciplinary approach to rehabilitation following the acute phase of medical treatment is needed by many TBI patients because of their complex needs (Box 39.3). Inpatient rehabilitation typically focuses on remediating impairments and reducing disability. This almost invariably involves focused one-to-one therapeutic intervention, the provision of physical aids and adaptations, and the development of compensatory strategies.[166,167] Following discharge

Box 39.3 Case 3

A 30-year-old woman sustained a severe TBI in a car accident. She was unconscious on arrival at hospital, her skull was fractured, and CT showed frontal and parietal haemorrhage with diffuse axonal injury. Her consciousness normalized across a week in ICU. After a month she was physically mobile but restless and still lacked continuous memory. She showed poor initiation, concentration, and insight, and was highly disinhibited. Her speech was fluent but verbose and tangential. Her PTA persisted, and after three months she was transferred to specialist inpatient rehabilitation.

The multidisciplinary team focused on independence in self-care and domestic activities. She learned to plan and undertake supermarket shopping, staying within her budget. Her memory was poor, as was her road-safety awareness, so the OT accompanied her on trips within her home area. Her support was decreased progressively until she was considered safe. Her communication skills improved but were limited by her persisting distractibility and variable comprehension. She had a tendency to make inappropriate, and often highly derogatory or abusive comments, and had inadequate self-monitoring. Her impaired insight and difficulty in accepting feedback raised concerns about her social vulnerability, and she was over-friendly and tactile with men. The team therefore liaised with the insurance company to arrange a support package and case management.

After two months she was discharged to the flat where she lived on her own, initially with support workers spending eight hours a week with her. Her case manager arranged sessions with a clinical psychologist (CP) to focus on her anger, frustration, and low mood, which she valued. The CP also advised the support workers on strategies for managing her disinhibited behaviour.

Over the next two years, she became independent in basic activities of daily living but remained extremely impulsive and stimulus-driven with impaired memory and reasoning. She depended on others for help with complex matters, and was placed under the Court of Protection. She was sociable and could be engaging, but her frequent antagonism alienated friends and family. Her emotional volatility and immaturity made her vulnerable: at one point she was having sex with exploitative local men in return for alcohol. She rejected attempts by the support workers to engage her in constructive social activities.

She reluctantly agreed to spend four months in a specialist inpatient rehabilitation centre. Here she responded well to a behavioural management programme which rewarded her for taking part in constructive activities and for inhibiting socially inappropriate behaviours. On returning home she accepted an increase in support input, and the team used the incentive programme with her effectively under the CP's guidance. Although she declined to participate in voluntary work, she agreed to visit a Headway day centre. She thoroughly enjoyed the social aspects of this, and began attending twice weekly; her mood improved, and her risky socializing in the evenings stopped.

home, interventions typically focus primarily on optimizing aspects of psychosocial functioning including independence in personal and domestic activities, family and social relationships, and participation in social and work-related activities.

For patients with pronounced cognitive or behavioural disturbances, successful intervention will usually require a combination of one-to-one input to help them develop new coping or compensatory strategies, and work with family members, carers, employers, etc., to ensure that appropriate support is provided. For example, enabling a disinhibited and cognitively impaired patient to resume social activities usually entails training other people in specific behavioural management techniques and adjusting task demands. The emotional and practical strain imposed on family members typically need to be addressed, both in its own right and because this is key to sustaining their support to the brain-injured person.

Broad-spectrum interventions after brain injury are often referred to as 'holistic' or 'cognitive' rehabilitation. This reflects the importance of understanding and addressing cognitive impairments. Whether gross or subtle, these often impact on the individual's ability to function in a range of settings and to engage with therapy.[168] Rehabilitation generally needs to be multifaceted if it is to yield major functional gains.[169] Training individuals to utilize effective compensatory cognitive or behavioural approaches to particular activities has been found in some cases to increase their self-confidence and thus to produce more generalized benefits; it may also be associated with potentially beneficial changes in brain connectivity.[170] There is some evidence for the efficacy of this broad-based approach to TBI rehabilitation,[167,171,172] though one recent systematic review concluded that there are as yet insufficient high-quality studies using the same outcome indices to draw firm conclusions.[173]

Numerous studies have focused on the remediation of specific cognitive abilities including attention, memory, insight, or problem-solving. Approaches include extensive practice, the utilization of preserved cognitive processes to compensate for impairments elsewhere, and the use of adaptive aids such as electronic reminder systems for people with memory problems. These highly specific techniques typically improve performance on experimental tasks that resemble those used in training sessions, but on the whole there is as yet a lack of persuasive evidence from high-quality studies that they translate to marked improvements in day-to-day functioning,[174] unless—as is often the case with adaptive aids—they are incorporated into a well-supported rehabilitation programme.[175,176] Thus, recent guidelines concluded that 'in the post-acute setting interventions for cognitive deficits should be applied in the context of a comprehensive / holistic neuropsychological rehabilitation programme. This would involve an interdisciplinary team using a goal-focused programme which has the capacity to address cognitive, emotional and behavioural difficulties with the aim of improving functioning in meaningful everyday activities.'[167]

Cognitive and behavioural enhancement with drugs

Various drugs produce beneficial effects on cognition and behaviour after TBI, although there is wide variability in the way they are used in practice.[177] Several catecholaminergic agents have been used as cognitive enhancers. These can be classified broadly into stimulants (e.g. methylphenidate (MP) and dextroamphetamine) and dopamine-enhancing agents (e.g. amantadine, bromocriptine, and levodopa).[22] There is good basic science and clinical evidence

that MP can improve certain outcomes after TBI.[22,178,179] MP is a dopaminergic and noradrenergic re-uptake inhibitor that inhibits the dopamine transporter (DAT), and is commonly used to treat attentional impairment in attention deficit/hyperactivity disorder (ADHD). In animal models, the drug reverses reductions in dopaminergic neurotransmission produced by the TBI,[180,181] and also improves the associated behavioural impairments.[182,183] In humans, 17 trials (10 RCTs) have investigated its effect on cognition following TBI, although all are relatively small (n = 40 or less). The majority indicate that it leads to faster information processing.[178,184,185] Less consistently, improvements in functional outcomes and attentional measures have been reported.[178,184,186] There is also meta-analysis evidence that MP can improve anger, aggression, and psychosocial function.[177] Few trials have investigated whether these improvements persist on stopping the medication.

Amantidine is both an indirect dopamine agonist and NMDA antagonist, and two double-blind RCTs support its use in the first six months after severe TBI.[187,188] A recent large multi-centre international RCT n = 184 showed it accelerated recovery over the first four months after TBI,[187] with improvements across all behavioural measures including sustained attention, command following, and object recognition. As with MP, its efficacy might be mediated through enhanced activity in dopamine dependent mesolimbic, mesostriatal, and frontostriatal circuits. Bromocriptine, a selective D_2 dopamine receptor agonist, has also been used with mixed success in moderate/severe TBI, and there is a little evidence for benefit on executive dysfunction at low doses.[189,190] There is weak evidence that the cholinergic agent donepezil, widely used to treat memory disturbance in Alzheimer's disease, can enhance memory and attention following TBI.[192] It inhibits acetylcholinesterase, thereby increasing synaptic acetyl choline levels. A recent meta-analysis concluded that it had produced 'very large' improvements in attention, memory and general cognition assessed with the MMSE.[177] Other cholinergic agents appeared to be ineffective.

Aggressive behaviour is a common and problematic long-term problem after TBI.[165] American guidelines have recommended the first line use of β-blockers, either propranolol at a maximum dose 420–520 mg/day or pindolol 40–100 mg/day.[165] However, a recent RCT n = 76 provides evidence that amantadine improves both irritability and aggression in the chronic phase after TBI.[191] Methylphenidate,[192] valproate, or SSRIs are alternative treatments. Any drug treatment should be monitored carefully and stopped if ineffective. Polypharmacy should be minimized as drug interaction effects are unpredictable, and benzodiazepines should be avoided given the risk of dependency. Anticonvulsants are often used briefly as a prophylactic against post-traumatic seizures and may affect cognitive state. Phenytoin has been well studied and generally found to be benign,[193] whilst others may have adverse effects; for example, levetiracetam may exacerbate psychiatric problems and worsen aggression.[194]

A stratified approach to selecting cognitive enhancers is likely to improve treatment response. As TBI patients are heterogenous and there are various causes for cognitive impairment, there is likely to be a wide range of response to any particular treatment. In part this is because endogenous levels of neurotransmitters will vary across patients, and a nonlinear relationship between neurotransmitter levels and cognition will affect treatment effects. For example, dopamine level shows an inverted U-shaped relationship with concentration and cognitive effects, such that too much as well as too little can cause impairment.[195] Hence, quantifying neurotransmitter levels after TBI in an individual should allow the principled use of different agents. This is not attempted routinely but in principle it is possible using neuroimaging techniques such as PET and SPECT. An additional limitation of current approaches to cognitive enhancement concerns the lack of psychopharmacological specificity in the agents used. For example, animal studies suggest that enhancing prefrontal function may require selective D1 agonists. Such agents are not widely available clinically, but assessing the cognitive effects of drugs that are more selective for neurotransmitter receptor subclasses is likely to be a promising future direction.

Cognitive and behavioural enhancement with brain stimulation

One exciting new approach to treatment is the use of electrophysiological techniques to stimulate or inhibit brain function after TBI. This is currently used only in research settings but it has the potential for clinical application. Invasive deep brain stimulation to the thalamus has already been shown to benefit patients in minimally conscious states after TBI,[196] possibly by enhancing corticocortical interactions. However, this invasive approach will always be difficult to use extensively. Non-invasive types of brain stimulation such as transcranial magnetic stimulation (TMS), transcranial direct current stimulation (tDCS), and transcranial alternating current stimulation (tACS) provide attractive alternatives. These methods use scalp stimulation to induce electrical changes in the underlying cortex and so need to be applied at a particular location. TDCS and TACS are portable and relatively safe techniques that have the potential to be used outside a hospital setting. Preliminary data suggest that these noninvasive approaches may enhance cognition.[197,198]

Who should be involved in managing TBI?

Although patients with complex problems after TBI benefit from timely specialist input from many disciplines, many patients do not receive this. Initial inpatient rehabilitation efforts are often focused, understandably, on patients with severe problems. This can be effective[171] and is often reasonably well resourced. However, the vast majority of TBI patients are not thought to require inpatient rehabilitation, despite many having significant problems that lead to long-term disability. Injury severity categorizations are imprecise and can be falsely reassuring about whether patients will require ongoing support; and some patients develop long-term difficulties after mild TBI, particularly if they have sustained multiple injuries. Most health systems lack an integrated and comprehensive care pathway for following up patients with TBI, making the management of ongoing problems in the majority vulnerable to neglect.

Neurologists should embrace the challenge of accurately diagnosing the causes of persistent cognitive problems after TBI and help to drive the development of specific new interventions to enhance functional recovery and cognitive function. This is best achieved in the context of a multidisciplinary team, and systematic outpatient follow-up has already been shown to be beneficial for functional outcome after moderate/severe TBI.[199] There is wide variation in the extent to which neurologists are involved in TBI care. In many healthcare systems, including the UK, most TBI patients never see a neurologist. This is problematic because there are good arguments for a neurological approach to the management of TBI, both in the acute and chronic phases. Fundamentally, TBI is a disorder of the brain, and neurologists have significant diagnostic expertise in this area. As discussed in this chapter, TBI produces highly complex and diverse problems that have a multitude of pathophysiological causes and different treatments. Precise and accurate diagnosis of the cause of ongoing symptoms is of paramount importance in guiding treatment decisions. Terms like 'post-concussional syndrome' are unhelpful, as they describe problems rather than underlying disease mechanisms.

Future directions

This is an exciting time to be engaged in the care of TBI patients. Recent major advances in our understanding of brain structure and function are illuminating the bases of cognitive impairment following TBI. Future work should allow treatments to be tailored for individuals. Advances in network science are clarifying how TBI affects brain function, how network abnormalities influence behaviour, and how pathological processes are triggered and affect long-term outcome. Network abnormalities are correlated with cognitive impairments after TBI, and diagnostic tests based on network integrity have the potential to improve prognostication and guide the development of new treatments. The continued evaluation of treatments, using RCTs, is needed to provide a solid evidence base for guiding management. This will be assisted through advances in information technology which enable patients' progress to be tracked remotely allowing detailed, frequent, and cost-effective follow-up. This could be coupled with online computer-based cognitive rehabilitation techniques, which may allow some patients to engage in intensive treatments that are currently too expensive to deliver on a one-to-one basis. The greatest restorative benefits may well occur when behavioural training is coupled with treatments that promote brain plasticity. For example, neuronal activity and growth is regulated by the extracellular matrix. Drugs that target matrix proteins can influence recovery from animal models of spinal cord injury when their administration is coupled with an enriched environment that encourages appropriate activity.[200] This suggests that neuronal plasticity might be manipulated in the future to amplify the functional effects of behavioural rehabilitation.

Acknowledgements

The authors would like to thank Jessica Fleminger for her help in preparing the manuscript.

References

1. Gustavsson A, Svensson M, Jacobi F, et al. Cost of disorders of the brain in Europe 2010. *European Neuropsychopharm.* 2011;21:718–79.
2. Langlois JA, Rutland-Brown W, and Wald MM. The epidemiology and impact of traumatic brain injury: a brief overview. *J Head Trauma Rehab.* 2006;21:375–78.
3. Chesser G. Afghanistan Casualties: Military Forces and Civilians. in *Congressional Research Service.* 2012, pp. 7–5700:5701–708.
4. Schretlen DJ and Shapiro AM. A quantitative review of the effects of traumatic brain injury on cognitive functioning. *Int Re Psychiatr.* 2003;15:341–49.
5. Whitnall L, McMillan TM, Murray GD, et al. Disability in young people and adults after head injury: 5–7 year follow up of a prospective cohort study. *J Neurol Neurosur Ps.* 2006;77:640–45.

6. Oddy M, Moir JF, Fortescue D, et al. The prevalence of traumatic brain injury in the homeless community in a UK city. Brain Injury. 2012 26:1058–64.

7. Williams H. Repairing shattered lives: brain injury and its implications for criminal justice. Barrow-Cadbury Trust. 2012.

8. Graham DI, McIntosh TK, Maxwell WL, et al. Recent advances in neurotrauma. J Neuropathol Exp Neurol. 2000;59:641–51.

9. Gurdjian ES. Re-evaluation of the biomechanics of blunt impact injury of the head. Surg Gynecol Obstet. 1975;140:845–50.

10. Bigler ED. Anterior and middle cranial fossa in traumatic brain injury: relevant neuroanatomy and neuropathology in the study of neuropsychological outcome. Neuropsychology. 2007;21:515–31.

11. Kinnunen KM, Greenwood R, Powell JH, et al. White matter damage and cognitive impairment after traumatic brain injury. Brain. 2011;134:449–63.

12. Hellyer PJ, Leech R, Ham TE, et al. Individual prediction of white matter injury following traumatic brain injury. Ann Neurol. 2012; Apr;73(4):489–99.

13. Adams JH, Doyle D, Ford I, et al. Diffuse axonal injury in head injury: definition, diagnosis and grading. Histopathology. 1989;15:49–59.

14. Smith DH, Meaney DF, and Shull WH. Diffuse axonal injury in head trauma. J Head Trauma Rehab. 2003;18:307–16.

15. Sharp DJ, Scott G, and Leech R. Network dysfunction after traumatic brain injury. Nature Neurol. 2014;Mar;10(3):156–66.

16. Scheid R, Preul C, Gruber O, et al. Diffuse axonal injury associated with chronic traumatic brain injury: evidence from T2*-weighted gradient-echo imaging at 3 T. Am J Neuroradiol. 2003;24:1049–56.

17. Basser PJ and Pierpaoli C. Microstructural and physiological features of tissues elucidated by quantitative-diffusion-tensor MRI. J Magn Reson B. 1996;111:209–19.

18. Mac Donald CL, Dikranian K, Bayly P, et al. Diffusion tensor imaging reliably detects experimental traumatic axonal injury and indicates approximate time of injury. J Neurosci.2007;27:11869–76.

19. Sidaros A, Engberg AW, Sidaros K, et al. Diffusion tensor imaging during recovery from severe traumatic brain injury and relation to clinical outcome: a longitudinal study. Brain 2008;131:559–72.

20. Donnemiller E, Brenneis C, Wissel J, et al. Impaired dopaminergic neurotransmission in patients with traumatic brain injury: a SPECT study using 123I-beta-CIT and 123I-IBZM. European J Nucl Med. 2000;27:1410–414.

21. Wagner AK, Scanlon JM, Becker CR, et al. The influence of genetic variants on striatal dopamine transporter and D2 receptor binding after TBI. Journal of Cerebral Blood Flow and Metabolism. 2014 Aug;34(8):1328–39.

22. Bales JW, Wagner AK, Kline AE, et al. Persistent cognitive dysfunction after traumatic brain injury: A dopamine hypothesis. Neurosci Biobehav Rev. 2009;33:981–1003.

23. Salmond CH, Chatfield DA, Menon DK, et al. Cognitive sequelae of head injury: involvement of basal forebrain and associated structures. Brain. 2005;128:189–200.

24. Mesulam MM. From sensation to cognition. Brain. 1998;121 Pt 6:1013–52.

25. Damoiseaux JS, Rombouts SA, Barkhof F, et al. 2006 Consistent resting-state networks across healthy subjects. P Natl Acad Sci USA. 2006;103:13848–853.

26. Smith SM, Fox PT, Miller KL, et al. Correspondence of the brain's functional architecture during activation and rest. P Natl Acad Sci USA. 2009;106:13040–45.

27. Bonnelle V, Leech R, Kinnunen KM, et al. Default Mode Network Connectivity Predicts Sustained Attention Deficits after Traumatic Brain Injury. J Neurosci.2011;31:13442–451.

28. Bonnelle V, Ham TE, Leech R, et al. Salience network integrity predicts default mode network function after traumatic brain injury. P Natl Acad Sci USA. 2012;109:4690–695.

29. Adams JH, Graham DI and Jennett B. The neuropathology of the vegetative state after an acute brain insult. Brain. 2000;123 Pt 7:1327–338.

30. Sharp DJ, Beckmann CF, Greenwood R, et al. Default mode network functional and structural connectivity after traumatic brain injury. Brain. 2011;134:2233–47.

31. Smith DH, Johnson VE, and Stewart W. Chronic neuropathologies of single and repetitive TBI: substrates of dementia? Nature Neurol. 2013;9:211–21.

32. McMillan TM, Teasdale GM, and Stewart E. Disability in young people and adults after head injury: 12-14 year follow-up of a prospective cohort. J Neurol Neurosur Ps. 2012;83:1086–91.

33. Mayeux R, Ottman R, Maestre G, et al. Synergistic effects of traumatic head injury and apolipoprotein-epsilon 4 in patients with Alzheimer's disease. Neurology. 1995;45:555–57.

34. McKee AC, Stern RA, Nowinski CJ, et al. The spectrum of disease in chronic traumatic encephalopathy. Brain. 2013;136:43–64.

35. Goldman SM, Kamel F, Ross GW, et al. Head injury, alpha-synuclein Rep1, and Parkinson's disease. Ann Neurol. 2012;71:40–48.

36. Nemetz PN, Leibson C, Naessens JM, et al. Traumatic brain injury and time to onset of Alzheimer's disease: a population-based study. Am J Epidemiol 1999;149:32–40.

37. Lye TC and Shores EA. Traumatic brain injury as a risk factor for Alzheimer's disease: a review. Neuropsychol Rev. 2000;10:115–29.

38. Goldstein LE, Fisher AM, Tagge CA, et al. Chronic traumatic encephalopathy in blast-exposed military veterans and a blast neurotrauma mouse model. Science Translational Medicine. 2012;4:134ra160.

39. Mauri M, Sinforiani E, Bono G, et al. Interaction between Apolipoprotein epsilon 4 and traumatic brain injury in patients with Alzheimer's disease and Mild Cognitive Impairment. Funct Neurol. 2006;21:223–28.

40. Ramlackhansingh AF, Brooks DJ, Greenwood RJ, et al. Inflammation after trauma: Microglial activation and traumatic brain injury. Ann Neurol. 2011;70:374–83.

41. Johnson VE, Stewart JE, Begbie FD, et al. Inflammation and white matter degeneration persist for years after a single traumatic brain injury. Brain. 2013;136:28–42.

42. Mathias JL and Wheaton P. Changes in attention and information-processing speed following severe traumatic brain injury: a meta-analytic review. Neuropsychology. 2007;21:212–23.

43. Kinsella G, Murtagh D, Landry A, et al. Everyday memory following traumatic brain injury. Brain Inj. 1996;10:499–507.

44. Scheid R, Walther K, Guthke T, et al. Cognitive sequelae of diffuse axonal injury. Arch Neurol. 2006;63:418–24.

45. Draper K and Ponsford J. Cognitive functioning ten years following traumatic brain injury and rehabilitation. Neuropsychology. 2008;22:618–25.

46. Levin H and Kraus MF. The frontal lobes and traumatic brain injury. J Neuropsychiatr Clin Neurosci. 1994;6:443–54.

47. Gentleman SM, Roberts GW, Gennarelli TA, et al. Axonal injury: a universal consequence of fatal closed head injury? Acta Neuropathologica. 1995;89:537–43.

48. Dehaene S and Changeux JP. Experimental and theoretical approaches to conscious processing. Neuron. 2011;70:200–27.

49. Laureys S, Lemaire C, Maquet P, et al. Cerebral metabolism during vegetative state and after recovery to consciousness. J Neurol Neurosur Ps. 1999;67:121.

50. Laureys S, Owen AM, and Schiff ND. Brain function in coma, vegetative state, and related disorders. Lancet Neurol. 2004;3:537–46.

51. Sitt JD, King JR, El Karoui I, et al. Large scale screening of neural signatures of consciousness in patients in a vegetative or minimally conscious state. Brain. 2014;137:2258–70.

52. Monti MM, Vanhaudenhuyse A, Coleman MR, et al. Willful modulation of brain activity in disorders of consciousness. N Engl J Med. 2010;362:579–89.

53. Prigatano GP and Altman IM. Impaired awareness of behavioral limitations after traumatic brain injury. Arch Phys Med Rehab. 1990;71:1058–64.

54. Ham TE, Bonnelle V, Hellyer P, et al. The neural basis of impaired self-awareness after traumatic brain injury. Brain. 2014 Feb;137(Pt 2):586–97.

55. Ponsford J and Kinsella G. Attentional deficits following closed-head injury. *J Clin Exp Neuropsychol.* 1992;14:822–38.

56. Ruttan L, Martin K, Liu A, *et al.* Long-term cognitive outcome in moderate to severe traumatic brain injury: a meta-analysis examining timed and untimed tests at 1 and 4.5 or more years after injury. *Arch Phys Med Rehab.* 2008;89:S69–76.

57. Stuss DT, Stethem LL, Hugenholtz H, *et al.* Reaction time after head injury: fatigue, divided and focused attention, and consistency of performance. *J Neurol Neurosur Ps.* 1989;52:742–48.

58. Robertson IH, Manly T, Andrade J, *et al.* 'Oops!': performance correlates of everyday attentional failures in traumatic brain injured and normal subjects. *Neuropsychologia.* 1997;35:747–58.

59. Whyte J, Polansky M, Fleming M, *et al.* Sustained arousal and attention after traumatic brain injury. *Neuropsychologia.* 1995;33:797–813.

60. Dockree PM, Kelly SP, Roche RA, *et al.* Behavioural and physiological impairments of sustained attention after traumatic brain injury. *Brain Res Cogn Brain Res.* 2004;20:403–14.

61. Singh KD and Fawcett IP. Transient and linearly graded deactivation of the human default-mode network by a visual detection task. *Neuroimage.* 2008;41:100–12.

62. Weissman DH, Roberts KC, Visscher KM, *et al.* The neural bases of momentary lapses in attention. *Nat Neurosci.* 2006;9:971–78.

63. Leech R and Sharp DJ. The role of the posterior cingulate cortex in cognition and disease. *Brain.* 2014;137:12–32.

64. Shallice T and Burgess PW. Deficits in strategy application following frontal lobe damage in man. *Brain.* 1991;114 Pt 2:727–41.

65. Damasio H, Grabowski T, Frank R, *et al.* The return of Phineas Gage: clues about the brain from the skull of a famous patient. *Science.* 1994;264:1102–105.

66. Duncan J. The structure of cognition: attentional episodes in mind and brain. *Neuron.* 2013;80:35–50.

67. Duncan J. The multiple-demand MD system of the primate brain: mental programs for intelligent behaviour. *Trends Cogn Sci.* 2010;14:172–79.

68. Stuss DT and Alexander MP. Is there a dysexecutive syndrome? *Philos Trans R Soc Lond B.* 2007;362:901–15.

69. Jilka SR, Scott G, Ham T, *et al.* Damage to the salience network and interactions with the default mode network. *J Neurosci.* 2014;34:10798–807.

70. Shores EA, Lammel A, Hullick C, *et al.* The diagnostic accuracy of the Revised Westmead PTA Scale as an adjunct to the Glasgow Coma Scale in the early identification of cognitive impairment in patients with mild traumatic brain injury. *J Neurol Neurosur Ps.* 2008;79:1100–106.

71. Levin HS, O'Donnell VM, and Grossman RG. The Galveston Orientation and Amnesia Test. A practical scale to assess cognition after head injury. *J Nerv Ment Dis.* 1979;167:675–84.

72. McMillan TM, Jongen EL, and Greenwood RJ. Assessment of post-traumatic amnesia after severe closed head injury: retrospective or prospective? *J Neurol Neurosur Ps.* 1996;60:422–27.

73. Ahmed S, Bierley R, Sheikh JI, *et al.* Post-traumatic amnesia after closed head injury: a review of the literature and some suggestions for further research. *Brain Inj.* 2000;14:765–80.

74. Zangwill OL. Neuropsychology of disorders of memory. In: MSaOL Zangwil (ed.). *Handbook of Psychiatry: General Psychopathology,* vol 1. Cambridge: Cambridge University Press, Cambridge, pp. 97–113.

75. Box O, Laing H, and Kopelman M. The evolution of spontaneous confabulation, delusional misidentification and a related delusion in a case of severe head injury. *Neurocase.* 1999;5(3):251–62.

76. Fleminger S. Head injury In: AS David, S Fleminger, MD Kopelman, *et al.* (eds). *Lishman's Organic Psychiatry: A Textbook of Neuropsychiatry,* 4th edn. Oxford: Wiley-Blackwell, pp. 181–2.

77. Godfrey HP, Partridge FM, Knight RG, *et al.* Course of insight disorder and emotional dysfunction following closed head injury: a controlled cross-sectional follow-up study. *J Clin Exp Neuropsychol.* 1993;15:503–15.

78. Wilson BA. *Memory Rehabilitation: Integrating Theory and Practice.* New York, NY: Guildford Press, 2009.

79. Teasdale G and Jennett B. Assessment of coma and impaired consciousness. A practical scale. *Lancet.* 1974;2:81–84.

80. Shores EA. Comparison of the Westmead PTA Scale and the Glasgow Coma Scale as predictors of neuropsychological outcome following extremely severe blunt head injury. *J Neurol Neurosur Ps.* 1989;52:126–27.

81. Perrin PB, Niemeier JP, Mougeot JL, *et al.* Measures of injury severity and prediction of acute traumatic brain injury outcomes. *J Head Trauma Rehab.* 2015 Mar-Apr;30(2):136–42.

82. Sandhaug M, Andelic N, Vatne A, *et al.* Functional level during sub-acute rehabilitation after traumatic brain injury: course and predictors of outcome. *Brain Inj.* 2010;24:740–47.

83. Fleming J, Tooth L, Hassell M, *et al.* Prediction of community integration and vocational outcome 2–5 years after traumatic brain injury rehabilitation in Australia. *Brain Inj.* 1999;13:417–31.

84. Asikainen I, Kaste M, and Sarna S. Predicting late outcome for patients with traumatic brain injury referred to a rehabilitation programme: a study of 508 Finnish patients 5 years or more after injury. *Brain Inj.* 1998;12:95–107.

85. Sigurdardottir S, Andelic N, Roe C, *et al.* Identifying longitudinal trajectories of emotional distress symptoms 5 years after traumatic brain injury. *Brain Inj.* 2014;28(12):1542–50.

86. Malec JF, Brown AW, Leibson CL, *et al.* The mayo classification system for traumatic brain injury severity. *J Neurotrauma.* 2007;24:1417–24.

87. McMillan TM, Teasdale GM, Weir CJ, *et al.* Death after head injury: the 13 year outcome of a case control study. *J Neurol Neurosur Ps.,* 2011;82:931–35.

88. McCrory P, Meeuwisse WH, Aubry M, *et al.* Consensus statement on concussion in sport: the 4th International Conference on Concussion in Sport held in Zurich, November 2012. *B J Sport Med.* 2013;47:250–58.

89. Lezak MD. Living with the characterologically altered brain injured patient. *J Clin Psychiat.* 1978;39:592–98.

90. Tate RL. Executive dysfunction and characterological changes after traumatic brain injury: two sides of the same coin? *Cortex.* 1999;35:39–55.

91. Burgess PW and Wood RL. Neuropsychology of behaviour disorders following brain injury. In: RL Wood (ed.). *Neurobehavioural Sequelae of Traumatic Brain Injury.* New York, NY:Taylor & Francis, 1990, pp. 110–33.

92. Fleminger S. Mental health is central to good neurorehabilitation after TBI. *Brain Impairment.* 2013;14(1):2–4.

93. Fazel S, Wolf A, Pillas D, *et al.* 2014 Suicide, fatal injuries, and other causes of premature mortality in patients with traumatic brain injury: a 41-tear Swedish population study. *JAMA Psychiat.* 2014 Mar;71(3):326–33.

94. Gould KR, Ponsford JL, Johnston L, *et al.* Relationship between psychiatric disorders and 1-year psychosocial outcome following traumatic brain injury. *J Head Trauma Rehab.* 2001;26:79–89.

95. Gould KR, Ponsford JL, Johnston L, *et al.* The nature, frequency and course of psychiatric disorders in the first year after traumatic brain injury: a prospective study. *Psychological Medicine.* 2011;41:2099–109.

96. Jorge RE, Robinson RG, Moser D, *et al.* Major depression following traumatic brain injury. *Arch Gen Psychiat.* 2004;61:42–50.

97. Tsaousides T, Ashman TA, and Gordon WA. *et al.* Diagnosis and treatment of depression following traumatic brain injury. *Brain Impairment* 2013;14.01: 63–76.

98. Kreutzer JS, Seel RT, and Gourley E. The prevalence and symptom rates of depression after traumatic brain injury: a comprehensive examination. *Brain Inj.* 2001;15:563–76.

99. Holsinger T, Steffens DC, Phillips C, *et al.* Head injury in early adulthood and the lifetime risk of depression. *Arch Gen Psychiat.* 2002;59:17–22.

100. Homaifar BY, Brenner LA, Gutierrez PM, *et al.* Sensitivity and specificity of the Beck Depression Inventory-II in persons with traumatic brain injury. *Arch Phys Med Rehab.* 2009;90:652–56.

101. Geuze E, Vermetten E, and Bremner JD. MR-based in vivo hippocampal volumetrics: 2. Findings in neuropsychiatric disorders. *Molecular Psychiatry*. 2005;10:160–84.

102. Knight RG, Devereux R, and Godfrey HP. Caring for a family member with a traumatic brain injury. *Brain Inj*. 1998;12:467–81.

103. Rapoport MJ, McCullagh S, Shammi P, et al. Cognitive impairment associated with major depression following mild and moderate traumatic brain injury. *J Neuropsychiat Clin Neurosci*. 2005;17:61–65.

104. Stulemeijer M, Andriessen TM, Brauer JM, et al. Cognitive performance after mild traumatic brain injury: the impact of poor effort on test results and its relation to distress, personality and litigation. *Brain Inj*. 2007;21:309–18.

105. Horsfield SA, Rosse RB, Tomasino V, et al. Fluoxetine's effects on cognitive performance in patients with traumatic brain injury. *Int J Psychiat Med*. 2002;32:337–44.

106. Fann JR, Uomoto JM and Katon WJ. Cognitive improvement with treatment of depression following mild traumatic brain injury. *Psychosomatics*. 2001;42:48–54.

107. Bedard M, Felteau M, Marshall S, et al. Mindfulness-based cognitive therapy reduces symptoms of depression in people with a traumatic brain injury: results from a randomized controlled trial. *J Head Trauma Rehab*. 2014;29:E13–22.

108. Vasterling JJ, Brailey K, Proctor SP, et al. Neuropsychological outcomes of mild traumatic brain injury, post-traumatic stress disorder and depression in Iraq-deployed US Army soldiers. *Brit J Psychiat*. 2012;201:186–92.

109. Sumpter RE and McMillan TM. Misdiagnosis of post-traumatic stress disorder following severe traumatic brain injury. *Brit J Psychiat*. 2005;186:423–26.

110. Sumpter RE and McMillan TM. Errors in self-report of post-traumatic stress disorder after severe traumatic brain injury. *Brain Inj*. 2006;20:93–99.

111. Drag LL, Spencer RJ, Walker SJ, et al. The contributions of self-reported injury characteristics and psychiatric symptoms to cognitive functioning in OEF/OIF veterans with mild traumatic brain injury. *JINS*. 2012;18:576–84.

112. Soo C and Tate R. Psychological treatment for anxiety in people with traumatic brain injury. *Cochrane Database Syst Rev*. 2007;CD005239.

113. Bryant RA, Moulds M, Guthrie R, et al. Treating acute stress disorder following mild traumatic brain injury. *Am J Psychiat*. 2003;160:585–87.

114. Tiersky LA, Anselmi V, Johnston MV, et al. A trial of neuropsychologic rehabilitation in mild-spectrum traumatic brain injury. *Arch Phys Med Rehab*. 2005;86:1565–74.

115. Molloy C, Conroy RM, Cotter DR, et al. Is traumatic brain injury a risk factor for schizophrenia? A meta-analysis of case-controlled population-based studies. *Schizophrenia Bull*. 2011;37:1104–10.

116. Malaspina D, Goetz RR, Friedman JH, et al. Traumatic brain injury and schizophrenia in members of schizophrenia and bipolar disorder pedigrees. *Am J Psychiat*. 2001;158:440–46.

117. Dikmen S, Machamer J, Fann JR, et al. Rates of symptom reporting following traumatic brain injury. *JINS*. 2010;16:401–11.

118. Lagarde E, Salmi LR, Holm LW, et al. Association of symptoms following mild traumatic brain injury with posttraumatic stress disorder vs postconcussion syndrome. *JAMA Psychiat*. 2014 Sep;71(9):1032–40.

119. Smith-Seemiller L, Fow NR, Kant R, et al. Presence of post-concussion syndrome symptoms in patients with chronic pain vs mild traumatic brain injury. *Brain Inj*. 2003;17:199–206.

120. Tiersky LA, K. C, Natelson BH, and DeLuca J. Neuropsychological functioning in chronic fatigue syndrome and mild traumatic brain injury: a comparison. 1988;12:503–12.

121. Hou R, Moss-Morris R, Peveler R, et al. When a minor head injury results in enduring symptoms: a prospective investigation of risk factors for postconcussional syndrome after mild traumatic brain injury. *J Neurol Neurosur Ps.*, 2012;83:217–23.

122. Ponsford J. Factors contributing to outcome following traumatic brain injury. *NeuroRehabilitation*. 2013;32:803–15.

123. Binder LM and Rohling ML. Money matters: a meta-analytic review of the effects of financial incentives on recovery after closed-head injury. *Am J Psychiat*. 1996;153:7–10.

124. Tsanadis J, Montoya E, Hanks RA, et al. Brain injury severity, litigation status, and self-report of postconcussive symptoms. *The Clinical Neuropsychologist*. 2008;22:1080–92.

125. Lange RT, Iverson GL, Brooks BL, et al. Influence of poor effort on self-reported symptoms and neurocognitive test performance following mild traumatic brain injury. *J Clin Exp Neuropsych*. 2010;32:961–72.

126. Belanger HG, Curtiss G, Demery JA, et al. Factors moderating neuropsychological outcomes following mild traumatic brain injury: a meta-analysis. *JINS*. 2005;11:215–27.

127. Ponsford J, Whelan-Goodinson R, and Bahar-Fuchs A. Alcohol and drug use following traumatic brain injury: a prospective study. *Brain Inj*. 2007;21:1385–92.

128. Ponsford JL, Parcell DL, Sinclair KL, et al. Changes in sleep patterns following traumatic brain injury: a controlled study. *Neurorehabil Neural Repair*. 2013;27:613–21.

129. Baumann CR, Werth E, Stocker R, et al. Sleep-wake disturbances 6 months after traumatic brain injury: a prospective study. *Brain*. 2007;130:1873–83.

130. Verma A, Anand V, and Verma NP. Sleep disorders in chronic traumatic brain injury. *Journal of Clinical Sleep Medicine*. 2007;3:357–62.

131. Baumann CR, Bassetti CL, Valko PO, et al. Loss of hypocretin (orexin) neurons with traumatic brain injury. *Ann Neurol*. 2009;66:555–59.

132. Mathias JL and Alvaro PK. Prevalence of sleep disturbances, disorders, and problems following traumatic brain injury: a meta-analysis. *Sleep Medicine*. 2012;13:898–905.

133. Johns M and Hocking B. Daytime sleepiness and sleep habits of Australian workers. *Sleep*. 1997;20:844–49.

134. Buysse DJ, Reynolds CF, 3rd, Monk TH, et al. The Pittsburgh Sleep Quality Index: a new instrument for psychiatric practice and research. *Psychiatry Res*. 1989;28:193–213.

135. Bloomfield IL, Espie CA, and Evans JJ. Do sleep difficulties exacerbate deficits in sustained attention following traumatic brain injury? *JINS* 16:17–25.

136. Ponsford JL, Ziino C, Parcell DL, et al. Fatigue and sleep disturbance following traumatic brain injury—their nature, causes, and potential treatments. *J Head Trauma Rehab*. 2012;27:224–33.

137. Shekleton JA, Parcell DL, Redman JR, et al. Sleep disturbance and melatonin levels following traumatic brain injury. *Neurology*. 2010;74:1732–38.

138. Kaiser PR, Valko PO, Werth E, et al. Modafinil ameliorates excessive daytime sleepiness after traumatic brain injury. *Neurology*. 2010;75:1780–85.

139. Larson EB and Zollman FS. The effect of sleep medications on cognitive recovery from traumatic brain injury. *J Head Trauma Rehab*. 2010;25:61–67.

140. Ouellet MC and Morin CM. Efficacy of cognitive-behavioral therapy for insomnia associated with traumatic brain injury: a single-case experimental design. *Arch Phys Med Rehab*. 2007;88:1581–92.

141. Behan LA, Phillips J, Thompson CJ, et al. Neuroendocrine disorders after traumatic brain injury. *J Neurol Neurosur Ps*. 2008;79:753–59.

142. Schneider HJ, Kreitschmann-Andermahr I, Ghigo E, et al. Hypothalamopituitary dysfunction following traumatic brain injury and aneurysmal subarachnoid hemorrhage: a systematic review. *JAMA*. 2007;298:1429–38.

143 Bondanelli M, De Marinis L, Ambrosio MR, et al. Occurrence of pituitary dysfunction following traumatic brain injury. *J Neurotrauma* 2004;21:685–96.

144. Baxter D, Sharp DJ, Feeney C, et al. Pituitary dysfunction after blast traumatic brain injury: UK BIOSAP study. *Ann Neurol*. 2013 Oct;74(4):527–36.

145. van Dam PS, Aleman A, de Vries WR, et al. Growth hormone, insulin-like growth factor I and cognitive function in adults. *Growth Horm IGF Res*. 2000;10 Suppl B:S69–73.

146. Monson JP. Indications for GH replacement in adolescents and young adults. *J Endocrinol Invest.* 2005;28:52–55.

147. Ho KK. Consensus guidelines for the diagnosis and treatment of adults with GH deficiency II: a statement of the GH Research Society in association with the European Society for Pediatric Endocrinology, Lawson Wilkins Society, European Society of Endocrinology, Japan Endocrine Society, and Endocrine Society of Australia. *Eur J Endocrinol.* 2007;157:695–700.

148. Ghigo E, Masel B, Aimaretti G, et al. Consensus guidelines on screening for hypopituitarism following traumatic brain injury. *Brain Inj.* 2005;19:711–24.

149. Lorenzo M, Peino R, Castro AI, et al. Hypopituitarism and growth hormone deficiency in adult subjects after traumatic brain injury: who and when to test. *Pituitary.* 2005;8:233–37.

150. Klose M and Feldt-Rasmussen U. Does the type and severity of brain injury predict hypothalamo-pituitary dysfunction? Does post-traumatic hypopituitarism predict worse outcome? *Pituitary.* 2008;11:255–61.

151. Leon-Carrion J, Leal-Cerro A, Cabezas FM, et al. Cognitive deterioration due to GH deficiency in patients with traumatic brain injury: a preliminary report. *Brain Inj.* 2007;21:871–75.

152. Bavisetty S, Bavisetty S, McArthur DL, et al. Chronic hypopituitarism after traumatic brain injury: risk assessment and relationship to outcome. *Neurosurgery.* 2008;62:1080–93; discussion 1093–94.

153. Kreitschmann-Andermahr I, Poll EM, Reineke A, et al. Growth hormone deficient patients after traumatic brain injury—baseline characteristics and benefits after growth hormone replacement—an analysis of the German KIMS database. *Growth Horm IGF Res.* 2008;18:472–78.

154. Fuller G, Bouamra O, Woodford M, et al. Temporal trends in head injury outcomes from 2003 to 2009 in England and Wales. *Brit J Neurosur.* 2011;25:414–21.

155. Kolias AG, Guilfoyle MR, Helmy A, et al. Traumatic brain injury in adults. *Practical Neurology.* 2013;13:228–35.

156. Cooper DJ, Rosenfeld JV, Murray L, et al. Decompressive craniectomy in diffuse traumatic brain injury. *N Engl J Med.* 2011;364:1493–502.

157. Hutchinson PJ, Corteen E, Czosnyka M, et al. Decompressive craniectomy in traumatic brain injury: the randomized multicenter RESCUEicp study. *Acta Neurochirurgica.* 2006;Supp 96:17–20. <http://www.RESCUEicp.com>.

158. Andrews PJ, Sinclair HL, Battison CG, et al. European society of intensive care medicine study of therapeutic hypothermia (32–35 degrees C) for intracranial pressure reduction after traumatic brain injury (the Eurotherm3235Trial). *Trials.* 2011;12:8.

159. Roberts I, Shakur H, Coats T, et al. The CRASH-2 trial: a randomised controlled trial and economic evaluation of the effects of tranexamic acid on death, vascular occlusive events and transfusion requirement in bleeding trauma patients. *Health Technology Assessment.* 2013;17:1–79.

160. Azzopardi D and Edwards AD. Magnetic resonance biomarkers of neuroprotective effects in infants with hypoxic ischemic encephalopathy. *Semin Fetal Neonatal Med.* 2010;15:261–69.

161. Young J, Murthy L, Westby M, et al. Diagnosis, prevention, and management of delirium: summary of NICE guidance. *BMJ.* 2010;341:c3704.

162. Brooke MM, Questad KA, Patterson DR, et al. Agitation and restlessness after closed head injury: a prospective study of 100 consecutive admissions. *Arch Phys Med Rehab.* 1992;73:320–23.

163. Corrigan JD. Development of a scale for assessment of agitation following traumatic brain injury. *J Clin Exp Neuropsychol.* 1989;11:261–77.

164. Fleminger S, Greenwood RJ, and Oliver DL. Pharmacological management for agitation and aggression in people with acquired brain injury. *Cochrane Database Syst Rev.* 2006;CD003299.

165. Warden DL, Gordon B, McAllister TW, et al. Guidelines for the pharmacologic treatment of neurobehavioral sequelae of traumatic brain injury. *J Neurotrauma.* 2006;23:1468–501.

166. Medicine BSoR. *Rehabilitation following acquired brain injury: National Clinical Guidelines.* London: Royal College of Physicians, 2003.

167. SIGN. *Brain injury rehabilitation in adults.* Edinburgh: SIGN, 2013.

168. Spitz G, Ponsford JL, Rudzki D, et al. Association between cognitive performance and functional outcome following traumatic brain injury: a longitudinal multilevel examination. *Neuropsychology.* 2012;26:604–12.

169. Wilson B. Towards a comprehensive model of cognitive rehabilitation. *Neuropsychological Rehabilitation.* 2002;12:97–110.

170. Cicerone KD. Facts, theories, values: shaping the course of neurorehabilitation. The 60th John Stanley Coulter memorial lecture. *Arch Phys Med Rehab.* 2012;93:188–91.

171. Turner-Stokes L, Disler PB, Nair A, et al. Multi-disciplinary rehabilitation for acquired brain injury in adults of working age. *Cochrane Database Syst Rev.* 2005;CD004170.

172. Cicerone KD, Langenbahn DM, Braden C, et al. Evidence-based cognitive rehabilitation: updated review of the literature from 2003 through 2008. *Arch Phys Med Rehab.* 2011;92:519–30.

173. Brasure M, Lamberty GJ, Sayer NA, et al. Participation after multidisciplinary rehabilitation for moderate to severe traumatic brain injury in adults: a systematic review. *Arch Phys Med Rehab.* 2013;94:1398–420.

174. Chung CS, Pollock A, Campbell T, et al. Cognitive rehabilitation for executive dysfunction in adults with stroke or other adult nonprogressive acquired brain damage. *Cochrane Database Syst Rev.* 2013;4:CD008391.

175. Krasny-Pacini A, Chevignard M and Evans J. Goal Management Training for rehabilitation of executive functions: a systematic review of effectiveness in patients with acquired brain injury. *Disability Rehab.* 2014;36:105–16.

176. Wilson BA, Emslie H, Quirk K, et al. A randomized control trial to evaluate a paging system for people with traumatic brain injury. *Brain Inj.* 2005;19:891–94.

177. Wheaton P, Mathias JL, and Vink R. Impact of pharmacological treatments on outcome in adult rodents after traumatic brain injury: a meta-analysis. *J Psychopharmacol.* 2011;25:1581–99.

178. Whyte J, Hart T, Vaccaro M, et al. Effects of methylphenidate on attention deficits after traumatic brain injury: a multidimensional, randomized, controlled trial. *Am J Phys Med Rehab.* 2004;83:401–20.

179. Wagner AK, Drewencki LL, Chen X, et al. Chronic methylphenidate treatment enhances striatal dopamine neurotransmission after experimental traumatic brain injury. *J Neurochem.* 2009;108:986–97.

180. Wagner AK, Sokoloski JE, Chen X, et al. Controlled cortical impact injury influences methylphenidate-induced changes in striatal dopamine neurotransmission. *J Neurochem.* 2009;110:801–10.

181. Wagner AK, Sokoloski JE, Ren D, et al. Controlled cortical impact injury affects dopaminergic transmission in the rat striatum. *J Neurochem.* 2005;95:457–65.

182. Wagner AK, Kline AE, Ren D, et al. Gender associations with chronic methylphenidate treatment and behavioral performance following experimental traumatic brain injury. *Behav Brain Res.* 2007;181:200–209.

183. Kline AE, Yan HQ, Bao J, et al. Chronic methylphenidate treatment enhances water maze performance following traumatic brain injury in rats. *Neuroscience Letters.* 2000;280:163–66.

184. Kim J, Whyte J, Patel S, et al. Methylphenidate modulates sustained attention and cortical activation in survivors of traumatic brain injury: a perfusion fMRI study. *Psychopharmacology.* 2012;222:47–57.

185. Willmott C and Ponsford J. Efficacy of methylphenidate in the rehabilitation of attention following traumatic brain injury: a randomised, crossover, double blind, placebo controlled inpatient trial. *J Neurol Neurosur Ps.* 2009;80:552–57.

186. Pavlovskaya M, Hochstein S, Keren O, et al. Methylphenidate effect on hemispheric attentional imbalance in patients with traumatic brain injury: a psychophysical study. *Brain Inj.* 2007;21:489–97.

187. Giacino JT, Whyte J, Bagiella E, *et al.* Placebo-controlled trial of amantadine for severe traumatic brain injury. *N Engl J Med.* 2012;366:819–26.

188. Meythaler JM, Brunner RC, Johnson A, *et al.* Amantadine to improve neurorecovery in traumatic brain injury-associated diffuse axonal injury: a pilot double-blind randomized trial. *J Head Trauma Rehab.* 2002;17:300–13.

189. Whyte J, Vaccaro M, Grieb-Neff P, *et al.* The effects of bromocriptine on attention deficits after traumatic brain injury: a placebo-controlled pilot study. *Am J Phys Med Rehab.* 2008;87:85–99.

190. McDowell S, Whyte J, and D'Esposito M. Differential effect of a dopaminergic agonist on prefrontal function in traumatic brain injury patients. *Brain.* 1998;121 Pt 6:1155–64.

191. Hammond FM, Bickett AK, Norton JH, *et al.* Effectiveness of Amantadine Hydrochloride in the Reduction of Chronic Traumatic Brain Injury Irritability and Aggression. *J Head Trauma Rehab.* 2014 Sep-Oct;29(5):391–9.

192. Wheaton P, Mathias JL, and Vink R. Impact of pharmacological treatments on cognitive and behavioral outcome in the postacute stages of adult traumatic brain injury: a meta-analysis. *J Clin Psycho Pharmacol.* 2011;31:745–57.

193. Torbic H, Forni AA, Anger KE, *et al.* Use of antiepileptics for seizure prophylaxis after traumatic brain injury. *Am J Health Syst Pharm.* 2013;9:759–66.

194. Wieshmann UC and Baker GA. Self-reported feelings of anger and aggression towards others in patients on levetiracetam: data from the UK antiepileptic drug register. *BMJ Open.* 2013;19:3.

195. Goldman-Rakic PS, Muly EC, 3rd, and Williams GV. D(1) receptors in prefrontal cells and circuits. *Brain Res.* 2000;31:295–301.

196. Schiff ND, Giacino JT, Kalmar K, *et al.* Behavioural improvements with thalamic stimulation after severe traumatic brain injury. *Nature.* 2007;448:600–603.

197. Ulam F, Shelton C, Richards L, *et al.* Cumulative effects of transcranial direct current stimulation on EEG oscillations and attention/working memory during subacute neurorehabilitation of traumatic brain injury. *Clinical Neurophysiology.* 2014.

198. Angelakis E, Liouta E, Andreadis N, *et al.* Transcranial direct current stimulation effects in disorders of consciousness. *Arch Phys Med Rehab.* 2014;95:283–89.

199. Wade DT, Filippov MA, Dityatev A, *et al.* Does routine follow up after head injury help? A randomised controlled trial. *J Neurol Neurosur Ps.* 1997;62:478–84.

200. Soleman S, Filippov MA, Dityatev A, *et al.* Targeting the neural extracellular matrix in neurological disorders. *Neuroscience.* 2013;253:194–213.

CHAPTER 40

Neurosurgery for cognitive disorders

Tom Foltynie and Ludvic Zrinzo

Space-occupying lesions including haematomata

Pressure effects from extra-axial/intra-axial space-occupying lesions (SOLs) can inevitably impact on cognitive function. The cognitive effects of any such lesions may reflect direct disruptions to specific cortical regions, their connections, or blood supply, the effects of increased intracranial pressure, or indeed seizure activity. Whether surgical intervention of an SOL is appropriate and if so how best it should be performed clearly needs to be made on a case-by-case basis and will depend on many factors including the nature of the lesion, its anatomical site, and the potential benefits and risks to cognition and other cerebral functions.

Hydrocephalus

Before the introduction of valve shunting systems, mortality from hydrocephalus was around 50 per cent and only 20 per cent of children with congenital hydrocephalus lived beyond the first decade. With the introduction of modern shunting procedures in the second half of the twentieth century, both survival and outcome in terms of independence improved; however, it remains far from normal.[1]

Hydrocephalus causes mechanical brain distortion and impaired cerebral blood flow resulting in changes in metabolism and neurotransmission. Shunting reduces intracranial pressure, decreases ventricular size, and improves neurochemical and cognitive functioning. However, surgery only incompletely reverses this damage and the potential for reversal fades with time. Timing of surgery is therefore an important factor.

External ventricular drainage provides a means of confirming cerebrospinal fluid (CSF) drainage in the acute phase. A third ventriculostomy or shunt procedure, most commonly to the peritoneal cavity but occasionally to the pleural space or right atrium, provides a more permanent solution when required (Figs 40.1 and 40.2).

Patients with adequately treated hydrocephalus nevertheless suffer from associated mild neuropsychological deficits, predominantly in visuospatial and motor functions, and other non-language skills.[2,3] In addition to the direct effects of hydrocephalus described earlier, other factors may contribute to this observation. Concomitant abnormalities (cerebral palsy, epilepsy, intraventricular haemorrhage, low birth weight, and asphyxia) all have a significant impact. Complications of CSF diversion can also have a significant effect on cognition. Shunt infections are associated with a higher risk of future shunt malfunction or infection, seizure, and reduced IQ and school performance.[4–6]

Normal pressure hydrocephalus

In 1965, Hakim and Adams first described a syndrome of gait disturbance, dementia, and urinary incontinence in patients with ventricular enlargement in the absence of elevated intracranial pressure.[7] This entity of normal pressure hydrocephalus (NPH) may be primary (so-called idiopathic NPH) or secondary, subsequent to diverse pathologies such as trauma or subarachnoid haemorrhage.

The diagnosis and management of NPH has been the subject of considerable controversy. Inaccurate diagnosis, overlap with comorbidity with similar clinical presentation in the elderly population, and variability in surgical complication rates have led to inconsistent results. Publication of international guidelines in 2005 established diagnostic criteria, diagnostic tests, surgical management, and outcome measures for idiopathic NPH.[8]

Diagnosis requires convergent evidence from the clinical history, examination, and investigations. Documentation of ventricular enlargement is required but not sufficient for the diagnosis. Although an Evans' index (the ratio of the transverse diameter of the anterior horns of the lateral ventricles to the greatest internal diameter of the skull adapted for measurement using computed tomography, CT) of ≥0.3 has been proposed, it is an unreliable means of measuring ventricular volume.[9]

Large-volume spinal taps (50 ml), prolonged external lumbar drainage, and infusion tests are often used to predict those who will benefit from shunt placement. Whilst positive results on these tests do predict a favourable response to shunt placement, high false negative rates with single spinal taps suggest that that it should not be used to exclude patients from surgery.[10] Conversely, patients responding well to shunt placement may have other diseases, including progressive supranuclear palsy, and CSF diversion has been proposed as a treatment for Alzheimer's disease, perhaps acting to clear abnormal proteins from the central nervous system.[11,12]

Study of the CSF proteins taken from patients with NPH shows broad decreases in the amyloid precursor protein-derived proteins (Aβ38, Aβ40, Aβ42) in contrast to the specific decreases seen in Aβ42 in Alzheimer's disease. This has been interpreted as either reflecting a reduced production of these proteins or their reduced clearance from the extracellular fluid space. Furthermore, CSF from ventricular shunts at the time of surgery compared with CSF sampled six months later suggested that a greater increase in these

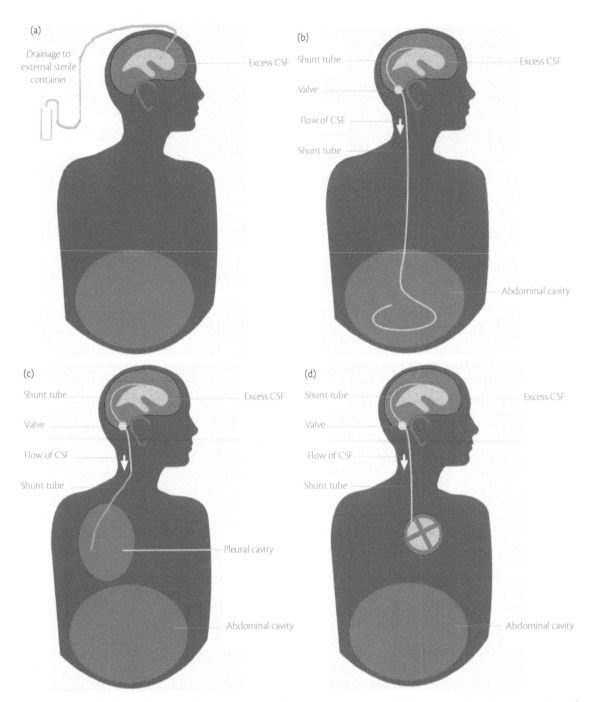

Fig. 40.1 Cerebrospinal fluid (CSF) diversion procedures. (a) External ventricular drainage involves drainage of CSF to an external sterile container. It is usually employed in the acute setting as a temporary measure when CSF is heavily blood-stained or infected. It allows close observation and tight control of CSF drainage as well as convenient access for administration of intrathecal antibiotics. (b) Ventriculoperitoneal shunt diverts excess CSF to the peritoneal cavity where it is subsequently absorbed. It is the most commonly used internalised CSF diversion procedure. Many different types of shunt valve are now commercially available to prevent over-drainage of CSF. (c) CSF diversion to the pleural cavity (ventriculopleural shunt) is an alternative that is used in patients with contraindications to peritoneal shunting (e.g. severe bowel adhesions) (d) Ventriculoatrial shunts divert CSF into the cardiovascular system via the right atrium. These are less commonly used because of their higher incidence of complications including septicaemia and shunt nephritis.

proteins was associated with greater clinical improvement perhaps indicating normalization of extracellular fluid (ECF) clearance to the CSF space.[13]

There is no clear evidence on the type of shunt that should be implanted for NPH. However, shunts with an anti-siphon device and adjustable valve may offer some advantages.[14] Class I outcome data are limited to a small trial in which 14 patients with extensive

vascular white matter disease and normal CSF dynamics were randomized to receive open or ligated shunts.[15] Patients and clinical examiners were blinded to group status. At three months, patients in the open shunt group improved significantly in their psychometric performance both when compared to their own baseline and when compared with patients with ligated shunts (p < 0.05). Patients with ligated shunts showed no change in psychometric

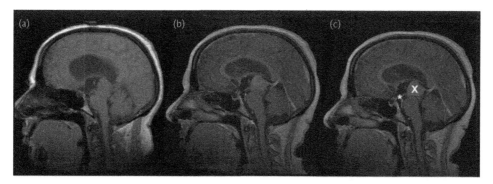

Fig. 40.2 Sagittal T1 weighted MRI scan before (a) and after (b&c) endoscopic third ventriculostomy (ETV). A pineal region tumour (x) was causing obstructive hydrocephalus. An endoscope introduced into the frontal horn of the lateral ventricle and, via the foramen of Munro, into the third ventricle. A small hole was placed in the floor of the third ventricle anterior to the mammillary bodies (*) to allow CSF to flow from the intraventricular to the subarachnoid space, thus bypassing the obstruction and allowing a reduction in ventricular size.

outcome. At three months, all patients underwent a further procedure: either removal of the ligature or sham surgery with a superficial incision over the shunt tubing. At six month follow-up, patients randomized to open shunts retained psychometric improvement; psychometric scores improved significantly between the three- and six-month assessment in those whose shunts were opened after the three-month follow-up.

Unfortunately, this promising early improvement in cognition is mitigated by open-labelled data that suggests that the longer-term prognosis for cognitive outcome is poor, even in patients who exhibit an initial improvement in gait, memory, or urinary continence.[16] Furthermore, surgery is not without complications, especially in the elderly. Infection, shunt malfunction, seizures, and subdural haematoma are among the possible complications.

In conclusion, NPH is a poorly understood clinical syndrome with variable outcome after shunt surgery. Nevertheless, it is one of the few conditions where significant reversal of cognitive decline has been observed in individual patients. Surgery should only be considered after judicious risk/benefit analysis. Further class I evidence is required to inform the surgical decision process better.

Epilepsy surgery

Epileptic seizures have a negative impact on cognitive development in childhood with evidence that the earlier the onset and the greater the resistance to pharmacotherapy, the greater the influence on cognition.[17] Pharmaco-resistant epilepsy also has a negative impact on cognition even when occurring in adulthood, affecting both attention and visual/verbal memory domains.[18] Furthermore, a long duration of epilepsy and an increased frequency of seizures are both associated with atrophy of both grey and white matter.[19]

Resective neurosurgery is increasingly used as treatment for refractory focal epilepsy following careful patient selection using detailed clinical, physiological, and imaging assessments. Most commonly this involves anterior temporal lobe resection although lesionectomies, extra temporal resections, and hemispherectomies are also sometimes performed. Long-term follow-up indicates that 52 per cent of individuals undergoing resective surgery for focal epilepsy become seizure-free at 5 years, and 47 per cent at 10 years.[20]

Data from a meta-analysis suggest that the memory outcome is linked to the seizure outcome,[21] and reduction in antiepileptic

drugs (AEDs).[22] It appears that patients achieving seizure freedom are more likely to have improvements in memory and non-memory cognitive performance over time, the surgery being most likely of benefit if accompanied by improvement in subclinical electro-encephalography (EEG) activity.[23] Unsuccessful surgery (with respect to seizure freedom) tends to have a negative impact on cognition.

While the overall evidence is favourable in well-selected individuals, there remain potential risks for cognition as a result of anterior temporal lobe resection surgery; these typically include impairments in verbal memory following left, and visual memory following right anterior temporal lobe resection. Using functional magnetic resonance imaging (fMRI) and a battery of neuropsychological tasks before and after resective surgery, it has been shown that patients that have effective pre-operative reorganization of verbal memory function to the ipsilateral posterior medial temporal lobe fare better in terms of verbal memory than those who reorganize verbal memory to the ipsilateral posterior temporal lobe structures post operatively. This was not true, however, for visual memory in the context of right temporal lobe resection largely explicable by the fact that in the series studied, only one patient suffered any visual memory deficit following surgery.[24]

Conclusions regarding the relative benefits and risks for cognition of epilepsy surgery requires appropriate measurement tools, detailed assessment of pre-operative cognitive status, and acknowledgement that impact may not be static but more likely fluctuates over time.[25] This said, the impact of cognition on quality of life is the most important issue and the majority of studies suggest that it is seizure freedom that predicts the overall quality of life regardless of cognitive outcome.[26]

Deep brain stimulation for cognitive disorders

Background

Deep brain stimulation (DBS) involves the precise delivery of focal electrical stimulation to either discrete nuclei or diffuse neuronal structures deep within the brain substance. The principles of DBS have existed for many years. The pioneers of functional neurosurgery demonstrated that the use of intra-operative high-frequency stimulation could usefully predict beneficial or unwanted effects in advance of producing an irreversible brain lesion for the treatment of pain or movement disorders.[27,28] Following recent improvements in technology, the ability to implant electrodes and pulse generators safely that can chronically deliver high-frequency stimulation has led to the near disappearance of lesional surgery such as pallidotomy and thalamotomy, and the widespread use of deep brain stimulation techniques.[29] The advantage of the DBS approach is that in many aspects it is a reversible therapy, and adverse events produced by stimulation can be avoided or ameliorated by changing the intensity of the current, or by choosing an alternative electrical contact on the implanted electrode for stimulation delivery.

While it is thought that high-frequency stimulation mimics the effect of a lesion (i.e. disrupts abnormal neuronal firing patterns), it is believed that low-frequency stimulation can excite local cell bodies/axons/dendrites and 'drive' activity both orthodromically and antidromically through discrete circuits. Low-frequency stimulation delivered to the sensory thalamus can be an effective treatment for some forms of chronic pain, while there has been significant interest in the use of low-frequency stimulation of the pedunculopontine nucleus (PPN DBS), known to be a key generator of locomotor activity, as a treatment for gait difficulties in Parkinson's disease (PD).[30]

Chronic high-frequency stimulation of the subthalamic nucleus (STN) or globus pallidus pars interna (Gpi) is now an accepted treatment for the motor complications of chronic PD,[31,32] and can lead to substantial improvements in motor function, and in the complications of chronic oral PD treatment, and the quality of life of the patient.[33] Disturbance of the activity in functional circuits explains why stimulation of the STN (the most common target to treat the motor complications of PD) leads to deterioration in verbal fluency and executive function among patients with limited cognitive reserves, because of the cognitive cortical-subcortical projections that pass through the associative territory of the STN.[34]

The observation that DBS can influence cognitive performance has sparked interest in the possible role of DBS to *improve* cognition. Cognitive processing involves the intact functioning of cortical-subcortical neuronal loops. Detailed knowledge regarding the circuitry underlying memory encoding and retrieval has been revealed as a result of lesioning experiments and functional imaging, and involves temporal lobe structures including the hippocampus and the adjacent perirhinal, entorhinal, and parahippocampal cortices. Manipulation of the neuronal circuitry underlying not only episodic memory but also attention and working memory, as well as further understanding of the circuitry involved in memory encoding and retrieval, represents not only a subject of great scientific interest but also has possible therapeutic potential in patients with mild cognitive impairment and early dementia syndromes.

Neurosurgical manipulation of structures involved in cognition

Hippocampus

The long-known importance of the hippocampus in memory circuits[35] has led to early studies investigating whether electrical stimulation of the hippocampus might influence memory functions. Rodent studies have demonstrated that low frequency stimulation (6 Hz) applied to the hippocampus can activate neocortical areas and indeed the contralateral hippocampus. In contrast,

high-frequency stimulation (130 Hz) does not recruit distal areas, confirming the distinction between presumed excitatory and inhibitory effects according to stimulation frequency.[36]

Human studies are difficult because of ethical concerns regarding experimental interventions with possible side-effects in either healthy volunteers or in individuals with deficits in cognition. A useful opportunity to evaluate the effects of stimulation to the hippocampus arises in the context of resective surgery for patients with medication resistant epileptic seizures. Ahead of resective surgery, the effects of electrical stimulation on temporal lobe structures including the hippocampus with respect to learning and recall have been examined, as this can serve as reassurance that the degree of surgical brain resection will be tolerated. Stimulation applied simultaneously to multiple medial temporal lobe structures was explored in the 1980s and found to disrupt memory rather than enhance memory irrespective of the timing of stimulation either during memory encoding or retrieval.[37]

Further studies have confirmed that stimulation of the hippocampus above the threshold which elicits activation of downstream structures (detected on the EEG), generally results in memory impairments rather than improvements. While unilateral stimulation of the hippocampus with single 1 ms pulses seemingly had no effects during a recognition memory task, pronounced deficits in memory were seen when bilateral stimulation was applied during the encoding phase.[38] This is consistent with clinical observations from subjects with isolated hippocampal lesions who are generally spared from cognitive damage, whereas subjects with bilateral lesions generally have severe memory deficits (see chapter 13). In contrast, another group reported that unilateral left hippocampal electrical stimulation delivered during memory encoding produced word recognition memory deficits, whereas right hippocampal stimulation delivered during memory encoding produced face recognition memory deficits.[39]

Despite the minor inconsistencies, the results of direct electrical stimulation of the hippocampus in humans have generally shown a disruptive effect on memory. It follows, therefore, that currently hippocampal stimulation is not considered likely to be useful as a therapeutic means of memory enhancement. The major inputs to the hippocampus are from the entorhinal cortex via the perforant pathway, as well as from the hypothalamus, mammillary body, and the medial septal area via the fornix. The possibility of manipulating these inputs to the hippocampus using electrical stimulation has been the subject of further studies.

Entorhinal cortex and perforant pathway

The entorhinal cortex (EC) is known to play a role in spatial memory and visual recognition memory based on *in vivo* recordings from the EC in non-human primates during standard cognitive tasks.[40,41] The EC projects to the hippocampus via the perforant pathway. The effect of electrical stimulation of the perforant pathway has been explored in rabbits. Short bursts of either low- or high-frequency stimulation led to long-term potentiation of the synaptic connections between cells within the hippocampus tested 30 minutes to 10 hours later.[42] Whether this alteration in hippocampal cell activity following EC stimulation might translate to clinically relevant effects has been studied in mice, with the demonstration that this improved spatial learning.[43] Of further interest was the observation that the improvements in learning were accompanied by an increase in dentate granule cell neurogenesis in the hippocampus. Although this may or may not be directly related to the mechanism of action of electrical stimulation, there is increasing interest in the role of hippocampal dentate gyrus neurogenesis and the normal processes of spatial learning,[44] and this remains an area of great interest.

The effect of electrical stimulation on other neurophysiological mechanisms influencing memory processing has also been explored in further rodent studies. The hippocampus is known to have high-amplitude neuronal activity in the theta (θ)-frequency, and it has been speculated that this θ-activity may be reset in response to presentation of environmental stimuli relevant to the encoding of new memories. In a rodent model, and after training on a visual discrimination task, stimulating electrodes were placed in the perforant pathway and in the fornix, accompanied by recording electrodes placed in the hippocampi. In response to a novel visual stimulus, resetting of θ-activity was recorded in the hippocampi. Furthermore, θ-resetting was reproducible through the delivery of stimulation to the perforant pathway or the fornix,[45] lending further evidence to support the possibility that memory processes might be amenable to manipulation by electrical stimulation.

Using a similar opportunity afforded by the study of human patients undergoing resective surgery for epilepsy, Suthana and colleagues combined neurophysiological assessments with a spatial memory task (a virtual maze) to see if DBS of the EC or hippocampus (using an amplitude below the threshold for eliciting an after-discharge) would improve memory.[46] Bilateral DBS of the EC during the learning phase of the task consistently improved performance during the test phase. Consistent with previous results, direct DBS of the hippocampus was not effective.

The impact of EC DBS on spatial memory seen to date is therefore encouraging, however whether these observations can be extended to patient groups with memory deficits needs further evaluation and will depend, at the very least, on the extent to which components of and connections between relevant circuitry are intact.

Fornix

The fornix is the main bidirectional pathway from the hippocampal complex to subcortical structures and carries the principal axonal projection from the hypothalamus to the hippocampus. Lesion studies in rodents have demonstrated that damage to the fornix results in spatial memory deficits. Transection of the fornix in non-human primates reveals that encoding of new spatial memory and long-term recall can remain intact despite fornix transection,[47] and this structure may indeed be rather more important for rapid acquisition of spatial memory.[48] Nevertheless, neurosurgical teaching has long since advised on avoidance of damage to the fornix because of postoperative declines in memory and motivation,[49] and a case report has documented a method of awake intraoperative stimulation of forniceal fibres to provide reassurance during tumour resection that the resection margins did not involve fibres necessary for memory. In this report, bipolar electrical stimulation of the fornix transiently disrupted memory encoding, although the authors did not detail the frequency of stimulation used.[50]

Human data of a potential beneficial use of DBS to the fornix for the amelioration of cognition also exist. The original observations surrounding the possible use of the fornix as a DBS target were somewhat serendipitous and were the subject of a case report (Fig. 40.3).[51] A gentleman with morbid obesity considered refractory to conventional treatments underwent an experimental

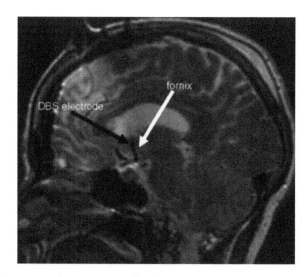

Fig. 40.3 Deep brain stimulation of the fornix: Sagittal magnetic resonance image (MRI) of DBS lead positioned immediately anterior and parallel to the vertical segment of the fornix within the hypothalamus.
Reproduced from *Ann Neurol.* 68(4), AW Laxton, DF Tang-Wai, MP McAndrews, *et al.* A Phase I Trial of Deep Brain Stimulation of Memory Circuits in Alzheimer's Disease, pp. 521–34, Copyright (2010), with permission from John Wiley and Sons.

procedure of hypothalamic DBS as an attempt to treat his obesity. His cognition was considered normal at baseline. During the surgical procedure the patient reported strong sensation of déjà vu accompanied by a perception of being in a familiar scene some years previously that reproducibly accompanied stimulation. (While the patient did later progress to have a generalized seizure, these observations were not considered to be epileptic in origin.)

Subsequent double-blind evaluation of memory with the stimulation either switched on at 130 Hz or off revealed improved recognition memory performance with the DBS switched on. Electromagnetic tomography demonstrated an increase in activity in medial temporal lobe structures when the DBS was switched on at 3 Hz (130 Hz stimulation was not used because of artefact produced on the electromagnetic tomogram).

Despite the difficulty interpreting the data with respect to high-/low-frequency stimulation, these observations formed the inspiration for the same group to evaluate the use of DBS of the fornix in six patients with early Alzheimer's disease. High-frequency stimulation was used through the most ventral contacts in the hypothalamus adjacent to the fornix. At 6 months, 4 of the 6 patients were improved compared to baseline using the ADAS–Cog scale; however, this was maintained in only 1 of the 6 patients at 12 months. No randomized controls were recruited to compare the natural history of decline in Alzheimer's disease but the authors observed a slowing in the decline in the mini-mental state examination (MMSE) in the 12 months following surgery compared to the 12 months prior to surgery.[52]

Again, electromagnetic tomography was used to examine activation patterns as a result of the stimulation. Given the artefacts associated with high-frequency stimulation, low-frequency stimulation was used for this aspect of the study. At a latency of 38–52 ms after stimulation, activation was seen in the ipsilateral hippocampus and parahippocampal gyrus. At 102–256 ms, activation was seen in the ipsilateral cingulate gyrus and precuneus suggestive of trans-synaptic transmission occurring in response to stimulation (at low frequency).

The chronic responses to high-frequency DBS were evaluated using fluorodeoxyglucose (FDG) positron emission tomography (PET) imaging, demonstrating that at baseline the patients had decrease FDG uptake in the temporoparietal regions compared with healthy controls. Increases in FDG uptake in these same areas were seen following one month and one year of high-frequency DBS.

Most importantly, the authors were able to confirm the safety and tolerability of surgery in this vulnerable patient group. All patients were discharged from hospital between 1 and 3 days following surgery, there were no hardware associated adverse events, and none required hospitalization in the 12 months following surgery.

Nucleus basalis of Meynert

The nucleus basalis of Meynert (NBM), the medial septum, and the diagonal band of Broca represent the major sources of cortical and limbic acetylcholine (Ach). There is extensive evidence of the importance of the NBM and ACh in the cognitive deficits of Alzheimer's disease and Parkinson's disease in which this nucleus undergoes degeneration. Furthermore, the cholinesterase inhibitors represent the most effective group of agents currently available for the relief of the early memory deficits seen in Alzheimer's disease and Parkinson's disease dementia.[53] It is thought that activation of the NBM is involved in directing attention to novel stimuli.[54]

It has been confirmed that lesions in this NBM area result in deficits in cognitive function in rodent models.[55] When the NBM is electrically stimulated in the rodent, it has been shown by several groups that cortical ACh is released,[56,57] there is EEG activation,[58] and there is an increase in regional cerebral blood flow (rCBF).[59,60] These and other *in vivo* experiments have thus added weight to the hypothesis that the basal forebrain cholinergic system can be manipulated and have positive effects on memory processes. Indeed, NBM electrical stimulation has been associated with facilitation of a range of cognitive tasks in rodent models including behavioural associative memory,[61,62] and acquisition of memory during aversively motivated conditioning.[63]

The cortical changes resulting from NBM stimulation can be blocked by the co-administration of atropine which blocks muscarinic ACh receptors,[64] confirming the relevance of cholinergic neuronal activity in the effects of NBM stimulation. While cholinergic manipulation is likely to be related to any beneficial response to NBM stimulation, it has also been observed that NBM stimulation can induce 'vasodilatation-independent' increase in blood flow to the cortex accompanied by prevention of delayed death of cortical neurons as seen in a model of cortical ischaemia in the rat.[65]

The extent to which subtle changes of cognitive performance that may accompany NBM stimulation can be judged in any rodent model is of course limited, as is the temptation to extrapolate any perceived effects to those which might be achievable in the human brain. Considerable work has also evaluated the basal forebrain cholinergic system using experiments in nonhuman primates (NHP) with a far more complex and relevant battery of neuropsychological measures. NHP studies provide consistent support for the role of the basal forebrain cholinergic structures in cognition. NBM neurons have been shown to be involved in decision making processes in a go/no-go task in the NHP, which can thus distinguish firing patterns that might be otherwise related to sensory or motor processes.[66]

The impact of NBM lesions on NHP cognition has been evaluated using MRI-guided ibotinic acid injections targeting the NBM, diagonal band of Broca, and medial septum. This approach has been used to destroy the cholinergic neurons originating from the basal forebrain with serial evaluation of the impact on object discrimination, delayed non-matching to sample task and an attention task. While there was no impact of the lesioning on the former tasks, attentional focusing was clearly impaired in the lesioned animals.[67,68]

Despite the extensive data on lesioning, the effects of electrical stimulation of the NBM in NHP is to our knowledge yet to be studied. Despite this major void in the translational pipeline, the possibility of influencing cognition in human subjects using DBS to the NBM has already prompted neurosurgical intervention in two patients.

The NBM was investigated as a possible target for chronic DBS in a human patient as early as 1985. A unilateral DBS electrode was placed in the NBM in a single 74-year-old patient with a 4-year history of memory problems consistent with Alzheimer's disease. FDG-PET scanning pre-operatively had shown widespread diminished utilization of glucose. Longitudinal assessments of clinical progression including neuropsychological tests were conducted, but after eight months of unilateral stimulation, the authors concluded that there had been no clinical response to the stimulation. Follow-up FDG-PET imaging after electrode implantation did, however, demonstrate that on the side of stimulation there was either an increase or lesser decrease in glucose activation in comparison to the non-operated side, indicating a possible biological effect of the stimulation.[69]

The NBM has also been of interest in the treatment of patients with Parkinson's disease (PD) and dementia. It is known that up to 80 per cent of PD patients will ultimately develop dementia, and the natural history of the progression of specific cognitive impairments to dementia in PD has been the subject of detailed population based studies.[70,71] The pathophysiological causes of cognitive impairment in PD are diverse being influenced by neurodegeneration occurring in subcortical dopaminergic and cholinergic neurons, non-physiological dopamine replacement and/or anticholinergic medications, comorbid conditions affecting brain function, and neurodegeneration of cortical neurons themselves due to α-synuclein-positive Lewy body pathology.[72]

At the time of writing, there has been a single report of a patient with cognitive impairment in association with PD who had DBS electrodes inserted into the NBM. Having had a 22-year history of L-dopa responsive PD, he developed widespread cognitive deficits over 2 years including problems with memory, concentration, executive function, and praxis. This patient had conventional bilateral electrodes placed in the STN at the same time and introduction of NBM stimulation only after a stable response to STN DBS had been achieved. The authors reported immediate improvements in attention, concentration, and alertness as a result of low-frequency stimulation delivered through the NBM electrodes, which were sustained for the subsequent two months. Further cognitive tests were performed one day after NBM stimulation was switched off, showing a rapid and marked decline in cognitive function that was restored with reintroduction of NBM stimulation (Fig. 40.4).[73,74]

There are therefore limited but encouraging data on the possibility of using DBS as a treatment for cognitive impairments in PD, in particular stimulation of the NBM. As a result there are several teams of investigators now evaluating the effects of NBM DBS in double-blind crossover trials.

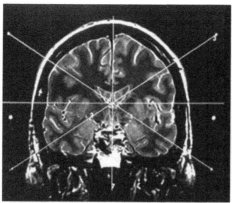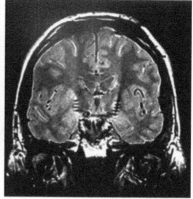

Fig. 40.4 Left: Coronal proton density stereotactic MRI prior to DBS lead implantation. The surgical plan aims to place the deepest contact of the quadripolar DBS lead within the nucleus basalis of Meynert that lies immediately inferior to the globus pallidus pars interna, around 8 mm posterior to the anterior commissure. Right: Coronal proton density stereotactic MRI following DBS lead implantation confirming accurate placement of the distal contact within the visualized anatomical target.

Deep brain stimulation as a treatment for cognitive deficits?

Ahead of any therapeutic extension of these observations, several major issues emerge.

1) Studies based on animal models can offer insights into neuronal processes that can follow electrical stimulation but are limited by the difficulty of detailed cognitive assessment. Nevertheless, animal models allow more detailed evaluation of possible mechanisms of action. It has been proposed that the effects of fornix lesions may lead to loss of transcription of the immediate–early gene *Arc* which is related to engagement of hippocampal synaptic plasticity,[75] and thus it is tempting to speculate that fornix DBS may facilitate/reinstate this. Separately, the proposed effects of electrical stimulation on neurogenesis in the dentate gyrus[43] or upon θ-resetting[45] require further study.

2) It is unclear whether DBS can be a positive influence on cognition only in individuals with intact brain anatomy, or whether stimulation may in fact assist cognitive processes in the context of cortical damage, or in the presence of ongoing neurodegeneration. The work from the neurosurgical epilepsy teams has given great insights into the potential for deep brain stimulation as a possible treatment for disorders of cognition, however many questions remain. The effects of stimulation in a healthy brain albeit in the presence of a seizure tendency (e.g. on processes of synaptic plasticity) may not apply in the presence of degenerating pathology such as due to accumulation of β-amyloid or α-synuclein.

Although DBS has been linked with neurogenesis in some animal models, few people believe that DBS offers a neuroprotective option. More likely is the possibility that deleterious abnormal activity emerging in an important neuronal circuit as a result of neurodegeneration might be overcome or replaced by the use of electrical stimulation. This would suggest that there might be only a narrow therapeutic window when electrical stimulation might help well-selected individuals. Further experimental studies should accurately document the long-term follow-up of patients to allow reliable estimates of the duration of any response to be made.

3) If stimulation is shown to be helpful in patients with neurodegeneration, whether the optimal application of stimulation is continuous (night and day), as is the case for stimulation of the STN or Gpi in patients with PD, or intermittent stimulation (e.g. switched on during periods of learning or encoding of new memory), or used sparingly to prevent tolerance occurring, as is the case of VIM thalamus DBS used for the treatment of tremor.

4) It remains unclear whether any differential effects may occur according to laterality of stimulation (i.e whether left hemisphere stimulation may have greater effects for verbal memory deficits while right hemisphere stimulation may have greater effects for non-verbal deficits), or whether bilateral stimulation is necessary for any therapeutic effect.

5) The use of electrical stimulation for patients with cognitive deficits will remain an experimental treatment option for the time being, therefore there are issues regarding consent and the capacity to provide informed consent which will potentially limit the patients that are eligible for participation in trial projects. Approaches to overcome this difficulty is the suggestion of performing tandem DBS (i.e. those patients already considered to be good DBS candidates for perhaps their motor symptoms in PD), undergoing the placement of additional brain electrodes at the same sitting. This of course is not free of additional risk given that every brain penetration carries a potential risk in its own right.

Conclusions regarding surgery in patients with cognitive impairment

Individuals with cognitive impairment deserve the same opportunities for clinical intervention as individuals with physical disabilities. In the context of life-threatening pathology such as lesions causing raised intracranial pressure, there is rarely any question about the appropriateness of surgical interventions as treatment options, even when altered consciousness or confusion impact on the normal processes of obtaining informed consent. In contrast, however, insidious processes leading to cognitive decline that occur over many years raise issues of consent and capacity, and are an appropriate source of concern in the development of any techniques that remain experimental rather than of proven efficacy. In the absence of effective long-term treatments for patients with degenerative dementias, the possible role of neurosurgery during a specific window of the dementia process is an appropriate consideration. It is unlikely that functional neurosurgery will be of use once dementia pathological processes are very widespread and significant atrophy has already occurred, however the parallels between the movement disorder of Parkinson's disease and the fluctuating cognitive deficits seen in PD dementia/dementia with Lewy bodies where a neurochemical disturbance causes downstream abnormalities of electrical function is appealing.

Such work needs to proceed with great caution, with parallel work collecting data in *in-vivo* models to support mechanistic insights, as well as in human subjects with safety remaining of paramount importance, and the collection of robust long-term clinical data together with neurophysiological and imaging biomarkers all being properly exploited.

References

1. Hirsch JF. Surgery of hydrocephalus: past, present and future. *Acta Neurochir (Wien)*. 1992;116:155–60.
2. Hoppe-Hirsch E, Laroussinie F, Brunet L, *et al*. Late outcome of the surgical treatment of hydrocephalus. *Childs Nerv Syst*. 1998 Mar;14(3):97–9.
3. Topczewska-Lach E, Lenkiewicz T, Olański W, *et al*. Quality of life and psychomotor development after surgical treatment of hydrocephalus. *Eur J Pediatr Surg*. 2005 Feb;15(1):2–5.
4. Kanev PM and Sheehan JM. Reflections on shunt infection. *Pediatr Neurosurg*. 2003;39:285–90.
5. Lindquist B, Carlsson G, Persson EK, *et al*. Learning disabilities in a population-based group of children with hydrocephalus. *Acta Paediatr*. 2005;94:878–83.
6. Mataro M, Junque C, Poca MA, *et al*. Neuropsychological findings in congenital and acquired childhood hydrocephalus. *Neuropsychol Rev*. 2001;11:169–78.
7. Hakim S and Adams RD. The special clinical problem of symptomatic hydrocephalus with normal cerebrospinal fluid pressure. Observations on cerebrospinal fluid hydrodynamics. *J Neurol Sci*. 1965;2:307–27.
8. Marmarou A, Black P, Bergsneider M, *et al*. Guidelines for management of idiopathic normal pressure hydrocephalus: progress to date. *Acta Neurochir Suppl*. 2005;95:237–40.
9. Toma AK, Holl E, Kitchen ND, *et al*. Evans' index revisited: the need for an alternative in normal pressure hydrocephalus. *Neurosurgery*. 2011;68:939–44.
10. Marmarou A, Bergsneider M, Klinge P, *et al*. The value of supplemental prognostic tests for the preoperative assessment of idiopathic normal-pressure hydrocephalus. *Neurosurgery*. 2005;57:S17–S28.
11. Schott JM, Williams DR, Butterworth RJ *et al*. Shunt responsive progressive supranuclear palsy? *Mov Disorders*. 2007;22(6):902–3.
12. Magdalinou NK, Ling H, Smith JD, *et al*. Normal pressure hydrocephalus or progressive supranuclear palsy? A clinicopathological case series. *J Neurol*. 2013 Apr;260(4):1009–13.
13. Jeppsson A, Zetterberg H, Blennow K, *et al*. Idiopathic normal pressure hydrocephalus: pathophysiology and diagnosis by CSF biomarkers. *Neurology*. 2013 Apr 9;80(15):1385–92.
14. Bergsneider M, Black PM, Klinge P, *et al*. Surgical management of idiopathic normal-pressure hydrocephalus. *Neurosurgery*. 2005;57:S29–S39.
15. Tisell M, Tullberg M, Hellstrom P, *et al*. Shunt surgery in patients with hydrocephalus and white matter changes. *J Neurosurg*. 2011;114:1432–8.
16. Koivisto AM, Alafuzoff I, Savolainen S, *et al*. Poor cognitive outcome in shunt-responsive idiopathic normal pressure hydrocephalus. *Neurosurgery*. 2013;72:1–8.
17. Berg AT, Zelko FA, Levy SR, *et al*. Age at onset of epilepsy, pharmacoresistance, and cognitive outcomes: a prospective cohort study. *Neurology*. 2012 Sep 25;79(13):1384–91.
18. Baker GA, Taylor J, and Aldenkamp AP. Newly diagnosed epilepsy: cognitive outcome after 12 months. *Epilepsia*. 2011;52:1084–91.
19. Coan AC, Appenzeller S, Bonilha LM, *et al*. Seizure frequency and lateralization affect progression of atrophy in temporal lobe epilepsy. *Neurology*. 2009;73:834–42.
20. de Tisi J, Bell GS, Peacock JL, *et al*. The long-term outcome of adult epilepsy surgery, patterns of seizure remission, and relapse: a cohort study. *Lancet*. 2011 Oct 15;378(9800):1388–95.
21. Tellez-Zenteno JF, Dhar R, Hernandez-Ronquillo L, *et al*. Long-term outcomes in epilepsy surgery: antiepileptic drugs, mortality, cognitive and psychosocial aspects. *Brain*. 2007;130(Pt. 2):334–45.
22. Skirrow C, Cross JH, Cormack F, Harkness W, *et al*. Long-term intellectual outcome after temporal lobe surgery in childhood. *Neurology*. 2011;76:1330–37.
23. Helmstaedter C, Kurthen M, Lux S, *et al*. Chronic epilepsy and cognition: a longitudinal study in temporal lobe epilepsy. *Ann Neurol*. 2003;54:425–32.
24. Bonelli SB, Thompson PJ, Yogarajah M, *et al*. Memory reorganization following anterior temporal lobe resection: a longitudinal functional MRI study. *Brain*. 2013 Jun;136(Pt 6):1889–900.
25. Baxendale S. The impact of epilepsy surgery on cognition and behavior. *Epilepsy Behav*. 2008;12:592–9.
26. Langfitt JT, Westerveld M, Hamberger MJ, *et al*. Worsening of quality of life after epilepsy surgery: effect of seizures and memory decline. *Neurology*. 2007;68:1988–94.
27. Wycis HT and Spiegel EA. Ten years' experience with stereotaxic operations on the basal ganglia. *Clin Neurosurg*. 1958;6:240–52.
28. Hassler R, Riechert T, Mundinger F, *et al*. Physiological observations in stereotaxic operations in extrapyramidal motor disturbances. *Brain*. 1960;83:337–50.
29. Limousin P, Pollak P, Benazzouz A, *et al*. Effect of parkinsonian signs and symptoms of bilateral subthalamic nucleus stimulation. *Lancet*. 1995;345:91–95.
30. Zrinzo L, Zrinzo LV, Tisch S, *et al*. Stereotactic localization of the human pedunculopontine nucleus: atlas-based coordinates and validation of a magnetic resonance imaging protocol for direct localization. *Brain*. 2008;131:1588–98.
31. Limousin P, Krack P, Pollak P, *et al*. Electrical stimulation of the subthalamic nucleus in advanced Parkinson's disease. *N Engl J Med*. 1998;339:1105–11.
32. Foltynie T and Hariz MI. Surgical management of Parkinson's disease. *Expert Rev Neurother*. 2010;10:903–14.
33. Foltynie T, Zrinzo L, Martinez-Torres I *et al*. MRI-guided STN DBS in Parkinson's disease without microelectrode recording: efficacy and safety. *J Neurol Neurosur Ps*. 2010.
34. Witt K, Daniels C, Reiff J, *et al*. Neuropsychological and psychiatric changes after deep brain stimulation for Parkinson's disease: a randomised, multicentre study. *Lancet Neurol*. 2008;7:605–14.
35. Drewe EA, Ettlinger G, Milner AD, *et al*. A comparative review of the results of neuropsychological research on man and monkey. *Cortex*. 1970;6:129–63.
36. da Silva JC, Amorim H, Scorza FA, *et al*. Brain electrical activity after acute hippocampal stimulation in awake rats. *Neuromodulation*. 2013 16(2):100–4.
37. Halgren E, Wilson CL, and Stapleton JM. Human medial temporal-lobe stimulation disrupts both formation and retrieval of recent memories. *Brain Cogn*. 1985;4:287–95.
38. Lacruz ME, Valentin A, Seoane JJ, *et al*. Single pulse electrical stimulation of the hippocampus is sufficient to impair human episodic memory. *Neuroscience*. 2010;170:623–32.
39. Coleshill SG, Binnie CD, Morris RG, *et al*. Material-specific recognition memory deficits elicited by unilateral hippocampal electrical stimulation. *J Neurosci*. 2004;24:1612–16.
40. Suzuki WA, Miller EK, and Desimone R. Object and place memory in the macaque entorhinal cortex. *J Neurophysiol*. 1997;78:1062–81.
41. Suh J, Rivest AJ, Nakashiba T, *et al*. Entorhinal cortex layer III input to the hippocampus is crucial for temporal association memory. *Science*. 2011;334:1415–20.
42. Bliss TV and Gardner-Medwin AR. Long-lasting potentiation of synaptic transmission in the dentate area of the unanaesthetized rabbit following stimulation of the perforant path. *J Physiol*. 1973;232:357–74.

43. Stone SS, Teixeira CM, Devito LM, *et al.* Stimulation of entorhinal cortex promotes adult neurogenesis and facilitates spatial memory. *J Neurosci.* 2011;31:13469–84.

44. Clelland CD, Choi M, Romberg C, *et al.* A functional role for adult hippocampal neurogenesis in spatial pattern separation. *Science.* 2009;325:210–13.

45. Williams JM and Givens B. Stimulation-induced reset of hippocampal theta in the freely performing rat. *Hippocampus.* 2003;13:109–16.

46. Suthana N, Haneef Z, Stern J, *et al.* Memory enhancement and deep-brain stimulation of the entorhinal area. *N Engl J Med.* 2012;366:502–10.

47. Kwok SC and Buckley MJ. Long-term visuospatial retention unaffected by fornix transection. *Hippocampus.* 2010;20:889–93.

48. Kwok SC and Buckley MJ. Fornix transection selectively impairs fast learning of conditional visuospatial discriminations. *Hippocampus.* 2010;20:413–22.

49. Hodges JR and Carpenter K. Anterograde amnesia with fornix damage following removal of IIIrd ventricle colloid cyst. *J Neurol Neurosur Ps.* 1991;54:633–8.

50. Brandling-Bennett EM, Bookheimer SY, Horsfall JL *et al.* A paradigm for awake intraoperative memory mapping during forniceal stimulation. *Neurocase.* 2012;18:26–38.

51. Hamani C, McAndrews MP, Cohn M *et al.* Memory enhancement induced by hypothalamic/fornix deep brain stimulation. *Ann Neurol.* 2008;63:119–23.

52. Laxton AW, Tang-Wai DF, McAndrews MP, *et al.* A phase I trial of deep brain stimulation of memory circuits in Alzheimer's disease. *Ann Neurol.* 2010;68:521–34.

53. Emre M, Aarsland D, Albanese A *et al.* Rivastigmine for dementia associated with Parkinson's disease. *N Engl J Med.* 2004;351:2509–18.

54. Yu AJ and Dayan P. Uncertainty, neuromodulation, and attention. *Neuron.* 2005;46:681–92.

55. Hasselmo ME and Sarter M. Modes and models of forebrain cholinergic neuromodulation of cognition. *Neuropsychopharmacology.* 2011;36:52–73.

56. Casamenti F, Deffenu G, Abbamondi AL, *et al.* Changes in cortical acetylcholine output induced by modulation of the nucleus basalis. *Brain Res Bull.* 1986;16:689–95.

57. Kurosawa M, Sato A, and Sato Y. Stimulation of the nucleus basalis of Meynert increases acetylcholine release in the cerebral cortex in rats. *Neurosci Lett.* 1989;98:45–50.

58. Jimenez-Capdeville ME, Dykes RW, *et al.* Differential control of cortical activity by the basal forebrain in rats: a role for both cholinergic and inhibitory influences. *J Comp Neurol.* 1997;381:53–67.

59. Adachi T, Inanami O, Ohno K, *et al.* Responses of regional cerebral blood flow following focal electrical stimulation of the nucleus basalis of Meynert and the medial septum using the [14C]iodoantipyrine method in rats. *Neurosci Lett.* 1990;112:263–8.

60. Hotta H, Uchida S, Kagitani F, *et al.* Control of cerebral cortical blood flow by stimulation of basal forebrain cholinergic areas in mice. *J Physiol Sci.* 2011;61:201–9.

61. McLin DE, III, Miasnikov AA, and Weinberger NM. Induction of behavioral associative memory by stimulation of the nucleus basalis. *Proc Natl Acad Sci USA.* 2002;99:4002–7.

62. Miasnikov AA, Chen JC, and Weinberger NM. Behavioral memory induced by stimulation of the nucleus basalis: effects of contingency reversal. *Neurobiol Learn Mem.* 2009;91:298–309.

63. Montero-Pastor A, Vale-Martinez A, Guillazo-Blanch G, *et al.* Effects of electrical stimulation of the nucleus basalis on two-way active avoidance acquisition, retention, and retrieval. *Behav Brain Res.* 2004;154:41–54.

64. Goard M and Dan Y. Basal forebrain activation enhances cortical coding of natural scenes. *Nat Neurosci.* 2009;12:1444–9.

65. Hotta H, Uchida S, and Kagitani F. Effects of stimulating the nucleus basalis of Meynert on blood flow and delayed neuronal death following transient ischemia in the rat cerebral cortex. *Jpn J Physiol.* 2002;52:383–93.

66. Richardson RT and DeLong MR. Context-dependent responses of primate nucleus basalis neurons in a go/no-go task. *J Neurosci.* 1990;10:2528–40.

67. Voytko ML, Olton DS, Richardson RT, *et al.* Basal forebrain lesions in monkeys disrupt attention but not learning and memory. *J Neurosci.* 1994;14:167–86.

68. Voytko ML. Cognitive functions of the basal forebrain cholinergic system in monkeys: memory or attention? *Behav Brain Res.* 1996;75:13–25.

69. Turnbull IM, McGeer PL, Beattie L, *et al.* Stimulation of the basal nucleus of Meynert in senile dementia of Alzheimer's type. A preliminary report. *Appl Neurophysiol.* 1985;48:216–21.

70. Williams-Gray CH, Foltynie T, Brayne CE, *et al.* Evolution of cognitive dysfunction in an incident Parkinson's disease cohort. *Brain.* 2007;130:1787–98.

71. Williams-Gray CH, Evans JR, Goris A, *et al.* The distinct cognitive syndromes of Parkinson's disease:5 year follow-up of the CamPaIGN cohort. *Brain.* 2009;132:2958–69.

72. Farlow MR and Cummings J. A modern hypothesis: The distinct pathologies of dementia associated with Parkinson's disease versus Alzheimer's disease. *Dement Geriatr Cogn Disord.* 2008;25:301–8.

73. Freund HJ, Kuhn J, Lenartz D, *et al.* Cognitive functions in a patient with Parkinson-dementia syndrome undergoing deep brain stimulation. *Arch Neurol.* 2009;66:781–5.

74. Barnikol TT, Pawelczyk NB, Barnikol UB *et al.* Changes in apraxia after deep brain stimulation of the nucleus basalis Meynert in a patient with Parkinson dementia syndrome. *Mov Disord.* 2010;25:1519–20.

75. Fletcher BR, Calhoun ME, Rapp PR, *et al.* Fornix lesions decouple the induction of hippocampal arc transcription from behavior but not plasticity. *J Neurosci.* 2006;26:1507–15.

CHAPTER 41

Cognition in severe mental illness
Schizophrenia, bipolar disorder, and depression

Philip D. Harvey and Christopher R. Bowie

Background

While schizophrenia is notable for its florid psychotic symptoms, including delusions and hallucinations, and negative symptoms associated with emotional blunting, amotivation, and anhedonia, cognitive impairments are a central feature of the illness.[1] Mood disorders are also defined by their clinical symptoms which include depression and elevated mood states such as mania or hypomania. Although there has been a long-term debate about the differences between mood disorders and schizophrenia in terms of cognitive functioning, cognitive impairments appear to be more strongly associated with disability and reduced quality of life than other symptoms of the illness across both schizophrenia and severe mood disorders.[2] Despite the fact that schizophrenia has long been characterized as a brain disorder with dementia-like features (e.g. its historical name, dementia praecox), the appreciation of the importance of cognitive deficits has often been minimal on the part of clinicians treating the illness and the importance of cognitive impairments in mood disorders is even less well appreciated.

One of the major controversies in the study of cognition impairments in mood disorders is their state-relatedness.[3] In an individual with significant depressive or manic symptoms, it seems quite logical to believe that poor performance on cognitive tests is a *secondary* feature of the condition, based on the state-related inability or unwillingness to generate optimal performance. This issue has most likely led to the reduced attention paid to cognitive impairments and their implications in mood disorders compared to schizophrenia. However, recent developments in the study of mood disorders, including several substantial meta-analyses, have clarified the nature and course of mood symptoms and suggested that substantial cognitive deficits are present even during relatively asymptomatic mood states.[4-5] As described later in this chapter, impairments in cognitive performance are most prevalent, both during psychosis and remission, for people with schizophrenia. In both major depression and bipolar disorder, cognitive impairments are more common during mood states but are also prevalent during periods of relative symptomatic remission. It appears that cognitive impairments in the absence of mood symptoms are approximately twice as common in bipolar disorder compared to major depression.

In this chapter, we discuss the course and profile of cognitive impairments in schizophrenia and severe mood disorders and relate these to their functional implications and potential treatments. Our evaluation of the cognitive impairments includes a description of the profile and severity of impairments, the timing of onset of impairments, and their course after diagnosis. We will evaluate the similarities of these impairments to those seen in other conditions where the neurobiology is better understood and will also present evidence that allows for rejection of certain possible causes for these impairments. We focus our discussion of mood disorders on bipolar disorder and major depression, both of which have received the majority of research attention.

Profile of cognitive impairment

Schizophrenia

Cognitive impairments in schizophrenia involve most of the ability domains identified in clinical neuropsychology, including episodic learning and memory for verbal and nonverbal information, working memory, attention, executive functioning, processing speed, and reasoning and problem-solving.[6] Performance in these ability areas is typically at levels that are over 1.0 standard deviation (SD) worse than would be expected on the basis of premorbid intellectual functioning. Premorbid functioning in schizophrenia is itself reduced compared to general population standards, although these reductions are of the order of 0.5–0.75 SD below general population expectations.[7]

There are some *spared* cognitive domains including long-term memory for verbal and nonverbal information learned previously and some (but not all) elements of basic perceptual functioning. In particular, one specific form of long-term memory, word-recognition reading performance, is spared to the extent that it is routinely used as an estimate of premorbid intellectual functioning much as with dementia.[8-9] Across large-scale studies of cognitive deficits,[10] the recent conclusion has been that there is a pattern of *global* impairments affecting nearly all ability areas, with some domains somewhat more impaired than others. Areas with more impairment include processing speed (typically indexed with coding tests such as Wechsler scale digit symbol), episodic memory (indexed with serial verbal learning tests), reasoning, and problem-solving tests, and working memory.[11] Compared to individuals with focal lesions, such as medial temporal lesions leading to anterograde amnesia, in schizophrenia the differences between impairments across the most impaired domains are small, of the order of 0.75 SD or less compared to the background levels of average impairment.

Bipolar disorder

The cognitive impairment profile in bipolar disorder is quite similar to the pattern observed in schizophrenia, although group comparisons find the magnitude of deficits tends to be approximately one-half as severe. Most severe deficits are often observed in verbal learning and executive functions (particularly those that involve either sustained attention or inhibition), while some domains such as visual processing and verbal skills are typically in the average or above-average range.[12–13] The study of cognition in bipolar disorder has certainly lagged behind schizophrenia. Although the field is now very actively examining the profile of impairment in bipolar disorder, and some researchers have suggested that there may be important lessons to be learned from schizophrenia research,[2] some methods are probably too closely aligned with schizophrenia research and possibly imperfect for research in bipolar illness.

As with the limitations found in borrowing from brain injury concepts methods earlier in research on the neuropsychology of schizophrenia,[14] this tendency to view bipolar disorder as a close relative of schizophrenia on the basis of similar profiles on relatively nonspecific tests could hamper our ability to understand its neuropsychological signature fully. Recent attempts to address this have been initiated, with suggested batteries of tests that differ slightly from those used in schizophrenia research.[15] New tools might need to be developed to reveal the true picture of the profile of impairment, similar to previous efforts in schizophrenia. Nonetheless, it is entirely possible that the determinants of cognitive deficits in both conditions are similar and perhaps unrelated to the aetiology of the primary symptoms of the disorder.

Major depression

Major depression is also accompanied by cognitive impairments that are generally believed to be greater during periods of depression. As with schizophrenia and bipolar disorder, deficits in verbal learning, working memory, and executive functions are noted and like bipolar disorder, minimal impairments are seen in verbal skills and visual processing.[16] It is estimated that about 25 per cent of people with major depression manifest residual cognitive impairment in the context of remission of their depressive symptoms and there are areas of statistically significant impairment even in remission.[17,18] On average, however, patients with major depression have considerably more limited impairments compared to people with schizophrenia[19] and many, even when depressed, do not have either objective or subjective cognitive impairments, at least compared to normative standards.[20]

Prevalence of cognitive impairment

This has been a controversial topic and is very relevant to comparisons between people with mood disorders and schizophrenia. While there are clearly some individuals with schizophrenia whose cognitive performance is within the 'average' range of performance (e.g. +/– 1.0 SD from the population average, consistent with an 'average' IQ), this is typically a small subset of cases, in the range of 15–30 per cent.[21–23] It has been persuasively argued, however, that the individuals whose performance is in this range are also quite

likely to have pre-illness levels of performance that were above average to superior.[23]

With a putatively smaller degree of impairment, a much greater proportion of individuals with bipolar disorder would be considered to have normal or 'intact' cognition. In fact, a follow-up study with an epidemiological sample found only about 60 per cent of those with bipolar disorder who had sustained remission displayed evidence of intact cognition.[13] The cyclical nature of this disorder, coupled with the more selective impairments that are often overlooked in these group comparisons, complicate the picture. It is possible, for example, that more selective impairments in bipolar disorder would be found with broader measurement or comparison with estimated premorbid deficits. A further issue is the well-known superiority in cognitive performance during the premorbid period on the part of people with bipolar illness.[24] It might be the case that bipolar illness is associated with greater longitudinal cognitive decline during developmental periods compared to people with schizophrenia, even if current performance appears superior.

Major depression seems more similar to bipolar disorder than schizophrenia in terms of prevalence of cognitive impairments. The study by Reichenberg and colleagues[13] reported that persistent cognitive deficits were present in the same proportion of cases with major depression and bipolar disorder in remission after their first episode. The evidence in terms of the premorbid functioning seems similar. Data from large-scale Israeli conscript studies demonstrate that currently asymptomatic cases who later developed major depression had less impairment compared to individuals who later developed schizophrenia.[25]

Profile of cognitive impairments

When evaluating the overall profile of impairment in schizophrenia, there have been attempts to compare performance to that seen in various forms of dementing condition with well-characterized neuropathology. In specific, the cross-sectional profile of cognitive deficits in schizophrenia has been characterized as resembling that seen in frontostriatal conditions such as Huntington's disease[26] as opposed to classical 'cortical dementias', for example, the prominent medial temporal lobe involvement of typical Alzheimer's disease. Impairments in rate of verbal and spatial learning, free recall without prompts or cures, and processing speed are common in similarly aged patients with schizophrenia compared to Huntington's disease conditions across levels of severity of Huntington's disease.[27] In contrast to dementias with prominent medial temporal involvement, impairment in delayed recognition and cued recall are less substantial in both schizophrenia and Huntington's disease. Direct comparative studies have also shown that people with possible Alzheimer's disease have impaired in delayed recognition memory that are more severe than those seen in people with schizophrenia, whether or not the schizophrenia and Alzheimer samples were matched on age, educational attainment, and the severity of overall impairment as indexed by the mini-mental state examination.[28,29]

In bipolar disorder and major depression, the preservation of more basic perceptual and bottom-up processes points toward the possibility of disruption being centered on cognitive control mechanisms. These top-down abilities are essential for strategy formation and freedom from distraction, skills that are impaired in mood disorders and can contribute to impairments in skills not traditionally considered frontal executive tasks, such as verbal declarative memory, where patients with more severe symptoms have a difficult time with organizational strategies.[30] The ability to regulate emotion and the ability to manage conflict appear in both the clinical manifestation of the disorder and performance on cognitive tests. Both of these skills are associated with frontal functioning in a number of neuropsychiatric conditions, and suggest the possibility of these cortical structures having key roles in the pathology of the illness. Functional imaging studies of bipolar disorder also point to a key role for frontal structures, although not surprisingly abnormalities are not restricted to these regions.[31]

Course of cognitive impairments

Course of impairments in schizophrenia

Studies of individuals who later developed schizophrenia who were assessed prior to the onset of their illness have indicated consistent reductions in cognitive performance. Both meta-analyses[7,32] and large-scale studies[25] have yielded relatively consistent findings of impairments of about 0.5 SD in premorbid intellectual functioning relative to the population as a whole. While these findings are consistent, they are also very nonspecific and not informative for prevention because about 30 per cent of the general population performs at or below this level.

Studies of the intellectual performance of individuals who were examined at the time of their *first episode* of illness have suggested impairments of approximately 1.0 SD, suggesting decline in cognitive functioning some time between the premorbid and first episode stage.[33,34] Identifying this decline has been challenging, however, and it is not clear when it takes place. Studies of individuals who are identified as experiencing the prodromal phase of schizophrenia have indicated that those who go on to develop the full psychotic syndrome already manifest substantial cognitive impairments at the time their prodromal psychosis has been detected.[35] Thus, the exact timing of the occurrence of decline is still to be determined.

Studies of patients experiencing their first diagnosable schizophrenia episode have suggested that their impairments in cognitive functioning are similar in profile and severity to patients with extended illness histories.[33] These findings suggest that cognitive impairments are not associated with treatments for the illness because they are similarly present in chronically treated and untreated patients, and that there is minimal progression in the early to middle course of the illness.[36,37] Most of these studies have also shown that symptomatic stabilization is not associated with improvements in cognitive functioning and that most patients are still significantly impaired after their symptoms have resolved from their first episode.[13]

It is a challenge to follow first episode patients for periods long enough to determine if there are progressive cognitive changes, even in subgroups. Such long-term follow-ups require large samples and extended funding. The subgroup of patients who would be expected to decline is quite small, given the fact that many studies have shown that, on average, outpatients with schizophrenia who are in late middle age do not perform on average any more poorly when compared to demographic norms than younger patients. Thus, it is likely that if there is cognitive decline over the course of the illness, it may be limited to a subgroup of patients.

The results of longitudinal studies have been reviewed in detail elsewhere,[37] but a brief overview can highlight the key findings. Changes in cognitive performance over periods of time as brief

as 18 months have been detected in these patients[38], with these changes clearly exceeding those expected in normal ageing.[39,40] The cognitive changes are found to occur across the different cognitive ability areas that are impaired in first episode patients;[41] the profile of impairment in these older patients is quite similar to that reported in younger samples. Also, the rate of change is not consistent with that seen in patients with Alzheimer's disease with similar demographic characteristics. Longitudinal changes appear to be more substantial in individuals with schizophrenia older than age 65, whereas in the same study Alzheimer patients showed no differences in the extent of 6-year cognitive decline as a function of their age at the beginning of the follow-up period.[40] Correlates of these declines, beyond older age, included more severe baseline negative and psychotic symptoms, lower levels of education, and more severe psychosis during the follow-up period.[37]

Course of impairments in bipolar disorder

Recent interest in the prodromal period of bipolar disorder has not yet revealed any important differences in the deficits in cognition compared to those seen in people who later develop schizophrenia. A small study[42] failed to find differences between clinical high-risk psychosis groups that converted to bipolar disorder or schizophrenia on a global measure of cognition. Larger-scale studies are underway and might help determine if earlier diagnostic prediction can be facilitated by cognitive assessment. After the onset of the disorder, cognitive functioning appears much less stable than the steady severe impairment observed during the early course of schizophrenia.

One might expect this condition, with a more cyclical pattern of symptoms, to have more temporal variability in cognitive functions; however, changes in symptoms are actually poor predictors of changes in cognition.[43] Impairments in sustained attention are the most reliable, with continued deficits observed even during periods of euthymia. Although change scores correlate poorly, the severity of the illness, particularly the number of manic episodes[44,45] and history of psychosis,[46] are associated with greater cognitive deficit. Interestingly, this same correlation is found in schizophrenia. Late-life bipolar disorder is understudied but there is some evidence for greater than expected age-associated decline even in clinically stable outpatients.[47] This might suggest that the trajectories of cognition in bipolar disorder are more variable than in schizophrenia and tied to possible toxic effects of severe repeated episodes,

Course of impairments in major depression

Cognitive performance does improve to an extent in the majority of patients who recover from major depression, something we noted earlier. As reviewed in detail by Hammar and Ardal,[48] there is much less information available about the course of cognitive deficits in major depression compared to schizophrenia or bipolar disorder although at least one study has indicated that greater numbers of episodes of major depression leads to greater cognitive impairment.[49] Patients with 'treatment-resistant' depression (TRD)—those who fail to show clinical improvement after effective antidepressant treatment—have poorer psychosocial functioning than patients whose symptoms respond. There is little published information available on cognition in TRD. One study compared cognition in TRD across patients with diagnoses of bipolar I and bipolar II disorders[50] and found substantial impairments in both groups, with slightly greater impairments in cases with bipolar

I disorder. What cannot be determined from these data, however, are whether extended depressive episodes cause deterioration in cognitive functioning or whether impairments in cognitive functioning are a risk factor for failure to response to treatment. In a recent study,[51] cognitive deficits in TRD could be improved with cognitive remediation therapy. Interestingly, although improvements in cognition were associated with improvements in everyday functioning, there were no changes in mood state variables.

Functional implications

Disability is ubiquitous in schizophrenia, with prevalence estimates for impairments in social, vocational, and residential domains close to 80 per cent at any point in time. Lifetime rates of achievement may be somewhat higher but a recent study of ambulatory patients with schizophrenia found that the number of patients currently employed, living independently, and functioning adequately on a social basis was about 6 per cent.[52] When lifetime achievement was substituted for current achievement, the rates of accomplishment across functional domains were still less than 20 per cent.

In bipolar disorder, rates of functional achievement are about twice as high as seen in schizophrenia, but attainment of functional milestones is still the exception rather than the rule.[53] These rates of functional disability seem to apply to patients early in their illness as well, with some studies estimating only a 40 per cent rate of functional recovery following the first mixed or manic episode.[54] While the condition is often popularly associated with high functioning and creativity, selective impairments in neurocognitive processes make it quite difficult to function in spite of previous or intermittent achievements, and the association between cognitive deficits and functional impairments has been demonstrated in a variety of systematic reviews and meta-analyses.

In major depression, there is a huge illness burden, but the research on disability and burden in depression has often not separated the impact of symptoms from the impact of other aspects of the illness. In contrast to schizophrenia and bipolar disorder, where there is considerable research examining functioning during and between episodes of illness, much of the research on major depression is more global. It is possible to examine the impact of cognitive deficits on functioning from a subset of the literature. Patients with major depression are more likely to have a history of employment than people with schizophrenia. Depression has a major impact on work functioning and work functioning does not recover along with depression,[55] with evidence suggesting that persistent cognitive deficits correlate with continued employment disability after remission.[56]

Across all three conditions, it seems clear that cognitive impairments are potent predictors of functional disability. In a recent meta-analysis in bipolar disorder[57] cognitive impairments across multiple domains were associated with everyday functioning. There were 22 studies and 1344 patients with bipolar disorder in the meta-analysis and primary findings from this meta-analysis of were that 1) cognitive abilities account for a significant, albeit moderate, proportion of variation in everyday functioning, 2) all but one cognitive domains were significantly related with everyday functioning and there was modest effect size variation among these relationships, 3) somewhat more variation was seen among functional measurement approaches, and 4) no sample or study design characteristics significantly modified effect sizes. Thus, there is considerable similarity to the findings seen in meta-analyses of the impact of cognition on functioning in schizophrenia. To date, there is no similar meta-analysis in major depression, largely because there have been few studies and most efforts to understand disability have focused entirely on symptoms.

Social cognition

Social cognition refers to the cognitively demanding skills that are required for socially relevant activities.[58] These include the perception, processing, and interpretation of emotional displays, the ability to infer intentions, and judge facial and nonfacial gestures. While there are some methodological limitations to date in the study of social cognition, these are important abilities. Meta-analyses have shown that social cognition and standard neuropsychological measures are minimally related to each other[59] and that social cognition is more consistently associated with social outcomes.[60] This is consistent with some of our most recent work, where we have found that neuropsychological test performance was minimally associated with social outcomes in people with schizophrenia when other factors, such as negative symptoms, were considered.[61]

Cognitive enhancement as a therapeutic strategy

Ten years ago, Hyman and Fenton[62] set the stage for the development of consensus cognitive assessments for clinical treatment studies aimed at cognitive enhancement in schizophrenia. This initiative led to a project entitled Measurement and Treatment Research for Improving cognition in schizophrenia (MATRICS).[63] The MATRICS initiative led to the eventual selection of a consensus cognitive assessment battery (i.e. the MATRICS consensus cognitive battery, MCCB)[64] endorsed as the standard performance-based cognitive assessment measure for treatment outcomes studies. This battery is presented in Table 41.1 and the premises on which this battery is based are presented in the following section.

In the development process of the MCCB, the initial consensus was that cognitive functioning in general was composed of separable cognitive domains and that schizophrenia was marked by the presence of impairments in most of these domains. Thus, the development process was based on the selection of important domains of functioning (e.g. verbal memory, processing speed, etc.) and then selection of representative and psychometrically useful exemplars of those domains. It was further designated that unless otherwise specified by the entity conducting the study, the outcome measure would be the composite, which is an unweighted average of the cognitive domains. Thus, despite the focus on selection of tests from domains, *global cognitive functioning* is the default treatment target.

Cognitive enhancement research design

As described in the following, there are potential interventions for cognition and functional capacity that are delivered through both pharmacological and behavioural methods. As result of the MATRICS process, a consensus research design has been endorsed by the US Food and Drug Administration (FDA)[65,66] and with additional acceptance by the European Medicines Agency (EMEA). This design would apply to studies of pharmacological cognitive

Table 41.1 MATRICS consensus cognitive battery

Speed of Processing
Category Fluency
Brief Assessment of Cognition in Schizophrenia (BACS)—Symbol-Coding
Trail Making A

Attention/Vigilance
Continuous Performance Test—Identical Pairs (CPT–IP)

Working Memory
Verbal: University of Maryland—Letter–Number Span
Nonverbal: Wechsler Memory Scale (WMS)—III Spatial Span

Verbal Learning
Hopkins Verbal Learning Test (HVLT)—Revised

Visual Learning
Brief Visuospatial Memory Test (BVMT)—Revised

Reasoning and Problem Solving
Neuropsychological Assessment Battery (NAB)—Mazes

Social Cognition
Meyer–Solovay–Caruso Emotional Intelligence Test

enhancement as well as for software or other computer programs aimed at computerized cognitive remediation. The FDA has previously allowed attempts to develop a treatment indication for features of illness not well treated with existing therapies, as long as it could be proved that these other features were not improved by previously approved treatments. Beyond these issues, the FDA has in the past required that treatments aimed at cognitive enhancement be supported by evidence of clinical benefit beyond improvements in performance-based assessments.

Cognitive remediation in severe mental illness

Behavioural treatments for cognitive impairments in schizophrenia have a long history, originating with behavioural modification techniques and borrowing largely from the drill and practice restorative philosophy behind neuropsychological rehabilitation for traumatic brain injury. Although contemporary approaches—variously referred to as cognitive remediation therapy, cognitive enhancement, or cognitive training (among others)—differ, a commonality includes the recognition that in order to be viewed as a successful intervention, the treatment-related changes in cognition should manifest in improved everyday functioning and/or quality of life. In the past ten years new treatments provide substantial evidence for neurobiological mechanisms of action as well as improvements in functioning. Some approaches rely heavily on therapist involvement to modify strategies and facilitate the bridging of cognitive gains to everyday behaviours exercises.[67]

Drill and practice exercises have been used with[68] and without[69] computer software to present and modify the complexity of stimuli. Treatment programs that can be quite labour-intensive include several non-cognitive and social cognitive aspects.[70,71] Improvements in functioning have also been found with compensatory strategies. Most recently, 'neuroplasticity-based treatment' has emerged (this term should not confuse the fact that all the above treatments

presuppose the treatments operate on the malleability of the organism's brain) for schizophrenia.[72] The philosophy behind this is that manipulation of early sensory processing is critical to improve the signal-to-noise ratio in schizophrenia. The only direct comparison between approaches published to date found more robust improvements in sensory gating indexed by an evoked potential paradigm and neurocognitive abilities with early sensory training compared to an older and graphically primitive software package that was not specifically developed for schizophrenia.[73]

Although cognitive remediation studies appeared in the 1960s, it was only in 2002 that Wykes and colleagues[74] first demonstrated changes in brain function for schizophrenia patients who received cognitive remediation. Following 40 hours of paper and pencil drill and practice techniques coupled with strategic monitoring, patients had increased activation in the frontal cortex during a verbal working memory task. In a series of recent studies, the neuroplasticity based cognitive remediation strategies targeting early auditory processing produced normalization in serum levels of brain-derived neurotrophic factor, which provides an indirect measurement of neuroplasticity,[75] and a normalization in electrophysiological markers of auditory stimuli.[76] Finally, normalization of a linked cortical network related to reality monitoring (the process of identification of the origin of information in short-term memory) was also found with this same treatment.[77]

Further evidence for the validity of cognitive remediation to produce neurobiological changes comes from the reduced gains that are found in cases who carry genetic polymorphisms associated with overly rapid degradation of dopamine (highly active catechol-O-methyltransferase)[78] and in patients receiving high doses of anticholinergic medication, which inhibits new learning.[79] One of the most encouraging findings for long-term prognosis comes from a study that used a two-year social and neurocognitive training program and found that, compared to a placebo group, the treatment effectively reduced the common structural grey matter loss in brain regions that is common during the early course of schizophrenia.[80]

Cognitive remediation alone may not be enough to cause functional gains, however. A meta-analysis[81] found larger-effect size changes in distal measures such as social functioning when cognitive remediation was used within a larger psychosocial treatment framework. Similarly, a meta-analysis[82] also found that combined therapy was required to induce functional gains, although gains in cognitive abilities are routinely found with cognitive remediation alone, a finding recently confirmed with a prospective study comparing cognitive remediation alone or combined with skills training.[83] The very small and non-significant effects on functioning when cognitive remediation is used in isolation suggest that the likelihood of these transferring to real-world functional behaviour is greatly diminished and perhaps not likely without other interventions.

Pharmacological cognitive enhancement

Target selection for pharmacological cognitive enhancement is complicated and has been reviewed elsewhere.[84,85] Developing targets for cognitive enhancement requires the decision as to whether to attempt to increase activity by stimulation of receptors (agonist), reducing activity by blocking receptors (antagonist), modifying the endogenous processes of down regulation of activity, either through stimulating autoreceptors, blocking re-uptake (transport), or reducing degradation of transmitters. While many of these actions would seem to lead to the same result, the complexities of neurotransmission suggest that the situation is not that simple. For instance, stimulating serotonin receptors directly with an agonist has no impact on depression, but increasing serotonin activity through blocking transport is a very effective antidepressant strategy (serotonin reuptake inhibition; SRI). There have been multiple recent studies on pharmacological cognitive enhancement with somewhat disappointing results that have been reviewed elsewhere.[86] These treatment failures include procholinergic medications used for the treatment of Alzheimer's and Parkinson's disease dementias, as well as medications targeting glutamate (NMDA; AMPA), serotonin, norepinephrine, and dopamine.

Neuroscience discoveries have identified pharmacological compounds that have effects other than transmitter manipulation/modulation. These include compounds that have other central nervous system effects, for example, promotion of neurogenesis or other brain growth processes. In a single study examining davunetide, a neuroactive peptide that appears to promote neurite outgrowth in animal models, in schizophrenia, intranasal administration davunitide led to statistically significant improvements in a performance-based measure of everyday living skills compared to placebo treatment.[87] As interventions such as davunitide bypass some of the shortcomings of transmitter-based interventions, this may be a promising compound and even more promising cognitive enhancement strategy.

Bipolar disorder and major depression

There have been few studies of cognitive treatments in bipolar disorder. There has been one pilot study on cognitive remediation[88] and one overall negative study using a dopamine agonist, pramipexole, for pharmacological treatment.[89] While the authors of the pramipexole study suggested that the results might have some promise, in the treatment of schizophrenia, similar partially positive results led to no follow-up studies with positive outcomes to date. As noted earlier, one study[51] found promising results for cognitive remediation therapy (CRT) in treatment-resistant depression (TRD), but in general there have been remarkably few attempts to study these interventions in mood disorders.

Conclusion

Cognitive impairment in severe mental illness seems to be quite similar in many of its features. Profiles of impairment are similar while levels of severity vary as a function across the diagnosis. This may be due to differences in pre-illness levels of cognitive functioning. Cognitive impairments are functionally relevant and share a common profile. Treatment efforts have shown success with cognitive remediation in patients with schizophrenia but have been understudied in other conditions. All preliminary results suggest excellent potential for good outcomes. Pharmacological treatments have been receiving substantial attention, but success has been limited to date. However, the level of attention to this topic suggests a high potential for future success.

References

1. Heinrichs RW. The primacy of cognition in schizophrenia. *Amer Psychol* 2005;60:229–42.
2. Harvey PD, Wingo AP, Burdick KE, *et al*. Cognition and Disability in Bipolar Disorder: Lessons from Schizophrenia Research. *Bipol Disord*. 2010;12:364–75.
3. Wingo AP, Harvey PD, and Baldessarini RJ.Neurocognitive impairment in bipolar disorder patients: functional implications. *Bipolar Disord*. 2009;11:113–25
4. Malhi GS, Ivanovski B, Hadzi-Pavlovic D, *et al*. Neuropsychological deficits and functional impairment in bipolar depression, hypomania and euthymia. *Bipolar Disord*. 2007;9:114–25.
5. Martinez-Aran A, Vieta E, Reinares M, *et al*. Cognitive function across manic or hypomanic, depressed, and euthymic states in bipolar disorder. *Am J Psychiatry*. 2004;161:262–70.
6. Bowie CR and Harvey PD. Cognition in schizophrenia: impairments, determinants, and functional importance. *Psychiatr Clin N Am*. 2005;28:613–33.
7. Woodberry KA, Giuliano AJ, and Seidman LJ. Premorbid IQ in schizophrenia: a meta-analytic review. *Am J Psychiatry*. 2008;165:579–87.
8. Harvey PD, Moriarty PJ, Friedman JI, *et al*. Differential preservation of cognitive functions in geriatric patients with lifelong chronic schizophrenia: less impairment in reading scores compared to other skill areas. *Biol Psychiatry*. 2000;47:962–8.
9. Harvey PD, Friedman JI, Bowie CR, *et al*. Validity and stability of performance-based estimates of premorbid educational functioning in older patients with schizophrenia. *J Clin Exper Neuropsychology*. 2006;28:178–92.
10. Keefe RS, Bilder RM, Harvey PD, *et al*. Baseline neurocognitive deficits in the CATIE Schizophrenia Trial. *Neuropsychopharmacology*. 2006;31:2033–46.
11. Dickinson D and Harvey PD. Systemic hypotheses for generalized cognitive deficits in schizophrenia: a new take on an old problem. *Schizophr Bull*. 2009 Mar;35(2):403–14.
12. Bowie CR, Depp C, McGrath JA, *et al*. Prediction of real-world functional disability in chronic mental disorders: a comparison of schizophrenia and bipolar disorder. *Am J Psychiatry*. 2010;167:1116–24.
13. Reichenberg A, Harvey PD, Bowie CR, *et al*. (2009). Neuropsychological function and dysfunction in schizophrenia and psychotic affective disorders. *Schizophr Bull*. 2009;35:1022–9.
14. Goldberg T, Hyde TM, Kleinman JE, *et al*. Course of schizophrenia: neuropsychological evidence for static encephalopathy. *Schizophr Bull*. 1993;19:787–804.
15. Yatham LN, Torres IJ, Malhi GS, *et al*. The International Society for Bipolar Disorders-Battery for Assessment of Neurocognition (ISBD-BANC). *Bipol Disord*. 2010;12:351–63.
16. Stordal KI, Lundervold AJ, Mykletun A, *et al*. Frequency and characteristics of recurrent major depressed patients with unimpaired executive functions. *World J Biol Psychiatry*. 2005;6:36–44.
17. Weiland-Fiedler P, Erickson K, Waldeck T, *et al*. Evidence for continuing neuropsychological impairments in depression. *J Affect Disord*. 2004;82:253–8.
18. Neu P, Bajbouj M, Schilling A, *et al*. Cognitive function over the treatment course of depression in middle-aged patients: correlation with brain MRI signal hyperintensities. *J Psychiatr Res*. 2005;39:129–35.
19. Rund BR, Sundet K, Asbjørnsen A, *et al*. Neuropsychological test profiles in schizophrenia and non-psychotic depression. *Acta Psychiatr Scand*. 2006;113:350–9.
20. Kessler RC, Berglund P, Demler O, *et al*. The epidemiology of major depressive disorder: results from the National Comorbidity Survey Replication (NCS-R). *JAMA*. 2003;289:3095–105.
21. Palmer BW, Heaton RK, Paulsen JS, *et al*. Is it possible to be schizophrenic and neuropsychologically normal? *Neuropsychology*. 1997;11: 437–47.
22. Leung WW, Bowie CR, and Harvey PD. Functional implications of neuropsychological normality and symptom remission in outpatients diagnosed with schizophrenia: A cross-sectional study. *J Int Neuropsychol Soc*. 2008;14: 479–88.
23. Wilk CM, Gold JM, McMahon RP, *et al*. No, it is not possible to be schizophrenic yet neuropsychologically normal. *Neuropsychology*. 2005;19:778–86.

24. O'Connor JA, Wiffen BD, Reichenberg A, *et al*. Is deterioration of IQ a feature of first episode psychosis and how can we measure it? *Schizophr Res*. 2012;137:104–9.

25. Reichenberg A, Weiser M, Rabinowitz J. *et al*. A population-based cohort study of premorbid intellectual, language, and behavioral functioning in patients with schizophrenia, schizoaffective disorder, and nonpsychotic bipolar disorder. *Am J Psychiatry* 2002; 159, 2027–35.

26. Paulsen JS, Heaton RK, Sadek JR, *et al*. The nature of learning and memory impairments in schizophrenia. *J Int Neuropsychol Soc*. 1995;1:88–99.

27. Paulsen JS, Salmon DP, Monsch A, *et al*. Discrimination of cortical from subcortical dementias on the basis of memory and problem-solving tests. *J Clin Psychol*. 1995;51:48–58.

28. Heaton RK, Paulsen JS, McAdams LA, *et al*. Neuropsychological deficits in schizophrenics. Relationship to age, chronicity, and dementia. *Arch Gen Psychiat*. 1994;51:469–76.

29. Davidson M, Harvey PD, Welsh K, *et al*. Cognitive impairment in old-age schizophrenia: A comparative study of schizophrenia and Alzheimer's disease. *Am J Psychiatry*. 1996;153:1274–9.

30. Chang JS, Choi S, Ha K, *et al*. Differential pattern of semantic memory organization between bipolar I and II disorders. *Prog Neuropsychopharmacol Biol Psychiatry*. 2011;35(4):1053–8.

31. Whalley HC, Papmeyer M, Sprooten E, *et al*. Review of functional magnetic resonance imaging studies comparing bipolar disorder and schizophrenia. *Bipol Disord*. 2012;14:411–31.

32. Mesholam-Gately RI, Giuliano AJ, *et al*. Neurocognition in first-episode schizophrenia: a meta-analytic review. *Neuropsychology*. 2009;23:315–36.

33. Saykin AJ, Shtasel DL, Gur RE, *et al*. Neuropsychological deficits in neuroleptic naive patients with first episode schizophrenia. *Arch Gen Psychiat*. 1994;51:124–31.

34. Bilder RM, Goldman RS, Robinson D, *et al*. Neuropsychology of first-episode schizophrenia: initial characterization and clinical correlates. *Am J Psychiat*. 2000;157:549–59.

35 Seidman LJ, Giuliano AJ, Meyer EC, *et al*. Neuropsychology of the prodrome to psychosis in the NAPLS consortium: relationship to family history and conversion to psychosis. *Arch Gen Psychiat*. 2010;67:578–88.

36. Hoff AL, Sakuma M, Wieneke M, *et al*. Longitudinal neuropsychological follow-up study of patients with first-episode schizophrenia. *Am J Psychiat*. 1999;156:1336–41.

37. Harvey PD. *Schizophrenia in late life: Aging effects on symptoms and course of illness*. Washington, DC: American Psychological Association, 2004.

38. Harvey PD, Silverman JM, Mohs RC, *et al*. Cognitive decline in late-life schizophrenia: A longitudinal study of geriatric chronically hospitalized patients. *Biol Psychiatry*. 1999;45:32–40.

39. Bowie CR, Reichenberg A, Rieckmann N, *et al*. Stability and functional correlates of memory-based classification in older schizophrenia patients. *Am J Geriatr Psychiatry*. 2004;14:376–86.

40. Friedman J, Harvey PD, Coleman T, *et al*. A six year follow-up study of cognitive and functional status across the life-span in schizophrenia: A comparison with Alzheimer's disease and healthy subjects. *Am J Psychiat*. 2001;158:1441–8.

41. Harvey PD, Reichenberg A, Bowie CR, *et al*. The course of neuropsychological performance and functional capacity in older patients with schizophrenia: Influences of previous history of long-term institutional stay. *Biol Psychiatry*. 2010;67:933–9.

42. Olvet DM, Stearns WH, McLaughlin D, *et al*. Comparing clinical and neurocognitive features of the schizophrenia prodrome to the bipolar prodrome. *Schizophr Res*. 2010;123:59–63.

43. Arts B, Jabben N, Krabbendam L, *et al*. A 2-year naturalistic study on cognitive functioning in bipolar disorder. *Acta Psychiatrica Scand*. 2011;123:190–205.

44. Elshahawi HH, Essawi H, Rabie MA, *et al*. Cognitive functions among euthymic bipolar I patients after a single manic episode versus recurrent episodes. *Journal of Affective Disorders*. 2011;130:180–91.

45. López-Jaramillo C, Lopera-Vásquez J, Gallo A, *et al*. Effects of recurrence on the cognitive performance of patients with bipolar

46. Glahn DC, Bearden CE, Cakir S, *et al*. Differential working memory impairment in bipolar disorder and schizophrenia: effects of lifetime history of psychosis. *Bipol Disord*. 2006;8:117–23.

47. Depp CA, Moore DJ, Sitzer D, *et al*. (2007). Neurocognitive impairment in middle-aged and older adults with bipolar disorder: comparison to schizophrenia and normal comparison subjects. *J Affective Disord*. 2007;101:201–9.

48. Hammar A and Ardal G. Cognitive functioning in major depression: A summary. Front Hum Neurosci 2009, VOl 3, article 26.

49. Sweeney JA, Kmiec JA, and Kupfer DJ. Neuropsychologica impairments in unipolar and bipolar mood disorders o the CANTAB neuropsycognitive battery. *Biol Psychiatry*. 2000; 48: 674–684.

50. Kessler U, Schoeyen HK, Andreassen OA, *et al*. Neurocognitive profiles in *treatment-resistant bipolar* I and bipolar II disorder depression. *BMC Psychiatry* 2013; 13:105.

51. Morimoto SS, Wexler BE, Liu J. *et al*. Neuroplasticity-based computer-ized cognitive remediation for treatment-resistant geriatric depression. *Nat. Comm.* 2014; 5: 4579.

52. Harvey PD, Sabbag S, Prestia D., *et al*. Functional Milestones and Clinician Ratings of Everyday Functioning in People with Schizophrenia: Overlap Between Milestones and Specificity of Ratings. *J Psychiatric Res*, 2012; 46:1546–1552.

53. Huxley N and Baldessarini RJ. Disability and its treatment in bipolar disorder patients. *Bipolar Disord*. 2007;9:183–96.

54. Tohen M, Zarate CA, Jr, Hennen J, *et al*. The McLean-Harvard First-Episode Mania Study: prediction of recovery and first recurrence. *Am J Psychiat*. 2003;160:2099–107.

55. Adler DA, McLaughlin TJ, Rogers W H. *et al*. Job performance deficits due to depression. Am J Psychiatry 2006; 163, 1569–1576.

56. Jaeger J, Berns S, Uzelac S. *et al*. Neurocognitive deficits and disability in major depressive disorder. Psychiatry Res.2006 145, 39–48.

57. Depp CA, Mausbach BT, Harmell AL, *et al*. Meta-analysis of the association between cognitive abilities and functional outcomes in bipolar disorder. *Bipol Disord*. 2012;14:217–26.

58. Harvey PD and Penn D. Social cognition: The key factor predicting social outcome in people with schizophrenia? *Psychiatry (Edgmont)*. 2010;7:41–4.

59. Fett AK, Viechtbauer W, Dominguez MD, *et al*. The relationship between neurocognition and social cognition with functional outcomes in schizophrenia: A meta-analysis. *Neurosci Biobehav Rev*. 2011;35:573–88.

60. Ventura J, Wood RC, and Hellemann GS. Symptom domains and neurocognitive functioning can help differentiate social cognitive processes in schizophrenia: A meta-analysis. *Schizophr Bull*. 2013;39(1):102–11.

61. Leifker FR, Bowie CR, and Harvey PD. Determinants of everyday outcomes in schizophrenia: the influences of cognitive impairment, functional capacity, and symptoms. *Schizophr Res*. 2009;115:82–87.

62. Hyman SE and Fenton WS. What are the right targets for pharmacotherapy? *Science*. 2003;299:350–1.

63. Marder SR and Fenton W. Measurement and treatment research to improve cognition in schizophrenia: NIMH MATRICS initiative to support the development of agents for improving cognition in schizophrenia. *Schizophr Res*. 2004;72:5–9.

64. Nuechterlein KH, Green MF, Kern RS, *et al*. The MATRICS Consensus Cognitive Battery: test selection, reliability, and validity. *Am J Psychiat*. 2008;165:203–13.

65. Buchanan RW, Davis M, Goff D, *et al*. Summary of an FDA-NIMH-MATRICS workshop on clinical trial design for neurocognitive drugs for schizophrenia. *Schizophr Bull*. 2005;31:5–19.

66. Buchanan RW, Keefe RS, Umbricht D, *et al*. The FDA-NIMH-MATRICS guidelines for clinical trial design of cognitive-enhancing drugs: What do we know 5 years later? *Schizophr Bull*. 2011;37:1209–17.

67. Medalia A, Revheim N, and Herlands T. *Cognitive Remediation for Psychological Disorders, Therapist Guide*. New York, NY: Oxford University Press, 2009.

68. Bell B, Bryson G, and Wexler BE. Cognitive remediation of working memory deficits: durability of training effects in severely impaired and less severely impaired schizophrenia. *Acta Psychiatr Scand.* 2003;108:101–9.

69. Wykes T, Reeder C, Comer J, *et al.* (1993). The effects of neurocognitive remediation on executive processing in patients with schizophrenia. *Schizophr Bull.* 1993;25:291–307.

70. Brenner HD, Hodel B, Roder V, *et al.* (1992). Treatment of cognitive dysfunction and behavioral deficits in schizophrenia. *Schizophr Bull.* 1992;18:21–6.

71. Hogarty GE, Flesher S, Ulrich R, *et al.* Cognitive enhancement therapy for schizophrenia: effects of a 2-year randomized trial on cognition and behavior. *Arch Gen Psychiatry.* 2004;61:866–76.

72. Fisher M, Holland C, Subramaniam K, *et al.* Neuroplasticity-based cognitive training in schizophrenia: an interim report on effects 6 months later. *Schizophr Bull.* 2010;36:869–79.

73. Popov T, Jordanov T, Rockstroh B, *et al.* Specific cognitive training normalizes auditory sensory gating in schizophrenia: a randomized trial. *Biol Psychiatry.* 2011;69:465–71.

74. Wykes T, Brammer M, Mellers J, *et al.* Effects on the brain of psychological treatment: cognitive remediation therapy: functional magnetic resonance imaging in schizophrenia. *Br J Psychiatry.* 2002;181:144–52.

75. Vinogradov, S., Fisher, M., Holland, C., *et al.* Is serum brain-derived neurotrophic factor a biomarker for cognitive enhancement in schizophrenia? *Biological Psychiatry.* 2009;66:549–53.

76. Fisher M, Holland C, Merzenich MM, *et al.* Using neuroplasticity-based auditory training to improve verbal memory in schizophrenia. *Am J Psychiat* 2009;166:805–11.

77. Subramaniam K, Luks TL, Fisher M, *et al.* Computerized cognitive training restores neural activity within the reality monitoring network in schizophrenia. *Neuron.* 2012;73:842–53.

78. Bosia M, Bechi M, Marino E, *et al.* Influence of catechol-O-methyltransferase Val158Met polymorphism on neuropsychological and functional outcomes of classic rehabilitation and cognitive remediation in schizophrenia. *Neurosci Lett.* 2007;417:271–4.

79. Vinogradov S, Fisher M, Warm H, *et al.* The cognitive cost of anticholinergic burden: decreased response to cognitive training in schizophrenia. *Am J Psychiat.* 2009;166:1055–62.

80. Eack SM, Hogarty GE, Cho RY, *et al.* Neuroprotective effects of cognitive enhancement therapy against gray matter loss in early schizophrenia: results from a 2-year randomized controlled trial. *Arch Gen Psychiatry.* 2010;67:674–82.

81. McGurk SR, Twamley EW, Sitzer DI, *et al.* A meta-analysis of cognitive remediation in schizophrenia. *Am J Psychiat.* 2007;164:1791–802.

82. Wykes T, Huddy V, Cellard C, *et al.* A meta-analysis of cognitive remediation for schizophrenia: methodology and effect sizes. *Am J Psychiat.* 2011;168:472–85.

83. Bowie CR, McGurk SM, Mausbach BT, *et al.* Combined cognitive remediation3and functional skills training for schizophrenia: effects on cognition, functional competence, and real-world behavior. *Am J Psychiat.* 2012;169:710–18.

84. Geyer MA and Tamminga CA. Measurement and treatment research to improve cognition in schizophrenia: Neuropharmacological aspects. *Psychopharmacology.* 2004;174:1–2.

85. Harvey PD and Bowie CR. Cognitive enhancement in schizophrenia: Pharmacological and Cognitive Remediation Approaches. *Psychiatric Clin North Am.* 2012;35:683–98.

86. Harvey PD. Pharmacological cognitive enhancement in schizophrenia. *Neuropsychol Rev.* 2009;19:324–35.

87. Javitt DC, Buchanan RW, Keefe RS, *et al.* Effect of the neuroprotective peptide davunetide (AL-108) on cognition and functional capacity in schizophrenia. *Schizophr Res.* 2012;136:25–31.

88. Deckersbach T, Nierenberg AA, Kessler R, *et al.* Cognitive rehabilitation for bipolar disorder: an open trial for employed patients with residual depressive symptoms. *CNS Neursci Ther.* 2010;16:298–307.

89. Burdick KE, Braga RJ, Nnadi CU, *et al.* Placebo-controlled adjunctive trial of pramipexole in patients with bipolar disorder: targeting cognitive dysfunction. *J Clin Psychiatry.* 2012;73:103–12.

Index